Orthopaedic Nursing

Orthopaedic Nursing

THIRD EDITION

Ann Butler Maher, MS, RN, APNC, ONC

Family Nurse Practitioner
Sussex Family Practice
Sussex, New Jersey

Susan Warner Salmond, EdD, RN

Professor and Chairperson, Department of Nursing
Kean University
Union, New Jersey

Teresa A. Pellino, PhD, RN, ONC

Clinical Nurse Research Specialist
University of Wisconsin
Madison, Wisconsin

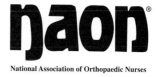

National Association of Orthopaedic Nurses

W.B. SAUNDERS COMPANY
An Imprint of Elsevier Science
Philadelphia   London   New York   St. Louis   Sydney   Toronto

W.B. SAUNDERS COMPANY

An Imprint of Elsevier Science

The Curtis Center
Independence Square West
Philadelphia, Pennsylvania 19106

Vice President and Publishing Director: Sally Schrefer
Executive Editor: Robin Carter
Associate Developmental Editor: Barbara Cicalese

NOTICE

Nursing is an ever-changing field. Standard safety precautions must be followed, but as new research and clinical experience broaden our knowledge, changes in treatment and drug therapy become necessary or appropriate. Readers are advised to check the most current product information provided by the manufacturer of each drug to be administered to verify the recommended dose, the method and duration of administration, and contraindications. It is the responsibility of the treating licensed prescriber, relying on experience and knowledge of the patient, to determine dosages and the best treatment for each individual patient. Neither the publisher nor the editor assumes any responsibility for any injury and/or damage to persons or property.

Library of Congress Cataloging-in-Publication Data

Orthopaedic nursing / [edited by] Ann Butler Maher, Susan Warner Salmond, Teresa A. Pellino.—3rd ed.

p.   ;   cm.

Includes bibliographical references and index.

ISBN 0–7216–9302–4

1. Orthopedic nursing.   I. Maher, Ann Butler.   II. Salmond, Susan Warner.   III. Pellino, Teresa A.
[DNLM: 1. Musculoskeletal Diseases—nursing.   2. Orthopedic Nursing—methods.
WY 157.6 O769 2002]

RD753 .M34 2002   610.73′677—dc21   2001049299

ORTHOPAEDIC NURSING, THIRD EDITION   ISBN 0–7216–9302–4

Printed in the United States of America

Last digit is the print number: 9   8   7   6   5   4   3   2   1

Contributors

Sue Addamo, BS

Preceptor, Physical Therapy Program, University of
Wisconsin–Madison; Center Coordinator of Clinical
Education and Physical Therapist, William S.
Middleton Memorial V.A. Hospital, Madison,
Wisconsin
Modalities for Mobilization

Maryann Alexander, MS, RN, ONC

Assistant Professor, Rush University College of Nursing;
Clinical Nurse Specialist, Rush–Presbyterian St. Lukes
Medical Center, Chicago, Illinois
Congenital and Developmental Disorders

Nancy Bell, RN, ADN, RVT

Manager, Vascular Lab, University of Wisconsin Hospital
and Clinics, Madison, Wisconsin
Complications of Orthopaedic Disorders and Orthopaedic Surgery

Carolyn L. Blue, PhD

Associate Professor, School of Nursing, Purdue University, West Lafayette, Indiana
Ergonomics

Sharon G. Childs, MS, CRNP-CS, ONC

Assistant Professor, Department of Orthopaedic Surgery,
Bayview Campus, The Johns Hopkins University;
Adult Nurse Practitioner, Concentra Medical Centers,
Baltimore, Maryland
*Anatomy and Physiology of the Musculoskeletal System; Athletic Perfor-
mance and Injury*

Margaret O. Doheny, PhD, RN, ONC

Associate Professor, Kent State University College of
Nursing, Kent, Ohio
Metabolic Conditions

Cynthia Fine, RN, MSN, CIC

Infection Control Consultant, Catholic Healthcare West,
Oakland, California
Infections of the Musculoskeletal System

Debra B. Gordon, BSN, MS

Clinical Assistant Professor, University of
Wisconsin–Madison, School of Nursing; Senior Clinical
Nurse Specialist, University of Wisconsin Hospital and
Clinics, Madison, Wisconsin
Assessment and Management of Pain

Kathleen Hansen, RN, MSN

Nursing Instructor, Madison Area Technical College,
Madison, Wisconsin
Complications of Orthopaedic Disorders and Orthopaedic Surgery

Kim Haynes, RN, MS, CS, ONC

Clinical Nurse Specialist, Mid-America Sarcoma Institute, Overland Park, Kansas
Neoplasms of the Musculoskeletal System

Marianne Genge Jagmin, PhD, RN, ONC

Complemental Faculty, Assistant Professor, Rush University College of Nursing, Chicago, Illinois
Assessment and Management of Immobility

Cathleen E. Kunkler, BSN, RN, ONC, CNA

Instructor of Practical Nursing, Northern Tier Career
Center, Towanda, Pennsylvania
Fractures

Tina Kurkowski, MS, RNFA, ONC, CNOR

Rice Medical Center, Stevens Point, Wisconsin
Perioperative Considerations for the Orthopaedic Client

Dale Halsey Lea, MPH, RN, FAAN

Adjunct Professor, Brandeis Genetic Counseling Program, Brandeis University, Waltham, Massachusetts; Assistant Director, Southern Maine Genetics Services, Foundation for Blood Research, Scarborough, Maine
Genetics

Pamela F. Levin, PhD

Deputy Director, Great Lakes Center for Occupational and Environmental Health and Safety, University of Illinois at Chicago, Chicago, Illinois
Ergonomics

Patricia A. MacDonald, BSN, RN, NP

Director, Arthritis Research, Rheumatology Associates SC, Rush–Presbyterian St. Lukes Medical Center, Chicago, Illinois
Autoimmune and Inflammatory Disorders

Ann Butler Maher, MS, RN, APNC, ONC

Family Nurse Practitioner, Sussex Family Practice, Sussex, New Jersey
Assessment of the Musculoskeletal System

Nancy E. Mooney, MA, RN, ONC

Director of Nursing, Nursing Hands, New York, New York
Computers As a Resource for Education

Monica J. Newton, MS, RN, CS

Clinical Nurse Specialist-Trauma Coordinator, University of Wisconsin Hospital and Clinics, Madison, Wisconsin
Complications of Orthopaedic Disorders and Orthopaedic Surgery

Teresa A. Pellino, PhD, RN, ONC

Clinical Nurse Research Specialist, University of Wisconsin, Madison, Wisconsin
Assessment and Management of Pain; Complications of Orthopaedic Disorders and Orthopaedic Surgery

Mary Ann S. Preston, BSN

Nurse Clinician, University of Wisconsin Hospital and Clinics, Madison, Wisconsin
Complications of Orthopaedic Disorders and Orthopaedic Surgery

Sarah Redemann, RN, MSN

Orthopedic Trauma Nurse Practitioner, University of Wisconsin Hospital and Clinics, Madison, Wisconsin
Modalities for Immobilization

Dottie Roberts, MSN, MACI, RN, ONC

Medical–Surgical Clinical Educator, Providence Hospital/Northeast, Columbia, South Carolina
Degenerative Disorders

Mary Faut Rodts, RN, MS, MSA, ONC

Assistant Professor, Rush University College of Nursing, Rush–Presbyterian St. Lukes Medical Center, Chicago, Illinois
Disorders of the Spine

Susan Warner Salmond, EdD, RN

Professor and Chairperson, Department of Nursing, Kean University, Union, New Jersey
Orthopaedic Wellness; Psychosocial Care of Clients and Their Families; Infections of the Musculoskeletal System

Carol A. Sedlak, PhD, RN, ONC

Associate Professor, Kent State University College of Nursing, Kent, Ohio
Metabolic Conditions

Jane E. Smith, MHSA, RN, C, ONC

Nursing Educator, Saint Clare's Hospital, Denville, New Jersey
Diagnostic Modalities for Orthopaedic Disorders

JoAnn Spears, BSN

Quality Assurance Specialist, Division of Mental Health Services, Trenton, New Jersey
Psychosocial Care of Clients and Their Families

Verdell Williamson, MS, RN, ONC

Advanced Practice Nurse, Northwestern Memorial Hospital, Chicago, Illinois
Amputation

Reviewers

Eugene E. Berg, MD, FACS
New Hampshire Bone & Joint Institute, Bedford, New Hampshire

Joie Davis, MSN, CPNP
NIH/National Human Genome Research Institute, Bethesda, Maryland

Dorothy B. Liddel, MSN, RN, ONC
Columbia Union College (Associate Professor, Retired), Takoma Park, Maryland

Joan Shurbet, RN
Senior Director Clinical Services, Christie Clinic, Champaign, Illinois

Alan Quittenton, MS, RN, ONC
University of Rochester Medical Center, Rochester, New York

Foreword

During my nursing career, which spans over 30 years, the body of nursing knowledge has increased exponentially. As a result of this ever-expanding body of knowledge, nurses have tended to gravitate to individual specialties and to concentrate their expertise in one area. Because of this trend to specialization, a text such as *Orthopaedic Nursing* is important to the nurse on several levels. This text is valuable in the educational setting as a basic text on orthopaedic nursing. As the nurse progresses in skills, this text becomes a ready reference on orthopaedic diagnoses and nursing interventions. Perhaps more important in this ever-changing health care environment, *Orthopaedic Nursing* is an essential resource for the nurse who is normally not considered an orthopaedic nurse, but who finds himself or herself caring for individuals with orthopaedic diagnoses, whether this occurs within the hospital, in ambulatory care settings, at schools, or in the home.

This edition presents care of the orthopaedic client across the life span, from congenital orthopaedic disorders through autoimmune disease to sports injuries to musculoskeletal neoplasms and infections to fractures. The breadth of data in this volume makes it a welcome, if not essential, addition to orthopaedic nursing literature for the nursing faculty member and for the nurse who cares for those with orthopaedic conditions, regardless of practice setting.

The editors of *Orthopaedic Nursing* are all seasoned nurses with a broad range of experiences in orthopaedics, including domestic violence, clinical practice, advanced practice, education, and nursing research. One has served as a past editor of the *Orthopaedic Nursing* journal; one has experience as the National Association of Orthopaedic Nurses (NAON) director of education; and one is a past president of NAON, as well as the research director of the *Orthopaedic Nursing* journal. They have always demonstrated their willingness to mentor young nurses and to enhance the knowledge of nurses who have been practicing for years. Their dedication is clearly authenticated in this text. I am proud to value all of them as mentors during my career in orthopaedic nursing.

This book advances the practice of orthopaedic nursing and should serve nurses in a wide variety of settings as a welcome tool to improve the care they provide for their clients. I commend Ann Butler Maher, Susan Warner Salmond, and Teresa A. Pellino for their efforts in the production of this welcome addition to the body of knowledge on orthopaedic nursing.

Sharon V. Stormer, RN, BSPA, ONC
President, National Association of
Orthopaedic Nurses, 2001–2002

Preface

The art and science of orthopaedic nursing practice require nurses to possess a comprehensive knowledge and skill base and a caring, humanistic, compassionate approach to nursing care. The third edition of *Orthopaedic Nursing* provides a comprehensive source of information needed for state-of-the-art orthopaedic nursing practice. This in-depth text includes an examination of orthopaedic wellness and disorders, with presentation of pathophysiology, interrelationships of the musculoskeletal system with other body systems, diagnostic modalities, and therapeutic interventions. This knowledge is further translated into the art and science of nursing with content addressing orthopaedic wellness and risk reduction, orthopaedic disorder management, assessment, nursing care management, and client teaching and counseling. Biophysical, social, cultural, and psychological perspectives are presented to capture the complexity of client care management. Life span considerations and attention to changing needs across wellness, acute illness, chronic illness, and disability capture the dynamic nature of illness and coping responses to illness.

OVERVIEW

This book's first 13 chapters provide the breadth of core knowledge necessary to provide care to orthopaedic clients with varying diagnoses. Information from these chapters can be applied to the orthopaedic client with any type of disorder. Chapters cover topics such as orthopaedic wellness, psychosocial dimensions of illness, ergonomics, immobility, pain, anatomy and physiology, genetics, assessment, diagnostic modalities, complications, perioperative care, immobilization, and mobilization. The in-depth content in these chapters provides the foundation of knowledge necessary for orthopaedic nursing practice.

The remaining chapters address specific orthopaedic disorders. Chapters cover topics such as autoimmune and inflammatory disorders, metabolic conditions, degenerative disorders, disorders of the spine, congenital and developmental disorders, fractures, amputations, athletic performance and injury, neoplasms of the musculoskeletal system, and infections of the musculoskeletal system. The chapters follow a similar format. Each chapter begins with an introduction to the disorder, including definition, incidence, and epidemiology. The pathophysiology of the condition is then described, followed by assessment and diagnostic evaluation. Treatment modalities are presented inclusive of medical, surgical, and pharmacologic management. Concluding the narrative section is nursing management incorporating the common nursing diagnoses and nursing interventions from the Nursing Interventions Classification (NIC) system.

This edition updates key orthopaedic content, providing timely information on diagnostics, treatment, and management. With awareness that practice should be grounded in research, each chapter presents key research evidence on particular topics or questions relevant to that chapter. This can be found incorporated into the narrative and in tables entitled "Examining the Evidence: Moving Toward Evidence-Based Practice."

Also new to this edition are chapters on orthopaedic wellness and genetics. The orthopaedic wellness chapter highlights the nurse's role in prevention and risk reduction and prevention of musculoskeletal conditions. The genetics chapter provides a foundation in basic genetic principles and genetic counseling, emphasizing their applicability to orthopaedics.

As information explodes on the Internet, the nurse must be aware of how to access and evaluate information relevant to orthopaedics. Chapter-relevant Internet sites and an appendix on computers for client and staff education are also included, providing the nurse with critical information on the use and evaluation of Internet sources for professional and client education. Every effort was made during the production of this book to ensure that all URLs were operational. However, URLs change and websites move. Therefore, to help aid the reader, we have also included the name of the site or sponsoring organization. Should the URL change, this should allow the reader to search for the new website.

The editors thank all of the authors and reviewers who have contributed to this or previous editions and who have made *Orthopaedic Nursing* the classic reference for orthopaedic nurses. We also thank Robin Carter and Barbara Cicalese at W.B. Saunders and Suzanne Kastner at Graphic World Publishing Services for their expertise and assistance.

ANN BUTLER MAHER
SUSAN WARNER SALMOND
TERESA A. PELLINO

Contents

1

Orthopaedic Wellness

SUSAN WARNER SALMOND

Orthopaedic nursing is devoted to the prevention and care of musculoskeletal disorders, that is, any disease, injury, or significant impairment to muscles, bones, joints, and supporting connective tissue. Musculoskeletal disorders cross all age ranges and may result from congenital, developmental, traumatic, metabolic, degenerative, or infectious processes. Musculoskeletal disorders or injuries will affect almost every individual at one time or another in their lifetime. Some conditions are minor and transient, but many cause lifelong disability. Musculoskeletal disorders place serious burdens on one's health, quality of life, finances, physical comfort, and psychological health.

THE BURDEN OF MUSCULOSKELETAL DISEASE

The burden of musculoskeletal disease refers to a combination of the incidence and prevalence, impact (in terms of quality of life and disability), and cost of musculoskeletal disorders to the individual and to society. Musculoskeletal disorders are a major cause of morbidity throughout the world and have a substantial influence on health and quality of life. It is the most common cause of severe long-term pain and physical disability affecting hundreds of millions of people worldwide, at a huge cost to society. In the United States alone, musculoskeletal conditions are the number one category of reported chronic impairment and also the number one reason for visits to physicians accounting for more than 131 million client visits to health care providers and 7.3 million musculoskeletal procedures performed annually. Musculoskeletal conditions, including back disorders, arthritis, and orthopaedic impairments, rank in the top five reported causes of activity limitation and work disability in the United States. Similarly, arthritis and back disorders rank among the top five reasons for requiring assistance with personal

care. The direct and indirect costs (mortality and morbidity) of musculoskeletal disease are estimated to be $215 billion per year (Bone and Joint Decade, 2000). Table 1-1 provides evidence of the burden of orthopaedic disease on clients and society. Despite this evidence, the amount of time spent teaching and counseling on orthopaedic prevention and risk reduction is minimal.

To promote musculoskeletal health, an international initiative, launched by the World Health Organization, the *Bone and Joint Decade 2000–2010,* has been established to improve the health-related quality of life for people with musculoskeletal disorders throughout the world. The goals of the Bone and Joint Decade are to reduce the social and financial burden of musculoskeletal conditions to society; to improve prevention, diagnosis, and treatment for all clients; to advance research on prevention and treatment; and to empower clients to make decisions about their care. The United States National Action Network will be the umbrella organization in which partnering of orthopaedic organizations, client advocacy groups, government, industry, and researchers interested in musculoskeletal care can work together to fulfill the goals of the Bone and Joint Decade initiative and to maximize musculoskeletal health for the population.

With a growing recognition that musculoskeletal disease is a worldwide concern consuming billions of dollars, greater attention is being paid to preventing musculoskeletal disorders and maximizing musculoskeletal health across the life span. This focus on health, prevention, and risk reduction requires that nurses in all settings provide pertinent counseling and education related to minimizing risks of musculoskeletal injuries and disorders and decreasing problems and complications, including pain, impaired physical mobility, self-care deficits, activity intolerance, impaired skin integrity, infection, peripheral neurovascular dysfunction, im-

TABLE 1–1. *The Burden of Musculoskeletal Disease*

In the United States, musculoskeletal conditions rank first among diseases according to measures of disability and on the basis of visits to physicians' offices.

Approximately 36.4 million community-dwelling and 0.5 million residents of nursing homes (1 in every 7 Americans) have musculoskeletal impairments resulting in disability.

Musculoskeletal conditions, including back disorders, arthritis, and orthopaedic impairments, rank in the top five reported causes of activity limitation and work disability in the United States.

Musculoskeletal impairments account for 488 million restricted-activity days and 153 million bed-days annually.

Arthritis is the leading chronic condition reported by older adults, affecting 1 of every 8 Americans of all ages and almost 50% of people who are 65 years of age or older.

Arthritis is a more common cause of limitation of activity than heart disease, cancer, or diabetes.

About 1% of the U.S. population is chronically disabled because of back pain, and an additional 1% are temporarily disabled.

Osteoporosis affects 10 million Americans, and 18 million more are at risk.

Fractures related to osteoporosis have almost doubled in number in the last decade, with almost 1.3 million fractures reported annually. Forty percent of all women older than 50 years will suffer from an osteoporotic fracture.

Two thirds of people who have a hip fracture do not return to their prefracture level of functioning.

The number of individuals older than the age of 50 is expected to double by 2020, with estimates that the absolute prevalence of musculoskeletal conditions will increase in the United States from 37.9 million to 59.4 million; the prevalence rate is estimated to increase from 15.0% to 18.2% of the population, and the prevalence rate of activity limitation will rise from 2.8% to 3.6% during this time.

Crippling diseases and deformities continue to deprive children of their normal development.

The severe injuries caused by traffic accidents and war produce a tremendous demand for preventive and restorative help. It is anticipated that 25% of health expenditure of developing countries will be spent on trauma-related care by the year 2010.

Sources: www.boneandjointdecade.org; Weinstein, 2000; and Yelin, Trupin, & Sebesta, 1999.

paired adjustment, disturbed body image, ineffective role performance, situational low self-esteem, and post-trauma syndrome when orthopaedic conditions exist. A focus on orthopaedic well-being and health will achieve these goals.

WELL-BEING AND HEALTH

Health relates to all aspects of life, from physical well-being to social interactions, mental and emotional capacities, and spiritual well-being. In the past, most literature dealing with health focused almost exclusively on disease or illness. Good health meant absence of illness and was conceived as a relatively passive, homeostatic state. The concept of wellness was a reaction to the preconceived preoccupation with illness. Health is seen as a state of being that can be characterized by any degree of illness or wellness or combination of both. High-level wellness is a dynamic, holistic, integrated state of functioning that is oriented toward maximizing the individual's potential toward a higher level of functioning and fuller potential. The World Health Organization defines *health* as a "state of complete physical, mental, and social well-being and not merely the absence of disease or infirmity" (World Health Organization, 1998).

From a systems perspective, health is enmeshed in cultural, social, biophysical, and psychological contexts over the life span (Fig. 1–1). In Western medicine, the emphasis has been predominantly on achieving homeostasis (stability) in the biophysical realm. The broader conceptualization of health and wellness is more consistent with the Chinese interpretation of health as a balance of yin and yang. Wellness is a balance of the biophysical, psychological, sociologic, and cultural systems. There is a dynamic, continuing process within human beings to

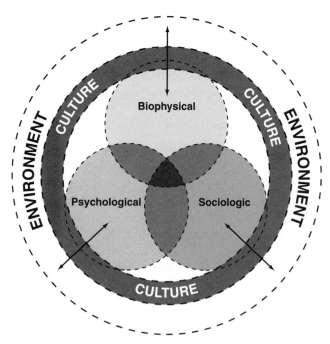

FIGURE 1–1. Systems view of the human being. The human is viewed as a total system with four interrelated subsystems (cultural, biophysical, psychological, and sociologic) that are in a dynamic state of continuous interaction with the environment. The cultural system is the initial system through which input from the environment is filtered and permeates the other three systems supplying the perceived input. Culture grounds the remaining three systems, and output leaving the system filters back through the cultural system.

maintain a positive balance of biophysical, psychological, sociologic, and cultural forces that tend to disturb their health equilibrium. Health is not simply the absence of disease or infirmity but is a process by which a *balance* is achieved between and within the forces of the biophysical, psychological, sociologic, and cultural systems and which results in a sense of stability and comfort. Table 1–2 summarizes wellness goals, assessment areas, and common nursing diagnoses within each subsystem.

Biophysical System

The biophysical system includes all mechanical, structural, and physiologic functions from cellular to organ system levels, as well as the interaction between organ systems. Expert orthopaedic nursing care requires a sound knowledge of the anatomic structure of bones, cartilage, muscles, ligaments, and tendons and their synergistic effects in providing the biomechanics of movement. An understanding of the effect of musculoskeletal conditions on these structures and on the biomechanical processes of movement enables the nurse to diagnose, plan, and intervene effectively to alleviate problems in the musculoskeletal system.

Assessment of orthopaedic wellness requires not only a focus on the musculoskeletal system (activity/exercise patterns, mobility, gait, strength, range of motion, balance, and behavioral/lifestyle activities associated with injury risk and orthopaedic disorders) but also assessment of other biologic systems that are affected by alterations in musculoskeletal function. For example, musculoskeletal immobility affects the cardiovascular, pulmonary, integumentary, gastrointestinal, and renal subsystems (see Chapter 4). Nursing interventions to promote orthopaedic wellness within the biophysical system are directed toward maximizing function, preventing cellular breakdown, maintaining homeostasis, and restoring function to damaged areas.

Psychological System

The psychological system includes the client's self-concept, attitudes toward illness and life, previous experience with illness and hospitals, cognitive functioning, personality, emotional states, spirituality, and coping strategies typically used when faced with stress. Failure to attend to the psychological system can result in anxiety, hopelessness, depression and despair, use of maladaptive coping mechanisms, denial of illness or injury, and inability to implement a therapeutic regimen. Orthopaedic wellness is maximized by a psychological approach characterized by hardiness, resiliency, tolerance of uncertainty, and connectedness. These factors generally promote emotional well-being and participation in health-promoting activities and injury prevention.

In addition to assisting the client and family in coping with the stress of dealing with illness and the health care system, the orthopaedic nurse can anticipate common alterations within the psychological system in the presence of orthopaedic disorders. Impaired mobility restricts a client's sense of independence and autonomy, often leading to discouragement and depression. Reliance on others may cause further emotional distress, frequently demonstrated as resentment, guilt, and helplessness. Degenerative, inflammatory, and traumatic orthopaedic conditions often result in body image and self-concept changes. Furthermore, clients experiencing acute catastrophic trauma are likely to experience the emotional sequelae of the post-trauma syndrome. Table 1–2 highlights the wellness goals, assessment areas, and diagnoses within the psychological realm. Nursing interventions in this system have three major foci: (1) educating the client and family about the disease, therapeutic regimen, and health care system; (2) facilitating client communication about anxiety and fears and the meaning and significance of the illness to his or her self-concept; and (3) assisting the client to learn or strengthen coping mechanisms.

Sociologic System

The sociologic system represents a person's functioning in roles and groups within the larger social system. It includes the individual's roles and relationships with family and friends; positions and roles within the workplace and community; economic status; and available supports, including insurance benefits, family support, community support, occupational safety and health, and medical care support. Nursing care in this system emphasizes the family and community as the unit of care, as well as the living and working conditions that affect the health of the individual, key populations, and society as a whole. Health and well-being from a sociologic perspective encompasses role competence, safe and productive work and family environments, adequate support systems, and community activities targeting wellness and injury prevention.

Table 1–2 describes wellness goals, assessment areas, and nursing diagnoses for the sociologic system. Nursing interventions are targeted toward strategies that are congruent with the system's social and cultural values and that assist the client to maintain role competence and/or return to previous role functions, adapt to role changes, and maintain or renegotiate relationships and supports within the social system. Specific social concerns faced by the orthopaedic client often revolve around dealing with workplace issues (work safety, work readiness, need for job retraining, or job strengthening programs), responding to the stigma of other people's responses to visible handicaps, and coping with altered financial and role requirements. From a community perspective, population-based care targeting sports and recreation safety for all age groups and reduction of high-risk behaviors that contribute to injury are important to orthopaedic wellness.

TABLE 1–2. *Nursing Care Using a Systems Model*

SUBSYSTEM	WELLNESS GOALS	ASSESSMENT AREAS	COMMON NURSING DIAGNOSES IN THE ORTHOPAEDIC CLIENT
Biophysical	Maximize function Prevent cellular breakdown Maintain homeostasis Restore function to damaged areas	Biologic system review Mobility and movement Exercise patterns Gait Balance Range of motion Skin turgor and intactness Neurovascular assessment Pain assessment Swelling Deformity Weight	Activity intolerance Hypothermia and hyperthermia Constipation Disuse syndrome Fatigue Growth and development, delayed High risk for falls Infection, risk for Injury, risk for Pain Perioperative positioning injury Peripheral neurovascular dysfunction Physical mobility, impaired Self-care deficit Skin integrity, impaired Sleep pattern, disturbed Transfer ability, impaired Trauma, risk for Walking, impaired
Psychological	Maintain and strengthen coping mechanisms Promote control by educating client and family about the illness, the therapeutic regimen, and other areas in which information is lacking	Coping styles Stress levels Emotional status Level of hope Knowledge of illness and therapeutic regimen Body image Self-esteem Sexuality Spirituality Previous experience with illness and health care system	Adjustment, impaired Anxiety Body image, disturbed Confusion Fear Grieving: anticipatory, dysfunctional Individual coping, ineffective Knowledge deficit Personal identity disturbance Post-trauma response Self-esteem: disturbance, situational low Powerlessness Management of therapeutic regimen: ineffective Sexuality patterns, ineffective Spiritual distress, risk for Therapeutic regimen: management of
Sociologic	Adequate support systems available Support systems used to promote wellness Assist client and family to evaluate therapeutic regimen within the context of sociocultural priorities Maintain role function or adapt to role change Promote workplace health and well-being Promote community safety	Support systems and resources: personal, interpersonal, community, organizational Role function Occupational stress and risk factors Client's perceptions of priority needs Cultural beliefs and traditions Financial stress	Caregiver role strain Community coping: readiness for enhancement Decisional conflict Family coping: compromised, disabling, potential for growth Therapeutic regimen, family management of Health maintenance, altered Role performance, ineffective Social interaction, impaired Social isolation

TABLE 1–2. *Nursing Care Using a Systems Model* Continued

SUBSYSTEM	WELLNESS GOALS	ASSESSMENT AREAS	COMMON NURSING DIAGNOSES IN THE ORTHOPAEDIC CLIENT
Cultural	Cultural care preservation and maintenance Cultural care accommodation and negotiation Cultural care repatterning and restructuring	Significant groups that client identifies with Cultural patterns of identified group: time orientation, preferred communication style, human to nature orientation, power distance, gender role definition Interpretation of health, healing, illness and regimen efficacy: What do you think caused your problem? Why do you think it started when it did? What do you think your sickness does to you? How does it work? How severe is your sickness? Will it have a short or long course? What kind of treatment do you think you should receive? What are the most important results you hope to receive from your treatment? What are the chief problems your sickness has caused for you? Valued caregivers and decision-makers Cultural sanctions and restrictions Use of traditional interventions: amulets, prayers, herbs, sacrifices Use of alternative approaches: massage, acupuncture, manipulation, herbology Spirituality Food preferences	Value or decisional conflict* Impaired verbal communication Nonadherence Spiritual distress Spiritual well-being, potential for enhanced

*Use of terms implying impairment or deficits when referring to cultural differences is controversial because it implies a judgment from the nurse's perspective. These diagnoses should be used only with awareness that the client's viewpoint is another way of seeing the world and should not be judged as lesser than the dominant viewpoint. The impairment (i.e., communication impairment) should not necessarily be judged as the client's problem because there is just as significant an impairment on the part of the nurse in the inability to understand the client.

Cultural System

Culture is the set of shared beliefs, customs, values, and attitudes that guide the behavior of a particular group. Within society, there is a general or dominant culture as well as different subcultures with varying worldviews based on differences in such factors as ethnicity, religion, education, occupation, age, sex, and health or illness.

Many references to systems theory combine the social and cultural systems into the sociocultural system. This approach fails to capture the depth of the cultural system and the extent to which it permeates all of the systems. Figure 1–1 more accurately portrays the influence of culture on the whole individual. Culture is the system that serves to interpret both input and output. It permeates each individual system influencing interpretation and response.

An understanding and appreciation of how different worldviews and experiences influence perception, cognition, and behavior are critical to effectively interacting with diverse clients. It must be stressed that the meaning of health, wellness, well-being, illness, and the cause of illness are culturally defined and consequently important components of assessment. The variety of specific, native, cultural theories of illness—and thus of curing—is wide. These beliefs are typically embedded in overarching native religious systems. Among the causes of disease that are commonly described are loss of one's soul(s) in whole or part; spirit possession; supernatural forces; intrusion of illness-causing spirit; violation of taboos—especially those having to do with correct relations to deities, including one's ancestors; spirit attack, including capricious "jokester" spirits; homeopathic and/or contagious magic; and disturbances or violation of social rules and relationships. It may be necessary to call in an alternative medical practitioner (e.g., a guru, shaman, curandero) to promote healing.

Assessment is designed to first gain an understanding of the individual and family's emic (inside) perspective regarding their interpretation of the event (e.g., condition, illness, disease), followed by an understanding of preferred cultural patterns (time orientation, preferred communication style, orientation to humans over nature, traditional approaches to treating the problem). Wellness goals are oriented to interventions that promote cultural maintenance, cultural accommodation, or cultural repatterning.

The Environment

The human being as an open system is in constant interaction with his or her environment. The majority of health intervention and policy has targeted biophysical factors and individual responsibility in prevention and disease management. However, health of populations must address the physical environment, the social environment, lifestyle factors, and health care services environment. This expanded view emphasizes interaction with the environment and the complexity of health issues.

The environment has many dimensions that influence wellness and adaptability. Physical environmental issues encompass the areas of environmental hazards in the immediate and broader living areas, the impact of environmental conditions on disease and symptoms, and those factors in the environment supportive of healing and wellness. For orthopaedic clients, physical environmental issues manifest in such things as the interplay of atmospheric conditions on arthritis or low-back pain symptoms, home and occupational hazards that can place the person at risk for injury, and adaptive aids that support the person's functional abilities.

Social environmental issues include factors such as access to care, trust and belief in the medical system, living and lifestyle conditions, educational issues, economic issues, and relationships to those social structures (e.g., family, community, church) that socialize a person into society. For the orthopaedic nurse, examples of social environmental issues that are important to practice include incidence of trauma in urban areas; trust and belief of the community in the medical system, a factor critical to support regimens such as long-term antibiotic use; and accommodations available to support individuals with disabilities.

Psychological components of the environment include the emotional tone created by the people, objects, animals, technology, and information within the environment. This tone can sway the individual's motivation to participate in wellness behaviors; to select appropriate, culturally relevant therapeutic regimens when illness exists; and to strive for optimal functional independence when disability is present.

The health care systems environment is a culture in itself, consisting of common values, beliefs, communication styles, and practices. This system is confusing and overwhelming to many clients and even unfriendly and hostile to some. For many, the unfamiliar language, sound, technology, and tone of the traditional health care system creates anxiety, fear, and discomfort. These reactions are intensified when the client has previous negative experiences with the system or when the individual's cultural background is not consistent with the values common to Western medicine. The nurse's role is to advocate for the client by being supportive of clients' health beliefs while assisting them to understand and negotiate the health care environment.

Maximizing Health

"Health is created and lived by people within the settings of their everyday life: where they learn, work, play and love" (Kickbusch, 1996). Achieving better health for the population requires actions that transcend traditional organizational definitions and involves many services that can assist in creating the systems and environments needed for maximizing health. Wellness promotion requires that the focus be on maximizing potential. Health promotion, risk reduction, prevention, and population-focused care are strategies to facilitate wellness.

Healthy People 2010 (U.S. Public Health Service, 1998) is the current set of national health objectives for the United States to achieve over the first decade of the new century. Focusing on health promotion and disease prevention, its goals are to (1) increase quality and years of healthy life and (2) eliminate health disparities. *Healthy People 2010* offers a roadmap to better health for all and can be used by states, communities, professional organizations, and groups to improve health. The Leading Health Indicators (LHIs) representing the 10 high-priority areas for the nation's health are (1) physical activity, (2) overweight and obesity, (3) tobacco use, (4) substance use, (5) responsible sexual behavior, (6) mental health, (7) injury and violence, (8) environmental quality, (9) immunization, and (10) access to health care. The focus areas for these leading health indicators that are especially relevant to orthopaedic nurses include arthritis, osteoporosis, chronic back conditions, disability and secondary conditions, educational and community-based programs, injury and violence prevention, physical activity and fitness, occupational safety and health, and nutrition.

Informational resources on health and staying healthy with disease conditions are growing exponentially with access to the worldwide web. At the end of this chapter are Internet resources that can be used to gather more information on topics of health, health promotion and disease prevention, orthopaedic illness, and disability. Throughout the text, other Internet resources are included on specific orthopaedic topics.

Maximizing Musculoskeletal Health

Musculoskeletal health is evidenced by safe interaction with the environment, the prevention of accidental injuries, and the adoption of a lifestyle that maintains the integrity of the musculoskeletal system (Table 1–3). Musculoskeletal health is associated with overall health, greater functional ability, and independence.

Lifestyles that promote optimal musculoskeletal health include adequate intake of nutrients essential for bone health (calcium, vitamin D, protein, and phosphorus); regular weight-bearing exercise programs that increase the stress load on the skeletal system, thereby stimulating production of stronger bones; safety-conscious behaviors, such as use of seat belts and safety helmets; use of other protective gear in the occupational, recreational, and home environments; and use of positive strategies to control stress (Chapter 2 contains a complete discussion of coping with stress).

The lessons of orthopaedic wellness need to begin in childhood. Rapid bone acquisitions occurs before, but also at and after, puberty. This two-decade period is crucial in skeletal development and critical for the prevention of osteoporosis later in life. Along with adequate calcium intake, children must understand and begin to practice routine weight-bearing activity programs, which maximizes skeletal development and minimizes bone loss in later years. Children and adults should engage in 30 minutes of moderate-intensity exercise on most and preferable all days of the week. This can include yard work, brisk walking, cycling, swimming, and home repair. Exercise does not have to be done in block periods to be beneficial. Intermittent periods of exercise are also efficacious (Pate et al., 1995). Walking stairs instead of using an elevator, walking short distances instead of driving, parking in the rear of parking lots and walking, pedaling a stationary bike while watching television, and performing housework or dancing at an intensity equivalent to a brisk walk are all strategies that can be easily

incorporated for maximum benefit. Importantly, evidence supports that lost fitness can be regained with regular physical activity, even in extreme old age.

Another component of orthopaedic health is awareness of potential musculoskeletal hazards and active strategies to prevent their occurrence. Preventing unintentional injury and maximizing safety in workplace, home, and recreation environments are critical approaches to maintaining musculoskeletal health.

Public health initiatives as well as anticipatory guidance by nurses and other health professionals are needed to send the message that routine intake of adequate calcium beginning in childhood maximizes bone strength and that routine exercise is associated with greater levels of overall health as well as greater levels of functional ability in individuals diagnosed with musculoskeletal disorders. An overall effort to encourage adequate calcium intake, optimal weight maintenance, regular weight-bearing activities, abstinence from or moderation in alcohol consumption, and the discouragement of smoking across the life span are important to maintaining optimal bone health.

Several public health campaigns regarding musculoskeletal health are currently aimed at the U.S. consumer. The Osteoporosis and Related Bone Diseases National Resource Center (ORBD-NRC), The National Osteoporosis Education Campaign, and the Milk Matters initiative are designed to increase calcium consumption and activity among all people, with a special emphasis on children and teens.

Many public health initiatives target increased safety awareness and prevention of unintentional injury. The Centers for Disease Control and Prevention (CDC), in conjunction with the National Institutes of Health (NIH), has prepared the *Guidelines to Clinical Preventive Services* (U.S. Preventive Services Taskforce, 1996), which emphasizes prevention of unintentional injury as a prime strategy in orthopaedic wellness. The American Academy of Pediatricians has initiated the TIPPS program (The Injury Prevention Program), designed to provide a systematic method to counsel parents and children about adopting behaviors to prevent injuries. To the same end, the National Safety Council has many programs to disseminate the message that seat belts save lives and that bicycle helmets prevent serious injury and death.

ORTHOPAEDIC DISORDERS

Orthopaedic disorders can be classified as acute, chronic, or disabling. The goal of health promotion efforts within the states of health (i.e., acute illness, chronic illness, and disability) is to move the person toward the optimal level of wellness. Each specific health or illness state has different priorities and intensities of health care needs within the biophysical, psychological, sociologic, and cultural systems.

Text continued on page 16

TABLE 1–3. *Population-Based Health Promotion and Disease Prevention*

INJURY AND CONDITION DATA	EVIDENCE	PREVENTION
Maximizing Orthopaedic Mobility and Bone Health ***Exercise, Activity, Functional Ability*** Fitness levels of young Americans are declining or failing to improve The most rapid reduction in physical activity levels occur between the ages of 18–24 years 56% of men and 61% of women do not participate in physical activity or do so only irregularly Sedentary lifestyle in 58% of the population Rates of inactivity are higher in subgroups of Mexican Americans, black women, and older adults	Program of regular aerobic physical exercise has measurable and substantial benefit for the health of each individual It will be cost-effective to change the lifestyle of children to optimize the skeleton during growth and adolescence by increasing calcium intake, improving overall nutrition, and encouraging exercise People who exercise have decreased mortality rates Physical activity and fitness reduce morbidity and mortality associated with osteoporosis, obesity, and impact on joints Resistance exercise improves mobility of the very old, increases muscle strength and mass, increases habitual gait velocity, improves the ability to climb stairs, and produces an overall increase in physical activity Weight-bearing exercise may slow the rate of bone loss in older women Balance exercise training and tai chi reduce the rate of falls in older adults For the population older than 65 years of age of both genders, exercise programs have been strongly associated with maintenance of functional capacity, the ability to live independently, and the reduction of risk for falls Lost fitness can be regained with regular physical activity, even in extreme old age There is insufficient evidence to recommend for or against counseling clients to exercise to prevent low-back pain Arthritis and fatigue may affect sexual functioning Multiple aspects of the social situation can influence functional ability, so gather data on recent changes in living arrangements, finances, and activities Ability to perform activities of daily living is a convenient way of assessing the level of supportive assistance required	Activity and exercise regimens Adult: Moderate intensity aerobic exercise for 30–40 minutes most days, if not every day of the week; resistance training as an adjunct to the aerobic exercise program 2 days per week Moderate physical activity comprises activities that can be comfortably sustained for at least 60 minutes (e.g., walking, slow biking, raking leaves, cleaning windows, performing light restaurant work) Vigorous activity describes those of an intensity sufficient to result in fatigue within 20 minutes (e.g., shoveling snow) For older adults, progressive resistance training of the hip and knee extensors For older adults, programs that incorporate mild aerobic activity and emphasize strength, flexibility, and proprioceptive training are beneficial; strength programs are associated with both enhancement and maintenance of activities of daily living and include activities such as progressive resistance with weights and elastic bands Flexibility and proprioception is needed for balance and is achieved through programs such as tai chi, stretching, and yoga Recognize that yard work, housework, and other "light" activities are an important source of activity for the older adult—do not attempt to take over all activities leaving the individual without a source of exercise Openly address sexuality and provide guidance on safe and pain-free positioning Social functioning assessment ADL Evaluation

TABLE 1–3. *Population-Based Health Promotion and Disease Prevention* Continued

INJURY AND CONDITION DATA	EVIDENCE	PREVENTION
Maximizing Orthopaedic Mobility and Bone Health *Continued* ***Promote Bone Mineralization, Prevent Demineralization and Accompanying Fracture*** It is imperative to build bone across the life span, beginning at a very young age Most children and teens are not getting adequate levels of calcium during the critical period when bones grow and incorporate calcium most rapidly Eating disorders are clustered uniquely in adolescent populations adding to the risk of bone demineralization More than ⅓ of high school students perceive themselves as being overweight and are attempting weight loss	Rapid bone acquisitions occurs before, but also at and after, puberty; this period is crucial in skeletal development and critical for the prevention of osteoporosis later in life Goal is to optimize calcium intakes not only to prevent deficiency diseases but also to build a better skeleton and to preserve it throughout life Poor eating habits continue or even worsen in late adolescence Osteoporosis does not need to be a consequence of aging; it is largely a preventable disease Fractures can be prevented and bone loss reduced, even in older individuals Physical activity and fitness reduce morbidity and mortality associated with osteoporosis, obesity, and impact on joints After menopause, bone loss accelerates because of the decline in estrogen production by the ovaries Osteoporosis is responsible for 70% of fractures that occur in older adults More than 12% of women older than 60 years of age sustain a hip fracture 15%–20% of these women die as a result of their injury Estrogen replacement has been shown to improve bone density and thus far is the most effective strategy for lowering the risk of osteoporotic fractures Routinely screen HIV-infected clients receiving antiretroviral treatment for osteopenia and osteoporosis	Assessment Assess and counsel about risk factors (men and women) Obtain bone mineral density testing baseline at age 50 Obtain bone mineral density testing for all postmenopausal women with a fracture Dietary and risk factor reduction Target children and adolescents to consume calcium at recommended levels because window of opportunity to add bone to the skeleton is limited To slow bone loss: counsel to consume an adequate intake of dietary calcium (at least 1200 mg per day, including supplements if necessary) and vitamin D (400 to 800 IU per day for persons at risk of deficiency) Avoid smoking and limit alcohol intake to moderate levels Activity and exercise regimen Participation in regular weight-bearing and muscle strengthening exercise decreases bone loss and reduces the risk of falls and fractures Implement fall prevention strategies in the older adult Pharmacologic treatment Bisphosphonates or selective estrogen receptor modulators (Evista) may be indicated to prevent bone mineral density from declining further in older women who have already sustained an osteoporosis-related fracture Hormonal replacement: counsel on benefits and risks of estrogen replacement therapy (ERT) Community education programs Assure that schools have routine programs on bone health stressing calcium intake and weight-bearing activity Support campaigns such as Milk Matters, designed to bring the message that increased calcium and weight-bearing exercise during the first two decades of life can be critical to good health as an adult

TABLE 1–3. *Population-Based Health Promotion and Disease Prevention* Continued

INJURY AND CONDITION DATA	EVIDENCE	PREVENTION
Maximizing Orthopaedic Mobility and Bone Health *Continued* **Promoting Joint Health** 9% of U.S. population age 30 or older has clinical osteoarthritis (OA) of the hip or knee OA is more prevalent in women	Physical activity and fitness reduce morbidity and mortality associated with osteoporosis, obesity, and impact on joints The Framingham Study data showed about a 60% reduction in incidence and progression of OA in older white women using ERT Optimal nutrition may play a role in slowing of the progression of OA Low levels of vitamin D may increase the risk of hip OA development and new OA progression Antioxidants, both natural and supplemental, may protect against OA progression; this is particularly true for vitamin C and may be true for vitamin E Stress placed on the joint from excessive weight or from repeated motions from certain occupations or sports contributes to OA Obesity increases the risk of knee OA and, to a lesser extent, hip OA Greater incidence of OA in joints previously injured with dislocations or sprains The mechanical process of joint movement is critical to cartilage regeneration and joint mobility Repetitive, low-impact joint use, as in jogging, does not cause degeneration; other sports (e.g., football, soccer, rugby, baseball pitching, volleyball) may increase the risk of OA through direct joint impact loading, repetitive indirect impact, and torsional loading	Nutritional and activity counseling Reducing excess weight, strengthening the quadriceps, and improving overall fitness may help reduce the impact of OA Eliminating obesity may prevent 25%–50% of knee OA and 25% of hip OA Antioxidant supplements Moderate recreational exercise decreases both the likelihood of developing OA and the progression of arthritic symptoms Reduce risk of OA in sports participants Evaluate risk factors before participating Decrease direct contact with other players Wear braces, pads, and proper shoes Play on appropriate surfaces Train Obtain early diagnosis and treatment of injury Complete a rehabilitation program after joint injury Hormonal replacement Counsel on benefits and risks of ERT
Preventing Unintentional Injuries **Motor Vehicle Accidents** Motor vehicle accidents (MVAs) are the leading cause of death of all ages from 1–34 years They are the 8th leading cause of death across all ages For child in booster, if shoulder straps are too high: risk of strangulation in accident For child in booster, lap belt across abdomen risks severe internal injury in accidents Major injuries are to head and lower extremities with motorcycle accidents	No matter what the age, rear seats are safer than front seats Risk of death in an accident is 35% lower with child riding in rear versus front seat 1998 NHTSA data showed only 4% of 5-year-olds in fatal crashes were in any form of child restraint The efficacy of child safety seats may be reduced by improper use; such misuse has been reported in up to ⅔ of children Use of helmets for motorcyclists decreases head injury rates by about 40%–75%	Occupant restraint devices Proper use of lap and shoulder belts can decrease the risk of moderate to serious injury to front seat occupants by up to 55% and can reduce crash mortality by 40%–50% Proper car seat use Infants ≤20 pounds up to 1 year: backward-facing seat strapped in the back seat; straps should be in the lowest slots until the child's growth places the shoulders above the slot

TABLE 1–3. *Population-Based Health Promotion and Disease Prevention* Continued

INJURY AND CONDITION DATA	EVIDENCE	PREVENTION
Preventing Unintentional Injuries *Continued* **Motor Vehicle Accidents** Continued	Half of fatal MVAs are alcohol related Cutoff point for blood alcohol levels is generally 0.1 g/dL (100 mg/dL); however, must recognize that risk begins to increase at levels of 0.02 g/dL and increases significantly at 0.05 g/dL The risk of a fatal crash among drivers with blood alcohol levels of 0.05–0.09 g/dL is nine times greater than among those with no alcohol in their blood Alcohol-impaired drivers are less likely to use seat belts than other drivers Alcohol remains the most commonly abused drug in America; an estimated 10% of the general population may have an alcohol abuse disorder, and alcohol abuse complicates medical care in as many as 20% of primary care hospitalized clients Long-distance truck drivers, especially those driving at night, are high risk for sleep deprivation, which has been reported as a cause in numerous accidents Adolescents have the highest rate of MVAs Older adult drivers drive relatively few miles and tend to be law abiding and account for a small proportion of total road accidents By age 85 and older, the accident rate is three times that of other drivers and is only exceeded by that of teenage drivers	Infants >20 pounds up to 1 year: use an infant seat approved for higher weight, in back, facing rear Children >1 year between 20–40 pounds (9–18 kg): child safety seat facing forward and fastened in back seat Children 4–8 who are too big for safety seat but too small for adult safety belt (40–50 pounds): belt positioning booster seat with lap and shoulder belts; shoulder harness should cross child's chest and lap belt to fit across the thighs Children 8–12 (>50 pounds): regular seating using seat belts; back seat positioning preferred; if in front seat, push seat as far back as possible to avoid injury if the airbag deploys Alcohol and drug avoidance education Should begin at an early age Designated driver awareness Families should anticipate and discuss with teens avoidance of alcohol and drugs but also to have transportation alternative for social activities in which alcohol and other drugs are used Motorcycle helmet use Lobby for mandatory helmet legislation Transportation safety regulations Requirement that operators of trucks and airplanes receive designated rest and sleep Many states and countries have restricted teen licenses that limit nighttime driving and set limits on the number of teen passengers allowed in the car while driving on a teen license Periodic screening of the older adult driver

Table continued on following page

INJURY AND CONDITION DATA	EVIDENCE	PREVENTION
Preventing Unintentional Injuries *Continued* **Bicycle Injuries** Head injuries cause 75% of bicycle-related deaths and serious disability	Case-control studies have demonstrated that bicycle helmets reduce the risk of head injury by 63%–85% and protect against upper face and midface injuries Multiple time-series studies show that mandatory bicycle helmet use laws and community-based education programs have been associated with substantial increase in helmet use and reduction in bicycle-related fatalities, head injuries, and hospitalizations	Bicycle safety training and counseling Educate parents about the risk of head and face injury for small children on all wheeled toys and the need for helmets Helmets for children <6 years of age should include safe and comfortable fit, low weight, and a lower face guard to protect the mouth and chin Adult role modeling to children as to the merits of bicycle helmets Avoiding riding near motor vehicle traffic Educational campaigns and legislative approaches to promote mandatory bicycle helmet use laws and enforcement of same
Recreational Vehicle Accidents Snowmobile injuries The most common sites of injury are the extremities and the head, neck, and face Predominance of lower extremity injuries in both adults and children Head and neck injuries are commonly reported to be a leading cause of death Boating injuries Head injury is the most common boating injury	The predominate mechanism in fatal snowmobile crashes is striking a stationary object Being pulled in a sled or inner tube behind a snowmobile has a significant mechanism of injury Helmets reduce the risk of death by about 42% in all-terrain vehicles (ATVs) Inner tubes being pulled behind boats has been identified as an emerging source of injury in young people	Safety precautions Avoid alcohol use when operating recreational vehicles Legislative action Lobby legislators to prohibit dangerous practices of pulling sleds/tubes behind motorized land and water vehicles Helmet laws and age restrictions similar to those enacted for motorcycle riders are necessary and appropriate Driving age restrictions for boating and ATV licenses
Sports and Recreation Injuries Most sports injuries involve the lower extremities, with fractures, sprains and strains, tendinitis, and overuse injuries being the most common conditions The knee is the most frequently injured joint Sports such as hockey, basketball, soccer, and lacrosse are associated with orofacial and dental injuries Football, wrestling, and soccer have the highest injury rates at the high school level In-line skating injuries have increased to involve more than 23 million people, and the number of in-line related injuries has been estimated as high as 99,500 There is a 140% increase in trampoline injuries since 1990, with 85,000 acute care visits secondary to trampoline use	Sports injuries are an important cause of long-term and temporary disability in adolescents Last two decades have seen a dramatic reduction in fatalities, predominantly because of community prevention programs and better training of coaches Relatively poor muscular strength has been shown to be associated with higher rates of injury The most common cause of injury in in-line skating is a simple fall, often related to difficulties in stopping—this mechanism leads to a fall on to the arm and wrists, which is the area most commonly injured Female athletes, especially gymnasts and dancers, should be evaluated for the female athlete triad: eating disorder, amenorrhea, and osteoporosis The incidence of this disorder ranges from 15%–62%	Evaluation and rehabilitation Preseason examination is an opportunity to diagnose and rehabilitate old injuries and thereby prevent reinjury Rehabilitation efforts to focus on: improving strength and flexibility of the injured structures, improvement in strength, flexibility, proprioception, and endurance of the injured structures Education and safety Proper stretching and coaching in technique associated with the sport is essential Physical conditioning is a major factor in reducing injuries; target conditioning exercises (i.e., neck strengthening in football) effective in reducing risk of injury

TABLE 1–3. *Population-Based Health Promotion and Disease Prevention* Continued

INJURY AND CONDITION DATA	EVIDENCE	PREVENTION
Preventing Unintentional Injuries *Continued* ***Sports and Recreation Injuries*** Continued	In amenorrheic athletes, bone density has been shown to be decreased not only in the spine and proximal femur but in many other sites, including cortical weight-bearing bone	Proper technique of instructing on sports safety (i.e., tackling and hitting to block with the head up and the head not to be the initial point of contact), teaching falling techniques for in-line skating Compliance with safety standards: helmet standards set by NOCSAE* with proper fitting of the helmet, use of protective mouth guards, wrist splints for in-line skating Nutritional strategies Encourage proper intake of calcium and balanced caloric intake Exercise Aerobic exercise develops an optimally functioning cardiovascular-respiratory system and develops muscular fitness, endurance, tone, strength, and flexibility Community strategies Proper field maintenance and repair Teaching and licensing of parent coaches Use of trainers or medical personnel in high school athletics Prohibit trampolines in school-based physical education programs
Falls In children younger than 5, falls are a common cause of injury, although without a large degree of mortality or permanent sequelae Falls are the leading cause of nonfatal injuries and unintentional injury deaths in older persons in the United States Each year, about 12,000 Americans, primarily older persons, die as a result of falls	Baby-walkers are an important cause of injuries in young children, many of which result from falls down stairs Children can fall from windows even when there are screens in place Falls are the second leading cause of unintentional injury death in the United States (after motor vehicle injuries) and the leading cause of nonfatal injuries One half of falls are caused by gait problems, and one third are caused by balance problems The annual incidence of falls in clients older than 65 years of age who live independently is about 25%; this rises to 50% in clients older than 80 years of age One third of clients with confirmed falls may not recall falling Among the risk factors associated with injury after falls are osteoporosis, syncope, impaired cognitive function, use of diuretics or vasodilators, and falling on hard surfaces such as concrete	Environmental safety precautions Collapsible gates have been advocated as a means of protecting children from stairways There is evidence that window guards can reduce child falls from windows Make sure hallways and stairwells are well lit Remove or repair things that could cause tripping, such as loose rugs, electric cords Put handrails and traction strips on stairways and in bathtubs Always lower toilet seats Secure foot wear Exercise and activity Exercise programs to enhance strength, balance, and mobility In the presence of postural hypotension, ankle pumps, hand clenching, and elevation of the head of the bed are helpful

Table continued on following page

TABLE 1–3. *Population-Based Health Promotion and Disease Prevention* Continued

INJURY AND CONDITION DATA	EVIDENCE	PREVENTION
Preventing Unintentional Injuries *Continued* ***Falls*** Continued	Randomized, controlled trials of exercise programs for older persons have generally shown improved strength and mobility; effects on balance have been less consistent Tai chi improves mobility, enhances stability, improves kinesthetic sense, and strengthens knee extension	Gait training in presence of impairment Use of appropriate assistive devices With impaired balance or transfer skills: balance exercises and training in transfer skills With impairment in leg or arm muscle strength or impaired range of motion: exercises with resistive bands and putty; resistance training 2–3 times per week Tai chi mediation/exercise as a low-stress activity to promote mobility Measures to increase bone density Intake of 1000–1300 mg of calcium per day Avoid smoking Avoid excess intake of alcohol Assess and respond to additional risks for falls Assessment of cognition Assessment of sensory deficits: Snellen chart Screening for alcohol abuse, polypharmacy Screening for sleep problems and nonpharmacologic treatment of sleep problems
Preventing Infectious Disease Immunizations	U.S. guidelines for polio vaccinations changed in 1999 The two initial doses should be inactivated polio vaccine (IPV) For the third and fourth doses, IPV or oral polio vaccine (OPV) may be used In Canada, IPV is recommended for all four doses to prevent the rare cases of paralytic polio that may follow administration of OPV	Obtain polio vaccinations
Lyme disease Found predominantly in New England, the Mid-Atlantic region, the Southeast, small endemic areas of Wisconsin and Minnesota, and to a lesser extent on the Pacific Coast	Prophylactic antibiotic therapy is probably not indicated even after tick bites in endemic areas because of the low transmission rate Risk of infection in an endemic area is estimated to be about 1.4% Most deer ticks (70%–80%), even in highly endemic areas for Lyme disease, are not infected with *B. burgdorferi* Efficacy rates of the OspA Lyme disease vaccine have been reported as 75% and 76% Vaccine preparation was less immunogenic in subjects older than 60 years of age	Avoid tick-infested habitats when in endemic areas When in endemic areas, use repellents, wear light-colored clothes: long sleeves and long pants that are tight at the wrists, ankles, and waist or pants tucked into socks; regularly check for and removed attached ticks In endemic residential areas, remove habitats suitable for ticks and their reservoir hosts: clear brush and trees, remove leaf litter and woodpiles, keep grass mowed Exclusion of deer from residential yards by fencing and maintaining tick-free pets

TABLE 1–3. *Population-Based Health Promotion and Disease Prevention* Continued

INJURY AND CONDITION DATA	EVIDENCE	PREVENTION
Preventing Unintentional Injuries *Continued* **Preventing Infectious Disease** Continued Lyme disease		Considerations for use of Lyme disease vaccine to persons who are 15 years of age or older who reside, work, or recreate in geographic areas of high or moderate risk and whose activities result in frequent or prolonged exposure to vector ticks
Preventing Workplace Injury Approximately one third of all injuries in the United States are occupational in nature Approximately 6.6 million workplace injuries and illnesses reported annually, with nearly 50% resulting in lost work days Occupational groups with the highest estimated prevalence of low-back pain (10%) are nurses and operators of heavy machinery and construction equipment	The National Safety Council estimates the cost of workplace injuries to be about $120 billion per year Aggressive multidisciplinary rehabilitation programs have been shown to achieve return-to-work rates as high as 50%–88% The longer persons are away from work, the less likely they are to ever return Occupational back injury is related to lifting and repeated activities Association between greater fitness or higher levels of physical activity and reduced prevalence of low-back pain or injury Inconsistent data regarding the effect of greater strength or flexibility on low-back pain—effects are modest and of uncertain duration Research on the efficacy of education (e.g., proper body mechanics, lifting) shows that only a small percentage consistently follow the recommendations once taught, therefore having little effect on minimizing back pain Research on the efficacy of lumbar supports to reduce back pain and injury shows that less than half of persons adhere to wearing the support Disability status of persons with musculoskeletal conditions is one of the strongest predictors of whether they leave or enter employment Evidence that musculoskeletal conditions can be prevented is slight; only two clear risk factors, other than age, have been identified, and these are obesity and overuse of joints, the latter principally result from occupational exposures There is evidence that the disability rates can be reduced through medical treatment, exercise programs, self-care, or a combination of these strategies	Assessment Individual limitations and job demands Exercise and activity Strengthening back extensors or flexors and general fitness exercises Increasing back flexibility to reduce injury risk Physical and occupational therapy Work conditioning Work hardening Workplace prescriptions Specialized equipment requirements Duty and work hour limitations Workplace wellness programs Nutritional counseling to address obesity

*National Operating Committee on Standards for Athletic Equipment.

Sources: American Academy of Pediatrics, 2000; American Academy of Pediatrics, Committee on Sports Medicine and Fitness, 2000; American College of Sports Medicine (www.acsm.org); CDC, 1996; Marshall, 2000; Miller, Zylstra, & Standridge, 2000; Mouton & Espino, 1999; National Institute of Arthritis and Musculoskeletal and Skin Diseases, 1999; National Safety Council, 1997; Rice, Alvanos, & Kenney, 2000; USPSTF, 1996; Van Poppell et al., 1998; Warshafsky et al., 1996; Wormser, 1999; and Yelin, Trupin, & Sebesta, 1999.

Acute Illness

The state of acute orthopaedic illness or injury is marked by a sudden onset of biophysical stressors. Acute orthopaedic illness states are either traumatic or nontraumatic. Acute traumatic episodes may be localized, as with a fractured femur or meniscal tear, or may involve several body systems, as with complex motor vehicle injuries or boating injuries. Nontraumatic acute episodes include periods of acute biophysical instability associated with infectious, inflammatory, metabolic, and degenerative types of disorders.

Acute orthopaedic illness is generally unanticipated and brings normal activity to a halt, with a focus on the illness. The biophysical alterations compromise the client's ability to provide self-care, achieve activity and mobility regimens, and maintain role functions. Consequently, the person must rely on varying degrees of assistance from health caregivers for resolution of the biologic crisis and assistance with self-care. The outcome in acute episodes may be a return to the wellness state with full function or a shift into the chronic or disabled state.

Biophysical care is generally the focus and the priority of the acute illness state. The initial period is characterized by acute physiological imbalance. The nurse attends to the biophysical needs of the client while remaining alert and responsive to the psychological and sociocultural needs as well as to the effect of these needs on the biophysical system. It is important to note that for many cultural groups, Western biophysical interventions are supplemented or dominated by traditional approaches that may involve spiritual practices and traditional remedies. Failure to appreciate and accommodate these cultural practices may result in lack of follow-through with the prescribed biophysical intervention.

During the acute state, the nurse ensures implementation of the medical regimen necessary for biophysical stabilization and supports the biophysical system with independent nursing strategies designed to support homeostasis, prevent further cellular breakdown, and restore function to damaged areas. As the biophysical state is stabilized, the nurse encourages the client to describe his or her interpretation of the cause and severity of the illness and perception of effectiveness of strategies to manage the illness (the emic view of the problem). Assessment of the emotional responses to the acute episode, available coping resources, and the presence of social supports guides nursing care designed to assist the individual to respond to and adapt to the biophysical threat.

Chronic Illness

Chronic orthopaedic disorders are marked by diseases that can be controlled but not cured. Rheumatoid arthritis, osteoporosis, degenerative disc disease, and systemic lupus erythematosus are examples of chronic diseases. They are characterized by the persistence of symptoms, in which severity changes unpredictably. The severity can range from acute episodes to chronic situations (in which symptoms are stabilized with a therapeutic regimen) to disability (in which functional deficits are ongoing). In the chronic state, the focus of care is assisting the client to develop an understanding of the illness and its therapeutic regimen and to develop coping mechanisms such that the disease is integrated as part of the self-concept, rather than its dominant focus.

Control of a chronic illness requires adopting therapeutic behaviors and coping strategies that promote selection and implementation of culturally responsive therapeutic regimens designed to maximize wellness within chronic illness. Chronic illness does not indicate the absence of health. A person can be well with a chronic illness. In this situation, the person has implemented a therapeutic regimen and coping response that enables the client and family to be healthy (in a state of wellness), with a sense of stability and comfort.

Because chronic illness, by definition, cannot be cured, lifestyle changes and coping strategies become the hallmark of this state, thereby making the cultural and psychological systems a priority. Nursing strategies are aimed at educating the client and family; helping them with problem-solving strategies; and strengthening their coping mechanisms, which are supportive of cultural maintenance or are supportive in the cultural negotiation or repatterning process. Biophysical instability remains a consideration so that the illness can be prevented from becoming acute. Sociocultural perspectives must also be considered when developing therapeutic regimens, when developing adequate support structures, and when evaluating a client's response to role disruption. Biophysical needs are continuous as the client attempts to eliminate or control the symptoms of illness. At times, the client may move into the acute state with exacerbations of the chronic illness. Chronic illness is often accompanied by disability.

Disability

The efficacy of modern medicine in treating acute and chronic illness and injury has had the effect of increasing the population of people living with a disability. It is estimated that more than 49 million Americans have disabling conditions. Minorities, people from lower socioeconomic backgrounds, and older adults are all affected disproportionately by disabilities.

Disability is characterized by limitations in functional performance and activity and refers to the loss of ability to perform self-care tasks and fulfill usual social roles and normal activities. A person may be in the disabled state with an accompanying acute or chronic process or may have no further acute or chronic illness but have remaining functional deficits. Functional deficits can lead to varying degrees of social disability. For example, the professional athlete with a meniscal tear is more disabled than the teacher with the same injury is. The athlete is unable to fulfill the role in relation to work, whereas the teacher could continue to carry out the usual teaching functions.

Disability may be temporary or permanent, reversible or irreversible, and progressive or regressive. Disabilities can be classified as emotional, intellectual, sensory, or physical. Disability is a far-reaching social and public health issue in the United States. The national cost of disabilities totals more than $190 billion each year (CDC, 1996). In a response to these issues, the *Disabilities Prevention Program,* part of the National Center for Environmental Health at the CDC, provides a national focus for the prevention of disabilities to build capacity at the state levels to conduct and evaluate prevention activities and to conduct surveillance to increase the knowledge base about disabilities (CDC, 1996). In addition, the CDC hosts the website Kid's Quest on Disability and Health, which is designed for children and targets education and sensitivity about disabilities.

Historic legislation, the Americans with Disabilities Act (ADA) of 1990, was passed with the intent of removing the barriers that deny individuals with disabilities an equal opportunity to share in and contribute to the vitality of American life. It gives civil rights protections to individuals with disabilities similar to those provided to individuals on the basis of race, color, sex, national origin, age, and religion. The ADA ensures access to jobs, public accommodations, government services, public transportation, and telecommunications. Ergonomics, or the interdisciplinary study of the fit between the design of the living and work environment and human behavioral and biologic capabilities and limitations, is a growing field in health care that is responsive to the intent of the ADA.

Clients undergoing rehabilitation for disabilities should be working toward the achievement of functional goals. Medicare Part B requires progress toward measurable functional goals for coverage of rehabilitation services. Functional goals define expected outcomes of performance of real-world activities that are realistic and reachable within a reasonable amount of time.

The focus of care for the disabled is to seek ways to enable the client to tap the various resources available. Understanding cultural groups' interpretation of the disability, the meaning of the disability, and the expectations regarding rehabilitation must be achieved to provide culturally relevant care. Nursing interventions focus on the social system and are targeted toward maximizing available support systems, maintaining functional roles, assisting the client in coping with societal attitudes, and overcoming structural and functional barriers to achieve maximum function. The disabled client's psychological needs center on coping with the functional deficits, and the biophysical needs focus on maintaining maximal functioning.

POPULATION-BASED CARE: PREVENTION AND RISK REDUCTION

Evidence shows that certain orthopaedic injury and orthopaedic illness (i.e., osteoporosis) can be prevented by improving personal health habits. Eating right, staying physically active, ensuring proper protective measures in sports and recreation, using occupant restraints, and avoiding alcohol when driving are major factors contributing to orthopaedic wellness. Awareness of prevalence rates and risk factors allows care to be focused on preventing problems in targeted populations. Epidemiologic and preventive strategies aimed at target population groups by condition and age are addressed in this chapter and summarized in Table 1–3 and the Clinical Pathway for Orthopaedic Wellness.

Counseling and screening guidelines for all age groups have been promulgated by the United States Preventive Services Task Force (USPSTF) and the Agency for Healthcare Research and Quality (AHRQ). These guidelines present epidemiologic data on more than 80 conditions, with evidence-based support for screening tests, counseling, immunizations, and chemoprophylactic regimens. Conditions addressed that are of special interest to the orthopaedic nurse include counseling to prevent household and recreational injuries, counseling to prevent low-back pain, counseling to promote physical activity, and counseling to prevent motor vehicle accidents. These recommendations are on the AHRQ website (www.ahrq.gov).

For children and adolescents, the American Academy of Pediatrics has promulgated prevention guidelines through TIPP. TIPP is designed to provide a systematic method for pediatricians to counsel parents and children about adopting behaviors to prevent injuries—behaviors that are effective and may be accomplished by most families. These guidelines are available on the Academy website (www.aap.org).

Preventing Unintentional Injury

Unintentional injuries rank as the fifth leading cause of death overall, the leading cause of death in all age groups from 1 to 34 years of age, and the leading cause of years of potential life lost before age 65 (USPSTF, 1996). Routine anticipatory guidance and counseling of children, parents, adults, and older adults to reduce the risk of unintentional household and recreational injuries has been shown to be efficacious in risk reduction. Unfortunately, research demonstrates that although unintentional injury is a leading cause of morbidity and mortality, prevention counseling is typically underemphasized (Baker, O'Neill, Ginsburg, & Li, 1992).

CLINICAL PATHWAY: *Orthopaedic Wellness*

INITIALLY AND RECOMMENDED ON ALL ENCOUNTERS	0–10 YEARS	11–24 YEARS	25–64 YEARS	≥65 YEARS
Assessment				
Goals: Determine level of homeostasis. Evaluate for congenital and degenerative process; if any, reason acquired: because of metabolic, mechanical, genetic, and other influences. Determine potential for restoring function to damaged areas.				
History and Physical Examination Complete baseline initially; then every 1–3 yr Assess cultural and religious views on health care, development, parenting, caretaking, and treatment	Head circumference in children <2 yr Assess for congenital disorders: club foot, developmental dysplastic hip, rotational problems	Assess for variations in physical growth and development Body image	Possible estrogen/calcium imbalance: hysterectomy, anorexia, inadequate calcium intake, subtotal gastrectomy, major organ transplant, malabsorption, menopause	Vital signs: blood pressure (orthostatic changes) Gait assessment for functional ability and detection of peripheral neuropathy and degenerative joint disease Presence of antalgic gait Joint limitations and functional ability Sensory changes with aging: visual acuity, glaucoma, cataracts, macular degeneration, hearing loss Signs and symptoms of osteoporosis: gradual loss of height, curvature of upper spine, fractures of hips or wrists, predominant abdominal bulge with no weight gain Depression screening
Dietary and Nutritional Patterns General nutritional pattern and calcium intake Cultural and religious factors influencing nutritional intake	No. of glasses milk intake per day	Fast food and soda intake Willingness to drink milk	Assess changing weight patterns related to metabolic and role changes	Weight changes Dental/gum changes influencing nutrition Income and nutritional intake
Activity Patterns and Fitness Level of activity Overuse/underuse injuries Functional ability ADL and developmental milestones Safety: seat belt use, bike helmet use	Assess parental enforcement and child use of safety interventions	Eating disorders (anorexia nervosa, bulimia) Assess for the female athlete triad: disordered eating, amenorrhea, and osteoporosis	Inconsistent activity (weekend athlete) and sedentary lifestyle	Fall risk: mobility, polypharmacy or medications that increase risk of falls, balance, endurance Changes in cognitive functioning Functional status changes should be assessed and tracked
High-Risk Patterns Stress levels Coping styles Risk factors: cigarette smoker, alcohol user, inactivity, obesity Signs of abuse/neglect	Parent-child interactions: signs of abuse, neglect, dysfunction	Individual teen use of safety interventions: Scoliosis screening High-risk excessive exercise patterns Use or potential use of nonprescribed steroids (usually male teen and young adult) Risk-taking behavior	Use of corticosteroids	Home safety screen Refusal to use assistive devices when indicated

CLINICAL PATHWAY: *Orthopaedic Wellness* Continued

INITIALLY AND RECOMMENDED ON ALL ENCOUNTERS	0–10 YEARS	11–24 YEARS	25–64 YEARS	≥65 YEARS

Diagnostics
Goals: Determine whether any congenital/traumatic injury. Determine whether any bone loss. Assess for side effects of treatment.

Periodic testing: ASA or NSAID use: CBC, renal function tests, stool for occult blood Trauma: x-ray films, MRI Malignancy: bone scan			Serum calcium and phosphate if at risk for osteoporosis Measurements of bone density with symptoms or risk of osteoporosis	Serum calcium and phosphate if at risk for osteoporosis Measurements of bone density with symptoms or risk of osteoporosis

Occupational/Recreational Assessment
Goals: Preventive measures to reduce orthopaedic hazards

Assess home/work environment for ergonomic hazards (chair height, use of computers, lighting, positioning of joints, strenuous activity) Determine participation in activities requiring repetitive motion, lifting, awkward postures, long periods of standing or stooping while working Assess recreation patterns Evaluate safety measures used during work and recreational activities (i.e., lumbar support belts, helmet and goggle use)	Potential for falls, recreational injuries: bicycling, sports, swimming/diving	Participation in contact sports, recreational vehicle use, recreational activities Evaluate workplace for potential areas creating physical strain Incorrect posture Underlying physical abnormalities Computer use	Recreational vehicle activities Evaluate workplace Computer use	Evaluate use of stairs Evaluate home environment and need for adaptive devices

Teaching and Counseling
Goals: Goal of health promotion efforts is to move the person toward the optimal level of wellness. Promote healthful lifestyles.

When and how to access health care
Behavioral change interventions
Positive coping mechanisms
Nutritional counseling
Body mechanics, including back care
Regular moderate weight-bearing exercise: increase exercise intensity and duration gradually
Always stretch before and after exercise
Hazards of immobility or sedentary lifestyle
Use of appropriate footwear
Injury prevention: safety belts, helmets, occupational hazards, recreational hazards, domestic violence
	Establish good eating habits from the start to build strong bones
	Injury prevention
	  Child safety car seats (age <5 yr) every time
	  Lap/shoulder belts (age ≥5)
	  Stair gate use
	  Window guards
	  Removal of sharp-edged furniture
	  Caution with use of baby-walkers
	  Use of bicycle helmet always
	  Too young to ride in street safely
	  Ensure that car safety seats are correctly installed
	  Never put an infant in the front seat of a car with a passenger-side airbag
	  Activity programs
		Prevention and risk reduction efforts for smoking, alcohol/drug abuse and avoidance of high-risk activities (e.g., driving, boating, swimming) while impaired
		Use of appropriate protective equipment according to sport
		Appropriate physical conditioning for specific sport
		Effects of nonprescription steroid use
		Injury prevention
		  Lap/shoulder belts
		  Bicycle/ATV helmets
		  High-risk patterns
		  Firearm safety
		  Regular physical exercise regimens
		  Diet regimens
			Behavioral change interventions with smoking cessation, alcohol moderation
			Injury prevention
			  Strategies for preventing repetitive strain injuries
			  Prevention of low-back pain
			  Back strengthening exercises
			Risks and benefits of hormone replacement and use of calcium supplements
			Exercise regimens
				Injury prevention
				  Identify treatment and environmental factors increasing propensity to fall and strategies to prevent fall
				Recommend adequate calcium intake
				Recommend consistent activity program
				Balance of rest and activity

Box continued on following page

CLINICAL PATHWAY: *Orthopaedic Wellness* **Continued**

INITIALLY AND RECOMMENDED ON ALL ENCOUNTERS	0–10 YEARS	11–24 YEARS	25–64 YEARS	≥65 YEARS

Nutritional Guidelines
Goals: Develop strong bones. Reduce bone loss. Help achieve or maintain optimal weight.

INITIALLY AND RECOMMENDED ON ALL ENCOUNTERS	0–10 YEARS	11–24 YEARS	25–64 YEARS	≥65 YEARS

Proper diet; should be individualized by height and weight, age, amount of activity, presence of disease (DM, heart disease, HTN, GI concerns)
Adequate caloric intake
Adequate calcium, vitamins, and minerals
Nutritional counseling
  Risks of low-calcium diets
  Avoidance of excess alcohol (no more than 1–2 drinks per day)
  Modest caffeine consumption
  Risks of being overweight
  Adequate intake of vitamin C and zinc supplements to aid in healing of bone fractures
	Diet history should be taken
	Adequate vitamins, minerals
	Calcium RDA:
	
	Age (mg)
	Birth–6 mo 210
	6 mo–1 yr 270
	1–3 yr 500
	4–8 yr 800
	9–10 yr 1300
		Calcium RDA:
		Age (yr) (mg)
		11–18 1300
		19–24 1000
		Caloric intake when pregnant: 2500–2700 kcal/day
		Calcium intake during pregnancy:
		  age 14–18: 1300 mg/day;
		  age > 19: 1000 mg/day
		Balanced diet
		  Limit fat and cholesterol
		  Maintain caloric balance
		  Emphasize grains, fruits, vegetables
			Average adult caloric intake is 1500–2500 kcal/day
			Calcium RDA:
			Age (yr) (mg)
			25–50 1000
			51–64 1200
			Calcium intake during pregnancy: minimum 1000 mg/day
			Increase calcium intake to 1200 mg after menopause (depending on presence of estrogen)
			Balanced diet
			  Limit fat and cholesterol
			  Maintain caloric balance
			  Emphasize grains, fruits, vegetables
				Average adult intake is 1500–2500 kcal/day
				Calcium RDA: 1200 mg/day

Medications and Special Considerations
Goals: Minimize discomfort and maximize ADLs. Prevent onset of osteopenia.

INITIALLY AND RECOMMENDED ON ALL ENCOUNTERS	0–10 YEARS	11–24 YEARS	25–64 YEARS	≥65 YEARS
Evaluate medication history, including over-the-counter and prescriptions, with specific attention to calcium supplements Therapeutic exercise Heat or cold therapy RICE (rest, ice, compression, and elevation) Evaluate for use of anti-inflammatory medications, steroids, thyroid or asthma medications			Hormone replacement in women and men Review hormone-free treatment for osteoporosis Calcium replacements	Polypharmacy risks Hormone replacement in women and men Calcium replacement

Causes of Death and Morbidity
Goals: Reduce morbidity and mortality through preventive measures and education.

INITIALLY AND RECOMMENDED ON ALL ENCOUNTERS	0–10 YEARS	11–24 YEARS	25–64 YEARS	≥65 YEARS
See individual age groups for causes of morbidity and death	Congenital disorders Motor vehicle accidents Unintentional injuries: fall-related injuries, bicycle injuries	Motor vehicle and other unintentional injuries Homicide Suicide	Motor vehicle and other unintentional injuries Homicide Suicide Orthopaedic deformities and impairments (including back and upper and lower extremities) Hearing and vision impairments	Accidents Osteoporosis, arthritis, or both Injuries (musculoskeletal and soft tissues) Hearing and vision impairments

ADLs, activities of daily living; ASA, aspirin; CBC, complete blood count; DM, diabetes mellitus; GI, gastrointestinal; HTN, hypertension; NSAID, nonsteroidal anti-inflammatory drug; ROM, range of motion.

Injury prevention is the single most important aspect of trauma care. We are reaching a critical point in the history of trauma care in which most of the deaths seen are caused by unsurvivable injuries, and hence the only way to decrease trauma-related mortality further is to prevent the injuries from occurring. Injuries are not random events; they follow predictable patterns and hence are susceptible to preventive interventions. Knowledge and attitudes are crucial determinants of injury prevention, and there is a continuing need for programs to increase knowledge of injuries and safety. Table 1–3 addresses varying injuries that can be predicted across the life span, the evidence to support the predictability of the injury, and/or the efficacy of the intervention.

Preventive strategies can be broadly classified into three categories: education, legislation, and cost subsidization (providing high-risk individuals with required safety equipment at reduced rates). Experience from bicycle helmet interventions suggests that an integrated approach combining all three types of strategies maximizes success of preventive measures (Shafi & Gilbert, 1998).

Motor Vehicle Accidents

Motor vehicle accidents account for half of unintentional deaths and are the eighth leading cause of death in the United States. Motorcycle occupant fatality rate is nearly 20 times higher than for passenger car occupants (USPSTF, 1996). The motor vehicle fatality rates for males are more than twice that for females. Alcohol use remains an important risk factor for motor vehicle injuries.

Motor vehicle fatality rates are highest for young and older adults. The high mortality rate in older adults reflects a high case fatality rate, probably attributable to increased likelihood of developing serious complications after motor vehicle injuries because drivers 65 years of age and older have the lowest rate of crashes per 100,000 licensed drivers.

Use of occupant restraints has been shown to reduce the risk of motor vehicle injury and death. The efficacy of safety belts has been demonstrated in a variety of studies. Child safety seats are also effective. They can reduce serious injury by up to 67% and mortality by as much as 71% (USPSTF, 1996). The efficacy of child safety seats may be reduced by improper use; such misuse has been reported in up to two thirds of children.

Airbags have been shown to further reduce the risk of injury and death. Parents must be cautioned against permitting children younger than 12 years to sit in the front seat. A number of childhood fatalities have been reported from deployment of the airbag when the child was sitting in the front passenger seat, particularly when unrestrained or in a rear-facing child safety seat.

Counseling all clients and the parents of young clients to use occupant restraints (lap/shoulder safety belts and child safety seats), to wear helmets when riding motorcycles, and to refrain from driving while under the influence of alcohol or other drugs is recommended.

Bicycle Injuries

Bicycle riding is a common leisure activity. Nearly half of all Americans and 80% to 90% of children ride bicycles. The consumer product safety commission (CPSC) estimates that there are about 33 million bicycle riders younger than age 20, with about 45% of this group riding for a total of about 10 billion hours each year (Sosin, Sacks, & Webb, 1996).

Medical care for bike injuries is estimated at $8 billion per year, with most injuries occurring in those 15 years or younger. Head injuries cause 75% of bicycle-related deaths and serious disability (Sosin, Sacks, & Webb, 1996).

Bicycle helmets reduce head injury between 74% and 85%, yet the majority of children still do not routinely use a helmet when riding a bicycle. Helmet use is lowest in the adolescent group. Only 7% of adolescents and 18% of all bicyclists wear bicycle helmets sometime or always (USPSTF, 1996). Barriers to helmet use include peer influences, helmet unattractiveness, helmet discomfort, lack of awareness of head injury risk and helmet effectiveness, and cost.

Additional interventions to reducing bicycle injury include bike safety training and avoidance of riding near motor vehicle traffic.

Sports Injuries

Approximately 30 million children and adolescents participate in organized sports in the United States, and many more participate in recreational sports. There are approximately 3 million annual injuries (time lost from sports participation) incurred during children's and teens' sports participation. Of these injuries, 777,000 require physician visits and 45,000 to 90,000 require hospitalization (Hergenroeder, 1998). The estimated direct and indirect costs are $1.3 billion for the evaluation and acute management of these clients.

Despite these high injury rates, the prevalence of sports injuries has been reduced in the last decade with increased safety regulation of the sport environment. Nurses and other health professionals should be involved on local community boards in setting policy and developing educational programs for youth sports. Mechanisms to reduce sports injuries that have been identified as successful include thorough preseason examinations with attention to need for conditioning and/or strengthening, medical/trainer coverage at sporting events, proper coaching, adequate hydration, proper officiating, and proper equipment and field or surface conditions.

In the area of recreational injuries, the greatest increases have been noted in in-line skating and home trampoline use. In-line skating accidents approach 100,000 per year (American Academy of Pediatrics, 1998). The majority of in-line skating injuries are to the upper extremity and are associated with lack of skill in stopping. The large increase in trampoline injuries (fractures and dislocations of the upper extremities and soft tissue injuries of the lower extremities) is a clear indicator that current prevention strategies are not sufficient. Community-wide education programs as well as anticipatory guidance by health practitioners should stress use of helmets and knee and wrist pads for skating and recommendations *not* to purchase home trampolines.

Falls

Each year, about 12,000 Americans, primarily older persons, die as a result of falls. Falls are the second leading cause of unintentional injury death in the United States (after motor vehicle injuries) and the leading cause of nonfatal injuries (USPSTF, 1996). Physiologic changes with age (postural instability, gait disturbances, diminished muscle strength and proprioception, poor vision, cognitive impairment, number of medications, and the use of psychoactive and antihypertensive drugs) and environmental agents (stairs, pavement irregularities, slippery surfaces [including loose rugs], inadequate lighting, unexpected objects, low chairs, and incorrect footwear) are the principal risk factors for falls in older clients. Interventions focus on exercise or activity regimens to enhance strength, balance, and mobility; the correction of environmental hazards; and measures to increase bone density.

Workplace Injury

Approximately one third of all injuries in the United States are occupational in nature, with estimates of 6.6 million workplace injuries and illnesses annually and nearly 50% of these injuries resulting in lost work days (Wyman, 1999). Musculoskeletal conditions rank in the top three workplace injuries and have a dramatic impact on employment, particularly when such conditions lead to disability.

Injury prevention and productive return-to-work strategies are needed to minimize the personal and economic consequences of these injuries. The evidence suggests that prevention strategies (teaching, use of protective and preventative gear) are not consistently effective in prevention, primarily a result of lack of personal adherence and lack of organizational system attention. Aggressive multidisciplinary rehabilitation programs have been shown to be more effective, with return-to-work rates as high as 50% to 88% (Wyman, 1999). Preventive workplace strategies incorporating ergonomic principles have been shown to reduce injury and disability (see Chapter 3).

ORTHOPAEDIC HEALTH SCREENINGS

Health screenings for musculoskeletal concerns should be an ongoing process in health promotion and disease prevention. Maintaining function necessitates screening for conditions that could lead to disability. The Wellness Clinical Pathway provides guidelines for screening for orthopaedic conditions and risk factors that cause significant morbidity and mortality across the life span.

Infants and Children

Key to orthopaedic health in this population is injury prevention. Prevention of falls, sports injuries, and other recreational injuries is a major concern in this age group. The parental role in teaching and reinforcing safety habits is critical at this stage. Parents must serve as role models and demonstrate consistent protective habits of wearing seat belts, using bike helmets, safely crossing at cross walks, and so forth.

TABLE 1–4. *SAFE TEENS—A Mnemonic Screen of Adolescent Clients*

S	= Sexuality
A	= Accident, abuse
F	= Firearms, homicide
E	= Emotions (suicide, depression)
T	= Toxins (tobacco, alcohol, drugs)
E	= Environment (school, sports, home, friends)
E	= Exercise
N	= Nutrition
S	= Shots (immunization status, school performance)

It is during young childhood that parents and children alike should be counseled on the role that adequate calcium intake and weight-bearing activity has on skeletal development and subsequent osteoporosis development. Encouraging adequate intake of milk and milk products is paramount.

Adolescents

Approximately three fourths of adolescent and young adult deaths are considered preventable. The developmental stage of adolescence is characterized by peer pressure influence, resistance to parental and societal advice, active sexuality, a sense of invulnerability, and the tendency toward high-risk behavior. In terms of orthopaedic wellness, a focus on screening and counseling in regard to accidents and violence is a priority. The four leading causes of all deaths among teens and young adults are motor vehicle accidents (30%), other unintentional injuries (12%), homicide (19%), and suicide (11%). Preventable injuries are also the leading cause of productive years of life lost; for every death that occurs, there are about 100 injuries (Grace, 1998).

Ideally, children are advised before adolescence on the importance of calcium and weight-bearing activity on skeletal development. This counseling should continue, and teens should be further advised on the risk factors of caffeine, smoking, and excess alcohol intake on bone health and general health.

The Guidelines for Adolescent Preventive Services (GAPS) provide 24 recommendations that encompass health care delivery, health guidance, screening, and immunizations for adolescents (Montalto, 1998). The hypothesis (requiring further evidence) is that if high-risk behaviors and negative lifestyle patterns can be identified at an early age, subsequent interventions can reduce premature morbidity and mortality in this population. Table 1–4 presents a commonly used mnemonic for the screening and counseling needs of adolescents.

Adolescent athletes should be screened for high-risk problems. In the male athlete, there is an increased use of anabolic steroids. In the female athlete, there is an elevated risk of developing what is known as the *female athlete triad*. This is a combination of disordered eating, amenorrhea, and osteoporosis. The disorder often goes unrecognized, with the devastating consequences of lost bone mineral density and premature osteoporotic fractures. Instituting an appropriate diet and moderating the frequency and intensity of exercise may result in the natural return of menses. Hormonal replacement therapy should be considered early to prevent the loss of bone density.

Adults

In the adult population, maintenance of healthful diets and physical activity regimens along with workplace and recreational safety are the mainstay of orthopaedic wellness. Because up to 60% of adults report at least one musculoskeletal complaint, with low-back pain being the most common, it is critical to assess activity and mobility patterns and to counsel adults on the need for consistent physical activity programs.

Older Adults

The number of older clients will increase dramatically in the upcoming years, from 34 million in 1998 to 69 million in 2020 (Hendrickson, 2000). Therefore, health practitioners must be cognizant of strategies to maintain wellness and maximal ability in this target population. A philosophical and management approach that proactively embraces healthy aging by continuing to reinforce health patterns of avoiding cigarette smoking, maintaining normal weight, and consistently participating in exercise and activity routines is predicted to decrease the level of disability and dependence often assumed to be part of old age.

Wellness goals for this age group include initiating or continuing healthful dietary and activity patterns and maximizing independence, functional ability, and quality of life. Screening for osteoporosis, risks for falls, activity levels, sensory alterations, and cognitive and affective disorders is important in this age group.

Functional status should be screened routinely so that improvements or deteriorations can be evaluated. Many office-based practices are using generic measures of functional status and quality of life, such as the Short-Form 36 (SF-36) Health Survey. The SF-36 has eight subscales (physical functioning, role-physical, bodily pain, general health, vitality, social functioning, role-emotional, and mental health) that are combined to give measures of physical health and emotional health (Ware, 2000). The SF-36 has well-documented reliability and validity and periodic measurements of functional well-being can detect changes (deterioration and improvement) in overall functional status and health. Thus, it is a useful tool in assessing outcomes of treatment.

Additional self-report questionnaires include the Activities of Daily Living (ADL) Scale and the Instrumental Activities of Daily Living (IADL) Scale (Mouton & Espino, 1999). The ADL index is moderately reliable and valid in evaluating behaviors that are predictive of the independent living ability of older adults. Ongoing use of the instrument can identify persons who may benefit from

assisted living or increased levels of care. Similarly, the IADL index has been shown to be reliable and valid in older populations. Impairment identified by this scale should trigger the development of a plan for supporting the continuation of independent living.

Performance-based tests are used to objectively measure functional status. The Get Up and Go Test and the Gait and Balance Evaluation are two simple measures of assessing gait. These tests evaluate a core physical activity: the ability to stand without assistance, maintain balance, and ambulate. In the Get Up and Go Test, the client is observed as he or she rises from a sitting position, walks 10 feet, turns, and returns to the chair to sit. The effectiveness of the test for predicting falls can be enhanced by timing the process, with more than 16 seconds suggesting an increased risk for falling (Miller, Zylstra, & Standridge, 2000). The Timed Manual Performance Test assesses upper extremity function as determined by the client's ability to open a sequence of locks (Mouton & Espino, 1999). Dexterity can be further evaluated by the ability to perform fine motor activities such as buttoning and writing.

An estimate of physical disability can be screened for by asking a series of questions related to common role activities. Morre and Siu (1996) suggest that questioning begin with more complex, strenuous activities and proceed downward to basic ADLs. Suggested questioning includes ability to do strenuous activities (fast walking, bicycling), ability to do heavy housework (washing windows, walls, or floors), ability to shop for groceries and food, ability to get to places that are out of walking distance, ability to bathe (sponge bath, tub bath, or shower), and ability to dress (put on a shirt, button and zip clothes, or put on shoes). A response to any of these questions that is indicative of lack of ability calls for a more thorough history and physical examination.

Fall assessment screening is accomplished by consideration multiple factors: affective state, cognition, gait and balance status, medication use, alcohol use or abuse, exercise and activity status, and environmental hazards. Table 1–5 lists medications associated with increased risks for falls.

TABLE 1–5. *Medications Associated with an Increased Risk of Falls in the Older Adult*

Antiarrhythmics	Laxatives
Antihistamines	Monoamine oxidase inhibitors
Antihypertensives	Muscle relaxants
Antipsychotics	Narcotics
Benzodiazepines and other sedative-hypnotics	Tricyclic antidepressants and selective serotonin reuptake
Digoxin (Lanoxin)	inhibitors
Diuretics	Vasodilators

Adapted with permission from Reuben, D. B., Herr, K., Pacala, J. T., Potter, J. F., Semla, T. P., & Small, G. W. (2001). *Geriatrics at your fingertips: 2001 edition* (p. 50). Belle Mead, NJ: Excerpta Medica, Inc., for the American Geriatrics Society.

Falls present a great risk in the person with osteoporosis. The fall can lead to a fracture and long-term disability. In addition, osteoporosis itself is an intrinsic factor that leads to falls. Risk factors for osteoporosis are presented in Chapter 16. Osteoporosis screening and adequate calcium and vitamin D intake are needed in the high-risk population.

Because alcohol use is a major factor in unintentional injuries and because it represents a significant health issue (especially in men older than 65 years of age), screening for alcohol abuse should be done. Using the short, four-item CAGE questionnaire acronym, ask: "Do you ever feel the need to **c**ut back on your drinking?" "Do you ever feel **a**ngry when people ask you about your drinking habits?" "Do you feel **g**uilty when you drink?" "Do you ever have an **e**ye-opener in the morning?" Further information can be solicited by asking about the frequency of drinking, number of drinks taken on a typical day, and frequency with which the person has five or more drinks on one occasion.

BEHAVIORAL CHANGE

Behavioral change is key to orthopaedic wellness and risk reduction; however, achieving this change is no easy task. It is clear that the American public is aware of the health

TABLE 1–6. *Stages of Behavioral Change*

STAGE	CHARACTERISTICS OF CLIENT	STRATEGIES TO SUPPORT CHANGE

Precontemplation	Not prepared to change
	May verbalize an inability to change
	May view that the cons outweigh the pros
		Identify risk factors and potential benefits in change
		  Discuss the targeted behavior—what in their life contributes to it, what meaning does the activity have for the client/family?
		  Discuss the risks of the current behavior (e.g., smoking, sedentary lifestyle, insufficient calcium intake)
		  Dialogue about the reasons for change, especially in relation to client's own life ways, support system

Contemplation	Seriously contemplating changing behavior in next 2–6 months but not within next month
	May verbalize an understanding of the risk but not the energy or readiness to change the behavior
	May verbalize "I know I should, but I can't"
		Assist client to have realistic expectations reinforced by small success
		  Encourage short-term, limited trials of change
		  Encourage a component of behavioral change (e.g., instead of initiating a daily walking regimen, park the car at the end of the lot rather than the front)
		  Discuss and strategize two or three choices of what could be started and have the client chose; this not only begins the process of change but also empowers the person because he or she has a choice; if successful, this engenders confidence to possibly move toward a more permanent program (e.g., could delay the first cigarette of the morning by 30 minutes, cut the daily consumption by 5 cigarettes, or refrain from smoking for 24 hours)

Preparation	Have a plan they expect to implement within the next month
	Fear failure
		Set practical goals congruent with cultural and life values
		  Help formalize details of plan
		  Discuss congruency of plan with life patterns
		  Support self-confidence
		  Facilitate involving supportive others

Action	The behavioral activity is consistently begun
	The stage takes approximately 6 months
	Relapses are frequent if client lets down their guard after just 2–3 months
		Identify sources for and provide support
		Initiate strategies for self-monitoring
		  Frequent positive reinforcement for a job well done
		  Encourage client to tell others what he or she is doing because it draws in more social support
		  Mobilization of social supports to participate with the process or reinforce the process

Maintenance	For most behavioral changes, it takes at least 5 years before risk of relapse becomes relatively low	Maintain self-monitoring strategies and support
		  Vigilance is required
		  Continued social support

Termination	A theoretical stage in which there is no risk of relapse May never be reached, prolonged maintenance is the reality for most	

benefits of maintaining a normal weight and a routine exercise program, yet obesity and underactivity are endemic. Clearly, behavior is complex, and nurses should be guided by social cognitive theory to tailor counseling and educational programs to the unique needs and circumstances of the individual, family, and community.

Client and family education should emphasize self-management plus regular review by the health care provider to assist with problem solving and adjustment. Gibson, Coughlan, Wilson, Abramson, Bawman, Hensley, and Walters (1999) performed a meta-analysis on educational interventions targeting individuals with asthma. Planned self-management programs consisting of a written action plan, use and adjustment of medications, self-monitoring of symptoms, and regular review by a caregiver resulted in improved outcomes of lower hospitalization rates, fewer unscheduled medical visits, and fewer days off from work and school. Similar programs need to be established for musculoskeletal wellness and management of chronic orthopaedic conditions.

Behavioral change is an extraordinarily difficult thing for clients and families to do. It is a *process that takes time*, not simply a strategy where the client is given information or a prescription and then expected to follow it. The nurse's role is to partner with the client and family and to facilitate understanding, dialog, and decision making regarding what particular strategies would be possible considering the context of that person's life ways.

Prochaska (1995) identifies six stages in the behavioral change process (Table 1-6). An awareness of each stage allows for more focused strategies, thereby facilitating movement from one stage to the next. This approach embraces the complexity of the change process. Interventions associated with higher rates of success target the following goals:

1. Facilitating awareness of current risk factors and benefits associated with the target change
2. Assisting the client to develop realistic expectations based on small success
3. Identifying sources of support and providing support
4. Assisting the client to set behavioral change goals congruent with cultural and life values
5. Initiating and maintaining self-monitoring approaches

SUMMARY

Orthopaedic conditions, although usually not life-threatening, are associated with high degrees of burden because of the need for medical care and the occurrence of disability. The nurse is in a unique position to maximize orthopaedic wellness through a prevention—risk reduction—health screening approach. Across all states of health and illness, the nurse maintains a philosophy of rehabilitation or restoration of the client to the fullest physical, mental, and social capabilities.

INTERNET RESOURCES

The Administration for Children and Families: www.acf.dhhs.gov/
Administration on Aging: www.aoa.dhhs.gov/
Agency for Healthcare Research and Quality: www.ahrq.gov
American Academy of Orthopaedic Surgeons: www.aaos.org
American Academy of Orthopaedic Surgeons: Prevent Injuries America: http://orthoinfo.aaos.org/prevention.cfm?category=Prevention
American Association of People with Disabilities: www.aapd.com/
American Disability Association: www.adanet.org/
American Public Health Association: www.apha.org
The Bone and Joint Decade: www.boneandjointdecade.org
Centers for Disease Control and Prevention (CDC): www.cdc.gov
CDC National Center for Chronic Disease Prevention and Health Promotion: www.cdc.gov/nccdphp
CDC National Center for Environmental Health: www.cdc.gov/nceh
CDC National Center for Health Statistics: www.cdc.gov/nchs
CDC National Center for Injury Prevention and Control: www.cdc.gov/ncipc
CDC National Center for Injury Prevention and Control: Acute Care, Rehabilitation Research, and Disability Prevention: www.cdc.gov/ncipc/dacrrdp/dacrrdp.htm
CDC National Institute for Occupational Safety and Health: www.cdc.gov/niosh/homepage.html
The Council on Quality and Leadership in Supports for People with Disabilities: www.accredcouncil.org/
Departments of Health and Human Services and Agriculture: Nutrition and Your Health: Dietary Guidelines for Americans: http://odphp2.osophs.dhhs.gov/dietaryguidelines/
Environmental Health Clearinghouse: www.infoventures.com/e-hlth/
Health Resources and Services Administration: www.hrsa.dhhs.gov
Healthfinder: www.healthfinder.gov/
Healthtouch: www.healthtouch.com/
Healthy People 2010: http://odphp2.osophs.dhhs.gov/healthypeople/
HealthWeb: healthweb.org
Job Accommodation Network: http://janweb.icdi.wvu.edu
Magic Stream: Emotional Wellness Journal: http://fly.hiwaay.net/~garson/
Mobility International USA: www.miusa.org/
Morbidity and Mortality Weekly Report: www.cdc.gov/mmwr/
National Health Information Center: http://nhic-nt.health.org

The National Information Center for Children and Youth with Disabilities: www.nichcy.org/

National Institutes of Health (NIH): www.nih.gov/

National Organization on Disabilities (NOD): www.nod.org/

National Osteoporosis Foundation: www.nof.org

The National Parent Network on Disabilities (NPND): www.npnd.org/

NIH National Institute on Aging: www.nih.gov/nia

NIH National Institute of Arthritis and Musculoskeletal Diseases and Skin Diseases (NIAMS): www.nih.gov/niams/

NIH National Institute of Environmental Health Sciences: www.niehs.nih.gov

NIH National Institute of Nursing Research (NINR): www.nih.gov/ninr/

Occupational Safety and Health Administration (OSHA): www.osha.gov/

Office of Disease Prevention and Health Promotion: www.odphp.osophs.dhhs.gov

Office of Minority Health: www.omhrc.gov/

OSH-Link: An Online Resource Summarizing Current Literature on Occupational Safety and Health: www.infoventures.com/osh/

United Nations: The UN and Persons with Disabilities: www.un.org/esa/socdev/enable/

The Virtual Hospital: www.vh.org

The Virtual Office of the Surgeon General: www.surgeongeneral.gov/sgoffice.htm

The World Health Organization: www.who.int

REFERENCES

American Academy of Pediatrics. (1998). In-line skating injuries in children and adolescents. *Pediatrics, 101,* 720–722.

American Academy of Pediatrics (2000). Prevention of Lyme disease. *Pediatrics, 105,* 142–147.

American Academy of Pediatrics, Committee on Sports Medicine and Fitness. (2000). Injuries in youth soccer: A subject review. *Pediatrics, 105,* 659–661.

Baker, S. P., O'Neill, B., Ginsburg, M. J., & Li, G. (1992). *The injury fact book.* Oxford: Oxford University Press.

Bone and joint decade 2000–2010: For prevention and treatment of musculoskeletal disorders. Executive summary. [Online]. Available at www.boneandjointdecade.org

Centers for Disease Control and Prevention, National Center for Environmental Health. (1996). *Disabilities prevention program.* Atlanta: Author.

Gibson, P. F., Coughlan, A. M., Wilson, A. J., Abramson, M., Bawman, A., Hensley, M. J., & Walters, E. H. (1999). The effects of self management education and regular practitioner review in adults with asthma. *Western Journal of Medicine, 170,* 266.

Grace, T. (1998). Health problems of late adolescence. *Primary Care: Clinics in Office Practice, 25,* 237–252.

Hendrickson, R. M. (2000). Health assessment of the geriatric patient. *American Family Physician, 61,* 949–950.

Hergenroeder, A. (1998). Prevention of sports injuries. *Pediatrics, 101,* 1057–1063.

Kickbush, I. (1996, November). *Setting health objectives: The health promotion challenge.* Keynote presentation at Healthy People 2000 Consortium Meeting, New York.

Marshall, K. (2000). *Family practice sourcebook.* St Louis: Mosby.

Miller, K., Zylstra, R., & Standridge, J. (2000). The geriatric patient: A systematic approach to maintaining health. *American Family Physician, 61,* 1089–1104.

Montalto, N. (1998). Implementing the guidelines for adolescent preventive services. *American Family Physician, 57,* 2181–2190.

Morre, A., & Siu, A. L. (1996). Screening for common problems in ambulatory elderly: Clinical confirmation of a screen instrument. *American Journal Medicine, 100,* 438–443.

Mouton, C., & Espino, D. (1999). Health screening in older women. *American Family Physician, 59,* 1835–1842.

National Institute of Arthritis and Musculoskeletal and Skin Disorders. (1999). *Conference summary: Stepping away from OA.* [Online]. Available at www.nih.gov/niams/reports/oa/oaconfsumsc.htm

National Institute of Arthritis and Musculoskeletal and Skin Disorders. (1999). *Statement by Stephen I. Katz, M.D., Ph.D. before Subcommittee on Labor, Health and Human Services: Osteoporosis.* [Online]. Available at www.nih.gov/niams/reports/may20jam

National Safety Council. (1997). *Accident facts.* Itasca, IL: Author.

Pate, R., Pratt, M., Blair, S. N., Haskell, W. L., Macera, C. A., Bouchard, C., Buchner, D., Ettinger, W., Heath, G. W., King, A. L., Kriska, A., Leon, A. S., Marcus, B. H., Morris, J., Paffenbarger, R. S., Jr., Patrick, K., Pollock, M. L., Rippe, J. M., Sallis, J., & Wilmore, J. H. (1995). Physical activity and public health, a recommendation from the Centers for Disease Control and Prevention and the American College of Sports Medicine. *Journal of the American Medical Association, 273,* 402–407.

Prochaska, J. O. (1995). Why do we behave the way we do? *Canadian Journal Cardiology, 11*(Suppl A), 20–25.

Reuben, D. B., Grossberg, G. T., Mion, L. C., Pacala, J. T., Potter, J. F., & Semla, T. P. (1999). *Geriatrics at your fingertips.* Dubuque, IA: Kendall Hunt.

Rice, M. R., Alvanos, L., & Kenney, B. (2000). Snowmobile injuries and deaths in children: A review of national injury data and state legislation. *Pediatrics, 105,* 615–619.

Shafi, S., & Gilbert, J. (1998). Pediatric surgery for the primary care pediatrician, Part I: Minor pediatric injuries. *Pediatric Clinics of North America, 45,* 831–851.

Sosin, D. M., Sacks, J. J., & Webb, K. W. (1996). Pediatric head injuries and deaths from bicycling in the United States. *Pediatrics, 98,* 868–870.

U.S. Preventive Services Task Force (USPSTF). (1996). *Guide to clinical preventive services* (2nd ed.). Baltimore: Williams & Wilkins.

U.S. Public Health Service Office of Disease Prevention and Health Promotion. (1998). *Healthy people 2010: National health promotion and disease prevention full report.* Atlanta: Author.

Van Poppell, M. N., Loes, B. W., van der Ploeg, T., Smid, T., & Bouter, L. M. (1998). Lumbar supports and education for the prevention of low back pain in industry: A randomized controlled trial. *Journal of the American Medical Association, 279,* 1789–1794.

Ware, J. E. (2000). SF-36 health survey update. *Spine, 25*(24), 3130–3139.

Warshafsky, S., Nowalowski, J., Nadelman, R. B., Kamer, R. S., Peterson, S. J., & Wormser, G. P. (1996). Efficacy of antibiotic prophylaxis for prevention of Lyme disease. *Journal of General Internal Medicine, 11,* 329–333.

Weinstein, S. (2000). 2000–2010: The bone and joint decade. *Joint and Bone Journal of Surgery, 82A*(1), 1–3.

World Health Organization. (1998). *Definition of health* [Online]. Available at www.who.ch/aboutwho/definition.htm

Wormser, G. (1999). Vaccination as a modality to prevent Lyme disease. *Infectious Disease Clinics of North America, 13,* 135–148.

Wyman, D. (1999). Evaluating patients for return to work. *American Family Physician, 59,* 844–848.

Yelin, E., Trupin, L., & Sebesta, D. (1999). Transitions in employment, morbidity, and disability among persons ages 51–61 with musculoskeletal and non-musculoskeletal conditions in the U.S., 1992–1994. *Arthritis and Rheumatism, 42,* 769–779.

2

Psychosocial Care of Clients and Their Families

SUSAN WARNER SALMOND and JoANN SPEARS

The dominant approach to client care in Western medicine has been the biomedical model. This model, with its primary emphasis on biophysical symptoms, often neglects the cultural, social, psychological, and behavioral dimensions of illness. This chapter explores the variety of psychosocial issues that influence the client's response to illness or disability. Failure to address the psychosocial dimensions of illness may have long-term sequelae that are as detrimental if not more detrimental to quality of life and well-being than the biomedical deficit itself.

CONCEPTUALIZING DISEASE AND ILLNESS

Disease, the focus of the biomedical model, refers to the physical, objective, and measurable aspects of a condition. Nursing's focus of practice includes the physical response to disease but also extends beyond to include other human responses to the condition. This focus of nursing targets the illness. *Illness* encompasses the subjective, unmeasurable experience of the disease, or the sum of the suffering. Lyon (2000) defines illness as the subjective experience of somatic discomfort (emotional or physical or both) that is accompanied by some degree of functional decline below the person's perceived capability level. Based on this definition, illness can result from disease factors (e.g., pathology, bacteria, viruses) as well as non–disease-based factors. Non–disease-based factors that influence illness include the number and type of stressors imposed, inadequate knowledge, inadequate self-care, deconditioning, inadequate nutrition, insufficient sleep or rest, ineffective use of support systems, and ineffective coping strategies, as well as a host of other factors. Both disease and nondisease factors are amenable to intervention. Nursing's emphasis is with nondisease factors.

Adaptation to illness or injury implies a *healing*—not necessarily of the biophysical system but of the psychological, sociologic, and cultural systems that influence an individual's sense of well-being in the presence of disease or disability.

Illness As a Family and Community Affair

Disease or injury strikes an individual; however, the illness or the response to the disease or injury has a ripple effect that extends outward from the client to family and friends and into the community itself. Although the individual has the disease, caregiving responsibilities rest primarily with the family and with resources or support drawn from the community. Consequently, the nurse must define the client as the individual and family within the community in which they reside. This broader focus is imperative for effective and efficient use of resources that support the whole individual trying to adjust to disease and illness.

Adaptation to illness is influenced not only by individual personality and coping factors but also by the family's response to the situation. The family is central to and influential in the expression of illness. Family encompasses those people involved in providing the support and care of the client and transcends relationships based on blood or marriage. The client must define who these supportive people are and which of them the client would like to involve in the disease/illness care process.

Care must be further understood in terms of the broader context of community. Population-focused care requires an understanding of the health needs of different groups of people within the community and the resources present within the community to assist client groups. Addressing health care concerns from a population-based perspective allows a more comprehensive understanding of common needs and concerns.

DISEASE AND ILLNESS AS STRESS

A *stressor* refers to conditions of threat, demands, and structural constraints that, by their very occurrence or existence, cause strain and threaten the operating integrity of the organism (Kaplan, 1996). Disease and illness factors act as stressors. Coping is the usual response to stress; however, the stressor can affect the organism without activating a specific coping response.

Categorizations of Psychosocial Stress

Stress does not have one definition. In understanding stress and in reading research on stress, the definition that is being used must be clear. There is no clear-cut division of stressors, and in fact, a particular stress may appear to fit different categories. The reason for categorization is to recognize variations in stressors and to critically analyze outcomes in relationship to the types of stress that may be occurring.

Life Events. Life events are discrete, observable events that represent significant life changes. They have a relatively well-defined onset and offset and, once in motion, a fairly well-defined set of subevents describing the "normal" progress of the event (Kaplan, 1996). Marriage, divorce, and job loss are examples of life events. *Health- and illness-related life events* are classified as events, situations, conditions, or cues that are related to health or to illness and/or to treatment for these. These events are generally unpredictable, are usually uncommon, and often result in dire consequences in addition to requiring adjustment and adaptation. Examples of health- and illness-related catastrophic events are hospitalization, surgery, death of a spouse, and diagnosis of a severe or functionally limiting illness or disability. These may remain as discrete events or become chronic stressors.

Chronic Stressors. In contrast to life events, chronic stressors do not necessarily start as an event; rather, they develop slowly and insidiously as a continuing problematic condition in people's social environments and roles and have a longer time course than life events from onset to resolution (Kaplan, 1996). Chronic stressors are continuous in nature and occur as part of the regular enactment of daily roles and activities. As such, chronic stressors are open-ended and use up coping resources, but they do not promise resolution. Chronic illness, chronic time pressures, ongoing fear of crime or personal assault, and long-term unmet needs (wanting to have children when you cannot or not being in a relationship when you want to) are all forms of chronic psychosocial stress. Clearly chronic stressors may have trajectories, which appear more as discrete events, and

some discrete events have periods that appear more like chronic problems. The categorization is not mutually exclusive.

Daily Hassles. Minor stress is sometimes referred to as *daily stressors* or *daily hassles*. These stressors are daily, often ongoing and repetitive, which have been appraised as salient to an individual. Macnee and McCabe (2000) summarize that hassles and uplifts are day-to-day irritants and momentary joys that reflect the stress of daily living in relation to how the individual psychologically and subjectively experiences a situation. Often, they occur along with other ongoing stressors. Whether an event is perceived as a daily hassle varies by individuals, but generally for adults, these events involve domains of work, finance, home maintenance, family, friends, personal life, social issues, and health. Kaplan (1996) argues that some theorists have conceptualized daily hassles too broadly to include both measures of distress and some life events. He argues that daily hassles should be carefully defined to encompass the mundane realities of daily life that, when experienced cumulatively, may be annoying and stressful. In this definition, hassles include things such as remembering to take medications, dealing with troublesome neighbors, misplacing or losing things, caring for a pet, repairing things around the house, having to wait, preparing meals, and waiting in traffic.

Nonevents. Stress related to nonevents occurs when a desired or anticipated event whose occurrence is normative does not occur. Examples of such stress include an anticipated promotion that does not come through and a medication regimen that does not produce the desired response of successfully controlling a disease. Nonevents have the unique characteristic of seeming like events or chronic stress. Within chronic illness, the disease may impose limitations that prevent normative transitions from occurring and these nonevents cause stress.

Traumas. Traumas, by their very nature, are severe and overwhelming in their impact, necessitating differentiation from life events. Lepore and Evans (1996) refer to this type of stressor as a *cataclysmic event*. This type of stress is sudden, tumultuous, deeply disturbing, and irrevocable, and in general, only a relative few experience it. There are many different forms that traumas can take, including natural disasters such as floods, earthquakes, and hurricanes; man-made disasters such as war or sexual abuse during childhood; and disease-related disasters such as the death of a child, amputation, or quadriplegia. The differentiating factor of trauma is the level of imputed seriousness of the stressor, an order of magnitude beyond what is included on life event or role event scales (Kaplan, 1996), as well as the infrequency of occurrence in the general population. It is often difficult to differentiate between trauma and critical life events.

IMPACT OF STRESS

Stress affects the biophysical, psychological, and social systems, as evidenced by biophysical, cognitive, emotional, and behavioral changes. Table 2–1 illustrates the range of effects that stress has on the individual.

The General Adaptation Syndrome

The stress response is universal and prepares the individual for "fight or flight." Selye (1956) pioneered early stress research and examined the role of the sympathetic-adrenal medullary system in emergent and threatening situations. Seyle described a three-stage reaction to stress that he categorized as the "general adaptation syndrome," which prepares the body for fight or flight. The first stage, the alarm reaction, is characterized by strong physical arousal and severe emotional upheavals. Here, the sympathetic portion of the autonomic nervous system is stimulated. Through the release of epinephrine, energy in the form of sugars and fat is made available to the cells to cope with the stressors. Typical symptoms of the alarm reaction include palpitations; shallow, fast

TABLE 2–1. *Common Signs and Symptoms of Stress*

BIOPHYSICAL CHANGES	COGNITIVE CHANGES
Circulation	**Mild Stress**
Increased heart rate	Increased alertness
Increased blood pressure	Attention to detail
Peripheral vessel constriction	Increased problem-solving ability
Fluid retention	Increased learning
Respiration	**Moderate Stress**
Increased depth	Decreased problem-solving ability
Increased rate	Narrowing of focus
Digestion/Eating	**Severe Stress**
Decreased secretions	Tunnel vision
Decreased peristalsis	Vacillating between decisions
Abdominal distention	Impulsive decisions
Nausea and vomiting	Clinging to ideas
Appetite changes	**Feelings**
Elimination	Tenseness
Frequency of urination	Anxiety
Gas and constipation	Fear
Diarrhea	Depression
Healing and Repair	Irritability
Decreased healing	Inappropriately directed anger
Decreased inflammation	Decreased self-esteem
Musculoskeletal	Malaise
Headaches	Suspicion
Clenching of jaw	Panic attacks
Grinding of teeth	**Behavior**
Backache	Tasks not completed
Muscle atrophy	Errors common
Decreased bone density	Change in activity
Joint swelling	Talk about self
Metabolism	Rapid speech
Energy burns at a higher rate	Scattered thoughts
Increased blood sugar	Aggression with little provocation
Fat mobilized	Purposeless or random activity
Neuropsychologic	Absenteeism at work, school
Anxiety	Strained interpersonal relations
Sweating	
Twitching	
Sleep	
Insomnia	

breathing; muscle tension (especially lower back, neck, and shoulders); dryness of the throat; nausea; anxiety; dizziness and light-headedness; sweating; and numbness of the limbs.

If the alarm reaction by itself is not effective in coping with the stress, the individual enters the resistance stage, in which the focus is to adapt to the stressor and neutralize or destroy the threat. Thus, the resistance stage is a "survival" strategy. Physiologic processes present in the alarm reaction now diminish through cycles of negative feedback. Coping mechanisms are used to adapt, and strategies chosen may be adequate or inadequate. When the body is successful in its fight against the threat, the general adaptation syndrome ends with the stage of resistance.

If coping is not successful, hormonal reserves become depleted, fatigue sets in, and the individual enters the stage of exhaustion. The stage of exhaustion occurs when demands on the body and mind are too high and cannot be met in an adaptive way. The individual experiences a general feeling of tiredness, lack of energy, and weakness. Sleeping difficulties and changes in eating habits are common at this point. Depression, anxiety, and physical disorders such as migraines, irritable bowel syndrome, impaired resistance, potentiation of asthma, dermatitis, psoriasis, backache, gastritis, and high blood pressure are outcomes of the stage of exhaustion. Emotional symptoms of exhaustion relate to depression and frustration and include uncontrollable crying; lack of interest in friends and family; general indifference; and reduced attention to personal issues such as exercise, clothes, and eating. Mental dysfunction in the exhaustion state presents as lack of concentration and coordination, which leads to impaired performance and judgment as well as negative attitudes and indecisiveness.

Impact of Stress Relative to Orthopaedic Concerns

Stress and the Immune System. For centuries, the apparent relationship between stress, illness, and health has been recognized. However, it was not until the 1960s that the immune system became a focus of study. Robert Adler first coined the term *psychoneuroimmunology* in 1980. He defined this field of study as the examination of interactions among behavior, neural, endocrine (neuroendocrine), and immunologic processes of adaptation. The premise of this approach is that the individual's response and adaptation to the environment is an integrated process involving interactions among the nervous, endocrine, and immune systems (Witek-Janusek & Mathews, 2000). In other words, thoughts, emotions, and behavior activate anatomic and biochemical pathways, and these pathways in turn modulate immune function. Likewise, altered immune function is known to mediate sickness behavior such as fatigue, lethargy, and decreased appetite associated with illness. With this as the underlying premise, interventions that target biobehavioral strategies

may be as important as medical interventions in strengthening immune competence. Nursing plays an important advocacy role in prescribing and/or teaching clients about holistic treatment plans that contribute to maximal functioning.

Similar to the description of the general adaptation syndrome, the effect of stress on the immune system is thought to vary depending on whether it is acute or chronic stress. Acute stress (time-limited, fight-or-flight phenomenon) mobilizes natural killer (NK) cells in response to adrenergic stimulation and glucocorticoid release. This response is thought to trigger allergic and autoimmune responses. In contrast, repeated or chronic stress suppresses immune responsiveness, particularly cell-mediated immunity, and increases susceptibility to infectious challenge and tumor cells (Witek-Janusek & Mathews, 2000).

Stress and Wound Healing. Stress-induced neuroendocrine activation is believed to impair healing and delay recovery. Stress-induced elevation in glucocorticoids prevents the early part of wound healing in which macrophages move into the area to remove cellular debris and secrete growth factors, cytokines, and chemotactic factors needed for tissue repair (Witek-Janusek & Mathews, 2000). Studies have demonstrated markedly delayed wound healing in individuals under stress compared with matched controlled samples. This evidence suggests the need for stress reduction programs before surgery as well as with individuals in high-risk categories—certainly those individuals diagnosed with acute and chronic illness as well as caretakers in these situations.

Stress and Surgery. Greater fear and distress before surgery is associated with a slower and more complicated postoperative recovery (Huddleston, 1996; Kiecolt-Glaser, 1998). Surgical stress has been shown to negatively affect immune function. Higher anxiety and anxious preoccupation have been linked to lower numbers and depressed functioning of lymphocytes, polymorphonuclear cells, and monocyte functions (Dahanukar, 1996; Kremer, 1999; Tjemsland, 1997). In addition, pain also has deleterious effects on immune function. Psychoneurologic phenomena, such as stress, depression, and pain, influence immune system functioning through neuroendocrine pathways (Kremer, 1999). These findings suggest the need to consecutively consider biologic and behavioral processes and aggressively respond to preoperative and postoperative anxiety and pain. More effective management of perioperative pain improves immune status and health outcomes (Kremer, 1999; Page, 1997).

Stress and Rheumatic Diseases. Since the first studies in the field of stress and rheumatic diseases, stress has been suspected to act as an initiating factor for rheumatoid arthritis (RA). In examining the cause of disease and disease flare, one must appreciate the multi-factor nature of genetic, gender-related, hormonal, immunologic, socioeconomic, and psychological factor interaction.

The role of stress as a provoking factor in RA is equivocal. Hermann, Scholmerich, and Straub (2000) in reviewing literature since 1949, reported on nine studies that supported the premise that stress is a *provoking factor* for the onset of RA and five studies that found that stress does not provoke the onset of RA. They concluded that the studies that support stress as a provoking factor found that major stress (e.g., life events, trauma) is more important than minor stress (e.g., chronic stress, daily hassles). In contrast, an examination of the literature on emotional stress provoking juvenile chronic arthritis (JCA) found stronger evidence demonstrating the link between stress and juvenile arthritis (Hermann, Scholmerich, & Straub, 2000). Major life stress events were found to be important for the initiation of JCA in all 10 studies examined. Major stress events consisted of divorce, separation, death, and adoption. In addition, many of the studies found that chronic minor stress in the form of chronic family difficulties also played a role in JCA occurrence. In other rheumatic conditions, stress was not found to be a provoking factor in systemic lupus erythematosus (SLE) but was found to be influential in fibromyalgia syndrome (FS).

The examination of the effects of stress as a *modulating factor* during the course of RA, SLE, and FS provides strong evidence that stress functions as a modulating factor. Hermann, Scholmerich, and Straub (2000) summarized 31 studies of clients with RA and found that 27 studies supported the modulating effect of stress and 4 did not. Ten studies examined the role of stress as a modulating factor in persons with SLE, and all found a positive relation. Similarly, the majority of studies of individuals with FS found that stress was related to functional status of these individuals. Of the 31 studies examining stress as a modulating factor, 19 were prospective studies.

In the studies examining the modulating impact of stress, chronic stress (e.g., negative spouse behavior, depression, lack of emotional support or a supportive environment) was noted to influence disease activity level. Persistent minor stress aggravates pain, joint inflammation, and tenderness and is often responsible for flares. Interpersonal stress was associated with higher levels of immune-stimulating hormones, which results in greater disease activity. Some studies subdivided rheumatoid clients into those who are seronegative and those who are seropositive. Seronegative clients were found to have higher preonset and postonset levels of minor stress. Thus, seronegative individuals may derive more benefit from psychological techniques to enhance stress management skills. Minor stress or chronic stress was also found to be a modulating factor in SLE and FS.

In summarizing the research on stress as a modulating effect, Hermann, Scholmerich, and Straub (2000) reported that the evidence regarding the role of major stress as a modulator is not as clear as the evidence of the role of chronic stress. Some studies found that short-lived major life events that do not provide a maximum of stress (e.g., change in work or residence) are related to disease flares and increased disability and general symptoms of RA. However, periods of severe major stress (e.g., death of a loved one and bereavement) seem to temporarily alleviate the symptoms of RA and inflammation. These findings were explained by their effect in weakening the immune system.

Stress and Bone Density. At the Third International Conference for the Society for Neuroimmunomodulation, the effect of stress on bone density was presented. In a comparison of two groups of women, half suffering from depression and half with a normal emotional state, the depressed women were found to have high levels of stress hormones; in addition, although the women were 40 years old, they had bone densities like those of 70-year-old women (Michelson, Stratakis, Hill, Reynolds, Galliven, Chrousos, & Gold, 1996; National Institutes of Health, 1996). In persons with depression, higher urinary free cortisol (UFC) is associated with lower bone mineral density. Greendale, Unger, Rowe, and Seeman (1999), using data from the MacArthur study of successful aging, found that higher levels of overnight UFC excretion predicted the occurrence of future fracture in a population of high-functioning, community-dwelling older adults. This relationship between fracture risk and UFC was even strong in men.

COPING AND STRESS

Lazarus and Folkman (1984) define *coping* as "constantly changing cognitive and behavioral efforts to manage specific external and internal demands that are appraised as taxing or exceeding the resources of the person" (p. 141). Thus, coping is anything the person does to change the situation or the way he or she feels or thinks about the situation. In addressing coping with disease and illness, it is important to recognize that a person does not cope with the disease in general but rather with the specific problems (stressors) experienced.

Figure 2–1 presents a model of coping proposed by Lyon (2000). The model is generally explained here and is followed by an explanation and summary of research on select pieces of the model. Using this model to guide assessment and intervention provides a comprehensive approach to management of the stress of disease and illness.

Antecedent variables, which affect the individual's response to stress, include a unique set of personal, environmental, and situational variables. The personal and environmental variables interact to produce situa-

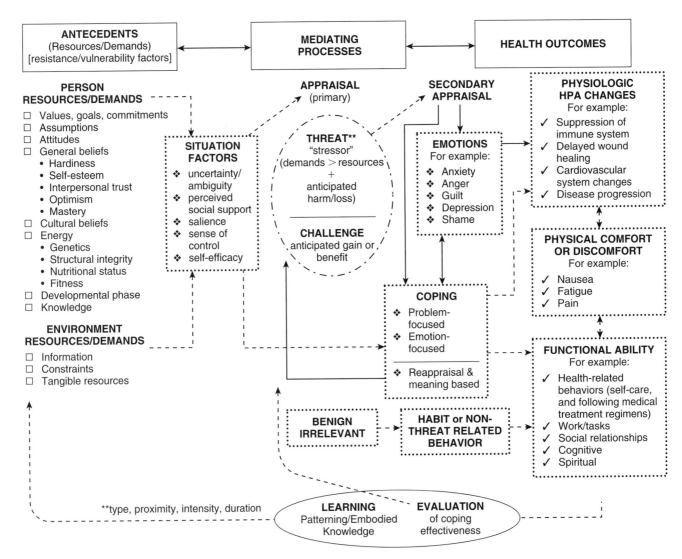

FIGURE 2–1. A conceptual model of stress-related factors and health outcomes. (From Rice, V. [Ed.]. [1999]. *Handbook of stress, coping and health: Implications for nursing research, theory, and practice* [p. 544]. Thousand Oaks, CA: Sage.)

tional variables. Together, the antecedent variables are mediators of stress and influence whether a person is resistant to or vulnerable to stress experiences.

Appraisal is a cognitive process in which the individual determines whether what is happening (or not happening) is relevant to his or her values, goal commitments, and beliefs about self and the world, thereby determining whether a situation represents a potential harm, loss, threat, or challenge. Whether the stressor is perceived to be a threat or a challenge affects the emotional and coping response. This initial appraisal process (primary appraisal) results in a judgment about whether what is happening is worthy of attention and, perhaps, mobilization. Appraisal continues from this point (secondary appraisal) to determine what can be done about the troubled person/environment relation-

ship. He or she evaluates the coping options available, decides which ones to choose, and decides how to set them in motion.

The outcome of the secondary appraisal process is an emotional response along with a coping response (action or inaction that the person takes in responding to the stressor). Reappraisal continues to determine effectiveness of coping behavior.

The effect of the stressor on health outcomes manifests as short-term physiologic effects, physical comfort or discomfort, and functional ability. Long-term effects are manifested as psychological well-being, social functioning, and somatic health or illness (Ryan-Wenger, Sharrer, & Wynd, 2000). The overall effectiveness of the stress coping process leaves individuals in a situation of relative resistance or vulnerability to additional stress.

Antecedent Factors: Personal Variables As Mediators of Stress

Antecedent personal factors include those aspects of the person that influence appraisal and coping resources. Select antecedent variables are discussed here.

Goal Hierarchy. A personal factor that is important to understanding appraisal of stress and the ultimate meaning of a stressful event is the person's goal hierarchy or goal commitments. If the perceived stressor touches upon an important personal goal, it will be perceived differently than one that is tangential to important life goals. Knowing the personal significance or meaning of the stressor to the individual is critical in understanding response to stress. Goal commitment implies that a person will strive hard to attain the goal despite discouragement and adversity (Lazarus, 2000).

Realistic goal setting and acceptance of small successes facilitate coping during rehabilitation. If the person can value modest effort as much as dramatic improvements, it is likely that he or she will feel more energized and hopeful. A person who sets unrealistic expectations or is rewarded only with the achievement of the final goal experiences a series of failures that undermine initiative, perceptions, and relationships.

Cultural Beliefs. The multicultural nature of American society mandates an appreciation for and understanding of cultural similarities and differences. *Culture* can be defined as the learned, shared, and transmitted values, beliefs, norms, and life practices of a particular group that guide their thinking, decisions, and actions in a patterned way (Leininger, 1988). Knowing the values, beliefs, and patterned expressions of a group of people is essential to assist, support, or enable them to maintain well-being; improve a human condition or way of life; or face death and disabilities. Leininger's theory of cultural care examines historical, cultural, and social contexts of human beings as they influence care expressions and patterns and practices of health and well-being. Because different cultural groups ascribe different attributions to disease and illness, awareness of the meaning of the illness is important to appraisal.

Health and *illness* refer to states of well-being and functioning that are culturally defined. There is no one definition for healthy and normal. Rather, cultures view health, health problems and illness, and their treatments differently. Often, nurses and other health care professionals operate with an ethnocentric viewpoint in which they impose their class and cultural viewpoint onto the person without regard for his or her particular beliefs and worldview. This is a major stressor for the client and family and may become a barrier to care all together.

Care can be effective only if the nurse is aware of cultural differences and plans and intervenes with respect for the individual's culture. Leininger (1988) proposes three major modalities to guide nursing judgments, decisions, or actions to ensure the provision of culturally congruent care or care that fits with the client's cultural beliefs, values, and way of life. *Cultural care preservation* or *maintenance* are those actions that support the preservation of relevant care values so that people can maintain their well-being. Being allowed to wear an important amulet or other artifact that is important to the client's generic caring is an example of cultural care preservation. *Cultural care accommodation* or *negotiation* refers to those professional actions and decisions that assist nurses and/or clients to adapt to or negotiate for a satisfying health outcome. Making accommodations for a gypsy family to remain in a room close to their loved one who is hospitalized and setting up a system for visiting is an example of accommodation. Other accommodations involve culture food preferences, religious practices, kinship needs, and child care (Leininger, 1991). *Cultural care repatterning* or *restructuring* refers to those professional actions and decisions that help clients change their lifestyles for new or different patterns that are culturally meaningful and satisfying and that support healthful life patterns. With a strong foundation in cultural knowledge and care, the nurse partners with the individual to design a new or different care lifestyle for the health or well-being of the client (Leininger, 1991).

General Beliefs: Hardiness. Hardiness is a personality characteristic that influences how a person copes with stress, anxiety, and disease (Kobasa, 1979). The three crucial dimensions for hardiness are commitment, perception of control over events and outcomes, and experiencing change as challenge (Amerikaner, 1994). Hardy individuals interpret the stresses of life in such a way that the events are placed in a meaningful context and are seen as controllable, challenging, and less alienating. Hardiness acts as a buffer in the stress/illness relationship.

Hardiness is an internal resource that enables the person to surmount obstacles despite lack of support in other areas. The hardy individual typically has a proactive, often goal-directed, approach to stress. In addition, the hardy individual has a pervasive sense of optimism and feels that he or she will be successful in dealings with the world. Therefore, hardiness moderates stress by influencing both the cognitive and emotional appraisal of the stressful event and the selection of coping strategies.

Pollock (1986) found that hardiness was related to better adaptation to illness. She examined clients with diabetes and RA and hypothesized that hardy clients would exhibit greater adaptation in both the physiologic and psychosocial domains. Her results showed that hardy diabetic clients exhibited better physiologic and psychosocial adaptation. However, although the effects of hardiness on the adaptation of persons with RA correlated positively with psychosocial adaptation, there was no correlation with physiologic adaptation. Pollock suggested that these findings may indicate that hardiness did not have a stress-moderating influence on arthritic clients because they had insufficient control over their pain.

General Beliefs: Optimism and Pessimism.

Optimism and pessimism have been shown to be pervasive and important attributes of human thought and expression. *Optimism* is the tendency to look forward to the future and give precedence to positive interpretations of stressful events. Optimistic responses tend to see the best in people and circumstances. *Pessimism,* or cynicism, is the tendency to view situations in a negative light. According to adage, the optimistic person sees a glass of water as half full, whereas the pessimistic person sees the glass as half empty.

A pessimistic explanatory style has been found to be related to poor health, lower immune functioning, depression, and less effective coping with stressful events (McConnell & Christine, 1993). In contrast, optimism has been correlated with higher levels of happiness, improved activity outcomes, and health.

The ability to maintain optimism in the face of adversity is a significant factor in coping with the stress of illness and disability. Optimism is associated with a greater sense of control and initiative, whereas pessimism is associated with greater degrees of depression and anger. Optimism may serve as a foundation for perception in the hardy individual and contributes to resiliency and thriving.

General Beliefs: Self-esteem.

Self-esteem is an overall affective (as opposed to cognitive) evaluation of one's own worth. It is influenced by how a person feels valued by family and friends, as well as how he or she values himself or herself. Individuals with high self-esteem experience more positive feelings about themselves and their circumstances and have a higher sense of well-being.

Chronic illness, especially in older adults, is postulated to damage self-worth. Measures to restore self-esteem are critical to stress reduction and adaptation. The degree of positive self-esteem (also referred to as *self-regard* or *self-acceptance*) has been shown to be a more influential factor in coping with chronic illness and disability than has the severity of the illness or disability.

Attitude: Depression and Anxiety.

Attitudes manifested in depression and anxiety can lead to a loss of interest or pleasure in activities. This lack of interest is accompanied by somatic signs of sleep disturbance, appetite disturbance, and loss of energy. Furthermore, the individual with depression or anxious state experiences somatic sensations as more intense, thereby increasing

how sick a client feels physically. Cognitive distortions may be personified as guilt and feelings of worthlessness.

Depression is the most common psychological disturbance associated with medical illness (DeVellis, 1993). Depression and anxiety have been found to be more prevalent in individuals with rheumatic diseases and other chronic pain syndromes than in the general population, with frequencies ranging from 14% to 50% (Bradley, 1994; Frank, Beck, Parker, Kashani, Elliott, Haut, Smith, Atwood, Brownlee-Duffeck, & Kay, 1998). These frequencies are generally higher among clients with FM, with ranges reported between 26% and 71% (Bradley & Alarcon, 1997).

Research evidence suggests that higher levels of depressive and anxious symptoms are associated with higher levels of pain (Huyser & Parker, 1999; Keefe, 1999) and lower functional ability in persons with RA, osteoarthritis, and FM (Bradley, 1994; Bradley & Alarcon, 1997). In addition, psychological distress is associated with higher levels of medical service utilization in this population.

It is believed that persons who are depressed cognitively appraise the affective component of pain as something that they cannot deal with. Thus, emotions and pain symptoms become integrated into common cognitive schemas, and because of this integration, emotional experiences can exacerbate pain and vice versa.

Antecedent Factors: Environment, Resources, and Demands As Mediators of Stress

Accuracy and Clarity of Available Information.

One must assess the sources and types of information to which the individual has access to understand response to stress. What is the information available to the person? Where is the information coming from? Is this information offered in a form that is clear and understandable to the individual? Is there conflict between sources of information?

American society is multicultural and multilingual. For clients who are non-English speakers or speakers with limited English proficiency, the health care organization and practitioner must ensure language competency. Using the family as translators is often an unacceptable situation because the medical discussion may be developmentally inappropriate for young children or culturally inappropriate with opposite gender or hierarchical relationships.

In assessing information available, the nurse should seek information about use of traditional healing remedies: use of amulets, herbs, rituals of prayer or spirit worship, and consultation with indigenous healers. This is an important source of generic caring. Leininger (1991) defines *generic caring* as culturally learned and transmitted lay, indigenous (traditional), or folk (home care) knowledge and skills used to provide assistive, supportive, enabling, and facilitative acts (or phenomena). Knowledge of this information is critical to decision making regarding use of cultural care maintenance, accommodation, or negotiation.

Constraints. Constraints are social and material realities that create a disadvantage and limit the resources that the person has to draw upon. Constraints create situations in which there is a restriction of choice and access to means. Constraints may be openly apparent but are often invisible. Practices that are not inclusive, that provide little or no language interpretation, and that are judgmental of other lifestyles create invisible barriers to access of services. In situations of severe social disadvantage, the disjunction between goals and means may not be actively responded to because the individual sees no options for himself or herself or for his or her family. Although not responded to from a coping perspective, there is an impact on assumptions about personal self-worth and power, assumptions about personal control, and assumptions about roles or contributions that a person has to offer.

Tangible Resources. Response to stress is influenced by what resources the individual has access to. This may be in the form of money, insurance support, transportation, and housing. This ties in with social support, which is further elaborated upon in the discussion of situational factors.

Antecedent Factors: Situation Factors As Mediators of Stress

Self-efficacy. Self-efficacy (SE) is the belief or confidence that one can perform specific behaviors to achieve specific health-related goals. It is the mediator between knowledge and action, and it influences the selection of behavior, the environment in which the behavior occurs, and the amount of effort and perseverance expended on performing the behavior. Persons with higher levels of SE tend to persevere despite failures, work harder at tasks, and show less anxiety than those with lower levels of SE (Keefe & Bonks, 1999). Individuals with low SE for illness self-management may be less persistent and adherent with treatment regimens. SE is task specific, so a person's SE for performing one task may differ from another's SE. For example, an individual with a hip fracture may have high SE for managing pain with medications and non-pharmacologic interventions but low SE for ambulation.

The importance of SE is that it tends to predict outcome. High SE for pain is correlated with high pain threshold, high pain tolerance levels, and low frequencies of pain behavior after controlling for demographics and disease activity (Buckelew, Parker, Keefe, Deuser, Crews, Conway, Kay, & Hewett, 1994). In addition, increases in SE are associated with improvements in depression, pain,

and disease activity among RA clients (Bradley & Alberts, 1999). Kurlowicz (1998) reports that interventions to enhance older clients' perceived SE while hospitalized after elective total hip replacement surgery may enhance functional ability, which in turn may decrease the likelihood of depressive symptoms postoperatively.

Interventions designed to produce behavioral change have been found to be more effective if strategies to enhance SE are incorporated in their design and implementation. Efforts to enhance mastery as well as verbal persuasion and emotional arousal appear to be the most common methods of intervention to increase SE (Siela & Wieseke, 2000).

Personal Control. Control is the individual's perception of his or her ability to exercise direction in or over situations and events (Ruiz-Bueno, 2000) and has a moderating effect on coping with stressors. Locus of control and learned helplessness are discussed here.

Locus of control (LOC) refers to the individual's belief that forces within and outside of himself or herself are responsible for outcomes. If the outcome is perceived to be at least in part outside of internal control—that luck, fate, powerful others, or complexities beyond the individual's control influence the outcome—an *external* LOC dominates. Those who view the outcome as contingent on their own behavior have an *internal* LOC. LOC appears to be a predictor variable that is a relatively stable phenomenon and therefore not highly amenable to intervention.

Research suggests some support for LOC as a predictor of pain and mood distress and disability in chronic pain sufferers (Pellino & Oberst, 1992) and psychological health and life satisfaction in persons with osteoarthritis (Laborde & Powers, 1985). The research on LOC is limited, and more studies need to be done before predictions can be made about LOC and specific diagnostic conditions.

Internal control influences one's view that one's own behavior affects current and future health outcomes and serves as a motivator that leads one to engage in health promotion and health protection activities and to assume responsibility for one's own health. Individuals with an internal LOC are more apt to use task-centered coping strategies than emotion-centered strategies.

External attributions have been found to foster anxiety and dismal assessments of coping resources. Persons with an external LOC use more suppression-related and palliative coping behavior. These persons are believed to respond more readily to role modeling or to suggestions from others for engaging in health-promoting and health-protecting activities.

There are two major areas of conflict in the premise that internal LOC enhances coping. First, control may not always be positive. There are parts of living with chronic illness and disability that need to be accepted because no matter how internally controlled the person, the outcome cannot be changed. It is possible to hypothesize that a person with an external LOC would cope more effectively with this type of stress and be able to get on with living as compared with someone who focuses on trying to fix the problem.

Overlapping with the issue that control is not always positive is the fact that the concept of LOC may be culturally biased. The dominant orientation in the United States is that of "doing" and "control over nature," which signifies that the best approach is an active problem-solving strategy. Reviewing sample selection in many of the studies on LOC reveals that relatively homogeneous groups of Caucasians were used. Further research is needed to test these relationships among culturally diverse groups.

The phenomenon of *learned helplessness* is a state in which the individual believes there are no viable solutions available to eliminate or reduce the source of stress. High levels of helplessness are associated with high levels of pain, low functional ability, and greater depression. Persons who receive nursing care may be at risk for developing learned helplessness because they may either be placed in an environment in which they have little or no control or face a diagnosis that is progressive and uncontrollable.

Resiliency and Thriving. When an individual is faced with adversity, there are four potential consequences: continued downward slide, survival with a diminished or impaired response/functioning, return to preadversity levels of functioning, or a surpassing of previous levels of functioning. The return to preadversity levels of functioning is known as *resiliency;* the surpassing of preadversity functioning is termed *thriving.*

Carver (1998) proposes that resiliency may occur from desensitization. The more the stressor occurs, the lesser the downward response to the stress. Having experienced and dealt with the adversity once, the person has acquired an "immunity" or "partial immunity" to its next occurrence. In this explanation, the stressor itself has less impact on the person. The second explanation for resiliency is enhanced recovery potential or a change in the speed of recovery from the stressor. The initial exposure to adversity enhances a person's ability to recover from the adverse impact should the stressor recur. In this explanation, it is assumed that the stressor retains its disruptive character but that the person is rendered more efficient at repairing the disruption.

With thriving, something about the experience of the adversity and its aftermath takes the person to a higher plane of functioning (Carver, 1998). This can be seen in individuals who were sedentary and acquire physical fitness (now functioning at a higher level) or in people who come to appreciate fulfilling aspects of life on

continuing bases after a personal trauma. Following adversity, some individuals find meaning and purpose in life and become active in pursuits toward this meaning. Other outcomes of thriving may be greater acceptance of self or others, change in personal philosophy or orientation to life, changes in life priorities, acquisition of new skills and knowledge, a sense of mastery, or strengthened personal relations. Thriving is differentiated from growth in that it occurs in circumstances in which, on the face of it, growth is unexpected because the circumstances seem to push in the opposite direction.

Carver (1998) proposes that high-mastery or confident people are continually trying to succeed in efforts to overcome the adversity and that low-mastery people are vulnerable to giving up the attempt or turning away from efforts to be successful in the face of adversity. Carver's proposition is supported with the findings of Abraido-Lanza (1998), who examined thriving in Latinas with RA. She found that thriving was not correlated with illness characteristics or social or cultural resources; rather, thriving was associated with personal resources of competence (self-esteem and SE) and psychological well-being (positive and negative affect).

Social Support. Social support is a person's perception that an individual is a member of a complex network of affection, mutual aid, and obligation. Interestingly, the perception of received and offered social support is uniformly associated with improved survival in a wide variety of illnesses in which it has been assessed.

The role of social support in influencing coping is complex. However, it appears that in combination with certain personal factors, supportive relationships promote adaptation to disability and illness by buffering the deleterious effects of environmental stress. There is ample evidence to show that that people with spouses, friends, and family members (social network) who provide psychological (appraisal or affirmation) and material (instrumental) resources are in better health than are those with fewer social contacts. The literature examining social support in medical populations shows that medical populations benefit from having a network of relationships on which they can rely for support. Lower levels of social support are related to increased physical disability, lower functional outcomes, and deterioration in psychosocial and emotional functioning.

A *support network* is the number of people around the person who can be called on in need. Social support can emanate from a variety of network sources: spouse, parents, children, siblings, relatives, friends, co-workers, health care providers, clergy, and members of self-help groups. A *support system* refers to the psychosocial and tangible aid provided by the social network and received by a person. This support can be categorized as emotional (or appraisal), informational, and instrumental. Emotional (or appraisal) support is the caring, loving, and positive feedback that a person receives, which affirms self-worth. Affirmational support provides avenues for ventilation of feelings, which allows for the open expression of negative feelings. It affirms the person's importance and acknowledges the appropriateness of personal interpretation of events (Jalowiec & Dudas, 1991). Appraisal support can be given through feedback on behavior and the provision of information and advice. Informational support is the useful advice or information that helps a person solve problems. Instrumental support refers to tangible goods and services, such as loaning money, helping to prepare meals, baby-sitting, providing transportation, acting as an advocate, and providing help with duties and responsibilities.

Researchers have suggested that it is not necessarily the provision of social support that has the enabling effect but rather the person's perception that help is available if needed or the perception of the quality of this support system that may be equally, if not more, important (Keefe & Bonks, 1999). Thus, persons may not use the support system available, but their perception that it is accessible if needed is a valuable strength.

Ongoing assessment of social support is necessary to detect changes in patterns that may signal potential problems in coping. The way social support is assessed may vary and includes counting members in a client's social network, determining the client's perception of available support, finding out who would be there to help in various situations, determining who has actually provided support in different situations, and assessing the client's satisfaction with the extent of the support available or provided (Jalowiec & Dudas, 1991).

Uncertainty. "Uncertainty is part of life and is believed to be inherent in the stress, coping, and illness experience when persons lack an adequate explanatory framework for understanding their situations and predicting outcomes" (Barron, 2000, p. 517). When stimuli are perceived as uncertain, the person is unable to subjectively evaluate the disease, treatment, or health care experience. This inability to effectively explain or evaluate the situation hinders the person from adequately appraising the situation, thereby influencing subsequent behavior and decision making.

Individuals process information to determine symptom pattern, event familiarity, and event congruency. Factors that inhibit information processing, such as medications and information overload, may interfere with this process. To determine whether uncertainty may exist in a situation, the nurse should determine whether the individual is able to recognize a consistent patterns of symptoms, is familiar with the situation/event/environment, and believes that his or her expectations are congruent with the actual experience. Affirmative responses to these conditions suggest low

uncertainty, whereas negative answers indicate the presence of uncertainty.

Uncertainty has been linked to perceptions of illness severity (Braden, 1990a, 1990b) and the appraisal of danger (Bailey & Nielsen, 1993) in persons with RA. Danger appraisals have been linked with more emotion-focused coping, whereas opportunity appraisals were found to be associated with more problem-focused coping (Wineman, Durand, & Steiner, 1994).

In a population of persons with multiple sclerosis, Wineman (1990) found that uncertainty was positively correlated with perceptions of unsupportiveness or dissatisfaction with social support. Examination of the relationship between uncertainty and outcomes have found uncertainty to be related to poorer psychosocial adjustment, more depression and psychological distress, poorer quality of life, and lower sense of purpose in life (Barron, 2000). Mishel (1997) proposes that the most effective interventions to reduce uncertainty are educational in nature, providing information and skill building related to management of uncertainty.

Emotional Responses

Secondary appraisal results in almost simultaneous emotional and coping responses. Emotions flow from the way a person appraises what is happening in his or her life. As such, emotions follow logic when viewed from the standpoint of an individual's premises about self and world, even when the emotions themselves may not be realistic. A range of emotions can occur as a result of stress. The meaning of the stressor and the relation to a person's identity influences the type of emotion that emerges.

Coping Responses

There is no universal effective or ineffective coping strategy. "Efficacy depends on the type of person, the type of threat, the stage of the stressful encounter, and the outcome modality—that is, subjective well-being, social functioning or somatic health" (Lazarus, 2000, p. 202). Coping is adaptive when distress is kept at a manageable level, hope is generated, self-worth is maintained or restored, relationships with others are maintained, and a sense of well-being is enhanced.

Denial is examined to illustrate the concept of a coping strategy being potentially effective or ineffective. Denial can be ineffective when it prevents seeking assistance for an acute problem. However, once the problem is recognized and the individual is in the critical phase of diagnosis and treatment, denial may be effective in alleviating stress from fear, projection, and uncertainty. Continued denial during the ongoing management phase of the illness can again become ineffective because it may contribute to high-risk behaviors that jeopardize well-being and health. Lazarus (2000) captures the usefulness of denial in his explanation that denial may be beneficial when nothing can be done to alter the condition or prevent further harm but harmful when it prevents necessary adaptive action.

Coping is an integrated process that addresses the two major functions of dealing with the problem and dealing with the emotions surrounding the problem. Coping strategies assist the individual in managing the stressful situation and regulating the emotional distress accompanying the situation. There are several schemas used to categorize coping.

Problem-oriented and Affective-oriented Coping.
Problem-oriented coping strategies are situation specific. The person obtains information on which to act and mobilizes action for the purpose of changing the reality of the troubled person/environment relationship (Lazarus, 2000). It involves efforts aimed at different phases of the problem-solving process, whereby the individual is able to define the problem, break it into achievable pieces, set goals, and experiment with different strategies. Seeking information, requesting support, brainstorming, and altering the environment or patterns of behaviors are examples of problem-oriented coping.

Affective-oriented coping strategies, or emotion-focused strategies, are used primarily at the emotional level and are not targeted at solving the problem but rather at responding to or handling the emotions tied to the stressful situation. Distancing, escape avoidance, and reappraisal are all affective strategies.

Generally, a combination of problem-oriented and affective-oriented coping is most beneficial. There is some evidence that problem-oriented strategies produce better outcomes. Although this may be true in situations that are controllable and in which emotion-focused coping could not alter the problem itself, there are situations in which the event cannot be changed and emotion-focused coping is the preferred approach. In reality, for most stressful encounters, the individual draws on both functions—they are not distinct but overlapping and are both essential to the coping process with one facilitating the other (Lazarus, 2000).

Cohen and Lazarus: Five Coping Modes.
Stressors can occur within the biophysical, psychological, sociologic, and cultural aspects of self. Coping mechanisms must then target the cultural, physical, social, and psychological realms. Cohen and Lazarus (1983) identify five main coping modes: information seeking, direct action, inhibition of action, intrapsychic processes, and turning to others for support. Each one serves both problem-solving and emotional-regulating functions and is capable of being oriented to the self or the environment. Box 2-1 outlines these five coping modes as they apply to the client with joint disease and also describes how the same coping strategy applies to stressors within the different aspects of self in the physical, social, and psychological realms. Strategies taken within these three realms are mediated by cultural norms.

Information-seeking strategies are aimed at gathering facts specific to a current problem. These are part of the general problem-solving process and facilitate ultimate decision making. Direct actions are strategies a person uses to handle a stressful situation. These actions can be aimed at the self or the environment. Inhibition is a strategy for avoiding actions that are potentially harmful. Intrapsychic processes encompass all the cognitive processes designed to regulate emotions, including such defense mechanisms as denial, avoidance, and detachment and such strategies as relaxation, biofeedback, and cognitive transformation. Turning to others for support may reduce the likelihood of an undesirable event occurring or may buffer the situation, thereby reducing the degree of experienced stress.

Approach versus Avoidance Strategies.
Another framework for viewing coping strategies is that of approach versus avoidance. Examples of such strategies are listed in Table 2–2. Using this framework, it is clear that approach/avoidance strategies can deal with both the problem and the emotions. However, the effectiveness of their use differs. Avoidance strategies are considered beneficial in the short term, but prolonged use of avoidance strategies is generally maladaptive.

Coping Assessment.
Any of the preceding frameworks can be used to assess coping. In addition, coping strategies and resources can be assessed using both open-ended client and family interviews and scales designed to identify preferred strategies. The nurse interviewing a client can ask specific questions about which coping strategies are used. The client is asked to define the problem and evaluate how realistic or unrealistic the perception is. The client is questioned about what is happening in the present: "Why do you think you need help now?" "What are you doing to deal with this problem (or these emotions) at this point?" The client's past is explored: "Have you experienced any stress similar to this in the past?" "How did you cope with the stress at the time?" The client's perception of factors that facilitate coping is determined by asking, "What do you think would help you cope with the situation now?" When the client is asked, "How is this problem affecting others around you?" information about whether the person can perceive that the stressor affects others is provided. These questions are likely to provide the nurse with information about how the client or family is coping. Table 2–3 identifies factors that promote or hinder coping and that can be incorporated into the coping assessment.

Coping and Gender.
Coping strategies that are generally used appear to vary by gender. Beginning in adolescence, girls are reported to cope by engaging in

BOX 2-1.

Cohen and Lazarus' Five Coping Modes Applied to the Client with Arthritis

1. Information Seeking
Physical Self
Learn to read body cues for what intensifies and contributes to symptoms
Learn about one's illness
Examine lifestyles for possible alterations
Learn about medications
Get information on exercises and mobility constraints
Get information on nontraditional approaches: tonics, herbs, amulets, acupuncture, and shark cartilage, for example

Social Self
Learn about available community and health care resources
Learn to use adaptive aids
Get information on new occupational roles that may prevent symptom exacerbation
Seek information on insurance coverage, unemployment, and disability benefits

Psychological Self
Get information on clothing that might alleviate body image concerns
Get information on sexual positions that can be used to minimize joint stress

2. Direct Action Strategies
Physical Self
Take medications and other therapies
Carry out isometric exercises
Protect joints from strain and injury
Alter the environment to accommodate mobility deficits
 Ramps vs. stairs
 Grab bar in bathroom
 High, straight-back chairs
 Self-care appliances
Use of the strongest joint for all activities
Moist heat to joints

Social Self
Attempt altered roles
Use of adaptive aids to continue with previous roles
Energy conservation for role accomplishment
Activity scheduling to enhance role performance
Prioritization of roles and completion of high-priority roles
Open communication with family, employer, and friends concerning variability in symptoms
Taking a part in "reciprocal" social roles even if role is altered

Psychological Self
Open communication with family and friends concerning fears, moods, concerns
Continued use of makeup and dressing in clothes rather than pajamas
Continued activity in the areas that bring most positive self-feedback
Find situations in which expertise can be given to others

3. Inhibition of Action
Physical Self
Do not continue joint exercises beyond the point of mild nonpersistent pain
Avoid strenuous physical exercise
Avoid long periods of physical activity

Social Self
Avoidance of situations that expose the individual to role changes

Psychological Self
Avoidance of situations that expose the person to failure

4. Intrapsychic Processes
Physical Self
Mental relaxation during physical exercise
Use of self-talk with pain
Use of distraction for pain
Biofeedback
Use of control strategies

Social Self
Affirmations
Self-talk
Prethinking
Downward comparison
Cognitive restructuring

Psychological Self
Relaxation techniques
Affirmations
Downward comparison
Prayer
Imagery
Cognitive restructuring

5. Seeking Social Support
Physical Self
Accept physical help from others
Form partnerships with health care providers

Social Self
Examine extent and effectiveness of social network
Maintain and use resources
Participate in self-help groups

Psychological Self
Verbalize emotions, concerns, fears
Verbalize expectations
Accept emotional support

Based on information from Cohen, F., & Lazarus, R. S. (1983). Coping and adaptation in health and illness. In D. Mechanic (Ed.), *Handbook of health, health care, and the health profession.* New York: Free Press.

TABLE 2–2. *Approach/Avoidance Coping Strategies*

APPROACH	AVOIDANCE
Seeking of information	Denial
Strength through spirituality	Minimization of symptoms
Diversion of attention	Withdrawal
Expression of feelings	Passive acceptance
Maintaining control	Sleeping
Setting of goals	Delayed decision making
Relaxation exercises	Blaming of others
Verbalization of concerns	Refusal of treatment
Positive thinking and humor	Excessive dependence
Seeking of help	Unrealistic goals
Maintaining realistic independence	Use of drugs or alcohol
Maintaining social activities	

social relationships and creating change, whereas boys are found to rely on stress-reduction activities, physical exercise, or diversion (Copeland, 1995). In general, ventilation strategies used by girls tend to rely more on social support (e.g., crying, talking to a friend). In contrast, boys use ventilation strategies such as swearing, complaining, and taking their anger out on others (Bird & Harris, 1990). Golden's work (1996) with adult males experiencing loss support this difference. He reports that, in general, men tend toward action as a primary mode in healing their grief while using relating as a secondary mode, and women do the opposite.

Coping and Culture. Cultural background and influences also affect an individual's perception of and reaction to stressful life events (Phinney, Lochner, & Murphy, 1990). Members of group-oriented cultures are likely to rely more heavily on the use of social support networks in coping. Individuals with a present-time orientation are more likely to use relaxation as an adaptive coping strategy. Seeking spiritual support is also a coping strategy that varies with cultural background.

Coping in Children and Families. Coping strategies in children are often assessed by observing play, using play therapy, or interpreting and discussing drawings done by the child. Although some of the coping strategies used by children are similar to those used by adults (e.g., denial, mastery, setting realistic goals, normalization), children use the strategies of fantasy and rituals more than adults do. When faced with a stressful reality, children use fantasy to "undo" reality and make it more palatable (Rose & Thomas, 1987). In essence, it is a retreat into a safer, kinder world. Rituals are another mechanism often used by children to cope with a situation over which they have little control or that causes great anxiety. The child establishes a protocol or plan for how to handle the

difficult stressor and becomes very upset when those rituals are not honored.

Adolescents experiencing the stress of trauma or chronic illness may be particularly vulnerable. It is during adolescence that young people typically confront many different types of life stressors and may not yet have a wide variety of coping strategies to rely on. Pulled between dependence and independence, the adolescent may need focused support during stress associated with health problems. The use of music as a means of catharsis provides a medium for expression of feelings while maintaining a safe distance from conflicts.

Parents of a child with a chronic illness experience common stressors associated with day-to-day living and

TABLE 2–3. *Factors That Promote or Hinder Coping*

ENABLING FACTORS	HINDERING FACTORS
Personality Characteristics	
Hardiness	Passive, helpless
Humor	Inability to laugh at situations or self
Optimism or positive appraisal	Pessimism, depression, guilt
Sense of spirituality or religiosity	Lack of spirituality or religiosity
Perception of self-control	Perception of others in control, blaming
Personal Styles	
Problem solving	Denial, minimization of situation
Able to make decisions	Delayed decision making
Information seeking	Wishful thinking
Goal setting	Unrealistic goal setting
Positive comparison	Negative comparison
Positive self-esteem	Negative or vulnerable self-esteem
Ability to ask for help	Inability to ask for help
Open communication	Closed communication
Hopefulness	Despair or hopelessness
High self-efficacy	Low self-efficacy
Tolerance for ambivalence, ambiguity	Discomfort with ambivalence, ambiguity
Supports and Resources	
Large and accessible social network	Small or inaccessible social network
Affirmation from supports	Lack of affirmation from supports
Instrumental support	Lack of instrumental support
Health care providers supportive	Health care providers not supportive
One key person to confide in	Absence of confidant
Access to others with similar experiences	No contact with others having similar experiences
Role flexibility	Cemented roles

altered future paths. Parents and families caring for children living with chronic illness or disability must reorient their goals and expectations to change from a future focus to present orientation. It is a challenge as family members cope with the reality that change has been thrust upon them. Family dynamics are stressed as the family attempts to normalize and minimize family vulnerability. Developing and capitalizing personal strengths while learning to use support networks further facilitates adaptation. Maintaining family integration, cooperation, and an optimistic definition of the situation; maintaining social support, self-esteem, and psychological stability; and understanding the medical situation through communication with other parents and consultation with medical staff are major coping skills used by parents.

HELPING CLIENTS COPE WITH STRESSORS OF DISEASE, ILLNESS, AND THE HEALTH CARE SYSTEM

Although all forms of psychosocial stress must be considered when looking at a situation holistically, it is important for the nurse to understand specific stressors associated with health problems and the health care system itself so that these stressors can be anticipated and minimized. Doing this effectively will ease the stress experience caused by the disease and illness.

Initial assessment involves clarifying the particular stressors being experienced and then determining the meaning of the stressors to the individual. With this information, the nurse then helps the person examine coping mechanisms and resources already being used and plans interventions focused on strengthening or developing adaptive mechanisms to alleviate the experienced stress. The goal is to effectively manage the stress so that crisis is prevented.

Stressors of Acute Injury and Disease

Although there are similarities between acute and chronic illness, each has certain characteristics that influence the degree of stress a client experiences. Table 2–4 compares key factors in acute and chronic illness. Acute injury and illness do not give time for advance preparation or planning. The episode occurs amid the individual's typical life situation with all its ordinary pressures and must be responded to with coping patterns established before the injury took place. Because of the suddenness of the event, the individual and family have had little opportunity to ready themselves or to gather resources that would be helpful during the initial period after the injury. This inability to plan often results in a sense of extreme disorganization and vulnerability characteristic of crisis.

While the health care team responds to the emergency biophysical concerns, the family is left in a position of waiting. They must wait to visit the client, wait for

TABLE 2–4. *Characteristics of Acute and Chronic Disease*

ACUTE DISEASE OR INJURY	CHRONIC DISEASE AND DISABILITY
Suddenness of onset	Onset may be sudden or insidious
No time for planning	Must confront concept of "forever"
Waiting	
Uncertainty of outcome	Shattering of hopes and dreams
Shatters illusion of invulnerability	Changing course of disease
Powerlessness, helplessness	Emotional turmoil over losses
Fear	Losses are multiple and ongoing
Few sources of guidance	
Sense of ongoing danger may continue	Powerlessness, helplessness
Emotional response may outlast biophysical instability	Work of treatment regimen
	Must prepare for medical crisis
	Must redefine self-concept
	May struggle over control with health care providers

news of their loved one's condition, wait for results of tests, and wait to talk to nurses and doctors. Although the waiting time is necessary and may not even appear to be long to the health care provider, it is interminable for the family. During these periods of waiting, the family must confront not only their feelings of powerlessness and fear for their loved one but also the shattering of their own sense of invulnerability. This confrontation with personal illusions of invulnerability exposes the individual to the reality of the fragility of the fabric of life, which may further heighten the family members' sense of powerlessness and fear. Supportive nursing staff can understand the helplessness and powerlessness felt by the family during these periods of waiting and assist them by listening to their concerns; accepting their emotional responses; and providing consistent, repetitive, informational support.

There are few sources of guidance that the family can draw on during the client's initial period of acute physiologic instability. Bookstores have a plethora of books with information about coping with normative transitions and a growing supply of information about living with chronic illness, yet there are few informational sources the family can draw on to assist them in coping with this extremely stressful period of acute injury or illness. Often, an effective coping strategy is to turn to someone in their social network who has been through the experience and who can help guide them. Unfortunately, because few people have experienced the crisis of acute trauma or illness, the family may feel isolated and alone.

In the case of the trauma client, the acute crisis may be prolonged by ups and downs in biomedical stability. It often seems that the client and family have weathered one storm only to be suddenly faced with another crisis. Referred to as the *roller coaster phenomenon,* the client and family must swing with and adapt to the ups and downs in the acute illness trajectory. As the trauma trajectory often is one life-threatening event after another, this period is especially stressful. Family members during this period need to feel hope, see their loved one often, receive frequent and repetitive up-to-date information, and if possible, participate in the caregiving process. These interventions lead to confidence that their loved one is really cared for by the staff.

Throughout roller coaster episodes, the client and family experience a sense of helplessness and powerlessness because they are unable to modulate the progression of events. In addition to the feelings associated with helplessness, there is an acute sense of loss that may be felt. These losses, both actual and potential, create additional stress and emotional responses. Examples of losses felt at this time include loss of family relations, loss of health, possible loss of role function, and loss of social support. Significant anxiety is generated while coping with the uncertainty of final outcomes. The acute illness or injury may result in disability. However, the scope and extent of the disability are typically not known immediately, and the wait for actual outcomes may take days or months. Anxiety, fear, and desperation are common emotions associated with uncertainty. Clients must cope with these feelings as they struggle with questions, such as "Will I ever walk again?" and "Will I be the same person I was?"

The experience of ongoing danger, helplessness, powerlessness, uncertainty, and loss manifests itself in a wide array of emotional reactions, including fear, anxiety, denial, anger, sorrow, grief, remorse, depression, and hope. It is important to understand that the emotional response to a catastrophic event may last well past the period of biophysical instability.

Psychological Sequelae to Acute Injury and Disease

Acute Stress Disorder. Acute stress disorder is a time-limited anxiety disorder characterized by a cluster of dissociative and anxiety symptoms occurring within 1 month of a traumatic event. In this disorder, the person copes by "sealing off" some features of the trauma from conscious awareness. Emotional detachment, temporary loss of memory, depersonalization, and derealization are characteristics of the dissociative response. Anxiety symptoms include irritability, physical restlessness, sleep problems, inability to concentrate, and being easily startled. Antidepressants and short-term psychotherapy are common treatment approaches. Meditation, breathing exercises, and yoga are beneficial in managing the anxiety. If symptoms last longer than 1 month, the diagnosis may be changed to post-traumatic stress disorder (PTSD).

Post-traumatic Stress Disorder, Post-traumatic Response. A post-traumatic response formation (Koren, Arnon, & Kelin, 1999) can be anticipated when a person experiences, witnesses, or is confronted with an event or events that involve actual or threatened death or serious injury, or threat to the physical integrity of self or others, in which the individual responds with intense fear, helplessness, or horror. This event results in persistent re-experiencing of the trauma, avoidance of stimuli associated with it, and increased rates of arousal. Post-trauma response typically begins within the first 7 days of the event and its incidence gradually decreases over time. Symptoms of PTSD (a pathologic response to trauma) usually begin within the first 3 months after the catastrophic event but may not develop until years after the trauma.

Catastrophic-type events, which are associated with post-traumatic stress, may include war, rape, violent acts, life-threatening illness, trauma, earthquakes, and floods. An estimated 70% of adults in the United States have experienced a traumatic event at least once in their lives, and up to 20% of these people go on to develop PTSD. An estimated 5% of Americans—more than 13 million people—have PTSD at any given time. Approximately 8% of all adults—1 of 13 people in this country—will develop PTSD during their lifetime. Women are about twice as likely as men to develop PTSD, with about 1 in 10 women estimated to have PTSD at some time in their lives. This may be because women tend to experience interpersonal violence (e.g., domestic violence, rape, abuse) more often than men (PTSD Alliance), or it may be related to a gender response to stress.

Apart from war, motor vehicle accidents are the leading cause of PTSD. Butler, Moffic, and Turkal (1999) indicate that after a traffic accident, a variation of PTSD, referred to as *subsyndromal* or *partial PTSD,* may occur. These individuals experience high levels of hyperarousal and re-experiencing of symptoms but fewer symptoms of avoidance or emotional numbing than classic PTSD. Studies of both adults and children show that the incidence of PTSD in individuals involved in motor vehicle accidents ranges from 9% to 34%. The severity of the accident is not predictive of the emotional response; rather the appraisal that life is endangered or the personal meaning of the event is related to the development of PTSD. Women and persons with prior psychiatric disorders have higher incidences.

Figure 2–2 illustrates the normal post-trauma response to a catastrophic event compared with a pathologic response characteristic of PTSD. As the individual experiences the event and its aftermath, he or she may immediately go into denial; however, more commonly, people express extreme emotions, such as fear, sadness, and rage, before attempting to limit their awareness. As the individual becomes painfully aware of the impact of the event, a state of denial or numbing occurs. This protective mechanism limits the individual's awareness of

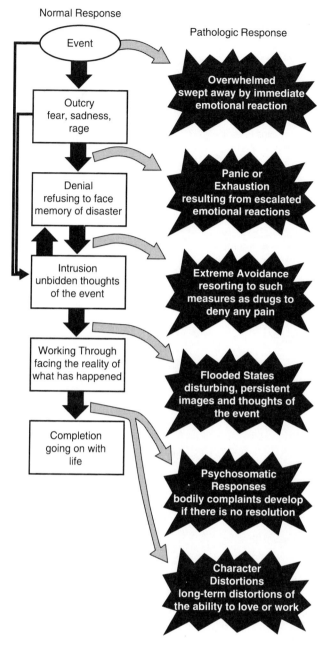

Normal Response

Pathologic Response

FIGURE 2–2. Normal and pathologic phases of poststress response. (From Horowitz, M. J. [1986]. *Stress response syndrome.* New York: Aronson.)

the scope and impact of the event and allows time for biophysical healing to occur. The denial can become pathologic when there is extreme avoidance of the painful event. This is accompanied by emotional blunting, which alters patterns of interaction with support systems, affecting family life, friendship, and work relationships (Horowitz, 2001). Repression of awareness and drug abuse to limit awareness are maladaptive strategies that some individuals use to inhibit their awareness and thus the pain of the event. In cases of extreme avoidance, the person avoids thoughts and feelings associated with the trauma, avoids activities that arouse recollections

of the trauma, and is unable to recall aspects of the trauma.

The denial is interspersed with periods of intrusion when unbidden thoughts of the event intrude by way of distressing recollections and dreams. This intrusion allows the client to begin to manage the psychological effect of the event in small doses of reality. The person unable to handle recollections of the event returns to denial. However, in a client who responds normally, this period of denial and intrusion usually progresses, so denial lessens and intrusion increases. The client attempts to work through the event. In an abnormal response, typical of PTSD, the intrusion period is characterized by flooded states of disturbing mental images in any sensory modality (visual, auditory, olfactory) that form as if they were the real perceptions, and the individual responds (acting or feeling) as if the traumatic event were recurring. This is known as a *flashback.* These unbidden images tend to occur most often when the person relaxes, lies down to sleep, or closer his or her eyes to rest. These frightening experiences may lead to anticipatory anxiety about their recurrence or to secondary anxiety and may result in sleep disturbances as the person tries to avoid the unpleasant experience (Horowitz, 2001).

The working-through phase begins when the person is able to begin to confront the emotions and effect of the traumatic event. In this phase, the client faces the reality of what has happened and invests energy into coping with the realities of the situation. The pathologic response is characterized by failure to reach the working-through phase, with consequent psychosomatic responses and character distortions. Biobehavioral symptoms include sleep disorders, difficulty concentrating, hypervigilance, and hyperalertness, as well as various psychosomatic complaints. One of the psychosocial consequences is that the client experiences a markedly diminished interest in normal activities. He or she may feel detached or estranged from others and exhibit a restricted range of affect, which interferes with personal relationships and the ability to work.

The key to treatment is early detection and prevention. Primary prevention involves measures to improve traffic safety and decrease acts of violence through measures such as gun control and educational efforts to prevent rape, child abuse, and domestic violence. Recognition by the practitioner of the association between traumatic events and PTSD is critical to early detection and thorough assessment. The efficacy of early debriefing, once considered standard therapy to prevent PTSD, has been questioned by recent randomized, controlled trials that show no different effect than observation and in some cases even detrimental effects. The clinical relevance of these trials as well as the difficulties in conducting rigorous, randomized, controlled trials of group debriefing creates further difficulty in interpreting the findings. An evidence-based practice table presents research on debriefing following traffic accidents.

EXAMINING THE EVIDENCE: Moving Toward Evidence-Based Practice

What Is the Efficacy of Debriefing Intervention Following Traffic Accidents As a Strategy to Prevent Post-traumatic Stress Disorder (PTSD)?

AUTHOR(S), YEAR	SAMPLE	DESIGN	OUTCOME VARIABLES	MAJOR FINDINGS
Hobbs, Mayou, Harrison, & Worlock, 1996	106 adults admitted to hospital following motor vehicle accidents Random assignment to intervention group (N = 54) or control group (N = 52)	Intervention: 1 hour debriefing combining a review of the traumatic experience, encouragement of emotional expression, and promotion of cognitive processing of the experience Reinforcement with a written pamphlet Measurement done at time of injury and 4 months later	Emotional distress: symptoms of post-traumatic stress disorder, mood disorders, anxiety, intrusive thoughts, travel anxiety Measured with Impact of Event Scale (IES), Brief Symptom Inventory (BSI) questionnaire	Emotional distress remained high in both groups at the initial and 4-month mark Higher but not statistically different scores on emotional distress in the intervention group at the 4-month mark No difference in travel anxiety between the 2 groups Conclusions: no benefit in debriefing and a suggestion of detrimental effects
Mayou, Ehlers, & Hobbs, 2000	Adults admitted to hospital following a motor vehicle accident	Intervention: 1 hour debriefing combining a review of the traumatic experience, encouragement of emotional expression, and promotion of cognitive processing of the experience Reinforcement with a written pamphlet Measurement done at 3 months and 3 years	Emotional distress: symptoms of post-traumatic stress disorder, mood disorders, anxiety, intrusive thoughts, travel anxiety Measured with IES, BSI questionnaire	The intervention group had a significantly worse outcome at 3 years in terms of general psychiatric symptoms (BSI), travel anxiety when being a passenger, pain, physical problems, overall level of functioning, and financial problems Clients who initially had high intrusion and avoidance symptoms (IES) remained symptomatic if they had received the intervention, but recovered if they did not receive the intervention Conclusions: psychological debriefing is ineffective and has adverse long-term effects
Conlon, Fahy, & Conroy, 1999	40 ambulant trauma clinic attenders following minor motor vehicle accident	Participants randomly assigned to intervention and monitoring groups Measurements at 7 days post-trauma and 3 months post-trauma	Emotional distress: symptoms of post-traumatic stress disorder	At 7 days, 75% reported significant levels of distress By 3 months, only 35% reported distress, 22% of which were significantly impaired Incidence of post-traumatic stress disorder over 3 months was estimated at 19% and reduced to 9% at the 3 month point No significant differences in outcome between intervention and monitoring groups at 3 months
Brown, 2000	Workers in a factory following a fatal accident who met for debriefing	3 groups held using 3 different intervention approaches Responses of group members qualitatively discussed	Emotional distress: evidence of anger	In the classic debriefing group (in which workers were warned that they may feel anger and other symptoms), participants had the greatest degree of anger Participants in the group that consisted primarily of support and comfort during the group session were told that the purpose was to wait comfortably for reactions to settle and they were prompted to share best memories of the man who died; no anger was expressed Conclusions: emotionally aroused people are suggestible; if we suggest that they might feel angry it is likely to come true Recommendations: consider elimination of the more confronting parts of the standard debriefing session
Rose, Wessely, & Bisson, 2001	Individuals who attended a single session of debriefing within 1 month of the traumatic stress	Synthesis of 8 trials to assess effectiveness of brief psychological debriefing for the management of psychological distress after trauma, and the prevention of post-traumatic stress disorder	Psychological distress Post-traumatic stress disorder	Single-session individual debriefing did not reduce psychological distress Single-session debriefing did not prevent onset of post-traumatic stress disorder Some evidence that debriefing increased the odds ratio for development of post-traumatic stress disorder Conclusions: no current evidence that psychological debriefing is a useful treatment for the prevention of post-traumatic stress disorder; compulsory debriefing of victims of trauma should cease

Assessment of the trauma client should include an emotional assessment and a targeted assessment for symptoms of the post-trauma response. Lange, Lange, and Cabaltica (2000) suggest using the mnemonic *DREAMS* to obtain relevant clinical data. The individual or family member should be questioned to determine whether signs of detachment are recognized. *D*etachment presents as aloofness from the event itself or in relationships with others. There is a general numbing of emotional responsiveness. The individual must be assessed as to whether he or she *re*-experiences the event in the form of nightmares, recollections or flashbacks, daydreams, slow-motion replays, and/or "freeze-frame" images. Information about the event itself, including whether the event involved substantial *e*motional distress, with threatened death or loss of physical integrity, and feelings of helplessness or disabling fear, must be obtained. The person should be questioned to determine whether there is evidence of ongoing *a*voidance of places, activities, or people that remind the person of the event. If a car accident was the precipitating event, the client should be questioned about any traveling difficulties as either the driver or the passenger. Duration of symptoms (longer than 1 *m*onth) and experiences of *s*ympathetic hyperactivity or hypervigilance that may manifest as insomnia, irritability, and difficulty concentrating should be elicited.

Intervention for PTSD involves a combination of behavioral and pharmacologic interventions. Debriefing must be questioned and critically examined as a routine intervention in the immediate post-traumatic period. Recent studies examining outcomes from these interventions have found conflicting results, with most studies suggesting that the intervention is not efficacious. Explanations for this finding have considered that the intervention occurred while people were still too numbed and distressed to be receptive, that early intervention may disturb natural psychological "defenses" against fear and distress, and that single interventions are inadequate for major emotional problems (Hobbs, Mayou, Harrison, & Worlock, 1996). Despite these findings, psychological debriefing remains the most widely used structured intervention following potentially traumatizing events, designed to reduce the incidence of long-term psychiatric morbidity. Further study and close clinical evaluation is critical to ensure therapeutic outcomes.

Relaxation techniques are taught to assist the individual in coping with the anxiety. Moderate physical exercise or activity may decrease hyperarousal symptoms. Those with sleep deficits should be encouraged to develop a daytime activity or exercise program that promotes fatigue.

Client education should inform individuals and families of the range of responses to trauma to facilitate recognition of the "normalcy" of the response. Learning about the disorder and recognizing cues or situations that trigger symptoms are invaluable. Psychotherapy and cognitive-behavioral therapy focus on breaking the person's pattern of self-defeat by reexamining the traumatic event and the person's response to it.

Selective serotonin reuptake inhibitors (SSRIs) have the broadest range of efficacy—being able to reduce all three clusters of PTSD symptoms. Tricyclic antidepressants have a more narrow effect and aid in lessening the symptoms of re-experiencing. Monoamine oxidase inhibitors can be used to treat both re-experiencing and avoidance symptoms but have little effect on the symptoms of hyperarousal. Antiadrenergic agents (clonidine, propanolol, and guanfacine) have successfully reduced nightmares, hypervigilance, startle reactions, and outbursts of rage. Benzodiazepines have questionable efficacy and are associated with a high frequency of comorbid substance dependence, so they are not commonly used (Lange, Lange, & Cabaltica, 2000).

Crisis: Stress Beyond the Ability to Cope. Acute disease, injury, or exacerbation of a chronic illness constitutes a highly stressful event with the potential for precipitating a major life crisis. A *crisis* can be defined as a situation which threatens to overwhelm the individual (Aguilera, 1994). It requires an appraisal that the event is stressful and is perceived to exceed the scope of the person's normal coping mechanisms. Crisis may be considered an acute variant of stress that is so severe that the individual reaches a state of disorganization in which ability to function deteriorates. Crisis occurs when the normal coping mechanisms are insufficient to alleviate the anxiety associated with the stress.

Crisis represents a state of severe disequilibrium. In the conceptual model of stress (see Fig. 2–1), crisis is a health outcome or functional ability outcome. The individual is in an acutely disorganized state, with an inability to solve problems and to carry out usual role responsibilities. Specific symptoms of severe stress as described in Table 2–2 vary from individual to individual. Because crisis is an extreme disequilibrium, it is time-limited, lasting up to 6 to 8 weeks.

According to Caplan (1964), a crisis has four developmental phases. Table 2–5 describes the phases, which are characterized by mounting anxiety and tension and failure of coping strategies to decrease the experienced stress. Crisis is not inevitable, however, and the emphasis in therapeutic intervention is on assisting the individual to strengthen or develop new coping mechanisms that will prevent him or her from moving into active crisis. Aguilera (1994) categorizes three groupings of balancing factors (perception of the event, situational supports, and coping responses) that can focus assessment and intervention, with the goal of helping the client to solve problems at an early stage. These three balancing factors are similar to the conceptual model of stress factors (see Fig. 2–1).

TABLE 2–5. *Phases of Crisis*

CRISIS PHASE	CHARACTERISTICS
Experience of the event	Rise in tension as the precipitating stressor continues
	More discomfort is felt
	Responds with familiar problem-solving mechanisms
Failure of normal coping mechanisms	Lack of success in coping with the precipitating stressor
	The stressor continues and more discomfort is felt
Emergency problem solving	Further increase in tension mobilizes internal and external resources
	Emergency problem-solving mechanisms are tried
	Willing to use new or unusual means to solve problem and reduce tension
	May redefine the problem
	May become resigned and give up certain aspects of the goal
Major disorganization "active crisis"	If problem is not solved with emergency problem solving, tensions and anxieties increase to an unbearable degree and a major disorganization occurs

Perception of the event is the subjective meaning that the client places on the event and results from the appraisal process in the conceptual model. When a threatening situation exists, the person makes a primary appraisal of it to judge its perceived outcome in relation to future goals and values. This is followed by a secondary appraisal, which analyzes the range of possible coping alternatives for dealing with the stressful event. Once coping strategies are initiated, appraisal continues. When a client's appraisal tells him or her that the event is too overwhelming or too difficult to be dealt with using available coping skills, he or she may use intrapsychic defense mechanisms. However, if his or her attempt to solve the problem is ineffective, tension will not be reduced. Situational supports provide the client with nurturance and the resources vital for coping. In Aguilera's model, situational supports are a combination of person resources and situation supports as presented in Figure 2–1. Situational supports play a major mediating role in the development or resolution of a crisis. Clients with fewer social supports are more susceptible to crisis. Other situational supports come from within the client. They are characteristics of personality or self-concept. Intact self-esteem, hardiness, and the ability to be optimistic are all characteristics that modulate the degree of stress that the client perceives and that assist in coping. Coping mechanisms (coping responses in Fig. 2–1) are

part of the client's repertoire and are the final category of modulating factors. Coping activities take a wide variety of forms and include all the diverse behaviors that people engage in to meet actual or anticipated challenges. Aguilera (1994) posits that crisis occurs when one or more balancing factors are absent (distorted perception of the event, inadequate situational support, or inadequate coping mechanisms). Without the necessary balancing factors the problem remains unresolved, disequilibrium continues, and the individual moves into crisis.

Crisis intervention is a short-term therapeutic intervention designed to assist the client in resolving the severe disequilibrium. Its focus is on immediate assessment, problem solving, and fostering of social support. Assessment focuses on determining the client's level of impairment with respect to affective, cognitive, and behavioral reactions to crisis. Affective categories include anger/hostility, fear/anxiety, sadness/melancholy, and exhaustion/hopelessness. Cognitive assessment focuses on the perception of the event as having the potential to harm or damage emotionally or physically; the degree of loss or perception of the irretrievability of an object, function, or relationship; and the level of transgression or perception of rights having been violated. Behavioral reactions to crisis include approach behaviors (overt or covert attempts to address the crisis event), avoidance behaviors (active attempts to ignore, evade, or escape the crisis event), and immobility (nonproductive, disorganized, or self-canceling attempts to address the crisis event).

The severity of the crisis determines the supportive strategy used with the client. In mild crisis, a nondirect approach to intervention is taken. Few suggestions are given to the client. Rather, the focus is to assist the client in identifying strengths and support systems. Moderate levels of crisis require a collaborative approach to intervention in which suggestions are made to assist clients in mobilizing coping skills yet encouraging them to take as much responsibility as they are able. For severe crisis, a direct approach requires active intervention, whereby the nurse or other supportive person assumes significant responsibility for determining what immediate actions need to be taken and how these will be initiated.

The Challenge of Chronic Illness and Disability

Chronic illness and disability have many similarities because they are ongoing conditions that cannot be cured. *Chronic illness* is an umbrella term encompassing "impairments or deviations from normal which have one or more of the following characteristics: are permanent, leave residual disability, are caused by nonreversible pathologic alteration, require special training of the patient for rehabilitation, may be expected to require a long period of supervision, observation, or care" (Mayo, 1956, p. 9). Chronic conditions are rarely cured but are managed through individual and family effort.

About 50% of Americans currently have one or more chronic illnesses, and 70% are expected to develop a chronic illness at some time during their lives. Chronic illness has replaced acute illness as the leading concern in both adults' and children's health. Approximately 15% of children (age 18 and younger) suffer from a chronic illness. Of this number, 1% to 2% have chronic illness severe enough to curtail normal activities.

Both acute and chronic illness can result in impairment and disability. Because American culture tends to use the term *disabled* in oppressively patronizing ways and distorts what people with disabilities are like, it is important to accurately define terms. *Impairment* refers to the residual limitation resulting from disease, injury, or a congenital defect. *Functional limitation* results from impairment and refers to loss of ability to perform self-care tasks and fulfill usual social roles and normal activities. *Disability* is the inability to perform some key life functions and is often used interchangeably with functional limitation. *Handicap* refers to the interaction of a person with a disability with the environment. Thus, the person who is paraplegic may be handicapped by not being able to climb stairs, but if elevators are available, that particular handicap has been eliminated.

The focus of care for the person with chronic illness and disability is on control of the therapeutic regimen and adaptation to the illness or disability. Two major areas of concern are biophysical stability/instability and psychosocial stability/instability. Biophysical instability is likely to occur at the time of diagnosis and during recurrent exacerbations of the disease (medical crisis). During these periods, the individual becomes aware of the diagnosis or of symptom progression and faces the reality of residual disability. Psychosocial instability is associated with periods of transition and ongoing management. During transition, the individual and family are challenged to do the work (learning, therapy, lifestyle alterations) associated with rehabilitation, recovery, and control of the illness or impairment. In ongoing management, the client and family must continue with the work of the therapeutic regimen, cope with the losses resulting from chronic illness and disability, and integrate the impairment and disability into a revised self-concept and way of life.

Biophysical Instability. The diagnosis phase of chronic illness may be similar to the experience of acute illness when the onset of illness begins with an acute episode, such as with osteomyelitis or SLE. For others with chronic illness, the period of diagnosis may be an ongoing process. In these cases, diagnosis may come as a relief in that it eliminates some of the stress of uncertainty and confusion present before the diagnosis.

In contrast to the client with acute injury, who must cope with uncertainty while waiting to determine the degree of permanent functional limitations, the person

with a diagnosis of chronic illness suddenly realizes the loss of health and the "foreverness" of the condition. This loss of health is often accompanied by an initial shattering of hopes and dreams that impaired health may now prevent. Consequently, the emotional reaction initially experienced by the client and family may seem to be greater than the client's acuity level warrants. The grief experienced at the time of diagnosis is not necessarily associated with the severity of illness but with the meaning of the illness to current and future plans. The expression of anxiety, anger, remorse, sorrow, grief, fear, and guilt is common during this phase. Assisting the client and family to remain in the present and to avoid excessive projection can be supportive during this period of diagnosis.

During periods of medical crisis, or biophysical instability, the client may be unable to control the biophysical response, necessitating dependence on others for care, a change in regimen, or possible hospitalization. This period is marked by the client's sense of powerlessness and frustration with the inability to control his or her body. It is therapeutic at this point to assist the client to exert control over factors he or she can in fact manipulate and not focus on factors outside his or her control. As the client enters or exits the period of diagnosis or medical crisis, a period of psychosocial adaptation occurs because the individual is now at a different point in the illness and must reintegrate the changed regimens, roles, relations, and self-concept.

A major role of the nurse during periods of biophysical instability is to provide support and education. Anxiety levels are extremely high during these times, and learning may be blocked. Calmness, simplicity, repetition, and culturally appropriate communication are the key. Although teaching is initiated during this time, it is unrealistic to plan to instruct clients and families about everything they need to know concerning the illness and therapeutic regimen. The emphasis during these periods should be to teach the skills and knowledge necessary to implement the regimen. Involving family in this process not only promotes adaptation but also is the preferred communication style for many cultural groups to express their care for another. Comprehensive education and understanding comes over time. Providing information may facilitate the defense mechanism of intellectualization. This allows the client to regain some of the control lost during the crisis of diagnosis and medical crisis and prepare for psychosocial adjustment.

Psychosocial Adaptation. In the transition phase of chronic illness or disability, the client must learn what the disease is or the meaning of disease progression, its effect on his or her life, the therapeutic regimen required to control the disease, the monitoring necessary to evaluate progress, and the work of physical therapy and occupational therapy necessary to maximize functioning.

Feeling overwhelmed with all of the information that must be processed, the skills that must be learned, and the routines that need to be established is quite common at this stage. There is often a honeymoon phase that begins at the stage of diagnosis and extends into early transition. At this point, there is a massive outpouring of support and understanding, and a positive outlook predominates. Because there is so much to learn and control in this stage, the client tends to deny the emotional response to illness. Denial provides the reduction in stress needed for effective learning. Clients and their families should be counseled, however, that a more intense emotional response may occur as they confront the meaning of the illness or disability in their lives.

For most clients, transition is faced at home, where there are fewer resource persons available to provide guidance and support. This phase can prove extremely stressful, but the stress can be somewhat alleviated by assuring clients in transition that there are people available to answer questions and concerns through either the acute care institution, their physician's office or clinic, a home care agency, or a support group. Clients should be advised that this period of learning and integration requires a significant amount of energy and time. They should be reminded that they will experience routine activities differently now and that things that were once done without thinking, such as getting up to go to the bathroom, may now be accompanied by fear and anxiety and may require a significant amount of energy. Helping the client and family to realistically plan for what will be involved can facilitate movement through this period and prevent the client and family from imposing unnecessary restrictions because they are afraid to do something.

The client with an impairment requiring rehabilitation meets the challenge of transition first in the rehabilitation setting and then in the home setting. This client invests a tremendous amount of energy into the work of rehabilitation. The rehabilitation setting attempts to be responsive to the biopsychosocial needs of the client. However, for many clients with orthopaedic disabilities, the emphasis is primarily on maximizing mobility and function. For some, there is little energy available to confront the issues of altered lifestyle.

The period of ongoing management marks the time when the client at home is no longer allowed the disorganization and dependency of the acute or early phases but must integrate the chronic illness into the daily routine and self-concept. Returning to or renegotiating role responsibilities and redefining a self-concept in which the illness or disability does not encompass the person's self-image are the major goals of this phase.

This period is fraught with emotional turmoil as the client faces the consequences of the disease or disability on body image, self-concept, role interactions, sexuality, and family and personal life. Nurses are in a key position to assist the client in coping with these stressors. Anticipatory planning by the nurse allows for identification of and discussion of potential stressors. Preparing the person for the range of responses and feelings that are normal in adapting to chronic illness and disability, the possible difficulties that will be encountered, and the problem-solving strategies that might be used strengthens the individual's adaptive mechanisms. Role-playing difficult situations such as how to tell the employer of functional impairment and what to tell friends and neighbors can prepare the individual for inevitable stressful encounters. The client should be encouraged to verbalize his or her feelings by being asked direct questions that elucidate his or her specific concerns; these concerns form the basis for supported problem solving. Education and counseling initiated in the hospital must extend into the home and community settings. Arranging contact with individuals who live with similar conditions or support groups can be very beneficial. This reduces the

TABLE 2–6. *Stressors Associated with Disease and Illness*

DISEASE STRESSORS	ILLNESS STRESSORS	HEALTH CARE SYSTEM STRESSORS
Lack of knowledge	Losses imposed by change in function	Strange, invasive tests
Lack of information and feedback	Management of symptoms	Esoteric language
Waiting	Breakdown of support network	Nothing routine to the client
Lack of control	Lack of control	Lack of control
Uncertainty	Normalizing	Depersonalization
Side effects of drugs	Role disruption	Locating community resources
Learning treatment regimen	Maintaining communications	Talks over client
Seeking help for regimen	Threat to self-esteem	Lack of privacy
Maintaining preparedness	Threat to body image	Insurance benefits
Recognizing and treating medical crisis	Fear of loss of love	Aloneness
	Fear of dependence	Care by strangers
	Fear of pain	Disruption of client rituals
	Fatigue or energy loss	
	Responding to stigma	
	Changing course of disease	

sense of isolation and promotes coping by observing others who have mastered the therapeutic regimen and by having the opportunity to ask questions of someone who has had similar experiences and feelings.

Stressors Associated with Chronic Illness and Disability

Table 2-6 categorizes chronic illness stressors as disease, illness, and health care system stressors.

Disease and Treatment Stressors. *Disease* and *treatment stressors* refer to the biophysical stressors of the disease and the treatment required to stabilize their effect. Disease and treatment stressors can include learning about how the disease occurs in the person, how to implement a therapeutic regimen, and how to recognize biophysical instability that requires new management interventions.

Knowledge Deficit about the Disease. A primary health care need is receiving ongoing and accurate information about the disease or injury and an interpretation of the significance of that information to the client's own condition. The nurse should be aware that clients have differing interpretations as to why the illness occurred, and this should be explored. Asking the client, "What do you think caused this problem?" may reveal causation stress associated with the belief that the disease is a punishment or a result of the person's being envious or exposed to the evil eye. The nurse must understand these differing interpretations of disease and not try to refute them, but rather accept them and integrate them into a discussion that may include what is actually happening in the body at this time. Treatment decisions in cases in which the client has a different interpretation of the cause of the disease should include use of traditional remedies and medical interventions.

Diagnosis of the disease or of changing trajectories of the disease as well as some therapies prescribed may involve unfamiliar diagnostic tests or treatment modalities that may be frightening. Jean Johnson's research (Backer, Bakas, Bennett, & Pierce, 2000) on nursing intervention for stress reduction in adults and children experiencing threatening health care events has clearly shown that the effects of preparatory information on clients' coping outcomes differ with the content that is included in the information. Generally, two types of information have been studied: procedural and sensory information. Procedural information focuses on the sequence and types of events that a client is likely to encounter. Sensory information describes the sensations that clients typically experience during a procedure or operation, including what they may see, hear, feel, or smell. Procedural information alone has been found to have limited effects on indices of postoperative recovery, although there has been a lack of consistency in these

TABLE 2–7. *Assessing Preferences for Information: Information Seekers versus Avoiders*

Ask the client to agree or disagree with each of the following statements:

1. I usually don't ask a doctor or nurse many questions about what they are doing as they examine me.
2. I'd rather have doctors and nurses make decisions about what is best than for them to give me a whole lot of choices.
3. Instead of waiting for them to tell me, I usually ask the doctor or nurse about my health immediately after they've finished examining me.
4. I usually ask the doctor or nurse lots of questions about what they are doing and why they are doing it while they examine me.
5. It is better to trust the doctor or nurse in charge of a medical procedure rather than to question what they are doing.
6. I usually wait for the doctor or nurse to tell me the results of a medical examination rather than asking them immediately.
7. I'd rather be given many choices about what's best for my health than to have the doctor or nurse make decisions for me.

From Morgan, J., Roufeil, L., Kaushik, S., & Bassett M. (1998). Influence of coping style and precolonoscopy information on pain and anxiety of colonoscopy. *Gastrointestinal Endoscopy, 48*(2), 120.

research findings. Provision of sensory information has been found to be more effective than simply direct procedural information in decreasing postoperative anxiety.

Later research examined type of preparatory information according to preferred coping styles of the person. These studies have shown that the key is to provide information congruent with the coping style. Thus, if an individual typically copes by seeking information, his or her adjustment is facilitated by providing both sensory and procedural information. In contrast, if the person is an information avoider, his or her adjustment is facilitated by providing procedural information alone. The following evidence-based practice table summarizes some of the research on preparatory information. Table 2-7 provides a list of questions the nurse can use to determine whether the person is an information seeker or information avoider.

Laboratory tests should be explained in relationship to their significance to the course of the illness. Giving accurate, timely information decreases the stress of uncertainty and waiting and provides the client and family with the foundation of knowledge on which to begin to assume more and more control. Even when information is not available, it is important to keep the client and family informed about what is happening in the evaluation process and when further information will be available. Providing this information further minimizes the uncertainty and stress associated with waiting.

EXAMINING THE EVIDENCE: Moving Toward Evidence-Based Practice
Preparatory Information for Diagnostic and Treatment Procedures

AUTHOR(S), YEAR	SAMPLE	DESIGN	OUTCOME VARIABLES	MAJOR FINDINGS
Fuller, Endress, & Johnson, 1978	24 women undergoing a routine pelvic examination	4 groups: sensory, sensory plus relaxation, health education, and health education plus relaxation	Radial pulse, overt distress behaviors, and fear self-report	The sensory group had significantly fewer distress behaviors ($p < .02$) and less pulse rate change ($p < .02$)
Gammon, 1996a, 1996b	82 individuals undergoing total hip replacements	Quasi-experimental design using non-random selection techniques Experimental group given procedural, sensory, and coping information Control group received only advice and support typically given to clients by staff	Anxiety and depression Self-esteem Sense of control Perception of coping Functional outcomes: pain, mobilization, length of stay	Providing information had positive effects on the psychological coping outcomes measured Experimental group had significantly less anxiety and depression with a high self-esteem and sense of control Participants in experimental group had significantly less postoperative intramuscular analgesia, mobilized sooner and had a 2-day shorter length of stay
Hartfield & Carson, 1981	24 hospitalized clients undergoing barium enema	Quasi-experimental with 3 groups: sensation, procedure, and control	Anxiety using Spielberger's State-Trait Anxiety Inventory	Significantly less state anxiety reported by sensation group than by the other two groups ($p < .05$)
Hill, 1982	40 hospitalized clients undergoing first-time cataract surgery	Experimental with 4 groups: behavioral instruction, sensation information, behavioral plus sensation information, and general information	Postoperative confusion, mood, functional performance	No difference in outcomes in behavioral or sensation groups Combination group (behavioral plus sensation) had significantly lower number of days after discharge when leaving their homes
Johnson, Kirchoff, & Endress, 1975	89 children undergoing cast removal	Experimental with 3 groups: sensations, procedure, and control	Radial pulse, Minor and major distress	Sensation group had no significant pulse rate changes during procedure whether or not child had fear of procedure
Johnson, Morrissey, & Leventhal, 1973	99 inpatients and outpatients undergoing an endoscopic examination	Quasi-experimental with 3 groups: sensations, procedure, control	Dose of sedation Heart rate changes Hand and arm movements Gagging Restlessness	Sensation group had significantly less sedation used ($p < .05$) and fewer hand and arm movements ($p < .02$)
McDaniel, 1998	20 women receiving chemotherapy for breast cancer	Pilot testing with one group Women reviewed a 20-minute preparatory sensory information videotape	Anticipatory coping	The intervention helped prepare the women for the sensory experiences associated with chemotherapy and was helpful in developing anticipatory coping and self-care behaviors
Mitchell, 1997	150 women undergoing minor gynecologic same-day surgery	Survey design to compare health locus of control with preferred level of preparatory information	Health locus of control Attitude to health	No correlation was established between the health locus of control measures and the selected level of preparatory information
Morgan, Roufeil, Kaushik, & Bassett, 1998	80 consecutive adult clients undergoing initial colonoscopy	Initial purposive assignment based on coping style (information seekers vs. information avoiders) then random assignment into 2 groups: standardized information and standardized information plus sensory information	Anxiety (self-report, physiologic and behavioral indices) Pain Recovery time	Clients given information congruent with coping style experienced significantly less self-report anxiety and spent less time in recovery Clients given information not congruent with coping style maintained their preintervention anxiety level Clients given information congruent with coping style scored lower on behavioral indices of pain but no difference in self-report or dosage of drugs used

The client and family are challenged to learn about the disease: what it is and the symptoms associated with it. This is more than a cognitive process and requires connecting cue recognition of biophysical symptoms as they are subjectively experienced to an interpretation of the disease process. The nurse can facilitate this process of symptom awareness or cue recognition by highlighting the client's objective and subjective symptoms and findings in relation to the disease process itself. For example, an individual newly diagnosed as having arthritis can be taught to assess the involved joints and describe what he or she sees and feels. The symptoms of a red, warm, swollen joint can be the symptoms of inflammation and extra fluid in the joint that causes pain and stiffness. The client can then follow the treatment and observe the changes in both the biophysical signs and the functional signs of pain and stiffness. It is through this association that the client and family become expert in knowing how the disease manifests itself.

Knowledge Deficit about Treatment. In addition to understanding disease and monitoring for symptoms, the client must become knowledgeable about the treatment regimen. Planned therapies should be described in terms of what the expected outcome should be. With time-limited acute disease, simply a cognitive understanding of what is happening may be required. For ongoing sequelae of acute illness or chronic disease, it is necessary to acquire not only the knowledge of the regimen but also the skills necessary to implement it. This may require practice in specific skills, such as range-of-motion exercises, splint application, and cast care, but it also requires planning of when and how these regimens are to be carried out.

Assessing past strategies used to cope with or manage symptoms is an important step in determining the array of approaches (traditional and conventional) used in health management. The use of herbs or amulets to prevent illness or minimize symptoms, the managing of hot and cold balance, and other approaches can be integrated with the medical regimen if the nurse is sensitive to cultural differences. This approach is likely to be associated with greater feelings of respect and with adherence to the medical regimen.

There is often a difficult transition between the hospital or rehabilitation center and home. Although the client and family may have demonstrated skills in performing the regimen while in the health care facility, it is particularly stressful when the regimen must be implemented at home. The nurse can decrease some of this likely stress by working with the client and family in planning. Asking questions aids in the development of a plan for the "who, what, where, and when" of the treatment regimen. Possible questions include the following: "When do you think you can fit in the range-of-motion exercises?" "Who will need to assist you?" "When

is it feasible for this person to be available?" "What supplies will you need in the house to make it easier for you?" "When will you schedule the necessary tests?" "Where will you go for these tests?"

Given the necessary education, adult clients are generally able to understand the link between the treatment and the disease and how the treatment is necessary for the cure or control of the disease. A child is less able to connect cause and effect and therefore may have difficulty understanding the link between painful or restrictive treatments and beneficial outcomes. For the young child, treatment may be perceived as a punishment. Parental and health care personnel reassurance is important. For the toddler and preschool child who cannot cognitively connect the injury and treatment, it is helpful to restrict painful treatments to certain areas and to have other areas that are considered safe.

Knowledge about Biophysical Instability. Another major disease or treatment stressor requires the individual and family to recognize the signs of impending medical crisis or imbalance and to initiate the appropriate evaluation and treatment. For example, individuals with myasthenia gravis need to recognize that swallowing difficulties and excessive muscular weakness in the middle of the day may be more critical than if these symptoms are experienced in the early morning before taking medication. Individuals with SLE must be on the alert for signs of urinary, skin, and respiratory infections that could send the illness into a downward course. The nurse can assist the client and family in developing the needed awareness of and preparation for a medical crisis. This can be accomplished through anticipatory role-playing, keeping records or charts that are easily accessible at home, and postcrisis evaluation of readiness and understanding.

Illness Stressors. Illness stressors are those events, changes, and losses that result from the effect of the disease on the client and family. Stressors specific to an illness are often anticipated by health care providers but may not be responded to because of the acuity of the illness while in the hospital setting. This means that the individual and family try to cope with these stressors at home without additional support. Illness stressors can be categorized as biophysical, psychogenic, and sociocultural.

Biophysical Illness Stressors. Biophysical stressors include the symptoms of the disease as well as the side effects experienced as part of the treatment. Sensations such as pain, nausea, spasms, and fatigue must be coped with. Management of energy deficit, pain management, and mobility deficits are common orthopaedic biophysical illness stressors. Health care outcomes should target symptom management as a priority intervention strategy.

Minimizing these discomforts as well as coping with the psychological and sociocultural stressors imposed by these symptoms is the challenge of illness.

Psychogenic Illness Stressors. Psychogenic stressors of illness are linked to the losses experienced by the client. The presence of disease or disability creates many losses that must be grieved for and coped with. These may include loss of health or wellness status, loss of control over biophysical and psychological symptoms, loss of a body part or change in body image, loss of independence, loss of self-esteem, loss of role function, loss of dreams and expectations, and loss of intimacy and relationships. These losses will be grieved for, and an understanding of the grief process is imperative for the nurse, the client, and the family.

Clients living with chronic illness should be counseled about the experience of loss and the grief reaction that accompanies it. Helping clients and their families become familiar with typical responses of grief assists them through the process and allows for a greater degree of acceptance of differences in response. The therapeutic goals of coping with loss stressors include mourning the loss; acknowledging remaining assets or abilities; and taking measures to actively cope with the stressors, drawing on the assets, abilities, and supports available.

Sociocultural Illness Stressors. Sociocultural stressors common to the illness experience may include role disruption, role renegotiation, social isolation, social stigma, social handicaps, and maintenance of intact family and personal resources. Patterns of living that were second nature to the family are challenged by illness. The client may be unable to continue all previous role responsibilities because of mobility deficits, energy deficits, or other symptoms. Skills in role negotiation are integral to avoiding exhaustion. If the family normally is flexible, role negotiation may produce little stress. However, in a rigid family structure, having to change role responsibilities may be associated with resentment, withdrawal, and rejection.

Different cultural responses to illness may impose barriers between the nurse and client because of a lack of understanding. Culture influences how feelings are expressed and what verbal and nonverbal expressions are appropriate. If the nurse is unfamiliar with a particular culture, a trusting relationship can be established if the nurse encourages the client to communicate cultural interpretations of health, illness, and health care.

With chronic illness and disability, some degree of social isolation is typically experienced. Part of this isolation may stem from the client's own insecurity in venturing back into typical social situations, and part is generally due to other people not knowing how to handle the situation. If the disability is visible, there may be more hesitation surrounding interpersonal interactions and the social isolation may be intensified.

Individuals with disabilities must deal with the stressors of a community environment that may not be prepared for the disability. This may result in situations in which the individual with a disability finds himself or herself handicapped. Although the United States has made progress in the last decade toward providing access for persons with disabilities, the reality is that a person with a disability is often barred from activities because of lack of facilities. This causes significant anger and hostility and sometimes withdrawal. In addition, the individual with a disability must cope not only with the handicap but also with the stigma associated with the disability or disease.

To respond to illness stressors, the client often invests a tremendous amount of energy into normalizing. Normalizing can be regarded as efforts an individual makes to maintain a sense of normalcy. This effort stems not only from the person's own demands but from the demands of significant others and demands of society, which has little tolerance for chronic illness and disability. The goal in normalizing is to live as normal a life as possible despite daily therapy and obvious symptoms. Common strategies used to normalize include covering up, keeping up, justifying inaction, pacing, eliciting help, and balancing options.

Stressors Associated with the Health Care System. Although the purpose of the health care system is to treat the client and alleviate concerns, the health care system often imposes additional stressors.

Hospitalization, surgical interventions, and medical visits themselves may be appraised as a major stressor. To health care providers, the routines, noises, appearances, and odors of the facility are rarely given a second thought. They are part of our everyday lives. However, to the client and family, the health care facility is a frightening setting in which they feel intimidated, anxious, and often alone, without the necessary knowledge to interpret the incoming stimuli.

Hospitalization, Same-Day Surgery. Hospitalization creates a crisis that signifies that the biophysical system is so threatened that the individual can no longer be helped at home or in the outpatient setting. Hospitalization signals a seriousness of the disease that may be terrifying. It requires that the individual and often the family drop their role in society and face their own mortality. Similarly, surgery, whether it be same-day surgery or require an overnight stay in the hospital, requires a surrendering of control, which can be very stressful.

Table 2–6 highlights many of the stressors associated with hospitalization and the health care system. On entry into the hospital or same-day surgical facility, the client surrenders most of his or her control and is placed in the hands of a variety of health care providers whom he or she does not even know. Clients undergo a variety of strange and painful diagnostic tests and must endure the seemingly endless wait to receive results, answers, or opinions. Communication is often rushed, leaving the client and family feeling like outsiders even though they are the focus of the care. Communication is further hampered by lack of a common language when speaking of the disease and treatment, leaving the client and family trying to decipher the meaning of it all by themselves.

Entry into the hospital can be even more stressful for the very young, the very old, and nondominant cultural groups. For the older client, removal from the home environment can be associated with confusion and disorientation. The effects of sleeping medication, darkness, and unfamiliar surroundings can produce further disorganization, placing a once independent, secure older individual into a high-risk, frightening situation. Additional stress can be produced when an alert and oriented older person places his or her well-being in the hands of a stranger, who might be 40 years younger and refers to the client as "Gramps" or "Granny." This disrespect can have a lasting effect on well-being and level of despair. On admission, the nurse should ask how the client wishes to be addressed, and this information should be recorded.

For children, the response to hospitalization is influenced by age and developmental levels as well as parental behavior. The toddler and preschool child may relate hospitalization to personal behavior. Their lack of understanding of what is happening makes them more resistive to treatment. Separation anxiety is a major stressor, with the child feeling alone and abandoned. The school-aged child may feel singled out and express feelings of guilt and self-blame. The child can be supported by reassurances that he or she is not responsible for the onset of the disease or the severity of the present condition. Adolescents may vary in their response to hospitalization, depending on the presence of symptoms and their social support, but they often feel isolated, alone, and different. These feelings are associated with a significant degree of anxiety.

The nurse can play a major role in alleviating much of the anxiety experienced. First, nothing should be considered routine. The nurse supports the client by providing information and meaningful communication about the "who, what, where, when, and how" of the daily hospital regimen or surgical same-day area. By decreasing the stress imposed on them from the physical environment and allowing flexibility with visiting and personalization of the area, the nurse maximizes the energy and resources the individual needs to cope with the disease and illness.

Regard for the individual is another vital nursing strategy. Health care interventions, especially surgery, often are accompanied by depersonalization, lack of privacy, and lack of regard. Health care providers should always introduce themselves and ask permission to deliver care. The client should not be called by the medical diagnosis, and his or her concerns regarding bodily exposure should be attended to. Empathic listening and consistent explanations are essential to establishing a trusting therapeutic relationship. The presence of a trusting relationship facilitates the client's ability to comfortably turn over control of the disease to the health care provider, a factor that promotes coping during the experience.

Another major nursing intervention for supporting the client during health care intervention is to assist the person to remain in control. Powerlessness is a common response to hospitalization and is associated with significant emotional discomfort. Although the individual may not be able to control biophysical phenomena at this point, giving them control over when and how care is to be administered and other decision-making opportunities maximizes the sense of control, thereby decreasing some of the fear and anger associated with powerlessness.

Generally speaking, client and family passivity is fostered by health care providers who are accustomed to a position of authority and control. In families skilled in managing chronic illness, a struggle for control may occur between the client and family and the nurse. The nurse can minimize this struggle by respecting the client's and family's expertise in caring for the condition, by respecting the family as a unit, and by listening to the knowledge and suggestions offered by the family. Clients and families consider it a priority to be thought of as members of the health care team and not simply as an object for provider discussion and intervention.

Outpatient Services. The client with a chronic disease or disability must learn to negotiate the health care maze to receive the services available. This is no easy task. In the absence of community case managers, clients and families must determine accessible, reliable, and affordable health care services. Unfortunately, this may be complicated by the client's type of health care plan. Many insurance plans necessitate geographically dispersed services because of preapproved providers. Case managers serve a central role in helping the client negotiate this maze. An additional stressor for many individuals with chronic orthopaedic illness or disability is accessing these services because many clients are limited both by their mobility deficits and by lack of transportation to the services.

As the health care system becomes more responsive to the needs of the client with a chronic illness or disability and with the general trend to provide care on an outpatient basis, it can be anticipated that more outreach and home-based programs will become available. Programs that target symptom management (e.g., handling of pain, altered mobility, fatigue, stress) have the potential of increasing the client's and family's ability to control the symptoms at home and effect improvements in general health outcomes and adaptation.

COPING WITH LOSS: THE GRIEF RESPONSE

Grief, or *bereavement,* is typically defined as the physical, emotional, and mental responses to loss. The presence of acute illness, chronic illness, or disability generally represents multiple losses for the individual and family (Box 2–2), which must be mourned if healing is to occur. A specific loss may have many dimensions and may be grieved for because of its physical, intrapsychic, interpersonal, or socioeconomic meaning. The types of loss and the manifestation of the grief response are uniquely individual lived experiences.

Death is a large, encompassing loss that is irretrievable and non-negotiable. The grief associated with loss in chronic illness or disability typically occurs on an ongoing basis with either the experience of new loss or the trigger of emotions around a previous loss. The grief in chronic illness or disability often reappears in situations when the illness takes a downward course, when the client is reminded of limitations, when hoped for goals are blocked because of the limitations of the chronic illness or disability, or when additional losses occur. The nurse provides support by explaining to clients and family that the grief response is normal and a needed part of healing. Fisher and Hanspal (1998) examined the presence of phantom pain, anxiety, and depression in clients with amputated limbs and found that those persons encouraged to express grief over their loss experienced less pain and emotional sequelae.

Stages of Grief

Grief is not a stable phenomenon but is a holistic process that affects people physically, emotionally, and spiritu-

---

BOX 2–2.
Losses Associated with Illness and Disability

Loss of independence
Loss of control
Loss of values
Loss of friends, family
Loss of self-concept
Loss of illusion of invulnerability or immortality
Loss of opportunities
Loss of familiar surroundings
Loss of valued personal belongings
Loss of valued others
Loss of valued roles played
Loss of physical faculties
Loss of memory

---

ally. It is represented in their thought processes, perceptions, and behaviors. When grief begins, the aching and terror are insistent. Figure 2–3 depicts a model of the grief process, illustrating four phases of grief and five realms in which these phases may be experienced: physical, cognitive, emotional, spiritual, and behavioral. The phases have no specific time frames, and may occur, reoccur, or co-occur in any sequence; however, in most cases, grief is particularly insistent and intense when it first begins.

Initial Awareness. Initial awareness typically marks the beginning of the grief process. This is a time when the reality of the loss first enters the conscious mind. Initial awareness may be immediate or delayed. The initial effect of the loss may be so powerful as to imprint itself on the client's memory such that years afterward recall of the event can stimulate vivid, painfully fresh feelings. With initial awareness, the person suddenly realizes the meaning of the illness or disability to his or her life.

Awareness is often experienced as shock and may be accompanied by complete disruption of daily routine and ability to function. Painful emotional turmoil and physiologic symptoms, such as feelings of choking, shortness of breath, emptiness in the stomach, and lack of muscular strength, may occur. Emotional responses may include disbelief, detachment, anxiety, fear, and anger. Initial awareness of the loss may precipitate a loss of meaning and purpose in the person's life. Daily routines are seen as meaningless and trivial. Life seems out of balance.

The initial awareness phase of grief is highly stressful; most persons cannot tolerate remaining in this phase for prolonged periods and seek ways to modulate their degree of distress.

During this phase, the individual is vulnerable. Vulnerable persons are extremely sensitive to the comments and actions of others. Use of clichés, such as "You wouldn't be given anything you couldn't handle," "God must have a plan in all of this," "You will learn to accept this," and "You shouldn't feel that way" are likely to be greatly resented and have the potential for disrupting interpersonal relations. At this stage, there are no solutions or advice that can resolve the mourner's situation or make the loss go away. There is no way to effectively address the client's feelings about the perceived meaninglessness in life. The individual may feel stopped in his or her tracks and unable to express the extent of emotions and experiences. Nonverbal actions are more supportive than words at this point. The importance of a "disciplined presence" in which the nurse is able to connect empathetically with the other is therapeutic.

Holding On and Letting Go. Holding on and letting go are defensive coping mechanisms that limit awareness as a way of modulating distress. Their use may precede the initial awareness phase of grieving or occur subse-

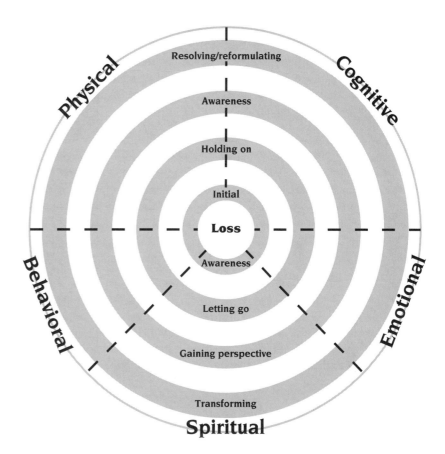

FIGURE 2–3. Bereavement: a holistic framework. (From Schneider, J. [1984]. *Stress, loss and grief* [p. 67]. Rockville, MD: Aspen.)

quent to it. These strategies can be protective if used on a limited basis, but if used unconsciously or habitually, they can have serious consequences.

Holding-on strategies are coping behaviors aimed at preventing, overcoming, or reversing loss by "holding on" to the actions, hopes, and desires of the past. A certain amount of denial, typically about the future, is inherent in this behavior, as is selective processing of information, with rejection of any information that confirms or validates the loss. The belief that "I can overcome anything" or "I can be like I was" can be an asset initially, prompting the person to make the maximum personal investment and get the greatest possible benefit from rehabilitative therapies. Holding on can be detrimental in cases in which the "I can overcome" attitude leads persons to nonadherence with their medical regimen in the belief that they can overcome the loss or disease without it.

Letting-go behaviors modulate distress with attempts to escape or minimize the loss itself or reminders of the loss, thereby denying its significance and making grief avoidable. In the short term, such behaviors can be therapeutic by buying some recovery time. Letting-go strategies include passivity, objectivity, repression, and helplessness; the person may demur to fate, God, or health care providers.

Both holding-on and letting-go behaviors may persist unhealthily if persons are fearful of "admitting defeat" or of being overwhelmed by the enormity of their loss and its implications. Overlong persistence of avoidance strategies can result in long-term failure to adapt to chronic illness or disability.

Awareness. Awareness is the phase of response to loss that is most readily recognized as grieving. It is the point at which holding-on and letting-go strategies are relinquished (possibly intermittently at first) and processing of the realities of the loss begins. Emotions are intense in response to awareness; helplessness, hopelessness, anger, fear, sorrow, and guilt may be experienced. Related somatic symptoms can include sleeplessness, malaise, energy deficit, tightness in the throat, heaviness throughout the body, difficulty sleeping, sighing, weeping, and sobbing.

As the person begins to confront the implications and extent of the loss, concentration and energy are focused and directed on the self. This emotional "knuckling down" to the work of recovery is healthy. However, the person may see himself or herself as the "ill victim" or egocentrically view the world with the self and the loss as the only points of reference. As a result, the person may be unable at this point to recognize or acknowledge that family members are also experiencing pain and grief. Families should be educated to anticipate rather than misinterpret this normal phase of the grieving process, to support the recovery of both the client and family.

Anger. Because anger is an emotion people are often taught to bury or avoid, it is perhaps the most difficult emotion for people to handle. Both genders experience anger; however, men are more likely to experience grief through anger than women, who typically experience grief through sadness (Golden, 1996). It is important to understand the objects, manifestations, and channeling of anger in dealing with anger and grief.

The client grieving a loss is usually angry about the loss itself, or the life effects of the loss. This anger may manifest in silence, negativity, sarcasm, exaggerated upset over trivial happenings, or the manipulation and upsetting of others. This anger may be vented at the client's significant others, or at caregivers.

Clients can be supported in dealing with anger by being guided to focus on the loss itself and the accompanying hurt and broken expectations rather than on the quality or nature of the angry emotions themselves. Families can be supported by education about anger, which helps them to understand that the anger is "better out than in" and that it is not about them even if it is being vented at them for the time being.

Sadness. Sadness is part of grief, and tears are part of sadness. Crying is healing, but in American culture, certain social parameters affect crying behavior. For example, many people feel uncomfortable when others cry in their presence; typically, crying by women is more acceptable than crying by men.

Because American culture values male independence and autonomy, a man may find it difficult to acknowledge the powerlessness over a situation that tears and sadness confirm. Therefore, men often use action, rather than sadness, to heal grief. Such actions might include keeping a journal, meditating, dedicating oneself to work to a cause through activism or advocacy, or setting up memorial funds. Women are more likely to use social support and intimacy as coping mechanisms and therefore may be more responsive to sadness.

Gaining Perspective. Persons who move forward in the grieving process begin a process of healing and acceptance by gaining perspective. This period is a contemplative rather than an active one; rest and recuperation slowly lead to revitalization and renewed energy. As with physical healing after trauma, emotional healing must be allotted adequate time and not hurried along.

Generally, the intensity and acuity of the pain of loss lessen during this phase of grief. However, the cyclical nature of the grief process described earlier may lead to periodic exacerbation in grief; this does not necessarily represent regression or overreaction. Clients and families benefit when the nurse educates them about this aspect of the grief process.

Gaining perspective is characterized by self-searching, solitude, and questioning, through which the client begins to understand the loss and integrate it into his or her life by reassessing values and reformulating the self-concept. This process can be supported by providing the client with adequate time and privacy for contemplation and by limiting additional responsibilities or obligations for a time. Some people end the grieving process here; others move on to a higher level of growth.

Resolving and Transforming Loss. The resolution of loss allows for the energy that has been devoted to grieving to be directed toward nongrieving life activities; the client detaches from the grief and moves on. Although situations may occur in which grief resurfaces, this grief is more "limited" because the client's psychological resources have been strengthened by the process of resolving the grief. Clients who have resolved loss may redirect their energies toward activities such as journal-keeping, service to support groups, or other new pursuits.

Transforming or reformulating of the loss may occur after the loss has been resolved. The client centers on the self during this time and focuses on the potential, opportunities, and possibilities associated with the new situation; the client not only accepts the loss but grows through it. New energies are available for loving, creating, and risking. Life continues with a deeper awareness of interdependency and feelings.

Shared Grief over Multiple Losses

With a chronic illness or disability, there is not one loss but rather a series of losses. Although there is an identified "client," the loss is typically shared by many persons central to the client's support system. These persons may be at different phases in their grief over different losses. Each person has a different sense and meaning of the loss and moves through the grieving process in his or her own way. Consequently, it is possible that in one family there may be similar losses but different perceptions of the meaning of the loss, and family members may be at different stages of grief. It is therefore important to gather information on what losses are in fact being mourned and where in the grief process the individual is at.

These differences in grief may cause conflict when interpreted as another person not caring or not understanding. Although it may not always be possible to change the grieving process, open communication about what is happening creates a level of understanding. The goal should be for all concerned parties to understand that movement through the grieving process occurs at different levels and that tolerance and acceptance of one another serve as a foundation for mutual efforts later on in the working phase.

Anticipatory Grieving

Anticipatory grieving occurs when there is awareness that a loss is imminent. The grieving process commences before the actual loss. From an adaptive point of view, anticipatory grieving allows the person to prepare emotionally for the loss so that when it is experienced, it may not be as overwhelming. Anticipatory grieving and anticipatory rehearsal help the person cope with predictable stressors and can prepare him or her so that the event does not overwhelm his or her coping resources and put him or her into crisis.

Chronic Sorrow

The term *chronic sorrow* was adopted by Olshansky (1962) to describe a natural response to a tragic, long-term fact. *Chronic sorrow* has often been used to describe the parental response to a child's chronic disability or illness. It is characterized by a continuing, cyclical experience of grief that is triggered by an event reminding the individual of the tragedy. These events may include exacerbation of a physical condition, requiring the person to face new limitations or new indignities in reaching what was anticipated to be important developmental milestones; deviation from milestones; and social barriers that remind the person of the illness or disability. Chronic sorrow is not mentioned frequently in the literature any longer because grief work now recognizes that grief is not a process that finishes but rather is revisited in response to triggering events, such as memories, birth dates, hearing a favorite song, or watching a familiar movie.

PSYCHOSOCIAL NURSING DIAGNOSES COMMON WITH ACUTE AND CHRONIC ILLNESS

Powerlessness

Oliver Wendell Holmes said, "The secret to longevity is to have a chronic, incurable illness and take good care of it." In this saying, the key is being in control and being able to do something to take care of the illness. Unfortunately, illness is often accompanied by numerous reminders of one's lack of control. Powerlessness occurs when the individual perceives that his or her own action will not significantly affect an outcome. The manifestation of powerlessness may vary from client to client but often mimics depression and is commonly accompanied by passivity, dissatisfaction, apathy, and lack of self-regulation.

Powerlessness can occur secondary to an accumulation of stressors resulting from hospitalization as well as from illness-related stressors. With acute illness and hospitalization, the person is often forced to relinquish control to strangers and cope with hospital routines and practices that make little sense. Restrictive dressings and equipment, as well as the physiologic condition itself, may limit mobility and sensory stimulation. Pain, fatigue, and sleeplessness intensify the experience of powerlessness. Lack of information about what is happening and lack of input regarding what they think is right for them

leaves individuals feeling like outsiders in their own bodies. This sense of psychological powerlessness or loss of control is intensified with depersonalization and lack of involvement in decision making.

Affleck, Tennen, Pfeiffere, and Fifield (1987) examined the relationship between the perception of control and predictability in adapting to RA. In a sample of 92 clients, the investigators found that perception of greater personal control over symptoms and treatment was associated with positive mood and psychosocial adjustment. Negative mood was associated with the belief that health care providers had greater control over the client's daily symptoms than the client did. Of interest is the differentiation between control over the disease and control over the daily symptoms. It appears that individuals who accept a certain lack of control over the disease but who exert and perceive control over their daily symptoms may demonstrate greater psychosocial adaptation to the illness. This suggests that strategies that promote participatory control are beneficial to the client with a chronic illness or disability. The rise in cognitive-behavioral approaches to disease management reflects the interest in returning control to people coping with disease and illness.

Miller (2000) suggests that maximizing individual and family power resources facilitates coping with illness. Power resources, as defined by Miller, include physical strength, psychological stamina (emotional outlook), support network, positive self-concept, energy, knowledge, motivation, and hope rooted in a belief system. The overlap of power resources is evident in this model. For example, it is difficult for a client to feel in control when he or she lacks the physical reserve or energy necessary to feel motivated. Nursing strategies that assist the client to maintain optimal wellness and to balance rest and activity facilitate physical strength and energy. Strategies that support the grieving process, provide access to and care for the client's social support system, stimulate hope, eliminate as many unpredictable events as possible, and develop mastery in knowledge and skills all facilitate power resources in the psychological and sociocultural domains.

In responding to powerlessness or helplessness, the nurse should determine the contextual events that led to this emotional response. Examples may include a downward course of the disease despite compliance with treatment regimens; lack of opportunity to engage in previous, reinforcing activities; being assigned a label that connotes inferiority to other persons; being uncertain about what energy resources will be available from day to day; and being uncertain about what the progression of the disease might be.

Strategies to overcome powerlessness target maximizing power resources. Clients and families should be provided with the information and resources they need to feel in control of symptoms and to make decisions about their care. Efforts should be made to avoid common stressors of hospitalization. The client and family should be included as active partners on the health care team. Teaching how to negotiate the health care system and how to be self advocates can enhance the sense of competence and power.

Situational Low Self-esteem

Self-concept is the individual's total thoughts and feelings about himself or herself. It is sometimes described as the cognitive gestalt of what people think about themselves. Self-concept may be further divided into distinct but interrelated subcomponents. Although different authors use various classifications, the commonly accepted subcomponents include body image or physical self (appearance, health), role performance or functioning—achieving self (cognitive ability, creativity, mastery, role function), personal self or moral self (values, ethics, conscience, spirituality), interpersonal self (relations with others in society), and self-esteem or self-worth (feelings about self). People place a value on each part of their self-concept based on how close it comes to an ideal. The composite of these values then determines how satisfied or unsatisfied they are with what they perceive they have.

The presence of illness or disability may promote a sense of being different, which can affect a client's sense of self-worth or self-esteem. Self-esteem is the affective component of how a person feels valued by family, friends, and eventually by himself or herself. Perhaps more than any other factor, self-esteem is fundamental to a person's perception of well-being and thus to a person's mental health. It represents the extent to which the individual believes himself or herself capable, significant, and worthy. Roy (1986) defines self-esteem as the extent to which a person feels he or she lives up to personal expectations and to the expectations of people whose opinion he or she values.

Self-esteem develops through a series of reflected appraisals from self and valued others. Reflected appraisals from others can be understood through the idea of the looking-glass self, in which perceptions of others are like mirrors that reflect images of the person back to himself or herself. Reflected appraisals from self are related to how effective a person is within society (accomplishments, relationships) or by a self-measure of how much control or power that person possesses. The presence of illness or disability affects the reflected appraisals from self and from others.

For children and adolescents, self-esteem is influenced by feelings of security, positive identification, belonging, and sense of purpose. During adolescence, self-esteem depends on how the individual believes that he or she is seen by others. Adolescents who have a chronic illness or disability, depending on its severity, may remain more dependent on their families than do their healthy peers. For young and middle-aged adults,

the perceived level of success in their jobs, interpersonal relations with others, and parenting roles serve as key standards against which self-esteem may be measured.

For many persons with a chronic illness, one of the biggest threats to self-esteem is the ongoing challenge of accomplishing what were once considered the simple activities of daily living. Preparing meals, getting to work, doing the grocery shopping, or completing yard work may all become a struggle. Lack of strength in a person's hands may cause him or her to drop cans in the grocery store or be unable to hold a rake. Fatigue and pain may interfere with a person's ability to complete his or her work, especially if strenuous activity is required. Inability to maintain independence and his or her role in work and family threatens a client's self-esteem.

Learning to do tasks differently to conserve energy and minimize pain is a crucial strategy for maintaining self-esteem as a person copes with the challenges of chronic illness and disability. Changing the concept of what is normal is one of the keystones to making the most of life with illness and disability. If the person can make peace with more conservative, more realistic new norms, there is a greater chance of maintaining self-esteem and positive self-concept.

Self-esteem alteration is also associated with role alteration and the need to depend on public assistance. Often, people with disabilities are more than capable of doing a job but are perceived by others to be incapable. This devaluing of the person with a disability can have a devastating effect on self-esteem.

Positive self-esteem is important because it helps clients feel worthy, effective, and productive. They respond to others and themselves in healthful, positive, growing ways. Chronic pain has been identified as a factor that lowers self-esteem. Helping individuals to master pain through cognitive-behavioral processes is critical to maintaining self-esteem.

The nursing diagnosis of self-esteem disturbance is characterized by negative feelings or a negative evaluation about self or self-capabilities that may be directly or indirectly expressed. Causes for this deficit include loss of significant roles, unrealistic self-expectations, learned helplessness, stress, loss of loved ones or objects, inconsistent behaviors, and loss of function. Assessment should include listening for self-negating verbalization ("I'm no good," "I'll never make it," "I'm ugly," or "I'm useless"), probing for behaviors that may signal self-esteem disturbances (fear of new experiences, exaggerated reactions to failure, social isolation, inability to take pride in accomplishing goals), observing for an unusual sensitivity to criticism or the presence of a strong need for positive reinforcement, and watching for a tendency to feel guilty about how the client thinks he or she "should" behave.

Strategies to enhance self-esteem require a valuing of the continued abilities of the client, with an emphasis on self-knowledge and self-understanding. This can be accomplished by recognizing function and ability along with any dysfunction or disability. Persons can be helped to develop an awareness that their feelings of self are composed of more than just one frame of reference. In this regard, they can be helped to acknowledge both strengths and weaknesses and can also be aided in guiding their thinking and feeling from the past or future into the present. This redirection helps the person to see the self more completely and recognize that one failure, one deficiency, or one alteration does not make the person "all bad." Emphasis is placed on strengths and a nurturing environment. To this end, the nurse provides a supportive environment in which the person can discuss feelings without fear of degradation. The nurse also offers praise in the form of positive reflected appraisal and assists the person to identify strengths and positive attributes.

Disturbed Body Image

Clients coping with chronic illness or disability are often confronted with disturbances in their body image. In American society, individuals who deviate from normal feel stigmatized. American culture values physically attractive, intact, healthy, and fully functional individuals. An individual with a chronic illness or disability may fail to live up to these socially accepted standards and may experience both a body image disturbance and social stigma. The extent of body image disturbance depends not only on the meaning of the alteration to the person but also on the visibility of the change to others and by the reaction of others to the change. People experiencing outwardly visible body image disturbances often comment that they "want people to look at them and see past their looks and see who they really are." This type of comment exemplifies the reality that disturbances in body image interfere with interpersonal relations and societal relations, with a potential for diminishing self-esteem.

Body image is the mental picture people use to distinguish themselves from others. It is both a conscious and an unconscious process, is both reality bound and fantasy directed, and is dependent on external and internal promptings. It is a dynamic state that changes and fluctuates. Variables contributing to body image include culture, physiologic disturbances, energy levels, internal drives, dependency needs, motivational states, and objects attached to the body. A person's body image includes not only the physical, living body but also inanimate objects, such as eyeglasses, cane, crutches, makeup, jewelry, and other things that are part of the person's daily concept of who he or she is. Body image, which develops from early childhood, is associated with freedom of movement and autonomy.

Body image disturbances are negative feelings or perceptions about the body or body parts and can be associated with loss of body integrity and control, altered body function, and physical alterations. Psychological changes, such as dealing with the illness itself, the hospital experience, and the reactions of others, can also alter a client's body image.

Integral to being human is the ability to be mobile. Mobility enables people to exert control over their environment. In children (especially toddlers and preschool children), mobility is integral to the learning experience of exploring and reaching out. The limitations imposed by immobilization influence the efficacy with which a client is able to interact with the environment. Part of what society requires of the fully functioning, healthy person is mobility. Therefore, immobility is likely to affect a person's body image. The nurse's goals in working with a person who is experiencing body image alterations because of immobility include helping the person obtain and learn how to use the necessary adaptive aids, working with the person until he or she has a sense of balance with body movement, reducing or eliminating phantom sensation, and encouraging the person to participate in normal interests and resume normal pleasurable sexual relations.

Mobilization aids can be incorporated into the person's body image. Referring to these devices and ascribing human qualities to them (as in giving a name to an artificial leg) often occur. Attending to the person's verbal messages and tone of voice can alert the nurse when negative alterations are present.

Severe pain in any body part can create body image distortions. The painful part receives an inordinate degree of attention and, consequently, is often perceived to increase in size so that it occupies the most prominent position in the body image. Although the hands are only a small portion of the total body, the person with RA may see his or her hands as the center of the body image. Such persons often take active measures to hide their hands from others.

The nurse should assess the value the person places on the altered or missing part; the meaning of the altered body to both the person and significant others; the person's current physical status, support system strength, and reaction to the alteration; and the person's current activities and plans for the future that may be affected by the body image alteration. In addition, the nurse should assess for a negative self-concept, as manifested by a refusal to participate in care, refusal to discuss the care, withdrawal from social contacts, and avoidance of intimate relationships.

Failure to integrate a changed body image is associated with long-term depression, difficulty with interpersonal interactions, social isolation, and a generally lower quality of life. A well-developed body image permits a person to enter into social interactions with confidence. The nurse can assist the person in the integration process by helping him or her think through the meaning of the change, proposing alternative meanings not previously considered, providing positive feedback, helping friends and family members examine the meaning of the changes, and communicating acceptance of the changes to the person (Burns & Holmes, 1991).

The nurse can become an integral part of the support system by demonstrating both positive regard and acceptance of the changed physical structure and function. Because persons often do not confront body image disturbance until some time after the acute crisis, the nurse can also provide anticipatory counseling to help prepare for a possible emotional reaction as well as provide guidance on how to deal with the reactions of others.

Stigma. Lack of understanding on the part of the community often leads to fear, avoidance, revulsion, and belittlement when dealing with the disabled or chronically ill. Visibility of symptoms and degree of role dysfunction correlate with the degree of stigma.

The disabled, chronically ill, and aged are often the victims of stereotyping and discrimination. A person with a physical disability is often assumed to be mentally handicapped as well. The aged individual is assumed by some to have a hearing deficit. Such people react not only with unnecessary shouting but also with demeaning, childish conversation.

It is hard for the able-bodied to imagine that there is similar joy or meaning in the lives of the disabled. Disabled individuals identify pity and unwanted attempts to help as major stressors. Persons with disabilities experience frustrations, society-imposed limitations, and feelings of self-devaluation and insecurity (Fraley, 1992). *Stigma* is the term given to social intolerance of differences in behavior or physical appearance.

Many persons experiencing musculoskeletal disorders face stigmatizing reactions by others. The child with cerebral palsy or muscular dystrophy is visibly different in both appearance and such observable behavior as walking. Individuals with RA or ankylosing spondylitis have body image alterations that set them apart from others. Persons requiring mobility devices, such as crutches, braces, or wheelchairs, are instantly set apart from others. Immobilization devices, such as halo vests and external fixators, with their unusual appearance set up immediate social barriers and accompanying stigma.

A hallmark of stigmatization is strained social interactions. Typically, the person is avoided, or when unavoidable, distinct social discomfort or strain is present. The stigma extends from the "impaired" individual to the family—a phenomenon known as *courtesy stigma*. Some of this social awkwardness occurs because friends and family do not know what to say, and social withdrawal seems safer. Avoidance tactics include minimal eye contact or refusal to address the person directly in conversation. One adult client diagnosed with SLE described how friends would telephone and limit conversation with her but would ask for her husband and begin asking questions about "how she really is." She described her reaction to this as feeling as if she did not exist and commented on how it seemed so condescending. These types of attitudes may erode self-worth and inhibit social development. Nurses can assist clients and their families in coping with stigmatization by giving them strategies to reduce the social awkwardness. Once individuals can comfortably say, "I know it's hard to talk about, but let me tell you what is happening," barriers often break down, minimizing the intensity of the stigmatization reaction.

Ineffective Sexuality Patterns

All people are sexual beings and have sexual desires. Sexuality is as much a part of the lives of children, adolescents, and adults with chronic conditions as it is in the "normal" population. Unfortunately, many persons with chronic medical conditions are assumed to be asexual, and little effort is directed toward helping individuals with disability and chronic illness reestablish positive sexual identities.

Sexuality may refer to sexual role, sexual identity or image, or sexual function. The term *sexual role* refers to a person's ability to perform in typical gender roles, such as husband and father or wife and mother. *Sexual identity* refers to a person's perception and comfort with herself or himself as feminine or masculine. Characteristics that constitute sexual identity may include expressiveness, intimacy, caring, independence, self-confidence, and assertiveness or aggressiveness. What constitutes sexual identity is strongly influenced by culture.

The development of a comfortable sexual identity may be a particularly difficult task for disabled and chronically ill adolescents for a number of reasons. For the adolescent with a physical disability, the opportunities to interact with peers in social relationships in which they can learn, practice, and perfect the social skills and roles necessary to form a sexual identity may be lessened. Furthermore, chronically ill adolescents may have limited opportunities for normal sexual experimentation because of their social isolation and because of possible parental overprotectiveness and ongoing parental monitoring. Sexuality is rarely discussed with chronically ill adolescents as compared with their healthy peers.

Problems in sexual identity and functioning can arise from many different sources. Therapeutic modalities, including hospitalization, may affect the sexuality of the client. Pharmacologic agents (e.g., long-term use of steroids) and physiologic alterations (e.g., fatigue, pain, limited range of motion) may decrease the client's libido and interfere with the ability to engage in sexual intercourse. The anxiety associated with fear of failure and the fear of pain may also interfere with a client's sexual desire, as can problems in interpersonal relationships. Alterations in body image, diminished self-esteem, role changes, and depression may all affect sexuality.

Lamb (1991) suggests the following three open-ended questions for gathering information for a brief assessment addressing sexual role, identity, and functioning: Has being ill interfered with your being a (husband, lover, mother, wife)? Has your illness changed the way you see yourself as a man (woman)? Has your illness affected your sexual functioning?

The nurse's awareness of common illness-related factors that interfere with sexual health can serve as the framework for assessment. For the orthopaedic client, pain, stiffness of joints or muscles, tremors, spasms, fatigue, and depression may all affect sexuality. The nurse in caring for the orthopaedic client can ask, "Have limitations in range of motion or pain interfered with your sexual relations with your partner?" Framed in terms of the presenting symptom, the question is easily pursued or disregarded by the client.

Communication about sexual history can be enhanced if the nurse ensures the individual's privacy and confidentiality and provides an uninterrupted period of discussion. A nonjudgmental attitude is essential for a successful discussion. The discussion can be initiated by introducing less sensitive topics ("Sometimes with a lack of energy, clients experience diminished sexual desire. Has this been a concern for you?") before moving into more sensitive ones.

Although many nurses are comfortable dealing with physiologic issues and their effect on sexuality, few nurses are comfortable discussing such practical issues as coital alternatives or the effect of decreased libido and impotency on the sexual relationship. This does not diminish the fact that, for many persons affected with musculoskeletal disorders, the inability to have sexual intercourse combined with the inability to establish satisfying alternatives for maintaining a sexual relationship is a problem.

Openness and willingness to talk honestly with the partner is critical to dealing with sexual difficulties. The existence of pain, fatigue, and limited mobility make it necessary to discuss and plan for sex ahead of time. Guidance and counseling about planning for and the timing of sexual intercourse to maximize comfort and enjoyment should be given. This need to plan upsets many persons because of the lack of spontaneity. However, planning does not mean that their enjoyment will be reduced.

Persons experiencing pain and discomfort may benefit from relaxation techniques, biofeedback, self-hypnosis, or the application of hot and cold to the affected areas to alleviate discomfort. Taking medications before an intimate dinner can alleviate some concerns related to the possible experience of pain. Couples should be encouraged to experiment to discover comfortable sexual positions. Pillows can be used to support the joints and assist in positioning for minimal exertion. Massage can be used not only to reduce pain but also as an arousal technique.

For some persons, despite sexual dysfunction, sexual desires are still present. These clients and their partners need to be provided with the information, insight, security, and support needed to explore alternatives. Alternative ways of expressing physical love should be explored if the couple's usual methods of sexual gratification are no longer feasible because of discomfort. Literature regarding sexual alternatives is available through the Arthritis Foundation and in most bookstores. The literature addresses not only different coital positions but also alternative forms of intimacy, such as autoerotic activities, mutual arousal techniques, and coital alternatives.

Although illness may compromise the client's ability to have intercourse, it generally does not diminish any previous desire to be held and touched. Sensuality and sexuality serve to corroborate the specialness of a person and often become more important when illness creates challenges to normal functioning. Most individuals desire to be touched to feel that they are loved and wanted.

For many persons, alterations in their sexuality with the loss of intimacy and touch are accompanied by an unverbalized fear of possible abandonment. Illness creates an internal desire for affection and physical closeness that is often countered by fear, depression, and miscommunication. Unmet needs and driving fears increase the anxiety about possible abandonment. Encouraging open communication about these fears between the client and partner can provide an avenue for clarification of misperceptions or for problem solving when problems do exist.

Many partners and loving friends and family ask the nurse while the client is in the hospital, "What can I do to help?" The nurse can seize this opportunity to suggest that touch can be a potent medicine and that the presence of a caressing hand or a loving kiss can promote healing. Physical contact reinforces a client's sexual identity and provides hope that the sexual role will not be disrupted.

The nurse can enhance body image and sexual identity by attending to personal appearance needs. Even though a client is sick, appearance continues to influence how he or she feels about self. Recognizing the effect of an altered physical appearance on self-esteem, interpersonal relationships, and general satisfaction with life, some health care institutions are providing innovative services to assist clients, in which personalized advice and instruction on the use of makeup by a licensed cosmetologist, specially designed turbans for clients with alopecia, and information describing community resources are provided. Attention to these needs is likely to benefit many clients who are experiencing body image changes and threats to their sexual identity.

Ineffective Role Performance

Role performance is the ability to carry out those behaviors appropriate to particular roles in life. Role performance requires that a person know what the appropriate behaviors are and has the psychomotor and emotional capacity to carry them out. Illness and disability often alter how a person approaches and contributes to different roles. This alteration and redefinition may be accompanied by anxiety, anger, guilt, powerlessness, and decreased self-esteem.

Role transition is a period in which the person experiences a change in role relationships, expectations, or abilities. To make this change, the person must assimilate new knowledge, change behaviors, and redefine self-concept. Role enhancement interventions are designed to assist clients, significant others, and family members to improve relationships by clarifying and supplementing specific role behaviors. It is a deliberate process in which actual or potential role insufficiency is identified. This is followed by role clarification, in which the specific information and cues required to enact a role are discussed by the client and a significant other (Bulechek & McCloskey, 1996).

Role taking is the next component of role supplementation. In role taking, the client imaginatively assumes the positions or points of view of another person through role modeling, role rehearsal, and reference group interactions. The outcome of these efforts is not only greater understanding and skills but also general flexibility about what can realistically be expected from different people. This flexibility is integral to role negotiation strategies and task division within the family system.

Sick Role. A role is associated with a set of expected behaviors. The client role is closely related to the sick role as defined by Parsons (1951). The sick role is assumed to be a set of adaptive behaviors in the person's relationship with a physician during illness. The role behaviors associated with the sick role and the client role include dependency, cooperation in the process, motivation to get well, conformity, and receptivity to care. Although these roles may be adaptive during acute illness, they are not adaptive with chronic illness and disability. Assertiveness, aggressiveness, attempts at self-reliance, and active participation are crucial to coping with long-term illness and disability and to preventing the sense of powerlessness and helplessness that can accompany illness. However, the sick role must be assessed in light of cultural expectations. Many cultures view dependency as an accepted and valued way of being. Caring for the person who is ill and allowing dependency may represent love and respect.

Personal and Role Dependency. Sally Tisdale (1987), nurse author of the book *Harvest Moon,* addressed the fears of older adults in saying, "We all die, and most of us grow old, and for a certain inevitable number of us, age brings its sisters: dependence, frailty and a gut wrenching perishability."

Trauma and other chronic and disabling orthopaedic conditions often incapacitate a person, necessitating that the client alter his or her typical roles and be dependent on others for basic self-care needs. This can create a sense of shame or humiliation because independence and self-reliance are key values of American society. Autonomy and respect for human dignity and an active approach to discuss and strengthen role contributions are important interventions.

Ineffective Family Coping. In addition to being aware of the typical stressors and coping patterns facilitative of effective family functioning, the nurse should be aware of common dysfunctional role patterns that may emerge.

Family responses may include overprotectiveness and overcompensation; strained parental relations; uncertainty; state of crisis for a family; and feelings of frustration, fear, isolation, and insecurity. As the family comes to grips with the reality of the illness or the disability, they must deal with their grief. Feelings of anger, inadequacy, guilt, and helplessness may lead the family into a pattern of helping the client avoid pain through their overprotectiveness and overindulgence. This is especially true of parents responding to children with a chronic illness. A pattern may become established in which more attention is focused on the disability than is warranted, and the needs of other children or family members are minimized or unrecognized. The person with the illness may become the center of attention in the family, demanding attention and help without trying to delay gratification or acknowledge the needs of others. This focus limits opportunities for successful interpersonal experiences outside the overindulgent family unit, ultimately robbing the child of the potential for growth and learning.

Opposite to the phenomenon of overprotectiveness is that of rejection. Rejection is usually not expressed overtly but in rather subtle behavioral patterns. Unreasonable demands are made of the client, or promises are extracted that cannot be kept. Small accomplishments are minimized while waiting for the "promised goal," leaving the client feeling useless, worthless, and unworthy of efforts or attention. Research suggests that mothers of congenitally disabled children tend to be afraid of getting close to their children because they are afraid the children will die. This rejection contributes to the child's sense of uselessness and unworthiness.

Studies examining factors contributing to adaptation in pediatric chronic illness have noted that although children themselves bear the major psychosocial burden of their chronic health condition, there is documented increased psychological risk among their parents. The psychological and social needs of children and families must be identified in cognitive-behavioral interventions to prevent family dysfunction and maladaptive coping.

Social Isolation. The social networks that provide support and the quality of the support that they provide may be affected by long-term illness and disability. Social isolation is a common phenomenon found with chronic illness and disability. It is characterized by a deficit in the social network or withdrawal from social relationships, inappropriate and extreme loneliness, expressions of loneliness or rejection, sadness or withdrawn feelings, and statements of dissatisfaction with the amount of interaction with others.

Social isolation may be precipitated by biophysical discomfort, social discomfort of others about the disease or illness, inability to function in previous roles, altered body image, emotional lability, or depression. There is usually more than one factor and more than one person contributing to the social isolation. For example, discomfort on the part of others about what to say and how to act toward the client may keep supportive persons away. This is interpreted by the client to mean lack of caring or lack of interest, and the client feels abandoned and alone. To defend against these uncomfortable emotions, the client may respond with a disinterested stance or may even minimize others' attempts to interact by defining actions as merely obligatory responses rather than true caring. This becomes a vicious cycle by further pushing away needed support network members.

Often, the individual with a chronic illness or disability does not feel he or she fits into relationships any longer. A friendship that was based on playing tennis may be disrupted because of osteoarthritis of the knee. The person may interpret the situation to mean that the friendship no longer continues. In these cases, it is important to reinforce that although the person's body and physical abilities have changed, the shared thoughts, feelings, and interests that created the friendship still remain. Proactive responses on the part of the person can be the impetus needed to maintain social contacts.

The individual with a chronic illness or disability may become very egocentric, or limitations in role function may necessitate that social activity be designed around the chronically ill person's schedule or desires. These demands can strain social relationships, and it is not uncommon to find that the social network becomes smaller. In addition, the individual with a chronic illness may be unable to reciprocate the support received, placing further strain on relationships. Clients should be assisted to redefine the ways in which they can reciprocate the support they receive rather than relying on methods used when function was not impaired. Again, this proactive approach minimizes the social isolation that may ultimately cause increased stress and decreased quality of life.

Assessment of social isolation can include such questions as the following: "Do you participate in activities with family or friends?" "Have these activities changed since your condition was diagnosed?" "How satisfied are you with the amount of contact you have with other people?" "How often do you feel lonely?" The client can be observed for the ability to initiate social activity as well as the response when engaged in activities with others.

To promote and maintain social interactions, clients should be encouraged to provide information to their family and friends about the disease and what they can and cannot do. The emphasis should be on what still can be done. Individuals with disabilities or chronic illnesses must be encouraged to be tolerant of behavior that may appear condescending or overbearing and must be urged to assert themselves in letting others know what they can do for themselves. An open discussion of the effect of the disease on a friendship helps to clarify issues.

The individual experiencing social isolation should reflect on his or her own behavior and how it may influence the situation. Does the person dominate conversation by discussing only his or her illness? Does the person take time to reflect on how someone else is doing, or is he or she completely absorbed by his or her own problem? Does the person make active efforts to participate and to be flexible in social activities? Does the person need to make sure that everyone is aware of problems? The first step toward altering behavior patterns is when the client becomes aware of his or her own contribution to social strain and social isolation.

Active involvement and denial of symptoms in favor of social interaction can facilitate more effective social interactions. However, this can be taken too far. A person must stay attuned to the signals or body cues that he or she is receiving and be comfortable with the need to occasionally decline activities to promote comfort or rest. This is especially difficult when the illness or disability is not visible to others (chronic low-back pain, some joint pain). A person's attempts at normalizing in order to maintain social interactions may cause others to forget about the realities of the illness.

Planning to balance rest and activity and to manage symptoms before a social activity can make things easier. For people with severe joint disease, days of rest before and after a planned social event may be necessary to maintain comfort.

PSYCHOLOGICAL AND BEHAVIORAL INTERVENTIONS FOR SYMPTOM MANAGEMENT AND ADAPTATION

The multifactor nature of biopsychosocial needs of clients and families coping with illness and disability have necessitated multifocal intervention strategies designed to alter perceptions of helplessness, SE beliefs, and coping strategies to improve pain and other health status factors. In the research examining disease activity and disability outcomes, cognitive factors have been found to be stronger predictors of pain and disability than disease activity (Broderick, 2000). Strategies aimed at maximizing cognitive control through education and other cognitive modalities are critical components of chronic illness therapy.

Cognitive-behavioral therapies directly focus on altering cognitive, behavioral, and emotional patterns. They teach persons to reappraise their thoughts and the events in their environment in more realistic and less irrational ways to reduce the experience of threat and subsequent physiologic arousal (Broderick, 2000). These interventions generally encompass education, training in relaxation and other coping skills, rehearsal of these newly learned skills in the home and work environment, and relapse prevention (Bradley & Alberts, 1999). These programs have been evaluated for efficacy and have been found to enhance perceptions of control or SE, improve pain ratings or displays of pain behavior, and improve perceptions of functional ability. Active spouse participation in programs produces the greatest improvements in pain, pain behavior, marital adjustment measures, psychological disability, and SE ratings.

Coping Strategies

Programs to facilitate adaptation and coping should determine in advance the direct action or palliative strategies that may be used to successfully manage symptoms. Direct action strategies are behaviors that contribute to the removal of the stressor and palliative strategies are responses that diminish the negative impact of the stressor. The person with carpal tunnel syndrome may seek treatment from the physician and/or wear a brace (direct action) and use relaxation or other cognitive distracters (palliative) to better control the effect of the pain.

Positive coping skills that may be incorporated into these intervention approaches include assisting the person to find meaning from the illness experience; to seek information about the disease; to learn to use distracting maneuvers (relaxation and stress management); to set behavioral goals; to desensitize to painful stimuli; and to use relaxation, positive reinforcement, and focusing on positive thoughts. In addition, programs should discuss coping strategies that have been found to be ineffective. For example, passive coping strategies, such as catastrophizing (e.g., believing that if medication is not effective, no other coping strategy will effectively control pain and other symptoms) and escapist fantasies (e.g., hoping that pain will get better someday) have been found to correlate with high levels of pain and psychological distress in clients with RA, osteoarthritis, and FS (Keefe, Brown, Wallston, & Caldwell, 1989; Keefe, Caldwell, Baucom, Salley, Robinson, Timmons, Beaupre, Weisberg, & Helms, 1996; Martin, Bradley, Alexander, Alarcon, Triana-Alexander, Aaron, & Alberts, 1996).

Stress management includes a number of therapeutic techniques to improve clients' behavioral coping strategies when faced with a stress or challenge. Problem solving in stressful situations to gain greater mastery over the environment is the cornerstone of this approach. Homework assignments that include increased assertiveness, exercises, and social contacts are often used.

Education

The educational component presents a credible rationale for the treatment intervention and elicits active collabo-ration of caregivers, clients, and families. Arthritis self-management programs and other similar cognitive-behavioral therapies are designed to increase the belief that the individual can learn the skills needed to cope better with pain and other illness-related problems. Informational areas covered commonly include the nature of the disease, use of medications, mobilization and exercise, relaxation techniques, joint protection, nutrition, interaction of clients with physicians and other providers, and evaluation of nontraditional treatments. It is important to note that information alone, the long-standing approach to care, has little effect on pain and other symptoms.

Cognitive and Behavioral Rehearsal

Coping skills training is aimed at helping clients and families engage actively in the process of learning new behaviors taught in informational sessions, which will help them better manage their symptoms. Giving time to rehearse and reflect on these new behaviors in the home and work environments and returning to the cognitive-behavioral therapy sessions to discuss their efficacy as well as the ease or difficulties in use are important components of long-term success. Rehearsal leads to mastery and mastery is associated with higher SE and self-esteem and fewer depressive symptoms. Rehearsal assignments are often supplemented by self-reflection using symptom diaries.

Relapse Prevention

The goal of relapse prevention is to help people retain their newly learned coping skills and to avoid increases in pain or other unpleasant symptoms following treatment, thereby diminishing the personal sense of control. Keefe and Van Horn (1993) found that relapse occurs most when perception of helplessness increases and the person begins to experience psychological distress. By identifying high-risk situations that are likely to tax coping resources as well as early signs of relapse, programs can target early recognition and intervention. Interventions to minimize relapse include rehearsal of cognitive and behavioral skills for coping with early relapse signs and provision of self-rewards for effective performance of coping responses to potential relapse (Bradley & Alberts, 1999). Evaluation studies of cognitive-behavioral programs have shown that relapse prevention training should occur at multiple points in the protocol rather than simply at the end.

COMPLEMENTARY AND ALTERNATIVE MEDICINE IN SYMPTOM MANAGEMENT

The inability of traditional Western medicine to effectively control symptoms and promote adaptation has led to a widespread interest in complementary and alternative medicine approaches. Interventions such as aromatherapy, hypnosis, meditation, guided imagery, stress management, and biofeedback are examples of these strategies. Yocum (2000) found that programs using alternative therapies, such as tai chi and meditation, in combination with prescribed medications appear to be more beneficial for clients with arthritis.

Distraction

For short-term painful procedures, simple distraction techniques, including using a party blower, blowing bubbles, or counting, have been used with children. For older children or adults, distraction can be achieved by discussing non–procedure-related topics such as movies, work, or school. Other distraction techniques include the use of music, artwork, or other engaging activities likely to shift attention away from the uncomfortable symptom.

Imagery is another distraction technique. Imagery teaches the individual to shift attention from the pain or other uncomfortable symptom by focusing on a self-determined pleasant scene such as being in the mountains, playing in a park, or being at the ocean. While focusing on the favorite place, the individual is encouraged to involve all of the senses in the imagery (e.g., the sounds of the waves lapping or crashing against the shore, seagulls flying above, the smell of salt air, the feel of the wind against the skin). Another variant of imagery encourages children to imagine themselves as their favorite superhero and then incorporate pain sensations into a self-designed "challenge episode" in which they are battling for a worthy cause (Schanberg & Sandstrom, 1999).

Relaxation Techniques

Relaxation exercises, meditation, and imagery all have the practice of inducing a more relaxed physiologic state by systematically redirecting the focus on a person's mind, thereby reducing physiologic arousal. Relaxation can be taught fairly easily. Two common features of the approach include (1) the repetition of a word, sound, prayer, thought, phrase, or muscular activity, and (2) the passive return to the repetition when other thoughts intrude. Providing preprinted copies of relaxation scripts or a tape recording of the exercise allows for practice of the technique at home once or twice per day.

Progressive relaxation training (PRT) is designed to teach persons how to reduce tonic levels of muscle activity. A series of exercises in which a person first tenses and then relaxes several major groups of muscles in the body is taught. Through practice, the individual gradually learns to focus on the difference between tense and relaxed sensations and to cue themselves to relax upon early warning signs of increased tension. In addition to PRT, diaphragmatic breathing exercises stressing slow, regular, deep breaths are taught. Persons are taught to exhale as if they were a leaky bike tire that is slowly losing air. This helps them break out of more shallow, rapid, and thoracic breathing styles as well as reduce other symptoms of heightened autonomic arousal such as rapid

heart rate, excessive perspiration, and anxious sensations (Schanberg & Sandstrom, 1999).

Hypnosis has been used successfully to minimize the pain and anxiety associated with uncomfortable procedures. It involves helping the individual focus attention away from the feared components of a procedure by instead focusing attention on an imaginative experience that is viewed as comforting, safe, fun, or intriguing. This helps take the focus off of the procedure and can be used to enhance sense of mastery through imaginative experience (Chen, Joseph, & Zeltzer, 2000). The primary goals of hypnotherapy are to capture attention, reduce distress, reframe pain experiences, and help dissociate from pain.

Spiritual Interventions

There is mounting evidence that spiritual practices are an important therapeutic process in adaptation and healing. Healing prayer seeks to direct an unseen power toward healing the visible condition of the client. Ritual aims to restore balance between the client, the community, and the larger universe.

Prayer has been found to be one of the most commonly used strategies in coping with chronic illness. Matthews, Marlowe, and MacNutt (1998) assessed the effects, in conjunction with standard medical treatment, of experimental intercessory prayer for healing on the clinical course of clients with RA. Particular attention was paid to the effect of prayer on symptoms (pain and functional impairment), physical signs (tender and swollen joints), and laboratory findings (acute-phase reactants). Clients with long-standing moderately severe RA were shown to derive significant short- and long-term physical benefits from in-person intercessory prayer ministry. Because of the multimodal nature of the intervention (prayer, education, support), the specific therapeutic agent of healing could not be proved definitively.

Spiritual and religious beliefs and actions have been shown to have a wide variety of effect on illnesses and stressors. These mechanisms include eliciting the relaxation response; enhancing immune functioning; providing hope and transcendence; overcoming depression and anxiety; providing meaning, purpose, and connection; augmenting instrumental social networks; and reducing unhealthful behaviors such as excessive use of alcohol, nicotine, and drugs (Matthews, 2000). Koenig (2001) reported on a review of more than 1200 studies of religion and health. At least two thirds of the studies evaluated showed significant associations between religious or spiritual activities and better mental health, better physical health, or lower use of health services.

Anandarajah and Hight (2001) emphasize that a spiritual assessment is the first step in facilitating spirituality as a coping mechanism. A spiritual assessment should include determination of spiritual needs and resources, evaluation of the impact of beliefs on medical outcomes and decisions, discovery of barriers to using spiritual resources, and encouragement of healthful spiritual practices. They present the acronym *HOPE* as a guide. *H* stands for sources of hope, strength, comfort, meaning, peace, love, and connection. *O* represents the role of organized religion for the person. *P* is the personal spirituality practices, and *E* is the effects on medical care and end-of-life decisions.

Based on the assessment, different strategies for intervention can be taken. Underlying all interactions should be to offer one's presence, understanding, acceptance, and compassion. These psychospiritual interventions enhance the connection between client and provider and maximize self-esteem and comfort. Spirituality can also be incorporated into the client's preventive health care or personal resources. This may include prayer, meditation, yoga, tai chi, walks in the country, or listening to soothing music. Spirituality may also be included in adjuvant care. A person may say the rosary while taking medication or may listen to music or read Scripture before surgery.

Herbal Remedies

Ancient Egyptians used herbs for the treatment of disease as early as 3000 BC The ancient Greeks also used herbal remedies, but it was the Romans who brought herbal medicine to Northern Europe. Herbs were also commonly used to treat disease in colonial America. However, as science became more established, people came to believe that synthetic ingredients were more effective than those found in nature and the use of herbal remedies quickly diminished, especially in the United States. Today, herbs are widely used in Europe and are again gaining popularity in the United States (Steyer, 2001). It is estimated that 1 in 3 Americans have used an herbal medication in the past year. Canedy (1998) estimates annual herbal regimen sales of $4 billion a year, with an annual increase of 20% per year.

About 25% of modern pharmaceuticals are derived from plants. Clients are often unaware of the similarities between medicinal herbs and prescription drugs, and they may mistakenly believe that these "natural" substances do not contain powerful bioactive ingredients. Because herbs may be sold and marketed without U.S. Food and Drug Administration (FDA) approval, there are concerns about the limited evidence on herbal side effects, drug interactions, and product consistency (Mar & Bent, 1999). The nurse or other health care provider who talks with the client about possible treatments should stress the importance of reading product labels.

The Dietary Supplement Act of 1994 determined that herbal products were not drugs but would be more loosely regulated as supplements. According to the act, an herbal product can carry no specific claims on its label but only a statement of structure and function in the body. A supplement cannot make a statement that it "reduces the pain and stiffness associated with arthritis" or "reduces joint pain." It can claim only that it "supports healthy joints." The FDA also requires manufacturers to provide a "Supplement Facts" panel similar to the information offered on food labels. Very little is otherwise prohibited or required on supplement labels, leaving the manufacturer free to choose words that suggest but do not get too specific. The client should be cautioned against believing any label or brochure that promises a "cure" for the illness.

There is also no guarantee that a herbal product is formulated to ensure that the same amount of active ingredient is present in each tablet. When using herbal therapies, finding a reputable manufacturer is essential to help ensure safety, appropriate use, and response.

The top 10 most commonly used herbs reported by Mar and Bent (1999) include those for general health promotion (ginseng, Siberian ginseng), mood (St. John's wort, valerian), cognition (*Gingko biloba*), prevention of upper respiratory infections and colds (Echinacea, Goldenseal), garlic for hypertension and hypercholesterolemia, saw palmetto for benign prostatic hyperplasia, and aloe for topical application for dermatitis.

Specific to orthopaedic conditions, herbs such as devil's claw (*Harpagophytum procumbens*) and willow bark extract have been found to be effective and safe in the treatment of osteoarthritis pain and low-back pain, respectively. Receiving the most attention is the use of glucosamine (see Chapter 16). Results of studies evaluating the efficacy of glucosamine suggest that it is effective and that it is at least as good as ibuprofen for treating osteoarthritis of the knee, albeit more expensive.

INTERNET RESOURCES

Arthritis and Sexuality: http://arthritis.about.com/ health/arthritis/library/weekly/aa072299.htm

Center for Loss and Life Transition: www. centerforloss.com/

Coping with Illness and Disability: www.soon.org.uk/ problems/disability.htm

Coping with Major Illness: www.susankramer.com/ coping.html

Crisis, Grief, and Healing: www.webhealing.com/

ElderWeb: www.elderweb.com

GriefNet: www.rivendell.org/

Integrative Medicine Reference Suite: www.library.ucsf. edu/sc/altmed/

International Society for Traumatic Stress Studies: www. istss.org/

Magic Stream: Emotional Wellness Site: http://fly. hiwaay.net/~garson/

Mental-Health-Matters.com: www.mental-health-matters.com/loss.html

National Center for Complementary and Alternative Medicine: http://nccam.nih.gov/

National Center for PTSD: www.ncptsd.org/

National Mental Health Association: www.nmha.org/

Online Resources for Coping with Chronic Illness:
    http://victorian.fortunecity.com/cezanne/518/
    copinglinks.htm
Psych Web: www.psychwww.com/
PTSD Alliance: www.ptsdalliance.org/home2.html
PTSTD.com (Post traumatic stress disorder resources):
    www.ptsd.com/
Prescription for Power: Coping with Chronic Illness:
    http://members.core.com/~echoes/
Selfhelp Magazine: www.shpm.com/
Sexual Health.com: www.sexualhealth.com/
Sexuality and People with Disabilities:
    www.iidc.indiana.edu/~cedir/sexuality.html

REFERENCES

Abraido-Lanza, A. (1998). Psychological thriving among Latinas with chronic illness. *Journal of Social Issues, 54,* 405–425.

Affleck, G., Tennen, H., Pfeiffer, C., & Fifield, J. (1987). Appraisals of control and predictability in adapting to a chronic disease. *Journal of Personality and Social Psychology, 53*(2), 273–279.

Aguilera, D. (1994). *Crisis intervention: Theory and methodology.* St. Louis: Mosby.

Amerikaner, M. (1994). Family interaction and individual psychological health. *Journal of Counseling and Development, 72,* 614.

Anandarajah, G., & Hight, E. (2001). Spirituality and medical practice: Using the HOPE questions as a practical tool for spiritual assessment. *American Family Physician, 63,* 81–89.

Backer, J. H., Bakas, T., Bennett, S., & Pierce, P. K. (2000). Coping with stress: Programs of nursing research. In V. H. Rice (Ed.), *Handbook of stress, coping, and health: Implications for nursing research, theory, and practice* (pp. 223–263). Thousand Oaks, CA: Sage.

Bailey, J. M., & Nielsen, B. I. (1993). Uncertainty and appraisal of uncertainty in women with rheumatoid arthritis. *Orthopaedic Nursing, 12*(3), 63–67.

Barron, C. (2000). Stress, uncertainty, and health. In V. Rice (Ed.), *Handbook of stress, coping and health: Implications for nursing research, theory, and practice* (pp. 517–539). Thousand Oaks, CA: Sage.

Bird, G. W., & Harris, R. L. (1990). A comparison of role strain and coping strategies by gender and family structure among early adolescents. *Journal of Early Adolescence, 10,* 141–151.

Braden, C. J. (1990a). Learned self-help response to chronic illness experience: A test of three alternative learning theories. *Scholarly Inquiry for Nursing Practice, 4*(1), 23–41.

Braden, C. J. (1990b). A test of the self-help model: Learned response to chronic illness experience. *Nursing Research, 39*(1), 42–47.

Bradley, L. A. (1994). Psychological dimensions of rheumatoid arthritis. In F. Wolfe & T. Pincus (Eds.), *Rheumatoid arthritis: Pathogenesis, assessment, outcomes & treatment.* New York: Marcel Dekker.

Bradley, L. A., & Alarcon, G. S. (1997). Fibromyalgia. In W. J. Koopman (Ed.), *Arthritis and allied conditions* (13th ed.). New York: Lippincott.

Bradley, L. A., & Alberts, K. (1999). Psychological and behavioral approaches to pain management for patients with rheumatic disease. *Rheumatic Diseases Clinics of North America, 25,* 215–232.

Broderick, J. E. (2000). Mind-body medicine in rheumatologic disease. *Rheumatic Disease Clinics of North America, 26,* 161–176.

Brown, D. (2000). Time could be the active ingredient in post-trauma debriefing. *British Medical Journal, 320,* 943a–943.

Buckelew, S. P., Parker, J. C., Keefe, F. J., Deuser, W. E., Crews, T. M., Conway, R., Kay, D. R., & Hewett, J. E. (1994). Self-efficacy and pain behavior among subjects with fibromyalgia. *Pain, 59,* 377–384.

Bulechek, G., & McCloskey, J. (1996). *Nursing interventions: Treatments for nursing diagnoses* (2nd ed.). Philadelphia: WB Saunders.

Burns, N., & Holmes, B. (1991). Alterations in body image. In S. Baird,

M. G. McCorkle, & M. Grant (Eds.), *Cancer nursing: A comprehensive textbook.* Philadelphia: WB Saunders.

Butler, D. J., Moffic, H. S., & Turkal, N. W. (1999). Post-traumatic stress reactions following motor vehicle accidents. *American Family Physician, 60,* 524–531.

Candey, D. (1998, July 23). Real medicine or medicine show? Growth of herbal sales raises issues about value. *New York Times,* pp. D1–D4.

Caplan, G. (1964). *Principles of preventive psychiatry.* New York: Basic Books.

Carver, C. (1998). Resilience and thriving: Issues, models, and linkages. *Journal of Social Issues, 54,* 245–267.

Chen, E., Joseph, M. H., & Zeltzer, L. K. (2000). Acute pain in children. *Pediatric Clinics of North America, 47,* 513–525.

Cohen, F., & Lazarus, R. S. (1983). Coping and adaptation in health and illness. In D. Mechanic (Ed.), *Handbook of health, health care, and the health professions.* New York: The Free Press.

Conlon, L., Fahy, T. J., & Conroy, R. (1999). PTSD in ambulant RTA victims: A randomized controlled trial of debriefing. *Journal Psychosomatic Research, 46,* 37–44.

Copeland, R. (1995, May). Differences in young adolescents' coping strategies based on gender and ethnicity. *Journal of Early Adolescence, 15,* 203.

Dahanukar, S. A. (1996). The influence of surgical stress on the psychoneuro-endocrine-immune axis. *Journal of Postgraduate Medicine, 42,* 12–14.

DeVellis, B. M. (1993). Depression in rheumatological diseases. In S. P. Newman & M. Shipley (Eds.), *Psychological aspects of rheumatic disease. Baillieres Clinical Rheumatology, 2,* 241–257.

Fisher. K., & Hanspal, R. S. (1998). Phantom pain, anxiety, depression, and their relation in consecutive patients with amputated limbs: Case reports. *British Medical Journal, 316*(7135), 903–904.

Fraley, A. M. (1992). *Nursing and the disabled: Across the life span.* Boston: Jones and Bartlett.

Frank, R. G., Beck, N. C., Parker, J. C., Kashani, J. H., Elliott, T. R., Haut, A. E., Smith, E., Atwood, C., Brownlee-Duffeck, M., & Kay, D. R. (1998). Depression in rheumatoid arthritis. *Journal of Rheumatology, 15,* 920–925.

Fuller, S. S., Endress, M. P., & Johnson, J. E. (1978). The effects of cognitive and behavioral control on coping with an aversive health examination. *Journal of Human Stress, 4,* 18–25.

Gammon, J. (1996a). Effect of preparatory information prior to elective total hip replacement on post-operative physical coping outcomes. *International Journal of Nursing Studies, 33,* 589–604.

Gammon, J. (1996b). Effect of preparatory information prior to elective total hip replacement on psychological coping outcomes. *Journal of Advanced Nursing, 24,* 303–308.

Golden, T. (1996). *Swallowed by a snake: The masculine side of healing.* Kensington, MD: Tom Golden.

Greendale, G., Unger, J., Rowe, J., & Seeman, T. (1999). The relation between cortisol excretion and fracture in healthy older people: Results from the MacArthur studies. *Journal of the American Geriatrics Society, 47,* 799–802.

Hartfield, M. J., & Carson, C. L. (1981). Effect of information on emotional responses during barium enema. *Nursing Research, 30,* 151–155.

Hermann, M., Scholmerich, J., & Straub, R. (2000). Neuroendocrine mechanisms in rheumatic diseases. *Rheumatic Disease Clinics of North America, 26,* 737–763.

Hill, B. J. (1982). Sensory information, behavioral instructions and coping with sensory alteration in surgery. *Nursing Research, 31,* 17–21.

Hobbs, M., Mayou, R., Harrison, B., & Worlock, P. (1996). A randomized controlled trial of psychological debriefing for victims of road traffic accidents. *British Medical Journal, 313,* 143–149.

Horowitz, M. J. (2001). *Stress response syndromes* (4th ed.). Northvale, NJ: Jason Aronson.

Huddleston, P. (1996). *Prepare for surgery, heal faster: A guide of mind-body techniques.* Cambridge, MA: Angel River.

Huyser, B., & Parker, J. (1999). Negative affect and pain in arthritis. *Rheumatic Disease Clinics of North America, 25,* 105–120.

Jalowiec, A., & Dudas, S. (1991). Alterations in patient coping. In S. Baird & M. Grant (Eds.), *Cancer nursing: A comprehensive textbook* (pp. 806–820). Philadelphia: WB Saunders.

Johnson, J. E., Kirchhoff, K. T., & Endress, M. P. (1975). Altering children's distress behavior during orthopedic cast removal. *Nursing Research, 24,* 404–410.

Johnson, J. E., Morrissey, J. F., & Leventhal, H. (1973). Psychological preparation for an endoscopic examination. *Gastrointestinal Endoscopy, 19,* 180–182.

Kaplan, H. (Ed.). (1996). *Psychosocial stress: Perspectives on structure, theory, life-course, and methods.* New York: Academic.

Keefe, F. J. (1999). Psychosocial assessment of pain in patients having rheumatic diseases. *Arthritis Care Research, 12*(2), 101–111.

Keefe, F. J., & Bonks, C. (1999). Psychosocial assessment of pain in patients having rheumatic diseases. *Rheumatic Diseases Clinics of North America, 25,* 81–103.

Keefe, F. J., Brown, G. K., Wallston, K. A., & Caldwell, D. S. (1989). Coping with rheumatoid arthritis pain: Catastrophizing as a maladaptive strategy. *Pain, 37*(1), 51–56.

Keefe, F. J., Caldwell, D. S., Baucom, D., Salley, A., Robinson, E., Timmons, K., Beaupre, P., Weisberg, J., & Helms, M. (1996). Spouse-assisted coping skills training in the management of osteoarthritic knee pain. *Arthritis Care and Research, 9*(4), 279–291.

Keefe, F. J., & Van Horn, Y. (1993). Cognitive-behavioral treatment of rheumatoid arthritis pain: Maintaining treatment gains. *Arthritis Care Research, 6*(4), 213–222.

Kiecolt-Glaser, J. K. (1998). Psychological influences on surgical recovery. Perspectives from psychoneuroimmunology. *American Psychologist, 53,* 1209–1218.

Kobasa, S. C. (1979). Stressful life events, personality, and health: An inquiry into hardiness. *Journal of Personality and Social Psychology, 37,* 1–11.

Koenig, H. G. (2001). Spiritual assessment in medical practice. *American Family Physician, 63,* 30, 33.

Koren, D., Arnon, I., & Kelin, E. (1999). Acute stress response and posttraumatic stress disorder in traffic accident victims: A one-year prospective, follow-up study. *American Journal of Psychiatry, 156,* 367–373.

Kremer, M. J. (1999). Surgery, pain, and immune function. *CRNA, 10*(3), 94–100.

Kurlowicz, L. H. (1998). Perceived self-efficacy, functional ability, and depressive symptoms in older elective surgery patients. *Nursing Research, 47,* 219–226.

Laborde, J., & Powers, M. (1985). Satisfaction with life for patients undergoing hemodialysis and patients suffering from osteoarthritis. *Research in Nursing and Health, 3,* 19–24.

Lamb, M. (1991). Alterations in sexuality and sexual functioning. In S. Baird, M. G. McCorkle, & M. Grant (Eds.), *Cancer nursing: A comprehensive textbook* (pp. 831–849). Philadelphia: WB Saunders.

Lange, J. T., Lange, C. L., & Cabaltica, R. B. G. (2000). Primary care treatment of post-traumatic stress disorder. *American Family Physician, 62,* 1035–1040, 1046.

Lazarus, R. (2000). Evolution of a model of stress, coping, and discrete emotions. In V. Rice (Ed.), *Handbook of stress, coping and health: Implications for nursing theory, research, and practice* (pp. 195–222). Thousand Oaks, CA: Sage.

Lazarus, R. S., & Folkman, S. (1984). *Stress, appraisal, and coping.* New York: Springer.

Leininger, M. (1988). Leininger's theory of nursing: Culture care diversity and universality. *Nursing Science Quarterly, 1*(4), 152–160.

Leininger, M. (1991). *Culture care diversity and universality: A theory of nursing.* New York: NLN Press.

Lepore, S. J., & Evans, G. W. (1996). Coping with multiple stressors in the environment. In M. Zeidner & N. S. Endler (Eds.), *Handbook of coping.* New York: Wiley.

Lyon, B. (2000). Stress, coping, and health. In V. Rice (Ed.), *Handbook of stress, coping, and health: Implications for nursing research, theory, and practice* (pp. 3–26). Thousand Oaks, CA: Sage.

Macnee, C. L., & McCabe, S. (2000). Microstressors and health. In V. Rice (Ed.), *Handbook of stress, coping, and health: Implications for nursing research, theory, and practice* (pp. 125–142). Thousand Oaks, CA: Sage.

Mar, C., & Bent, S. (1999). An evidence-based review of the 10 most commonly used herbs. *Western Journal of Medicine, 171,* 168–171.

Martin, M. Y., Bradley, L. A., Alexander, R. W., Alarcon, G. S., Triana-Alexander, M., Aaron, L. A., & Alberts, K. R. (1996). Coping strategies predict disability in patients with primary fibromyalgia. *Pain, 68*(1), 45–53.

Matthews, D. A. (2000). Prayer and spirituality. *Rheumatic Diseases Clinics of North America, 26,* 177–187.

Matthews, D. A., Marlowe, S. M., & MacNutt, F. S. (1998). Intercessory prayer ministry benefits rheumatoid arthritis patients. *Journal General Internal Medicine, 13*(Suppl 1), 17.

Mayo, L. (Ed.). (1956). *Guides to action on chronic illness.* New York: National Health Council.

Mayou, R. A., Ehlers, A., & Hobbs, M. (2000). Psychological debriefing for road traffic accident victims: Three-year follow-up of a randomised controlled trial. *British Journal of Psychiatry, 176,* 589–593.

McConnell, A., & Christine, B. (1993). Personality through metaphor: Optimism, pessimism, locus of control, and sensation seeking. *Current Psychology, 12*(9), 195.

McDaniel, R. W. (1998). Development of a preparatory sensory information videotape for women receiving chemotherapy for breast cancer. *Cancer Nursing, 21,* 143–148.

Michelson, D., Stratakis, C., Hill, L., Reynolds, J., Galliven, E., Chrousos, G., & Gold, P. (1996). Bone mineral density in women with depression. *New England Journal of Medicine, 335,* 1176–1181.

Miller, S. (2000). *Coping with chronic illness: Overcoming powerlessness.* Philadelphia: FA Davis.

Mishel, M. H. (1997). Uncertainty in acute illness. *Annual Review of Nursing Research, 15,* 57–80.

Mitchell, M. (1997). Patients' perceptions of preoperative preparation for day surgery. *Journal of Advanced Nursing, 26,* 356–363.

Morgan, J., Roufeil, L., Kaushik, S., & Bassett M. (1998). Influence of coping style and precolonoscopy information on pain and anxiety of colonoscopy. *Gastrointestinal Endoscopy, 48,* 119–127.

National Institutes of Health. (1996, November). Neuroimmunomodulation Congress. Bethesda, MD.

Olshansky, S. (1962). Chronic sorrow: A response to having a mentally defective child. *Social Casework, 43,* 190–193.

Page, G. G. (1997). The immune-suppressive nature of pain. *Seminars in Oncology Nursing, 13,* 10–15.

Parsons, T. (1951). *The social system.* New York: Free Press.

Pellino, T. A., & Oberst, M. (1992). Perceptions of control and appraisal of illness in chronic low back pain. *Orthopaedic Nursing, 11,* 22–26.

Phinney, J. S., Lochner, B. T., & Murphy, R. (1990). Ethnic identity development and psychological adjustment in adolescence. In A. R. Stiffman & L. E. Davis (Eds.), *Ethnic issues in adolescent mental heath* (pp. 53–72). Thousand Oaks, CA: Sage.

Pollock, S. (1986). Human responses to chronic illness: Physiologic and psychosocial adaptation. *Nursing Research, 35,* 90–95.

PTSD Alliance. Available at www.ptsdalliance.org/home2.html

Rose, M., & Thomas, R. (1987). *Children with chronic conditions: Nursing in a family and community context.* Orlando: Grune & Stratton.

Rose, S., Wessely, S., & Bisson, J. (2001). Brief psychological interventions ("debriefing") for trauma-related symptoms and prevention of post traumatic stress disorder. *The Cochrane Library, 2.*

Roy, D. J. (1986, Winter). Caring for the self-esteem of the cosmetic patient. *Plastic Surgical Nursing, 6,* 138–141.

Ruiz-Bueno, J. B. (2000). Locus of control, perceived control, and learned helplessness. In V. Rice (Ed.), *Handbook of stress, coping, and health: Implications for nursing research, theory, and practice* (pp. 461–481). Thousand Oaks, CA: Sage.

Ryan-Wenger, N., Sharrer, V., & Wynd, C. (2000). Stress, coping, and health in children. In V. Rice (Ed.), *Handbook of stress, coping, and health: Implications for nursing research, theory, and practice* (pp. 265–293). Thousand Oaks, CA: Sage.

Schanberg, L. E., & Sandstrom, M. J. (1999). Causes of pain in children with arthritis. *Rheumatic Disease Clinics of North America, 25*(1), 31–53.

Seyle, H. (1956). *The stress of life.* New York: McGraw-Hill.

Siela, D, & Wieseke, A. W. (2000). Stress, self-efficacy, and health. In V. Rice (Ed.), *Handbook of stress, coping, and health: Implications for nursing research, theory, and practice* (pp. 495–516). Thousand Oaks, CA: Sage.

Steyer, T. E. (2001). Complementary and alternative medicine: A primer. *Family Practice Management, 8*(3), 37–42

Tisdale, S. (1987). *Harvest moon.* New York: Holt.

Tjemsland, L. (1997). Preoperative psychological variables predict immunological status in patients with operable breast cancer. *Psychooncology, 6,* 311–320.

Wineman, N. M. (1990). Adaptation to multiple sclerosis: The role of social support, functional disability, and perceived uncertainty. *Nursing Research, 39,* 294–299.

Wineman, N. M., Durand, E. J., & Steiner, R. P. (1994). A comparative analysis of coping behaviors in persons with multiple sclerosis and their spouses. *Journal of Neuroscience Nursing, 25,* 356–361.

Witek-Janusek, L., & Mathews, H. (2000). Stress, immunity and health outcomes. In V. Rice (Ed.), *Handbook of stress, coping, and health: Implications for nursing research, theory, and practice* (pp. 47–68). Thousand Oaks, CA: Sage.

Yocum, D. E. (2000). Exercise, education, and behavioral modification as alternative therapy for pain and stress in rheumatic disease. *Rheumatic Disease Clinics of North America, 26,* 149–159.

3

Ergonomics

CAROLYN L. BLUE and PAMELA F. LEVIN

Ergonomics is the scientific study of human work. The term *ergonomics* is derived from two Greek words: *ergos,* meaning work, and *nomos,* meaning laws. Ergonomics (also called human factor engineering) may be defined as the interdisciplinary study of the interrelationships among the work environment, job demands, work methods, and the human behavioral and biologic capabilities and limitations (Keyserling, 2000). It is a basic premise of ergonomics that *all* work imposes physical and mental demands on the worker. The goal of ergonomics is to reduce job demands so that the worker's health and well-being are maintained.

Ergonomic risk factors include repetitive, forceful, or prolonged exertions; frequent or heavy lifting; pushing, pulling, or carrying heavy objects; fixed or awkward work postures; contact stress; localized or whole-body vibration; cold temperatures; and poor lighting (which can lead to awkward body postures). These risk factors can be intensified by work organization characteristics that include inadequate work-rest cycles; stressful working conditions resulting from demanding, boring, frustrating, or socially alienating working conditions; excessive work pace or duration or both; unaccustomed work; lack of task variability; machine-paced work; and piece rate. Work-related musculoskeletal disorders typically result from multiple exposures to risk factors. A work-related musculoskeletal disorder may result from a single episode of overexertion, cumulative overuse of anatomic structures, or a combination of both. Sudden-onset injuries, resulting from a single episode of overexertion, may be classified as an "accident," but the category may be somewhat arbitrary because the individual may have had exposure to cumulative overuse before the single incident that triggered the current symptoms. Therefore, identifying the underlying risk factor(s) may be a complex task. Nevertheless, these underlying risk factors should be assessed, taking into account the duration and frequency of the exposure during the work shift.

As an applied science, ergonomics strives to fit workplace conditions and job demands to the physiologic, anatomic, and psychological capabilities and limitations of the worker (Cohen, Gjessing, Fine, Bernard, & McGlothlin, 1997). A proactive approach to ergonomics involves designing work processes such as job tasks, equipment, and workplace layout and designing work strategies such as the use of mechanical assist devices or assembly line designs. Simply put, ergonomics strives to adapt the workplace to fit the workers rather than the other way around.

A work environment that does not fit the behavioral and biologic characteristics of the worker can lead to musculoskeletal injuries. Musculoskeletal injuries are among the 10 leading work-related diseases and are the leading cause of worker disability. Although the incidence rate for injuries and illnesses resulting in lost work time has declined since 1992, a total of 1.7 million persons with injuries and illnesses required recuperation away from work (U.S. Department of Labor, 2000). Sprains and strains (44%) were the leading nature of injury, followed by bruises and contusions (9%) and fractures (7%). Three occupations—nursing assistants, truck drivers, and nonconstruction laborers—accounted for 1 in 5 musculoskeletal injuries. Many of these injuries are a result of work-related ergonomic hazards and therefore can be effectively reduced with proactive ergonomic considerations.

The primary focus of ergonomics is to create tolerable and acceptable living and work conditions that improve health and enhance worker productivity (Keyserling, 2000). A higher-level goal of ergonomics is to achieve an environment that is so well adapted to humans that physical and psychosocial well-being is enhanced to improve both worker performance and health and safety (Carayon & Smith, 2000). Because ergonomics focuses on work environment and human physiology and psychology, the spectrum of study includes items such as accident prevention, static and dynamic human body biomechanics, forceful exertions, repetitive exertions, environmental temperature extremes, vibration, lighting, equipment and process design, circadian rhythm, and physical and psychological job demands. Applied ergonomics, then, is the application of this knowledge to modify the design of equipment and task to maintain, promote, and enhance health and well-being. This applied science incorporates knowledge from the disciplines of engineering, psychology, anatomy, physiology, anthropology, and statistics (Kroemer, 1996; Wilson, 2000).

IMPORTANCE OF ERGONOMICS TO NURSES

The nurse often cares for clients who have orthopaedic problems resulting from unsatisfactory living and work environments. The nurse is in a unique position to assess injuries presented in the clinical setting as well as to plan necessary interventions that may prevent or control musculoskeletal risks. A detailed history may reveal hazardous situations that not only contributed to the illness or injury but also will most certainly contribute to a poor prognosis if allowed to continue after treatment. Ergonomics is also important to nurses because the practice of nursing requires an environment that is not always ergonomically optimal. Data from the National Bureau of Labor Statistics (2001) revealed that workers employed in acute care and long-term care facilities were two to five times more likely to develop a musculoskeletal disorder compared with other service industries. As a member of a health care team, the nurse can be proactive in identifying both environmental and human factors that can be improved or controlled so that injury does not present itself.

Ergonomic considerations are critical to compliance with the Americans with Disabilities Act of 1990. The Americans with Disabilities Act of 1990 became effective in 1992 and is designed to protect persons with disabilities from discrimination. The focus of the act is on employee accommodations with respect to job function and placement rather than on employee selection. This is important to orthopaedic nurses in that it is now difficult, if not impossible, to select workers for a job based on their physical characteristics. Nurses can counsel workers regarding strength training and overall physical fitness. However, the primary focus of ergonomics is to match the environmental conditions of work, job and workstation design, and work demands to the worker rather than fitting the worker to the job.

There are five basic elements for ergonomic hazard control: work site analysis, hazard prevention and control, health management, training and education, and

management commitment and employee involvement (U.S. Department of Labor, 1990). The National Institute for Occupational Safety and Health (NIOSH) developed a practical stepped-approach to controlling work-related musculoskeletal disorders (Cohen et al., 1997) (Box 3–1). Basically, the *Pathway to Controlling Work-Related Musculoskeletal Disorders* can fit the nursing process. Assessment involves assessing the worker (i.e., looking for signs of musculoskeletal problems in the workplace), the stage for action (i.e., determining management commitment and employee involvement in addressing possible problems), and the work environment (i.e., identifying jobs or work conditions that contribute to musculoskeletal problems). Planning involves identifying effective options for (1) reducing risks and establishing health care management to emphasize the importance of early detection and treatment of musculoskeletal disorders and (2) creating a proactive ergonomics program with an accent on training and education to prevent ergonomic problems. Evaluation of the ergonomic program involves an evaluation of the worker, management and worker commitment to an ergonomic program, and effectiveness of controls for reducing musculoskeletal problems. Generally, occupational health nurses are involved with work site analysis and hazard prevention and control at the work site as well as in primary care treatment and case management. However, all nurses involved with persons who may have illnesses or injuries relating to ergonomic hazards in their occupations are in key positions to assist in the management of these conditions and reduce ergonomic risks through worker education.

ERGONOMIC ASSESSMENT

A systematic assessment of both the worker and workplace characteristics is needed to identify specific work hazards that contribute to potential injuries or to the worker's present physical condition. Human, tool, task, workstation, and environment form a complex system of interacting components that are the basis of an ergonomic assessment. Box 3–2 lists an overview of items to consider when conducting an ergonomic assessment. Because worker capabilities are a factor in fitting the workplace to the worker, workforce characteristics, such as body size, physical condition, and disabilities of the workers, are included in the assessment.

Illnesses and injuries are often difficult to attribute to an occupation because of several factors. One factor is that a history of work exposures is difficult to secure or interpret. Another factor is that occupational illnesses and injuries are often associated with a variety of types of exposures. In addition, risk evaluation of some exposures has not been adequately defined. Finally, heredity, current medical problems (e.g., diabetes, rheumatoid arthritis, systemic lupus erythematosus), personal lifestyle, and psychosocial factors may also contribute to the current

BOX 3–1.

Pathway to Controlling Work-Related Musculoskeletal Disorders

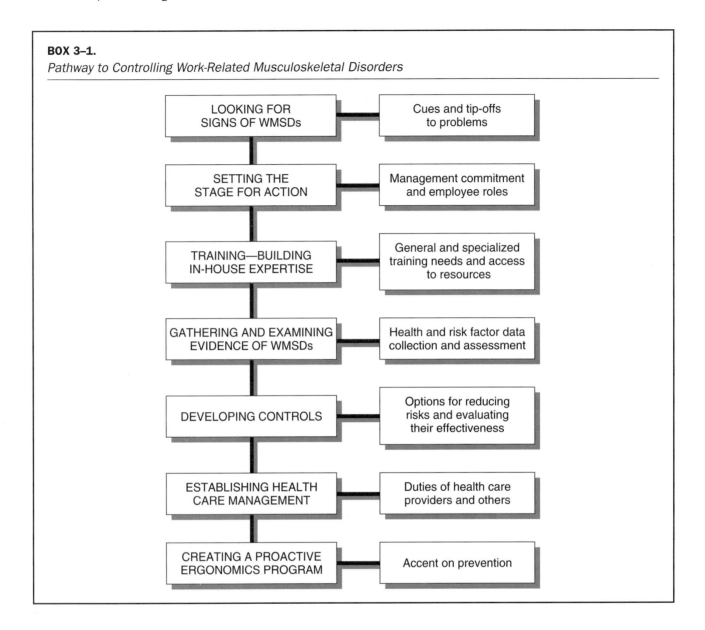

LOOKING FOR SIGNS OF WMSDs	Cues and tip-offs to problems
SETTING THE STAGE FOR ACTION	Management commitment and employee roles
TRAINING—BUILDING IN-HOUSE EXPERTISE	General and specialized training needs and access to resources
GATHERING AND EXAMINING EVIDENCE OF WMSDs	Health and risk factor data collection and assessment
DEVELOPING CONTROLS	Options for reducing risks and evaluating their effectiveness
ESTABLISHING HEALTH CARE MANAGEMENT	Duties of health care providers and others
CREATING A PROACTIVE ERGONOMICS PROGRAM	Accent on prevention

condition (Hagberg, Silverstein, Wells, Smith, Hendrick, Carayon, & Pérusse, 1995; Westgaard, 2000). A symptoms survey used in the workplace, such as the one in Figure 3-1, is helpful in identifying the location, frequency, and duration of discomfort associated with the current medical problem. The identification and comparison of work demands and symptoms may provide important clues to ergonomic hazards.

Much of the worker assessment is done to gather necessary information for determining potential risks. A person's physical tolerance for work can be determined by examining that person's physical capabilities and the job's physical requirements. If the physical requirements equal or exceed the physical capabilities of the worker, the job will create strain on both specific anatomic structures and the respiratory and cardiovascular systems. Strain causes not only damage to anatomic structures but also fatigue and a decrease in physical functioning. When

continuous fatigue-induced low performance is not restored by rest, chronic fatigue will result. However, physical tolerance for work is achieved when the demands of the job task and environment are lower than the worker's physical capabilities.

Anthropometry

Designing the workplace to fit the worker can be achieved only through understanding the characteristics, capabilities, and limitations of the human body. No two people are built alike. People may be the same height but have a different range of arm reach or different leg length. People may also vary in muscle strength and joint flexibility. A workplace with a good ergonomic design should accommodate at least 90% of the population (National Safety Council, 1993). For example, the fifth percentile woman who is standing with arms at the side has an elbow-to-floor height of 36.5 inches, whereas 95%

of the female population has an elbow-to-floor height of 45.3 inches (Kroemer, 1996).

Body size has become a matter of interest to human factor engineers. Physical characteristics of the worker are determined through anthropometry, which is a measurement of the human physical form (e.g., height, girth, breadth, reach, range of motion, curvatures, circumferences). Often presented in terms of *population percentiles,* anthropometric data provide an expedient means of describing the range of body dimensions to be accommodated.

Most anthropometric information has come from military research. Consequently, the data ranges or norms apply to young, healthy, male soldiers. As a result, many of the home and work environments designed from anthropometric norms fit a sample of the male population and most likely do not represent the same proportion of the adult female population. In addition, some male body proportions do not fit the normal distribution

of the standard measurements. However, it is common practice to design equipment, workspaces, and tools so that they fit the small body (e.g., women at the 5th percentile) as well as the large body (e.g., men in the 95th percentile). The point of this discussion is that workplace and home designs generally fit no person because no one is average in every body dimension. In addition, population dimensions have changed and will probably continue to change. People are larger and heavier than in the past. In addition, the current workforce is made up of a larger proportion of women, older persons, and people with disabilities.

Biomechanical Measures

Whereas anthropometry defines humans in terms of body measures of structure, biomechanical measures have to do with the mechanical condition of the human body. Because some jobs and job tasks are difficult to redesign, reliance on the physical fitness of the human body is

---

BOX 3–2.
Potential Ergonomic Hazards in the Workplace

I. General Work Environment
Workforce characteristics
  Age, anthropometrics (body size and proportions)
  Strength, endurance, fitness
  Disabilities
  Diminished senses
  Communication/language problems (e.g., non–English speaking or illiterate workers)
  Lighting
  Cold temperatures
  Noise level
  Health and safety safeguards (e.g., presence of transfer aids)
  General housekeeping (e.g., slippery surfaces)

II. Job and Workstation Design
Location of controls, displays, equipment, stock
  Accessibility (e.g., special patient conditions)
  Visibility
  Legibility
  Efficiency of sequence of movements during operation or use (e.g., restricted toileting or bathing areas)
  Use of pedals
  Posture of workers
    Sitting, standing, or a combination
    Possibility for variation
    Stooping, twisting, or bending of the spine (e.g., lifting a patient from a wheelchair to a bed)
  Chair availability, adjustments
  Room to move about (e.g., few obstructions, such as medical equipment)
  Work surface height

Uneven work surfaces (e.g., transfer from a wheelchair to a bed)
Predominantly dynamic or static work
  Job rotation
  Unpredictable or shifting loads (e.g., combative patient)
  Use of devices such as clamps or jigs to avoid static work
  Availability of supports for arms, elbows, hands, back, feet

III. Muscle Workload Task Demands
Repetitiveness
  Frequency (e.g., multiple lifts or transfers per shift)
  Force
  Availability of rest pauses
  Possibility for alternative work
  Skill, vigilance, perception demands
  Efficiency of organization (supplies, equipment)
Use of hand tools
  Hand and wrist posture during use
  Work surface height
  Size and weight of tool
  Necessity, availability of supports
  Shape, dimensions, and surface of handgrip
  Vibratory or nonvibratory

IV. Strength Requirements
Strength capabilities
Working pulses/respiratory rate
Loads lifted, carried, pushed, or pulled
  Manner in which handled (e.g., type of patient transfer)
  Weight and dimensions of objects handled
  Distance of load transfer

Adapted from Frederick, L., Habes, D., & Schloemer, J. (1984). An introduction to the principles of occupational ergonomics. *Occupational Health Nursing, 32,* 643–645.

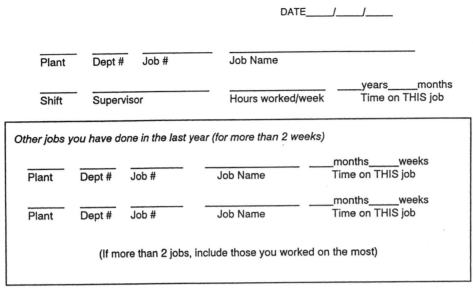

DATE_____/_____/_____

_____ _____ _____ _____
Plant Dept # Job # Job Name

_____ years_____months
Time on THIS job

_____ _____ _____
Shift Supervisor Hours worked/week

Other jobs you have done in the last year (for more than 2 weeks)

_____ _____ _____ _____ _____months_____weeks
Plant Dept # Job # Job Name Time on THIS job

_____ _____ _____ _____ _____months_____weeks
Plant Dept # Job # Job Name Time on THIS job

(If more than 2 jobs, include those you worked on the most)

Have you had any pain or discomfort during the last year?
❏ Yes ❏ No (If NO, stop here)

If YES, carefully shade in the area of the drawing which bothers you the MOST.

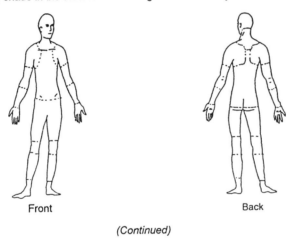

Front   Back

(Continued)

FIGURE 3–1. Worker symptoms survey. (From Hales, T. R., & Bertsche, P. K. [1992]. Management of upper extremity cumulative trauma disorders. *AAOHN Journal, 40,* 120–121. Copyright 1992 by SLACK Incorporated. Reprinted by permission of the American Association of Occupational Health Nurses.)

necessary to reduce ergonomic risks. Physical fitness includes optimal muscle strength and endurance, flexibility of joints and surrounding tissues, and total aerobic fitness.

Muscle Strength. There are more than 200 skeletal muscles in the human body. The only active action of a muscle is contraction, brought about by muscle filaments that slide along each other. Muscular strength can be defined as the maximum ability to apply or to resist force (Pollock & Wilmore, 1990). A model developed to predict biomechanical responses to strenuous exertions associated with common manual handling tasks take in to account the worker's anthropometry (height and body weight), working posture (angles at the ankles, knees, hip,

trunk, shoulders, and elbows), and the magnitude and direction of the external forces. The muscles at each joint must have sufficient strength to create an equal and opposite reactive moment; therefore, strength is characterized as the ability to create a mechanical moment (Chaffin & Andersson, 1991). Related to muscle strength are the terms *muscle power* and *endurance,* both of which are dependent on the strength of a muscle or group of muscles. Power is the product of strength and speed, and muscular endurance is the capacity of a muscle group to sustain repeated contractions over time until muscular fatigue develops.

Flexibility. *Flexibility* refers to one's ability to move a joint through its maximum range of motion. Flexibility is joint specific and reflects the interrelationships among muscles, tendons, ligaments, skin, and the joint itself. Flexibility is affected by the temperature of the joint and surrounding tissue, with warmth increasing the ability to move a joint through its full range of motion. In addition, women are generally more flexible than men.

Total Aerobic Fitness. A person's physical tolerance for physical work is usually determined by the capacity of the respiratory and cardiovascular systems to deliver oxygen to the working muscles and to transform calories into working energy. The balance of energy capacity and the energy demands of work are largely determined by the

(Complete a separate page for each area that bothers you)

Check Area: ☐ Neck   ☐ Shoulder   ☐ Elbow/Forearm   ☐ Hand/Wrist   ☐ Fingers
☐ Upper Back   ☐ Low Back   ☐ Thigh/Knee   ☐ Low Leg   ☐ Ankle/Foot

1. Please put a check by the word(s) that best describe your problem

☐ Aching   ☐ Numbness (asleep)   ☐ Tingling
☐ Burning   ☐ Pain   ☐ Weakness
☐ Cramping   ☐ Swelling   ☐ Other
☐ Loss of Color   ☐ Stiffness

2. When did you first notice the problem? _____(month) _____(year)

3. How long does each episode last? (Mark an X along the line)

_____/_____/_____/_____/_____
1 hour   1 day   1 week   1 month   6 months

4. How many separate episodes have you had in the last year?_____

5. What do you think caused the problem?_____
_____

6. Have you had this problem in the last 7 days?   ☐ Yes   ☐ No

7. How would you rate this problem (mark an X on the line)
   NOW

   _____
   None   Unbearable

   When it was the WORST

   _____
   None   Unbearable

8. Have you had medical treatment for this problem?   ☐ Yes   ☐ No
   8a. If NO, why not_____

   8b. If YES, where did you receive treatment?_____
      1. Company Medical ☐   Times in past year_____
      2. Personal doctor ☐   Times in past year_____
      3. Other ☐   Times in past year_____
   8c. If YES, did the treatment help?   ☐ Yes   ☐ No

9. How much time have you lost in the last year because of this problem?_____days

10. How many days in the last year were you on restricted or light duty because of this problem?
    _____days

11. Please comment on what you think would improve your symptoms
_____
_____
_____
_____

FIGURE 3–1 *Continued*

total aerobic fitness of the individual. If the job demand exceeds physical capabilities, the individual will be under much strain and either will not be able to perform the task or will perform the task but be at risk for sustaining an injury. Fatigue is caused by overexertion that leads to a temporary decrease in physical performance. It is commonly associated with a buildup of lactic acid in the body. Although the lactic acid reduces to carbon dioxide and water during lessened activity and rest, fatigue may contribute to perceptions of declining motivation and mental and physical activities. We all are able to perceive the strain generated in the body by overexertion and can make a judgment about the perceived effort the task requires, so our perceived effort can be used to determine the balance among job, job strain, and resulting fatigue. Whenever the job leads to judgments about excessive strain and fatigue, the job demand is too great for the person's aerobic fitness.

Assessment of the Workplace

Health threats from poor workplace design, repetitive movements, awkward body postures, inadequate rest, and other hazards affect workers in all types of work settings. A detailed and organized assessment of the workplace is necessary to determine potential exposure to ergonomic hazards associated with jobs and workstations. Insight into the client's condition is obtained by understanding potential work site stressors. Generally, ergonomic risk factors can be reduced by eliminating awkward positions, prolonged static postures, repetitious and forceful movements, vibration, and other environmental risks.

Manual Material Handling. Prevention of physical injury requires that loads lifted, carried, pushed, or pulled in the workplace be matched to the physical strength capabilities of the worker. NIOSH uses a lifting equation as a guideline for permissible loads for a person to safely lift, move, or carry (U.S. Department of Health and Human Services, 1994). The general intent of the NIOSH lifting equation is to identify ergonomic solutions that reduce the physical stresses associated with manual lifting. This is accomplished by identifying the features of the lifting task that contribute most to the risk for low-back injuries. The amount of weight to be handled is determined by several factors, including the weight or force to be handled, the object's location, posture used to perform the lift, the frequency and duration of the lifting task, the stability of the object, grip, and environmental conditions (e.g., friction).

The NIOSH guidelines recommend that, under optimal conditions, engineering or administrative controls be required in work settings where employees lift weights heavier than 51 pounds (Waters, Putz-Anderson, & Garg, 1994). This 51-pound maximum recommended weight for lifting would be acceptable to only 75% of female workers and 90% of male workers. In addition to the weight of the load, the NIOSH lifting formula considers horizontal and vertical lifting, distance, frequency, grasp, and asymmetrical lifts. However, the NIOSH guidelines are not intended for lifting or lowering people or for unpredictable conditions. Furthermore, the guidelines assume that environmental work factors are ideal. Because of these restrictions, the NIOSH lifting guidelines are not appropriate for workers such as nurses, firefighters, physical therapists, or emergency medical technicians, who often are faced with lifting people under poor environmental conditions with poor footing and often unpredictable conditions.

Physical Work Demands. Physical work demands affect the incidence, severity, and potential disability of the individual performing the work. The assessment guide presented in Box 3-3 can be used to define work factors that contribute to potential or current injuries. The checklist offers a broad view of the workplace and can be used as a guide when conducting individual assessments to define the source of exposure to work demands. A worker's description of operations performed on the job may reveal potential ergonomic hazards not suggested by the individual's job title. It may also be helpful to ask whether co-workers have similar complaints of injury and to determine the demands of job tasks the individual performs while at home. In assessing physical work, it may also be useful to examine videotapes of people at work and examine various postures and other risk factors. If many employees from the same company are exhibiting similar symptoms, a work site walk-through survey can be conducted to identify hazards and activities of workers and to become familiar with work processes that are ergonomic triggers to musculoskeletal injury.

Job Design. An effective work practice program includes an approach to work in a safe manner. Management commitment is essential to an ergonomic program. Administrative controls are important for reducing the duration, frequency, and severity of the exposure to ergonomic hazards. For example, jobs that have high exposure to repetitive movements could be rotated among employees so that workers could spend some of the work time doing nonrepetitive jobs. Repetition can also be reduced by substituting mechanization and automation for human work, combining or sequencing job components, increasing the number and variety of tasks, expanding available work time, and self-pacing work demands. For example, the repetitive work of the operating room instrument nurse could be rotated with the more dynamic work of the circulating nurse. Similarly, work assignments could be made so that job tasks vary among the workers. Workers in jobs that require awkward or static positions should be provided more frequent rest periods or breaks.

BOX 3–3.

An Ergonomic Checklist for Physical Work Demands

[ ] Does the task require strenuous two-hand lifting?

[ ] _____ Lifting at too great a horizontal distance?

[ ] _____ Lifting more than once per minute?

[ ] _____ Lifting over too great a vertical distance?

[ ] Does the task require strenuous one-hand lifting and reaching (such as too long a reach when feeding parts into a machine)?

[ ] Are lifts awkward because they are near the floor, above the shoulders, or too far from the body?

[ ] Does the job require twisting while lifting?

[ ] Must the worker handle difficult-to-grasp items? (Are the items difficult to reach? Is the hand-hold poor?)

[ ] Does the job require continual manual handling of materials?

[ ] Does the job require handling of oversized objects?

[ ] Does the job require two-person lifting?

[ ] Must force be exerted in an awkward position (e.g., to the side, overhead, or at extended reaches)?

[ ] Is help for heavy lifting or exerting force unavailable?

[ ] Does the job involve peak loads of muscular effort? How often do peak loads occur? How long do they last?

[ ] Can the job be designed to alternate periods of exertion and rest?

[ ] Can the job be designed to alternate periods of static effort and movement?

[ ] Is the pace of material handling determined by a machine (e.g., feeding machines, conveyors)?

[ ] Does the job lack material handling aids, such as air hoists or scissor tables?

[ ] Does the job involve static muscle loading, such as holding or carrying?

[ ] Is there a high level of hand tool vibration?

[ ] Must the worker stand on a hard surface for 45% or more of the work shift?

[ ] Is there frequent daily stair or ladder climbing?

From National Safety Council. (1993). Workplace checklist. In *Ergonomics: A practical guide* (2nd ed., p. 96). Itasca, IL: Author. Used by permission of the National Safety Council.

Workplace Design. Engineering controls are the best method for reducing or eliminating ergonomic hazards because the basis of ergonomics is to fit the workplace to the worker rather than compelling the worker to fit the job. Workplace design includes workstations, tools, and equipment that accommodate movement, safe postures, and use by each individual worker. The work comfort zone (Fig. 3-2) is generally 2 to 4 inches (5 to 10 cm) below the elbow. For more precise work, the zone should be 2 to 4 inches above the elbow, whereas for heavier work, the zone is 4 to 5 inches below the elbow (Putz-Anderson, 1988). For example, equip-

ment and supplies should be arranged so that the worker does a minimum of lifting, twisting, and reaching. Workspace for the hands should be directly in front of the torso, between hip and chest height. This location should be lower in jobs that require heavy manual work and higher in jobs requiring close visual observation. Workplace design that promotes keeping the elbow at the side of the body, the forearm semipronated, and the wrist straight reduces the risk of repetitive trauma in jobs in which upper extremity movements are intense.

Other workplace design measures that improve comfort and prevent injury include tool design and housekeeping measures. Tools designed to the size of the worker's hands prevent awkward gripping and strain on anatomic structures of the hand and wrist. Good housekeeping, such as floors that are clean and dry, helps prevent slips and falls. Walkways should be free from obstacles that can cause accidents and injuries. There is a lack of scientific evidence that antifatigue mats or antifatigue shoe inserts are helpful to workers who are subjected to prolonged standing (Hansen, Winkel, & Jørgensen, 1998).

Complaints related to unhealthful postures and vision have become common among computer operators and may originate from an improperly designed and poorly arranged workstation (Kroemer, 1996). The causes of these complaints may be interrelated. For example, problems associated with viewing the computer screen may result in attempts to compensate by straining the neck and lumbar region of the back. The ensuing awkward position causes fatiguing postures of the shoulders and arms. Workstations that include computer terminals should be designed so that the source document is in front of or off to the side and visual display screens are placed in front of the body and below eye level so that the line of sight is declined 10 to 40 degrees below the horizontal level (Kroemer, 1996) (Fig. 3-3). The keyboard should be adjusted so that the wrists are straight when it is being used. A chair that is padded and that can accommodate good working postures that maintain lordosis (forward curve) of the lumbar spine is healthier for the back. In essence, computer workstations should be designed with fully adjustable visual display terminals, keypads, chairs, and footrests to maintain healthful work postures and to prevent restricted and stressed work positions of the hands, wrists, and back.

Static and Dynamic Work. Muscular activity can be classified as either static or dynamic work. Fatigue can result from both static and dynamic types of work when stresses of mechanical work are excessive. Fatigue can be limited to a small number of muscles or may be generalized, affecting the entire body. In static work, muscles or a muscle group remains in a contracted state for a prolonged period. Muscle contraction leads to a rise in pressure in the muscle, compressing blood vessels, and

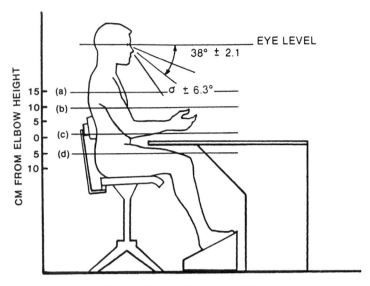

a. For fine work, exacting visual tasks
b. For precision work, e.g., mechanical assembly work
c. For writing or light assembly work
d. Coarse or medium manual work such as packaging

FIGURE 3–2. Comfort zones for correct height of work surfaces for sitting and standing work. (From Putz-Anderson, V. [1988]. *Cumulative trauma disorders: A manual for musculoskeletal diseases of the upper limbs* [p. 95]. Bristol, PA: Taylor & Francis. Copyright 1988 by Taylor & Francis.)

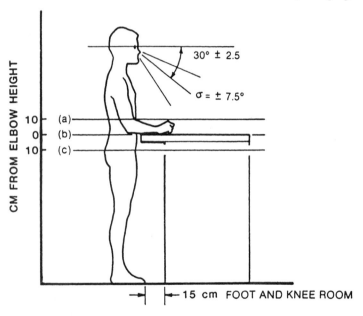

a. For precision work with supported elbows
b. For light assembly work
c. For heavy work

results in an insufficient supply of nutrients necessary to the surrounding tissue. If the muscle cannot relax periodically, the demand for metabolic nutrients exceeds the supply and metabolic wastes accumulate. Short-term static work, such as prolonged pinching or grasping a tool (e.g., holding an operating room clamp), can cause ischemic muscle pain and a reduced capacity to produce muscle tension. If prolonged and excessive, static work can lead to injury of the joints, tendons, and ligaments. In addition to the increased risk for tissue injury, static postures often are responsible for nonspecific aches and pains and muscular fatigue. Examples of static postures include sustained standing and sitting postures, forward reaching, crouching and holding objects, and working in a bent or twisted position. Work should be designed to reduce the intensity and duration of a static exertion.

The major difference between static and dynamic aspects of work is that during dynamic work, the body is partially moving. Dynamic work involves continual, cyclic contraction and relaxation of the working muscle and is generally preferable to static work. This pumping action promotes circulation of blood to the muscle and surrounding tissue. As a result, a muscle receives the necessary nutrients and rids itself of painful waste products. Examples of dynamic work include lifting and handling activities, walking, stooping, bending or rotating the trunk, and pulling and pushing. Dynamic work can be limited by the capacity of the cardiopulmonary system to deliver adequate supplies of oxygen and metabolic nutrients to the working muscles and to remove metabolic waste products. Although the use of large muscle groups can be maintained for prolonged durations with dynamic work, overexertion of a body not prepared for the intensity, duration, and frequency of activity can exceed the worker's aerobic capacity and lead to generalized fatigue. Generalized fatigue often results in tightening of muscle groups and consequent risk for musculoskeletal injury. The prevention of whole-body fatigue can be accomplished by designing the work to minimize body movements and the use of large muscles, for example, using mechanical equipment to perform the work. Frequent rest periods, particularly in hot, humid environments, are also needed to reduce the potential for whole-body fatigue.

Equipment Design. Much of the equipment used in work is meant to serve as an extension of the human hand, amplifying the hand's strength, extending the reach, protecting the delicate human tissue; it also is used to allow humans to perform tasks they are not otherwise capable of accomplishing. However, the interface of equipment and the hand can result in injuries to the hand, wrist, and arm when handheld equipment is poorly designed. Although the exact design desired is specific to the equipment and task to be performed, a few general principles can guide the safe use of equipment in the work setting. The preferred size of a cylindrical grip is about 1.5 inches (Kroemer, 1996). Handles should be large enough that the user does not maintain a static posture for long periods. In addition, it is recommended that handles accommodate the length of the hand in contact with it. Pressure points along the hand and fingers are avoided by using handles with smooth, rounded edges. The design of the equipment should result in keeping the wrist near a straight position with respect to the forearm.

Vibration. Workers who are continuously exposed to the vibration of equipment can sustain injuries to limbs, organs, or the whole body. Vibration is the mechanical oscillation of a surface transferred directly to a reference point (i.e., a person's body) (Leffler & Hu, 2000). Workers who are particularly vulnerable to vibration hazards are those who operate tools or machines that vibrate (e.g., sanders, weedeaters, jackhammers) or those who drive automobiles and trucks for long periods. The most common vibration injury is *white finger syndrome*, attributed to deterioration of the blood supply to the fingertip

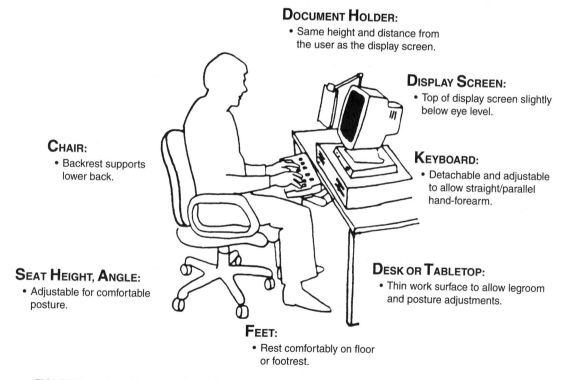

DOCUMENT HOLDER:
• Same height and distance from the user as the display screen.

DISPLAY SCREEN:
• Top of display screen slightly below eye level.

CHAIR:
• Backrest supports lower back.

KEYBOARD:
• Detachable and adjustable to allow straight/parallel hand-forearm.

SEAT HEIGHT, ANGLE:
• Adjustable for comfortable posture.

DESK OR TABLETOP:
• Thin work surface to allow legroom and posture adjustments.

FEET:
• Rest comfortably on floor or footrest.

FIGURE 3–3. Comfort zones for video display terminal workstation design. (From U.S. Department of Labor, Occupational Safety and Health Administration. [1991]. *Ergonomics: The study of work* [p. 13]. [OSHA 3125]. Washington, DC: U.S. Government Printing Office.)

area. White finger syndrome is characterized by numbness, tingling, and blanching of the fingertips. Of course, the best control to prevent injury from vibration is to eliminate the source. However, if elimination is not possible, vibration can be reduced by selecting tools and equipment that have low levels of vibration and that are in good working condition, using tool wraps or antivibratory gloves that minimize vibration, designing work so that the hands are not in direct contact with large surfaces of the tool, and controlling environmental conditions that magnify the response to vibration, such as cold (which causes vasoconstriction). For example, redesigning a riveting tool in a car foundry significantly reduced vibration to workers' hands (Laws, 2000). Such efforts as ensuring proper vehicle suspension and providing padded seats in vehicles can reduce the effects of whole-body vibration. Redistributing the work among workers is also helpful because the modification decreases the duration and thus exposure to the vibration.

Safe Lifting Practices. Lifting involves a complex combination of moving body parts, changing joint angles, tightening muscles, and loading the spinal column (Kroemer, 1996). Although safe lifting practices have been shown to reduce the number and severity of work-related injuries, workers continue to be exposed to overexertion because of poor lifting practices. This unfortunate result is attributable to stressful job requirements and a tendency of people to revert back to previous poor lifting habits. Furthermore, demands are placed on individuals when emergency situations arise in which quick, unsuspected movement occurs or in which the weight being lifted suddenly increases. Even normal lifting can overly strain a body that has impaired physical well-being. Proper training in lifting techniques and periodic reinforcement should reduce the number of injuries sustained from poor lifting practices.

Engineering designs are aimed at eliminating or reducing injuries from overexertion in persons who lift, carry, push, or pull loads. The best intervention is to eliminate the task. If the task cannot be eliminated, it may be mechanized or mechanical aids may be used to lessen the work demand on the individual. Other interventions may include reducing the load and, if this is not possible (as in lifting and moving people), reducing the distance and frequency of the lift or movement. It is important to recognize that eliminating or mechanizing the task will solve the problem of the ergonomic hazard. However, using aids, reducing the load, or reducing the distance and frequency of the task will only partially eliminate the potential hazard.

Some general guidelines that can be applied to safe lifting practices are listed in Box 3-4. The work should be designed so that lifting is accomplished by using mechanical lifting and transferring equipment rather than by direct handling. For example, much of the physical lifting

---

BOX 3–4.
Key Guidelines for Safe Lifting Practices

Always use lifting aids when possible.
Exercise regularly to maintain overall physical condition. Use muscles of the legs, arms, and abdomen to reduce stress on the back.
Begin the lift with the object between the level of the knuckles (when the arm is hanging at the side) and the shoulder.
Plan before attempting to lift. Place the object or patient within reach.
Have handling aids available. Make sure sufficient space is cleared.
Determine the safest, most efficient, and least difficult methods for movement.
Be realistic about your ability to lift the object or patient.
Get a good grip on the object or patient.
Bring the object or patient as close to your body as possible.
Maintain a broad base of support, with feet pointing in the direction of movement.
Move the object or patient in a straight line, avoiding twisting or sideways bending of the back.

From Blue, C. L. (1996). Preventing back injury among nursing personnel: The worker and the worksite. *Orthopaedic Nursing Journal, 15,* 12.

---

could be completely eliminated by using mechanical hoists or sliding boards.

People who are in good physical condition are less likely to be injured because the gap between the physical capabilities of the person and the work demands of lifting and moving is narrower. Safety involved with lifting requires that major muscle groups of the thighs, knees, upper and lower arms, abdomen, and pelvis have the strength and endurance to withstand the stresses placed on them. Generally, if the person is not used to lifting and vigorous exercise, difficult lifting and lowering tasks should not be attempted.

The height from which an object is to be lifted is also important to the safety of the lift. Lifting when the spine is bent or twisted causes additional stress on the structures of the spine and back muscles. Assuming the arms are held relaxed at the side of the body, lifting should occur with the object or person above the knuckles of the hand and below the shoulder.

A thorough assessment of the object to be lifted and the environment in which the lift will occur is necessary for smooth body movements and ensures enough workspace to use healthful lifting postures and body mechanics. When the object to be lifted is a person, the abilities and limitations of the person to be lifted should be assessed. Is the person willing and able to assist with the move, and if so, will the person experience pain when movement occurs? It is a normal human response to avoid painful situations. A patient who is normally cooperative may become less cooperative in a painful situation, such as when being moved or lifted. Consideration given to the patient's suggestions can greatly enhance the efficiency and safety of the movement.

Body mechanics are essential to maintaining the normal curvature of the back; that is, the natural curvature, particularly its lumbar lordosis, of the standing spine should be maintained whenever lifting, pulling, or pushing tasks are performed. The feet should be placed apart to allow the weight to be shifted from one foot to the other without sideways bending of the back. In addition, the wider base of support offers increased stability so that unexpected movement by the patient does not create a situation in which the nurse loses stability.

Bringing the object to be moved as close as possible to the body allows the weight to be close to the center of gravity and over the base of support. Bringing the weight closer to the base of support prevents adjustment of the body toward the opposite direction to reestablish the center of gravity over the feet. When an object is lifted farther away from the center of gravity, the head, shoulders, and spine move in the opposite direction to reestablish the center of gravity over the feet. Such compensating movements result in unhealthful body postures that place added strain on the musculoskeletal system.

In addition to the use of proper body mechanics, engineering or management interventions should be applied to facilitate carrying out the safe lifting practices. For example, loads being lifted should be a size and weight that can be lifted by straightening the legs. Loads, whether people or objects, should be in a position to lift in front of the trunk while maintaining a normal body posture. Enough space should be provided so that lifting or lowering tasks do not have to be carried out in awkward positions.

COMMON ORTHOPAEDIC PROBLEMS AND ERGONOMIC CONSIDERATIONS

The relationship of occupational etiologic factors with musculoskeletal disorders was recognized as early as the beginning of the 18th century, but the scientific evidence of work-related conditions has been collected only since the 1970s (NIOSH, 1997). There is controversy surrounding this relationship because of the multiple factors (e.g., physical, work organizational, psychosocial, individual, sociocultural) that contribute to these disorders (NIOSH, 1997). Traumatic injuries to the musculoskeletal system, such as fractures, dislocations, and tears, can result from a fall, direct blow, or other events that result in sudden tissue injury. However, occupational injuries related to ergonomic hazards are more commonly associated with repeated small injuries (i.e., microtears or microtrauma) that are related to the duration, frequency, and severity of exposures to ergonomic stressors. Table 3–1 lists occupational injuries and workers who are commonly affected by these injuries. As can be seen in Table 3–1, ergonomic-related injuries affect both the musculoskeletal system (e.g., carpal tunnel syndrome [CTS]) and systems outside the musculoskeletal system (e.g., hearing impairment). Because most work conditions occur over time, this discussion is limited to common cumulative trauma disorders involving orthopaedic problems.

Cumulative Trauma Disorders

Cumulative trauma disorders (also called repetitive strain injury or repetitive motion disorder) are associated with repetitive exertions and is currently the fastest growing cost concern in industry (Roughton, 1996). The cost in lost earnings and workers' compensation payments to industry is higher than any other health disorder (Zabel & McGrew, 1997). The tendons, muscles, and neurovascular system are the sites primarily affected by repeated trauma (Fig. 3–4). A number of specific associations of

TABLE 3–1. *Conditions Caused by Biomechanical and Environmental Stresses*

INJURY/SYMPTOMS	COMMONLY AFFECTED WORKERS
Back problems	Material handlers
Carpal tunnel syndrome or tendinitis	Clerical workers, assembly line workers, checkout workers, stamping job workers
Raynaud's phenomenon	Forestry workers, construction workers
Degenerative joint disease	Material handlers, forestry workers
Eyestrain resulting in fatigue	Clerical workers, foundry workers, high-precision assembly and inspection workers
Hearing impairment	Furnace operators, truck drivers, machinery operators, construction workers
Segmented vibratory diseases	Chainsaw, chipper, and jackhammer operators
Loss of strength, problems with hand-eye coordination, decreased mental capacity, fatigue	Most workers

From U.S. Department of Health and Human Services. (1991). *Occupational diseases: NIOSH instructional module* (No. 88-79896). Cincinnati: NIOSH, Division of Training and Manpower Development.

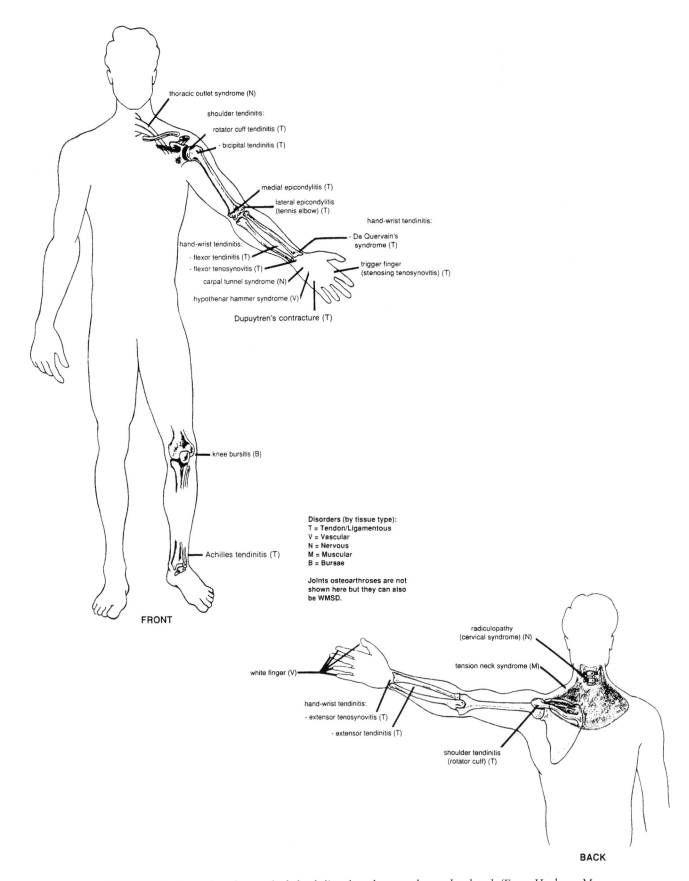

FIGURE 3–4. Examples of musculoskeletal disorders that may be work related. (From Hagberg, M., et al. [1995]. *Work related musculoskeletal disorders (WMSDs): A reference book for prevention* [pp. 22–23]. Bristol, PA: Taylor & Francis. Copyright 1995 by Taylor & Francis.)

cumulative trauma disorders with jobs and work-related activities that primarily involve the upper extremities, back and neck, and lower extremities are summarized in Table 3–2. Many of these conditions are seen together because work tasks involve an array of movements that increase the risk for multiple traumas. In addition, cumulative trauma disorders may be seen bilaterally. Although there may be several reasons for bilateral involvement, there are two more obvious reasons: First, people may be susceptible in both extremities. Second, discomfort in the affected extremity increases the risk for trauma in the opposite extremity because the worker uses the unaffected extremity while trying to protect the extremity with the problem.

Although an exact physiologic mechanism has not been identified, it is believed that repeated minor trauma with insufficient time for repair and recovery to specific body parts leads to irritation, swelling, pressure, tearing, and finally, scarring of tissue. Repetitive gripping, moving, static pinch or grip force, twisting, or reaching, especially in a forceful or awkward manner without sufficient rest, generally causes cumulative trauma disorders. The incidence of and emphasis on cumulative trauma disorders have increased in recent years because of

TABLE 3–2. *Common Cumulative Trauma Disorders*

DISORDER	TYPICAL JOB ACTIVITIES	MOVEMENTS TO AVOID
Upper Extremity Disorders		
Carpal tunnel syndrome	Belt conveyor or assembly work, bricklaying, carpentry, meat packing or butchering, typing and data input, using a cash register, sewing, cutting, packing, playing musical instruments, working in an operating room	Dorsal and palmar flexion, pinch grip, vibrations between 10 and 60 Hz
De Quervain's syndrome	Buffing and grinding, operating a punch press, sewing, cutting, packing, housekeeping, cooking, meat packing or butchering, working in an operating room	Combined forceful gripping and hard twisting
Lateral epicondylitis, or tennis elbow	Belt conveyor or assembly work, lumbering, construction	Wrist dorsiflexion and forceful wrist extension
Medial epicondylitis, or golfer's elbow	Belt conveyor or assembly work, lumbering, construction	Forceful rotation of the forearm, palm down, while bending or flexing the wrist at the same time
Rotator cuff tendinitis	Assembly work, food packing, clerical work	Inward or outward rotation or abduction of the arm
Trigger finger	Use of large tool handles that cause the phalanx of the finger to be flexed while the middle phalanx is straight	Flexion of distal phalanx alone
White finger syndrome, or Raynaud's phenomenon	Sanding, stone cutting, using handheld power tools, grinding, truck or bus driving	Vibrations between 40 and 125 Hz
Back and Neck Disorders		
Low-back pain	Handling materials, nursing, truck or bus driving	Poor postures, static postures, twisting, reaching
Tension neck syndrome	Operating video displays, welding, construction	Overhead reaching or static head, neck, and shoulder postures
Thoracic outlet syndrome	Carrying weights on shoulders and reaching behind the body (e.g., letter carriers, store checkout workers)	Overhead reaching, reaching behind, pushing or pulling, shoulder flexion, and arm hyperextension
Lumbar intervertebral disc syndrome	Material handlers, nursing, truck or bus driving	Poor postures, static postures, twisting, reaching
Lower Extremity Disorders		
Knee bursitis	Floor scrubbing, carpet laying, carpentry	Repeated kneeling
Achilles tendinitis	Ballet dancing, jumping	Repeated stretching and contraction of the tendon

media attention, increased production rates and computer use, and the increase of women and older workers in the workplace (Ostendorf, Rogers, & Bertsche, 2000). The only national source of data showing the magnitude of work-related musculoskeletal disorders is the Bureau of Labor Statistics (BLS) Annual Survey of Occupational Injuries and Illnesses. The BLS reported that cumulative trauma disorders accounted for nearly 66% of the work-related illness cases in 1998 (U.S. Department of Labor, 2000). Although each disorder has its own set of symptoms, a common aspect of all of them is that they develop gradually as a result of cumulative microtraumas rather than as a result of an acute macrotraumatic episode.

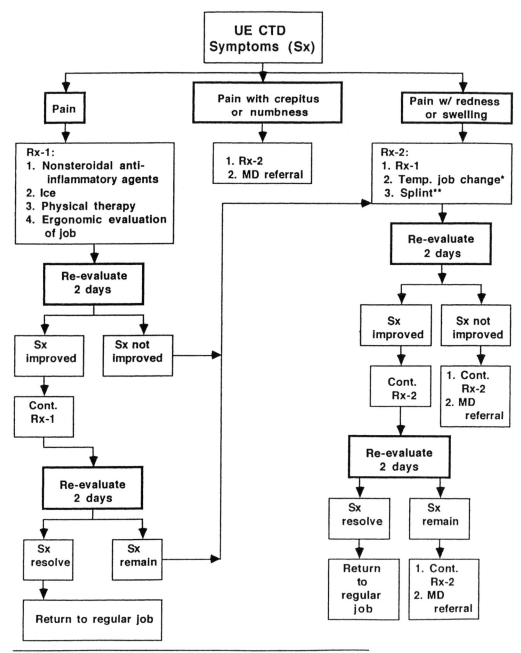

* *Transfer to a light duty job with no ergonomic risk factors.*
** *Use splint at work only if no wrist bending is required on the job.*
The splint should be used while the employee is not at work.

FIGURE 3–5. Algorithm of upper extremity (UE) cumulative trauma disorders (CTD). (From Hales, T. R., & Bertsche, P. K. [1992]. Management of upper extremity cumulative trauma disorders. *AAOHN Journal, 40,* 125. Copyright 1992 by SLACK Incorporated. Reprinted by permission of the American Association of Occupational Health Nurses.)

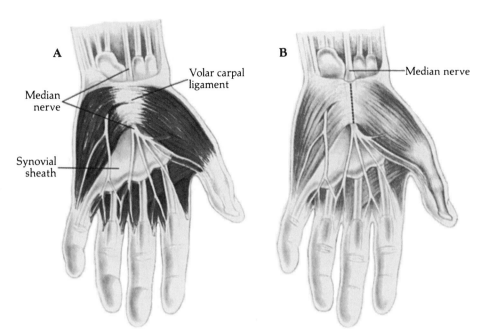

FIGURE 3–6. *A,* Wrist structures affected in carpal tunnel syndrome. *B,* Decompression of median nerve. (From Thompson, J. M. [1989]. *Mosby's manual of clinical nursing* [p. 435]. St. Louis: Mosby.)

The following sections review common cumulative trauma disorders of the upper extremities, back and neck, and lower extremities as they relate to ergonomics. Primary prevention of these disorders is considered in this chapter, but clinical management is discussed in the appropriate chapters of this book. Effective patient care requires coordination of patient and health management with workplace ergonomic considerations. Figure 3-5 gives an example of an algorithm combining these two considerations.

Upper Extremity Disorders

Carpal Tunnel Syndrome. A common site for cumulative trauma is the hand and wrist. Repetitive movements, such as wrist extension and flexion and ulnar and radial deviation of the wrist, are examples of postures that can affect the anatomic structures of the hand and wrist. CTS is the most common compression neuropathy affecting the hand. It is caused by increased pressure in the carpal tunnel resulting in compression of the median nerve, a relatively soft structure (Fig. 3-6). The carpal tunnel is a passageway in the wrist formed by the eight carpal bones and the transverse carpal ligament, stretching across the roof of the tunnel. Inside the carpal tunnel are nine flexor tendons to the digits as well as to the median nerve. The median nerve lies directly beneath the transverse carpal ligament and comes in contact with the ligament when bending or straightening the wrist or fingers. The tendons are structurally stronger than the median nerve. Inflammation of the tendons can restrict the space within the tunnel and cause the nerve to become pressed against the ligament forming the roof of the tunnel.

When the median nerve is pushed up against the ligament, blood flow to the nerve is restricted, causing pain, tenderness, numbness, tingling, or a feeling of "pins and needles" of the median nerve distribution (Fig. 3-7) (i.e., palmar side of the thumb and index and middle fingers and radial half of the ring finger). This numbness and tingling sensation often awakens the person at night, with relief obtained by hanging the hand in a dependent position or by shaking it. Often, there is a loss of grip strength. It is important to ask the patient what aggravates and what relieves the symptoms. Tinel's sign and Phalen's maneuver are important tests to be included in the assessment. There may be a positive Tinel's sign at the wrist, where the median nerve is located and compressed. A positive Phalen's maneuver, tingling of the fingers within 60 seconds with forced flexion of the wrist, is almost always present.

Therapeutic management of CTS is directed toward relieving the nerve compression. Conservative management usually involves rest of the hand and arm and avoidance of activities that may provoke further symptoms. Often, a splint that keeps the extremity in a neutral position is worn to prevent hyperextension and prolonged flexion of the wrist. Local injections of steroidal antiinflammatory agents are often helpful in reducing inflammation. Because CTS is also associated with conditions that cause an increase in fluid retention, such as diabetes, thyroid disease, or pregnancy, short-term treatment with diuretics can often relieve symptoms. Another conservative measure is the use of oral vitamins B_6 and C, although the relationship between vitamins and CTS symptom relief is conflicting (Franzblau, Rock, Werner, Albers, Kelly, & Johnston, 1996; Keniston,

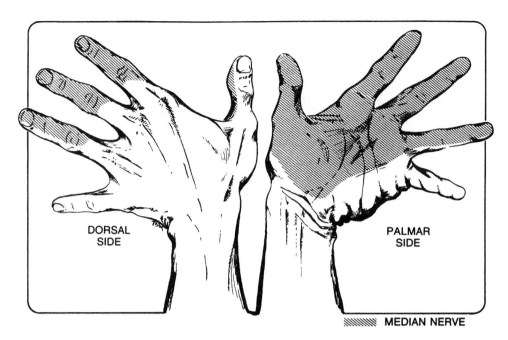

FIGURE 3–7. Median nerve distribution. Shaded areas typically affected by symptoms of carpal tunnel syndrome, which include tingling, numbness, and pain. (From Putz-Anderson, V. [Ed.]. [1988]. *Cumulative trauma disorders: A manual for musculoskeletal diseases of the upper limbs* [p. 19]. Bristol, PA: Taylor & Francis. Copyright 1988 by Taylor & Francis.)

Nathan, Leklem, & Lockwood, 1997). CTS is usually progressive, and when CTS does not respond to conservative measures, open carpal tunnel release (OCTR) to release the ligament forming the roof of the tunnel is indicated. Endoscopic carpal tunnel release (ECTR) was introduced in 1989 as an alternative to OCTR.

The best ergonomic solution for preventing CTS is to avoid the awkward, static positions and repetitive motions that create overloads to the muscular structures of the wrist. Designing tools and equipment so that the hand and wrist can be held in a neutral position while working can reduce awkward positions of the wrist (Carson, 1994). This is accomplished by ensuring that employees are at a proper height in relation to the task. Other approaches to reducing awkward positions of the wrist involve determining whether the work includes frequent reaching for items on a shelf or other work requiring static contractions of the muscles in the hand and wrist. The number of repetitions can be reduced by limiting work time, rotating employees, increasing the number of employees assigned to a particular task, providing mechanical assistance (e.g., automatic paper sorters and staplers), and encouraging employees to take frequent minibreaks for rest and to perform stretching exercises. One exercise approach is the seven-way stretch discussed by Pheasant (1991) (Box 3-5). Pheasant recommends holding each stretch for four deep breaths, slightly increasing the stretch with each breath.

Although the number of cases of CTS requiring days away from work has decreased since 1993, the median days away from work for CTS was 24 in 1998 (U.S. Department of Labor, 2000). A review of more than 30 epidemiologic studies revealed a positive association between highly repetitive or forceful work or work involving hand and wrist vibration and incidence of CTS (NIOSH, 1997). The association between CTS and extreme postures of the hand and wrist is insufficient based on the reviewed studies. Typists and other keyboard operators are particularly at risk of CTS developing. In addition, assembly line workers, carpenters, food preparers and packagers, and cashiers are also at risk (Andersson, Fine, & Silverstein, 2000; Kroemer, 1996).

Tendinitis and Tenosynovitis. The incidence of tendinitis (inflammation of a tendon) and tenosynovitis (inflammation of a tendon's lubricating sheath) has decreased since 1994 (U.S. Department of Labor, 2000). A review of several epidemiologic studies revealed a positive association between repetition, force, and posture and incidence of hand and wrist tendinitis; there is also strong evidence that jobs that require a combination of these risk factors increase the risk for hand and wrist tendinitis (NIOSH, 1997).

Several tendon disorders are associated with work, and each specific disorder is associated with the anatomic location of inflammation. Excessive friction occurs from thickening of the tendon sheath. The tendon sheath presses on the tendon, a condition known as stenosing tenosynovitis. *De Quervain's syndrome* is a stenosing tenosynovitis that involves the first dorsal compartment of

BOX 3–5.
Seven-Way Stretch Exercises

Stretch 1. Suboccipital Stretch

Clasp hands behind head. Bend head forward, gradually stretching out the upper part of the neck while breathing deeply, but keep the back and shoulder regions as straight as possible. Roll your head to one side, then the other, four times. This stretches the posterior neck muscles, particularly those in the suboccipital region (e.g., semispinalis capitis). The rotation at the end gives an additional stretch to the splenius.

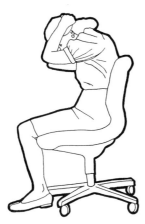

Stretch 2. Upper Trapezius Stretch

Grasp leg or seat of chair with right hand. Place palm of left hand above right ear (hand passes behind head). Pull head to left, laterally flexing neck. Repeat to the other side. This stretches the upper part of the trapezius muscle.

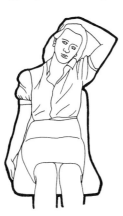

Stretch 3. Head and Neck Rotation

Balance head carefully with the shoulders dropped and arms folded behind your back. Turn head to left as far as it will go. Nod four times. Repeat to other side. This stretches the sternomastoid.

Stretch 4. Backward Shoulder Stretch

Clasp hands behind back. Reach out backward over chair back while expanding chest, arching back (hyperextension), and lifting hands. This stretches the muscles that protract the shoulders (e.g., pectorals).

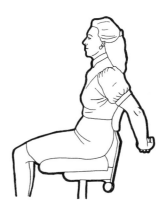

Stretch 5. Lumbar Twist

Cross left leg over right. Place outside of right elbow against outside of left knee. Place left hand behind back on left hip. Turn head, neck, and shoulders to the left as far as they will go, pressing with the right elbow. Hold for four breaths. Repeat other side. This stretches the back muscles, particularly multifidus lumborum.

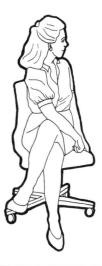

Courtesy S. Pheasant.

Box continued on following page

BOX 3–5.
Seven-Way Stretch Exercises Continued

Before Each of the Following Wrist Exercises, Shake the Hands Vigorously

Stretch 6. Wrist Extensor Stretch

Raise your left hand in front of your face and turn it into pronation (so that the palm faces away from you). Place the palm of your right hand on the back of your left hand and gently press your left wrist into full flexion, straightening your left elbow as you do so. This stretches the muscles of the extensor compartment of the forearm.

Stretch 7. Wrist Flexor Stretch

Place palms together as if praying. Raise elbows (thus extending wrists). Separate palms so that only fingertips are pressing together. This stretches the muscles of the flexor compartment of the forearm.

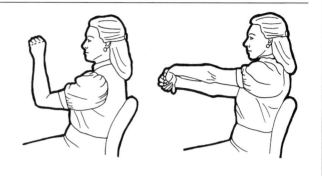

Courtesy S. Pheasant.

the wrist, affecting the tendons that help pull the thumb up and away from the hand. Another stenosing tenosynovitis is *trigger finger,* in which there is swelling of the finger tendon sheath or development of an enlarged nodule on the tendon. This results in the finger (or thumb) locking into position when bent because of the interference with normal motion.

The specific cause of tendinitis or tenosynovitis depends on the muscle-tendon system and the motion(s) that it controls. However, tendinitis and tenosynovitis are generally caused by repetitive, short-cycle tasks, such as those of the industrial assembly line, agricultural workers (e.g., cane cutters), typists, and keyboard users. *Epicondylitis* is caused by inflammation resulting from strain or overuse of the tendons of the wrist extensor muscles on the outer (lateral epicondylitis, or tennis elbow) or inner (medial epicondylitis, or golfer's elbow) side of the elbow. *Rotator cuff tendinitis,* or inflammation of one or all of the four rotator cuff muscles, results from repetitive or prolonged work with the arms at or above shoulder height. Both the elbow and shoulder tendons are unsheathed, and because of the imbalance between the large muscle size and small insertion area, the elbow and shoulder are particularly vulnerable to injuries caused by forceful and repetitious motions. The most damaging jobs are those that combine repetitive motions with forceful gripping actions with the wrist in a deviated position (e.g., butchering, meat packing).

Prevention of injury to the tendons and surrounding structures involves reducing exposure to the ergonomic risk factors by identifying high-risk jobs. Rapid or repetitive movements, forceful exertions, external mechanical force concentrations, awkward postures, vibration, and cold temperature should be avoided (Ranney, 1997).

Raynaud's Phenomenon. Raynaud's phenomenon, also known as *white finger syndrome* and *hand-arm vibration syndrome,* is a disorder resulting from direct injury to the blood vessels and nerves in the fingers (Hagberg et al., 1995). This disease is characterized by spasms of the digital arteries, which causes finger blanching. Attacks of vasospasm are more likely to occur with exposure to cold and can last for minutes to hours. Raynaud's phenomenon is caused by vibrations transmitted directly to the hands by tools, parts, or work surfaces. This injury is the most common example of an occupational injury caused by segmental vibration of the hands. Examples of tools that expose the hands to vibration include power saws, grinders, sanders, jackhammers, and other tools used in construction, mining, and industry. Redesign of the task or tool should be used to reduce or eliminate vibration exposure.

Back and Neck Disorders

Low-Back Pain. Low-back pain has been a complaint of humans since the times of the Egyptians 5000 years ago. It is estimated that up to 80% of adults will experience an episode of low-back pain requiring activity modification during their lifetime (Bigos, Bowyer, Braen, et al., 1994; NIOSH, 1997). According to the BLS, it is estimated that 56% of all workplace back injuries are caused by repeated trauma (U.S. Department of Labor, 1991). In 1998, back injuries accounted for 25.4% of occupational injuries and illnesses involving days away from work (U.S. Department of Labor, 2000). A review of more than 40 epidemiologic studies provided scientific evidence with respect to the relationship between low-back disorder and heavy physical work, lifting and forceful movements, bending and twisting (awkward postures), and whole-body vibration (NIOSH, 1997). The review provided insufficient evidence of a relationship of static work postures and low-back disorders. However, in the "Pathophysiology of Regional MSDs" in Appendix III of the *Proposed Ergonomics Standard* (Occupational Safety & Health Administration [OSHA], 2000), the point was made that maintenance of posture requires balancing of counteracting mechanical forces about the spine. Continuous static loading from prolonged postures may result in energy depletion and fatigue. Fatigued muscles result in additional load bearing by the intervertebral discs.

Back injury and pain result when the limits of maximal strain of the tissues (bone, cartilage, ligaments, and muscles) are exceeded. This may occur by a direct trauma, a single strenuous effort, or repeated or sustained loadings that add up to a cumulative overloading (Pope, Andersson, & Chaffin, 1991). Awkward, constrained postures produce muscle fiber spasm and consequent pain. The spasm is thought to constrict blood flow to the area, leading to a decrease in the supply of nutrients and oxygen to tissues and the buildup of toxic metabolic waste products that induce more spasm and pain (Herington & Morse, 1995). In most cases, low-back pain cannot be traced to one specific incident of overexertion (Kroemer, 1996).

Although degenerative joint disease of the spine occurs with normal aging, under some circumstances it may develop from and will definitely be aggravated by cumulative trauma. The compression force on the structures of the spine from weight bearing and excessive loading on the joints, vibration exposure, or continuous seated work may accelerate degeneration of the spine. Progression of the disease can be slowed or halted by preventing further repetitious and injurious movements and postures, as well as by providing proper seating for workstations. In addition, self-managed back protection, weight loss, and exercises designed to strengthen abdominal and back muscles and increase joint flexibility have been helpful in the prevention and relief of back pain in general.

Tension Neck Syndrome. Tension neck syndrome can be caused from prolonged sitting with the neck in a fixed or extreme position such as occurs with repetitive reaching without rest and repetitive or prolonged viewing that is too high or too low. A common complaint is constantly tilting the head up to see with bifocals (e.g., in video display terminal use). A possible solution to this problem is ordering bifocals with higher segment heights or progressive lenses. When the neck has been put in an extreme position or held flexed or extended over time, cervical degenerative disc disease can result (Herington & Morse, 1995). The most common complaint of workers is posterior neck pain or trapezius pain with some restriction of neck motion after prolonged sitting with the head fixed in one position. Workers should be instructed to avoid prolonged sitting with the neck in a fixed position

or holding the head or neck in extreme positions. Gentle range-of-motion exercises while at work should be taught (see Box 3–5 for exercise suggestions).

Thoracic Outlet Syndrome. One of the most common conditions involving the nerves and adjacent blood vessels is thoracic outlet syndrome. Like CTS, thoracic outlet syndrome involves peripheral nerve entrapment. Compression or irritation of the entire neurovascular bundle at the shoulder (subclavian vessels and the brachial plexus) causes pain at the neck and shoulder. The injury is caused from high static loads on the shoulders, neck, and back either directly or suspended from straps in satchels (e.g., letter carriers, students). Injury can also result from extreme postures of the shoulders, as in reaching overhead (e.g., ceiling painting) or reaching behind the body (e.g., supermarket checkout tasks). Anatomic anomalies of the thoracic inlet, such as cervical ribs, can increase one's risk of developing thoracic outlet syndrome. The risks involved for developing thoracic outlet syndrome can be reduced or eliminated by redesigning the job activities so that the body does not have to assume awkward or non-neutral postures, such as repeated reaching behind or holding the arms above the head for extended periods.

Lower Extremity Disorders

Repetitive friction or pressure between tendon or skin and bone may cause inflammation of these structures, with resultant swelling and thickening of the synovial wall. Jobs that require frequent kneeling, such as in carpet laying or domestic work, have been found to be associated with cumulative injuries, such as bursitis or tendinitis of the knee and hip. In addition to injuries of the tendons and surrounding structures, entrapment neuropathies can result from nerve compression at anatomically vulnerable sites. Repetitive motions or stressful, prolonged postures, such as crouching, squatting, or kneeling, can lead to stretching and subsequent ischemia of the nerve as it is squeezed between muscle edges. In addition, entrapment may result from direct compression against work surfaces or by wearing constrictive clothing. Although common sites of peripheral nerve entrapment are the sciatic, femoral, peroneal, posterior tibial, and interdigital nerves, the sciatic nerve is especially vulnerable to prolonged sitting on a hard surface or repeated hip extension (Castorina & Deyo, 1994). Ergonomic interventions are aimed at reducing the intensity, duration, and timing of exposures to the postures and work conditions that contribute to pressure on the nerves of the lower extremities.

Summary of Interventions

Musculoskeletal stress and strain result from static holding positions and static body positions. Workstations and work itself should be designed to avoid frequent and prolonged stooping, bending, and other extreme static work postures. Work activity should be rotated or interrupted by frequent rest periods. A simple intervention is to teach employees to do a stand-and-stretch exercise every 20 to 30 minutes to loosen the muscles, break up the constrained posture, and improve the blood flow and tendon lubrication in the affected area.

Exercises can be done at the workstation, take relatively little time to do, and can be helpful in preventing cumulative injuries. Micropauses as short as 1 to 2 minutes should be taken frequently over the workday during times when musculoskeletal stress builds up. Although specific exercises should be done based on the specific job demand, stretching exercises should be designed to relieve stress associated with awkward postures, highly repetitive tasks, and sedentary or static work. Exercises of the upper and lower extremities, shoulder, neck, and lumbar and thoracic regions of the back target the areas that become particularly stressed.

ERGONOMIC CONSIDERATIONS FOR PRACTICING NURSES

Musculoskeletal injuries, particularly back injuries, are highly prevalent in nursing. The reduction of ergonomic hazards associated with providing nursing care involves a proactive approach to safety. Because nurses do not work with people who have fixed sizes and shapes, the application of ergonomics to nursing is in many ways different from applications in other fields, where the focus of the work can be redesigned. The model in Figure 3–8 represents the interaction of the nurse, client, and equipment within the work organization, work environment, and workspace. In nursing, the interaction is not only with the equipment but also with a client, who may be interacting with the equipment as well. For example, bedside tables are designed for the client to use but often present limitations of workspace for nursing tasks. Because the interaction in nursing includes the client as well as the nurse, an unresolved ergonomic dilemma is presented that involves the needs of the client and the needs of the nurse. Therefore, in the nursing profession, consideration must be given to both nursing ethics and the health and safety of the client as well as the nurse.

Although health and safety and management personnel should be interested in and actively pursue approaches to providing safe working conditions, practicing nurses should also be aware of and offer solutions to ergonomic hazards. Attention to workplace design, job design, and worker capacity may not eliminate all injuries, but it can have a substantial effect in reducing the risk of many injuries.

Workplace Design

Space Limitations. Enough space should be provided to accommodate the full range of required movements needed to carry out nursing tasks. Postures should

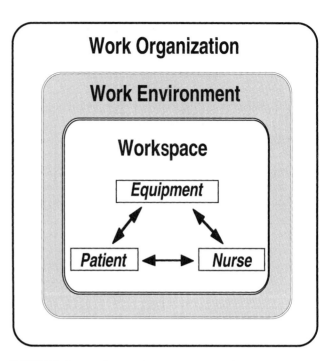

FIGURE 3–8. Work considerations in providing nursing care. (From Stubbs, D. A. [1987]. Introduction . . . ergonomics in healthcare. *International Journal of Nursing Studies, 24,* 287. Copyright 1987. With permission from Elsevier Science Ltd., The Boulevard, Langford Lane, Kidlington OX5, IGB, UK.)

be unrestricted so that motion is smooth and continuous. The layout of a building or room cannot be changed easily, but small changes in modifying the layout of furniture and equipment within the facility can improve safety for both nursing staff and clients. Bedside tables and chairs can be placed so that the posture of the nursing staff is unrestricted. In providing care for clients who need nursing assistance, additional equipment (e.g., wheelchairs, walkers) should be stored in a closet or other designated area rather than adding to the number of items already at the bedside. Bathrooms and toilet facilities are small areas in many nursing care facilities, adding to physical restrictions. The support equipment required by many clients further limits space. Although supportive equipment, such as monitors and ventilators, is smaller, it still takes space in an already restricted room. When clients need assistance in small areas, it is ergonomically desirable to use additional equipment for transfers that will ensure the safety of both client and nurse. Placement of needed items and equipment should be within easy reach of the nurse but out of the way when direct nursing care, such as turning, lifting, and transferring clients, is done. Equipment placed on wheels can be easily moved out of the way so that unrestricted nursing maneuvering can be performed.

Visual Considerations. Visual comfort and ergonomics may significantly affect working capacity and may lead to other injury risks from positioning the body to compensate for poor visual fields. Proper vision requires both sufficient quantity and quality of illumination. Visual comfort requires pleasant luminance levels that can be adjusted to accommodate the level needed for specific tasks of nursing care. Excessive illumination that causes glare can lead to eyestrain and general fatigue. For example, it is recommended that the illumination level at the computer workstation be lower to reduce glare from the monitor screen, or an antiglare screen can be used (Kroemer, 1996). A task lamp may be used to read the source document. Indirect lighting should therefore be used when greater levels of luminance are needed, such as when physically assessing a client, and concentrated luminance directed at a specific focus but away from the nurse's eyes could be used for such tasks as inserting a urinary catheter. While a client is being interviewed, soft lighting may have a relaxing effect on the client and may also provide a period when illumination is not contributing to the length of time the nurse is subjected to excessive luminance levels.

Visual targets, such as monitor displays, should be placed so that the head posture is comfortable, which means that surfaces to be viewed should be at eye level or lower. Not only does this result in a more healthful head posture, but also eye irritation from restricted blinking is reduced.

It is important for the nurse to pay attention to how the eyes feel during the course of work. Stressful working conditions cause tension around the eyes. Relaxation of the eye and facial muscles can be achieved by frequent exercises, such as blinking, rolling the eyes in gentle circles, or looking around and refocusing (Doheny, Linden, & Sedlak, 1995).

Staff Considerations. Understaffing, lack of peer support, and stress have been identified as contributors to nurses' lifting injuries (Laflin & Aja, 1995). Nursing staff working on understaffed units are exposed to repeated and more intense client lifting and transferring activities. Biomechanical stress created during repeated lifting and transferring of clients is believed to be a major contributing factor to back pain (Zhuang, Stobbe, Hsiao, Collins, & Hobbs, 1999). Exposure to other ergonomic hazards is also increased when patient units are understaffed. For example, nursing staff will undoubtedly be subjected to more reaching and bending activities.

Fatigue, involving both psychological and physiologic factors, has been defined as the transient inability to continue work at the same rate as previously, influencing an individual's motivation and capacity for work (Hagberg et al., 1995). General fatigue often accompanies prolonged strenuous physical efforts but can also result from physiologic and psychological stress and disruption of normal circadian rhythm (such as occurs in night workers). Localized muscle fatigue resulting from static and dynamic work depends on the frequency and intensity of muscular contraction (Astrand & Rodahl, 1986).

Although both prolonged dynamic work and static work cause localized muscle fatigue, the onset of localized muscle fatigue takes longer to develop with dynamic than with static work (Moore, 1994). Staffing patterns can have a positive effect on the development of both generalized and local muscular fatigue. During hours when work demands are the greatest, more staff is needed to reduce the psychological stress and to spread the strenuous activities among more individuals. In positions in which more static work and postures occur, such as in the operating room or emergency room, it is desirable to schedule staff so that jobs can be interchanged and static work can be interrupted by more dynamic work during a shift.

The occurrence of work-related stress is increasing, as is long-term exposure to work conditions that exceed workers' ability to meet or master the demands of work, such as excessive workload. Scientific evidence supports the relationship between occupational stress and a wide range of health effects, such as heart and cerebrovascular disease and musculoskeletal problems (Baker & Karasek, 2000). Nursing activities are determined by the clients' needs. In addition, sustained attentiveness and alertness are vital to the safety of that care. The inability of nursing staff to modify the pace or content of their activities is a major source of occupational stress. Stress can also be caused by monotony, in which the job demand is below the individual's capacity or in which the work environment has little change; by negative interpersonal aspects of work such as job security and growth opportunities; and by organizational characteristics such as climate, culture, and communications (NIOSH, 2000). Restructuring and reorganizing health care facilities can have a negative effect on work organization and ergonomics (Carayon & Smith, 2000). Choosing nursing staff to fill nursing jobs requires a good match between job demands and the individual's physical and mental capacity. In addition to maintaining numbers of staff necessary to fit the work demand to the nurse's work capabilities, several modest changes can be implemented to reduce occupational stress. These changes include increasing worker control in staffing decisions, restructuring work, implementing social support interventions, encouraging exercise, and providing problem-oriented coping in-services (e.g., time management and stress reduction methods).

Work-related disruption of the body's normal physiologic balance may also contribute to occupational stress. A prerequisite for human health is a state of balanced control, called *homeostasis*. Many of the body's physiologic functions occur in rhythmic cycles, or circadian rhythms, rather than at a constant steady state. Many nursing jobs, especially those in hospitals and extended care facilities, require shift work. Shift work includes working long-term night shifts or rotating among day, evening, and night shifts. When shift work extends into hours that would normally be spent sleeping, the worker's circadian rhythms may be disrupted. Working the night shift has been found to be disruptive of circadian rhythms and has been associated with increased errors, illnesses, and injuries (Åkerstedt & Knutsson, 2000; Coburn & Sirois, 1999; Kawachi, Colditz, Stampfer, Willett, Manson, Speizer, & Hennekins, 1995).

Nursing staffing patterns have recently included a compressed work week, in which staff typically work 10- or 12-hour shifts 3 or 4 days per week, allowing workers to have 3 or 4 days off work each week. Because of nursing shortages, mandatory overtime is increasingly necessary. There have been concerns about fatigue from long work periods and resulting reduced cognitive ability, performance, and safety because of long workdays (Institute of Medicine, 1996; Lipscomb & Borwegen, 2000). Kroemer, Kroemer, and Kroemer-Elbert (1994) recommend that work duration not be more than 8 hours (especially in physically demanding jobs), that the number of consecutive night shifts be as small as possible, and that each cycle of night shift work be followed by at least 24 hours of free time. Because it is easier to adjust to a delay in sleep rather than to a shorter period of wake time, rotating shifts should be scheduled in the direction of the delay of rhythms (i.e., working later each day). Workers who are assigned to a permanent shift may adjust their internal rhythms to accommodate the shift. However, it should be emphasized that for workers working the night shift, the arrangement is not entirely permanent. Days off from work interrupt the work/rest pattern of the night shift sleep/wake routine. Some individuals appear to be more able to adjust to these deviations in the work/rest pattern than other workers. Åkerstedt and Knutsson (2000) recommend good sleep hygiene (e.g., using ear plugs; sleeping in a cool, dark room; turning the ringer on the phone off) and strategic sleeping between 2 and 9 PM or morning sleep with a 2-hour nap in the evening.

Flextime, a somewhat more flexible arrangement of work time, has been used in industry and allows the worker to distribute hours of working time over a specified period. Although flextime requires cooperation between the nursing manager and staff nurse, the staffing arrangement has generally been appealing in other occupational settings (Kroemer et al., 1994). In addition to reducing worker fatigue, flextime has increased job satisfaction and productivity and has reduced tardiness, absenteeism, and employee turnover. The workforce size can adjust to short-term fluctuations in work demand by using flextime staffing patterns. This advantage is particularly appealing in hospital settings where there are seasonal fluctuations in the demand for nursing staff.

Job Design

Work (re)organization and work (re)design are important ergonomic considerations in recognizing and alleviating potentially injurious activities and conditions. Often, employee selection and training are used to reduce the frequency of injury from ergonomic job hazards. Al-

though employee selection and training have been useful approaches for safer and more efficient work, these approaches focus on fitting the person to the job. The best method for reducing injury uses the ergonomic approach of fitting the job to the workers. One of the challenges of using this ergonomic approach is to design jobs that fit multiple workers. Knowledge of the specific job tasks and the employees' capabilities and limitations is necessary to redesigning jobs to fit the worker(s). Accessible equipment and supplies, chair designs to promote more healthful postures, and the use of mechanical lifting aids are all ergonomic interventions that lead to a reduction in acute and cumulative injuries to nurses and their assistants.

Accessibility. *Accessibility* refers to the ease of obtaining materials used to provide nursing care. This factor includes both clearance for accomplishing work and reach of supplies and equipment. Adequate clearance considers legroom, headroom, elbowroom, and access to confined spaces. The region or arc of healthy reach is determined by the length of an arc made by the arm as it rotates about the shoulder joint. Nurses spend a large portion of their time in postural stress, such as stooping or rotated trunk positions, because they must reach for objects that are beyond the zone of normal convenience. In a study examining anthropometric aspects of workstation design, Pheasant (1987) found several design problems associated with nursing, including inadequate space for task performance; seated workstations with inadequate legroom; and the need to reach over obstacles, equipment, controls, and working surfaces that were too high or too low. Because nurses are primarily women, who are shorter than men, sinks, cabinets, and working surfaces may need to be lower than that for the average person.

The hospital bed in many ways can be considered a workstation for the performance of nursing tasks. Most hospital beds have adjustable heights. The nurse's choice of an acceptable working height of a hospital bed depends on the task to be performed, keeping work within the comfort zone (see Fig. 3–2). Generally, height is measured using the fingertips, knuckle, elbow, and shoulder as anatomic landmarks when the arm is held at the side of the body. Pheasant (1987) summarizes acceptable bed heights for the performance of nursing tasks. For heavy lifting and handling tasks involving clients, the surface of the mattress should be somewhere between knuckle and elbow height. Below knuckle height, lifting and handling tasks would need to be performed with the nurse in a stooped position. In a study of client handling activities, Lee and Chiou (1994) found that nurses' strength was greatest when the bed surface height was at the level of the nurse's iliac crest. Delicate tasks, such as inserting an angiocatheter, may be performed with the nurse sitting in a chair at the bedside, with the height of the bed high enough that the nurse's knees are under the bed. Considering client safety, the bed is adjusted to its lowest position after the task is completed.

Sitting Posture and Chair Design.
Energy consumption and circulatory strain are lower when the body is in a sitting position as opposed to standing. Because the chair seat supports most of the body's weight, strain is generally limited to the torso and upper extremities. The posture of the seated person depends on the individual's sitting habits, the design of the chair, and the task to be performed. Good sitting posture requires that the weight of the spinal column, torso, and head be kept on the pelvis. The spinal column is straight from the front view but maintains the natural S-curve in the side view. That is, lordosis (forward curve) is maintained in the cervical and lumbar regions, and kyphosis (backward curve) is maintained in the thoracic region of the spine. However, good sitting posture is a dynamic process, not a static position. Because muscle tension, discomfort, and fatigue result from maintaining the trunk posture over long periods, the sitting posture should be changed frequently. Doing standing stretches; walking; and moving the head, trunk, arms, and legs can accomplish this.

The seat designed with a forward slope, low-back support, and armrests promotes the normal curves of the back and reduced disc pressure. This is probably because some of the upper body weight is transferred to the back and armrests of the chair (Andersson, Chaffin, & Pope, 1991). The chair height should be adjusted so that the elbows are about even with the work surface. Leg support, with the feet resting firmly on the floor (or on a small stool for shorter people), is critical to the distribution and reduction of weight on the buttocks and back of the thighs.

Manual Lifting Considerations.
Musculoskeletal injuries continue to be a serious problem for nurses and nursing assistants. The frequency and cumulative nature of biomechanical stress from manual handling tasks make back injuries a particularly important problem (Owen, Welden, & Kane, 1999). Box 3-6 identifies the

---

BOX 3–6.

Basic Nursing Situations Involving the Transfer of Clients

Lifting a client from a wheelchair to a bed, and vice versa
Lifting a client from the floor to a bed
Lifting a client from a stretcher to a bed, and vice versa
Adjusting the position of a client lying in bed
Supporting a client above the bed
Removing a client from a bathtub
Assisting a client from a commode to a chair

---

lifting and transfer situations common to nursing practice.

The frequency and intensity of client handling are associated with the incidence and prevalence of back pain and injury in nursing (Collins & Owen, 1996; Smedley, Egger, Cooper, & Coggon, 1995). Specific client handling tasks associated with back injuries have been transferring, lifting, and bathing clients (Owen et al., 1999). Because of excessive static loading on the spine, particularly harmful is the use of the underaxilla method of lifting (Garg, Owen, & Carlson, 1992; Owen, Keene, Olson, & Garg, 1995; Owen et al., 1999). There is scientific evidence that training in the correct use of body mechanics does not reduce the incidence of occupational back injuries of health care personnel (Daltroy, 1997; Lagerstrom & Hagberg, 1997). These findings may reflect the fact that nurses often perform lifts and other tasks in confined work environments (e.g., bathrooms or rooms where space is reduced because of equipment), where the situation inhibits proper body mechanics. Lifting stress is magnified because of awkward body postures assumed because of limited space and consequent inability to move the feet. Therefore, the nurse must identify potential client and environmental obstacles to moving and lifting clients in each lifting situation. Kjellberg, Johnsson, Proper, Olsson, and Hagberg (2000) developed a reliable and valid observation instrument for assessment of client transfers. Box 3-7 lists the considerations from Kjellberg et al.'s instrument for the preparation phase, starting position, and actual performance in transferring clients.

Often, nurses have another person assist in lifting. Some may believe that this practice divides the weight to be lifted in half, but this assumption is not true. Although the load to be lifted may be more stable and balanced when two or more persons assist in lifting, the timing of lifting is not exactly the same, particularly when the load is a person and difficult to grasp and handle (Kroemer et al., 1994). The safe limit of two people is only about two thirds of their combined individual total strengths in dynamic lifting and less if lifting uses static exertion or when more than two persons cooperate in the lift (Karawowski & Pongpatanasuegsa, 1988). Even if teamwork had an additive effect, two-person manual lifting of most clients has been found to exceed the spinal compressive force limits set by NIOSH (Laflin & Aja, 1995; Owen & Garg, 1993).

The ideal ergonomic solution to prevent back and other musculoskeletal injuries from lifting tasks is for an organization to adopt a no-lift policy. Client lifting, transferring, and repositioning would be done with mechanical aids, such as hydraulic or electric lifts (Fig. 3-9), gait or transfer belts (Fig. 3-10), and slide or transfer boards (Fig. 3-11). Turning sheets are also helpful for positioning people in bed. Researchers have found that low-back pain and injury were not associated with man-

BOX 3–7.

Considerations for Client Transferring and Lifting

Preparation Phase
1. The nurse encourages the client to cooperate.
2. The nurse creates enough space around the transfer.
3. The nurse corrects positions of objects that client is transferred between.
4. The nurse corrects the height of the bed.
5. The nurse uses a transferring aid.
6. The nurse corrects positions of transferring aids.
7. The nurse carries out the transfer alone.

Starting Position
8. Feet distance
9. Feet position
10. Gait position
11. Left knee bending
12. Right knee bending
13. Back sagittal bending
14. The nurse has a curved back.

Actual Performance
15. The nurse(s) start(s) after a starting sign.
16. The nurse stimulates the client verbally during the transfer.
17. Effort direction
18. Back motion
19. Main motor components
20. If legs are the motor component, in what way are they used?
21. Does the nurse move the feet in the direction of the movement?
22. The quality of motion
23. Performance of transfer
24. Is there a sudden loss of balance?

Adapted from Kjellberg, K., Johnsson, C., Proper, K., Olsson, E., & Hagberg, M. (2000). An observation instrument for assessment of work technique in patient transfer tasks. *Applied Ergonomics, 31,* 139–150. With permission from Elsevier Science.

ual handling activities when mechanized client transfers were used (Elford, Straker, & Strauss, 2000; Smedley et al., 1995; Zhuang, Stobbe, Collins, Hsiao, & Hobbs, 2000). The choice of product will depend on its suitability for the task. Shape, size, weight, and stability of the load; available space; and the individual needs of the client should also be considered. Finally, training in the correct use of the equipment is essential.

If manual lifting cannot be avoided, the object or person to be lifted could be raised so that the nurse does not have to bend to lift. Relying on principles of leverage rather than muscle strength reduces injury risk when lifting and transferring clients. Canadian nurses have decreased their musculoskeletal injury rates by combining the transfer belt with a transfer technique that uses the nurse's body as a lever (Haley, 1994) (Fig. 3–12). In this one-person lifting technique, the nurse's center of mass is matched to the client's center of mass, and leverage counterbalances the client's weight. The method can be adapted for two-person transfers, getting a fallen client off the floor, and routine nursing lifting and moving tasks, such as moving a client up in bed or from a lying to a sitting position.

It is the nurse's responsibility to know his or her individual lifting and handling capabilities and limitations. In addition, nurses need to assess information about the load, such as the weight of the client, the client's physical and mental condition, and the amount of cooperation that can be expected from the client. For example, a client who has been cooperative lying in bed may experience pain with moving and suddenly become uncooperative with a transfer because of the natural protective reactions to the pain. Nurses can reduce the episodes of unexpected situations that put them at risk for injury by thoroughly assessing the client and situations that involve moving and transferring. Measures nurses may take to help make lifting and transferring activities safer for the client and the nurse include explanations to the client about how he or she is to be moved, what equipment will be used to provide assistance, what the client is expected to do to help, and what the potential for pain is.

Rogers (1994) identifies key elements of an ergonomically safe working environment to include "proper work techniques, employee conditioning, regular monitoring, feedback, maintenance, adjustments and modifications, and enforcement" (p. 145). More attention by nurses to the principles of ergonomics is essential so that they can better assess and plan interventions with ergonomic solutions to their recovery and protection from future hazards. In addition, the practice of nursing has a number of ergonomic hazards, and nurses must be more proactive in deciding how they will effect changes to make a safer workplace. The relatively favorable working conditions of today have not eliminated the risks imposed on the musculoskeletal system. Knowledge of ergonomic risk factors related to the workplace is necessary so that nurses can effectively evaluate the causes of musculoskeletal problems and assist in planning interventions that will prevent injuries in the future.

Worker Capacity

The ergonomic approach to employee health is to reorganize the workplace and job demands on the worker rather than attempt to improve worker capacity for the job. However, this approach overlooks consideration of the role of improved physical fitness in narrowing the gap between job demands and worker capabilities. Important worker characteristics that appear to be protective of job-related musculoskeletal injury include physical capabilities of the worker, weight control, and use of proper

EXAMINING THE EVIDENCE: Moving Toward Evidence-Based Practice
Can Back Stress from Transferring Patients Be Reduced through an Ergonomic Approach?

AUTHOR(S), YEAR	SAMPLE SIZE	ACTIVITY	DESIGN	OUTCOME VARIABLE	MAJOR FINDINGS
Charney, 1997	N = 9 acute care and 1 long-term care facilities	Professional patient movers as a "lift team" for all total body lifting Mechanical lifts were always used	Quasiexperimental Before and after team comparisons	Back injuries Number of lost work days Incidence rates	69% back injury reduction 62.5% incidence rate reduction 90% lost work day reduction
Garg & Owen, 1992	N = 57 nursing assistants	Multiple transferring tasks	Prospective quasiexperimental Before and after ergonomic intervention comparison	Perceived physical exertion Compression forces to the lumbar spine and mean forces exerted by the hands	Perceived exertion less after the intervention Back injury incidence reduced almost in half
Owen & Fragala, 1999	N = 13 nursing assistants	Transferring non-weight-bearing residents from bed to chair and chair to bed	Nonexperimental Comparison of methods	Perceived physical exertion of CNAs Perceived comfort and security of residents	CNAs perceived significantly decreased exertion using a friction-reducing transfer pad and ergonomically designed chair than traditional methods of transfer Residents reported feeling more secure and comfortable with the transfer pad and chair than with the traditional method
Owen & Garg, 1994	N = 6 female senior nursing students	Weighing a patient with a chair scale	Nonexperimental Comparison of methods	Perceived physical stress and biophysical measures of compressive forces for shoulder, upper and lower back, and whole body	Using a ramp scale and hoist with a digital scale resulted in reduced perceived physical stress than manually lifting a patient onto a scale Manual lifting resulted in greater compressive and shear force than the two ergonomic methods
Elford et al., 2000	N = 22 nurses	Chair-to-chair transfer	Nonexperimental Comparison of methods	Perceived physical stress and lifter preference Motion analysis to register angular displacement, velocity, and acceleration for lumbar motion	Biomechanical stress significantly greater in transfers using no patient handling sling than when one or two slings were used Total-body stress ratings for the one- and two-sling methods were less than half the ratings for the no-sling method First preference was using the patient handling sling
Zhuang et al., 1999	N = 9 nursing assistants	Transferring nursing home residents from a supine position on a bed to an upright position in a chair	Experimental Comparison of methods	Motion analysis to register body postures and joint angles of nursing assistants Compressive forces	Transfers without using assistive devices cause excessive biomechanical stress compared to using devices Compared with manual transfer, the use of basket-sling and overhead lifts significantly reduced back-compressive forces during transferring preparation stage (lifting/rolling/rotating) Basket-sling lifts required significantly larger pushing forces than other devices; sliding board required significantly larger pushing force than other devices; no statistical differences in turning forces among the basket-sling and stand-up lifts Resident weight was an important factor in hand force

CNAs, certified nurse assistants.

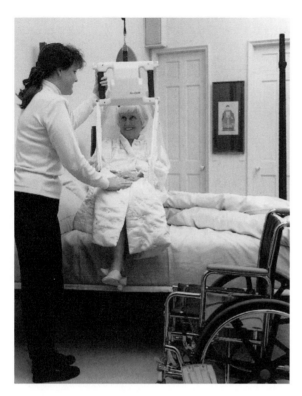

FIGURE 3–9. An electric lift for transferring client from bed to chair. (Courtesy Gaper Products Ltd., 18-4060 Ridgeway Drive, Mississauga, Ontario, Canada L5L 5X9.)

body mechanics (Blue, 1996). Proper body mechanics have been discussed throughout this chapter.

Physical Capabilities. An individual's capability may be limited by muscular strength, by the ability for movement of the body's joints, and by the ability to maintain work for prolonged periods without experiencing fatigue. The level, duration, and frequency of the loads imposed on tissues and the adequacy of recovery time determine a worker's tolerance or intolerance and determine whether the worker is susceptible for musculoskeletal injury (OSHA, 2000). For nurses, strength, flexibility, and coordination may be the most important aspects of physical fitness (Legg, 1987). Owen (1986) found that nurses who paticipated in aerobic physical activities and those who rated themselves to be in better physical condition were less likely to have back injuries than other nurses. The basic premise is that the risk of overexertion injury decreases as the worker's capacity to meet job demands increases. Although evidence supporting this suggestion is minimal, muscular strength and endurance may help prevent muscular strain and fatigue associated with prolonged static positions, as well as overall fatigue from prolonged strenuous labor (Blue, 1996). For specific exercises to increase joint flexibility and muscle strength, the reader is referred to Blue (1996).

Scientific evidence is insufficient at this time to conclude that overall physical health prevents work-related injuries (OSHA, 2000). However, a body that is generally in a healthy state reduces the gap between a person's capability and job demands. Because the physiologic stress from lifting or holding a given weight is directly proportional to the strength needed for these activities, enhancement of muscular strength and endurance would increase an individual's ability to perform such tasks with reduced physiologic stress (American College of Sports Medicine, 1991). In addition, adequate muscular performance is necessary for the maintenance of healthful postures.

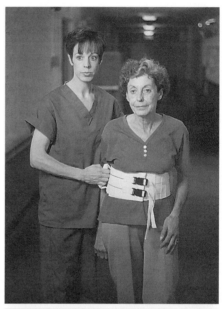

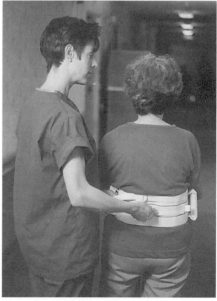

FIGURE 3–10. Example of an ergonomically designed gait/ transfer belt. (Courtesy J. T. Posey Company, Arcadia, California.)

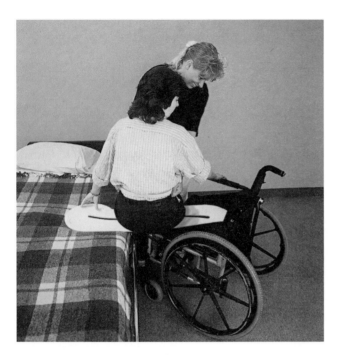

FIGURE 3–11. Example of a slide board for transferring clients. (Courtesy Beatrice M. Brantman, Inc., BeasyTrans Easy Transfer Systems, 207 E. Westminster, Lake Forest, IL 60045.)

Innovations and Future Trends

In recent years, there has been an increase in research dealing with the identification of ergonomic risk factors. For example, the most risky methods of transferring clients have been identified (Collins & Owen, 1996), and it has been found that work that creates intracarpal pressure is a causal factor in the development of CTS (OSHA, 2000). What is now needed are more studies that demonstrate the effectiveness of ergonomic interventions aimed at reducing the adverse health effects of the worker's environment.

The availability of scientific evidence pertaining to work-related musculoskeletal disorders has prompted OSHA to propose a national ergonomic standard targeting jobs in manufacturing and manual handling jobs in the general industry sector (OSHA, 2000). The standard is projected to prevent more than 4.6 million musculoskeletal disorders in 10 years, saving $9.1 billion annually. Under the OSHA proposal, employers will need to implement a "basic ergonomics program" that includes (1) job hazard analysis and control; (2) information to employees about the risk of injuries, signs and symptoms of musculoskeletal disorders, and importance of early reporting of injuries; (3) injury management; and (4) periodic program evaluation. Through thorough assessment, nurses can take an active role in identifying the role of work environment to injuries presented by clients. In addition, nurses are valuable resources to workers and their work sites in teaching aspects of injury prevention and rehabilitation with respect to ergonomic factors.

The increase in technology and informatics in our society will add to the already alarming rate of injuries, particularly to the upper extremities, neck, and hip, as more people use a computer workstation in the home and at work. Children and young adults, especially, are using computers during large proportions of their day. The long-term effect on their bodies is unknown. In addition, the computer has helped create a sedentary future workforce that may have physically inactive jobs. Their diminished physical fitness may affect their health if their physical capacity does not meet their future work demands.

The importance of ergonomics cannot be overemphasized. Modifying or redesigning the work site will optimize the use of energy and allow the working

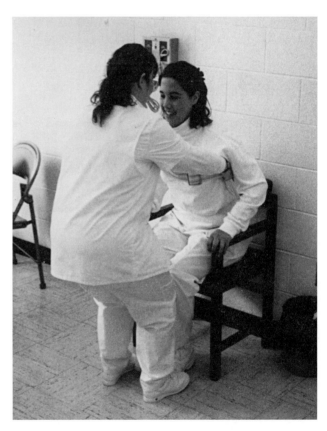

FIGURE 3–12. An approach to lifting using the body as a lever.
1. Place the transfer belt over the nipple line of the client.
2. Position your body directly in front of the client, and grasp the belt on either side of the client. Arms are kept straight and wrists kept in neutral position. The head should be straight with the chin held in.
3. Place your knees in front of and touching the client's knees to prevent the client from slipping or collapsing. This blocking provides the pivot point around which the leverage will act.

Straighten your arms under the client's shoulders, lower your pelvis (the center of mass), and then lean back, letting your body weight and leg muscles exert the lifting force on the client. You should not be using the muscles of your upper body.

population to perform their jobs safely. Worker training in initiated changes is imperative. Because we live in a technologically advanced society, more technical changes are being introduced into the work site than ever before. In addition, ergonomic research is revealing more scientific evidence with respect to work-related injuries. Occupational health nurses are vital to addressing ergonomic problems in the workplace. However, all nurses who have knowledge about ergonomic risk factors are valuable assets in assessing clients, assisting with changing the work environment, and rehabilitating injured workers. In addition, nursing is one of the highest-risk jobs for musculoskeletal injuries. An awareness of ergonomic factors in the nurse's own practice is essential to be proactive in preventing work-related injuries.

INTERNET RESOURCES

American Academy of Orthopaedic Surgeons: www. aaos.org

Cornell University Ergonomics Web: CUErgo: http:// ergo.human.cornell.edu/

Ergonomics Society: www.ergonomics.org.uk/

ErgoWeb: www.ergoweb.com/

Human Factors and Ergonomics: Usernomics: www. usernomics.com/hf.html

Human-Computer Interaction Resources on the Net: www.ida.liu.se/labs/aslab/groups/um/hci

Human-Computer Interaction Sites Links: www.hcibib. org/hci-sites

Injury Control Resource Information Network: www. injurycontrol.com/icrin/

National Institute of Occupational Safety and Health: www.cdc.gov/niosh/

Occupational Safety Engineering: http://turva.me.tut. fi/english/indexeng.html

REFERENCES

Åkerstedt, T., & Knutsson, A. (2000). Shift work. In B. S. Levy & D. H. Wegman (Eds.), *Occupational health: Recognizing and preventing work-related disease and injury* (4th ed., pp. 437–445). Philadelphia: Lippincott Williams & Wilkins.

American College of Sports Medicine. (1991). *Guidelines for exercise testing and prescription* (4th ed.). Philadelphia: Lea & Febiger.

Andersson, G. B. J., Chaffin, D. B., & Pope, M. H. (1991). Occupational biomechanics of the lumbar spine. In M. H. Pope, G. B. J. Andersson, J. W. Frymoyer, & D. B. Chaffin (Eds.), *Occupational low back pain: Assessment, treatment and prevention* (pp. 20–43). St. Louis: Mosby.

Andersson, G. B. J., Fine, L. J., & Silverstein, B. A. (2000). Musculoskeletal disorders. In B. S. Levy & D. H. Wegman (Eds.), *Occupational health: Recognizing and preventing work-related disease and injury* (4th ed., pp. 503–535). Philadelphia: Lippincott Williams & Wilkins.

Astrand, P., & Rodahl, K. (1986). *Textbook of work physiology*. New York: McGraw-Hill.

Baker, D. B., & Karasek, R. A. (2000). Stress. In B. S. Levy & D. H. Wegman (Eds.), *Occupational health: Recognizing and preventing work-related disease and injury* (4th ed., pp. 419–436). Philadelphia: Lippincott Williams & Wilkins.

Bigos, S. J., Bower, O., Braen, G., et al. (1994). *Acute low-back problems in adults. Clinical practice guideline number 14* (Publication #95-0642). Rockville, MD: Agency for Health Care Policy and Research, Public Health Service, U.S. Department of Health and Human Services.

Blue, C. L. (1996). Preventing back injury among nursing personnel: The worker and the worksite. *Orthopaedic Nursing, 15,* 9–20.

Carayon, P., & Smith, M. J. (2000). Work organization and ergonomics. *Applied Ergonomics, 31,* 649–662.

Carson, R. (1994). Reducing cumulative trauma disorder. *AAOHN Journal, 42,* 270–276.

Castorina, J. S., & Deyo, R. A. (1994). Back and lower extremity disorders. In L. Rosenstock & M. R. Cullen (Eds.). *Textbook of Clinical Occupational and Environmental Medicine* (pp. 364–388). Philadelphia: WB Saunders.

Chaffin, D. B., & Andersson, G. B. (1991). *Occupational biomechanics* (2nd ed.). New York: Wiley.

Charney, W. (1997). The lift team method for reducing back injuries: A 10 hospital study. *AAOHN Journal, 45,* 300–304.

Coburn, E., & Sirois, B. (1999). Working round-the-clock. *Occupational Health and Safety, 68,* 201–207.

Cohen, A. L., Gjessing, C. C., Fine, L. J., Bernard, B. P., & McGlothlin, J. D. (1997). *Elements of ergonomics programs: A primer based on workplace evaluations of musculoskeletal disorders.* Cincinnati, OH: National Institute for Occupational Safety and Health.

Collins, J. W., & Owen, B. D. (1996). NIOSH research initiatives to prevent back injuries to nursing assistants, aides, and orderlies in nursing homes. *American Journal of Industrial Medicine, 29,* 421–424.

Daltroy, L. (1997). A controlled trial of an educational program to prevent low back injuries. *The New England Journal of Medicine, 337,* 322–328.

Doheny, M., Linden, P., & Sedlak, C. (1995). Reducing orthopaedic hazards of the computer work environment. *Orthopaedic Nursing, 14,* 7–16.

Elford, W., Straker, L., & Strauss, G. (2000). Patient handling with and without slings: An analysis of the risk of injury to the lumbar spine. *Applied Ergonomics, 31,* 185–200.

Franzblau, A., Rock, C. L., Werner, R. A., Albers, J. W., Kelly, M. P., & Johnston, E. C. (1996). The relationship of vitamin B_6 status to median nerve function and carpal tunnel syndrome among active industrial workers. *Journal of Occupational and Environmental Medicine, 38,* 485–491.

Garg, A., & Owen, B. D. (1992). Reducing back stress to nursing personnel: An ergonomic intervention in a nursing home. *Ergonomics, 35,* 1353–1375.

Garg, A., Owen, B. D., & Carlson, B. (1992). An ergonomic evaluation of nursing assistant's job in a nursing home. *Ergonomics, 35,* 979–995.

Hagberg, M., Silverstein, B., Wells, R., Smith, M. J., Hendrick, H. W., Carayon, P., & Pérusse, M. (1995). *Work related musculoskeletal disorders (WMSDs): A reference book for prevention.* Bristol, PA: Taylor & Francis.

Haley, E. (1994). One approach to patient lifting. *Canadian Nurse, 90,* 57–58.

Hansen, L., Winkel, J., & Jørgensen, K. (1998). Significance of mat and shoe softness during prolonged work in upright position: Based on measurements of low back muscle EMG, foot volume changes, discomfort and ground force reactions. *Applied Ergonomics, 29,* 217–224.

Herington, T. N., & Morse, L. H. (1995). *Occupational injuries evaluation, management, and prevention.* St. Louis: Mosby.

Institute of Medicine. (1996). *Nursing staff in hospitals and nursing homes: Is it adequate?* Washington, DC: National Academy Press.

Karawowski, W., & Pongpatanasuegsa, N. (1988). Testing of isometric and isokinetic lifting strength of untrained females in teamwork. *Ergonomics, 31,* 291–301.

Kawachi, I., Colditz, G. A., Stampfer, M. J., Willett, W. C., Manson, J. E., Speizer, F. E., Hennekins, C. H. (1995). Prospective study of shift work and risk of coronary heart disease in women. *Circulation, 92,* 1–5.

Keniston, R. C., Nathan, P. A., Leklem, J. E., & Lockwood, R. S. (1997). Vitamin B$_6$, vitamin C, and carpal tunnel syndrome. *Journal of Occupational and Environmental Medicine, 39,* 949–959.

Keyserling, W. M. (2000). Occupational ergonomics promoting safety and health through work design. In B. S. Levy & D. H. Wegman (Eds.), *Occupational health: Recognizing and preventing work-related disease and injury* (4th ed., pp. 195–209). Philadelphia: Lippincott Williams & Wilkins.

Kjellberg, K., Johnsson, C., Proper, K., Olsson, E., & Hagberg, M. (2000). An observation instrument for assessment of work technique in patient transfer tasks. *Applied Ergonomics, 31,* 139–150.

Kroemer, K. H. E. (1996). Ergonomics. In B. A. Plog, J. Niland, & P. J. Quinlan (Eds.), *Fundamentals of industrial hygiene* (4th ed., pp. 347–401). Itasca, IL: National Safety Council.

Kroemer, K., Kroemer, H., & Kroemer-Elbert, K. (1994). *Ergonomics: How to design for ease & efficiency.* Englewood Cliffs, NJ: Prentice-Hall.

Laflin, K., & Aja, D. (1995). Health care concerns related to lifting: An inside look at intervention strategies. *The American Journal of Occupational Therapy, 49,* 63–72.

Lagerstrom, M., & Hagberg, M. (1997). Evaluation of a 3 year education and training program for nursing personnel at a Swedish hospital. *AAOHN Journal, 45,* 83–92.

Laws, J. (2000). A war on weight & vibration. *Occupational Health & Safety, 69,* 76, 78.

Lee, Y., & Chiou, W. (1994). Risk factors for low back pain, and patient-handling capacity of nursing personnel. *Journal of Safety Research, 25,* 135–145.

Leffler, C. T., & Hu, H. (2000). Other physical hazards. In B. S. Levy & D. H. Wegman (Eds.), *Occupational health: Recognizing and preventing work-related disease and injury* (4th ed., pp. 379–397). Philadelphia: Lippincott Williams & Wilkins.

Legg, S.J. (1987). Physiological ergonomics in nursing. *International Journal of Nursing Studies, 24,* 299–305.

Lipscomb, J., & Borwegen, B. (2000). Health care workers. In B. S. Levy & D. H. Wegman (Eds.), *Occupational health: Recognizing and preventing work-related disease and injury* (4th ed., pp. 767–778). Philadelphia: Lippincott Williams & Wilkins.

Moore, J. S. (1994). Ergonomics. In R. J. McCunney (Ed.), *A practical approach to occupational and environmental medicine* (2nd ed., pp. 396–417). Boston: Little, Brown.

National Bureau of Labor. (2001). Incidence rates for nonfatal occupational injuries and illnesses involving days away from work per 10,000 full-time workers by industry and selected events or exposures leading to injury or illness, 1998. Available at http://stats.bls.gov/case/ostb0799.pdf

National Institute for Occupational Safety and Health. (1997). *Musculoskeletal disorders and workplace factors: A critical review of epidemiologic evidence for work-related musculoskeletal disorders of the neck, upper extremity, and low back.* Cincinnati: National Institute for Occupational Safety and Health.

National Institute for Occupational Safety and Health. (2000). *Organization of work.* Available at www.cdc.gov/niosh

National Safety Council. (1993). *Ergonomics: A practical guide* (2nd ed.). Itasca, IL: Author.

Occupational Safety & Health Administration. (2000). Available at www.osha.gov

Ostendorf, J. S., Rogers, B, & Bertsche, P. K. (2000). Ergonomics: CTD management evaluation tool. *AAOHN Journal, 48,* 17–24.

Owen, B. D. (1986). Personal characteristics important to back injury. *Rehabilitation Nursing, 11,* 12–16.

Owen, B. D., & Fragala, G. (1999). Reducing perceived physical stress while transferring residents. *AAOHN Journal, 47,* 316–323.

Owen, B. D., & Garg, A. (1993). Back stress isn't part of the job. *American Journal of Nursing, 2,* 48–51.

Owen, B. D., & Garg, A. (1994). Reducing back stress through an ergonomic approach: Weighing a patient. *International Journal of Nursing Studies, 31,* 511–519.

Owen, B. D., Keene, K., Olson, S., & Garg, A. (1995). An ergonomic approach to reducing back stress while carrying out patient handling tasks with a hospitalized patient. In M. Hagberg, F. Hofmann, U. Stobel, & G. Westlander (Eds.), *Occupational health for health care workers* (pp. 298–301). Landsberg, Germany: ECOMED.

Owen, B. D., Welden, N., & Kane, J. (1999). What are we teaching about lifting and transferring patients? *Research in Nursing & Health, 22,* 3–13.

Pheasant, S. T. (1987). Some anthropometric aspects of workstation design. *International Journal of Nursing Studies, 24,* 191–198.

Pheasant, S. (1991). *Ergonomics, work and health.* Gaithersburg, MD: Aspen.

Pollock, M. L., & Wilmore, J. H. (1990). *Exercise in health and disease: Evaluation and prescription for prevention and rehabilitation* (2nd ed.). Philadelphia: WB Saunders.

Pope, M. H., Andersson, G. B. J., & Chaffin, D. B. (1991). The workplace. In M. H. Pope, G. B. J. Andersson, J. W. Frymoyer, & D. B. Chaffin (Eds.), *Occupational low back pain: Assessment, treatment and prevention.* St. Louis: Mosby.

Putz-Anderson, V. (1988). *Cumulative trauma disorders: A manual for musculoskeletal diseases of the upper limbs.* Bristol, PA: Taylor & Francis.

Ranney, D. (1997). *Chronic musculoskeletal injuries in the workplace.* Philadelphia: WB Saunders.

Rogers, B. (1994). *Occupational health nursing concepts and practice.* Philadelphia: WB Saunders.

Roughton, J. E. (1996). *Ergonomic problems in the workplace: A guide to effective management.* Rockville, MD: Government Institutes.

Smedley, J., Egger, P., Cooper, C., & Coggon, D. (1995). Manual handling activities and risk of low back pain in nurses. *Occupational and Environmental Medicine, 52,* 160–163.

U.S. Department of Health and Human Services. (1994). *Applications manual for the revised NIOSH Lifting Equation* (DHHS [NIOSH] Publication No. 94-110). Cincinnati: National Institute for Occupational Safety and Health.

U.S. Department of Labor. (1990). *Ergonomics program management guidelines for meatpacking plants* (OSHA Publication No. 3123). Washington, DC: Author.

U.S. Department of Labor. (1991). *Annual published release.* (USDL 91-600). Washington, DC: Bureau of Labor Statistics.

U.S. Department of Labor. (2000). *Lost-worktime injuries and illnesses: Characteristics and resulting time away from work, 1998.* (USDL 00-115). Washington, DC: Bureau of Labor Statistics.

Waters, T. R., Putz-Anderson, V., & Garg, A. (1994). *Applications manual for the revised NIOSH lifting equation* (DHHS Publication No. 94-110). Cincinnati: National Institute for Occupational Safety and Health.

Westgaard, R. H. (2000). Work-related musculoskeletal complaints: Some ergonomic challenges upon the start of a new century. *Applied Ergonomics, 31,* 569–580.

Wilson, J. R. (2000). Fundamentals of ergonomics in theory and practice. *Applied Ergonomics, 31,* 557–567.

Zabel, A. M., & McGrew, A. B. (1997). Ergonomics: A key component in a CTD control program. *AAOHN Journal, 45,* 350–359.

Zhuang, Z., Stobbe, T. J., Collins, J. W., Hsiao, H., & Hobbs, G. R. (2000). Psychophysical assessment of assistive devices for transferring patients/residents. *Applied Ergonomics, 31,* 35–44.

Zhuang, Z., Stobbe, T. J., Hsiao, H., Collins, J. W., & Hobbs, G. R. (1999). Biomechanical evaluation of assistive devices for transferring residents. *Applied Ergonomics, 30,* 285–294.

4

Assessment and Management of Immobility

MARIANNE GENGE JAGMIN

The human body was meant to be mobile as is evident by the detrimental effects of immobility. Mobility facilitates physiologic processes in the body, but immobility can impede these processes. Specifically, ambulation provides the stress on joints, muscles, tendons, and bone to allow proper functioning of the musculoskeletal system. Although immobility decreases stress on the musculoskeletal system, which in turn decreases tension in injured tissues, enhances healing, and decreases pain, immobility may also cause joint contractures, muscle wasting, and bone weakening. Other body systems also face the hazards of immobility (Table 4–1). Thus thorough objective and subjective initial assessments of the immobilized client are essential (Table 4–2). Although varying degrees of immobility may be required for efficient healing, mobility is encouraged and vital. The detrimental effects of immobility on all of the body's physiologic systems far outweigh the positive effects of bed rest.

INTEGUMENTARY SYSTEM

The negative effect of immobility is often first and most easily visible in the integument. Its impact on this system is often more severe and lasting, both physiologically and monetarily, than its impact on any other body system A pressure sore prevalence study noted that 10.8% of hospital clients at a given time are afflicted with pressure ulcers (Barczak, Barnett, Childs, & Bosley, 1997). Clients with pressure ulcers have a longer hospital stay than clients without pressure ulcers. The cost of pressure ulcers in hospitals is conservatively $55 billion per year (The National Decubitus Foundation, www.decubitus. org). The mortality rate for hospitalized clients with pressure ulcers is between 23% and 27% (The National Decubitus Foundation, www.decubitus.org).

Pressure causes and fosters pressure ulcers. A constant pressure of 60 mm Hg on the skin causes irreversible tissue damage within 1 to 2 hours. Pressures of 40 to 100 mm Hg have been documented over the ischial, posterior trochanter, and thigh areas when clients are sitting in a wheelchair, even when using wheelchair cushions. Bony prominences such as the sacrum, heels, spine, hips, knees, costal margins, and occiput are especially at risk for increased pressure in the lying position. The site and duration of pressure; the individual's health status, nutritional status, and ability to change position; and whether or not the individual is incontinent determine the amount and severity of tissue damage.

Tissue damage initiates with pressure over a bony prominence, altering the pressure gradient within the underlying capillaries of the skin and subcutaneous tissues. Interstitial fluid pressure increases until it exceeds venous pressure, leading to fluid retention in the area and a concomitant further increase in tissue pressure. Blood flow is diminished, and poor tissue oxygenation leads to cell death.

Shearing forces and friction contribute to the development of pressure ulcers. Gravitational forces (sliding down in bed when the head of the bed is raised) and repositioning may cause direct injury to the skin.

Risks and Assessment

The Agency for Health Care Policy and Research (AHCPR) generated a pressure ulcer prediction and prevention algorithm that begins when a client is admitted to a health care program (Fig. 4–1). Knowledge of the client's immediate past experience with immobility and pressure loads is also important. A study conducted on 24 clients who had undergone fairly long surgical procedures suggested that the body's failure to increase blood

TABLE 4–1. *Adverse Effects of Immobilization*

SYSTEM AND TISSUE	EFFECTS	SYSTEM AND TISSUE	EFFECTS
Integumentary	Pressure sores	Musculoskeletal	
Cardiovascular	Orthostatic intolerance	Bone	Calcium resorption
	Risk for thromboembolism		Osteoporosis
	Decreased work capacity	Muscle	Atrophy
Blood	Hypercalcemia		Decreased strength
	Increased venous volume (early)		Decreased endurance
	Decreased volume (late)	Joints	Ligaments shorten or ligament laxity
Heart	Decreased stroke volume		Tendons shorten
	Decreased cardiac output		Intra-articular degeneration
	Increased heart rate		Connective tissue fibrosis
	Systole longer than diastole		Contractures
Peripheral vessels	Decreased venous return	Body part	Decreased range of motion
	Increased blood viscosity		Joint instability
Respiratory	Decreased lung volume		Muscle atrophy
	Ventilation/perfusion mismatch		Pressure sores
	Secretion stasis	Psychosensory	Altered perception
Gastrointestinal	Constipation		Slowed EEG waves
	Anorexia		Sleep disturbance
Urinary	Urinary stasis		Role disturbance
	Renal calculi		
Metabolic	Increased nitrogen excretion		
	Decreased protein intake		

EEG, electroencephalogram.

TABLE 4–2. *Subjective and Objective Assessments*

SUBJECTIVE ASSESSMENT	OBJECTIVE ASSESSMENT
Integumentary System	
History of incontinence, neurologic deficits, or nutritional deficit	Inspection
Symptoms of pressure: pain, tingling, or numbness	Tissue hydration
	Presence of moisture
	Causes of skin irritation: friction, shear, or immobilization devices
Cardiovascular System	
History of hypertension, congestive heart failure, thrombophlebitis, vascular injuries, clotting abnormalities, or recent surgery	Vital signs
	Peripheral edema
	Auscultate heart sounds
	Orthostatic vital signs
	Lower leg assessment
Respiratory System	
Dyspnea	Full pulmonary assessment
Preexisting pulmonary disease	
Medications	
Gastrointestinal System	
Bowel pattern	Full abdominal assessment
Food and fluid intake (recent)	Bowel record
Usual dietary intake	
Medications	
Urinary System	
Ability to empty bladder	24-hr intake and output
Prostate history	Urine inspection for odor, cloudiness, and color
Volume of voiding	Bladder distention
Pain (including flank)	
Burning	
Frequency	

Table continued on following page

TABLE 4–2. *Subjective and Objective Assessments* Continued

SUBJECTIVE ASSESSMENT	OBJECTIVE ASSESSMENT
Metabolic System	
Protein intake	24-hr diet history
Appetite	Peripheral edema
Musculoskeletal System	
Usual activity level	Gait
Ability to perform activities of daily living	Posture
Use of assistive devices	Coordination
Previous musculoskeletal disorders	Ease of movement
Symptoms include fatigue, weakness, paralysis, decreased joint range of motion, decreased strength, decreased muscle mass, anorexia, lethargy, nausea, headache, abdominal cramping, pain, and stiffness	Joint range of motion Measure muscle mass Observe muscle tone Test muscle strength
History of compression fracture	Test activity endurance
Risk factors for osteoporosis	
Psychosensory System	
Social and ethnic background	Signs of withdrawal, depression, or anxiety
Experience with sick role	Neurologic status of extremities
Medication history	
Life stressors	
Life roles	
History of depression	
Signs of withdrawal	
Support system	

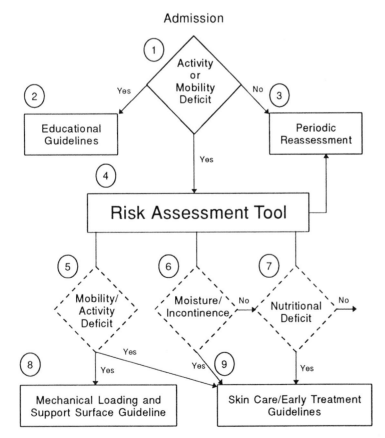

FIGURE 4–1. Pressure ulcer prediction and prevention algorithm. (From Agency for Health Care Policy and Research. [1992, May]. *Pressure ulcers in adults: Prediction and prevention.* [Clinical Practice Guideline. Quick Reference Guide for Clinicians No. 3. AHCPR Pub. No. 92-0047]. Rockville, MD: Public Health Service, U.S. Department of Health and Human Services.)

flow in response to the long period of pressure experienced during surgery might have contributed to the development of pressure ulcers (Sanada, Nagakawa, Yamamoto, Higashidani, Tsuru, & Suzamo, 1997).

Skin breakdown usually occurs at bony prominences. Skin should be assessed as frequently as possible, with particular attention to skin under and near immobilization devices, casts, braces, or traction. Pressure ulcers are staged based on the degree of tissue damage noted. A four-point staging system is the most appropriate to use in staging pressure ulcers (Box 4–1). These staging definitions acknowledge the following limitations: (1) stage I ulcers may be superficial, or they may be a sign of deeper tissue damage; (2) stage I pressure ulcers are not always reliably assessed, especially in clients with darkly pigmented skin; (3) when eschar is present, a pressure ulcer cannot be accurately staged until the eschar is removed; and (4) it may be difficult to assess pressure ulcers in clients with casts, other orthopaedic devices, or support stockings, so the nurse must be especially vigilant in assessing and documenting skin integrity (AHCPR, 1994). The Braden Scale (Table 4–3) is a recommended risk assessment tool.

BOX 4–1.
Staging Pressure Ulcers

Stage I

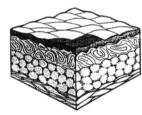

Nonblanchable erythema of intact skin, the heralding lesion of skin ulceration. In individuals with darker skin, discoloration of the skin, warmth, edema, induration, or hardness may also be indicators.

Stage II

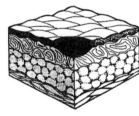

Partial-thickness skin loss involving epidermis, dermis, or both. The ulcer is superficial and appears clinically as an abrasion, blister, or shallow crater.

Stage III

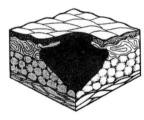

Full-thickness skin loss involving damage to or necrosis of subcutaneous tissue that may extend down to, but not through, underlying fascia. The ulcer appears clinically as a deep crater with or without undermining of adjacent tissue.

Stage IV

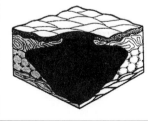

Full-thickness skin loss with extensive destruction, tissue necrosis, or damage to muscle, bone, or supporting structures (e.g., tendon, joint capsule). Undermining and sinus tracts also may be associated with stage IV pressure ulcers.

The staging of pressure ulcers recommended for use here is consistent with the recommendations of the National Pressure Ulcer Advisory Panel Consensus Development Conference.

From Agency for Health Care Policy and Research. (1994, December). *Pressure ulcer treatment.* [Clinical Practice Guideline. Quick Reference Guide for Clinicians No. 15. AHCPR Pub. No. 95-0653]. Rockville, MD: Public Health Service, U.S. Department of Health and Human Services.

TABLE 4–3. *Braden Scale of Risk Predictors for Skin Breakdown*

CLIENT'S NAME	EVALUATOR'S NAME			DATE OF ASSESSMENT
Sensory Perception Ability to respond to discomfort	*1. Completely Limited* Unresponsive to painful stimuli either because of state of unconsciousness or severe sensory impairment, which limits ability to feel pain over most of body surface	*2. Very Limited* Responds only to painful stimuli (but not verbal commands) by opening eyes or flexing extremities; cannot communicate discomfort verbally OR Has a sensory impairment that limits the ability to feel pain or discomfort over half of body surface	*3. Slightly Limited* Responds to verbal commands by opening eyes and obeying some commands, but cannot always communicate discomfort or need to be turned OR Has some sensory impairment that limits ability to feel pain or discomfort in one or two extremities	*4. No Impairment* Responds to verbal commands by obeying; can communicate needs accurately; has no sensory deficit that limits ability to feel pain or discomfort
Moisture Degree to which skin is exposed to moisture	*1. Very Moist* Skin is kept moist almost constantly by perspiration, urine, etc.; dampness is detected every time client is moved or turned; linen must be changed more than once per shift	*2. Occasionally Moist* Skin is frequently but not always kept moist; linen must be changed two to three times in 24 hr	*3. Rarely Moist* Skin is rarely moist more than three to four times a week, but linen does require changing at that time	*4. Never Moist* Perspiration and incontinence are never a problem; linen changed at routine intervals only
Activity Degree of physical activity	*1. Bedfast* Confined to bed	*2. Chairfast* Ability to walk severely impaired or nonexistent and must be assisted into chair or wheelchair; is confined to chair or wheelchair when not in bed	*3. Walks Occasionally* Walks occasionally during day but for very short distances, with or without assistance; spends majority of each shift in bed or chair	*4. Walks Frequently* Walks a moderate distance at least once every 1–2 hr during waking hours
Mobility Ability to change and control body position	*1. Completely Immobile* Unable to make even slight changes in position without assistance	*2. Very Limited* Makes occasional slight changes in position without help but unable to make frequent or significant changes in position independently	*3. Slightly Limited* Makes frequent although slight changes in position without assistance but unable to make or maintain major changes in position independently	*4. No Limitations* Makes major and frequent changes in position without assistance

Nutrition Usual food intake pattern	1. Very Poor Never eats a complete meal; rarely eats more than half of any food offered; intake of protein is negligible; takes even fluids poorly; does not take a liquid dietary supplement OR Maintained on clear liquids or IV	2. Probably Inadequate Rarely eats a complete meal and generally eats only about half of any food offered; protein intake is poor; occasionally takes a liquid dietary supplement OR Receiving less-than-optimal amount of liquid diet supplement	3. Adequate Eats more than half of most meals; eats moderate amount of protein source once or twice daily; occasionally refuses a meal; usually takes a dietary supplement if offered OR Is on a tube-feeding regimen, which probably meets most of nutritional needs	4. Excellent Eats most of every meal; never refuses a meal; frequently eats between meals; does not require a dietary supplementation
Friction and Shear	1. Problem Requires moderate to maximum assistance in moving; complete lifting without sliding against sheets is impossible; frequently slides down in bed or chair, requiring frequent repositioning with maximum assistance; either spasticity, contractures, or agitation leads to almost constant friction	2. Potential Problem Moves feebly independently or requires minimum assistance; skin probably slides against bed sheets or chair to some extent when movement occurs; maintains relatively good position in chair or bed most of time but occasionally slides down	3. No Apparent Problem Moves in bed and chair independently and has sufficient muscle strength to lift up completely during move; maintains good position in bed or chair at all times	
			Total Score	

Generalizability across settings has not been established. Each institution must determine its own score for providing intervention.

From Braden, B. J., & Bergstrom, N. (1989). Clinical utility of the Braden scale for predicting pressure sore risk. *Decubitus, 2*(3), 44-51. © Copyright Barbara Braden, 1985. Reprinted with permission.

Alteration in Skin Integrity

Pressure Ulcer Prevention and Pressure Ulcer Care. To avoid pressure ulcers in immobilized clients, a regular turning schedule should be followed. The client should be repositioned every 2 hours, preferably to at least a 30-degree oblique position to relieve sacral pressure. Positioning devices such as footboards, cradles, trapezes, pillows, wheelchair cushions, and mattresses should be used. For clients who are incontinent, a toileting schedule should be followed. Care should be taken to thoroughly cleanse both the perineal area and buttocks with a nonirritating soap and water and to dry the area thoroughly.

Even when quality care is provided, there are situations in which an alteration in skin integrity can occur. An algorithm entitled "Management of Pressure Ulcers: Overview" (Fig. 4–2) might be individualized in the care of the client with skin breakdown. The algorithm starts with identification of the pressure ulcer and staging,

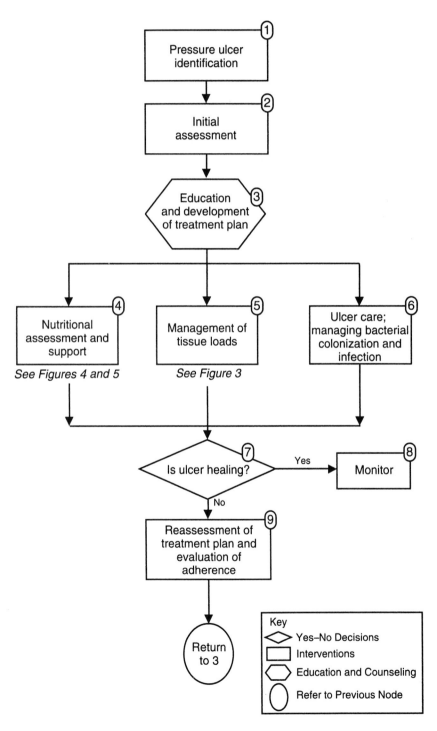

FIGURE 4–2. Management of pressure ulcers: overview. (From Agency for Health Care Policy and Research. [1994, December]. *Pressure ulcer treatment.* [Clinical Practice Guideline. Quick Reference Guide for Clinicians No. 15. AHCPR Pub. No. 95-0653]. Rockville, MD: Public Health Service, U.S. Department of Health and Human Services.)

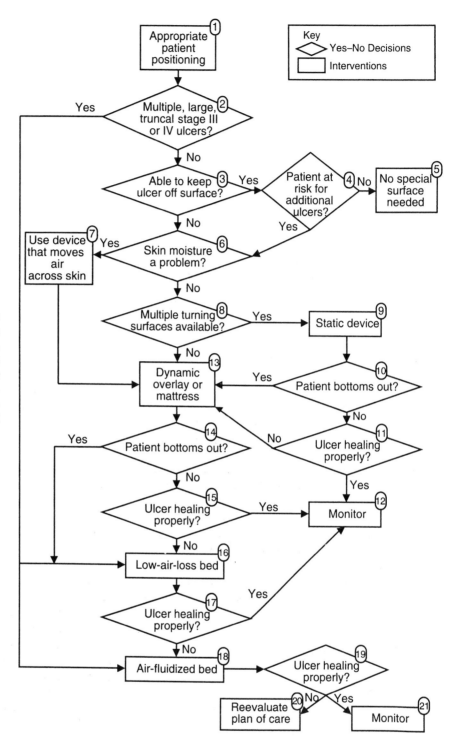

FIGURE 4–3. Management of tissue loads. (From Agency for Health Care Policy and Research. [1994, December]. *Pressure ulcer treatment.* [Clinical Practice Guideline. Quick Reference Guide for Clinicians No. 15. AHCPR Pub. No. 95-0653]. Rockville, MD: Public Health Service, U.S. Department of Health and Human Services.)

previously described. The initial assessment includes assessment of the pressure ulcer, a complete history and physical examination, assessment for complications and comorbidities, nutritional and pain assessments, psychosocial evaluation, and assessment of risk for developing additional pressure ulcers. Following assessment, the client and family caregivers are educated about the plan of treatment. This plan should include turning schedules,

positioning techniques, support surfaces, nutritional support, management of tissue loads, and management of bacterial colonization and infection. Nutritional support ensures that the client receives adequate supplements of protein, calories, vitamin C, iron, and zinc. Management of such tissue loads as pressure, friction, and shear is critical (Fig. 4-3 and Table 4-4). Debridement, wound cleansing, dressings, and infection control are covered.

TABLE 4–4. *Selected Characteristics for Classes of Support Surfaces*

PERFORMANCE CHARACTERISTICS	AIR FLUIDIZED	LOW AIR LOSS	ALTERNATING AIR	STATIC FLOTATION (AIR OR WATER)	FOAM	STANDARD MATTRESS
Increased support area	Yes	Yes	Yes	Yes	Yes	No
Low moisture retention	Yes	Yes	No	No	No	No
Shear reduction	Yes	?	Yes	Yes	No	No
Pressure reduction	Yes	Yes	Yes	Yes	Yes	No
Dynamic	Yes	Yes	Yes	No	No	No
Cost per day	High	High	Moderate	Low	Low	Low

From Agency for Health Care Policy and Research. (1994, December). *Pressure ulcer treatment.* [Clinical Practice Guideline. Quick Reference Guide for Clinicians No. 15. AHCPR Pub. No. 95-0653]. Rockville, MD: Public Health Service, U.S. Department of Health and Human Services.

Frequent monitoring of ulcers at all stages and reassessment of treatment are essential (AHCPR, 1994).

Dressing types vary and should be individualized to the type of wound or pressure ulcer. Dressing types include woven dressings, low-adherence dressings, thin polyurethane films, hydrocolloids, alginates, polyurethane foams, and hydrogels (Casey, 2000). Nurse wound care specialists as well as information from manufacturers, websites such as Surgical Materials Testing Laboratory (www.smtl.co.uk), and nursing research on wound care are all resources that may be used when choosing the appropriate dressing for various stages of pressure ulcers.

Nutrition Therapy. Malnutrition has been related to pressure ulcers. The algorithm "Nutritional Assessment and Support" (Fig. 4–4) clearly identifies how this contributing factor might be addressed. Clients should be assessed periodically using a form similar to that in Figure 4–5, entitled "Nutritional Assessment of Patient with Pressure Ulcer(s)." The reader is referred to the AHCPR's clinical practice guidelines (AHCPR, 1992, 1994) for more information on the prevention and treatment of pressure ulcers.

CARDIOVASCULAR SYSTEM

The major adverse effects to the cardiovascular system as a result of immobility are orthostatic intolerance, increased risk of thromboembolism, and diminished work capacity.

During the first few days of bed rest, the horizontal position causes a temporary increase in circulating blood volume. This increased volume causes a shift of extracellular fluid to the venous system. Increased venous volume stimulates volume receptors in the right atrium that inhibit antidiuretic hormone and aldosterone, leading to water and salt diuresis. Diuresis results in an 8% to 10% loss of plasma volume during the first few days and eventually results in a 15% to 20% loss of volume during 2 to 4 weeks of immobility. After an initial period of increase, resting cardiac stroke volume and cardiac output also decrease during bed rest. Resuming an upright position results in a significant increase in heart rate (because of a reduction in cardiac output and stroke volume), nausea, diaphoresis, and syncope. This most common manifestation of cardiac deconditioning following bed rest is orthostatic intolerance, or postural hypotension. It is a direct response to the decreased overall blood volume and pooling of blood in the lower extremities, which result in a cardiac stroke volume too small to maintain cerebral perfusion.

In healthy subjects, the ability to adjust to an upright position may be completely impaired after 3 weeks of bed rest. Blood pressure may drop 15 mm Hg or more when the person changes from a sitting to a standing position. In individuals with major trauma and systemic disease, even a few days of bed rest may cause orthostasis. Older people have an increased risk of developing orthostatic hypotension because of age-related changes in the cardiovascular system, multiple chronic diseases, and medications that predispose clients to hypotension. Persons with coronary artery disease may have anginal pain on arising because of reduced diastolic filling that causes an inadequate coronary blood supply.

There is a high rate of thrombophlebitis and deep vein thrombosis in paralyzed limbs as well as in physically compromised, immobilized individuals. In general, the classic factors that predispose to thrombus formation, Virchow's triad, include stasis of blood in the lower extremities, alteration of the vascular lining because of endothelial injury, and hypercoagulability. The immobilized individual experiences decreased use of lower leg muscles that facilitate venous return. The action of platelets and hypercalcemia experienced during immobility results in increased activation of the clotting chain, specifically prothrombin to thrombin, which converts fibrinogen to fibrin, resulting in blood that is more prone to clot.

Blood viscosity is increased in the immobile person because there is a greater reduction in plasma volume than in red cell mass. The decrease in circulating fluid volume and cardiac output causes diminished work capacity when the immobile individual returns to an active state. Decreased mobility sets up an imbalance in the autonomic nervous system, leading to sympathetic (adrenergic) control over parasympathetic (cholinergic) activity. Increased heart rate is one manifestation of this imbalance.

Elevated basal heart rates are common among individuals on prolonged bed rest. This increased heart rate

contributes to a diminished work capacity of the heart. An increased heart rate leads to a shorter diastolic filling time, smaller systolic ejection, and diminished capacity of the heart to respond to metabolic demands beyond the basal rate. At high rates, the systolic phase of the cycle is longer than the diastolic phase. Because the majority of coronary blood flow occurs during diastole, a shortened diastolic filling time decreases blood flow

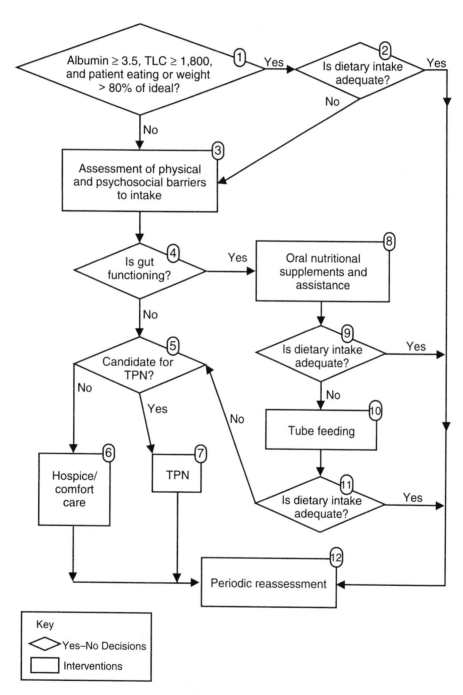

FIGURE 4–4. Nutritional assessment and support. TLC, total lymphocyte count; TPN, total parenteral nutrition. (From Agency for Health Care Policy and Research. [1994, December]. *Pressure ulcer treatment.* [Clinical Practice Guideline. Quick Reference Guide for Clinicians No. 15. AHCPR Pub. No. 95-0653]. Rockville, MD: Public Health Service, U.S. Department of Health and Human Services.)

Patient Name: _____ Date: _____ Time: _____

To be filled out for all patients at risk on initial evaluation and every 12 weeks thereafter, as indicated. Trends will document the efficacy of nutritional support therapy.

Protein Compartments

Somatic:

Current Weight (kg)   _____
Previous Weight (kg)   _____ (_____date)
Percent Change in Weight   _____

Height (cm)   _____
Height/Weight
Current Body Mass Index (BMI)   _____ [wt/(ht)^2]
Previous BMI   _____ (_____date)
Percent Change in BMI   _____

Visceral:

Serum Albumin   _____
  (Normal $\geq$ 3.5 mg/dL)
Total Lymphocyte Count (TLC)   _____ (optional)
  (White Blood Cell count x percent Lymphocytes/100)

  Guide to TLC:
   • Immune competence $\geq$ 1,800 mm^3
   • Immunity partly impaired   < 1,800 but $\geq$ 900 mm^3
   • Anergy   < 900 mm^3

State of Hydration

24-Hour Intake_____ mL   24-Hour Output _____ mL

Note: Thirst, tongue dryness in non-mouth-breathers, and tenting of cervical skin
may indicate dehydration. Jugular vein distension may indicate overhydration.

Estimated Nutritional Requirement

Estimated Nonprotein Calories (NPC) _____ /kg   Estimated Protein_____ (g/kg)
Actual NPC   _____ /kg   Actual Protein   _____ (g/kg)

Recommendations/Plan

1.

2.

3.

4.

FIGURE 4–5. Nutritional assessment of patient with pressure ulcer(s). (From Agency for Health Care Policy and Research. [1994, December]. *Pressure ulcer treatment*. [Clinical Practice Guideline. Quick Reference Guide for Clinicians No. 15. AHCPR Pub. No. 95-0653]. Rockville, MD: Public Health Service, U.S. Department of Health and Human Services.)

to the heart muscle, and heart muscle fatigues more readily.

Stroke volume and systolic time intervals following prolonged bed rest do not return to prior levels for up to 4 weeks, despite regular exercise. Athletes may take a greater amount of time to recover from the cardiac effects of bed rest than do clients who were sedentary before bed rest.

Risks and Assessment

Preexisting cardiovascular conditions may contribute to the effects of immobility, particularly hypertension, congestive heart disease, or thrombophlebitis. A history of vascular injuries or clotting abnormalities is a significant assessment finding in the individual to be immobilized. Predisposing factors for the development of thrombophlebitis include impaired venous return, hypercoagulability of the blood, and vessel wall injury. Slowed venous return in an immobilized older person combined with paralysis, heart disease, or recent surgery is a particularly problematic combination. Blood hypercoagulability is heightened in injured or surgical clients who are also immobilized, resulting in a decreased circulating blood volume. Vein wall injury can occur because of atherosclerotic plaque formation or microtears caused by venodilation.

Increased heart rate may indicate stress. Narrow pulse pressure is indicative of small stroke volume and diminished cardiac reserve. Impaired peripheral circulation may be evidenced by peripheral edema, and the presence of a third heart sound may raise suspicion of heart failure. Orthostatic hypotension combined with an increased heart rate is an indicator of orthostatic intolerance. The lower legs should be assessed for signs of thrombophlebitis (see Chapter 10).

Activity Intolerance/Alteration in Cardiac Function

Activity Promotion, Exercise Therapy, and Embolus Precautions. Elevation of the head of the bed, or Fowler's position, diminishes venous return and thereby decreases the workload on the heart that occurs with the supine recumbent position. Periodic alteration of body position helps prevent orthostatic intolerance through stimulation of the postural neural reflex. Elevation of the head of the bed, dangling, and ambulation are useful in preventing orthostatic intolerance. The individual's participation in the achievement of all position changes promotes venous return as well. Elevation of the legs may also be helpful in the prevention of venous stasis by promoting passive drainage of vessels in the lower leg.

The pulse and blood pressure should be assessed at least twice daily. Orthostatic blood pressure measurements should be taken before each attempt to ambulate the client till they have achieved readings near, or at, their baseline.

Clients who have severe postural hypotension may benefit from a tilt table when starting to mobilize. The angle is increased gradually, and the goal is to obtain a position of 75 degrees for 20 minutes without orthostatic changes.

The relaxation and contraction of muscle groups during isometric exercise provide changes in pressure required to increase venous flow. As described, caution must be taken with individuals with hypertension, and Valsalva's maneuver should be avoided.

Sequential pneumatic compression devices are special inflatable sleeves that simulate the pumping action of the muscle groups through the provision of external alternating pressure. The compression allows cyclic emptying and refilling of leg veins. Pneumatic devices may be helpful for individuals unable to exercise or may supplement exercises for individuals at high risk for deep venous thrombosis. Elastic support stockings may also promote venous return via the pressure gradient provided by the stockings. However, special care should be taken to prevent constriction of the extremity by the stocking bands. Stockings should be removed for about 30 minutes every 8 hours to assess the skin. Sequential pneumatic compression devices and elastic support stockings may be used together.

RESPIRATORY SYSTEM

Immobility results in decreased metabolic processes. The body also accomplishes work less efficiently in the immobilized state. Cells in the body require less oxygen, and less carbon dioxide is produced. Respiratory rate decreases and respirations become shallower to compensate for a lower oxygen need.

Overall, immobility affects lung volumes, distribution of ventilation, and blood flow to the lungs. The counter-resistance of the bed or chair may cause limitations in chest expansion by compression of the thorax by sitting or lying or by abdominal compression from distention or external devices. Chest movement during immobilization can be decreased as a result of muscle weakness and the use of central nervous system depressants. A change of position from upright to supine decreases all lung volume capacities except tidal volume. The side-lying position causes less of a change in the functional residual capacity (FRC) than the supine position.

The physiologic importance of decreases in lung volume is illustrated by the relationship of the CV and the FRC in each client. CV is the volume at which the net forces of gravity, elasticity of lung tissue, and airway properties are able to induce closure of small airways. When CV exceeds FRC, some airways remain closed during tidal breathing. Closed airways result in decreased ventilation to dependent lung zones. Because blood flow continues, ventilation/perfusion mismatch occurs, which leads to a fall in arterial oxygen levels. The CV is less than FRC in healthy young individuals. As aging or disease ensues, lung pliability decreases and CV increases.

Gravity directs blood flow toward dependent areas of the lung. Increased perfusion of dependent, underventilated lung zones leads to an even greater discrepancy in the ventilation/perfusion ratio. Secretory activity of mucous glands in the lungs continues at a normal rate even in collapsed alveoli. Stasis of these secretions in dependent lung zones leads to pneumonia and further atelectasis.

The airways of the lungs are dependent on the action of cilia, the production of mucus, and an intact cough reflex to rid themselves of pathogens. In the supine position, gravity works to pull mucus toward dependent areas of the lung. In the presence of dehydration or other pathologic condition, upper surfaces of the lung can become dry, thus inhibiting cilia movement. Dependent portions of the lung become covered with abnormal amounts of mucus, which also inhibits cilia motion. Muscle weakness from immobilization inhibits the individual's ability to produce an effective cough. Concomitant use of medications that depress central nervous system activity may lead to inhibition of the cough reflex itself, resulting in stasis of secretions and further contributing to the development of pneumonia.

Risks and Assessment

Older individuals are at an increased risk of developing respiratory complications, particularly pneumonia, from immobility because of the anatomic changes in the respiratory system that occur with age, such as loss of elastic recoil of the lungs and decreased mucociliary clearance. The presence of dyspnea or preexisting pulmonary disease significantly increases the risk of complications from immobility. Medications that may depress respiratory efforts should be noted.

Thorough pulmonary and vital sign assessments at least twice a day are essential in determining preexisting conditions that may affect individual responses to immobility. The nurse should assess for dyspnea, respiratory distress, and lung sounds. Temperature elevation, increased heart rate, and at times, confusion are initial signs of respiratory compromise. Decreased chest movement, dullness to percussion, reduced or absent lung sounds, and vocal fremitus over affected areas may indicate atelectasis. Pneumonia may be exhibited by decreased chest movement, dullness to percussion, bronchovesicular to bronchial lung sounds, egophony, and whispered pectoriloquy with lobar involvement. Late inspiratory crackles over the area of involvement are early auscultatory signs of pneumonia.

Ineffective Breathing Patterns

Airway Management. Proper positioning to prevent aspiration in clients with poor or lost pharyngeal or laryngeal reflexes is essential. Lateral recumbent and Trendelenburg's positions are helpful in promoting gravity drainage of respiratory secretions. Repositioning at regular intervals minimizes the effects of gravity on lung tissue and mobilizes lung secretions.

Deep breathing and coughing along with turning and repositioning on a regularly scheduled basis maintain maximum lung capacity and mobilize secretions. Deep breathing, or hyperinflation, is best done sitting, when possible, to allow for easier diaphragmatic movement. Each inspiration should be slow, with a pause between inspiration and expiration to allow for maximal inflation of the alveoli. Deep breaths should be alternated with several normal breaths. Several types of incentive spirometry devices that provide immediate feedback to

the individual and encourage independence in the deep-breathing routine are available. Deep breathing should be performed at least every hour and more frequently if the individual has an altered level of awareness, is receiving opioids, or has a previously existing respiratory condition. Individuals unable to assist with deep breathing can have involuntary or reflexive hyperventilation induced by movement of their limbs.

Coughing is effective in mobilizing secretions. If secretions are not present, however, coughing may be contraindicated. When an individual takes a deep breath and holds it, the glottis is closed and there is an increase in pressure in the trachea. Coughing causes a forceful exhalation, which may serve to collapse the smaller airways.

Adequate fluids, 30 to 40 mL/kg of body weight per day, should be provided to mobilize dry, tenacious respiratory secretions. If oxygen therapy is greater than 5 L/min, humidified air should be provided to prevent drying of mucous membranes and secretions.

Clients who are at high risk for developing respiratory complications or who are on prolonged bed rest, but do not have an unstable spinal cord injury or traction of arm abductors, may benefit from continuous lateral rotational therapy. This therapy involves a specialized bed that provides a continuous slow rotation along a longitudinal axis. Potential problems with the bed include inadvertent disconnection of intravenous lines, client intolerance, and adverse effects on intracranial pressure in clients with intracranial hypertension, arrhythmias, and hemodynamic instability.

GASTROINTESTINAL SYSTEM

Constipation is one of the major side effects of immobilization. Bowel elimination is an integrated process, involving smooth muscle and skeletal muscle activity as well as complex visceral reflex patterns. Interference with the mechanisms of elimination because of decreased muscle power and loss or suppression of reflexes leads to constipation. The adrenergic (sympathetic) state that exists with immobilization inhibits peristalsis and causes constriction of all gastrointestinal sphincter muscles, including the anal sphincter, leading to altered colonic motility patterns. Increased intestinal absorption of water and low dietary intake of fluids and fiber further contribute to constipation.

Overall skeletal muscle weakness affects abdominal and perineal muscles, which contributes to difficulty in defecation. Positions required for defecation during bed rest are altered from the normal physiologic posture. This position eliminates the postural and gravitational assistance, interferes with the ability of the abdominal muscles to increase intra-abdominal pressure, and makes it necessary for the individual to exert more than a normal amount of intrathoracic pressure to facilitate defecation.

The addition of an atmosphere that deprives the individual of privacy can lead to suppression of the urge to defecate, which may in itself lead to constipation. The simple problem of constipation is complex when all the contributing factors are considered.

Fecal impaction and fecalomas may develop after feces have been retained for long periods. The most significant symptom is passage of liquid stool around the impaction.

Risks and Assessment

Information related to preimmobilization bowel patterns and food and fluid intake during the previous 4 to 5 days is essential. Usual dietary and fluid intake should be assessed. Use of medications that contribute to constipation should be noted, as should the use of laxatives. Bowel sounds should be auscultated, and the abdominal area should be palpated for distention and masses. A record of frequency and consistency of bowel movements should be kept. Passage of flatus should also be noted.

Constipation

Constipation Management. The position that most closely approximates the normal position used during elimination is preferred. The semi-Fowler's position with the head elevated and knees flexed should be used when possible to assist with elimination. The sitting position in the bathroom or on a bedside commode is ideal.

Frequent repositioning facilitates motility of the bowel. High-fiber diets and adequate fluids facilitate bowel elimination. Suppositories and stool softeners may be indicated. Privacy is essential in promoting normal bowel habits.

URINARY SYSTEM

The human urinary tract is designed to work most efficiently in the upright position. The anatomy of the kidney in the erect position has the hilum located medially, facilitating urine flow out of the renal pelvis into the ureter with the aid of gravity. Only a small portion of the renal pelvis is in a dependent position to the ureter, where stasis of urine might take place. During recumbency, the hila are positioned superiorly and urine must be forced against gravity into the ureter. Peristaltic activity of the renal pelvis is not sufficient to overcome constant gravitational resistance, and the renal pelvis may fill completely before the urine is transmitted into the ureter. Similarly, bladder anatomy is such that in the recumbent position gravity impedes emptying of the bladder, resulting in urinary stasis in the renal pelvis and bladder. Decreased muscle tone resulting from immobility can affect the tone of the main muscle of micturition (detrusor) and further compromise bladder emptying.

The reclining position can also make it difficult for persons to achieve relaxation of the perineal muscles and external sphincter, thus inhibiting the detrusor muscle reflex and eliminating normal contraction and bladder emptying. If the sensation to void is not heeded, the bladder further distends, causing extensive stretch of the detrusor muscle and inhibiting the sensation to void. In males with prostatic hypertrophy, micturition difficulties are exacerbated.

Renal excretion of calcium also increases with immobility. Hypercalciuria as a result of immobilization has been shown to contribute to the formation of renal calculi in the renal pelvis or bladder. As opposed to the oxalate or urate stones that form in ambulatory individuals, calculi in immobilized individuals are composed of calcium phosphate. Paralyzed persons exhibit a typical triad of conditions (hypercalciuria, renal stasis, and urinary tract infection) that may lead to development of renal calculi of great magnitude.

Risks and Assessment

The ability to position the immobilized individual in a manner conducive to urination should be assessed. If the individual is feeling as though he or she is not fully emptying the bladder or if small amounts of urine are passed, the individual should be assessed using a bladder scanner or by catheterization after voiding to evaluate residual urine. The client should be assessed for symptoms of urinary tract infection, such as pain, burning, and frequency. Sharp flank pain may be indicative of urinary tract calculi.

Measurement of 24-hour fluid intake and output, urine specific gravity, and/or daily weights can be useful in determining the degree of hydration or dehydration present. Inspection of the immobilized individual's urine may indicate signs of infection, such as foul odor or cloudiness. Assessment of bladder distention is important in determining if urine stasis is present.

Alteration in Urinary Elimination

Urinary Elimination Management. The nurse should obtain subjective data of the person's usual voiding routine and assess for hematuria, dysuria, frequent voiding, and urgency. Repositioning facilitates drainage of the renal pelvis, thereby decreasing the incidence of renal calculi. Achieving a position conducive to urinary elimination, such as elevating the head of the bed or using a bedside commode, should be done when possible. A regular voiding schedule should be maintained. If retention is a problem, intermittent catheterization or a retention catheter may be necessary until the individual is able to assume a more natural voiding position.

Dietary intake plays a role in preventing urinary complications from immobility. Calcium intake in excess of daily requirements may contribute to higher renal excretion of calcium and concomitant risk of renal calculi. Fluctuation in fluid intake and output is to be avoided to prevent concentration of urine. Fluids are best taken evenly over the entire 24-hour period, with increased amounts during peaks of calcium excretion. Calcium excretion peaks occur during the middle of the day and for a period of 3 hours after each meal. Urine output ideally should average at least 30 mL/hr or more.

METABOLIC SYSTEM

Negative nitrogen balance as a result of muscle atrophy has been found in immobilized individuals as early as the 6th to 10th day of immobilization. Muscle is catabolized and nitrogen is excreted in urine as a byproduct. Nitrogen excretion in excess of nitrogen intake leads to depletion of protein stores essential for building muscle mass and for wound healing. Persons in negative nitrogen balance exhibit anorexia, which may reduce their intake of protein. Decreased demand for energy to perform daily activities during immobilization can also contribute to reduced calorie intake. Immobilized persons with severe discrepancies between their protein intake and nitrogen excretion may experience malnutrition.

Risks and Assessment

Dietary intake, particularly of protein, should be assessed. Decreased appetite may be a cause or effect of negative nitrogen balance. A 24-hour diet history may be helpful in assessing general nutritional status and adequacy of protein intake. The presence of peripheral edema may also be an indicator of negative nitrogen balance because of decreased protein in the system.

Alteration in Nutrition

Nutrition Management. Appropriate nutrition and fluid intake are the mainstays of preventing metabolic complications of immobility. Calorie intake should be maintained at a rate equal to the metabolic needs of the individual. An immobilized client's diet should include 1 g of protein per kilogram of body weight per day and 1 to 1.5 g of calcium to prevent hypoproteinemia and osteoporosis.

MUSCULOSKELETAL SYSTEM

Bones, muscles, and joints are all affected by immobilization. Although some degree of immobility can promote the healing of injured tissues, many detrimental effects on these tissues from prolonged immobility can occur.

Bone

Bone is a dynamic tissue that not only functions to support the body but also is a major component of the metabolic and endocrine systems that maintain mineral homeostasis. Bone is continually being resorbed and deposited. Nothing demonstrates this interdependence of systems better than the bone demineralization that occurs with immobilization.

Immobilization-induced bone demineralization is due to either the lack of stress experienced with weight bearing or altered mineral homeostasis. Stress placed on the bones from weight bearing is necessary for osteoblast function. Immobility is thought to lead to demineralization and loss of the osseous matrix of bone.

Bed rest leads to negative calcium balance and calcium mobilization from the bones, resulting in net resorption of bone. Increased calcium excretion is a result of imbalance between osteoblastic and osteoclastic activity, with osteoclasts breaking down bone at a rate much faster than osteoblastic buildup. This process results in a decrease in bone density, termed *bone demineralization* or *osteoporosis*.

Hypercalcemia may result from the loss of calcium from the bone during immobility. The primary factor that puts an individual at increased risk for hypercalcemia is a rapid bone turnover before immobilization. This may occur in adolescent males during a growth spurt, in individuals with Paget's disease, and in clients with hyperthyroidism.

Implications for the older individual whose bone density is marginally or truly osteoporotic before the immobilization are significant. Research has shown that high bone turnover in older adults may be a result of physical inactivity rather than hyperparathyroidism (Theiler, Stahelin, Kranzlin, Tyndall, & Bischoff, 1999). Even short-term immobility may greatly increase the risk of fracture because of bone calcium depletion in these individuals.

Muscle

Both muscle mass and strength are maintained by the balance of protein synthesis and degradation. Research indicates that muscle load and activity in some way regulate this balance. Contraction of a muscle at 20% to 30% of maximal strength is necessary to maintain a muscle's normal strength. Immobility decreases muscle load, activity, and protein synthesis and increases protein degradation, resulting in muscle, or disuse, atrophy. Disuse atrophy (the loss of muscle mass and strength secondary to inactivity) is an adaptive mechanism that allows the survival of cells in unfavorable conditions. Several factors may influence the degree of atrophy, including age and gender, duration of immobilization, length of stretch at which muscle was immobilized, degree of disuse compared with normal use, pretreatment, preexisting muscle weakness or atrophy, muscle fiber types, and type of muscle (e.g., extensor or flexor muscles). Although atrophy may be an adaptive mechanism, muscle strength and endurance may decrease as much as 20% during the first week of bed rest. The rate at which this decrease occurs depends on amount of muscle contractions during the period of immobilization.

Increased metabolic needs as a result of fever or trauma contribute to the rapid decline in muscle strength and endurance by accelerating protein catabolism. The greatest changes in muscle strength occur during the first week of immobilization. One to two months of immobility can decrease muscle size by half, with concomitant loss of function. Full function usually returns with resumption of mobility. However, after 4 months of immobility, degeneration of nerve fibers with replacement by fat and fibrous tissue has occurred, so full recovery of muscle function is impossible.

Joints

Joints are also adversely affected by immobility. Daily movement maintains full range of joint motion. Normally, there is continual breakdown and replacement of connective tissue in joints. Progressive degenerative changes in joint tissue during immobilization have been documented. Ligaments and tendons shorten, connective tissue changes occur, and intra-articular degeneration occurs. Fibrosis or increased density of the connective tissues develops because of improper alignment of tissue cells, resulting in decreased range of motion (ROM). A lack of full passive range of motion (PROM) of the joint because of either joint, muscle, or soft tissue limitations is termed a *joint contracture.*

The effects of aging on joints compound the effects of immobility. With age, the collagen content of connective tissue increases. Tissue becomes stiffer, decreasing joint mobility and making contracture more likely in older individuals. Hip and knee joints are particularly prone to contractures and may make the individual less stable when transferring and ambulating, thus increasing the risk of falling.

Joint motion also promotes the interchange of fluid between surface layers of articular cartilage and synovial fluid. Immobility prevents this fluid exchange, resulting in degenerative changes in cartilage.

Ligament laxity may be a consequence of immobility. If the joint is maintained in a stretched position or if muscle tension is not present, ligament laxity and instability of the joint may result. Both of these conditions predispose the client to instability in ambulating and to falls.

Effects of Immobilization of a Body Part

The systemic effects of immobility are not generally evident when immobilization is confined to a single body part. Decreased ROM, joint instability, muscle atrophy, and pressure sores can all be seen as a result of immobilization of a single body part.

Joint instability may occur in an individual who has had limited, short-term immobility imposed. Joint alignment and stability are aided by ligament and muscle activity. With significant muscle atrophy, which occurs

within 4 to 6 days of immobilization, considerable ligament laxity can develop.

The effects of pressure on a body part can be augmented by the apparatus used to maintain immobilization and can be further complicated by the presence of neurologic deficit. Casts and braces are hard surfaces that may compress the integument against bony surfaces, creating pressure areas where tissue necrosis would not normally be a problem. In addition, the apparatus may cover the limb in such a way that inspection of pressure areas is impossible, thus making it difficult to assess for tissue damage. Any neurologic deficit may make it difficult to identify areas of early tissue ischemia because of the lack of perceived pain by the individual.

Assessment

Subjective assessment of the musculoskeletal system includes client reports of declining muscle mass and strength; decreased joint ROM and contracture; and limitation of movement because of pain, fatigue, or depression. Assessment of pain is important because attempts to avoid or minimize pain can limit overall mobility or mobility of a body part. Stiffness and joint pain may result in diminished joint mobility. Symptoms of hypercalcemia may be present, including anorexia, lethargy, nausea, headache, and abdominal cramping. History of compression fracture or presence of risk factors for osteoporosis is noted.

Gait, posture, general coordination, and ease of movement should be assessed objectively. Joint ROM is measured with a goniometer, and muscle mass is measured with a tape measure for both upper and lower extremities. Muscle tone can be evaluated subjectively by observing the person in a relaxed position. Tautness of relaxed muscle indicates tone. Strength can be measured by the individual's ability to move a joint against varying degrees of resistance applied by the examiner. A more objective test of strength can be obtained using an ergometer. Activity endurance should also be measured.

Potential for Disuse Syndrome

Key points to remember with all exercises are to plan exercise periods at optimal energy times for the client (after rest and in early morning).

Exercise Management: Ambulation. Increasing mobility is the primary intervention for limiting the effects of immobility on muscles, bones, and joints. Interventions such as intermittent urinary catheterization and intermittent intravenous infusion devices may facilitate increased mobility in many clients.

Positioning. Normal body alignment is imperative in preventing the effects of immobility on joints. Joint contractures and deformities may result from joints being in improper alignment. The goal is to maintain the body in a posture as near as possible to the normal upright position. The spine should be straight, the head neutral, and all extremities in functional positions. Frequent repositioning also assists in preventing joint contractures. Appropriate devices should maintain the functional position of wrists, hands, fingers, and other body parts. The major joints should be positioned in extension to prevent hip and knee flexion contractures. A footboard or high-top sneakers to maintain the ankles flexed to 90 degrees helps prevent plantar flexion contractures, or foot drop. The footboard also provides a surface for performing isometric exercises of the lower extremities.

Exercise Management: Muscle Control.

Isometric muscle contraction is achieved by tensing the muscle without changing the length of the muscle. Therefore, no resulting joint movement occurs. (For more information on exercises, see Chapter 13.) Isometric exercise can be taught to individuals who are experiencing immobility by having them alternately contract and relax their antagonist muscle groups. Isometric exercise can be done within the confines of a cast or brace. These exercises can be helpful in preventing muscle atrophy. Caution must be taken with the individual with hypertension because there can be a marked increase in blood pressure and heart rate during the exercises. Blood pressure should be monitored when any individual starts these exercises. Further stress can be caused to the cardiovascular system through inadvertent use of Valsalva's maneuver during exercise. Emphasis should be placed on performing all exercises while breathing through the mouth and exhaling during the contraction phase of the exercise to minimize the occurrence of Valsalva's maneuver.

To isometrically exercise the lower extremities, the client should be taught to do quadriceps sets by tightening the kneecap and gluteal sets by tightening the buttocks. For upper extremity exercise, the client should be taught to make a strong fist with each hand for a few seconds with the arms extended. The client can do sets of five isometric contractions of 6 seconds each performed at 2-minute intervals, building up his or her tolerance. Exercise benefits are maximized when they are performed at periods when energy reserves are at their greatest, such as after a rest or early in the morning.

In isotonic, or resistive exercises, the length of the muscle is changed but the muscle tension is maintained in an unaltered state. Lifting weights is one example of isotonic exercise. Pushing or pulling against a stationary object, such as a tensed hand of the examiner, a trapeze, or a footboard, are other examples of isotonics. Examples of isotonic exercises for immobilized individuals are lifting up with the aid of a trapeze, pushing against the bed with the arms from a sitting position, pulling up to a sitting position with a rope attached to the foot of the bed, pushing up from the prone position, or pulling oneself up in bed by pulling on the headboard.

The benefits gained from isotonic exercise are several. Force transmitted across the bone during isotonic exercise is an effective means of preventing loss of bone mass and calcium. Muscle strength, mass, and general endurance are also maintained because of the active use of muscles.

Isotonic exercise may be contraindicated in individuals with cardiovascular compromise. Isotonic exercise raises the blood pressure, and the additional danger from the use of Valsalva's maneuver may contraindicate such exercise in some individuals.

Exercise Management: Joint Mobility.

Active range of motion (AROM) involves an isotonic exercise that moves each body joint through its complete ROM. The objective is to stretch all muscle groups to their maximum over the joint. The client should perform each exercise to the point of slight resistance—never to the point of discomfort.

At first, the nurse may need to assist the client in performing ROM exercises until the client is able to perform them independently. For individuals unable to perform active exercise, either isometric or isotonic, PROM exercises are indicated. PROM serves only to maintain joint mobility, whereas AROM also contributes to muscle strength. A regular schedule of ROM exercises should be established to assure maintenance of mobility in all joints regardless of the client's degree of immobility. The most convenient time to provide ROM exercises is during the bath. The nurse or family member should perform three to five full-range movements of each joint each day. A twice-daily regimen is preferable.

For the individual with a body part immobilized, isometric exercise of the limb immobilized by a cast or traction may aid in maintenance of muscle strength. Emphasis must be placed on providing AROM or PROM to the joints above and below the area of immobilization. Individuals who have experienced an injury may be afraid of mobilizing adjacent joints and may need encouragement or assistance to prevent complications to adjacent joints. Immobilized muscle or muscle groups may be stimulated electrically to help preserve muscle strength and bulk.

Body parts immobilized by paralysis or stroke require diligent isometric and ROM exercise to maintain joint mobility. When at rest, the body part must be maintained in a functional position. Long-term immobility may result in joint contracture; if the contracture is in a nonfunctional position, it may become a further obstacle to care. For example, an individual with paralysis of the lower extremities who experiences ankle contractures in the plantar-flexed position has difficulty sitting in a wheelchair or standing for transfers. In contrast, the individual who develops ankle contracture in the functional position of 90 degrees of flexion is able to place the feet flat on the floor or wheelchair footplates. Functional positioning performed in anticipation of ultimate contracture formation assists in maintaining as much function as possible.

Environmental Management: Safety. To reduce complications from osteoporosis (i.e., fractures), the limbs should be supported while bathing and moving the individual.

Electrolyte Management: Hypercalcemia. In clients who develop immobilization-related hypercalcemia, therapy with pamidronate, which reduces serum calcium levels, may be beneficial.

PSYCHOSENSORY SYSTEM

Personality is shaped, in part, by sensory and motor interactions with the environment and by integration of these interactions. Bed rest restricts physical activity and limits sensory stimulation. This may contribute to psychosocial changes in the individual. Underlying psychosocial maladjustments, hidden and controlled under usual circumstances, may be revealed under the stress of immobilization.

Immobility decreases the quantity and quality of sensory and social interactions available to the individual, thus limiting the ability to interact with the environment. This limited interaction contributes to alterations in perception of such aspects of the environment as time, temperature, and weight. The lack of social stimulation may cause disturbances in cognitive, perceptual, and motor processes.

Neurologic responses to immobility have been evidenced by the slowing of electroencephalographic (EEG) waves. Sleep-pattern disturbances have been linked with interruptions in the circadian rhythm as manifestations of immobility. Disturbing the natural cycles of work/rest and light/dark leads to decreased performance ability and increased psychosomatic complaints. The actual response observed is unique to the individual and depends partially on personality factors and ability to adapt to disturbances in sleep patterns and forced changes in circadian rhythm.

Limitation in social interaction may be the greatest deprivation imposed by immobility. Limited contact with family and friends can lead to decreased motivation to seek medical care as well as decreased potential for recovery. Individuals whose support systems exhibit caring attitudes toward them and ensure that needed care is obtained respond more quickly to treatment than do those without such caring contacts.

Alteration in social roles of the immobilized individual may contribute to feelings of depression and diminished self-worth. With decreased physical activity, inability to perform work, and decreased interpersonal interactions, the immobilized individual's capability to perform expected roles diminishes.

Risks and Assessment

Determination of social and ethnic behaviors or beliefs may reveal some potential contributing factors to the development of psychosocial problems related to immobility. An assessment of the medications the individual is receiving that may contribute to psychosensory impairment should also be done.

The presence or history of life stressors contributes to the individual's ability to cope psychologically with immobility. Information should be elicited about the individual's life roles and potential changes in those roles as a result of the illness or treatment. Concerns over the cost of the illness or issues related to sexuality may be exerting additional stress. A history of depression or signs of withdrawal should be assessed. Knowledge of available support systems, including friends, family, work, and religious resources, is important to developing a plan of care.

Psychosensory assessment includes observation for signs of possible withdrawal, depression, or anxiety. The neurologic status of all extremities supplies information about nerve conduction and the client's ability to receive sensory information for the purposes of maintaining both safety and mobility.

Self-esteem Disturbance and Social Isolation

Self-esteem Enhancement and Socialization Enhancement. One of the most effective means of counteracting the effects of sensory deprivation in immobilized individuals is to involve them in their own care. Active participation returns a sense of control to the client and allows purposeful thought and activity. Visits by family and friends and nursing staff provide information from the outside world and conversation. The more human contact an activity affords, the greater the intellectual and emotional stimulation. Television and reading are less effective but useful diversional activities. Clocks, calendars, and newspapers help maintain realistic time perception. Wearing clothes rather than gowns or pajamas and sitting at a table for meals are other activities that may promote a sense of normalcy.

Altered Role Performance

Role Enhancement. Discussion of client concerns about altered roles, finances, and other matters is essential. Social service and occupational therapy are important resources in assisting the individual to deal with alterations in home and self-care, family roles, and financial concerns.

CLINICAL PATHWAY: *Care of the Immobilized Client*

NURSING DIAGNOSIS AND ACTIVITY	INTERVENTIONS

Musculoskeletal System

Alteration in Physical Activity: Potential for Disuse Syndrome

Assessment	Assess active range of all pertinent joints with and without counter-resistance daily; record
	Grade strength of all pertinent muscle groups; record
	Assess passive range of motion of all pertinent joints daily; record
Treatments	Plan exercise periods at optimal energy times for client: after rest and in early morning
	Maintain normal body alignment: spine straight, head neutral
	Extremities in functional position: major joints in extension, footboard to maintain ankles flexed to 90 degrees
	Reposition frequently
	Active range of motion: body joints within imposed restrictions
	Passive range of motion: if client unable to participate in exercise, perform three to five ranges daily or twice daily
	Support limbs during activity
	Monitor blood pressure and pulse during isotonic and isometric exercise
	Isotonic exercises
Education	Teach client exercises
Clinical outcomes	Client will maintain muscle strength, endurance, joint flexibility, and mobility
Discharge planning	Teach family/significant other how to perform passive range of motion on client as needed, or arrange for physical therapist to see client daily to perform passive range of motion

Cardiovascular System

Alteration in Activity Tolerance: Decreased Cardiac Function

Assessment	Assess pulse and blood pressure twice daily
	Perform orthostatic blood pressure measurements before each ambulation until blood pressure is within normal limits
Treatments	Elevate head of bed
	Reposition frequently
	Dangle and ambulate when able
	Encourage client participation in positioning
	Tilt table with gradual increase of angle to upright position
	Use sequential pneumatic compression devices and elastic support stockings
	Elevate legs to promote passive drainage
Education	Teach client/significant other to do the following:
	Assess pulse and blood pressure twice daily
	Perform orthostatic blood pressure measurements before each ambulation until blood pressure is within normal limits
	Elevate head of bed
	Reposition frequently
	Dangle and ambulate when able
	Use sequential pneumatic compression devices and elastic support stockings
	Elevate legs to promote passive drainage
Clinical outcomes	Client will tolerate activity well, and cardiac function will remain at baseline or improved

Integumentary System

Potential for Impaired Skin Integrity

Assessment	Asses skin frequently; pay particular attention to skin under and near immobilization devices, casts, braces, or traction
Treatments	Reposition every 2 hr; use turning schedule
	Turn to at least 30-degree oblique position to relieve sacral pressure
	Use positioning devices: footboard, cradle, trapeze, wheelchair cushion
	For incontinence, use scheduled toileting, external urinary incontinence devices, disposable incontinence briefs
	Cleanse with nonirritating soap and water and dry thoroughly
Education	Teach client/significant other to do the following:
	Assess skin frequently; pay particular attention to skin under and near immobilization devices, casts, braces, or traction
	Reposition every 2 hr; use turning schedule
	Turn to at least 30-degree oblique position to relieve sacral pressure
	Use positioning devices: footboard, cradle, trapeze, wheelchair cushion
	For incontinence, use scheduled toileting, external urinary incontinence devices, disposable incontinence briefs
	Cleanse with nonirritating soap and water and dry thoroughly
Clinical outcomes	Skin is intact

Respiratory System

Potential for Ineffective Breathing Pattern

Assessment	Assess and record lung sounds twice a day
	Assess for productive cough
	Assess for dyspnea
	Assess for respiratory distress

CLINICAL PATHWAY: *Care of the Immobilized Client* **Continued**

NURSING DIAGNOSIS AND ACTIVITY	INTERVENTIONS

Respiratory System *Continued*

Potential for Ineffective Breathing Pattern Continued

Treatments	Use lateral recumbent and Trendelenburg's positions
	Deep breathe and cough; every 2 hr, in sitting position when able
	Fluid intake of 30–40 mL/kg of body weight/day
	Humidify oxygen, if used
	Continuous lateral rotation therapy if at high risk
Education	Teach client/significant other to do the following:
	Assess for productive cough, dyspnea, or respiratory distress and notify physician if any occur
	Use lateral recumbent and Trendelenburg's positions
	Have client deep breathe and cough; every 2 hr, in sitting position when able
	Have client drink fluid intake of 30–40 mL/kg of body weight/day
	Humidify oxygen, if used
	Continuous lateral rotation therapy if at high risk
Clinical outcomes	Respiratory rate is within normal limits
	Breath sounds are clear
	Client is afebrile
	Oxygenation is within normal limits

Gastrointestinal System

Constipation

Assessment	Inquire about usual bowel routine
	Assess for chronic use of laxatives
Treatments	Reposition frequently
	Use semi-Fowler's position or sit on commode seat or toilet to void
	Encourage high-fiber diet
	Encourage fluids
	Record and monitor bowel routine
Education	Teach client to do the following:
	Reposition frequently
	Use semi-Fowler's position or sit on commode seat or toilet to void
	Encourage high-fiber diet
	Encourage fluids
	Record and monitor bowel routine
Clinical outcomes	Client will have regular bowel movements

Urinary System

Altered Pattern of Urinary Elimination

Assessment	Inquire about usual voiding routine
	Assess for hematuria, dysuria, frequent voiding, and urgency
Treatments	Reposition frequently
	Use semi-Fowler's position or sit on commode seat or toilet to void
	Maintain regular voiding schedule
	Monitor for urine retention
	Offer fluid intake at regular intervals
	Increase fluid consumption midday and 3 hr after meals
Education	Teach client to do the following:
	Reposition frequently
	Use semi-Fowler's position or sit on commode seat or toilet to void
	Maintain regular voiding schedule
	Monitor for urine retention
	Take fluid at regular intervals
	Increase fluid consumption midday and 3 hr after meals
Clinical outcomes	Client will void adequate amounts at least every 6–8 hr without urinary retention

Psychosensory System

Alteration in Role Performance

Treatments	Encourage discussion of altered roles, finances, and concerns
	Social service referral
Clinical outcome	Client will cope effectively

Box continued on following page

CLINICAL PATHWAY: *Care of the Immobilized Client* **Continued**

NURSING DIAGNOSIS AND ACTIVITY	INTERVENTIONS
Psychosensory System *Continued*	
Social Isolation	
Treatments	Encourage visits by family and friends
Clinical outcome	Have client wear own clothes or pajamas
	Client will engage in social activities
Self-esteem Disturbance	
Assessment	Assess for orientation to person, place, and time
Treatments	Involve client in own care
	Occupational and recreational therapy for diversion
	Offer roommate for company
	Clock and calendar in room
Clinical outcome	Client will verbalize positive statement about self

ASSESSMENT OF RISK FOR COMPLICATIONS OF IMMOBILITY

Three important qualifying factors provide a reference for predicting the effects of immobilization on a particular individual: (1) control over mobility, (2) duration of immobility, and (3) degree of immobility. *Control* over mobility refers to the individual's ability to control physical movement. The presence of chronic illness, advancing age, or any condition that depletes physical resources compromises an individual's ability to meet and overcome the physical demands of immobility.

The *duration* of immobility is a measure of time and is relative to the type of immobilizing event and its potential for complications. For example, the healthy individual with a short-leg cast for a metatarsal fracture experiences immobility of that limb for approximately 6 to 8 weeks. The effects of such immobility in that individual are most likely limited to localized muscle atrophy, decreased joint mobility, and potential pressure areas under the cast. On the other hand, a frail, older woman in negative nitrogen balance on admission to the hospital for a fractured hip who is immobilized in bed with Buck's traction for 3 days before surgery has the potential for more severe complications from immobility. The duration of immobility may be less in the second situation, but the potential for serious effects is greater.

The *degree* of immobility refers to the extent or severity of the mobility limitations. Degree of immobility represents the individual's level of restriction in the ability to produce body movements and the constancy with which a body position is maintained without adjustment. Restrictions may be a result of decreased energy, motor paralysis, cast, or traction. The greater the physical immobility and the more constant the body posture, the greater the potential for complications to develop. Using the concepts of control, duration, and degree, the nurse can readily assess those indicators that place individuals at greatest risk for development of complications.

Determining Risk

Determining the risk for developing complications of immobility is complex. Currently available risk scales do not incorporate assessment parameters for development of general complications of immobility. Scales have been devised to determine an individual's risk for development of pressure sores (a single complication resulting from immobility) and may be generalized to determine the risk for development of other complications of immobility.

There are many individual variables to be taken into consideration when assessing the risks from immobility. A thorough knowledge of the potential complications of immobility, the individual's health history, and the current assessment findings (subjective and objective), as well as the pathologic process causing the immobilization, must all be weighed. Nursing judgment is used to determine risk and subsequent nursing interventions. Ongoing assessment includes evaluation of the effectiveness of preventive nursing interventions and detection of complication development in its early stages.

Diagnostic Evaluation

Baseline diagnostic studies, in conjunction with assessment parameters, can aid in determining the risk for complications of immobility. Diagnostics are also useful in determining the presence or absence of certain complications throughout the period of immobility. A summary of diagnostic findings is included in Table 4–5.

Increased serum calcium and phosphate levels and elevated urine calcium levels indicate bone demineralization. Bone densitometry is a noninvasive study that yields an actual measurement of bone density and is diagnostic for osteoporosis. Increases in blood urea nitrogen (BUN), serum hematocrit, urine pH, and urine specific gravity suggest dehydration, which is an indicator of decreased venous flow and possible orthostatic intolerance. Doppler studies help evaluate peripheral vascular status and venous and arterial blood flow to the extremities. Elevated white blood cell count, decreased Pao_2, and increased $Paco_2$ can signify respiratory compromise. Lung scans and pulmonary angiography are useful in diagnosing pulmonary embolus. Negative nitrogen balance is indicated by decreased serum protein and increased BUN. Excretion of urinary nitrogen in excess of protein intake is also indicative of negative nitrogen balance.

EVIDENCE-BASED PRACTICE

Nursing practice significantly affects the various hazards of immobility daily. The one hazard of immobility, which happens most quickly, is most obvious, often incurs the most cost, and has probably the longest recovery period,

TABLE 4–5. *Diagnostic Findings in Complications of Mobility*

TEST	FINDING
Laboratory	
Serum protein	Decreased in negative nitrogen balance
Serum calcium	Increased in bone demineralization
Serum phosphate	Increased in bone demineralization
Blood urea nitrogen (BUN)	Increased in negative nitrogen balance and dehydration
White blood cell count	Increased in respiratory compromise
Hematocrit	Increased in dehydration
Arterial blood gases	Decreased Pao_2 and increased $Paco_2$ in respiratory compromise
Urine calcium	Increased in bone demineralization
Urine pH	Increased in dehydration
Urine specific gravity	Increased in dehydration
Radiographic	
Chest x-ray film	Diagnostic in pneumonia
Lung scan, ventilation/ perfusion scan	Diagnostic in pulmonary embolus
Noninvasive Procedures	
Doppler studies	Diagnostic in deep vein thrombosis, thrombophlebitis
Bone densitometry	Diagnostic in bone demineralization

is the pressure ulcer. Assessment, prevention, and treatment are the three primary areas nursing research has concentrated on to limit the effect of pressure ulcers. Research on assessment has yielded the Braden Scale, which is currently used worldwide to single out clients at high risk for pressure ulcers. Utilization of this tool has aided in preventing many pressure ulcers from occurring. Nursing research continues on aspects of prevention and treatment of pressure ulcers. The search continues for the most appropriate support surface as well as the most appropriate dressing for the various stages of pressure ulcers. After a review of the literature on immobility, two practice questions can be identified:

1. In immobilized clients at risk for pressure ulcers, what is the effect of support surfaces such as pressure-relieving beds, mattresses and cushions, on the prevention and treatment of pressure ulcers?
2. In immobilized clients with pressure ulcers, which dressing technique is most effective in treating pressure ulcers?

Studies related to these questions are summarized in the evidence-based practice tables in this chapter.

INNOVATIONS AND FUTURE TRENDS

Various subsets of the client population will continue to require immobilization to some extent. How nursing deals proactively with the care of these clients will depend on the easy accessibility of current quality clinical research related to the hazards the clients are sure to experience. Evidence-based nursing practice is an essential tool to be thoroughly used in the near and distant future. Use of this research will legitimize reimbursement for preventative care of the immobilized client.

Utilization of quality support surfaces, dressing compounds, aggressive turning schedules and exercise regimens, as well as nutritional guidelines and toileting schedules, will continue to be the core of quality care of the immobilized client.

SUMMARY

The ability to move freely, purposefully, and without restriction is vital to maintaining life. The balance of human beings in their environment is based on a state of dynamic equilibrium that is maintained by mechanisms of autoregulation so broad that they affect virtually every body system. The ability to maintain mobility is a major factor on which autoregulation mechanisms are dependent for proper functioning. The nurse who is knowledgeable about the potential dangers of immobility and who is diligent in implementing preventive interventions becomes a key instrument in forestalling the complications of immobility. *Text continued on page 127*

EXAMINING THE EVIDENCE: Moving Toward Evidence-Based Practice
1. In Immobilized Clients at Risk for Pressure Ulcers, What Is the Effect of Support Surfaces Such As Pressure-Relieving Beds, Mattresses, and Cushions on the Prevention and Treatment of Pressure Ulcers?

AUTHOR(S), YEAR	SAMPLE	DESIGN/METHOD	OUTCOME VARIABLE	MAJOR FINDINGS
Aronovitch et al., 1999	N = 217 Surgical clients with minimum of 3-hr surgery	Comparative study Experimental alternating air device (experimental group) compared with tertiary care facility's conventional practice (control group)	Pressure ulcer incidence	Zero ulcers in experimental group; 11 ulcers in 7 patients in control group; (1 stage I; 4 stage II; 6 no stage because of eschar); 8.75% incidence rate with $p = .005$
Cooper, Gray, & Mollison, 1998	N = 100 orthopaedic clients	Randomized, controlled trial of 2 dry-flotation pressure-reducing surfaces	Pressure ulcer incidence	Not possible to determine any difference in effectiveness between mattresses because of low rate of pressure sore incidence in this high-risk group
Defloor & Grypdonck, 2000	N = 20 healthy volunteers	Interface pressures of 29 cushions and a sheepskin measured on each participant in upright posture with back against back of chair, hands on lap, knees at 90 degrees, and feet on floor	Interface pressure	13 cushions had pressure-reducing effect; gel cushions and sheepskins had no pressure-reducing effect; lowest interface pressures on air cushions and some foam cushions
Defloor & Grypdonck, 1999	N = 56 healthy volunteers	Interface pressures measured in volunteers in 8 postures using 4 cushions (designed for incontinent clients)	Interface pressure at seat surface	Lowest maximum pressure posture was sitting back with legs on a rest; less pressure if legs on floor Sliding down and slouching caused highest maximum pressure Thick air cushion had lowest maximum pressure and significantly better than other cushions at reducing high pressure because of sliding down or slouching
Fontaine, Risley, & Castellino, 1998	N = 11 healthy participants	Comparative study in laboratory setting 3 different Medicare-approved therapeutic support surfaces (on identical platforms): • Nonpowered fluid overlay • Powered, air-filled overlay • Powered air-filled mattress	Interface pressure and shear	Pressure on nonpowered fluid overlay lower than that on powered air-filled overlay at trochanter Pressure on both nonpowered fluid overlay and powered air-filled mattress lower than that on powered air-filled overlay at sacrum No pressure differences among surfaces at heels, supine sacrum, or scapula Shear on nonpowered fluid overlay was significantly lower than on either of the powered support surfaces
Wells & Karr, 1998	N = 22 volunteers N = 33 recruited clients	Interface pressure measured on 22 volunteers on nonpowered fluid mattress (study mattress) Pressure ulcer healing and cost of mattress evaluated for 36 stage I–IV pressure ulcers and 24 surgically repaired ulcers in 33 clients Client and practitioner satisfaction measured upon completion of study	Interface pressure, wound healing, client and practitioner satisfaction	Study mattress relieves pressure as well as present technology per direct comparison of interface pressures with air-fluidized and low-air-loss beds Wounds of clients on study mattress healed at rate of 31% per week Flapped wounds healed at rate of 7.7% per week No new ulcers reported among clients using study mattress Clients and practitioners satisfied with comfort and performance of study mattress, comparing it favorably with air-fluidized and low-air-loss surfaces

EXAMINING THE EVIDENCE: Moving Toward Evidence-Based Practice
1. In Immobilized Clients at Risk for Pressure Ulcers, What Is the Effect of Support Surfaces Such As Pressure-Relieving Beds, Mattresses, and Cushions on the Prevention and Treatment of Pressure Ulcers?
Continued

AUTHOR(S), YEAR	SAMPLE	DESIGN/METHOD	OUTCOME VARIABLE	MAJOR FINDINGS
Torra i Bou, Rueda López, & Ramón Cantón, 2000	$N = 3$ healthy volunteers	Experimental study Pressure measured before and after application of an Allevyn hydrocellular external application at sacrum, ischium, and heel of subjects (A, an 85-kg 170-cm male; B, a 54.3-kg 159-cm female; C, a 69.4-kg 164-cm male) Pressures measured on 2 surfaces: a viscoelastic foam mattress and a conventional hospital mattress at 0, 30, 45, and 60 degrees of inclination	Pressure	Total of 144 pressure readings Average pressure reduction after applying external hydrocellular application on all participants at all inclinations on all surfaces for each of the 3 zones was 19.5% in sacrum; 13.8% in ischium; and 20.15% in heel The external hydrocellular application studied does have a local reducing effect on pressure Although each external hydrocellular application has unique structure, results cannot be generalized to other types of external hydrocellular groups
Russell & Lichtenstein, 2000	$N = 198$ clients having cardiovascular surgery of at least 4 hr	Single center, prospective, randomized, controlled trial Participants assigned randomly before surgery to dynamic mattress system or conventional management beginning in OR and continuing for 7 days postoperatively Clients assessed daily using standardized scoring system	Evidence of pressure ulcers	Dynamic mattress group ($N = 98$) and conventional group ($N = 100$) similar at baseline Decreased pressure ulcers in dynamic group ($N = 2$) compared with conventional group ($N = 7$) Conclusion: multicell pulsating dynamic mattress system is safe and limits risks for and decreases incidence of pressure ulcers in cardiovascular surgery clients
Schultz et al., 1999	$N = 413$ surgical clients	Experimental design Subjects randomized to receive "usual perioperative care" or new mattress overlay Participants assessed over 6 postoperative days	Pressure ulcer incidence	89 clients (21.5%) developed pressure ulcers, mostly stage I; 2% developed stage II or IV ulcers Clients with ulcers were older, were diabetic, had smaller body mass and lower Braden scores on admission, and used the new mattress overlay ($p < .02$) Ecchymotic or "burnlike" ulcers did not progress to stage III or IV during the study Mattress overlay was not effective in preventing pressure ulcers
Pring & Millman, 1998a	$N = 20$	Evaluation	Interface pressures	Pegasus Airwave mattress had higher readings than Quattro DC2000 ($p = .021$, 95% confidence level) and Nimbus II ($p = .009$, 99% confidence level) No significant difference between pressures for Quattro DC2000 and the Nimbus II
Pring & Millman, 1998b	$N = 40$ clients with neurologic disorders who had Waterlow scores $\leq$ 15 and required pressure support	Mattresses evaluated	Effectiveness in relation to pain and discomfort	Pain and discomfort were rated significantly less with the Quattro DC2000 than the Nimbus II and Pegasus Airwave

Box continued on following page

EXAMINING THE EVIDENCE: Moving Toward Evidence-Based Practice
1. In Immobilized Clients at Risk for Pressure Ulcers, What Is the Effect of Support Surfaces Such As Pressure-Relieving Beds, Mattresses, and Cushions on the Prevention and Treatment of Pressure Ulcers?
Continued

AUTHOR(S), YEAR	SAMPLE	DESIGN/METHOD	OUTCOME VARIABLE	MAJOR FINDINGS
Nixon et al., 1998	N = 446 general, vascular, and gynecologic surgical clients	Two-center, double-triangular randomized, controlled trial Standard operating table mattress (N = 224) Experimental group, dry visco-elastic polymer pad (N = 222)	Pressure ulcer incidence postoperatively	Pressure ulcer incidence: Experimental group—11% (22/205) Standard group—20% (43/211) Significant reduction in odds of developing pressure ulcer on dry visco-elastic polymer pad as compared with standard mattress (95% confidence interval of [0.26, 0.82], p = .010)
Cullum et al., 2000		Search by two reviewers independently of 19 databases, hand searching of journals, conference proceedings, and bibliographies for randomized, controlled trials evaluating support surfaces for prevention or treatment of pressure ulcers No language or publication restrictions Trials with similar clients, comparisons, and outcomes pooled Other trials discussed		Conclusions: Regarding prevention: Good evidence of effectiveness of high specification foam over standard hospital foam, and pressure relief in OR Regarding treatment: Good evidence of effectiveness of air-fluidized and low-air-loss devices, but not possible to determine most effective surface for either prevention or treatment

In summary, a review of the most current, pertinent research related to the question of the effect of support surfaces used by immobilized clients on the prevention and treatment of pressure ulcers suggests that findings can be grouped into two groups based on the outcome variable. One group of studies has the incidence of pressure ulcers as the outcome variable, and the second group of studies has interface perfusion as the outcome variable. It is assumed that the higher the interface pressure, the greater the risk of pressure ulcers. Of the 13 studies reviewed, 5 had outcome variables of the incidence of pressure ulcers and 6 had interface pressure as the outcome variable. One study was a review of 19 research articles on support surfaces. Of the five studies done on the incidence of pressure ulcers, the participants were primarily surgical clients. The studies were primarily randomized, controlled trials. Major findings of the studies were that alternating air device had no incidence of pressure ulcers, mattress overlay was not effective in preventing pressure ulcers, and there is a significant reduction in chance of developing pressure ulcer on dry visco-elastic polymer pad. The review of 19 articles could not determine which was the best surface for prevention or treatment. The study that looked at both incidence and interface pressure reported no new ulcers with nonpowered fluid mattress.

The Agency for Health Care Policy and Research (AHCPR) has recommended that clients at risk for pressure ulcers be placed on some type of pressure-reducing support surface. Even though many types of support surfaces exist, few published researches articles exist that specifically compare the efficacy of one product to another (Day, Hayes, Kennedy, & Diercksen, 1997).

Andrychuk (1998) summarized qualities of various support surfaces for the bed and also addresses nursing interventions as well.

EXAMINING THE EVIDENCE: Moving Toward Evidence-Based Practice
2. In Immobilized Clients with Pressure Ulcers, Which Dressing Technique Is Most Effective in Treating Pressure Ulcers?

AUTHOR(S), YEAR	SAMPLE SIZE	DESIGN	OUTCOME VARIABLE	MAJOR FINDINGS
Baynham, Kohlman, & Katner, 1999	$N = 1$ with three wounds	Experimental Three stage IV wounds at right ischium ($7.5 \times 2.5 \times 2.5$ cm), left ischium ($8 \times 3.5 \times 2.5$ cm), and sacrum ($3.5 \times 2 \times 2$ cm) treated with a vacuum-assisted closure device (VAC) to speed wound healing Treatment began in August 1996 and consisted of insertion of sterile sponge into the wound bed connected to negative pressure of 125 mm Hg per suction hose with 5 min on and 2 min off cycle Dressings changes every 48 hr	Wound healing	Successful closure of sacral ulcer occurred in 3 months Ischial ulcers off VAC in 4 months
Banks et al., 1997	$N = 61$ clients	Prospective, stratified, randomized clinical trial Clients grouped according to wound type: 20 leg ulcers, 20 stage II or stage III pressure ulcers, and 21 other wounds Clients randomized to treatment and dressings changes Treatment for 6 wk or until wound exuding (absence of leakage with dressing in place for more than 4 days on two consecutive occasions) Wound photos and tracings done weekly	Performance and safety of dressing	Two dressings were similar in performance (could remain in place for about 2.5 days regardless of wound type) No statistically significant differences in surrounding skin condition, reduction in size, client comfort, or ease of application or removal
Thomas et al., 1998	$N = 30$ clients	Randomized, controlled trial Clients randomized to receive either daily topical application of hydrogel study dressing (acemannan hydrogel wound dressing) or a moist saline gauze dressing	Healing of wound	Complete wound healing in 19 of 30 clients (63%) during 10-week observation No difference in complete healing between experimental and control groups Study suggests acemannan hydrogel dressing is as effective as, but is not superior to, moist saline gauze for management of pressure ulcers
Burke et al., 1998	$N = 42$ (A, $N = 18$) (B, $N = 24$)	Clients in two acute care facilities with stage III or IV pressure ulcers All wounds mechanically debrided of necrotic tissue Then clients randomly assigned to either conservative treatment (group A) or conservative treatment plus whirlpool (group B) Conservative treatment included interventions to maximize pressure relief and wet-to-wet dressings using normal saline Dressings changed twice daily and when soiled Whirlpool for 20 min per day in group B clients Ulcer changes over time were compared between groups	Ulcer dimension	Group receiving conservative treatment plus whirlpool improved at a significantly faster rate then did the group receiving conservative treatment only ($p < .05$).

Box continued on following page

EXAMINING THE EVIDENCE: Moving Toward Evidence-Based Practice
2. In Immobilized Clients with Pressure Ulcers, Which Dressing Technique Is Most Effective in Treating Pressure Ulcers? Continued

AUTHOR(S), YEAR	SAMPLE SIZE	DESIGN	OUTCOME VARIABLE	MAJOR FINDINGS
Seeley, Jensen, & Hutcherson, 1999	$N = 40$	Comparison of adhesive hydrocellular dressing with a leading hydrocolloid dressing in management of pressure ulcer Clients had either stage II or III pressure ulcers and were randomized to either hydrocellular or hydrocolloid dressing Dressings done as required and ulcer assessed weekly Clients followed for 8 wk, until ulcer closed, or until client withdrawn from study		Hydrocellular dressing was found to compare favorably with hydrocolloid dressing Hydrocellular dressing easier to remove ($p > .001$) and quicker to change ($p < .001$) than hydrocolloid dressing No differences between dressing groups regarding mean wound pain, odor, and changes in ulcer appearance and ulcer area
Yamashita et al., 1999	$N = 40$ clinical cases	Clinical evaluation Allogeneic cultured dermal substitute (CDS) was applied to the debrided wound, over which a covering material and a conventional gauze dressing were applied to protect the CDS	Granulation tissue formation	93% (14/15) of burns, 100% (5/5) of pressure ulcers, 82% (9/11) of skin ulcers, and 89% (8/9) of traumatic skin defects had good or excellent results; that is, in the cases of deep skin defects, healthy granulation tissue was formed by 4 wk In the cases of chronic skin defects, granulation tissue formation and wound size reduction was noted at 4 wk Study suggests allogeneic CDS is able to provide effective therapy for clients with full-thickness skin defects
Alvarez et al., 2000	$N = 21$	To evaluate efficacy of two chemical debridement formulations: (1) a formulation with specific protease (collagenase) alone and (2) a formulation containing both enzymatic and nonenzymatic agents (papain/urea) Clients were screened for 2 wk to stabilize wound and to provide supportive therapies Then only clients with wounds stable or improving were included in the study Wounds were treated until debridement or for 4 wk	Efficacy assessments: type and amount of necrotic tissue, time to granulation, wound size, rate of closure, bacterial burden and overall wound improvement Safety assessments: wound infection, localized irritation, pain, and wound deterioration	Papain/urea debriding ointment significantly more effective than collagenase in reducing amount of nonviable tissue (68.3% vs. 22.3% at 2 wk, 86.5% vs. 37.3% at 3 wk, $p < .05$ and 95.4% vs. 35.8% at 4 wk, $p < .01$) Mean time to 50% granulation for papain/urea group was 6.8 days compared with 28 days for collagenase group Overall wound response to papain/urea was 4.1 times better than for collagenase ($p < .01$) No significant differences in bacterial burden or rate of wound closure between the two groups Both substances slightly better at dissolving black eschar than fibrin slough No adverse effects associated with either substance
Thomas et al., 1997	$N = 199$ (100 clients with leg ulcers, 99 clients with pressure sores in the community)	Randomized, controlled clinical study comparing a hydropolymer dressing (Tielle) and a hydrocolloid dressing (Granuflex)	Healing	Statistically significant differences in favor of hydropolymer dressing detected for dressing leakage and odor production No statistically significant differences recorded in number of clients with either leg ulcers or pressure sores who healed in each treatment group

EXAMINING THE EVIDENCE: Moving Toward Evidence-Based Practice
2. In Immobilized Clients with Pressure Ulcers, Which Dressing Technique Is Most Effective in Treating Pressure Ulcers? Continued

AUTHOR(S), YEAR	SAMPLE SIZE	DESIGN	OUTCOME VARIABLE	MAJOR FINDINGS
Bale et al., 1998	N = 50	Randomized, controlled, assessor-blind, clinical trial assessing efficacy of two hydrogel dressing in debridement of necrotic pressure sores Clients assessed weekly per computerized wound analysis for 4 wk or until debrided Debridement identified when 80% red granulation tissue present and no sign of necrosis	Comfort, wound odor, surrounding skin condition, time to debride	No statistically significant differences between groups in any of areas assessed
Bale et al., 1997	N = 61 clients with stage II or III pressure sores in 5 centers in United Kingdom	Randomized study comparing polyurethane foam dressing with a hydrocolloid dressing Dressings applied for up to 30 days, with assessments made at each dressing change	Ease of application and removal, adhesion, conformability, absorbency, and wear time	Both dressings easy and convenient to apply Absorbency and ease of removal were significantly better with polyurethane foam dressing than with hydrocolloid dressing Wear times were similar

In summary, a review of the most current research related to the most effective dressing choice for immobilized clients with pressure ulcers suggests that findings may be grouped as follows: Six studies looked at the outcome variable of wound healing, and four studies looked at the qualities of the dressings. In the studies related to wound healing, half were randomized, controlled trials. These studies found that (1) acemannan hydrogel dressing is as effective, but not superior to, moist saline gauze for management of pressure ulcers; (2) wounds provided conservative treatment plus whirlpool improved more quickly than wounds provided the use of only conservative treatment (increased pressure relief and wet-to-wet normal saline dressings); and (3) hydropolymer dressings were found to promote healing better than hydrocolloid dressings. The other three studies found that a vacuum-assisted-closure device assisted in faster closure of sacral ulcers, allogeneic cultured dermal substitutes provide effective therapy for clients with full-thickness skin deficits, and the use of papain/urea debriding ointment is more effective than collagenase in debriding wounds and thus speeding up the time to achieve granulation of the wound. Three of the four studies that looked at dressing qualities were randomized, controlled trials. All three studies found that dressings were all similar. One study looked at time to achieve granulation using two types of hydrogel dressings; one looked at ease of application, removal, adhesion, conformability, absorbency, and wear time comparing a hydrocolloid and a polyurethane dressing, and one looked at performance and safety of dressing.

Further information regarding wound debridement options and a dressing options guide for wounds may be found in an article by Andrychuk (1998). Although existing dressing research has improved the status of wound care, further research is essential to foster the best care of pressure ulcers at various stages.

INTERNET RESOURCES

The National Decubitus Foundation: www.decubitus.org
World Wide Wounds: www.worldwidewounds.com/
index.html
WoundCareNet.com: www.woundcarenet.com

REFERENCES

Agency for Health Care Policy and Research (AHCPR). (1994, December). *Pressure ulcer treatment.* (Clinical Practice Guideline. Quick Reference Guide for Clinicians No. 15. AHCPR Pub. No. 95-0653). Rockville, MD: Public Health Service, U.S. Department of Health and Human Services.

Agency for Health Care Policy and Research (AHCPR). (1992, May). *Pressure ulcers in adults: Prediction and prevention.* (Clinical Practice Guideline. Quick Reference Guide for Clinicians No. 3. AHCPR Pub. No. 92-0047). Rockville, MD: Public Health Service, U.S. Department of Health and Human Services.

Alvarez, O. M., Fernandez-Obregon, A., Rogers, R. S., Bergamo, L., Masso, J., & Black, M. (2000). Chemical debridement of pressure ulcers: A prospective, randomized, comparative trial of collagenase and papain/urea formulations. *Wounds—A Compendium of Clinical Research & Practice, 12*(2), 15–25.

Andrychuk, M. A. (1998). Pressure ulcers: Causes, risk factors, assessment, and interventions. *Orthopaedic Nursing, 17*(4), 65–83.

Aronovitch, S. A., Wilber, M., Slezak, S., Martin, T., & Utter, D. (1999). A comparative study of an alternating air mattress for the prevention of pressure ulcers in surgical patients. *Ostomy Wound Management, 45*(30), 42–44.

Bale, S., Banks, V., Haglestein, S., & Harding, K. G. (1998). A comparison of two amorphous hydrogels in the debridement of pressure sores. *Journal of Wound Care, 7,* 65–68.

Bale, S., Squires, D., Varnon, T., Walker, A., Benbow, M., & Harding, K. G. (1997). A comparison of two dressings in pressure sore management. *Journal of Wound Care, 6,* 463–466.

Banks, V., Bale, S., Harding, K., & Harding, E. F. (1997). Evaluation of a new polyurethane foam dressing. *Journal of Wound Care, 6,* 266–269.

Barczak, C. A., Barnett, R. I., Childs, E. J., & Bosley, L. M. (1997). Fourth national pressure ulcer prevalence survey. *Advances in Wound Care, 10*(4), 18–26.

Baynham, S. A., Kohlman, P., & Katner, H. P. (1999). Treating stage IV pressure ulcers with negative therapy: A case report. *Ostomy Wound Management, 45,* 28–30.

Braden, B. J., & Bergstrom, N. (1989). Clinical utility of the Braden scale for predicting pressure sore risk. *Decubitus, 2*(3), 44–51.

Burke, D. T., Ho, C. H., Saucier, M. A., & Stewart, G. (1998). Effects of hydrotherapy on pressure ulcer healing. *American Journal of Physical Medicine & Rehabilitation, 77,* 394–398.

Casey, G. (2000). Modern wound dressings. *Nursing Standard, 15*(5), 47–51.

Cooper, P. J., Gray, D. G., & Mollison, J. (1998). A randomized controlled trial of two pressure-reducing surfaces. *Journal of Wound Care, 7,* 374–376.

Cullum, N., Deeks, J., Sheldon, T. A., Song, F., & Fletcher, A. W. (2000). Beds, mattresses and cushions for pressure sore prevention and treatment. *The Cochrane Library (Oxford)*, (2), CD001735.

Day, D., Hayes, K., Kennedy, A. M., & Diercksen, R. M. (1997). Pressure ulcer prevention: review of literature. *Journal of the New York State Nurses Association, 28*(2), 12–17.

Defloor, T., & Grypdonck, M. H. F. (1999). Sitting posture and prevention of pressure ulcers. *Applied Nursing Research, 12*(3), 136–142.

Defloor, T., & Grypdonck, M. H. F. (2000). Do pressure relief cushions really relieve pressure? *Western Journal of Nursing Research, 22*, 335–350.

Fontaine, R., Risley, S., & Castellino, R. (1998). A quantitative analysis of pressure and shear in the effectiveness of support surfaces. *Journal of Wound, Ostomy, and Continence Nursing, 25*, 233–239.

The National Decubitus Foundation. [Online]. Available at www.decubitus.org

Nixon, J., McElvenny, D., Mason, S., Brown, J., & Bond, S. (1998). A sequential randomized controlled trial comparing a dry visco-elastic polymer pad and standard operating table mattress in the prevention of post-operative pressure sores. *International Journal of Nursing Studies, 35*(4), 193–203.

Pring, J., & Millman, P. (1998a). Measuring interface pressures in mattresses. *Journal of Wound Care, 7*, 173–174.

Pring, J., & Millman, P. (1998b). Evaluating pressure-relieving mattresses. *Journal of Wound Care, 7*, 177–179.

Russell, J. A., & Lichtenstein, S. L. (2000). Randomized controlled trial to determine the safety and efficacy of a multi-cell pulsating dynamic mattress system in the prevention of pressure ulcers in patients undergoing cardiovascular surgery. *Ostomy Wound Management, 46*(2), 46–51, 54–55.

Sanada, H., Nagakawa, T., Yamamoto, M., Higashidani, K., Tsuru, H., & Suzamo, J. (1997). The role of skin blood flow in pressure ulcer development during surgery. *Advances in Wound Care: The Journal for Prevention and Healing, 10*(6), 29–34.

Schultz, A., Bien, M., Dumond, K., Brown, K., & Myers, A. (1999). Etiology and incidence of pressure ulcers in surgical patients. *AORN Journal, 70*, 437–440, 443–444.

Seeley, J., Jensen, J. L., & Hutcherson, J. (1999). A randomized clinical study comparing a hydrocellular dressing to a hydrocolloid dressing in the management of pressure ulcers. *Ostomy Wound Management, 45*(6), 44, 46–47.

Surgical Materials Testing Laboratory. [Online]. Available at www.smtl.co.uk

Theiler, R., Stahelin, H. B., Kanzlin, M., Tyndall, A., & Bischoff, H. A. (1999). High bone turnover in the elderly. *Archives of Physical Medicine and Rehabilitation, 80*, 485–489.

Thomas, S., Banks, V., Bale, S., Fear-Price, M., Hagelstein, S., Harding, K. G., Orpin, J., & Thomas, N. (1997). Evaluation. A comparison of two dressings in the management of chronic wounds. *Journal of Wound Care, 6*, 383–386.

Thomas, D. R., Goode, P. S., LaMaster, K., & Tennyson, T. (1998). Acemannan hydrogel dressing versus saline dressing for pressure ulcers: A randomized, controlled trial. *Advances in Wound Care, 11*, 273–276.

Torra i Bou, J., Rueda López, J., & Ramón Cantón, C. (2000). Reducing the pressure in risk zones which develop bedsores by means of a hydrocellular external application; and experimental study [Spanish]. *Revista Rol de Enfermeria, 23*(3), 211–218.

Wells, J. A., & Karr, D. (1998). Interface pressure, wound healing, and satisfaction in the evaluation of a non-powered fluid mattress. *Ostomy Wound Management, 44*(2), 38–40, 42, 44–46.

Yamashita, R., Kuroyanagi, Y., Nakakita, N., Uchinuma, E., & Shioya, N. (1999). Allogeneic cultured dermal substitute composed of spongy collagen containing fibroblasts: Preliminary clinical trials. *Wounds—A Compendium of Clinical Research & Practice, 11*(2), 34–44.

5

Assessment and Management of Pain

DEBRA B. GORDON and TERESA A. PELLINO

Pain is like a symphony conducted by the brain with major input from various instruments within the body and mind sections. The sounds can be as varied as those from an orchestra, and too often it's hard to know exactly which instruments are playing, particularly when sweet healthy melodies turn into blaring nightmarish noises.

SCOTT FISHMAN, *THE WAR ON PAIN*, 2000

Orthopaedic nurses, whatever the developmental age or diagnoses of their clients or the environment in which they practice, face the challenges associated with pain management. Pain, whether acute or chronic, is a common symptom for many orthopaedic clients. A recent survey on the pain experience of nearly 10,000 ambulatory surgical clients showed that orthopaedic clients have the highest incidence of severe pain, with shoulder and elbow surgery being the most painful orthopaedic procedures (Chung, Ritchie, & Su, 1997). In a review of epidemiologic studies of chronic pain, Verhaak, Kerssens, Dekker, Sorbi, and Bensing (1998) found an estimated prevalence of chronic pain in 10% of the general population (from studies worldwide), with musculoskeletal pain being the most commonly reported type of pain. Because pain accompanies a variety of medical and surgical diagnoses in musculoskeletal disorders, the orthopaedic nurse must evaluate each client individually.

Over the past decade, a number of evidence-based clinical practice guidelines have become available to assist clinicians in the treatment of many painful conditions (Table 5-1). In January 2001, pain assessment and management were incorporated into the survey and accreditation process by the Joint Commission on Accreditation of Healthcare Organizations (JCAHO), making pain the first

evidence-based JCAHO standards. Pain assessment and management are now incorporated into all five patient function chapters (patient rights and organization ethics, assessment of patients, care of patients, education of patients, continuum of care) as well as the chapter on improving organization performance (Table 5-2), further outlining our responsibility to help clients manage pain.

DEFINITIONS

There are many definitions of pain. The most generally accepted definition, developed by Merskey and later put forth by the International Association for the Study of Pain (IASP) (1986) states, "Pain is an unpleasant sensory and emotional experience associated with actual or potential tissue damage, or described in terms of such damage. Pain is always subjective. Each individual learns application of the word through experiences related to injury early in life. . . . It is unquestionably a sensation in a part or parts of the body but it is always unpleasant and therefore an emotional experience" (Merskey, 1979, p. 250). This is an important definition because it recognizes both the biophysical and the cognitive-emotional aspects of the pain experience. Another well-accepted definition is, "Pain is whatever the patient says it is, wherever he/she says it is, as severe as he says it is, lasting as long as he says it lasts" (McCaffery, 1979, p. 8).

Because of the subjectivity and complexity of the pain experience, no one definition is used exclusively. Melzack and Wall (1983), generally thought to be pioneers in the pain management arena, describe pain as a category of experiences, signifying a multitude of unique experiences having different causes and being characterized by different qualities that vary along a number of sensory and affective dimensions.

CLASSIFICATION OF PAIN

Numerous methods of classifying pain exist, including definitions based on temporal aspects, neurophysiologic mechanisms, intensity, categories of clients with pain, and specific pain syndromes. Defined by time, acute pain usually has a recent, definable onset and is of short duration, whereas chronic pain is generally extended over time, beyond a period of healing—more than 6 months.

Neurophysiologic classifications of pain include somatic (skin, soft tissue, and bone), visceral, and neuropathic (arising from injured peripheral or central neural structures). Intensity is generally defined as mild (1 to 4 on a scale of 0 to 10), moderate (5 to 6), or severe (7 to 10) (Serlin, Mendoza, Nakamura, Edwards, & Cleeland, 1995). The National Institutes of Health (NIH) Consensus Development Conference (1986) classified pain into three types: acute, chronic malignant (cancer), and

TABLE 5–1. *Evidence-Based Consensus Statements, Guidelines, and Other Resources*

Agency for Healthcare Policy and Research (AHCPR). (1992). *Acute pain management: Operative or medical procedures and trauma: Clinical practice guideline No. 1.* AHCPR Publication No. 92-0032. Rockville, MD: Public Health Service, U.S. Department of Health and Human Services.

Agency for Health Care Policy and Research (AHCPR). (1994). *Management of cancer pain: Clinical practice guideline No. 9.* AHCPR Pub. No. 94-0592. Rockville, MD: Public Health Service, U.S. Department of Health and Human Services.

American Academy of Neurology. Silberstein, S. D. for the U.S. Headache Consortium. (2000). Practice parameter: Evidence-based guidelines for migraine headache (an evidence-based review). *Neurology, 55,* 754–763. Available at www.aan.com/public/practiceguidelines/hasummry.pdf

American Academy of Pain Medicine, American Pain Society, & American Society of Addiction Medicine. (2001). *Definitions related to the use of opioids for the treatment of pain.* Glenview, IL: Author. Available at www.ampainsoc.org/advocacy/opioids2.htm

American Academy of Pediatrics and Canadian Paediatric Society. (2000). Policy Statement: Prevention and management of pain and stress in the neonate. *Pediatrics, 105,* 454–461.

American Academy of Physical Medicine & Rehabilitation. Sanders, S. H., Rucker, K. S., Anderson, K. O., Harden, R. N., Jackson, K. W., Vicente, P. J., & Gallagher, R. M. (1996). Clinical practice guidelines for chronic non-malignant pain syndrome patients. *Journal of Back and Musculoskeletal Rehabilitation, 5,* 115–120.

American Academy of Physical Medicine & Rehabilitation. Sanders, S. H., & Rucker, L. (1996). Clinical practice guidelines for chronic non-malignant pain management. *Journal of Back and Musculoskeletal Rehabilitation, 7,* 19–25.

American Academy of Physical Medicine & Rehabilitation. Sanders, S. H., Harden, R. N., Benson, S. E., & Vicente, P. J. (1999). Clinical practice guidelines for chronic non-malignant pain syndrome patients II: An evidence-based approach. *Journal of Back and Musculoskeletal Rehabilitation, 13,* 47–58.

American Geriatric Society Panel on Chronic Pain in Older Persons. (1998). The management of chronic pain in older persons. *Journal of the American Geriatrics Society, 46,* 635–651.

American Medical Directors Association. (1999). *Chronic pain management in the long-term care setting.* Available at www.amda.com

American Pain Society Quality of Care Committee. (1995). Quality improvement guidelines for the treatment of acute pain and cancer pain. *Journal of the American Medical Association, 23,* 1874–1880.

American Pain Society and the American Academy of Pain Medicine. (1996). *Consensus statement on the use of opioids in chronic pain.* Available at www.ampainsoc.org and www.painmed.org

American Pain Society. (1999). *Principles of analgesic use in the treatment of acute pain and cancer pain* (4th ed.). Glenview, IL: Author. Available at www.ampainsoc.org

American Pain Society. (1999). *Guideline for the management of acute and chronic pain in sickle-cell disease.* Glenview, IL: Author. Available at www.ampainsoc.org

American Society of Anesthesiologists Task Force on Pain Management, Cancer Pain Section. (1996). Practice guidelines for cancer pain management. *Anesthesiology, 84,* 1243–1257.

American Society of Anesthesiologists Task Force on Pain Management, Acute Pain Section. (1995). Practice guidelines for acute pain management in the perioperative setting. *Anesthesiology, 82,* 1071–1081.

American Society of Anesthesiologists. (1997). Practice guidelines for chronic pain management. *Anesthesiology, 87,* 995–1004.

American Society of Clinical Oncology. (1992). Cancer pain assessment and treatment curriculum guidelines. *Journal of Clinical Oncology, 10,* 1976–1982.

Federation of State Medical Boards of the United States, Inc. (1998). *Model guidelines for the use of controlled substances for the treatment of pain.* Euless, TX: Author (817-868-4000).

Mersky, H., & Bogduk, N. (1994). *Classification of chronic pain: Descriptions of chronic pain syndromes and definitions of pain terms.* Seattle: IASP Press.

Society for Nuclear Medicine. (1999). *Procedure guideline for bone pain treatment* (Version 2.0). Reston, VA: Society of Nuclear Medicine.

Stanton-Hicks, M., Baron, R., Boas, R., Gordh, T., Harden, R. N., Hendler, N., Koltzenburg, M., Raj, P., & Wilder, R. (1998). Complex regional pain syndromes: Guidelines for therapy. *Clinical Journal of Pain, 14,* 115–116.

Woolfe, F. (1996). The fibromyalgia syndrome: A consensus report on fibromyalgia and disability. *Journal of Rheumatology, 23,* 534–539.

TABLE 5–2. *Joint Commission on the Accreditation of Healthcare Organizations*

Pain assessment and management standards can be printed from the JCAHO website: www.jcaho.org

For standards interpretation questions, contact the JCAHO Standards Interpretation Unit at: 630-792-5900, by e-mail: tmister@jcaho.org, or on the JCAHO website (www.jcaho.org) under "Contact us"

chronic nonmalignant. This classification is important because time elements are not considered in labeling pain. The term *pain syndromes* is used to characterize a number of symptoms occurring together in a specific disease or condition, such as fibromyalgia, diabetic neuropathy, and phantom limb pain. Orthopaedic nurses work with individuals who fit into all categories. These categories are not mutually exclusive and are practical because they capture the multidimensional aspects of pain. An individual who experiences chronic nonmalignant pain (e.g., osteoarthritis) can have concomitant acute pain (e.g., following a total hip arthroplasty).

THEORIES OF PAIN

Many explanations of pain have been proposed over the years, but fundamental questions remain unanswered. The word *pain* comes from the Latin word *poena,* which means punishment. Aristotle was one of the first to document the concept of pain and believed the experience of pain to be opposite that of pleasure: a negative passion. This idea was generally accepted until the 17th century, when Descartes proposed that the brain was the center of sensation and that pain is transmitted through vibrations in the skin resulting from noxious stimuli traveling to the brain with pathways to the pineal gland. As knowledge has increased in the science of pain management, a better understanding and appreciation of the complexity and multidimensional aspects of pain has emerged.

Although the specific cause for pain remains unclear, several theories have been proposed, including the specificity (or sensory), intensity (or pattern), and gate control theories.

The most influential theory remains the gate control theory. In simplistic terms, the gate control theory blended features of preceding theories to propose a gating mechanism that exists in the dorsal horn of the spinal cord (Melzack & Wall, 1965). Opening and closing of the gate is determined by the relative amount of activity of nerve fibers. Ascending, large-diameter fibers close the gate, inhibiting transmission of nociception, whereas activity of small-diameter nerve fibers opens it. The spinal gating mechanism is proposed to be modulated through descending fibers by a central control trigger system that is activated by selective cognitive processes. Wall (1996), commenting on gate control 30 years after its inception, stated "for its time, it was not a

bad guess" (p. 12); however, he called for further study of separate excitatory and inhibitory components as well as axes of time and space. Although the gate control theory does not offer all answers to the question of pain, it is extremely important because it ushered in a new view of the nervous system and a new era of pain research, specifically modulation. New ideas continue to be needed as possible testable solutions to the hugely puzzling questions about pain.

PAIN PHYSIOLOGY

Despite much research, more is unknown than known about the complexity of pain mechanisms. There are generally two classifications of pain structures: peripheral and central. In the periphery, primary afferent nerve fibers (nociceptors) are excited by mechanical, thermal, or chemical stimuli. These fibers are located in skin, joints, muscles, and viscera. In sufficient quantity, stimuli can activate biochemical mediators, resulting in a noxious or nociceptive response. Mediators include potassium, substance P, bradykinin, prostaglandin, and other substances. When the primary afferent nerve is stimulated, a process of depolarization, called *transduction,* occurs. An action potential is then generated, traveling the length of the neuron from the periphery to terminations of the fiber in the dorsal horn of the spinal cord in a process called *transmission.*

Peripheral nerve fibers have been classified based on the diameter of the nerve fiber and the speed of conduction of the impulse. A delta fibers, which are myelinated, are the largest and conduct impulses most rapidly. In contrast, C fibers are the smallest of the peripheral nervous system. They are unmyelinated, and their conduction rate is much slower. Although both A and C fibers transmit nociceptive impulses, the characteristic sensations carried are different. A fibers primarily transmit sharp pain, such as a pinprick, whereas C fibers carry dull or achy pain.

On reaching the dorsal horn, neuropeptides and other substances (e.g., substance P) are released from the terminals of the fiber. These peptides are thought to bind to secondary neuron receptors, eliciting an action potential in that neuron. Transmission of the nociceptive message crosses to the opposite side of the cord and ascends within the central nervous system (CNS) along secondary neurons in the spinothalamic tract (Fig. 5–1). An individual does not actually perceive the sensation of pain until transmission terminates in various areas of the brain, including the thalamus, midbrain, cortex, frontal lobe, and limbic system.

MODULATION

There are many opportunities for the nociceptive message to be inhibited as it travels along its route. One common treatment approach is to use nonsteroidal anti-

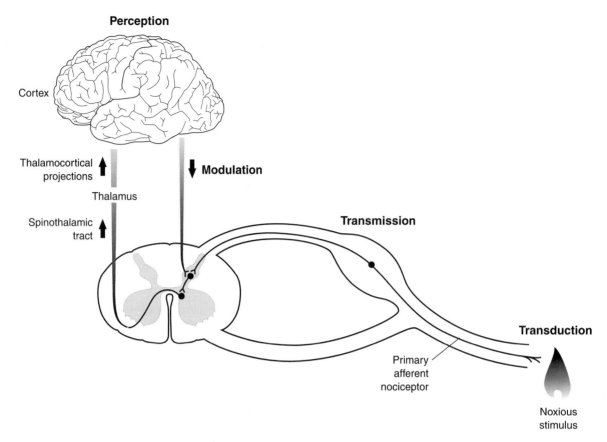

FIGURE 5–1. Nociception transmission and modulation, spinothalamic tract.

inflammatory drugs (NSAIDs), which inhibit the formation of the nociceptive mediator prostaglandin, thus inhibiting the pain message in the periphery. At the central level, administered opioids or the body's own endogenous endorphins and enkephalins bind to opioid receptors in the spinal cord and brain, inhibiting the release of nociceptive neuromediators. In addition, descending neurons in the spinal cord, known as the *modulatory system,* can release substances such as serotonin and norepinephrine to inhibit transmission of nociception in the dorsal horn.

However, pain is multidimensional and cannot be described or understood in solely physiologic terms. Sensory, cognitive, affective, and behavioral components that constitute the pain experience are important considerations and are discussed further in the assessment section.

ASSESSMENT OF PAIN

Whatever else philosophy or biomedical science can tell us about pain, the reporting of pain is a social transaction between caregiver and client (Agency for Health Care Policy and Research [AHCPR], 1992). Therefore, establishing a positive relationship with clients and families is key to successful assessment and control of pain. Finding out what the pain means to the client is of utmost

importance in the assessment of our client's pain. Communication is the basis of accurate assessment.

In keeping with the notion that pain is a subjective experience and can best be described by the client, it is important for the nurse to routinely ask clients about the presence of pain and when present perform a more comprehensive pain assessment. Research has shown that the most common reason for unrelieved pain in U.S. hospitals is the failure of staff to routinely assess pain and pain relief (American Pain Society [APS], 1999). When possible, the client's self-report should be the primary source of assessment. For people with more than one site or source of pain, proper evaluation includes thorough questioning about each site or source.

Perhaps the most difficult part of assessing pain is believing that the client's expression of pain is real. As McCaffery and Pasero (1999) point out, believing the client's pain is a professional responsibility of all health care workers. All clients deserve our trust. Every major position paper and clinical practice guideline on pain management include similar statements to the effect "Believe the client's complaint of pain" (APS, 1999; AHCPR, 1992, 1994a, 1994b; American Geriatric Society [AGS], 1998; American Society of Anesthesiologists [ASA], 1995).

It is generally recognized that pain is a complex phenomenon and incorporates the following dimensions:

1. Physiologic—the physical, neurologic, and biochemical aspects of pain
2. Sensory—the intensity, location, and quality of the pain
3. Affective—emotional responses, such as anger, mood changes, depression, anxiety, or relief
4. Cognitive—the manner in which pain influences a person's thought processes; how he or she views himself or herself; or the meaning of pain, coping strategies, attitudes, and beliefs
5. Behavioral—pain-related behaviors, such as overt manifestations of pain (grimacing, moaning), medication intake, or activity level
6. Sociocultural—various demographic, social, and cultural characteristics that are related to the experience of pain

Tables 5-3 and 5-4 outline the key areas of pain assessment and questions that elicit the needed data. Using standardized questions lessens the likelihood of missing pertinent information. Giving the client the tools (body diagrams, visual analogue scales [VAS]) to translate subjective experience into an objective form facilitates communication between client and nurse.

Research indicates that an attempt should be made to measure as many dimensions as feasible of all types of pain, although the relative importance of each dimension varies by pain type (NIH Consensus Development Conference Statement, 1986). For clients who are able to use self-report, a simple numeric 0-to-10 scale (0 = no pain, 10 = worst pain possible) has been shown to be both valid and reliable in studies of cancer clients across different language and cultural groups (Serlin et al., 1995). Importantly, researchers using the 0-to-10 scale have found significant correlations between various reported numerical ratings and interference with function, sleep, appetite, mood, and relations with others (Serlin et al., 1995). That is, as clients report higher levels of pain, there is a significant decline in quality of life. Although either VAS or verbal rating scales (VRS) can be used to assess pain intensity, VRS were found to be more practical and reliable in a study of 417 postoperative orthopaedic clients (Briggs, Closs, & Mphil, 1999). The 0-to-10 scale can be useful to help clients determine tangible goals for pain relief, particularly for acute pain (Gordon & Ward, 1995).

Special consideration must be given when communicating with people who have special needs: neonates and

TABLE 5–3. *Key Areas of Pain Assessment*

PHYSIOLOGIC	SENSORY	AFFECTIVE	COGNITIVE	BEHAVIORAL	SOCIOCULTURAL
Location	Intensity	Distress	Meaning of pain	Communication	Ethnocultural
Onset	Quality	Anxiety	Thought processes	Interpersonal	Family/social
Duration	Pattern	Depression	Coping strategies	Activities	Work/home
Etiology		Mood	Knowledge	Behaviors	Recreation/leisure
Syndrome		Suffering	Attitudes/beliefs	Medications	Environment
Type of pain		Mental state	Influencing factors	Sleep/fatigue	Attitudes/beliefs
Anatomy		Irritability/agitation			
Physiology		Relief			

From McGuire, D. B. (1992). Comprehensive and multidimensional assessment and measurement of pain. *Journal of Pain and Symptom Management, 7*, 312–319. Copyright © 1992 by the U.S. Cancer Pain Relief Committee. Reprinted by permission of Elsevier Science Inc.

TABLE 5–4. *Mnemonic QISS TAPE: Questions to Ask during Initial Pain Assessment*

Q = quality	Can you describe what the pain feels like? Is it dull, sharp, burning?
I = impact	How does the pain affect your ability to sleep, eat, or function? How does it affect your mood?
S = site	Can you show me where it hurts? Can you put your hand on it?
S = severity	On a scale of 0–10 with 0 being no pain and 10 being the worst pain imaginable, how much pain do you have now? What is the worst pain? What is the lowest it gets to after taking pain medication or using other strategies?
T = temporal characteristics	When did the pain first begin? Is it constant or intermittent? Is it predictable, or does it occur without warning? Is there any pattern to it?
A = aggravating and alleviating factors	What makes the pain better or worse?
P = past treatment and response, preferences	What have you used in the past to relieve the pain? How long did you use it? What has worked and not worked? Have you had any problems with side effects? What do you prefer to use?
E = expectations, meaning, and goals	What do you think is causing the pain? What kind of fears do you have? How do you cope with pain? What is your pain relief goal? What level of pain relief do you think we need to work toward so that you can sleep and function?

children, persons with developmental delays or cognitive impairments, comatose clients, psychotic clients, and people who do not speak the same language as the caregiver (AHCPR, 1992, 1994a, 1994b).

Because neonates and infants cannot verbally express pain, interpretation of behaviors and physiologic signs must be used. Younger children may lack the language skills to describe the pain experience. Tools that use cues such as facial expression, motor activity, crying, and consolability have been developed (Fuller & Neu, 2000; Soetenga, Frank, & Pellino, 1999). Using age-appropriate words or words that are identified by the parent or caregiver as being familiar to the child can promote more accurate pain assessment. Assessment and management strategies should be tailored to the child's developmental level, personality style, and emotional and physical resources and to the context. Several instruments have been developed specifically for use in pediatrics and are research based, including the Poker Chip Tool, Pain Affect Faces, Pain Experience History, Eland Color Scale Figures, and Word-Graphic Rating Scale (AHCPR, 1994a).

Older adult clients are another group requiring special attention to pain assessment. Older persons have a high prevalence of pain and are often undertreated because of incorrect assumptions about pain sensitivity, pain tolerance, and the ability to tolerate use of analgesics (AHCPR, 1994a). Often, older clients think that pain (e.g., soreness, aches) is a normal part of the aging process. A careful assessment of the complaints must be made and documented in the medical record. Cognitive impairment and dementia can cause serious impediments to assessment, although researchers have found that many clients in nursing home settings with mild to moderate cognitive impairment are able to reliably report pain (Ferrell, Ferrell, & Rivera, 1995). In another study, Herr and Mobily (1993) reported that older individuals were able to use a variety of commonly used pain assessment tools, including both verbal descriptor scales (VDS) and VAS, although they seemed to prefer VDS.

Puntillo and Wilkie (1991) differentiate between nociception and pain in the acutely ill client. *Nociception* is the stimulation of neural pathways by noxious stimuli, whereas *pain* requires perceptual activity for noxious stimuli to be interpreted by the client. This distinction is important in caring for a comatose client, who may be perceived as having no pain. These authors suggest a conservative and humanitarian approach to this type of client and recommend that all nociceptive stimuli be considered painful. Whether a client is conscious or not, there is clear evidence that pain can cause profound pathophysiologic changes that can increase both morbidity and mortality (Liebeskind, 1991). Investigation into methods of assessing critically ill clients for pain is ongoing (Carroll, Atkins, Herold, Mlcek, Shively, Clopton, & Glaser, 1999; Puntillo, Miaskowski, Kehrle, Stannard, Gleeson, & Nye, 1997).

Clients with chronic nonmalignant pain require a comprehensive pain assessment similar to that for clients with acute pain. Emphasis should be placed on the client's affective response to pain and any functional disabilities associated with the syndrome. With these clients, it is important to understand how much suffering is associated with the pain. Depression is a common comorbidity in clients with chronic pain. Often, a barrage of surveys is used to assess the overall impact of pain on the client's life. These surveys generally include measures of function or disability, assessment of coping with pain, and psychological health profiles. These individuals often have devised routines that work for them and that have great importance to their treatment regimen. For example, a client with arthritis may regulate pain with a specific schedule for medications, relaxation, and physical exercises. During the assessment of these clients, it is important to ask what works for them. They are usually the best judges of their pain and have lived with it for many years.

A variety of tools, ranging from a complete pain history to a simple numerical scale, can help the nurse in assessing a client's pain. JCAHO (2000) recommend the availability of more than one pain-intensity measure. For example, a hospital serving both children and adults selects a scale to be used with each of those client populations. Assessment of cognitively impaired clients may also require assessment of behavioral factors signaling pain or discomfort. Table 5–5 summarizes some of the current assessment tools for documenting pain.

Pain assessment is an ongoing process. Pain intensity varies, as does the level of distress or suffering that accompanies it. Re-evaluation and documentation of the amount of pain relief a person experiences after interventions are critical parts of assessment.

MANAGEMENT OF PAIN

Management of pain, like assessment, focuses on a variety of mechanisms of pain and therefore requires use of a multimodal approach, that is, a combination of medications, methods of analgesic delivery, and nonpharmacologic interventions. This multimodal approach may lead to a major reduction in undesirable sequelae of surgical stress with improved pain control. Combining techniques to provide a more "balanced" approach to pain management that facilitates early ambulation; reduction of nausea, vomiting, and ileus; and early enteral nutrition has been shown to result in improved surgical outcome and reductions in morbidity and costs (Kehlet, 1997, 1999; Kehlet, Werner, & Perkins, 1999; Moiniche, Hansen, Christensen, Dahl, & Kehlet, 1992; Weingarten et al., 1994). For the orthopaedic surgical client, this may involve use of an epidural or regional technique (opioids and/or local anesthetics) combined with nonopioid analgesics, intravenous (IV) or oral opioids, ice, and

TABLE 5–5. *Instruments for Measuring or Assessing Pain*

INSTRUMENT (REFERENCES)	DESCRIPTION	ADVANTAGES	DISADVANTAGES
Behavioral scales (Fuller & Neu, 2000; Soetenga, Frank, & Pellino, 1999)	Descriptions of behavior that may indicate discomfort/pain; primarily used for clients who cannot express pain (e.g., infants, those with cognitive impairment); components and ratings vary by scale but generally include facial expressions, movement, and vocalizations	Provides some structure to evaluating pain in clients who cannot self-report	Subjectivity on part of evaluator; individuality of pain expression; tested primarily on neonates and young infants
Brief Pain Inventory (Daut, Cleeland, & Flanery, 1983)	Rating of severity—worst, least, average, now; indicate location of pain on schematic diagram; pain descriptors, information about relief, interference with activities	Self-administered; simple; comprehensive sensory component	Does not measure psychological or sociocultural components
Faces scales	A series of faces with varying expressions that represent increasing intensity of pain; the number of faces and the type of drawing varies with the individual scale	Easily understood by children; do not require a numerical value by the child	Facial characteristics used (i.e., a smiling face or tears) may skew pain rating; may be affective rating rather than pain
McGill Pain Questionnaire (short form) (Melzack, 1987)	15 word descriptors; has sensory, affective, and overall evaluative descriptors; Present Pain Index (PPI) is rated as follows: 0 = no pain, 1 = mild, 2 = discomforting, 3 = distressing, 4 = horrible, 5 = excruciating	Self-administered; takes about 5 minutes to complete; sensory and affective components; can aid in diagnosis of clinical pain syndromes	Must be familiar with scoring system
Numerical rating scales	Use numbers, usually 0–10 (can use 0–5 or 0–100), where 0 = no pain and 10 (or highest number) = worst pain imaginable (pain as bad as it could be)	Brief, simple, more sensitive than verbal descriptor scale, less confusing than visual analogue scale; can be administered in written or verbal form	Unidimensional; may be less sensitive than the visual analogue scale
Verbal rating scales	List of adjectives that describe different levels of pain intensity (e.g., no pain to extremely intense pain); the number of descriptors varies depending on the scale	Brief, simple, usually easy to understand	Unidimensional; scoring assumes equal intervals between descriptors; may be difficult for clients with limited language skills
Visual analogue scale	Vertical or horizontal 10-cm line with verbal or pictorial anchors of no pain to severe pain (worst imaginable)	Brief, provides a sensitive measure; scores can be analyzed as interval level data	Unidimensional; may be difficult for some individuals; scoring is awkward in the clinical setting and may be a source of error

positioning. The treatment of chronic pain also involves use of a combination of interventions depending on the pain symptoms and the patient's response to treatment. These interventions may include nonopioid analgesics, antidepressants, neuromodulators, long-acting opioids, cognitive-behavioral therapy (CBT), and physical therapy.

Pharmacologic Management

Pharmacologic management is the cornerstone in the treatment of moderate to severe pain and includes opioids, nonopioid analgesics, and adjuvant drugs. An analgesic regimen should be based on the severity and nature of the pain. Nonpharmacologic techniques are also important in the treatment of pain but are rarely used alone, particularly for moderate and severe pain. Principles of pharmacologic management are listed in Box 5–1.

The older terms *narcotic analgesic* and *strong analgesic* are being phased out in favor of *opioid analgesic* because of a newer understanding of sites and mechanisms of pharmacologic action and the negative association of *narcotic* with the campaign against illegal drug use.

Nonopioid Analgesics. Nonopioid analgesics are generally prescribed for mild to moderate pain or as a coanalgesic for severe pain. Included in this category are aspirin, acetaminophen, and the NSAIDs (Table 5-6). These drugs differ from opioids in four ways; they are (1) antipyretic, (2) anti-inflammatory at higher dosages (except for acetaminophen), (3) limited by an analgesic ceiling (above which a further dose increase will not increase analgesia, only toxicity), and (4) believed to have different mechanisms of action than opioids. Although the mechanisms of action of aspirin and acetaminophen are not fully understood, NSAIDs inhibit the enzyme cyclooxygenase (COX), the first step in the conversion of arachidonic acid to prostaglandins and thromboxanes (Dahl, 1999). Prostaglandins sensitize peripheral pain receptors, induce fever, and are released in allergic and inflammatory processes. Thromboxanes are involved in platelet aggregation. Nonopioids appear to primarily have peripheral effects and do not activate opioid receptors. Hence, concurrent use of nonopioid and opioid agents often provides improved analgesia (AHCPR, 1994a, 1994b).

Acetaminophen is often used for clients with degenerative joint disease, yet aspirin remains the drug of choice for clients who can tolerate it. Hepatotoxicity has been associated with acetaminophen, and clients should avoid alcohol consumption while taking it. The maximum daily dose of acetaminophen is 4 g. This should be considered when clients are receiving combination opioid-acetaminophen analgesics; it may be necessary to change to a pure opioid to avoid exceeding the acetaminophen limits. Combining acetaminophen or aspirin with an NSAID usually provides little additional analgesia, and the side effects appear to increase in frequency and severity.

Aspirin remains the salicylate of choice in most cases. At dosages commonly prescribed, aspirin has a good safety profile in rheumatoid arthritis and is less costly than NSAIDs. When assessing a client's medications, one must be sure to include over-the-counter (OTC) medications as well as prescription medications because many OTC medications contain aspirin.

Nursing implications for NSAIDs are many. Adverse effects of NSAIDs are a particular concern and may appear at any time. They include renal failure, hepatic dysfunction, bleeding, and gastric ulceration. In addition to major gastrointestinal bleeding, NSAIDs have also been associated with dyspepsia, heartburn, nausea, and abdominal pain. Serious effects are not always preceded by minor gastrointestinal effects (AHCPR, 1994a, 1994b). Bronchospasm and urticaria may be precipitated by aspirin or NSAIDs (Rawlins, 1993). A history of this type of hypersensitivity reaction or asthma dictates caution because the sensitivity reaction may apply to all NSAIDs.

An exception to this is the COX-2–specific inhibitors. As mentioned previously, NSAIDs inhibit the enzyme COX. Two distinct COX isoforms (COX-1 and COX-2) have been identified. Although there is some overlap of activity, COX-1 is thought to be largely responsible for physiologic functions such as maintenance of gastrointestinal tract mucosal integrity, platelet aggregation, and kidney function, whereas COX-2–derived prostaglandins mediate the inflammatory process. By selectively inhibiting COX-2, one can theoretically obtain the therapeutic analgesic effect with less risk of adverse effects (Day et al., 2000). Although initial clinical studies support a significantly lower incidence of gastroduodenal ulceration from COX-2 inhibitors, these agents do not spare the kidney and are not recommended for clients with renal insufficiency (Laine et al., 1999; Rossat, Maillard, Nussberger, Brunner, & Burneir, 1999) and long-term effects of the drugs are not yet known. These drugs are becoming a first-line medication in osteoarthritis when simple analgesics are unsuccessful and the client is NSAID intolerant or on coumadin (Cannon et al., 2000; Goodman, 2000).

BOX 5–1.
Basic Principles of Pharmacologic Management

- Individualize the route, dosage, and schedule.
- Administer analgesics regularly (not only as needed) if pain is present most of the day.
- Become familiar with the dose and time course of several strong opioids.
- Give infants and children adequate opioid doses.
- Follow clients closely, particularly when beginning or changing analgesic regimens.
- When changing to a new opioid or a different route, first use the equianalgesic doses (see Table 5-7) to estimate the new dose. Then, modify the estimate based on the clinical situation and the specific drugs.
- Recognize and treat side effects.
- Be aware of the potential hazards of meperidine (Demerol) and mixed agonist-antagonists, particularly pentazocine (Talwin).
- Do not use placebos to assess the nature of pain.
- Watch for the development of tolerance and treat appropriately.
- Be aware of the development of physical dependence and prevent withdrawal.
- Do not label a client addicted (i.e., psychologically dependent) if you merely mean physically dependent on or tolerant to opioids (see Box 5-3).
- Be alert to the psychological state of the client.

Adapted from the American Pain Society. (1999). *Principles of analgesic use in the treatment of acute pain and cancer pain* (4th ed.). Skokie, IL: Author.

TABLE 5–6. *Salicylates, Acetaminophen, and Nonsteroidal Anti-inflammatory Drugs (NSAIDs)*

DRUG	AVERAGE ANALGESIC DOSE (mg)	DOSE INTERVAL (hr)	MAXIMAL DAILY DOSE	PEDIATRIC DOSE (mg/kg)	COMMENTS
P-Aminophenol Derivatives					
Acetaminophen (Tylenol)	500–1000	4–6	4000	10–15	Rectal suppository and sustained-release forms available
Salicylates					
Aspirin	500–1000	4–6	4000	10–15	Not recommended in children <12 yr because of risk of Reye's syndrome
Diflunisal (Dolobid)	1000 initial 500 subsequent	8–12	1500	—	Less GI toxicity than aspirin
Choline magnesium trisalicylate (Trilisate)	1000–1500	12	2000–3000	25 bid	Minimal GI toxicity, no effect on platelet aggregations; available as liquid
NSAIDs					
Propioinic Acids					
Ibuprofen (Motrin, Rufen, Nuprin, Advil, Medipren)	200–400	4–6	2400	10 q6–8h	
Naproxen (Naprosyn)	500 initial 250 subsequent	6–8	1250	5 bid	
Naproxen sodium (Anaprox, Aleve)	550 initial 275 subsequent	6–8	1375	5 bid	
Fenoprofen (Nalfon)	200	4–6	800	—	
Ketoprofen (Orudis, Actron)	25–50 12.5–25 OTC	4–6 6–8 OTC	800 300 OTC	—	
Acetic Acids					
Indomethacin (Indocin)	25	8–12	100	—	Not routinely used because of high incidence of side effects
Tolmetin	200	8	2000	—	
Sulindac (Clinoril)	150	12	400	—	Not recommended for prolonged use because of increased GI toxicity
Ketorolac (Toradol)	30 IV initial 15 subsequent	6	150 first day 120 after	—	Limit treatment to 5 days, may precipitate renal failure in dehydrated clients
Diclofenac (Cataflam, Voltaren)	25	8	150	—	
Oxicams					
Piroxicam	20	24	40	—	
Fenamates					
Mefenamic acid (Ponstel)	250	6	1000	—	In United States, use restricted to intervals of 1 wk
Pyranocarboxylic Acids					
Etodolac (Lodine)	200	8	1200	—	
Other nabumetone (Relafen)	1000	24	2000	—	Minimal effect of platelet aggregation
Cyclooxygenase-2 Inhibitors					
Celecoxib (Celebrex)	100	24	200	—	Less GI toxicity, no effect on platelet aggregation; not recommended for clients with history of sulfa allergy
Meloxicam (Mobic)	7.5	24	15	—	
Rofecoxib (Vioxx)	25	24	50	—	Less GI toxicity, no effect on platelet aggregation

GI, gastrointestinal; OTC, over-the-counter.

Adapted from McCaffery, M., & Pasero, C. (1999). *Pain: Clinical manual* (2nd ed., pp. 139–140). St. Louis: Mosby; and American Pain Society. (1999). *Principles of analgesic use in the treatment of acute pain and cancer pain* (4th ed.). Skokie, IL: Author. MicroMedix, 2001.

One of the most efficacious NSAIDs is ketorolac, the only available parenteral preparation in the United States at the time of this writing. Although it provides superior pain relief, careful consideration in client selection and a course of therapy less than 5 days are recommended (Syntex Laboratories, 1996) because of the risk of adverse reactions. An alternative approach to standard NSAIDs is to use nonacetylated salicylates (salsalate, choline magnesium trisalicylate) or the COX-2 inhibitors (rofecoxib, celecoxib, meloxicam), which have little effect on platelet function, thus reducing the risk of bleeding (Conaway, 1995). A parenteral COX-2 inhibitor has been developed and is undergoing testing.

Quantitative comparative information on NSAID toxicity is available to assist in drug selection. However, the choice of a particular NSAID does not depend on toxicity alone. The efficacy of NSAIDs has been shown to vary widely among individual clients and can be determined only by empirical treatment. Finding the best tolerated NSAID is often a matter of trial and error. The initial choice should be based on the efficacy, safety, and relative expense.

Opioid Analgesics. Opioid analgesics are indicated for moderate to severe pain. The prototype for opioid analgesics is morphine, which binds with opiate receptors at many sites in the CNS (brain, brainstem, and spinal cord), altering transmission and perception to pain. There has been some research to suggest that opioids may also exert some effect at peripheral sites (Hargeaves & Joris, 1993; Picard, Tramer, McQuay, & Moore, 1997; Stein, 1993). Other examples of opioids include hydromorphone, fentanyl, meperidine, codeine, oxycodone, hydrocodone, levorphanol, and methadone (Table 5-7). In general, opioids have a predictable and treatable side effect profile, with common side effects including sedation, nausea, constipation, and respiratory depression. Opioids (morphine in particular) can also cause histamine release, with resultant pruritus, exacerbation of asthma, or hypotension. Except for constipation, clients develop tolerance to side effects with chronic dosing. A preventive and creative approach to managing constipation is a primary nursing consideration with all clients who take opioids. Methods used to reduce side effects may include using drugs to counteract the adverse effect,

TABLE 5–7. *Equianalgesic Dose Table*

DRUG	PARENTERAL	PO	PARENTERAL/ PO RATIO	DURATION OF ACTION (hr)
Morphine	10	30	1:3	3–4
Hydromorphone (Dilaudid)	1.5	7.5	1:5	3–4
Oxymorphone (Numorphan)	1	10	1:10	3–4
Oxycodone* (Roxicodone, Roxicet, Percocet)	Not available in United States	20–30	—	3–4
Codeine	130	200 NA	1:1.5	3–4
Hydrocodone† (Vicodin, Vicoprofen, Lortab, Lorcet)	—	30 NA	—	3–4
Propoxyphene (Wygesic, Darvocet)	—	NA‡	—	4–6
Meperidine (Demerol)	75	300§	1:4	2–3
Levorphanol (Levo-Dromoran)	2	4	1:2	4–8
Methadone (Dolophine)	10	3–5‖	—	4–12
Fentanyl (Sublimaze) (Duragesic¶)	0.1¶	—	—	1–3**

*These products contain 5 mg oxycodone with some combination of aspirin or acetaminophen.

†These products contain 5, 7.5, or 10 mg of hydrocodone with some combination of aspirin, acetaminophen, or ibuprofen.

‡Long half-life. Accumulation of toxic metabolite (norpropoxyphene) is possible with repetitive dosing. Inappropriate for use in older adults.

§Avoid multiple dosing with meperidine (no more than 48 hours or at dosages greater than 600 mg/24 hr). Accumulation of toxic metabolite normeperidine (half-life, 12–16 hours) can lead to central nervous system excitability and convulsions. Contraindicated in patients receiving monoamine oxidase inhibitors.

‖Although many equianalgesic tables list 20 mg as the oral methadone equianalgesic dose, recent data suggest that methadone is much more potent with repetitive dosing. Ratios between PO morphine and PO methadone may range from 4:1 to 14:1.

¶Transdermal fentanyl 100 µg/hr is approximately equivalent to 2–4 mg/hr of IV morphine. A conversion factor for transdermal fentanyl that can be used for equianalgesic calculation is 17 µg/hr. Roughly, the dose of transdermal fentanyl in µg/hr is approximately ½ of the 24 hour dose of oral morphine.

**Single dose data. Continual intravenous infusion produces lipid accumulation and prolonged terminal excretion.

Note: Duration of action based on use of short-acting formulations.

NA, equianalgesic data unavailable. Codeine doses should not exceed 1.5 mg/kg because of an increased incidence of side effects with higher dosages.

Adapted from Cherny, N. I. (1996). Opioid analgesics: Comparative features and prescribing guidelines. *Drugs, 51,* 713–717; Pasero, C., Portenoy, R., & McCaffery, M. (1999). *Pain: Clinical manual.* St. Louis, Mosby; and UW Hospital and Clinics Authority Board. (1999). *Health Pain Reference Card* (5th ed.). Madison, WI: Author. Reprinted from Gordon, D. B., Stevenson, K. K., Griffie, J., Muchka, S., Rapp, C., & Ford-Roberts, K. (1999). *Journal of Palliative Medicine, 2,* 212.

BOX 5-2.
Respiratory Depression and the Use of Naloxone

Opioid administration by any route is associated with dose-related respiratory depression. Signs of respiratory depression are a respiratory rate below 6 to 8 breaths/min, progressive sedation, and somnolence. The treatment is to administer naloxone intravenously (an initial bolus followed by a continuous infusion if needed), administer oxygen with assisted ventilation as needed, transfer to the intensive care unit for observation if necessary, and intubate and ventilate if indicated.

Naloxone is classified as an opioid antagonist because of its high affinity for opioid receptors, especially the mu receptor, and its lack of intrinsic receptor activity. Naloxone is used in the treatment of untoward side effects associated with the use of opioids. Naloxone is often thought of as a drug devoid of side effects. However, care should be taken because several cases of cardiovascular complications have been associated with naloxone. Special care should be taken with opioid-dependent clients because symptoms ranging from anxiety and irritability to life-threatening tachycardia and hypertension have been reported. Incremental intravenous doses of 0.1 to 0.2 mg should be given at 2- to 3-minute intervals. Also note that the half-life of naloxone is much shorter (45 to 60 minutes) than that of most opioids (3 to 5 hours). Thus, care must be taken to prevent recurrent respiratory depression. Very-low-dose continuous infusions of naloxone may be used in some situations to prevent side effects such as pruritus.

changing the dosing or route regimen, or trying different opioids (APS, 1999). Treatment of respiratory depression and the use of naloxone are addressed in Box 5-2.

Several routes of administration are available with various opioids. This includes oral, parenteral (intramuscular, IV bolus, IV infusion, IV patient-controlled analgesia [PCA], subcutaneous), transdermal, oral transmucosal, sublingual, intra-articular (IA), rectal, epidural, or intrathecal routes. When changing drugs or routes or administration, it is important to consider equianalgesic dosing for maximal efficacy and safety (Rapp & Gordon, 2000) (Table 5-7). The oral route is preferable because of flexibility in dosing, ease of administration, and sustained serum levels. Often, the parenteral (IV) or spinal route is necessary in clients with acute and/or severe pain because of their inability to take oral preparations, the drug's shorter effect time, and the ability to titrate more rapidly than with oral analgesics. The intramuscular route is not recommended because of variability in drug absorption and tissue damage from the injection.

Extended-release tablets of both morphine and oxycodone (and, in development, hydromorphone) that allow the client to have up to 12 hours of analgesia are now available, and more recently, as long as 24 hours

(Maccarrone, West, Broomhead, & Hodsman, 1994) of analgesia is available. This method is important to the client with constant pain in that it allows valuable hours of pain-free sleep. Another long-acting opioid preparation is a transdermal patch of fentanyl. A small amount of drug is released through a rate-limiting membrane, allowing the client analgesia for up to 3 days. One advantage of these patches is that they can get wet with no loss of potency; therefore, the client may bathe or shower with them on. It is important to appreciate the pharmacokinetics of extended-release preparations, particularly transdermal fentanyl, because of the difficulty they pose in titration (Payne, Chandler, & Einhaus, 1995). These preparations are best used after an initial period of titration with a short-acting opioid to determine dosage requirements. Extended-release preparations are designed for the treatment of chronic, stable pain and should rarely be used with acute pain, particularly in the postoperative period. Many clients receiving long-acting preparations will continue to require an allowance of an adequate rescue dose with a short-acting opioid that can be taken as necessary for breakthrough pain.

A drug that deserves special consideration is meperidine. Perhaps one of the most commonly prescribed postoperative opioids at one time, meperidine has fallen out of favor for a number of reasons. Meperidine is a weak opioid with a short half-life, producing analgesia for only 2 to 3 hours and often resulting in underdosing. Meperidine has a long-acting metabolite (normeperidine) that can accumulate in chronic dosing, causing CNS toxicity, including irritability, hallucinations, myoclonus, and seizures (AHCPR, 1992). For this reason, its use should be avoided; in the rare instances when it must be used, the APS (1999) cautions that meperidine should not be used for more than 48 hours for acute pain in clients without renal or CNS disease or at dosages greater than 600 mg per 24 hours. For a summary of studies on the use of meperidine, see the evidence-based practice table in this chapter. The one condition in which the use of meperidine is recommended is for the treatment of amphotericin or postoperative rigors at subanalgesic doses.

In 1995, tramadol (Ultram) was released for use in the United States. This is a completely unique binary analgesic with both opioid and nonopioid mechanisms. In analgesic studies, tramadol has been shown to have analgesic efficacy comparable to that of codeine (Raffa, Friderichs, Reemann, Shank, Codd, & Vaught, 1992). Like codeine, tramadol seems best indicated for mild to moderate pain. Side effects of tramadol include nausea, constipation, dizziness, and somnolence (Lehmann, 1994).

Opioid use in chronic nonmalignant pain has received much attention over the past decade. Although use of chronic opioid treatment has risen in recent years, careful client selection, clear treatment goals, and monitoring of the impact of opioids on goals is warranted.

EXAMINING THE EVIDENCE: Moving Toward Evidence-Based Practice
Should Meperidine Be Used for Postoperative Analgesia?

AUTHOR(S), YEAR	SAMPLE	DESIGN/METHOD	OUTCOME VARIABLE	MAJOR FINDINGS
Radnay, Brodman, Mankikar, & Duncalf, 1980	40 patients undergoing elective cholecystectomy	Prospective, randomized trial Patients received equianalgesic doses of either fentanyl, morphine, meperidine, or pentazocine while under anesthesia	Common bile duct pressure measurements	The common bile duct pressures rose 99.5% after fentanyl, 52.7% after morphine, 61.3% after meperidine, and 15.1% after pentazocine Use of pentazocine must be monitored or may be contraindicated in patients with chronic opioid use because it is an agonist-antagonist
Kaiko et al., 1983	(1) 67 patients with postoperative or chronic pain receiving meperidine (2) 47 postoperative patients receiving meperidine and 29 patients receiving other analgesics	(1) Prospective descriptive study; patients were interviewed; blood levels of meperidine and normeperidine were drawn (2) Prospective, patients rated mood items	(1) CNS excitatory signs (2) Mood	(1) 48 of 67 (72%) patients experienced shaky feelings (N = 20), tremors or twitches (N = 9), multifocal myoclonus (N = 8), or grand mal seizures (N = 2); those with CNS disturbances received meperidine longer and at higher dosages than those without CNS problems and had higher serum levels of normeperidine (2) Significant changes in negative mood scores after administration of meperidine and no changes in mood for patients receiving other analgesics
Marcantonio et al., 1994	91 patients (>50 yr) who developed delirium during postoperative days 2 through 5 and 154 matched controls; 47% of patients underwent orthopaedic procedures	Prospective descriptive study Patients underwent preoperative evaluation and daily structured interviews on postoperative days 2–5 (or until discharge)	Delirium	Overall opioid use was not associated with delirium; however, the use of meperidine had a significant association with delirium
McHugh, 1999	N = 1 patient postoperative laparotomy and ileostomy formation	Case study	Seizures	Woman with normal renal function developed seizure postoperatively after meperidine use of 3000 mg IV PCA in past 24 hours Meperidine best avoided for PCA, especially in patients with anticipated high opioid need Early recognition of meperidine toxicity not always possible
Nadvi, Sarnaik, & Ravindranath, 1999	N = 73 pediatric patients (153 admissions) with sickle cell crisis hospitalized for at least 10 days	Retrospective chart review	Seizures	Authors report incidence of meperidine-related seizures, based on entire population of sickle cell patients followed on their service, to be 0.4% (2/510) and 0.06% of admissions (2/2921) If, however, the rate is calculated from the charts actually reviewed, it would be 2.7% of patients and 1.3% of admissions This figure is still conservative because it was not indicated how many of the patients whose charts were reviewed received meperidine
Hassan, Bastani, & Gellens, 2000	N = 1 patient with end-stage renal disease admitted for gangrenous left lower extremity	Case study	Seizures	Patient developed diffuse myoclonic muscle contractions, confusion, and grand mal seizure after 250 mg IV and 600 mg PO (equivalent to 150 mg IV) meperidine in 48 hours If CNS side effects develop, authors recommend withholding meperidine, providing alternative pain control, giving supportive care, and using hemodialysis in serious cases; naloxone is not effective in reversing CNS effects

Summary: The studies' references here are a sampling of the evidence regarding use of meperidine as an analgesic. Meperidine was originally developed as an anticholinergic and its properties as an analgesic were discovered. As the first synthetic opioid, it gained widespread use. In the 1970s and 1980s, several reports that outlined the risks of meperidine use, including the study by Kaiko and colleagues described previously, were published. Based on these reports, national guidelines (AHCPR, 1992; APS, 1999) have advocated limiting its use as an analgesic because of its relative limited duration of action compared with other opioids and its potential for side effects, particularly CNS excitability from its metabolite, normeperidine. Patients with compromised renal function are at particular risk for the development of these side effects. Naloxone does not reverse the hyperexcitability and may in fact increase it. There have been varying reports on the use of meperidine in patients with biliary colic and pancreatitis. There is no clear-cut evidence that meperidine is superior to other opioids in treating these patients. Meperidine is useful in treating rigors.

CNS, central nervous system; PCA, patient-controlled analgesia.

Studies of chronic opioid therapy have shown positive effects on pain and function for some clients; however, there is still a need for randomized, controlled, longitudinal trials of their efficacy to determine long-term efficacy and safety (Sanders, Harden, Benson, & Vicente, 1999). Client education, use of a controlled substance agreement form or contract, and close monitoring are recommended. The reader is referred to Portenoy (1994, 1996) for specific guidelines for management of opioid therapy for nonmalignant pain.

Adjuvant Drugs. Adjuvant drugs are used to enhance analgesia, treat concurrent symptoms that exacerbate pain, and provide independent analgesia for specific types of pain (AHCPR, 1994a, 1994b). Commonly used adjuvants include antidepressants, anticonvulsants, oral local anesthetics, muscle relaxants, corticosteroids, and topical counterirritants.

Tricyclic antidepressants are commonly used as adjuvant analgesics for a variety of pain syndromes. The most effective of this class appear to be those that potentiate both serotonin and norepinephrine in the CNS (e.g., amitriptyline) and the selective noradrenergic agents (e.g., desipramine, imipramine, nortriptyline) (Watson, 1994). These drugs appear to be most effective in relieving headaches, atypical facial pain, diverse types of neuropathic pain, and cancer pain. Their effectiveness in other orthopaedic disorders, such as low-back pain and arthritic disorders, is less certain.

Other adjuvants that may be used in the treatment of neuropathic pain include anticonvulsants, such as gabapentin (Neurontin), carbamazepine (Tegretol), or phenytoin (Dilantin), and oral local anesthetics (mexiletine). These neuromodulators may be particularly useful for pain that is described as burning, lancinating, or shock-like. A relatively high incidence of side effects, some of which may be life-threatening, have been reported with systemic administration of local anesthetics. These drugs should be administered only by persons experienced with their use.

Muscle relaxants can be helpful in reducing anxiety-related muscle tension associated with arthritis, vertebral disc protrusions, or bone metastasis (McCaffery & Pasero, 1999). Baclofen (Lioresal) and diazepam (Valium) are two effective antispastic agents; baclofen is preferred because it causes fewer sedative effects. Abrupt withdrawal of baclofen should be avoided because temporary hallucinations can occur and there may be a rebound in the severity of spasms.

Corticosteroids may be used to reduce pain from swelling and inflammation and can be taken systemically or injected into the joint. However, because of the potential for serious side effects, these drugs are reserved for specific situations, such as arthritis flares or tumor infiltration into nerve or bone.

Topically applied counterirritants, such as menthol or capsaicin cream and aspirin creams, may be a familiar therapy for orthopaedic clients. Capsaicin in concentrations of 0.025% to 0.075% has gained widespread use for various pain problems. Capsaicin is a pepper extract that causes transient burning on application but produces no known systemic side effects or drug interactions (Schnitzer, Posner, & Lawrence, 1995). It is believed to deplete substance P at the site, although there is controversy about the effect of placebo response. Schnitzer, Posner, and Lawrence (1995) found a 50% reduction in pain severity with capsaicin cream use in osteoarthritis clients.

Tolerance, Physical Dependence, and Addiction. A major concern with pain is undermedication, which may be the result of incorrect assessment, insufficient knowledge of the pharmacology of the prescribed drug, or personal attitudes of the caregivers and clients toward analgesics.

The literature is replete with authors who have suggested that some nurses tend to undermedicate clients with analgesics because of a fear of potential abuse or addiction (Drayer, Henderson, & Reidenberg, 1999; McCaffery & Ferrell, 1995). A clear understanding of the differences among psychological dependence (addiction), physical dependence, and tolerance is critical. Concern about the problems of addiction and respiratory depression is greater than the actual risk.

Box 5–3 clarifies the differences among psychological dependence (addiction), physical dependence, and toler-

---

BOX 5–3.
Clarification of Terms

Physical Dependence
A state of adaptation that is manifested by a drug class–specific withdrawal syndrome that can be produced by abrupt cessation, a rapid dosage reduction, decreasing blood level of the drug, and/or administration of an antagonist.

Tolerance
A state of adaptation in which exposure to a drug induces changes that result in a diminution of one or more of the drug's effects over time.

Addiction
A primary, chronic, neurobiologic disease, with genetic, psychosocial, and environmental factors influencing its development and manifestations. It is characterized by behaviors that include one or more of the following: impaired control over drug use, compulsive use, or continued use despite harm and craving.

From the American Pain Society. Available at www.ampainsoc.org/advocacy/opioids2.htm

ance of medication. *Tolerance* means that the client requires increasing doses of medication to maintain the same effect. Development of tolerance is variable and appears to be a problem in only a small subgroup of clients with pain (Cleary & Backonja, 1996). Often, the first indication of development of tolerance is decreased duration of analgesia. The client may notice that the medication is "not lasting as long." Treatment of tolerance involves ruling out disease progression as a source of lost pain control, increasing the dosage of opioid, or switching to another opioid.

Physical dependence is characterized by the development of withdrawal symptoms on abrupt discontinuance of an opioid. The development of physical dependence may occur as early as 2 weeks into opioid therapy (AHCPR, 1994a, 1994b). Typical symptoms of withdrawal include anxiety, irritability, chills and hot flashes, joint pain, lacrimation, rhinorrhea, diaphoresis, nausea, vomiting, abdominal cramps, and diarrhea. Symptoms of withdrawal can be prevented by gradually tapering the opioid dosage. Physical dependence is a normal physiologic response to chronic opioid therapy and is not synonymous with addiction.

Addiction is a psychological dependence on a drug. The incidence of addiction is unknown; however, opioids appear to account for a small part (less than 5%) of the national drug abuse problem, as measured by drug overdoses (Joranson, Ryan, Gilson, & Dahl, 2000). Addiction is defined as a pattern of compulsive drug use characterized by a continued craving for opioid and the need to use the opioid for effects *other* than pain relief (APS, 1999). A hallmark of addiction is persistent use despite declining quality of life. As discussed earlier, the risk of developing addiction when treated with opioids for pain control is extremely small. It is important for clinicians to understand that the trend of increasing medical use of opioid analgesics to treat pain over the past decade does not appear to have contributed to increases in opioid analgesic abuse (Joranson et al., 2000).

Specialized Techniques for Drug Administration

Intravenous Patient-Controlled Analgesia.

IV patient-controlled analgesia (IVPCA) is a system of administering analgesia designed to enable maintenance of optimal serum analgesic levels throughout a therapeutic course. This modality allows clients to self-administer their pain medication, giving them control over when they can have it. A physician prescribes the amount of medication, and through a computerized system, a preset amount of opioid is delivered via an IV line. Any analgesic that can be given intravenously can be given through a PCA device. Clients may receive a continuous low dose (basal rate), ordered to provide a continuous serum level of medication. This may be used at night when the client is asleep. For PCA doses, the client pushes a button (much like a call light) to provide analgesic. Clients might push

that button when getting out of bed or before turning or doing their exercises. A lockout system is also present to prevent the client from receiving more medication in a limited time than prescribed. This modality can be used for almost any surgical client.

Perhaps the most beneficial part of PCA is that it gives clients control over their pain management and allows individual titration. Unfortunately, meta-analysis of randomized, controlled trials of IVPCA used for postoperative pain showed only a small improvement in pain control compared with conventional therapy (Ballantyne, Carr, Chalmers, Dear, Angelillo, & Mosteller, 1993). Studies subjected to the meta-analysis did not provide evidence of statistically significant reductions in side effects, analgesic use, surgical morbidity, or hospital stay with the use of PCA. The authors concluded that little attempt has been made to take advantage of, and demonstrate, the finely tuned nature of analgesia produced by PCA. Concern regarding the consequences of taking opioids, self-image, and beliefs that "it is just not good to take more medication than necessary" may also limit that amount of opioid clients take when on PCA, thereby limiting its effectiveness (Pellino, Gordon, Bowers, & Norton, 1998).

Nursing responsibilities in caring for a client with PCA include careful client selection, appropriate client education, and continued assessment of pain status and side effects of the medication. Generally, clients must be selected based on their willingness to participate in this therapy, their ability to understand directions, and careful assessment of their drug allergies. Many postoperative orthopaedic clients are eligible for this therapy. The only major contraindication is confusion.

Client education is a critical component of PCA therapy and has been shown to positively affect pain control (Knoerl, Faut-Callahan, Paice, & Shott, 1999). Before surgery, clients should be given directions both verbally and in writing. Most companies who manufacture these machines have preprinted materials written in language clients can understand. Clients need to be reassured that they will not be given too much medication. Continued assessment and teaching during PCA therapy are vital. Clients need to be reminded to administer medications before therapies and before the pain becomes too intense. Careful evaluation of the client's level of sedation is important to monitor for potential respiratory depression, particularly in the opioid-naive client.

While the client is using the PCA machine, careful assessment of other potential complications is important (where the pain occurs is important; e.g., types of calf pain must be differentiated so that the client is not self-medicating for potentially lethal complications). Neurovascular status, response to pain medication, and documentation of the medication remain nursing responsibilities.

Local and Regional Analgesia

Local and regional analgesia, achieved by injecting a local anesthetic into tissues or in proximity to certain parts of the peripheral nervous system, to relieve pain has been used for nearly a century. The most commonly used nerve blocks are intercostal, peripheral nerve, and epidural blocks. Local anesthetics are chemicals that inhibit neural excitation by preventing membrane depolarization. Nerve blocks performed with local anesthetic agents (bupivacaine, ropivacaine, lidocaine, mepivacaine, prilocaine, and etidocaine) or neurolytic agents (phenol, ethyl alcohol, and chlorocresol) can be used for diagnostic or treatment purposes. The agents can last for hours (local anesthetics) or for days or weeks (neurolytic agents).

Regional or Local Infusions of Local Anesthetics.

A unique form of analgesia that can sometimes be offered to orthopaedic clients is the continuation of a regional block through use of PCA local anesthetic after major shoulder surgery. Interscalene PCA with a local anesthetic (e.g., ropivacaine, bupivacaine) following an interscalene brachial plexus block has compared favorably over IVPCA in terms of pain relief, side effects, and client satisfaction after open shoulder surgery (Borgeat, Perschk, Bird, Hodler, & Gerber, 2000; Singelyn, Sequy, & Gouverneur, 1999). Continuous local anesthetic infiltration of the wound is another option being explored. A disposable elastic pump that maintains a constant flow rate of local anesthetic into the wound via a catheter has been used with good results in initial studies of orthopaedic clients. Use of this method resulted in less opioid use following total knee arthroplasty and lower pain scores following anterior cruciate ligament reconstruction when compared with clients who did not have local anesthetic infiltration (Morris, Pulido-Thompson, Colwell, & Hoenecke, 2001).

An important nursing concern following a regional nerve block is the correct positioning of the body part (e.g., with an axillary block) and the safety of the individual. The onset and regression of a nerve block vary between different drugs. Clients and family members need reassurance that the numbness is temporary and that motor function and sensation will return in 4 to 8 hours, depending on the medication used. Communication (and documentation) between the nurse and the client is important in establishing a database for return of neurovascular function. Monitoring for adverse effects, such as localized tissue toxicity (nerve damage) and systemic toxicity (CNS and cardiovascular), is an important nursing role.

Several other regional techniques can be used in the treatment of chronic pain. The first is myofascial-trigger pain injections, in which saline or local anesthetics are injected into trigger points. It may produce long-lasting relief without systemic toxicity or myotoxicity. The second technique is subcutaneous infiltration, in which a mixture of a local anesthetic and a steroid is administered two to six times a week. This combination is helpful in the treatment of acute herpes zoster infection, causalgia, neuroma, and postherpetic neuralgia. The third technique is IV local anesthetic administration, which is systemic in nature. This technique is used with clients who have sustained burns and with those who have central pain, Raynaud's phenomenon, phantom limb pain, and other types of severe neuropathic pain such as complex regional pain syndrome (CRPS).

Spinal (Epidural and Intrathecal) Analgesia.

The epidural space is the area surrounding the neural tube and its coverings (dura mater, arachnoid, and pia mater). It contains fatty tissue, veins, spinal arteries, and spinal nerves. The space extends from the foramen magnum to the sacrococcygeal membrane. The spinal cord ends at approximately L1 in the adult, where it splits into the cauda equina (the lumbar and sacral nerve roots). Below the arachnoid membrane is the subarachnoid or intrathecal space, containing cerebrospinal (CSF). Figure 5–2 depicts spinal anatomy and correct positioning for an epidural catheter.

Pain reception in the periphery passes by impulse via afferent nerves through the dorsal root ganglion into the dorsal horn of the spinal cord, crosses to the contralateral spinothalamic tract, and ascends through the spinal cord to the thalamus and cortex. An opioid administered into the epidural space diffuses across the dural membrane into the CSF and then to the opioid receptors in the dorsal horn of the cord to inhibit pain transmission. Intrathecal drugs are administered directly into the CSF, requiring much smaller doses than epidural administration to achieve analgesia.

In addition to the receptor affinity, the lipid solubility of an opioid is an important property that determines the pharmacokinetic actions of the drug. The more lipophilic the opioid, the more rapid its diffusion across the dural membrane. This property is important in the diffusion into the lipid-rich areas of the spinal cord following administration of an epidural opioid. For example, meperidine and fentanyl are more lipophilic than morphine. Crews (1990) reports that the onset of analgesia of morphine exceeds 20 minutes, with maximal analgesia obtained 40 to 90 minutes after administration. Conversely, meperidine and fentanyl have a reported onset of 5 to 10 minutes, with maximal analgesia after 12 to 30 minutes. Agents that are more water soluble diffuse more slowly across the dura mater and tend to linger, spreading through the CSF rostrally to the respiratory brainstem. This rostral spread can cause a delayed-onset respiratory depression, usually occurring 6 to 12 hours after initial administration of the opioid.

The analgesic agents most commonly administered via the epidural route are morphine, hydromorphone, fentanyl, and sufentanil, with or without local anesthetic

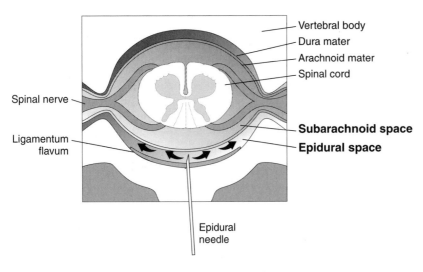

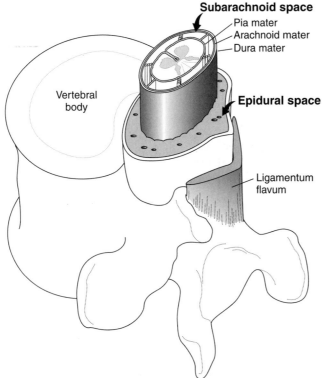

FIGURE 5–2. Spinal analgesia anatomy.

agents, such as bupivacaine or ropivacaine. Epidural and intrathecal analgesics may be given continuously using an infusion pump or may be given intermittently by bolus, usually by the anesthesiologist or via a PCA pump. For some procedures, a single dose may be given after surgery by the anesthesiologist. The spinal catheter may be removed before the client is brought to the postanesthesia care unit or, in many instances, left in for continuous analgesia after surgery.

Epidural analgesia has been used with clients having total joint replacements, ligament reconstructions, other procedures of the lower extremities, and abdominal and thoracic surgeries. It has also been used for postoperative

pain management after spine surgery. Lumbar epidural anesthesia is the most common regional analgesic technique for lower extremity surgery and has been shown to reduce the risk of thromboembolism and to facilitate rehabilitation (Peng & Chan, 1999). Contraindications for epidural analgesia in the orthopaedic client are coagulopathy, sepsis, shock or hypotension, some spinal cord diseases, increased intracranial pressure, procedures with a risk of rapid blood loss, and client refusal. Relative contraindications that must be individually evaluated are anticoagulation therapy and localized infection.

Complications of spinal analgesia include inadvertent dural puncture, spinal or IV injection of opioids, epidural hematoma or abscess, breakage of the epidural catheter, and backache. Dural punctures are usually manifested by headaches and treated by increasing fluids, maintaining IV fluid intake, imposing strict bed rest (with client flat in bed), administering analgesics for headaches, flushing the epidural catheter with a saline infusion, and administering caffeine to increase CSF production. If the dural leak and headaches continue, an epidural blood patch may be done after 24 hours to halt CSF leakage. Inadvertent intrathecal (spinal) injection of opioids is associated with respiratory depression. If such depression occurs, naloxone can be used to counteract the opioid's effect (see Box 5-2). The reported incidence of severe respiratory depression from epidural opioids is 1% (Wild & Coyne, 1992). Peak time for respiratory depression occurs approximately 1 hour after epidural administration (because of vascular absorption) and again between 6 and 12 hours after initial administration, when opioid in the CSF reaches the brain through rostral spread. Although respiratory depression usually occurs within the first 24 hours, it may occur later, is dose dependent, and may be position dependent or dilution dependent. Morphine is generally more commonly involved in respiratory depression than other drugs given by epidural infusion because of its higher water solubility and tendency to spread rostrally. Respiratory depression is also more common with increased age, adjunctive systemic opioids, and higher level (thoracic versus lumbar) epidurals.

The most common side effects with epidural injection of opioids are itching, nausea, vomiting, and urinary retention (Slowikowski & Flaherty, 2000). Nausea, vomiting, and itching may initially be controlled with prochlorperazine and diphenhydramine hydrochloride. If these problems continue, very low dosages of an opioid antagonist (naloxone) or an opioid agonist-antagonist (nalbuphine) may be given intravenously. Urinary retention is more common in males than in females and is difficult to treat. Bethanechol chloride (Urecholine) is generally ineffective in treatment. Increased dosages of naloxone may be used, but the best treatment is usually urinary catheterization. There is some controversy regarding the use of epidural analgesia in clients at high risk for compartment syndrome (see Chapter 10). Some authors report neurologic complications being more prevalent in patents with an epidural than when other forms of analgesia are used (Iaquinto, Pienkowski, Thornsberry, Grant, & Stevens, 1997), or epidural analgesia masking symptoms of compartment syndrome (Price, Ribeiro, & Kinnebrew, 1996) or delaying treatment of compartment syndrome (Dunwoody, Reichert, & Brown, 1997). There are no randomized trials that support these findings, and other authors raise questions about these reports (Mubarak & Wilton, 1997; Politis, 1998; Schmitz, Brown, Stoner, & Vollers, 1997). Mubarak and Wilton (1997) state that whatever mode of analgesia is used, a high index of clinical

suspicion, detailed examination, and compartment pressure measurements are the cornerstones for diagnosis and treatment of compartment syndrome.

Intra-articular Opioids. The use of IA opioids during joint surgery is generally accepted as a safe technique for analgesia, although its effectiveness is still under investigation. Clinical trials using IA morphine have suggested the possibility of analgesia mediated by local opioid action within the joint (Joshi, McCarroll, & Cooney, 1992). There is increasing evidence that inflammation in the joint results in an increase in the density and activation of opioid receptor sites (Kalso, Tramer, Carroll, McQuay, & Moore, 1997; Keates, Cramond, & Smith, 1999). In some studies of clients undergoing knee arthroscopy and arthroscopic anterior cruciate ligament reconstruction, IA morphine was shown to provide prolonged pain relief up to 24 hours when compared with bupivacaine or placebo (Brandsson, Karlsson, Morberg, Rydgren, Eriksson, & Hedner, 2000; Jauregito, Wilcox, Cohn, Thisted, & Reider, 1995). Clients in the morphine group tended to take less supplemental pain medication on the first postoperative day (Jaureguito et al., 1995). Other studies have shown no significant beneficial effect of IA opioids following knee arthroscopy or arthroplasty (Klasen, Opitz, Melzer, Thiel, & Hempelmann, 1999; Reuben, Steinberg, Cohen, Prasad, & Gibson, 1998). Authors of a systematic review of randomized, controlled trials of the use of IA morphine after knee surgery concluded that IA morphine may have some effect in reducing pain intensity and consumption of analgesics; however, better methodologic quality is needed in future studies to determine whether IA morphine is analgesic and whether the analgesia produced is clinically useful (Kalso et al., 1997). The use of IA morphine is also being investigated in the treatment of chronic inflammatory arthritis or osteoarthritis of the knee. Stein, Yassouridis, Szopko, Helmke, and Stein (1999) found IA morphine to have an effect similar to IA dexamethasone on pain-intensity ratings and synovial leukocyte counts.

Preemptive Analgesia. The use of preemptive analgesia has grown in popularity since the late 1980s. The idea is that analgesia given before a painful stimulus prevents or reduces the development of any memory of the pain in the nervous system, resulting in a subsequent lower analgesic requirement (McQuay, 1994). This theory is based on the observation that tissue injury may cause expansion of receptive fields and a decrease in the threshold of dorsal horn neurons (Dahl & Kehlet, 1993). The final result can be the development of allodynia (in which innocuous stimulation generates pain), hyperalgesia (increased pain), and prolonged changes in the nervous system. Based on experimental studies, it has been proposed that preinjury neural blockade can eliminate or reduce postinjury pain.

Clinical trials of preemptive analgesia have included administration of opioids, NSAIDs, or both; infiltration with local anesthetics; and nerve block before making an incision. Although the value of preemptive analgesia remains controversial, several studies have shown promising results (Bach, Noreng, & Tjellden, 1988; Ejlersen, Andersen, Eliasen, & Morgensen, 1992; Richmond, Bromley, & Woolf, 1993), with clients reporting prolonged analgesia. The most striking example in studies of preemptive analgesia is a lowered incidence of phantom limb pain following amputation after using preemptive epidural block. Preemptive analgesia for at least 24 to 48 hours before amputation is effective in reducing or preventing phantom limb pain. Postoperative efforts alone have no effect. See Chapter 20, Amputations Examining the Evidence table, for specific studies that address this topic. Although some studies of preemptive analgesia have reported some benefit, most have not, suggesting a need to extend the preemptive treatment into the postoperative period using a balanced, multimodal approach (Katz, 1995).

Nonpharmacologic Management

Nonpharmacologic interventions are an essential component to a multimodal approach to pain management. Any experience of pain has three components: physical, psychological, and cognitive. Medication management targets the physical dimension of pain and is only one intervention of many that can be used. The most therapeutic treatments may include repositioning an affected extremity, providing information, or just listening to the client. Although these measures are commonly discounted as pain management tools, they often are just what the client needs to deal with the stress of pain. Touch, holding, and rocking are especially therapeutic with infants and young children.

Health care consumers are increasingly requesting something other than analgesics for pain relief. The use of complementary therapies has grown tremendously over the past decade, and it is estimated that more clients are seen by alternative than conventional providers (Eisenberg et al., 1998). The primary reason for seeking these therapies is chronic pain related to conditions such as arthritis, back problems, and headaches (Astin, 1998; Eisenberg et al., 1998). Nonpharmacologic approaches to pain management are used widely by "conventional" practitioners. Ninety-four percent of pain specialists surveyed in 1997 used or referred clients to some type of nonpharmacologic therapy for pain management (Berman & Bausell, 2000). In 1995, the NIH held a 3-day Technology Assessment Conference to review the data on the relative merits of behavioral and relaxation interventions in the treatment of chronic pain and insomnia. The final report endorsed integrating behavioral and relaxation techniques, such as meditation, hypnosis, and biofeedback, with conventional treatment (Chilton, 1996).

Nonpharmacologic pain management strategies can be categorized as cognitive-behavioral and physical. Cognitive-behavioral approaches include techniques such as passive relaxation with mental imagery, distraction or focusing, progressive relaxation, biofeedback, hypnosis, and music therapy. Physical techniques include applications of heat and cold, massage, exercise, and transcutaneous nerve stimulation. The goal of these techniques is to reduce pain by altering the physiologic response and providing the client with some sense of control over the pain. Cognitive-behavioral strategies can help clients understand more about their pain, alter their pain behavior and coping skills, and change their perception of pain.

Cognitive-Behavioral Techniques. Cognitive-behavioral strategies attempt to inspire more positive patterns of thoughts and actions in response to perception of pain. Education, skills acquisition, cognitive and behavioral rehearsal, and generalization and maintenance are the four basic components of these interventions (NIH, 1996). Several mechanisms have been suggested for the usefulness of CBT in reducing pain. These include activation of the frontal-limbic attention system to inhibit pain impulse transmission from thalamic to cortical structures, reduction of depression and anxiety, alteration of expectations, and enhancement of a sense of self-control over their pain (and thereby, decreased helplessness) (NIH, 1996). More than 20 studies indicate that cognitive and behavioral interventions initiated preoperatively decrease anxiety before and after surgery, reduce postoperative pain intensity and intake of analgesics drugs, improve treatment compliance, improve cardiovascular and respiratory indices, and accelerate recovery (Carr & Goudas, 1999).

The educational component of treatment consists of the presentation of the cognitive-behavioral perspective on pain and the control of pain (e.g., role of cognition, affect, behavior, environmental factors, physical factors). The history of the client's pain is unraveled, including spoken and unspoken fears that he or she might have. Including the family and significant others is important because the client's pain affects those individuals also. Homework assignments may be given to the client to assist in identifying feelings, thoughts, and behaviors that increase or decrease pain.

The next step, skills acquisition, addresses the fact that not one technique works for all clients. Cognitive-behavioral therapists serve as coaches, helping clients learn new ways of behaving, learning, and thinking. Clients are encouraged to become active participants in their therapy, not helpless victims. Skills that might be taught are relaxation training, active physical therapy using paced mastery, problem-solving training, distraction training, rational restructuring, and communication training.

In cognitive-behavioral rehearsal, clients practice and consolidate the skills they have learned during the skills acquisition phase and learn to apply them in a natural situation. Using role-playing and rehearsal techniques, among other methods, the client interacts with the therapist to replicate a specific situation and the specific skills he or she must use in that situation.

In the final stage of treatment, the focus is on ways of predicting and avoiding or dealing with pain after treatment. Clearly, not all possible situations can be predicted, so clients are encouraged to use all of the skills and competencies within their repertoires. The focus of this stage is a reminder to clients that they are in charge of their lives and are capable of relearning techniques that can help in coping with pain.

Imagery. Imagery occurs spontaneously during periods of reverie, while listening to music or relaxing, or during a light sleep. It can be nonverbal or accompanied by the use of words. Guided imagery encourages clients to create images that are pleasant to them and to focus their attention on pleasant and peaceful thoughts. As with other modalities, imagery is an adjunct to analgesia and is never used in place of it. The reader is reminded that not all clients enjoy (or even permit) the use of this technique, but for many, it is of great benefit.

There are many published imagery exercises (Davis, Eshelman, & McKay, 2000, pp. 55-56). The exercise selected ideally should be congruent with the client's interests. Visualizing the ocean, for example, may not be appealing to all clients—they may prefer a mountain or valley image. Imagery can be taught individually or in a group. The client can then use the exercise independently as a technique to modulate anxiety and pain.

Distraction. Distraction involves assisting clients to focus their attention on something other than the pain. Music, reading, and television can assist the individual to refocus, even for a short time. Humor is another distraction technique that produces therapeutic results. It is important to discuss and select distraction techniques with the client. Favorite movies, shows, or even home movies may bring the client pleasant memories or thoughts.

One must be careful not to inaccurately assess a client as pain free when the client is using distraction technique. Remember also that the client who is unable to communicate may benefit from the nurse's continuing to converse with him or her about concerned people who have called, changing colors of the fall leaves, world events, and so forth.

Relaxation. Relaxation approaches involve two components: a repetitive focus on a word, sound, or muscular activity and a passive attitude toward introducing thoughts (Chilton, 1996). Passive relaxation involves

focusing attention on one's breathing, sense of warmth, or muscle tension. Progressive or active muscle relaxation involves the active tensing and relaxation of various muscle groups. Many scripts are available (Davis, Eshelman, & McKay, 2000, pp. 101-104) and are often combined with other techniques, such as imagery. In general, relaxation alters sympathetic activity, perhaps through alteration in catecholamines, and causes a decrease in oxygen consumption, respiratory rate, heart rate, and blood pressure (NIH, 1996).

Music Therapy. Music can elicit an array of physiologic responses, including changes in heart rate, blood pressure, electrocardiographic waves, and muscle contractions. Music therapy has been used to provide pain relief in a variety of situations, including after surgery and during procedures. Distraction and attentional factors associated with music, release of endorphins, and stimulation of the limbic system are proposed mechanisms of music-induced pain and anxiety reduction (Taylor, 1999).

Biofeedback. Biofeedback uses instrumentation to help clients monitor and enhance their ability to influence psychophysiologic responses. Electromyographic biofeedback is commonly used in combination with relaxation exercises for a variety of pain problems, including headaches, low-back pain, and temporomandibular joint pain. Obvious drawbacks are access to equipment and reimbursement issues.

Hypnosis. Hypnosis is a state of intense focused concentration and can be used to manipulate the perception of pain. Some individuals are more susceptible to hypnosis than others. Clients who are hypnotized may be able to alter sensations in a painful area by changing them to a more acceptable temperature sensation or a tingling. Hypnosis is thought to work through inhibition of pain impulses, not through endorphin production (NIH, 1996).

Physical Techniques. Cutaneous stimulation, such as application of heat, cold, or massage, can reduce pain by aiding in relaxation while exercise strengthens weakened muscles and stiff joints. (See Chapter 13 for additional information on these strategies.) These activities encourage participation in self-care and offer a variety of options. It is important to remember that like CBT, these methods should be used concurrently with drugs and other modalities to manage pain.

Heat and Cold. Application of heat increases the blood flow to the skin and superficial organs. Vasodilation increases oxygen and nutrient delivery to damaged tissue and also decreases joint stiffness by increasing the elastic properties of muscles. Heat can be applied by warm packs (dry or moist) and immersion into water. Application of heat to an injured area is not recommended within 24 to 48 hours of injury because of increased blood flow, which can cause increased edema. Client education and close monitoring for skin protection to prevent burns are important nursing responsibilities.

Conversely, application of cold causes vasoconstriction and local hypoesthesia. Cold is effective in reducing inflammation and edema soon after injury and is a common therapy for orthopaedic clients. Cold may often provide more effective and prolonged pain reduction than heat and is recommended when superficial heat is ineffective in reducing spasm. In a study of clients who had total hip or knee arthroplasty, cold therapy was associated with earlier ambulation and shortened hospital stays (Scarcella & Cohn, 1995). However, cold may increase or decrease joint stiffness and range of motion, warranting an individualized approach. If the site of pain is inaccessible, application of heat or cold proximally, distally, or to the contralateral site may provide effective pain reduction (McCaffery & Pasero, 1999). The duration of ice application is generally shorter than that of heat, usually lasting less than 15 minutes. Raynaud's phenomenon or other vascular or connective diseases in which vasoconstriction is contraindicated may preclude the use of cold therapy.

Massage. Massage and vibration are commonly used methods to aid in relaxation. Both techniques aid by increasing superficial circulation. Techniques include stroking, kneading, and rubbing with rhythmic circular, distal-to-proximal motions. Knowledge of acupressure or trigger points can be helpful in site selection. The comfort of touch is a powerful tool to reassure clients and also provides an opportunity to talk with them. It is important to find an acceptable method of touch for a client because not all clients may be open to massage.

Transcutaneous Electrical Nerve Stimulation. Transcutaneous electrical nerve stimulation (TENS) has obtained increasing acceptance as a noninvasive method for managing pain, such as that occurring in causalgia, peripheral nerve injuries, phantom limb pain, bursitis, cervical pain, postoperative pain, labor, reflex sympathetic dystrophy, and other pain syndromes. Beneficial effects have been maintained for longer than 6 months in the majority of clients who have shown an immediate favorable response (Meyler, de Jongste, & Rolf, 1994). No one knows exactly how electrical nerve stimulation helps reduce pain, but several mechanisms have been suggested. Possible mechanisms include interference with the pain messages carried in the A delta and C fibers, increasing skin and muscle microcirculation, and activation of endogenous opioids. The placebo effect may also play a role in the pain relief obtained with TENS treatment.

Clients need to be instructed in the use of TENS units, which have two pads that are placed close to the painful area. Insurance companies generally reimburse for the renting of TENS units, which are relatively inexpensive. This modality, as with all other modalities, is not always used alone. Sometimes, a combination of modalities, including medication, is the most effective for the client.

Acupuncture. Acupuncture is a traditional therapeutic method from Chinese medicine and is traditionally used not only to relieve pain but also to treat diseases. Individuals with a variety of pain syndromes, including osteoarthritis, back pain, and tennis elbow, have been treated successfully with traditional acupuncture (Taylor, 1999).

Acupuncture points are located on meridians. The energy, called *chi,* flows through a meridian to assist a person's health. An inhibitory effect on the adrenergic system is useful in acupuncture treatment (Murray, 1995). Recent data favor a neurohumoral explanation with activation of endogenous pain control, such as via the opioid or serotonergic pathways.

SUMMARY

Pain, acute and/or chronic, is prevalent in the orthopaedic client population. The adverse effects of undertreated pain are becoming more recognized. A comprehensive, empathic approach using multiple modalities is critical in the effective assessment and management of pain. Nurses are in a unique position to positively contribute to effective pain management on an individual client basis and on an institution-wide basis through incorporation of available guidelines (see Table 5–1) into daily practice and taking a leadership role in operationalizing these guidelines in the settings in which we work.

Consumer demand and incorporation of pain assessment and management into accreditation standards will serve as impetuses for system-wide changes in pain management. As outlined in the JCAHO Pain Assessment and Management Standards, all clients have the right to appropriate assessment and management of pain. To achieve this goal, systems must be in place that incorporate screening of all clients for pain, comprehensive assessments if pain is identified, education of providers in pain assessment and management, and policies and procedures to support appropriate prescription of analgesics. Client and family education, continuity of care for symptom management, and monitoring the quality of pain management are additional components to promote appropriate management of pain.

WEBSITES FOR PAIN MANAGEMENT

American Academy of Pain Medicine: www.painmed.org
American Pain Foundation: www.painfoundation.org
American Pain Society: www.ampainsoc.org

American Society of Pain Management Nurses: www. aspmn.org/

International Association for the Study of Pain: www. halcyon.com/iasp

Wisconsin Cancer Pain Initiative: www.wisc.edu/wcpi

REFERENCES

Agency for Health Care Policy and Research (AHCPR). (1992). *Acute pain management: Operative or medical procedures and trauma: Clinical practice guideline No. 1.* AHCPR Publication No. 92-0032. Rockville, MD: Public Health Service, U.S. Department of Health and Human Services.

Agency for Health Care Policy and Research (AHCPR). (1994a). *Management of cancer pain: Clinical practice guideline No. 9.* AHCPR Pub. No. 94-0592. Rockville, MD: Public Health Service, U.S. Department of Health and Human Services.

Agency for Health Care Policy and Research (AHCPR). (1994b). *Acute low back problems in adults: Assessment and treatment: Clinical practice guideline No. 14.* AHCPR Pub. No. 95-0643. Rockville, MD: Public Health Service, U.S. Department of Health and Human Services.

American Geriatric Society (AGS) Panel on Chronic Pain in Older Persons. (1998). The management of chronic pain in older persons. *Journal of the American Geriatrics Society, 46,* 635-651.

American Pain Society (APS). (1995). Quality improvement guidelines for the treatment of acute pain and cancer pain. *Journal of the American Medical Association, 274,* 1874-1880.

American Pain Society (APS). (1999). *Principles of analgesic use in the treatment of acute pain and cancer pain* (4th ed.). Skokie, IL: Author.

American Society of Anesthesiologists (ASA) Task Force on Pain Management, Acute Pain Section. (1995). Practice Guidelines for Acute Pain Management in the Perioperative Setting. *Anesthesiology, 82,* 1071-1081.

Astin, J. A. (1998). Why patients use alternative medicine: Results of a national study. *Journal of the American Medical Association, 279,* 1548-1553.

Bach, S., Noreng, M. F., & Tjellden, N. U. (1988). Phantom limb pain in amputees during the first 12 months following limb amputation, after preoperative lumbar epidural blockade. *Pain, 33*(3), 297-301.

Ballantyne, J. C., Carr, D. B., Chalmers, T. C., Dear, K. B. G., Angelillo, I. F., & Mosteller, F. (1993). Postoperative patient-controlled analgesia: Meta-analysis of initial randomized control trials. *Journal of Clinical Anesthesiology, 5,* 182-193.

Berman, B. M., & Bausell, R. B. (2000). The use of non-pharmacological therapies by pain specialists. *Pain, 85,* 313-315.

Borgeat, A., Perschk, H., Bird, P., Hodler, J., & Gerber, C. (2000). Patient-controlled interscalene analgesia with ropivacaine 0.2% versus patient-controlled intravenous analgesia after major shoulder surgery: effects on diaphragmatic and respiratory function. *Anesthesiology, 92,* 102-108.

Brandsson, S., Karlsson, J., Morberg, P., Rydgren, B., Eriksson, B. I., & Hedner, T. (2000). Intraarticular morphine after arthroscopic ACL reconstruction: A double-blind placebo-controlled study of 40 patients. *Acta Orthopaedica Scandinavica, 71,* 280-285.

Briggs, M., Closs, J. S., & Mphil, R. G. N. (1999). A descriptive study of the use of visual analogue scales and verbal rating scales for the assessment of postoperative pain in orthopedic patients. *Journal of Pain and Symptom Management, 18,* 438-446.

Cannon, G. W., Caldwell, J. R., Holt, P., McLean, B., Seidenberg, B., Bologenese, J., Ehrich, E., Mukhopadhyay, S., & Daniels, B. (2000). Rofecoxib, a specific inhibit of cyclooxygenase 2, with clinical efficacy comparable with that of diclofenac sodium. *Arthritis & Rheumatism, 42,* 978-987.

Carr, D. B, & Goudas, L. C. (1999). Acute pain. *The Lancet, 353,* 2051-2058.

Carroll, K. C., Atkins, P. J., Herold, G. R., Mlcek, C. A., Shively, M.,

Clopton, P., & Glaser, D. N. (1999). Pain assessment and management in critically ill postoperative and trauma patients: a multisite study. *American Journal of Critical Care, 8,* 105-117.

Chilton, M. (1996). Panel recommends integrating behavioral and relaxation approaches into medical treatment of chronic pain, insomnia. *Alternative Therapies, 2,* 18-24.

Chung, G., Ritchie, E., & Su, J. (1997). Postoperative pain in ambulatory surgery. *Anesthesia and Analgesia, 85,* 808-816.

Cleary, J., & Backonja, M. (1996). "Translating" opioid tolerance research. *APS Bulletin, 6*(2), 4-7.

Conaway, D. C. (1995). Using NSAIDs safely in the elderly. *Hospital Medicine, 31*(1), 1-9.

Crews, J. C. (1990). Epidural opioid analgesia. *Critical Care Clinics, 6,* 315-342.

Dahl, J. (1993). State cancer pain initiatives. *Journal of Pain and Symptom Management, 8,* 372-375.

Dahl, J. (1999). COX-2 Selective NSAIDs. *Cancer Pain Forum.* The Resource Center of the American Alliance of Cancer Pain Initiatives, Madison, WI. Available at www.wisc.edu/trc/ epf/fall99/COX-2.html

Dahl, J. B., & Kehlet, H. (1993). The value of pre-emptive analgesia in the treatment of postoperative pain. *British Journal of Anaesthesia, 70,* 434-439.

Daut, R. L., Cleeland, C. S., & Flanery, R. C. (1983). Development of the Wisconsin Brief Pain Questionnaire to assess pain in cancer and other diseases. *Pain, 17*(2), 197-210.

Davis, M, Eshelman, E. R., & McKay, M. (2000). *The relaxation & stress reduction workbook.* Oakland, CA: New Harbinger.

Day, R., Morrison, A. L., Castaneda, O., Stursberg, A., Nahir, M., Helgetveit, K. B., Kress, B., Daniels, B., Bolognese, J., Krupa, D., Seidenberg, B., & Ehrich E. (2000). A randomized trial of the efficacy and tolerability of the COX-2 inhibitor rofecoxib vs. ibuprofen in patients with osteoarthritis. *Archives of Internal Medicine, 160,* 1781-1787.

Drayer, R. A., Henderson, J., & Reidenberg, M. (1999). Barriers to better pain control in hospitalized patients. *Journal of Pain Symptom Management, 17,* 434-440.

Dunwoody, J. M., Reichert, C. C., & Brown, K. L. B. (1997). Compartment syndrome associated with bupivacaine and fentanyl epidural analgesia. *Journal of Pediatric Orthopaedics, 17,* 285-288.

Eisenberg, D. M., Davis, R. B., Ettner, S. L., Appel, S., Wilkey, S., Van Rompay, M., & Kessler, R. C. (1998). Trend in alternative medicine use in the United States, 1990-1997. *Journal of the American Medical Association, 280,* 1569-1575.

Ejlersen, E., Andersen, H. B., Eliasen, L., & Morgensen, T. A. (1992). A comparison between pre- and post-incisional lidocaine infiltration on postoperative pain. *Anesthesia and Analgesia, 74,* 495-498.

Ferrell, B. A., Ferrell, B. R., & Rivera, L. (1995). Pain in cognitively impaired nursing home patients. *Journal of Pain and Symptom Management, 10,* 591-598.

Fishman, S., & Berger, L. (2000). *The war on pain.* New York: Harper-Collins.

Fuller, B. F., & Neu, M. (2000). Validity and reliability of a practice-based infant pain assessment instrument. *Clinical Nursing Research, 9,* 124-143.

Goodman, S. B. (2000). Use of COX-2 specific inhibitors in operative and nonoperative management of patients with arthritis. *Orthopedics, 23,* S765-S768.

Gordon, D., & Ward, S. (1995). Correcting patient misconceptions about pain. *American Journal of Nursing, 95*(7), 43-45.

Hargeaves, L. M., & Joris, I. L. (1993). The peripheral effects of opioids. *American Pain Society Journal, 2*(1), 51-59.

Hassan, H., Bastani, B., & Gellens, M. (2000). Successful treatment of normeperidine neurotoxicity by hemodialysis. *American Journal of Kidney Diseases, 35,* 146-149.

Herr, K. A., & Mobily, P. R. (1993). Comparison of selected pain assessment tools for use with the elderly. *Applied Nursing Research, 6*(1), 39-46.

Iaquinto, J. M., Pienkowski, D., Thornsberry, R., Grant, S., & Stevens, D. B. (1997). Increase neurological complications associated with postoperative epidural analgesia after tibial fracture fixation. *American Journal of Orthopaedics, 26,* 604–608.

International Association for the Study of Pain. (1986). *Classification of chronic pain: Description of chronic pain syndromes and definitions of pain terms. Pain Supplement 3.* Amsterdam: Elsevier.

Jaureguito, J. W., Wilcox, J. G., Cohn, S. J., Thisted, R. A., & Reider, B. (1995). A comparison of intraarticular morphine and bupivacaine for pain control after outpatient knee arthroscopy. *American Journal of Sports Medicine, 23,* 350–353.

Joint Commission for Accreditation of Healthcare Organizations (JCAHO). (2000). *Accreditation manual for hospitals.* Oakbrook Terrace, IL: Author.

Joranson, D. E., Ryan, K. M., Gilson, A. M., & Dahl, J. L. (2000). Trends in medical use and abuse of opioid analgesics. *Journal of the American Medical Association, 283,* 1710–1714.

Joshi, G. P., McCarroll, S. M., & Cooney, C. M. (1992). Intra-articular morphine for pain relief after knee arthroscopy. *Journal of Bone and Joint Surgery, 74B,* 749–751.

Kaiko, R. F, Foley, K. M., Grabinski, P. Y., Heidrich, G., Rogers, A. G., Inturrisi, C. E., & Reidenberg, M. M. (1983). Central nervous system excitatory effects of meperidine in cancer patients. *Annals of Neurology, 13,* 180–185.

Kalso, E., Tramer, M. R., Carroll, D., McQuay, H. J., & Moore, R. A. (1997). Pain relief from intra-articular morphine after knee surgery: A qualitative systematic review. *Pain, 71,* 127–134.

Katz, J. (1995). Pre-emptive analgesia: evidence, current status and future directions. *European Journal of Anaesthesiology, 12*(Suppl 10), 8–13.

Keates, H. L., Cramond, T., & Smith, M. T. (1999). Intraarticular and periarticular opioid binding in inflamed tissue in experimental canine arthritis. *Anesthesia and Analgesia, 89,* 409–415.

Kehlet, H. (1997). Multimodal approach to pain control postoperative pathophysiology and rehabilitation. *British Journal of Anaesthesiology, 78,* 606–617.

Kehlet, H. (1999). Acute pain control and accelerated postoperative surgical recovery. *Surgical Clinics of North America, 79,* 431–443.

Kehlet, H., Werner, M., & Perkins, F. (1999). Balanced analgesia: What is it and what are its advantages in postoperative pain? *Drugs, 58,* 793–797.

Klasen, J. A., Opitz, S. A., Melzer, C., Thiel, A., & Hempelmann, G. (1999). Intraarticular, epidural and intravenous analgesia after total knee arthroplasty. *Acta Anaesthesiologica Scandinavica, 43,* 1021–1026.

Knoerl, D. V., Faut-Callahan, M., Paice, J., & Shott, S. (1999). Preoperative PCA teaching program to manage postoperative pain. *Medsurg Nursing, 8*(1), 25–33, 36.

Laine, L., Harper, S., Simon, T., Bath, R., Johanson, J., Schwartz, H., Stern, S., Quan, H., & Bolognese, J. (1999). A randomized trial comparing the effect of rofecoxib, a cyclooxygenase 2-specific inhibitor, with that of ibuprofen on the gastroduodenal mucosa of patients with osteoarthritis. *Gastroenterology, 117,* 776–783.

Lehmann, K. A. (1994). Tramadol for the management of acute pain. *Drugs 47* (Suppl 1), 19–32.

Liebeskind, J. C. (1991). Pain can kill. *Pain, 44,* 3–4.

Maccarrone, C., West, R. J., Broomhead, A. F., & Hodsman, G. P. (1994). Single dose pharmacokinetics of Kapanol a new oral sustained morphine formulation. *Clinical Drug Investigation, 7,* 262–274.

Marcantonio, E. R., Juarez, G., Goldman, L., Mangione, C. M., Ludwig, L. E., Lind, L., Katz, N., Cook, E. F., Orav, E. J., & Lee, T. H. (1994). The relationship of postoperative delirium with psychoactive medications. *Journal of the American Medical Association, 272,* 1518–1622.

McCaffery, M. (1979). *Nursing management of the patient with pain* (2nd ed.). Philadelphia: Lippincott.

McCaffery, M., & Pasero, C. (1999). *Pain: Clinical manual for nursing practice.* (2nd ed.). St. Louis: Mosby.

McCaffery, M., & Ferrell, B. R. (1995). Nurses' knowledge about cancer pain: A survey of five countries. *Journal of Pain and Symptom Management 10,* 356–369.

McGuire, D. B. (1992). Comprehensive and multidimensional assessment and measurement of pain. *Journal of Pain and Symptom Management, 7,* 312–319.

McHugh, G. J. (1999). Norpethidine accumulation and generalized seizure during pethidine patient-controlled analgesia. *Anaesthesia & Intensive Care, 27,* 289–291.

McQuay, H. J. (1994). Do preemptive treatments provide better pain control? In G. F. Gebhart, D. L. Hammond, & T. S. Jensen (Eds.), *Proceedings of the 7th world congress on pain* (pp. 709–723). Seattle: IASP Press.

Melzack, R. (1987). The short-form McGill Pain Questionnaire. *Pain, 30*(2), 191–197.

Melzack, R., & Wall, P. D. (1965). Pain mechanisms: A new theory. *Science, 150,* 971–979.

Melzack, R., & Wall, P. D. (1983). *The Challenge of Pain.* New York: Basic.

Merskey, H. (1979). Pain terms: A list with definitions and notes on usage. *Pain, 6,* 242.

Meyler, J. J., de Jongste, M. J., & Rolf, C. A. (1994). Clinical evaluation of pain treatment with electrostimulation: A study on TENS in patients with different pain syndromes. *Clinical Journal of Pain, 10*(1), 22–27.

Moiniche, S., Hansen, B. L., Christensen, S. W., Dahl, J. B., & Kehlet, H. (1992). Activity of patients and duration of hospitalization following hip replacement with balanced treatment of pain and early mobilization. *Ugeskrift for Laeger, 154,* 1495–1499.

Morris, B. A., Pulido-Thompson, P., Colwell, C. W., & Hoenecke, H. R. (2001). *The efficacy of continuous bupivacaine infiltration for pain management following orthopaedic surgery: ACL reconstruction and TKA.* Presentation at the American Society of Pain Management Nurses Annual Meeting, Houston.

Mubarak, S. J., & Wilton, N. C. T. (1997). Compartment syndromes and epidural analgesia. *Journal of Pediatric Orthopaedics, 17,* 282–284.

Murray, J. B. (1995). Evidence for acupuncture's analgesic effectiveness and proposals for the physiological mechanisms involved. *Journal of Psychology, 129,* 443–461.

Nadvi, S. Z., Sarnaik, S, & Ravindranath, Y. (1999). Low frequency of meperidine-associated seizures in sickle cell disease. *Clinical Pediatrics, 38,* 459–462.

National Institutes of Health (NIH) Consensus Development Conference Statement. (1986*). The integrated approach to the management of pain* (Vol. 6, No. 3). U.S. Department of Health and Human Services, U.S. Government Printing Office, 491-292:41148.

National Institutes of Health (NIH) Technology Assessment Panel. (1996). Integration of behavioral and relaxation approaches into the treatment of chronic pain and insomnia. *Journal of the American Medical Association, 276,* 313–318.

Payne, R., Chandler, S., & Einhaus, M. (1995). Guidelines for the clinical use of transdermal fentanyl. *Anti-Cancer Drugs, 6*(Suppl 3), 50–53.

Pellino, T. A., Gordon, D. B., Bowers, B., & Norton, S. (1998). *Hospitalized patients' experience of taking analgesics via intravenous patient-controlled analgesia.* Poster presented at the American Society of Pain Management Nurses, Orlando.

Peng, P. W. H., & Chan, V. W. S. (1999). Local and regional block in postoperative pain control. *Surgical Clinics of North America, 79,* 345–369.

Picard, P. R., Tramer, M. R., McQuay, H. J., & Moore, R. A. (1997). Analgesic efficacy of peripheral opioids (all except intra-articular): A qualitative systematic review of randomised controlled trials. *Pain, 72,* 309–318.

Politis, G. D. (1998). Postoperative epidural analgesia and neurologic complications. *American Journal of Orthopedics, 27,* 757–758.

Portenoy, R. K. (1994). Opioid therapy for chronic nonmalignant pain: current status. In H. L. Fields & J. C. Liebeskind (Eds.), *Progress in pain research and management. Vol. 1. Pharmacologic approaches to the treatment of chronic pain: New concepts and critical issues* (pp. 247–287). Seattle: IASP Publications.

Portenoy, R. K. (1996). Opioid therapy for chronic nonmalignant pain: A review of the critical issues. *Journal of Pain and Symptom Management, 11,* 203–217.

Price, C., Ribeiro, J., & Kinnebrew, T. (1996). Compartment syndromes associated with postoperative epidural analgesia. *Journal of Bone and Joint Surgery, 78A,* 597–599.

Puntillo, K., Miaskowski, C., Kehrle, K., Stannard, D., Gleeson, S., & Nye, P. (1997). Relationship between behavioral and physiological indicators of pain, critical care patients' self-reports of pain, and opioid administration. *Critical Care Medicine, 25,* 1159–1166.

Puntillo, K., & Wilkie, D. J. (1991). Assessment of pain in the critically ill. In K. A. Puntillo (Ed.), *Pain in the critically ill: Assessment and management* (pp. 45–64). Gaithersburg, MD: Aspen.

Radnay, P. A., Brodman, E., Mankikar, D., & Duncalf, D. (1980). The effect of equi-analgesic doses of fentanyl, morphine, meperidine and pentazocine on common bile duct pressure. *Anaesthesist, 29,* 26–29.

Raffa, R. B., Friderichs, E., Reemann, W., Shank, R. P., Codd, E. E., & Vaught, J. L. (1992). Opioid and nonopioid components independently contribute to the mechanisms of action of tramadol, an "atypical" opioid analgesic. *Journal of Pharmacology and Experimental Therapeutics, 260,* 275–284.

Rapp, C. J., & Gordon, D. B. (2000). Understanding equianalgesic dosing. *Orthopaedic Nursing, 19*(3), 65–72.

Rawlins, M. D. (1993). Nonopioid Analgesics. In D. Doyle, G. W. C. Hanks, & N. MacDonald (Eds.), *Oxford textbook of palliative medicine* (pp. 182–186). Oxford: Oxford University Press.

Reuben, S. S., Steinberg, R., Cohen, M. A., Prasad, K., & Gibson, C. (1998). Intraarticular morphine in the multimodal analgesic management of postoperative pain after ambulatory anterior cruciate ligament repair. *Anesthesia & Analgesia, 82,* 374–378.

Richmond, C. E., Bromley, L. M., & Woolf, C. J. (1993). Preoperative morphine pre-empts postoperative pain. *The Lancet, 342,* 73–75.

Rossat, J., Maillard, M., Nussberger, J., Brunner, H. R., & Burnier, M. (1999). Renal effects of selective cyclooxygenase-2 inhibition in normotensive salt-depleted subjects. *Clinical Pharmacology & Therapeutics, 66,* 76–84.

Sanders, S. H., Harden, R. N., Benson, S. E., & Vicente, P. J. (1999). Clinical practice guideline for chronic non-malignant pain syndrome patient II: An evidence-based approach. *Journal of Back and Musculoskeletal Rehabilitation, 13,* 47–58.

Scarcella, J. B., & Cohn, B. T. (1995). The effect of cold therapy on the postoperative course of total hip and knee arthroplasty patients. *American Journal of Orthopedics, 24,* 847–852.

Schmitz, M. L., Brown, R. E., Stoner, J. M., & Vollers, J. M. (1997). Compartment syndromes associated with postoperative epidural analgesia, commentary. *Journal of Bone and Joint Surgery, 79A,* 1271–1272.

Schnitzer, T. J., Posner, M., & Lawrence, I. D. (1995). High strength capsaicin cream for osteoarthritis pain: Rapid onset of action and improved efficacy with twice daily dosing. *Journal of Clinical Rheumatology, 1,* 268–273.

Serlin, R. C., Mendoza, T. R., Nakamura, Y., Edwards, K. R., & Cleeland, C. S. (1995). When is cancer pain mild, moderate or severe? Grading pain severity by its interference with function. *Pain, 61,* 277–284.

Singelyn, F. J., Sequy, S., & Gouverneur, J. M. (1999). Interscalene brachial plexus analgesia after open shoulder surgery: Continuous versus patient-controlled analgesia. *Anesthesia and Analgesia, 89,* 1216–1220.

Slowikowski, R. D., & Flaherty, S. A. (2000). Epidural analgesia for postoperative orthopaedic pain. *Orthopaedic Nursing, 19*(1), 23–33.

Soetenga, D., Frank, J., & Pellino, T. A. (1999). Assessment of the validity and reliability of the University of Wisconsin Children's Hospital pain scale for preverbal and nonverbal children. *Pediatric Nursing, 25,* 670–676.

Stein, A., Yassouridis, A., Szopko, C., Helmke, K., & Stein, C. (1999). Intraarticular morphine versus dexamethasone in chronic arthritis. *Pain, 83,* 525–532.

Stein, C. (1993). Peripheral mechanisms of opioid analgesics. *Anesthesia and Analgesia, 76,* 182–191.

Syntex Laboratories. (1996). Toradol package insert. Palo Alto, CA.

Taylor, A. G. (1999). Complementary/alternative therapies in the treatment of pain. In J. Spencer & J. Jacobs (Eds.), *Complementary/alternative medicine* (pp. 282–339). St. Louis: Mosby.

Verhaak, P. F. M., Kerssens, J. J., Dekker, J., Sorbi, M. J., & Bensing, J. M. (1998). Prevalence of chronic benign pain disorder among adults: A review of the literature. *Pain, 77,* 231–239.

Wall, P. D. (1996). Comments after 30 years of the gate control theory. *Pain Forum, 5*(1), 12–22.

Watson, C. P. N. (1994). Antidepressant drugs as adjuvant analgesics. *Journal of Pain and Symptom Management, 9,* 392–405.

Weingarten, S., Riedinger, M., Conner, L., Siebens, H., Varis, G., Alter, A., & Ellrodt, A. G. (1994). Hip replacement and hip hemiarthroplasty surgery: Potential opportunities to shorten lengths of hospital stay. *American Journal of Medicine, 97,* 208–213.

Wild, L., & Coyne, C. (1992, April). The basics and beyond: Epidural analgesia. *American Journal of Nursing, 92,* 26–36.

6

Anatomy and Physiology of the Musculoskeletal System

SHARON G. CHILDS

The musculoskeletal system consists of bones, which provide the structural architecture for the body, and other structures, soft tissues, or connective tissues that assist the bones to perform their many functions. These soft tissues include muscles, ligaments, tendons, and cartilage. The joint, the articulating juncture between two bones, provides synchronized movement of bones. For smooth and integrated functioning of the musculoskeletal system, several critical attributes are necessary. They are strong bone, healthy conditioned muscle, complete communication within the central nervous system between the cerebral and cerebellar components, neuromuscular intactness between neurotransmitter and receptor, and sufficient nutrition and energy reserves to meet metabolic demands.

The biophysical adaptability of the musculoskeletal system benefits the body's needs in two respects. In the short term, the fact that a bone or cartilage fractures on impact allows the affected structure to absorb the energy of impact. Thus, further injury to other body structures is minimized. In the longer term, the fact that physically active individuals tend to have greater bone and muscle mass enables the body to respond to the demands placed on it; increased demand (similar to muscles) causes hypertrophy. Cultural differences have produced variations in musculoskeletal structure (Table 6–1).

From an evolutionary stance, consider the structural and functional adaptations that have taken place over millennia. The upper and lower extremities are one such example. The upper limbs are capable of performing sophisticated, technical tasks over a wide range of movement. The lower limbs are more restricted in movement but are more robustly constructed. These characteristics allow for two features that characterize the human body: bipedal locomotion in an erect position and versatility to engage in innumerable activities requiring considerable dexterity and finite movements.

When normal musculoskeletal structure or function is disturbed, the consequences can be far reaching. The individual is affected physically, psychosocially, and financially. Alteration in the musculoskeletal system takes on greater significance if one considers that almost everyone who has reached later adulthood has been affected by some type of physical dysfunction.

The musculoskeletal system has several functions, including supporting the body; shielding of internal structures and organs; serving as a reservoir for minerals and hematopoietic functions; and coordinating voluntary muscle movement, which aids in activities related to work, play, and protection.

It logically follows that musculoskeletal dysfunction or injury results in maladaptive states. These dysfunctions include osteoporosis, consequences of immobility that affect all physiologic systems, pain, ineffective breathing patterns resulting from chest trauma (flail chest), and congenital maladies (e.g., pectus carinatum, pectus excavatum). The wide variety of musculoskeletal disorders thus becomes important from the standpoint of disruption in either the function or structure of muscles, bones, joints, ligaments, and other associated structures.

TISSUES OF THE MUSCULOSKELETAL SYSTEM

The musculoskeletal system is made up of two major types of tissue: connective tissue and muscle. The specific types of tissue that contribute to this system include dense connective tissue (tendon, ligament, fascia), cartilage (hyaline and fibrous), and osseous tissue (or bone). Voluntary muscle is the specific type of muscle tissue.

TABLE 6–1. *Biocultural Variations in the Musculoskeletal System*

	VARIATIONS

Bone

Frontal	Thicker in black males than in white males
Parietal occiput	Thicker in white males than in black males
Palate	Tori (protuberances) along the suture line of the hard palate
	Problematic for denture wearers
	Incidence (%)
	Blacks: 20
	Whites: 24
	Asians: up to 50
	Native Americans: up to 50
Mandible	Tori (protuberances) on the lingual surface of the mandible near the canine and premolar teeth
	Problematic for denture wearers
	Most common in Asians and Native Americans; incidence exceeds 50% in some Eskimo groups
Humerus	Torsion or rotation of proximal end with muscle pull
	Whites have a greater incidence than blacks
	Torsion in blacks is symmetrical; torsion in whites is greater on the right side than on the left side
Radius	Length at the wrist variable
Ulna	Ulna or radius may be longer
	Equal length (%)
	Swedes: 61
	Chinese: 16
	Ulna longer than radius (%)
	Swedes: 16
	Chinese: 48
	Radius longer than ulna (%)
	Swedes: 23
	Chinese: 10
Vertebrae	24 vertebrae (cervical, thoracic, lumbar) are found in 85%–93% of all people; racial and sex differences reveal 23 or 25 vertebrae in select groups
	Vertebrae *Population*
	23 11% of black females
	25 12% of Eskimo and Native American males
	Increased number is related to lower-back pain and lordosis
Pelvis	Hip width is 1.6 cm (0.6 inches) smaller in black women than in white women; Asian women have significantly smaller pelvises
Femur	*Curvature* *Population*
	Convex anterior Native American
	Straight Black
	Intermediate White
Second tarsal	Second toe longer than the great toe
	Incidence (%)
	Whites: 8–34
	Blacks: 8–12
	Vietnamese: 31
	Melanesians: 21–57
	Clinical significance for joggers and athletes, who reported increased foot problems
Height	White males are 1.27 cm (0.5 inches) taller than black males and 7.6 cm (2.9 inches) taller than Asian males
	White females have the same height as black females
	Asian females are 4.14 cm (1.6 inches) shorter than white or black females
Composition of long bones	Longer, narrower, and denser in blacks than in whites; bone density in whites is greater than in Chinese, Japanese, and Eskimos
	Osteoporosis incidence is lowest in black males; highest in white females

Table continued on following page

TABLE 6–1. *Biocultural Variations in the Musculoskeletal System* Continued

VARIATIONS

Muscle

Peroneus tertius   Responsible for dorsiflexion of foot
     Muscle absent (%)
        Asians, Native Americans, and whites: 3–10
        Blacks: 10–15
        Berbers (Sahara desert): 24
     No clinical significance because the tibialis anterior also dorsiflexes the foot

Palmaris longus   Responsible for wrist flexion
     Muscle absent (%)
        Whites: 12–20
        Native Americans: 2–12
        Blacks: 5
        Asians: 3
     No clinical significance because three other muscles are also responsible for flexion

From Jarvis, C. (1996). *Physical examination and health assessment* (p. 656). Philadelphia: WB Saunders.

Connective tissues develop from embryonic mesenchymal cells and later differentiate into specialized connective tissue cell types. Connective tissues consist of living cells and *matrix,* intercellular biochemical substances that surround the cells. The matrix has both fibrous and amorphous components. The fibrous component consists of two types of fibers: collagen and elastic. The connective tissue framework is depicted in Figure 6–1. The amorphous component, or ground substance, is the material in which the fibers and cells are embedded. The ground substance in tendon and ligament has the physical properties of a thin gel. In cartilage, the ground substance is more of a firm gel, whereas in bone, it is a solid substance. Substances such as proteoglycans, chondroitin sulfate, and hyaluronic acid control the deposition of calcium and phosphate salts, which are collectively referred to as *hydroxyapatites.* Other ions conjugated to hydroxyapatite are magnesium and carbonate.

The types of cells that predominate within the musculoskeletal system are fibroblasts, chondrocytes, and osteocytes. Fibroblasts proliferate along collagen or elastic fibers. The matrix of bone and cartilage contains only their respective cell types: osteocytes and chondrocytes.

Fat cells and synovial cells are also found in the musculoskeletal tissues. These cells form the adipose tissue and synovium, respectively, both of which fall into the classification of loose connective tissue. Fat cells are found in the marrow of bone, and synovial cells are found in joints, tendon sheaths, and bursae. Within the context of musculoskeletal tissue types, the existence of these cells is considered incidental.

Depending on the type of connective tissue, the matrix produced by the cells varies in density, compressional and tensile strength, plasticity, and elasticity. At the same time, the cells remain metabolically active. These cells, by virtue of their roles in secreting intercellular materials, have an important function in tissue regeneration and remodeling.

Collagen fibers (formed from the protein collagen) are white and nonextensible, with a high tensile strength, yet they are flexible. Defects in collagen production can result in a variety of musculoskeletal disorders, such as various connective tissue diseases and osteogenesis imperfecta.

Certain cells, macrophages and neutrophils in particular, are capable of secreting collagenases and lysosomes, which are enzymes capable of breaking down collagen. Oxidizing agents, which are also produced by neutrophils and macrophages, for example, superoxide (O_2^-), hydrogen peroxide (H_2O_2), and the hydroxyl ion (OH^-), not only kill bacteria but also are known to damage cartilage and synovial tissue. They are implicated in many autoimmune and connective tissue diseases. Thus, macrophages and neutrophils clearly play a role in certain inflammatory diseases.

Elastic fibers consist of the protein elastin. As the name implies, they exhibit elastic properties. When released after stretching, they return to their original length. Elastic fibers are produced by fibroblasts in tendons and ligaments and by chondroblasts in cartilage.

The ground substance contains water, noncollagenase protein, polysaccharides, and calcium salts, varying by the type of connective tissue. Compound structures, known as *proteoglycans,* are an important constituent of connective tissues because they largely define the different physical properties of these tissues. For example, proteoglycans rich in hyaluronic acid act as a lubricant and form an important constituent of synovial fluid.

Connective Tissue

Collagenous Tissue. Five types of connective tissue dominate the musculoskeletal system. Three of the five—tendon, ligament, and fascia—are derived from dense fibrous connective tissue constructed primarily of collagen fibers. *Tendons* attach muscle to bone, and *ligaments* attach bone to bone. Both of these types of connective tissue contain fibers arranged in the same direction and in the same plane, with this consistency of direction being greater in tendons.

This largely parallel arrangement of fibers within tendon and ligament imparts greater tensile strength to these tissues. This is functionally significant because it enables them to withstand pulling forces more effectively. Such forces are exerted on these structures during activity, with joint motion largely affecting ligaments and muscle contraction largely affecting tendons.

The orientation of fibers in *fascia*, which are intermeshed, is nonparallel. As a result, this tissue can withstand limited stretching in all directions. These

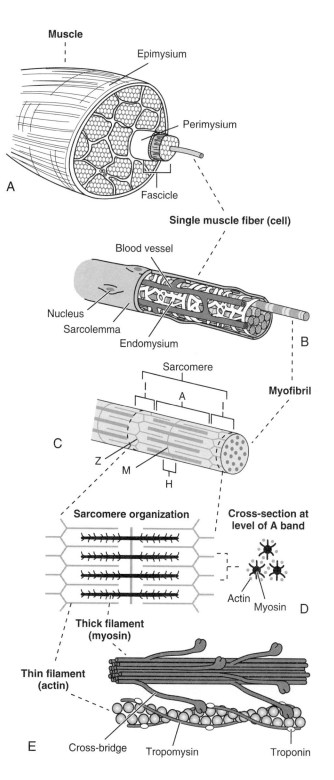

FIGURE 6–1. The structural organization of muscle consists of a connective framework and arranged muscle fibers. *A* and *B,* Connective tissue surrounds the epimysium, perimysium, and endomysium. *C,* Intricately arranged thick and thin filaments allow fibers to slide past each other in the sarcomere. *D,* Thick filaments are made up of a protein aggregate that consists of myosin, and thin filaments are made up of a protein aggregate that consists of actin, troponin, and tropomyosin. *E,* Bands and zones make up the sarcomere, enabling effective and efficient muscle contraction at the subcellular or molecular level. (Reproduced with permission from Pitman, M. I., & Peterson, L. [1989]. Biomechanics of skeletal muscle. In V. H. Frankel & M. Nordin [Eds.], *Basic biomechanics of the skeletal system* [ed. 2, p. 90]. Philadelphia: Lea & Febiger.)

factors make fascia more suitable for enveloping limbs and muscle compartments, among other structures.

The other two types of connective tissue that are of great importance to the musculoskeletal system are cartilage and bone. Both are highly specialized in their structure and represent forms of dense connective tissue.

Cartilage.   Cartilage is able to accommodate biomechanical stress and resist compressive forces to a considerable extent, but less so than bone. It is found in the body in three varieties: hyaline, fibrous (fibrocartilage), and elastic cartilage, depending on the nature of the matrix. Cartilage is relatively avascular, with a low rate of metabolism. Cartilage cells, or chondrocytes, receive nutrition by diffusion from the synovial fluid.

Hyaline Cartilage.   The most common type of cartilage, hyaline, constitutes many of the cartilages of the respiratory tract, costal cartilages, models of developing bones, growth plate cartilage, and articular cartilage. Unlike the other types of cartilage, hyaline cartilage is capable of being calcified. Avascularity is a characteristic often ascribed to cartilage when, in fact, it is a characteristic limited to articular cartilage (that lining the ends of bones in movable joints).

Fibrocartilage.   Fibrocartilage is found in certain ligaments, in intervertebral discs, and in articular discs. (Note that articular discs, as exemplified by the menisci of the knee, are found within joints, although they do not line articulating ends of bones. Thus, they do not technically fall into the classification of articular cartilage.) The proportion of this type of cartilage increases with age, and the transformation of hyaline cartilage into fibrocartilage may be one of the early signs of aging. Because aging is associated with diminished bone growth, it logically follows that the proportion of calcifiable cartilage moves in the direction of calcifiable (hyaline) to noncalcifiable (fibrous) cartilage.

Elastic Cartilage.   Also called yellow cartilage, elastic cartilage is characterized by the presence of elastic fibers. These fibers confer resiliency on the tissue and are found in such structures as the external ear and epiglottis.

For a more complete discussion of cartilage refer to the section, "Supporting Structures," later in this chapter.

Bone

Osseous connective tissue, or bone, has as its cellular component the osteocyte. Its complementary matrix consists predominantly of collagen (fibrous component) and calcium phosphate (amorphous component). Bone matrix is like hyaline cartilage in that it can be permeated with calcium salts. Unlike cartilage, however, bone is highly porous and highly vascular.

Two or more bones may come into close contact with each other at articulations known as *joints*. The joint, as a functional unit, serves to secure the bone ends together so that movement is possible.

Skeletal Muscle

Skeletal muscle tissue accounts for about half of the body weight in humans. A unique feature of muscle is its ability to contract, thus giving rise to its prime functions of producing or preventing movement of the body and its parts. Skeletal muscles have often been referred to as *voluntary* muscles because other types of muscle—cardiac and smooth—are not directly subject to voluntary control.

Structure.   All muscles and their subunits at each level are enveloped by connective tissue. The *epimysium,* a continuous layer of deep fascia, encloses the muscle as a whole and consequently defines it anatomically. It also facilitates muscles sliding on surrounding structures. Projections of this connective tissue extend into the substance of the muscle and subdivide it into fiber bundles, or *fasciculi.* The fasciculi are ensheathed by *perimysium.* The innermost sheath, the *endomysium,* surrounds the individual fibers that are the cellular units of skeletal muscle.

Blood Supply.   The blood supply to skeletal muscle is rich to meet the high metabolic demands of contractile tissue. Arteries and veins penetrate the epimysium, branch out in the perimysium, and are ultimately embedded in the endomysium, where they surround individual muscle fibers. Blood vessels enter the muscle usually at one or two well-defined points. The viability of muscles with two parent arteries is less threatened by injury than that of muscles with only one parent artery.

Nerve Supply.   Generally, one or two nerves supply each muscle, and each nerve contains both afferent and efferent fibers. On entering the epimysium, they gradually branch into nerve fibers, coursing through the endomysium. A motor neuron and all the muscle fibers supplied by it constitute the *motor unit,* the unit of contraction in skeletal muscle. Although afferent impulses may be received by a variety of sources, the *muscle spindle* is the distinctive receptor. By sensing the length of muscle fibers, it conveys a sense of position and contributes to coordination.

Microscopic Structure.   Cells highly specialized for contraction that constitute muscles are known as *muscle fibers.* They are long and cylindrical and contain many mitochondria as evidence of their high metabolic activity.

Myofibrils (*subcellular* units, which are not to be confused with muscle fibers, or the cells themselves) are the many fine fibrils of contractile protein that are embedded in the *sarcoplasm* (the cytoplasm of the muscle cell). They run the entire length of the muscle cell and consist of two types of subunits, thick filaments and thin filaments, that consist chiefly of myosin and actin, respectively. In addition, tropomyosin and troponin are proteins that assist in the control of muscle contraction through a series of complex biophysical events. Essentially, they prevent the interaction of myosin with actin, thus inhibiting a state of constant, uninterrupted contraction.

Muscle Contraction. Muscle contraction is accomplished when myosin thick filaments and actin thin filaments slide past each other. The appositional myosin and actin filaments define a *sarcomere*. During muscle contraction, the sarcoplasmic reticulum releases large amounts of calcium into the vicinity of the myofibrils. This sudden rise in calcium concentration within the sarcoplasm initiates muscle contraction by removing the tropomyosin-troponin block. Thus, the myosin and actin filaments are able to slide past each other, and myofibrillar contraction occurs, as evidenced by shortening of the sarcomere.

Metabolic Factors. Adenosine triphosphate (ATP) provides the direct energy source for muscle contraction. However, it is rapidly used up through conversion to adenosine diphosphate (ADP) and must be replenished. Reconversion of ADP to ATP is accomplished via three enzyme systems: (1) glycolysis, (2) mitochondrial oxidative phosphorylation, and (3) the phosphocreatine reservoir.

Glycolysis often serves as the source of ATP when oxygen delivery to muscle cells is inadequate to meet their metabolic demands. During this process, glucose or glycogen is broken down to pyruvic acid. If the lack of oxygen is severe, the pyruvic acid is further converted to lactic acid, which essentially makes more oxygen available. Lactic acid continues to accumulate and pass through other fluid compartments of the body. This process is important to the clinician in that it assists in understanding such phenomena as fatigue and shin splints.

Oxidative phosphorylation, also known as the *citric acid cycle,* produces great amounts of ATP relative to the amounts of substrate used for fuel. This process requires a continuously available supply of oxygen. Thus, the utility of this process may be limited during strenuous exercise.

Phosphocreatine acts as a rapid buffer for the resynthesis of ATP. However, in resynthesizing ATP, phosphocreatine is converted, in turn, to creatine. This means that creatine must now be recharged to phosphocreatine with ATP derived from either of the remaining two enzyme systems.

Ionic Factors. Muscle contraction arises from a change in the electrochemical gradient along the muscle cell membrane. This electrochemical gradient is largely defined by the predominantly intracellular potassium ion (K^+) and the predominantly extracellular sodium ion (Na^+) and is mediated by the release of acetylcholine. This neurotransmitter is released from the motor neuron's axon terminal and attaches to receptors in the subneural plate. Acetylcholine release requires the presence of calcium ions (Ca^{2+}). As a result, cell membrane excitability is influenced by calcium levels. When serum calcium is low, cell membranes are hyperexcitable, and tetany may occur.

Mechanical Properties. As the effectors for movement in the body, muscles possess special mechanical properties. For example, the force a muscle can generate depends on its length when a contraction is initiated. Generally, the longer the muscle, the less force it can generate. Obviously, tension is placed on muscle fibers during contraction. Muscle tone, or tonus, is present in resting and relaxed muscle. This tonus may be palpated when a relaxed muscle group is passively moved.

The speed at which a muscle contracts is also affected by the load applied to it. This principle is exemplified by an individual's ability to lift a weight faster if it is lighter, whereas a heavier weight takes longer to lift.

Muscle contraction can be classified on the basis of the mechanics involved. Two types are well recognized: isotonic and isometric. During an *isotonic* contraction, the length of the muscle changes while the force remains constant. During an *isometric* contraction, the force exerted by the muscle may change while its length remains constant. In reality, most contractions are both isotonic and isometric. When a load is moved, the contraction is first isometric until sufficient force has been developed to move the load. When movement occurs, the contraction then becomes isotonic, eventually returning to an isometric state. For a more detailed discussion of muscle function, see Chapter 13.

Other types of less-well-known contraction are the *auxotonic* and *isokinetic*. In an auxotonic contraction, force continually increases and motion continually occurs; the stretching of a rubber band is an example of this. The isokinetic contraction occurs when the load is continuously readjusted during movement to coincide with the length of the muscle to keep the amount of tension on the muscle fibers constant.

Muscles can be divided into two groups based on the mechanical activity they exhibit. These categories are referred to as *slow twitch* (type I) and *fast twitch* (type II). Slow-twitch muscle fibers contract and relax more slowly. These fibers support high levels of oxidative metabolism rather than produce energy by glycolytic processes. Large amounts of myoglobin potentiate the action of stored oxygen to provide continual energy. The slow fibers are modified for prolonged or continuous muscle activity (e.g., endurance marathon running) and support of the body against gravity (posture). Their higher content of myoglobin and cytochrome gives them a red color. By contrast, fast-twitch fibers rely on the release of energy that is supplied by the glycolytic process. Type II fibers are used for rapid muscle contraction, such as jumping, short-distance sprinting, or the blinking of the eye. These fibers are white because of the lack of myoglobin. Fast-twitch fibers tend to fatigue more easily than slow-twitch fibers.

Muscles increase in both bulk and strength developmentally as well as from placing physical demands on them. This phenomenon, known as *hypertrophy,* results from an increase in the number of myofibrils within each muscle fiber rather than an increase in the number of muscle cells. Enlargement of a muscle represents the aggregate effect of an increase in size of the many muscle fibers within it. After birth, the number of muscle cells does not increase, but growth hormone during childhood and testosterone during puberty foster muscular development. Anabolic steroids, which are similar to testosterone, have been misused by some athletes and body builders to produce hypertrophic muscular changes.

CONTROL OF MUSCLE ACTION

Various factors assist in the control of muscle action. These can be viewed from the standpoint of sensory mechanisms, reflexes, and nervous control.

Sensory feedback of muscle action is largely derived from *muscle spindles* and *Golgi tendon organs.* The muscle spindles are complex structures that can sense changes in the length of muscle fibers. Efferent feedback to these structures modulates their sensitivity to muscle length, after which they are capable of providing afferent feedback to the central nervous system. The Golgi tendon organs are capable of sensing tension at the myotendonal junction.

A few reflexes help control muscle action. One is the *stretch reflex,* also known as the *myotatic reflex.* When a load is applied to a muscle, it responds by sustaining contraction or, in a sense, resisting that motion. Postural muscles, for example, accommodate changes in position without conscious effort. Muscle tone itself is a consequence of the stretch reflex. The stretch reflex is mediated by the muscle spindle and the motor neurons that serve the particular muscle.

The *inverse myotatic reflex* exists to protect against tissue damage. The more a muscle is loaded, the greater is the tension on musculotendinous structures and the more forceful the contraction. However, once tension in the musculotendinous structures increases, the Golgi tendon organs become stimulated and they inhibit muscle contraction via neurologic reflex arcs. Thus, tension on the musculotendinous structures does not become so great as to damage them.

When an individual is exposed to noxious or harmful stimuli, the person reflexly pulls away. This defensive maneuver is known as the *nociceptive* or *pain reflex.*

Certain motor centers of the brain influence muscle action via various spinal reflexes. The *motor cortex* orches-

trates muscle activity during voluntary movement. The *brainstem* assists in postural reflexes. The *basal ganglia* modulate the activity of the motor cortex and may fine-tune many voluntary movements. The *cerebellum* is involved in motor coordination, especially smaller, more precise movements.

THE SKELETAL SYSTEM: BONE

Bone is dynamic tissue, with cell and matrix proliferation. Many processes occur in bone. Bone physiology is well documented in the literature. The phenomenon described by Wolff 100 years ago—that bone forms and remodels itself in response to the forces applied to it—has stimulated further exploration of bone physiology up to the present. This phenomenon is well recognized today as Wolff's law, which postulates that osteogenesis or bone formation is stimulated by the direction of loading (forces). Bone is deposited at sites subjected to stress and reabsorbed from areas where forces are absent (e.g., nongravitational osteoporosis sustained by astronauts during space flight).

It logically follows from Wolff's law that bone strength is greatest where maximal stress is applied from any area within a bony structure. Bone shape and histology reflect its function. Bones can be categorized as *flat* (innominate), *cuboidal* (vertebrae), or *long* (tibia) on the basis of shape (Fig. 6–2).

Classification of Bone

Bone can be classified in two other ways. On the basis of histologic orientation, bone is referred to as either *cancellous* (spongy) or *cortical* (compact). On the basis of embryonic development, bone can be classified as *intramembranous* or *endochondral.* Intramembranous bone is formed from a membrane template, such as the fontanels of an infant's skull. Endochondral bone is formed from a cartilage model, the method by which most of the bones of the human body are formed.

Structure

The human skeleton contains 206 bones. Figure 6–3 shows the anterior and posterior aspects of the skeleton. The typical long bone consists of epiphyses, physis, metaphyses, and diaphysis (Fig. 6–4). The epiphyses are the widened ends of the bone, composed largely of cancellous bone. The physis, or epiphyseal plate, is composed of hyaline cartilage and is where longitudinal growth takes place. The metaphyses, corresponding to the advancing fronts of ossification in the growing child, merge with the epiphyses after puberty following obliteration of the growth plate. Like the epiphyses, they are composed of cancellous bone. The middle half of a long bone represents the diaphysis, or shaft, and is composed of cortical bone. Subchondral bone provides the bone surface at its ends, and it is covered with articular cartilage.

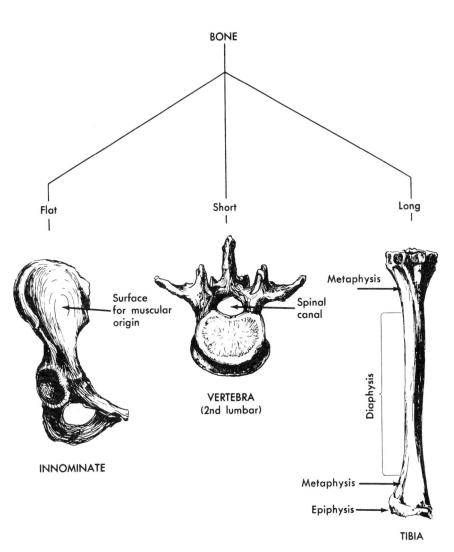

FIGURE 6–2. Bone types. (From Schneider, E. R. [1976]. *Handbook for the orthopaedic assistant* [2nd ed., p. 10]. St. Louis: Mosby.)

Epiphyses are widened to allow for greater weight distribution; that is, weight is distributed over a greater surface than if it were oriented around a single point. This weight distribution helps minimize friction and biomechanical wear. The thick, rigid, tubular structure permits the diaphysis to more easily withstand the bending, torsional, and compressive forces to which it is subjected.

Microscopically, bone exhibits the existence of haversian systems, which are also known as *osteons*. Haversian canals are those parts of the osteon represented by the long channels running parallel to the long axis of the bone (see Fig. 6–4). From the haversian canals, *canaliculi* are extended that serve to communicate with the *lacunae*, the little "lakes" in which the mature bone cells are embedded. The haversian canals are surrounded by a series of concentric rings known as *lamellae* that characterize mature bone. The term *lamellar bone* is sometimes used to refer to mature bone. By contrast, young bone is often called *immature, woven,* or *fibrous*.

The osteones serve as the vehicle for interstitial communication among bone cells. Fluid flow occurs within osteones rather than among them, except via the nutrient arteries in bone. Canaliculi are too small to permit the passage of red blood cells and therefore must rely on diffusion for oxygen delivery to the cells.

Periosteum is a dense connective tissue membrane covering the outer surface of bone except for joint surfaces that are encased in articular cartilage. Microcirculation penetrates through the periosteum to the bone surface, assisting with bone nutrition and healing postinjury. An extensive network of nociceptive fibers is embedded in the periosteum. Localized hemorrhage from damaged blood vessels and nerve irritation are two factors producing pain by bone fracture.

Bone Cellular Structure

Bone cells are generally of three types. *Osteocytes* are the mature bone cells found within the lacunae. *Osteoblasts* are formed in the periosteum and are essential for new bone formation. *Osteoclasts* are those cells capable of resorbing bone (either healthy or dead) and occasionally foreign materials within bone.

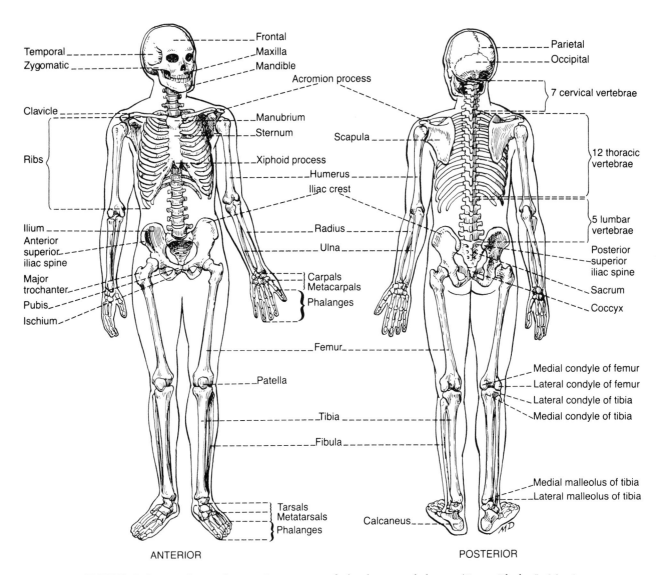

FIGURE 6–3. Anterior and posterior aspects of the human skeleton. (From Black, J. M., & Matassarin-Jacobs, E. [1993]. *Luckman and Sorensen's medical surgical nursing* [4th ed., p. 1866]. Philadelphia: WB Saunders.)

Cancellous bone differs from cortical bone in that it does not contain osteons. Furthermore, it represents a tremendously large surface area (thus enhancing its diffusion characteristics), which better enables it to respond to the metabolic demands of other body systems (e.g., fluid and ionic exchanges, discussed later). Both metabolic and remodeling processes occur at higher rates in cancellous bone. Despite these differences, cancellous and cortical bone are fundamentally similar in terms of their chemical composition and ultrastructure.

Bone Matrix

Bone matrix consists of organic and inorganic components. The organic matrix constitutes about 35% of the total weight of bone, which consists of collagen (the largest constituent), protein polysaccharide, and lipid (including phospholipid). The inorganic matrix, representing 65% of bone's total weight, consists largely of calcium and phosphate. In the adult, this mineral component exists as a crystalline structure, hydroxyapatite. Magnesium, sodium, and potassium are also found in lesser amounts in bone, and zinc, fluoride, and molybdenum can be identified as trace elements.

Mineralization

Bone formation occurs in two phases: matrix formation, which is the biosynthesis of collagen for the most part, and mineralization. The osteoblast is capable of collagen synthesis, and it also exerts control over the mineralization process. Initially, following protein synthesis in the osteoblast, protocollagen is produced from the protein and then converted into procollagen. Osteoblasts secrete the procollagen, after which it polymerizes and matures into collagen. At this point, calcium phosphate precipitates out of solution from the body fluids and becomes packed in and around the collagen fibers in crystalline form. This mineralization process is initiated by genetic encoding.

Bone resorption is the opposite of bone formation. During resorption, bone matrix, essentially collagen, is hydrolyzed, and crystalline bone mineral is dissolved. This process requires that osteoclasts secrete enzymes and acids capable of breaking down and decalcifying the collagen matrix. Once the breakdown is initiated, smaller, particulate bone matter can be taken into the cell (ingested), where lysozymes can further act on it. In essence, the subcellular structures known as *lysosomes*, which secrete the lysozymes, assist in the overall process of bone resorption. They are more adept at further hydrolyzing the smaller products of the breakdown process.

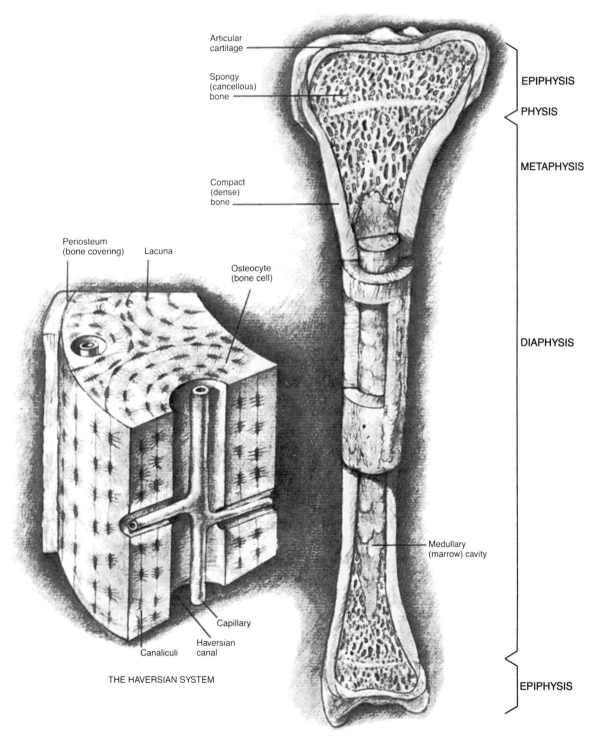

FIGURE 6–4. Long bone and the haversian system. (From Ignatavicius, D. D., & Bayne, M. V. [1991]. *Medical-surgical nursing: A nursing process approach* [p. 719]. Philadelphia: WB Saunders).

The well-developed endoplasmic reticulum of osteoblasts renders them well suited to the synthesis of protein and the production of cartilage. By contrast, osteoclasts are well endowed with lysosomes, suggesting their abilities for catalytic and hydrolytic breakdown. Both types of cells share a rich complement of mitochondria, indicative of high levels of metabolic activity in both cell types.

Osteocytes demonstrate a limited ability to synthesize collagen and resorb bone, although certainly not to the magnitude that osteoblasts and osteoclasts can perform these respective functions. The osteocyte also exerts some influence over bone mineralization. Contrary to earlier notions of osteocyte function, this cell is not inert or dormant (Gamble, 1988). The management of various metabolic bone diseases and disuse conditions may become more exact as more is learned about the osteocyte.

PHYSIOLOGIC PROCESSES IN THE SKELETAL SYSTEM

Five physiologic processes that occur within the skeletal system have been identified. Each of these basic processes serves a defined purpose for bone.

Growth

Growth is a process that results in an increase in a tissue's volume. The process is modulated by the endocrine system and influenced by genetic (phenotype) and environmental (climate, nutrition) factors. Growth is the process that allows the individual to achieve adult body size.

Being a tubular structure, bone achieves circumferential growth by bone formation (osteoblastic activity) on the outer surface, whereas bone resorption (osteoclastic activity) occurs on the inner surface. During the process, bone cortex becomes thicker and stronger. Longitudinal growth is achieved through the epiphyseal growth plate, whereby new bone tissue is laid down on existing bone tissue. Longitudinal growth usually continues in girls until age 15 and boys until age 16. However, bone maturation and shaping continue until age 21 in both sexes.

Bone formation begins during the second month of fetal life. Long bones in the fetus begin growing when diaphyseal perichondrium (the outer covering of cartilage cells) converts to an osteoblastic layer of tissue (now periosteum). This periosteum gradually becomes vascularized, and bone tissue is laid down along this outer layer, creating a primary ossification center. Hence, this bone nucleus represented by the ossification center gradually expands. For the most part, this same process occurs near either end of the developing cartilaginous bone. At birth, what remains is a shaft of bone covered at both ends by a large mass of cartilage cells, which will differentiate into cartilage, epiphysis, and epiphyseal growth plate.

Modeling

Modeling refers to the architectural patterning or organizing of tissue that occurs simultaneous with growth, thus influencing the shape of a bone. This process is influenced by the type and nature of forces applied to the bone because "form follows function." A slight deformation in bone initiates electric events (which are too low in intensity for the body to sense) that mediate osteoblastic activity. The bone produced is structured to resist forces causing the original deformation. Modeling occurs beginning in embryonic life and lasting through adult life and serves a biomechanical purpose. Bone may model in response to abnormal environmental forces (e.g., osteogenesis imperfecta, Paget's disease, vitamin-deficiency rickets). The inherent factors here are genetic and nutritional. Because modeling occurs in cartilage and fibrous tissue as well, these same phenomena explain such abnormal conditions as clubfoot, genu varum and genu valgum, achondroplasia, and scoliosis in the case of cartilage, and osteogenesis imperfecta and structural changes in the hand of a person with an inflammatory arthritic disease in the case of fibrous tissue.

Remodeling

Remodeling refers to the turnover of bone in microscopic packets mediated via special functional units (also microscopic) so that, qualitatively and quantitatively, bone remains unchanged. That is, the composition and total mass of the involved bone are unaffected along microscopically circumscribed areas of simultaneous resorption and formation. Thus, these two processes obviously must occur in balance with each other. Remodeling likely represents the mode of repair for microscopic bone damage, such as microfracture. In a sense, the follow-up or fine-tuning of the modeling process is accomplished through remodeling so that the physiologic and mechanical integrity of bone can be maintained. Disorders of bone remodeling underlie the pathophysiology of adult-acquired (involutional-type II) osteoporosis and osteomalacia.

Repair

Repair is the process that heals gross physical injury to restore function. Repair represents the macroscopic version of remodeling, a microscopic activity. As is true in other tissues, repair in bone also serves to isolate or confine local threats to tissue integrity, such as infection, foreign bodies, and various tumors.

Blood-Bone Exchange

Blood-bone exchange is the movement of certain ions, largely electrolyte and acid-base substances, between blood and the bone tissue via the interstitial fluids.

Hypercalcemia or hypocalcemia can be modulated by bone tissue. Levels of other ions (e.g., phosphate, sodium) in the blood may be subject to the influence of bone as well, but to a lesser extent. Bone may also possess limited activity as a buffer for the body fluids by providing a source of, or reservoir for, hydrogen ions (H^+) when acid-base fluctuations occur. The osteocyte probably plays the major role among the various cells in the freeing or depositing of ionic substances.

Besides these physiologic processes, another special and unique aspect of the biochemical nature of bone can be used for intraosseous fluid resuscitation. Bone marrow contains a dense meshwork of sinusoids that drain into large central medullary venous channels. These channels exit the bone through emissary and nutrient veins. Because of this rich network of vascular supply, a technique called *intraosseous infusion* may be used to infuse drugs and solutions as rapidly as those delivered through intravenous access. This technique may be implemented in emergent situations where venous access cannot be readily obtained. Resuscitating fluids, as well as antibiotics and drugs, may be administered via the intraosseous route. This method is used in pediatric and adult patients, but it may be used only for short-term periods.

BONE METABOLISM

The knowledge base necessary to practice contemporary orthopaedic nursing comprehensively is incomplete without some discussion of bone metabolism. This is particularly relevant at a time when new developments are taking place in the treatment and management of patients with metabolic bone disease. (For detailed discussion of metabolic bone disease, see Chapter 15.) Patient care outcomes are enhanced when the nurse has an understanding of basic bone metabolism and can use this knowledge when providing patient care.

Bone metabolism is modulated by a variety of systemic hormones. The complex process of bone replication directly affects the quality of bone matrix. Bone metabolism is regulated by hormones, polypeptides, steroids, and thyroid hormone. Local biochemical agents, such as growth hormone and prostaglandins, also affect bone remodeling (Table 6–2).

1,25-Dihydroxyvitamin D (Vitamin D)

Strictly speaking, vitamin D does not fit the description of a vitamin at all. Instead, it is more appropriately defined as a steroid hormone. The metabolic pathway for the production of vitamin D is summarized here.

The precursor to vitamin D is often called *cholecalciferol* (occasionally designated vitamin D_3). Cholecalciferol is available from two sources: the diet and the skin. Dietary sources include dairy products, liver, and fish. In skin exposed to sunlight, ultraviolet light (a component of sunlight) converts a derivative of cholesterol into cholecalciferol (a process known as *ultraviolet photolysis*).

Cholecalciferol then undergoes two conversions, one in the liver and one in the kidney, resulting in the biologically active form of vitamin D, known as *calcitriol*. To say that vitamin D is now in its biologically active form means that it can now act as a hormone on its target organs—specifically, the intestine and skeleton.

Calcitriol exerts its main effect on the intestinal tract, where it promotes calcium absorption. It also exerts two effects on bone. The first and probably most familiar is to facilitate mineralization of osteoid. When this process fails, rickets and osteomalacia result. The second is to work with parathyroid hormone (PTH) in the efficient mobilization of calcium from bone. Calcitriol is necessary for proper PTH function.

Vitamin D is a potent stimulator of osteoclastic bone resorption. Its effect on calcium is seen in those tissues that metabolize calcium (bone, kidney, and intestine).

TABLE 6–2. *Biochemical and Physiologic Factors Affecting Bone and Muscle in the Aging Musculoskeletal System*

STIMULATION (FORMATION)	RETARDATION (RESORPTION)	DUAL REGULATION (FORMATION AND RESORPTION)
Anabolic steroids	Anemia	Hormones
Bone marrow cells	Anticoagulants	Peptide
Calcitonin	Diabetes mellitus	Calcitonin
Chondroitin sulfate	Delayed stabilization after fracture	CGRP (calcitonin gene–related peptide)
Cytokines and growth factors	Denervation (secondary to muscle	Parathyroid hormone
Demineralized bone matrix	atrophy and loss of type II fast-	Steroid
Electromagnetic fields	twitch fibers)	Vitamins A and D
Exercise (load bearing)	Glucocorticoids	Estrogen
Growth factor/hormone	Hypoxemia	Testosterone
Hyaluronidase	Loss of estrogen/testosterone	Thyroid
Hyperbaric oxygenation	Prostaglandins/leukotrienes	Glucocorticoid (protein synthesis)
Insulin		
Thyroid hormone		
Vitamins A and D		

Parathyroid Hormone

PTH serves to increase serum calcium levels of the blood and is released by the parathyroid gland in response to hypocalcemia. PTH acts on its target organs to increase bone resorption, freeing stored calcium, and to increase distal tubular reabsorption of calcium in the kidney. This hormone also plays a role in the vitamin D metabolic pathway and, in this way, indirectly effects an increase in serum calcium. PTH has effects on the stimulation and inhibition of collagen-matrix synthesis.

Calcitonin

Calcitonin, a polypeptide hormone, is released by the perifollicular cells of the thyroid gland in response to high plasma levels of calcium. It is a potent inhibitor of bone resorption, but only for transient periods. Calcitonin may have a pharmacologic influence rather than a physiologic effect on bone metabolism.

Adrenocortical Steroids

The adrenocortical steroids act opposite to vitamin D. These substances decrease both the intestinal and the renal absorption of calcium. In addition, corticosteroids accelerate bone resorption. Glucocorticoids affect the metabolism of osteoblasts and effect the synthesis of insulin-like growth factor (IGF), thereby playing a part in the pathogenesis of steroid-induced osteoporosis. Individuals who have taken exogenous steroids over a long time develop osteoporotic bone and have an increased incidence of developing avascular necrosis.

Estrogens and Androgens

Sex hormones bring about bone loss by their effects on cytokines and by their influence on the production and regulation of vitamin D. They are also important for skeletal growth in child and adolescent development. Estrogen-depleted postmenopausal women who are not receiving estrogen replacement therapy may develop osteoporosis.

Thyroxine

Thyroxine influences bone calcium turnover and possibly the metabolism of vitamin D. Hyperthyroidism is associated with hypercalcemia, although bone metabolism becomes altered in either hyperthyroidism or hypothyroidism. Hyperthyroid patients as well as postmenopausal women receiving thyroid suppression may develop osteopenia.

Insulin-like Growth Factor (IGF)

The increased metabolic demand for calcium during developmental growth is mediated in part by vitamin D. Polypeptide growth factors, also known as IGF, are synthesized in various tissues, including osseous tissues. IGF affects tissue growth and enhances collagen synthesis. Matrix and osteoblast regeneration is also stimulated by IGF.

Insulin

Insulin has no direct effect on bone resorption, but it has a significant effect on the synthesis of bone matrix and on the formation of cartilage. Insulin is necessary for the process of bone mineralization. Individuals with diabetes mellitus have decreased bone mineralization and skeletal growth deficits.

BONE BIOMECHANICS

It is important to understand the biomechanics of bone when providing treatment and care to clients with musculoskeletal problems. Understanding the specifics of bone biomechanics related to static and dynamic forces (which are applied to musculoskeletal tissue during the time of injury or trauma) is necessary to nursing practice because if these forces are understood, client care can be more effectively planned and clinical consequences predicted. Preventive education and secondary education postinjury encompass theory-related bone biomechanics.

Material Properties

Some of the material, or physical, properties of bone that differentiate it from other physiologic tissues are discussed. The strength of bone depends on bone mineral density and the quality and quantity of collagen. In distinguishing these properties, the following terms are considered: nonhomogeneous, anisotropic, viscoelastic, brittle, and weak in tension.

Nonhomogeneous. Bones are nonhomogeneous in that they vary in composition, nature, and structure. To understand the properties of various bones within the body, the physiologic type (e.g., compact, cancellous, flat, long) and anatomic position of the particular bone must be known.

Anisotropic. Tensile, or pulling, forces can be applied to bone in different directions. Bone responds differently depending on the direction of pull. For example, a bone actually changes its shape slightly when a pulling force is applied at a right angle to its long axis. This type of force is referred to as *shear stress*. If this stress is strong enough, the movement of two perpendicular points may create an angular deformity. However, if the same pulling force is applied parallel to its long axis, the bone shape changes minimally. In other words, a long bone may bend slightly, but it cannot be stretched. Therefore, bone has anisotropic qualities.

Viscoelastic. The behavior of bone varies according to how rapidly forces (loads) are applied to it and how much strain (change in linear dimension) results from the application of the load. Such materials are known as *viscoelastic*. For example, a runner is more vulnerable to microfracture (fatigue or stress fracture) of the tibia the faster he or she runs over time.

Brittle. Cortical bone is capable of slight bending before breaking. However, it breaks before other musculoskeletal materials when deformed. Thus, it is more brittle than other structures in the body.

Weak in Tension. Bone is weaker under tension than compression. Consider when a long bone fractures from a force applied at a right angle to its long axis within the confines of its diaphysis. The bone tends to resist compressive force on the side where the force is applied, but it fails under tensile forces on the opposite side.

Structural Properties

The structural properties of bone address how size, shape, and configuration affect its strength. Terms used in discussing these properties include moment of inertia, stress concentration, and open and closed sections.

Moment of Inertia. The relationship between shape and resistance to bending is referred to as the *moment of inertia.* The structure of a bone dictates its strength along its different segments and under varying conditions. For example, the tubular structure of a diaphyseal long bone imparts greater resistance to both bending forces from all directions and torsional forces than if its same mass were in the shape of either a solid rod or a beam. Wolff's law becomes apparent here. Essentially all bones model to assume the shape that best resists external forces, and they remodel to rearrange their tissue structure to one that best accommodates the distribution of stresses within that structure. Any sudden change in shape alters the distribution of stresses within the structure.

Stress Concentration. When external force is applied to a solid object, any bending that occurs causes a redistribution of stress along its internal structure. Mechanically, stress lines, or a stress riser, are created within the object. An interruption in structural continuity may cause areas of stress concentration (exaggerated stress lines) within the object, resulting in an overall weakening. Examples of this weakness can be seen clinically in factors that interrupt bone continuity and the potential sequelae of factors such as the following:

1. Tumor: pathologic fracture
2. Callus: refracture near callus
3. Metallic implants: create a stress riser-potentiating fracture at the lower end of the implant
4. Holes from screws/pins/wires: transcending fracture

Open and Closed Sections. The concept of open and closed sections shares both mechanical and clinical significance. Consider a solid, hollow cylindrical object and the analogous structure of diaphyseal bone. In either case, symmetry and intact walls (characteristics of the cortical bone) allow for the dissipation of energy derived from external sources evenly over its surface. These characteristics represent a closed section. However, if a section is removed from its wall, the forces can no longer be dissipated evenly over the surface. The bone becomes weaker, representing an open section.

Behavior of Bone under Various Loading Modes

Bone is routinely subjected to a variety of forces, called *loading modes,* that produce expected responses. These loading modes are tension, compression, bending, torsion, and shear forces, or a combination thereof. Long bone, especially its diaphyseal structure, can be used as a model for discussion.

When under *tension* (pulling apart), bone failure occurs by debonding along microarchitectural lines that represent areas where one bone shape blends into another. Under *compression,* cracks develop that run obliquely to the haversian systems, ultimately leading to bone failure. With *shear forces,* loads are applied at right angles to the long axis but on opposite sides of the structure. Shear fractures are usually seen in cancellous bone because of the biomechanical behavior of this type of bone (it cannot represent a closed section) and because of its relative locations throughout the skeletal system (e.g., trochanteric area of the hip). During *bending,* tensile and compressive forces act on opposite sides of the bone's neutral axis. They may not be equal because of the bone's asymmetry. Failure begins on the tensile side. Cortical bone is weaker in tension than compression. Therefore, fracture may be incomplete, giving rise to a greenstick fracture. *Torsion* arises from shearing and tension forces (twisting) that result in a fracture that propagates around the shaft of the bone. Living bone is usually subjected to a combination of loads rather than any one type of load, and fracture patterns are defined by *combined loading phenomena.*

Fracture patterns correspond to load or force application. Consider the following fracture types and load stresses and strains:

1. Transverse fracture: bending
2. Spiral fracture: torsion
3. Butterfly fracture: compression and bending
4. Oblique fracture: compression and bending and torsion
5. Comminuted fracture: variable load(s)

The concepts of stress and strain are important to the discussion of loads. In mechanical terms, *stress* is the load per unit area that develops on a plane surface within a structure in response to externally applied loads. *Strain* is the deformation that occurs at a point in a structure under loading. Stress versus strain relationships can be used to describe the behavior of various materials, such as soft metal, glass, and bone.

At one extreme is soft metal, which when stressed exhibits elasticity, meaning that it does not permanently deform but returns to its prestress shape. It does this up to a certain point, after which if stress continues, the soft metal is permanently deformed. Such a material is called *ductile;* it undergoes a relatively large amount of deformation before failure. At the other extreme is glass. Glass deforms little before failure and is, by contrast, *brittle.* A ductile material that is pieced together after fracture does not conform to its original shape, but brittle material does. The pieces of the brittle material fit back together much better. Although not as brittle as glass, bone is a brittle material nonetheless. Its brittleness is an evolutionary adaptation. Bone segments after fracture can be made to fit back together like the pieces of a puzzle so that healing can take place. However, with age, bone becomes more brittle, and bone fracture tends to produce bone segments that are smaller and greater in number, making fracture repair more difficult.

JOINTS

Classification

Joints are commonly classified as immovable (the *synarthroses*), slightly movable (the *amphiarthroses*), or freely movable (the *diarthroses*) depending on the amount of movement they exhibit. The freely movable joints require

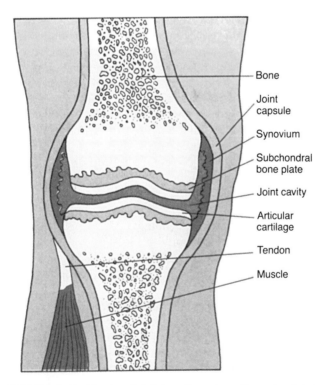

FIGURE 6–5. Diarthrodial joint. Synovium lines the joint capsule but does not extend into the articular cartilage. (From Ignatavicius, D. D., & Bayne, M. V. [1991]. *Medical-surgical nursing: A nursing process approach* [p. 720]. Philadelphia: WB Saunders.)

- Bone
- Joint capsule
- Synovium
- Subchondral bone plate
- Joint cavity
- Articular cartilage
- Tendon
- Muscle

TABLE 6–3. *Types of Synovial Joints*

JOINT TYPE	EXAMPLE
Plane (gliding)	Patellofemoral joint
Hinge	Tibiofemoral joint of the knee
Pivot	Radioulnar joint
Ellipsoid (condyloid)	Radiocarpal joint of the wrist
Saddle	Carpometacarpal joint at the base of the thumb
Ball and socket	Hip, shoulder

a lubricant to minimize friction between adjoining bones. This lubricant is provided to a large extent by synovial fluid (Fig. 6–5). Hence, joints can also be classified as synovial or nonsynovial. In *nonsynovial joints,* either fibrous or cartilaginous tissue exists between adjoining bones.

The *synovial joints* can be categorized into six types, ranging from the simpler plane joint to the complex ball-and-socket joint. These are summarized in Table 6–3 and pictured in Figure 6–6.

Factors in Stability

Stability among the various synovial joints of the body can vary, depending on three main factors: (1) the shape of the articulating surfaces, (2) the capsule and ligaments, and (3) the musculature. Clinically, factors that contribute to the stability of a joint and how they can be disrupted can become a prime concern. Total joint replacement is an excellent example of how such concerns arise because at least one of the aforementioned factors is affected in any given joint subjected to such a procedure.

The three most commonly replaced large joints—the hip, knee, and shoulder—can be compared with respect to their stability. The hip achieves its stability largely from the bony contours of its articulating surfaces (Fig. 6–7). In a sense, the ball and socket fit together rather well. However, the knee derives its stability mostly from its ligamentous structure (Fig. 6–8). That is why threats to knee stability, such as sports injuries, often involve one of the ligaments. By contrast, the shoulder achieves stability largely through its musculature (Fig. 6–9). Because muscle is characterized by greater elasticity than either ligament or bone, the shoulder exhibits a wider range of motion than any other joint, but at the expense of stability. Relative to other joints, shoulder dislocation tends to be more common.

The amount of friction generated within the freely movable joints is surprisingly small considering the magnitude of the load borne and the amount of movement occurring between opposing bones. Even in weight-bearing joints, the amount of friction is essentially negligible if those joints are healthy. Freedom of movement is fostered by a number of interrelated, complex lubricating mechanisms. However, as joints become diseased and joint function becomes disrupted, friction increases.

Of the nonsynovial joints, stability and friction involve only the slightly movable joints (amphiarthroses) and are dependent on the integrity of the cartilaginous structures that make up the joint (i.e., the intervertebral joint). The role of healthy cartilage in joint function is discussed later in this chapter, and the effect of diseased or eroded cartilage in joint function is addressed in Chapter 16.

The Freely Movable Joints (Diarthroses)

The diarthroses represent movable connections between bones across articular cavities (see Fig. 6–5). Essential to their function are the synovial membrane and synovial fluid.

The *synovial membrane* lines the inner aspect of bursa, ligaments, joint capsule, and the tendons. This membrane, together with the articular cartilages, forms the walls of the synovial cavity. It is a highly permeable vascular membrane and contains many mast cells and macrophages. The synovial membrane has excellent reparative and regenerative capabilities. Synovial tissue contains type A and type B cells. Type A cells make up 20% to 30% of synovial tissue. These cells line bursa, joints, and tendon sheaths. They have immunologic, inflammatory, and phagocytic capacities.

The *synovial fluid* (produced by type B cells) represents a dialysate, or ultrafiltrate, of the blood that contains a mucin of highly polymerized hyaluronic acid. This

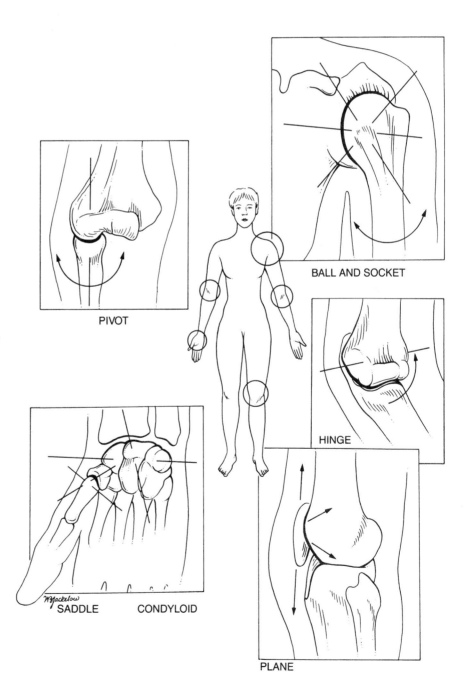

FIGURE 6–6. Types of synovial joints. (From Swartz, M. H. [1998]. *Textbook of physical diagnosis* [3rd ed., p. 449]. Philadelphia: WB Saunders.)

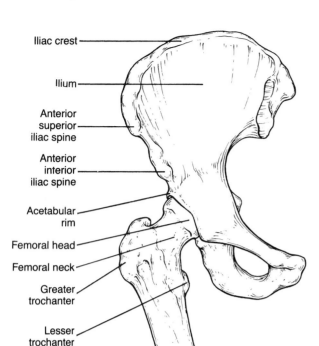

FIGURE 6–7. Hip joint.

chemical composition allows synovial fluid to achieve its major function, lubrication.

The synovial membrane and fluid represent an effective line of defense against the invasion of microbes and foreign bodies. Thus, it is also very immunogenically active. Even blood is recognized as a foreign body when introduced into the joint cavity. Within the joint space, blood does not clot well and is rapidly removed, often after being broken down by proteolytic enzymes released by the synovium. The initiation of fracture healing—clot formation—may be retarded by this mechanism. This is one reason why malunion develops after intra-articular fracture.

Specific joints are considered here for their clinically significant anatomic and biomechanical aspects. Joints discussed include the lower extremity joints—hip, knee, and ankle—and upper extremity joints—shoulder and elbow.

Hip. The hip is a ball-and-socket joint, of which the acetabulum faces obliquely forward, outward, and downward; its articulating surface is provided by the head of the femur (see Fig. 6-7). Activities of daily living require that the individual be able to flex hips to 120 degrees, abduct hips to 20 degrees, and externally rotate them to 20 degrees. Forces across the hip joint may be three to six times body weight during ambulation. During standing,

it is about 2.5 to 3 times body weight. When walking, an individual weighing 150 pounds exerts 900 pounds across either hip joint with each step. While standing, the joint force may be 450 pounds.

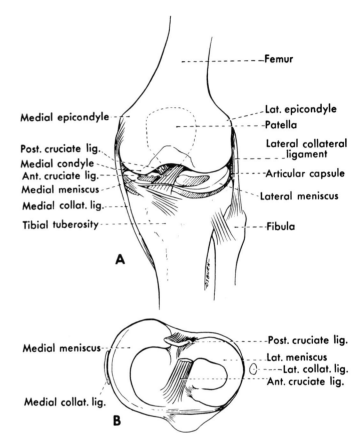

FIGURE 6–8. Knee joint with ligaments. (From Gartland, J. J. [1987]. *Fundamentals of orthopaedics* [4th ed., p. 365]. Philadelphia: WB Saunders.)

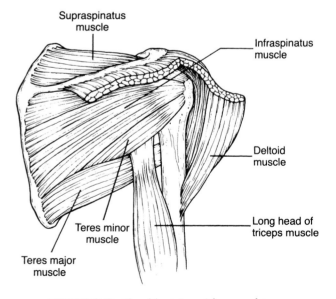

FIGURE 6–9. Shoulder joint with musculature.

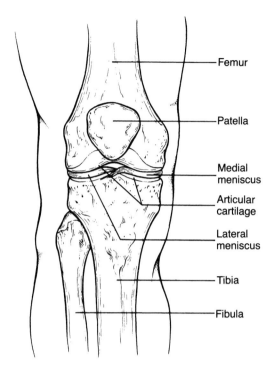

FIGURE 6–10. Knee joint.

The use of a cane decreases the joint force on the contralateral hip by reducing the amount of contraction of the abductor muscles needed to support body weight. This is why a cane is used on the opposite side from a painful hip. Compressive, torsional, shear, and bending loads are normally applied to the hip joint and help to explain common hip fractures, such as subcapital, intertrochanteric, and subtrochanteric.

Knee. The knee is actually a structure composed of two joints: the tibiofemoral and the patellofemoral (Fig. 6-10). Both joints are subjected to very high forces during normal activity. When an individual stands with knees slightly flexed, force across the tibiofemoral joint may exceed four times body weight, whereas force across the patellofemoral joint may exceed three times body weight. During weight bearing, most of the load is borne by the tibial plateau; but the cartilage, menisci, and ligaments also share some of the load. The function of the menisci (specialized articular cartilages of the knee) is to distribute the loading forces imposed on the tibial plateaus. The patellae serve to lengthen the lever arm of the quadriceps for better distribution of compressive forces on the femur.

Ankle. The ankle joint is actually three articulating structures: the tibiotalar, the fibulotalar, and the tibiofibular joints (Fig. 6-11). During standing, forces across the ankle joint can reach more than two times body weight, and during ambulation, they may exceed five

times body weight. Approximately one sixth of the load carried by the lower leg is borne by the fibulotalar joint.

Shoulder. The shoulder joint has a ball-and-socket configuration with three linkages to facilitate its mobility: the scapula, the clavicle, and the spine (Fig. 6-12). The primary movement occurs in the glenohumeral joint. This movement is assisted by three other joints: the scapulothoracic, the sternoclavicular, and the acromioclavicular. With the arm outstretched at 90 degrees, the amount of force across the glenohumeral joint has been estimated to be from one half to almost full body weight.

Elbow. The elbow actually involves three articulations: the humeroulnar, the humeroradial, and the proximal radioulnar (Fig. 6-13). This joint provides both hinging (flexion and extension) and forearm rotation

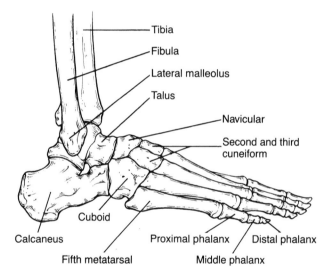

FIGURE 6–11. Ankle joint.

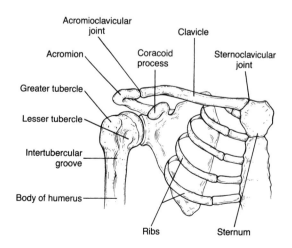

FIGURE 6–12. Shoulder joint.

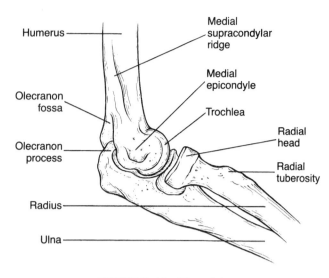

FIGURE 6–13. Elbow joint.

(pronation and supination). Significant fracture involving the elbow often results in loss of motion because of the high level of integration of muscular movement needed to use this joint.

SUPPORTING STRUCTURES

Aside from muscle and bone, other structures serve to support overall musculoskeletal functioning. They are cartilage and collagenous tissues.

Cartilage

Articular cartilage covers the opposing ends of bones within the synovial joint. It is largely avascular and consequently has a limited capacity for repair and regeneration. The function of articular cartilage is biomechanical. It serves to spread the loads applied to articulating bone ends over a larger area, thereby decreasing contact stresses, and to minimize friction and wear within the joint during movement.

Because of the very hydrophilic nature of its matrix, the water content of cartilage is 70%. Intercellular matrix in cartilage, largely collagen fibers, accounts for nearly all of the rest of its weight, for the cellular component of cartilage represents less than 2% of its weight.

Joint lubrication is provided by two methods. One mechanism is by the automechanics of joint physiology. When a load or weight-bearing force is applied to the articular cartilage, fluid is abstracted from the matrix, forming a lubricating coating between the surfaces. This transudation of fluid under pressure serves as a self-lubricating mechanism. The liquid from the matrix is reabsorbed by the cartilage once the load is removed. The second method is assisted by glycoprotein molecules that cover the cartilage and provide a lubricious surface. Both mechanisms work together to minimize friction during movement within the joint. Cartilage must have weight

bearing and joint movement to remain healthy. It shrinks and atrophies if the joint is not used because the cells are not nourished with nutrients from the synovial fluid.

Articular cartilage is subject to *wear* (i.e., the removal of material from solid surfaces by biomechanical action). Two types of wear act on cartilage: interfacial wear and fatigue wear. *Interfacial wear* may occur by either adhesive or abrasive action. *Fatigue wear* occurs from repeated deformation of the cartilage, which can cause microscopic damage. In reality, no one type of these wear mechanisms occurs in isolation. Cartilage wear, as seen in degenerative joint diseases, arises from a combination of these types of wear. However, once the cartilage microstructure is damaged, any one of these damage mechanisms becomes possible as an initiating factor in the progressive degeneration of cartilage. The other damage mechanisms quickly come into play.

This process means that cartilage subjected to large stresses, in both frequency and magnitude, suffers tissue damage (wear). Degeneration, now initiated, is further exacerbated by disruption of the joint lubrication process, rendering the cartilage highly vulnerable to further wear and, ultimately, to a degenerated joint.

Collagenous Tissues: Ligaments and Tendons

Collagen serves a supporting role in all body tissues and organs, but it is particularly important to the musculoskeletal system in the form of tendons, ligaments, and perhaps to a lesser extent, fascia. These collagenous tissues consist primarily of collagen and elastin fibers. As previously discussed, the behavior of these tissues under loading is largely influenced by the structural orientation of their fibers. The functions of the ligaments (joint capsules are also included here because they are ligamentous structures) are to stabilize the joints, guide joint motion, and prevent excessive motion. The functions of tendons are to attach muscle to bone or fascia and to transmit tensile forces among muscle, bone, and fascia. Fascia is the layer of connective tissue that serves to envelop and separate the various organs and their parts from one another. In this fashion, fasciae support the muscles of the body. Indeed, the collagenous nature of fascia imparts a great deal of strength to this tissue. Its inelasticity is often a contributing factor in the clinical entity *compartment syndrome* (see Chapter 10).

Collagenous tissues are capable of undergoing deformation—more so than bone—before failure. Like bone, they model in response to the mechanical demands placed on them.

THE PELVIS AND ACETABULUM

The pelvis is a ringlike structure composed primarily of cancellous bone, with a thin cortex (Fig. 6-14). This type of structure imparts great strength to the pelvis. The pelvis serves two functions: (1) It protects abdominal viscera, and (2) it provides the mechanical link for the support of the trunk on the lower extremities.

A component of the pelvis's mechanical function is that it serves as a shock absorber. It achieves its shock-absorbing qualities through its highly ligamentous structure and through its high composition of cancellous bone.

Fractures incurred by the pelvic ring vary in stability and can influence weight bearing. Acetabular fractures inevitably impair weight bearing.

THE SPINE

The human spine, or vertebral column, is a complex structure consisting of 24 vertebrae (7 cervical, 12 thoracic, and 5 lumbar) and 23 intervertebral discs that are held together by an arrangement of ligaments and muscles. It also contains two bony segments: (1) the sacrum, consisting of five fused vertebrae, and (2) the coccyx, consisting of four fused vertebrae (Fig. 6–15). On a lateral view, it is S-shaped—convex forward in the cervical and lumbar regions (lordosis) and convex posterior in the thoracic and sacral regions (kyphosis). The functional unit of the spine consists of two vertebrae and their intervening soft tissue. This unit is known as either the *motion segment* or the *spinal unit.*

The main functions of the spine are to protect the spinal cord and cauda equina and to transfer loads from

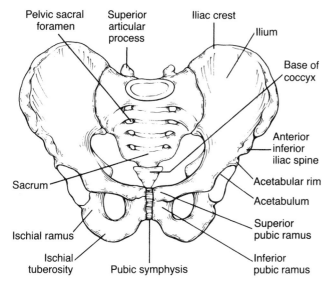

FIGURE 6–14. Bony pelvis, anterior view.

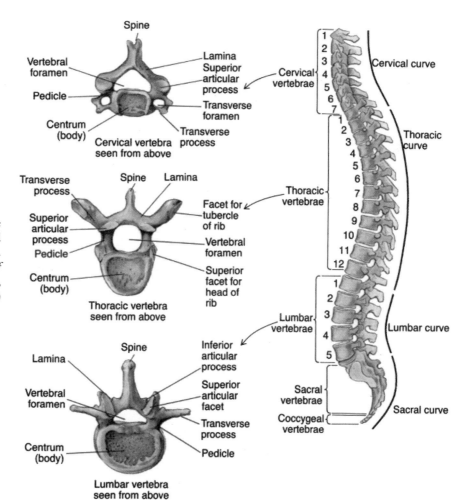

FIGURE 6–15. Lateral view of the spine showing normal lordosis and kyphosis. (From O'Toole, M. [1997]. *Miller-Keane encyclopedia & dictionary of medicine, nursing, & allied health* [6th ed., Plate 2]. Philadelphia: WB Saunders.)

Lumbar Vertebrae

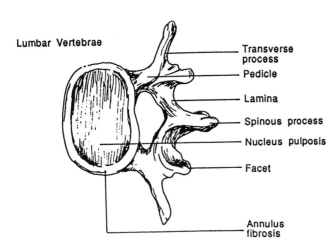

- Transverse process
- Pedicle
- Lamina
- Spinous process
- Nucleus pulposis
- Facet
- Annulus fibrosis

FIGURE 6–16. Anatomy of a vertebral body and disc. (From Chase, J. A. [1991]. An overview of the lumbar spine. In D. A. Slye & L. A. Theis [Eds.], *An introduction to orthopaedic nursing: An orientation module* [p. 75]. Pitman, NJ: National Association of Orthopaedic Nurses.)

head to trunk to pelvis. It also provides attachment for the ribs. Vertebrae are derived from cancellous bone, and they have two major components: the body and the vertebral arch. Also, vertebrae articulate with one another at two joints: a fibrocartilaginous joint (symphysis) between bodies and synovial joints (facet joints) between arches.

The symphysis between the vertebral bodies is the *intervertebral disc,* which acts to resist displacement of the vertebrae on one another while allowing some movement and to dissipate forces that are transmitted along the vertebral column (i.e., serves as a shock absorber in loading forces). The disc has two components, an outer fibrocartilaginous ring known as the *annulus fibrosus* and a pliable, inner, gelatinous mass known as the *nucleus pulposus* (Fig. 6–16). The disc is avascular in the adult. A *cartilaginous endplate* separates the nucleus pulposus and annulus fibrosus from the vertebral body.

The annulus fibrosus contains cartilage fibers arranged in a crisscross pattern radially about the nucleus pulposus. The annulus fibrosus is thicker anteriorly than posteriorly, giving rise to a relative weakness posteriorly. This predisposes humans to posterior herniations, which may lead to adjacent nerve root compression. Under normal circumstances, however, the nucleus pulposus is pressurized outward against the annulus fibrosus when force is applied to the spine, and the annulus is sufficiently strong to contain the nucleus within the intervertebral space.

A complex network of ligaments provides additional stability to the spinal column. The anterior longitudinal ligament lies along the ventral surface of the vertebral bodies, from the axis to the sacrum. The posterior longitudinal ligament closely adheres to the posterior body, which forms the anterior portion of the spinal canal. The ligamentum flavum, which helps constitute the posterior portion of the canal, is located between

vertebral segments. The interspinous ligament is found between each pair of spinous processes, and the supraspinous ligament is found posterior to the spinous processes, between vertebrae (Fig. 6–17).

Degenerative changes in the disc occur with aging. The hyaline cartilage that lines the vertebral bodies (cartilaginous endplate) becomes thinner. The nucleus pulposus loses much of its water content, with a concomitant decrease in pliability.

Intervertebral disc syndrome is a common cause of low-back pain. It is thought that repetitive, stressful, axial loading may create pressure within the nucleus pulposus that pushes against the annulus fibrosus. With time, the annulus weakens, allowing for disc herniation, protrusion, extrusion, and the most involved degree, sequestration (i.e., the escape of disc fragments within the intrathecal compartment). This phenomenon, as well as disc degeneration with age, results in disc narrowing, which may disturb the mechanics of the back and cause pain.

Various forces act on the spinal unit. Compression, or axial loading, is one of these forces. In the normal spine, such pressure causes the vertebral endplate to bulge, squeezing blood out of the cancellous bone. The normal nucleus pulposus does not change its shape under pressure; it is actually incompressible. In fact, the normal, healthy intervertebral disc is stronger than bone.

Flexion (forward bending) causes compression of the vertebral body and tension on the posterior ligaments of the spine. In injuries resulting from flexion, the vertebral body is crushed before the posterior ligaments rupture.

Extension (backward bending) increases tension anteriorly and compression posteriorly. The shape of the healthy intervertebral disc is unaffected. Extension injuries of the spine are typically limited to crush fractures of the neural arch.

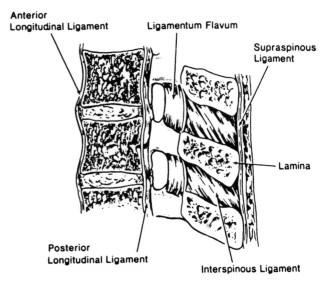

Anterior Longitudinal Ligament

Ligamentum Flavum

Supraspinous Ligament

Lamina

Posterior Longitudinal Ligament

Interspinous Ligament

FIGURE 6–17. Ligaments of the lumbar spine. (From Genge, M. L. [1988]. Epidural analgesia in the orthopaedic patient. *Orthopaedic Nursing, 7*[4], 13.)

Of the various loading mechanisms, the spine is least able to resist rotation. This movement, if done to the extreme, disrupts spinal ligaments and produces subsequent dislocation. Fracture of the vertebral body is also possible.

Distraction (tension) of the spine subjects the entire vertebral body and the neural arches to tensile stress. Such forces (traction) are applied therapeutically to patients with lumbar disc syndrome.

Translation (shear) is usually accompanied by other loading forces when applied to the spine. Translation is the loading mechanism responsible for most fracture-dislocation injuries to the spine.

Because of its high degree of mobility, the cervical spine is highly vulnerable to injury. For example, vertebral subluxation may result from flexion rotation of the neck, and burst fractures may result from compression.

The thoracic spine is unique in that the ribs serve as the stabilizing outriggers for this area, limiting lateral flexion and extension. However, there is less resistance to torsion in this area. The middle portion of the thoracic spine is most resistant to movement, for the trunk and back musculature serve to stabilize it. Because of its torsional stiffness, the area of T10 to T12 is a common site of spinal injury.

The lumbar spine is characterized by massive vertebral bodies and large facet joints. It carries the largest amount of weight in the spine, and the normal lordotic curve renders it more susceptible to biomechanical stresses, particularly shearing loads. Consequently, lumbar disc syndrome most commonly affects this segment of the spine. The lordotic configuration of the lumbar spine also requires that the facet joints in this area, particularly those of L5, provide greater assistance in supporting the lumbar joints on the sacrum.

PHYSIOLOGIC CHANGES IN THE AGING MUSCULOSKELETAL SYSTEM

Aging, an inevitable life process, can be somewhat standardized from one person to the next by normative changes. Multiple factors affect the aging process, including smoking, poor nutrition, chronic stress, and medical illness. Although some people appear to age more subtly than others do, the physiologic changes associated with the aging musculoskeletal system may be more apparent.

Several causes related to the physical changes of aging are biologic, functional, and pathologic. Flexibility is altered because of morphologic changes in supporting collagenous structures, disuse phenomenon from decreased activity, and disease that modifies the shape and function of tissues. Collagen undergoes maturational stabilization that increases the rigidity of collagen fibers. This leads to decreased tissue compliance and tension-resistant connective tissues.

Body composition changes with age. Lean body mass (bone and muscle) decreases as the deposition of fat generally increases. A slow, yet gradual loss of height is attributable to the loss of water content in intervertebral discs. Osteoporotic changes, especially in women, create brittle, less compact bones subject to compression and fracture. Tendons, ligaments, and cartilage are prone to calcification because of repeated biomechanical stressors, poor posture, and generalized deconditioning.

The effects of aging on the musculoskeletal system are many. The initial changes begin at the cellular level. Alteration in cellular function changes the shape and structure of collagen fibers. The fibers become compressed and larger. Biochemically, molecular bonding among macromolecular structures increases. Metabolically, collagen biosynthesis is altered, creating stiffer and less flexible fibers. In older people, there is less differentiation of mesenchymal cells into respective connective tissue cells. Healing of musculoskeletal structures in the older individual follows the same inflammatory, repair, and remodeling stages as in the younger individual. However, healing is slower and less effective, which may result in a greater incidence of malunion and nonunion after fracture.

Physiologic changes in the aging neuroendocrine system have widespread cumulative effects on many organ systems. The decline in mature B and T lymphocytes affects humoral responses, thereby altering host ability to mount an effective febrile as well as infection-fighting response. These neuroendocrine effects have an impact on the older person whose body undergoes stress, for example, from fracture, injury, or surgery.

Bone

Alterations in bone structure also occur. The architecture of collagen influences the osteons to become more dense and compacted, making them shorter and narrower. The nutrient canals become wider, leading to a decrease in the capacity of the entire haversian system. Following fracture in the older adult, callus contains increased collagen whereby bone remodeling is slower.

The long bone model can be used as an analogy in understanding the aging structural changes within bone. There is an inverse relationship to thickness of the diaphyseal cortex and density of bone mass in the endosteal (inner cortex) versus periosteal (outer cortex). This translates into loss of bone mineral density (BMD) within the interior of bone, with a reciprocal attenuation to the outer cortex.

By age 35 in women and 55 in men, BMD decreases by 1% per year. Involutional (type II) or normal age-related osteoporosis is associated with decreased osteoblastic function. Type I osteoporosis, or postmenopausal osteoporosis, is characterized by loss of BMD because of lowered serum estrogen levels. Cortical bone loss may rise to 2% to 3% per year after the first 5 years postmenopause. For a complete discussion of osteoporosis, see Chapter 15.

The intervertebral disc responds to the effects of aging. The increase in the size of collagen fibers and decrease in water content cause the nucleus pulposus and the annulus fibrosus to coalesce, losing structural differentiation and becoming fibrocartilage. The nucleus diminishes and displaces posteriorly within the confines of the disc. Associated with the change in disc shape, facet joints undergo biomechanical stress, particularly shear and torsional loading.

Changes in the water content of the disc and demineralization of the vertebral bodies often precipitate collapse and compression of the vertebral spine, causing nerve impingement, chronic pain, and loss of structural support. Classic skeletal changes associated with advanced osteoporosis are kyphosis, or dowager's hump, and loss of height because of compression of the vertebral bodies.

Biochemical and physiologic factors related to the stimulation or retardation of bone in the aging musculoskeletal system are listed in Table 6-2. The general slowing of tissue repair and healing is reflected in the quantity of the production of these factors.

Articular Cartilage

Articular cartilage remains fairly constant during the aging process. Cell count of articular cartilage is the same in the older individual, and elastic properties stay the same. Overall, the chemical components, histomorphometry, and physical attributes remain constant in the aging musculoskeletal system. In the reparative process associated with a traumatic injury or repetitive wear-and-tear situation (e.g., osteoarthritis), metabolic and remodeling processes are diminished. These effects alter the configuration of the joint.

Muscle

Lean muscle mass generally lessens with age. Disuse atrophy leads to muscle wasting. The number of muscle fibers decreases with age, as do important enzymatic activities within the mitochondria. Reduction in acetylcholine and increased resorption of calcium affect muscle contraction time, skeletal muscle function, fatigability, and endurance.

Associated with disuse of muscle, ligaments and tendons lose elasticity and resiliency. In the presence of trauma or repetitive stress, these soft tissue structures shorten, creating stiffness and loss of flexibility and range of motion. In the restoration phase postinjury, calcium hydroxyapatite crystals may be deposited in muscle and tendon-ligamentous structures, creating pain and further disrupting function.

The benefits of early mobilization after injury are replete in the literature. Musculoskeletal integrity can be enhanced and outcomes reached if the aging effects on the musculoskeletal system are appreciated and incorporated within client care.

INTERNET RESOURCES

Wheeless' Textbook of Orthopaedics: www. medmedia.com

BIBLIOGRAPHY

Bobb, J. (1994). Trauma in the elderly. In V. Cardona, P. Hurn, P. Bastnagel Mason, A. Scanlon, & S. Veise-Berry (Eds.), *Trauma nursing: From resuscitation through rehabilitation* (2nd ed., pp. 721–735). Philadelphia: WB Saunders.

Buckwalter, J. A., Einhorn, T. A., & Simon, S. R. (1999). *Orthopaedic basic science* (2nd ed.). Park Ridge, IL: American Academy of Orthopaedic Surgeons.

Cardona, V. D., Hurn. P. D., Basnagel Mason, P. J., Scanlon, A. M., & Beise-Berry, S. W. (1994). *Trauma nursing: From resuscitation through rehabilitation.* Philadelphia: WB Saunders.

Crowther, C. (1999). *Primary orthopaedic care.* St. Louis: Mosby.

Edwards, B., & Perry, H. (1994). Age-related osteoporosis. *Clinics in Geriatric Medicine, 10,* 575–588.

Favus, M. (1993). *Primer on the metabolic bone diseases and disorders of mineral metabolism* (2nd ed.). New York: Raven.

Gamble, J. G. (1988). *The musculoskeletal system: Physiologic basics.* New York: Raven.

Gates, S., & Mooar, P. K. (1999). *Musculoskeletal primary care.* Philadelphia: Lippincott.

Greene, W. (2000). *Essentials of musculoskeletal care* (2nd ed.). Rosemont, IL: American Academy of Orthopaedic Surgeons.

Gunby, M., & Morley, J. (1994). Epidemiology of bone loss with aging. *Clinics in Geriatric Medicine, 10,* 557–574.

Guyton, A., & Hall, J. E. (2000). *Textbook of medical physiology.* Philadelphia: WB Saunders.

Hoppenfeld, S. (1976). *Physical examination of the spine and extremities.* New York: Appleton-Century-Crofts.

Levy, D., Hanlon, D., & Townsend, R. (1993). Geriatric trauma. *Clinics in Geriatric Medicine, 9,* 601–620.

Mow, V. C., & Hayes, W. C. (1997). *Basic orthopaedic biomechanics* (2nd ed.). New York: Lippincott-Raven.

Rockwood, C., Green, D., & Bucholz, R. (1996). *Fractures in adults* (4th. ed., Vol. 1 & 2). Philadelphia: Lippincott.

Salter, R. (1970). *Textbook of disorders and injuries of the musculoskeletal system.* Baltimore: Williams & Wilkins.

Schenck, R. C. (1992). Biology of fracture repair. In B. D. Browner, J. B. Jupiter, A. M. Levine, & Trafton, P. G. (Eds.), *Skeletal trauma: Fractures, dislocations, ligamentous injuries* (pp. 31–75). Philadelphia: Lippincott Williams & Wilkins.

Schenck, R. C. (1999). *Athletic training and sports medicine.* Rosemont, IL: American Academy of Orthopaedic Surgeons.

Schoen, D. C. (2000). *Adult orthopaedic nursing.* Philadelphia: WB Saunders.

Schoen, D. (Ed.). (2001). *NAON core curriculum for orthopaedic nursing.* Pitman, NJ: National Association of Orthopaedic Nurses.

Simon, S. R. (1994). *Orthopaedic basic science.* Rosemont, IL: American Academy of Orthopaedic Surgeons.

Turek, S. (1994). *Orthopaedics: Principles and their application* (5th ed.). Philadelphia: Lippincott.

Wilmore, J. H., & Costill, D. L. (1999). Aging and the older athlete. In J. Wilmore & D. Costill (Eds.), *Physiology of sports and exercise* (2nd ed., pp. 544–569). Champaign, IL: Human Kinetics.

Windsor, R. E., & Lax, D. M. (1998). *Soft tissue injuries: Diagnosis and treatment.* Philadelphia: Hanley & Belfus.

Woo, S. L., & Buckwalter, J. A. (1991). *Injury and repair of the musculoskeletal soft tissues.* Park Ridge, IL: American Academy of Orthopaedic Surgeons.

7

Genetics

DALE HALSEY LEA

New genetic discoveries during the last decade have emerged primarily from the Human Genome Project, an international research effort to map and sequence the human genome in its entirety. These discoveries are providing a wealth of information about how genes function and how they contribute to human health and disease. There are now more than 10,000 identified genetic disorders recognized as being inherited in predictable patterns (OMIM, 2000). New opportunities for health promotion and prevention are becoming available as a result of using gene-based technologies. Individuals and families at risk for such common conditions as cancer and heart disease, for example, now have options for presymptomatic diagnosis using gene mutation testing. This information is being used to develop individualized prevention and intervention plans (Collins, 1999).

Nurses today are challenged by a need for genetic knowledge and skills. They must blend genetic knowledge and applications with their skills in health promotion, health maintenance, and restoration so that they can continue to participate fully in interdisciplinary partnerships in all practice settings and provide holistic and family-centered care. This includes identifying individuals who may have a genetic condition or predisposition and collaborating with genetic specialists to ensure that those individuals are able to access the most current genetic diagnostic, treatment, and management therapeutics. With this new knowledge, nurses can collect and record family history information; provide current and accurate genetic information and support; and participate in ongoing management of individuals, families, and communities as they assimilate new genetic health information into daily living (Lashley, 1998; Lea, Jenkins, & Francomano, 1998; Williams, Prows, & Lea, 2000).

This chapter provides orthopaedic nurses with general information about genetic aspects of health and disease—the structure and function of genes, chromosomal disorders, and the inheritance of genetic conditions in families. If offers a foundation for the clinical applications of genetic principles in orthopaedic nursing, resources for nurses and their clients including genetic counseling and evaluation, and emerging genetic technologies. Nursing participation in providing genetic services and important ethical, legal, and social implications for nurses are described. Specific emphasis is placed on how genetic discoveries and future web-based technologies are creating new pathways for community-based and individualized health care planning and delivery.

THE GENETIC BASIS OF HEALTH AND DISEASE
Gene Discovery

In 1865, Gregor Mendel, an Austrian monk, first described the basic elements of heredity—genes. Through his observations and analyses of the observable traits of garden peas, he concluded that specific traits, later to be called *genes,* were passed on unaltered from a parent plant to its offspring. In modern science and medicine, genes are recognized as a central component of human health and disease. In 1990, a research effort called the Human Genome Project was officially established as a joint project of the Department of Energy (DOE) and the National Institutes of Health (NIH). The term *genome* refers to the complete DNA sequence, containing the entire genetic information of a reproductive cell, an individual, a population, or a species (Nussbaum, McInnes, & Willard, 2001). Working together, DOE and NIH have been able to construct a genetic and physical map of the human genome and have also been able to sequence greater than 90% of this rough map. Progress has been considerably accelerated by the introduction of commercial companies seeking to be the first to map and sequence the human genome. As a result, gene mapping and sequencing was completed in the spring of 2000, some 5 years ahead of a projected finish time (Wolpert, 2000).

Work on the Human Genome Project has made clear just how basic human genetics is to human development, health, and disease. Knowledge that specific genes are associated with specific genetic conditions makes diagnosis possible, even in the unborn. Understanding the underlying causes of conditions points researchers toward finding and developing effective therapies and even cures.

Researchers say that each human being carries six to seven recessive genes with the potential for creating genetic conditions in their descendants if their partner has the same recessive gene(s). Many people carry genes that predispose them to conditions such as arthritis, diabetes, and cancer. The term *genetic disease,* therefore, no longer refers to rare syndromes and devastating illnesses. Advances in research continue to demonstrate how many common conditions have genetic causes. Many additional associations will no doubt emerge as scientists complete and refine human gene mapping and sequencing (Collins, 1999).

Genes and Chromosomes: What They Are and What They Do

Each human being's genome contains between 30,000 to 40,000 genes (Baltimore, 2001). An individual gene is conceptualized as a unit of heredity. Genes are packaged in a threadlike manner within chromosomes, and chromosomes are located within the cell nucleus (Fig. 7–1). Genes are arranged in a linear order along each chromosome. Each gene has an assigned genetic locus, that is, a chromosomal location that is consistent between individuals. Chromosomes can be distinguished by size and by unique banding patterns.

Every organism has a specific number of chromosomes. Humans have 46 chromosomes that occur in pairs in all cells of the body, except egg (oocytes) and sperm. In egg and sperm, there are only 23 chromosomes, or half the number found in all other body tissues. The chromosomes of each pair are said to be *homologous* to each other, meaning that genes on each of a chromosome pair have the same position and order. Twenty-two pairs of chromosomes—referred to as *autosomes*—are the same in females and males. The 23rd pair is referred to as the *sex chromosomes.* A female has two X chromosomes, and a male has one X and one Y chromosome. Each parent donates one chromosome of each pair to their children. Thus, children receive half of their chromosomes from their fathers and half from their mothers (Hartl & Jones, 1998; Lashley, 1998; Lea, Jenkins, & Francomano, 1998).

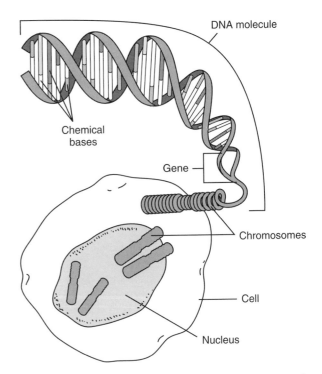

FIGURE 7–1. DNA, which carries the instructions that allow cells to make proteins, is made up of four chemical bases. Tightly coiled strands of DNA are packaged in units called *chromosomes,* which are housed in the cell's nucleus. Working subunits of DNA are known as *genes.* (From the National Institutes of Health and National Cancer Institute. [1995]. *Understanding gene testing.* [NIH Pub. No. 96-3905]. Washington, DC: U.S. Department of Human Services.)

Cell Division—Mitosis and Meiosis. As the human body grows and develops, worn out cells are replaced and wounds are healed through a process of cell division. Two distinctly different types of cell division—mitosis and meiosis—contribute to these processes.

Mitosis is the cell division process that occurs in all body cells except egg (oocytes) and sperm. Mitosis is involved in cell growth, differentiation, and repair. During mitosis, the chromosomes of each cell duplicate. The result is two cells (i.e., daughter cells), each containing the same number of chromosomes as the parent cell. The daughter cells are said to be *diploid* because they contain 46 chromosomes in 23 pairs.

Meiosis, on the other hand, is the cell division process by which reproductive cells (oocytes and sperm) are formed. Meiosis occurs only in reproductive cells. A reduction in the number of chromosomes takes place through a series of complex mechanisms during meiosis, resulting in oocytes or sperm that contain 23 chromosomes—half the usual number. Oocytes and sperm are thus said to be *haploid* because they contain a single copy of each chromosome compared with all other body cells that have two of each chromosome. During the initial phase of meiosis, a phenomenon called "crossing over" may take place. As the paired chromosomes come together in preparation for cell division, portions cross over and an exchange of genetic material occurs. The event of recombination of genetic material inherited from either the father or mother creates greater diversity in the makeup of oocytes and sperm.

During meiosis, a pair of chromosomes sometimes fails to separate completely, creating a sperm or oocyte that contains either two copies or no copy of a particular chromosome. This accidental event is called *nondisjunction.* An embryo created from a normal sperm fertilizing an oocyte that contains two copies of a chromosome will have 47 chromosomes with an extra chromosome of a particular chromosome pair. This is referred to as *trisomy.* Down syndrome is an example of a trisomy. A person who has Down syndrome has three number 21 chromosomes instead of the usual two. When a sperm or oocyte lacks one chromosome, the resulting embryo will have 22 pairs of chromosomes with a single chromosome that is missing its mate. This is called *monosomy.* The chromosomal disorder called Turner's syndrome is an example of monosomy. Girls who have Turner's syndrome usually have only one X chromosome, causing them to have short stature and infertility (Lashley, 1998).

DNA, RNA, and the Code for Proteins. Each individual gene consists of a segment of DNA. DNA is the chemical that holds the genetic instructions, or blueprint, for making human organisms. Genes provide the instructions to make proteins needed for healthy body functioning. Genes also control the rate at which proteins are made. Changes in gene structure—*mutations*—can alter the type and amount of protein produced. In the case of osteogenesis imperfecta, a genetic disorder of connective tissue, for example, there is an abnormality in either the *COL1A1* or *COL1A2* gene that encodes for both chains of type I collagen. Mutations in these genes cause abnormal collagen structure and function and result in characteristic connective tissue and bone defects seen in individuals with osteogenesis imperfecta such as bone fragility, blue sclerae, progressive bone deformities, and presenile hearing loss (Lashley, 1998).

The double-helix shape of DNA was identified in 1963 by Watson and Crick. DNA is made up of a sugar (deoxyribose), a phosphate group and one of four nitrogen bases: adenine (A), cytosine (C), guanine (G), and thymine (T). When a sugar group is combined with a phosphate group and one of the four bases, it is referred to as a *nucleotide.* DNA has two strands shaped like a spiral staircase, and each of these strands is made up of a number of nucleotides. The paired strands are held together by hydrogen bonds between the base pairs. The sugar/phosphate molecules are comparable to the railings on a spiral staircase, and the bases serve as a

backbone and are comparable to the stairs that hold the railings of the spiral staircase together (see Fig. 7-1). The bases on each strand of DNA are said to be complimentary and are referred to as base pairs. The formation of hydrogen bonds between bases is referred to as *basepairing,* and the bases are said to be complimentary.

RNA has a similar composition to DNA. RNA is made up of nitrogenous bases, a sugar (ribonucleic acid) and a phosphate group. RNA differs from DNA in that it is single stranded and has a base of uracil (U) instead of thymine (T). Three major types of RNA—messenger RNA (mRNA), ribosomal RNA (rRNA), and transfer RNA (tRNA)—have specific roles in protein production. mRNA carries the coded information transcribed from DNA and is the template for protein production. There are a number of genetic disorders that are caused by alterations in RNA that affect the protein made. Beta-thalassemia, an inherited chronic anemia among individuals of Mediterranean descent is one example. Beta-thalassemia is often caused by abnormalities that can reduce the amount of mRNA or its encoded protein, the beta chain of hemoglobin. Discovery of these gene abnormalities has lead to a better understanding of the cause of thalassemia, diagnosis, and treatments (Thompson, McInnes, & Willard, 1991).

Amino acids are the building blocks that make up human proteins. There are 22 amino acids in the human body. The sequence of amino acids needed to make up a specific protein is determined by a specific sequence of nucleotides or base pairs in DNA. Each of the 22 amino acids is created by a set of three bases called a *triplet,* or *codon.* Each triplet makes only one amino acid; however, amino acids can be specified by more than one triplet. As an example, the following triplets may specify the amino acid phenylalanine: UUG, UUU, UUC, UUA. The particular relationship of specific triplets to specific amino acids is called the *genetic code* (Lashley, 1998).

The Process of Protein Synthesis. Although genetic information contained in DNA and packaged in chromosomes is located in the cell nucleus, the actual production of proteins for which the DNA code is needed takes place outside of the nucleus in a portion of the cell called *cytoplasm.* Protein production or synthesis begins when DNA separates into two strands. One of the strands functions as the coding or *sense strand,* and the other is referred to as the *antisense strand.* The genetic information needed for protein synthesis is on the sense strand.

Transcription and translation are two central processes involved in protein synthesis. Transcription is the process in which mRNA is copied from the coding strands of DNA. Translation involves the assembly of amino acids into proteins as specified by the triplet sequences of the genetic code. Transcription of DNA to RNA and translation of RNA into a protein product are the central processes of molecular genetics (Lashley, 1998).

GENE MUTATIONS AND HUMAN DISEASE

Gene Mutations

Regulation and expression of the 30,000 to 40,000 genes in the human genome is complex and the result of many intricate interactions within each cell. Gene structure and function, transcription and translation, and protein synthesis are all involved. Alterations in any one of these essential processes may influence a person's health. Gene mutations—changes in gene structure—result from several types of alterations in DNA. Gene mutations involve a permanent change in the sequence of DNA. Changes in the normal sequence of bases can alter the characteristics of the proteins for which DNA codes. Table 7–1 provides examples of various types of mutations.

Codons are groups of triplet bases in nucleic acids specifying the amino acid placement that produces the final protein product. Because codons are read as triplets, an addition or deletion of only one nucleotide shifts the entire reading frame. For example, a *nonsense mutation* is a point mutation that creates a premature "stop" codon, which shortens the gene product; a *frameshift mutation* involves a deletion or addition of one, two, or any number of bases that is not a multiple of three. This disrupts the normal reading frame, resulting in premature termination of translation. A *missense mutation* involves a single base change that alters an amino acid in the gene product, resulting in an abnormal protein (Lashley, 1998; Lea, Jenkins, & Francomano, 1998).

Some mutations (e.g., silent mutations) have no significant effect on the protein product made, whereas other gene mutations result in partial or complete alterations in the protein produced. The way in which a protein is altered and the relative importance of the protein to proper body functioning determine the relative effect of the mutation. Gene mutations may occur in

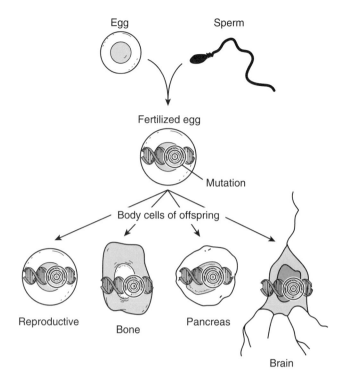

FIGURE 7–2. Hereditary mutations are carried in the DNA of the reproductive cells. When reproductive cells containing mutations combine to produce offspring, the mutation will be present in all of the offspring's body cells. (From the National Institutes of Health and National Cancer Institute. [1995]. *Understanding gene testing.* [NIH Pub. No. 96-3905]. Washington, DC: U.S. Department of Human Services.)

TABLE 7–1. *Gene Mutations: Examples That May Lead to Disease*

Gene mutations are changes in the normal sequence of bases that can alter the type and nature of proteins for which DNA codes. Below are examples of types of gene mutations using a sequence of three words—CAT ATE RAT

Normal base sequence	CAT	ATE	RAT
Deletion	CAT	AT	RAT
Point mutation	CAN	ATE	RAT
Insertion	CAT	ATE	RATS
Translocation	RAT	ATE	CAT
Amplification	CATTTTTT	ATEEE	RATTTTT

From Lea, D. H., Jenkins, J. F., & Francomano, C. A. (1998). *Genetics in clinical practice: New directions for nursing and health care.* Boston: Jones and Bartlett.

hormones or enzymes, important protein products. A gene mutation may cause a protein to be ineffective. Because hormones and enzymes are important regulators of most body functions, mutations in these have significant implications for health and disease (Hartl & Jones, 1998).

An example of a common gene mutation that may have a significant effect on protein structure involves a "misspelling" in the DNA sequence. The misspelling results in an alteration of a single base, such is the case with sickle cell anemia, a genetic disorder of hemoglobin structure. One nucleotide in the gene coding for the beta-globin chain of hemoglobin is mutated in sickle cell anemia. The mutation produces hemoglobin S. A person who inherits two copies of the gene mutation, hemoglobin S, has the condition sickle cell anemia and experiences the symptoms of severe anemia and thrombotic organ damage resulting from hypoxia.

Other gene mutations involve RNA processing, splicing, transcription, or regulatory mutations. Some are larger mutations involving a deletion (loss), an insertion (addition), a duplication (multiplication), or rearrangement (translocation) of a longer DNA segment. Duchenne muscular dystrophy, a common inherited form of muscular dystrophy affecting males, is caused by structural gene mutations such as deletions or duplications in the dystrophin gene. A more recently discovered type of gene mutation—triplet or trinucleotide repeats—involves the expansion of more than the usual number of a triplet (e.g., CTG) repeat sequence within a gene. Usually, there are fewer than 20 to 40 of any given repeat. When these nucleotides become unstable and expand or lengthen, which often occurs during meiosis, they may cause disease. Such is the case in the inherited muscular dystrophy, myotonic dystrophy, in which affected individuals have a significantly increased number of CTG repeats.

Gene mutations are either inherited or acquired. Inherited gene mutations are present in the DNA of all body cells and are passed on in reproductive cells from parent to child. Germ-line mutations are present in all daughter cells when body cells replicate (Fig. 7–2). The gene that causes Huntington's disease is one example of a germ-line mutation.

Spontaneous gene mutations occur in individual oocytes or sperm at the time of conception. These mutations are not inherited in other family members; however, the person who carries the new mutation may then pass on the gene mutation to his or her offspring. The genetic condition achondroplasia, a form of short stature, is caused by a mutation in the fibroblast growth receptor-3 gene (FGFR3). Achondroplasia is an example of a genetic condition that usually occurs in a single family member as a result of spontaneous mutation (Lashley, 1998; Rimoin, Connor, & Pyeritz, 1996).

An acquired, or somatic, mutation involves changes in DNA that occur during a person's lifetime (after conception). Somatic mutations, in contrast to germ-line mutations, develop as a result of cumulative changes in body cells other than reproductive cells (Fig. 7–3). Somatic gene mutations are passed on to the daughter cells derived from that particular cell line.

Gene mutations happen in the human body all of the time. Cells are able to recognize mutations in DNA and in most instances can correct the change before it is passed on via cell division. Body cells' ability to repair damage from gene mutations may diminish over time, leading to an accumulation of genetic changes that may ultimately result in disease. An accumulation of unrepaired gene mutations is often involved in the development of cancer and may be involved in other disorders of aging such as

FIGURE 7–3. Acquired mutations develop in DNA during a person's lifetime. If the mutation arises in a body cell, copies of the mutation will exist only in the descendants of that particular cell. (From the National Institutes of Health and National Cancer Institute. [1995]. *Understanding gene testing.* [NIH Pub. No. 96-3905]. Washington, DC: U.S. Department of Human Services.)

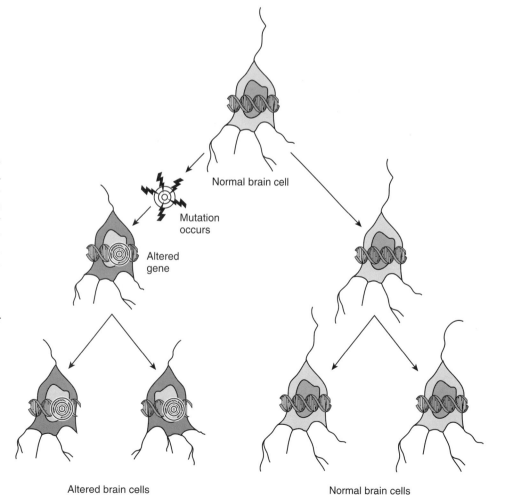

Alzheimer's disease (Thompson, McInnes, & Willard, 1991).

Mendelian Inheritance Patterns

Each person has a unique genetic constitution called a *genotype*. The observable characteristics of a person's genotype is said to be that person's *phenotype*. A person's phenotype includes physical appearance or other physiologic, molecular, or biologic traits. All phenotypes, including those with a major genetic component, are modified by environmental influences.

Human growth, development, and disease are generally believed to occur as a result of both genetic and environmental influences and interactions. The relative contribution of the genetic component may be either large or small. In a person with osteogenesis imperfecta or Down syndrome, for example, the genetic contribution is essential and significant. In contrast, a person's response to a major environmental influence such as an infection or an accidental injury may reside in the genetic component of that person's physiologic capacity for immune response and repair. This concept is illustrated in Figure 7–4.

Genetic conditions that are inherited in families in fixed proportions among generations are referred to as *mendelian* disorders after Gregor Mendel. Mendelian disorders are caused by gene mutations present on one or both chromosomes of a pair. In each of these instances, an individual gene in a single or double dose can cause a genetic condition. Mendelian disorders are classified according to their pattern of inheritance in families. Three classic patterns of mendelian inheritance are autosomal dominant, autosomal recessive, and X-linked. The terms *dominant* and *recessive* refer to the trait, disorder, or phenotype, but not to the genes or alleles that cause the observable characteristics.

GENES AND ENVIRONMENTAL INFLUENCES

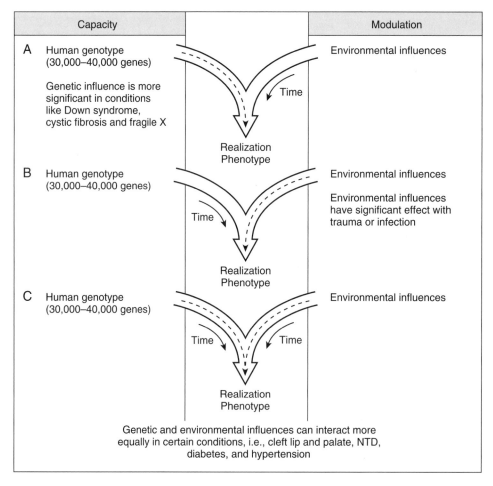

FIGURE 7–4. Human growth, development, and disease are generally believed to occur as a result of both genetic and environmental influences. The relative contribution of the genetic component may be either large or small. (From the National Institutes of Health and National Cancer Institute. [1995]. *Understanding gene testing.* [NIH Pub. No. 96-3905]. Washington, DC: U.S. Department of Human Services.)

Nursing assessment of clients' health includes obtaining and recording family history information. Family history assessment should be a central and ongoing component of every nurse's health assessment, used as a means of finding those families who may benefit from further genetic counseling, testing, and therapeutics. Family history evaluation is done by diagramming the genetic family health history in a genetic family pedigree. The pedigree is the first step in establishing a pattern of inheritance of a genetic condition in a family. It provides a visual schema of the connections between the client and his or her family, particularly with respect to heritable conditions. Medical elements captured on the genetic family pedigree include (1) all births; (2) all deaths and ages and causes of death; (3) miscarriages, stillbirths, elective pregnancy terminations; (4) infant deaths; (5) birth defects; (6) inherited and familial disorders; (7) diagnosis of other illness, including cancer; (8) age at diagnosis; and (9) confirmation by medical record or pathology report.

Nurses need to become familiar with the characteristics of mendelian patterns of inheritance and of pedigree construction and analysis so that they can participate in identifying those individuals and families at increased risk for inherited genetic conditions (Lashley, 1998; Lea, Jenkins, & Francomano, 1998).

Autosomal-Dominant Inherited Disorders. Genetic disorders inherited in an autosomal-dominant manner follow a vertical pattern of inheritance in families with someone usually having the disorder in each generation. Female and male family members are equally affected. A person who has an autosomal-dominant inherited disorder has a gene mutation for that condition located on one chromosome of a pair. Each of that person's children has a 50% chance to inherit the gene mutation for the condition and a 50% chance of inheriting the normal version of the gene. Children who do not inherit the gene mutation for the dominant disorder do not develop the disorder, nor do they have an increased risk for having children with the dominant condition (Fig. 7–5). Characteristics of disorders inherited in an autosomal-dominant pattern are given in Table 7–2, along with examples of genetic conditions illustrating the disorder.

Two important features of dominantly inherited disorders are the phenomena of variable expression and reduced penetrance. *Variable expression* refers to the varying degrees of severity of a disorder observed among family members and other individuals with the disorder. Some individuals with the condition may have significant symptoms, but others may have only mild features of the disorder. Genetic and environmental influences are related to variability in clinical presentation.

The presence of a gene mutation does not invariably mean that a person will have or develop the dominant disorder. As an example, when a woman has the *BRCA1* hereditary breast cancer gene mutation, the risk of breast

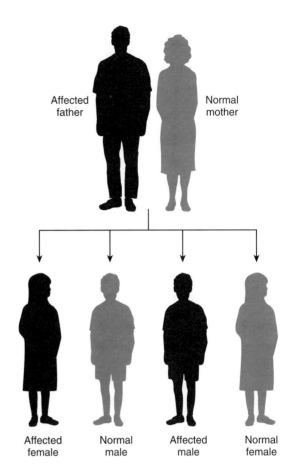

FIGURE 7–5. In dominant genetic disorders, if one affected parent has a disease-causing allele that dominates its normal counterpart, each child in the family has a 50% percent chance of inheriting the disease allele and the disorder. (From the National Institutes of Health and National Cancer Institute. [1995]. *Understanding gene testing.* [NIH Pub. No. 96-3905]. Washington, DC: U.S. Department of Human Services.)

cancer by age 65 is 80%, not 100%. This concept known as *reduced penetrance* indicates that there is a certain probability that a given gene will produce disease. Reduced penetrance refers to the situation in which a person inherits a gene mutation that causes an autosomal-dominant disorder but may not have any of the observable physical or developmental features of that disorder. Despite not showing any of the characteristics of the disorder seen in other affected family members, these individuals still carry the gene mutation and still have a 50% chance to pass it on to each of their children. Examples of genetic disorders with reduced penetrance include Marfan's syndrome and neurofibromatosis.

Autosomal-Recessive Inherited Disorders. Genetic disorders inherited in an autosomal-recessive pattern are commonly seen in specific ethnic groups and occur more often in children of parents who are related by blood (e.g., first cousins). The pattern of inheritance in autosomal-recessive inherited disorders is horizontal,

TABLE 7-2. *Mendelian and Complex Inherited Disorders*

CHARACTERISTICS OF MENDELIAN AND COMPLEX INHERITED DISORDERS	EXAMPLES OF GENETIC CONDITIONS INHERITED IN MENDELIAN AND COMPLEX PATTERNS
Conditions Inherited in an Autosomal-Dominant Pattern 1. Vertical transmission in families 2. Equal frequency of affected males and females 3. Variable expressivity 4. In some disorders, less or no expression of the condition—reduced penetrance	**Autosomal-Dominant Inherited Conditions** 1. Myotonic dystrophy 2. Marfan's syndrome 3. Stickler syndrome
Conditions Inherited in an Autosomal-Recessive Pattern 1. Horizontal transmission in families 2. Equal frequency of affected males and females 3. Associated with particular ethnic groups, parents related by blood (e.g., first cousins)	**Autosomal-Recessive Inherited Conditions** 1. Gaucher's disease 2. Osteogenesis imperfecta 3. Spinal muscular atrophy
Conditions Inherited in an X-linked Recessive Pattern 1. Transmission is vertical through females 2. Males are predominantly affected 3. X inactivation causes variable expression in females	**X-Linked Recessive Inherited Conditions** 1. Becker muscular dystrophy 2. Duchenne muscular dystrophy 3. Hemophilia
Conditions with Complex Inheritance Patterns 1. Tend to cluster in families 2. Do not demonstrate the same characteristic pattern of inheritance as is observed in mendelian inherited disorders	**Complex Inherited Conditions** 1. Club foot 2. Congenital hip dislocation 3. Neural tube defects (spina bifida)

From Lea, D. H., Jenkins, J. F., & Francomano, C. A. (1998). *Genetics in clinical practice: New directions for nursing and health care.* Boston: Jones and Bartlett.

with relatives of a single generation tending to have the condition.

In autosomal-recessive inheritance, each parent of an affected child carries a gene mutation on one chromosome of the pair and the normal working copy of the gene on the other chromosome. The parents are said to be carriers of the defective gene. Unlike autosomal-dominant inherited disorders, a carrier of a gene mutation for a recessive inherited disorder does not have symptoms or express the genetic condition. If two carrier parents have children, there is a 25% chance that their offspring will inherit one gene mutation from each parent and will have the disorder. Carrier parents also have a 50% chance of bearing a child who inherits the gene mutation from one parent, has the working healthy copy of the gene from the other parent, and like the parents, is a healthy carrier. Carrier parents have a 25% chance that their children will inherit the working copy of the gene from each parent and neither carry nor have the disorder (Fig. 7-6). Characteristics of autosomal-recessive inherited disorders and their associated conditions are found in Table 7-2.

X-linked Inheritance. X-linked disorders may be inherited in recessive or dominant patterns. The gene mutation is located on the X chromosome. All males receive an X chromosome from their mother and a Y chromosome from their father for a normal sex constitution of 46,XY. Because males have only one X chromosome, a gene mutation on their X chromosome confers the specific disorder when present in one copy. A female receives one X chromosome from each parent for a normal sex constitution of 46,XX. A female may be a heterozygous, healthy carrier of a recessive gene mutation or affected if the gene mutation is dominant. Either the X chromosome that a female inherits from her mother or the X chromosome she inherits from her father is passed on to her sons as a random event.

X-linked recessive inheritance is the most common pattern of sex-linked traits. A female carrier for an X-chromosome mutation has a 50% chance to pass it on to a son who will be affected or to a daughter who will carry the unexpressed trait like her mother. The female carrier also has a 50% chance to pass on the normal X chromosome to a son who would be normal and to a daughter who would not be a carrier. Duchenne muscular dystrophy, hemophilia, and deutan color blindness are classic X-linked recessive genetic disorders (Lashley, 1998).

An affected female with an X-linked dominant disorder has reproductive outcomes: a 50% chance for passing the gene mutation to a male or female child who will be affected and a 50% chance of giving the working copy of the gene to both who would not be affected. X-linked dominant inherited disorders may be lethal in males who tend to be more severely affected than females because they have only one X chromosome. A rare disorder that exemplifies X-linked dominant transmission is X-linked hypophosphatemia or vitamin D–resistant rickets, a disorder of renal tubular transport. Clinical symptoms include bowed legs, growth deficiency, rickets with ultimate short stature, and possible hearing loss.

The phenomenon of X inactivation—also referred to as *lyonization,* after Mary Lyon who first described it—is a characteristic of X-linked recessive inherited disorders in women (Lashley, 1998). Because female cells have two X chromosomes, one X chromosome is inactivated, or "turned off," to maintain a steady level of X-linked gene expression. Some genes on the X chromosome may escape this process, but most X chromosomes are expressed in only one copy in each cell. X inactivation leads to variations in trait expression among females, which depends on the proportion of cells in which the mutated gene has been inactivated. For example, some females

GENE CHANGES IN CYSTIC FIBROSIS

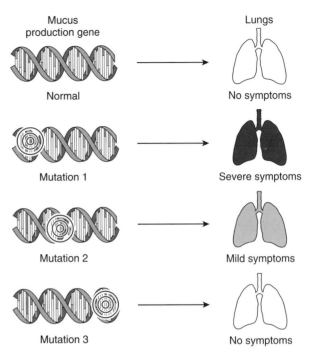

FIGURE 7–7. Different mutations in the same gene can produce a wide range of effects. In cystic fibrosis, for instance, the gene that controls mucus production can have more than 800 different mutations; some cause severe symptoms; some, mild symptoms; and some, no symptoms at all. (From the National Institutes of Health and National Cancer Institute. [1995]. *Understanding gene testing.* [NIH Pub. No. 96-3905]. Washington, DC: U.S. Department of Human Services.)

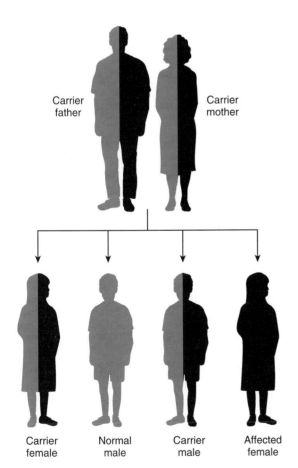

FIGURE 7–6. In diseases associated with altered recessive genes, both parents—although disease-free themselves—carry one normal allele and one altered allele. Each child has one chance in four of inheriting two altered alleles and developing the disorder, one chance in four of inheriting two normal alleles, and two chances in four of inheriting one normal and one altered allele and being a carrier like both parents. (From the National Institutes of Health and National Cancer Institute. [1995]. *Understanding gene testing.* [NIH Pub. No. 96-3905]. Washington, DC: U.S. Department of Human Services.)

who carry the gene for Duchenne muscular dystrophy experience muscle weakness if the normal working gene is predominantly inactivated. Table 7–2 provides characteristics and examples of X-linked inheritance.

Although mendelian inherited disorders can demonstrate a specific pattern of inheritance in some families, many genetic diseases do not follow these simple patterns. Many factors influence how a gene performs and is expressed. Different mutations in the same gene can produce a wide range of symptoms. Such is the case with cystic fibrosis of different severities (Fig. 7–7). Different mutations in several genes can lead to a similar outcome and has been observed with Alzheimer's disease. Some traits involve the simultaneous mutation of two or more genes. A recently observed phenomenon, imprinting, can determine which pair of genes—mother's or father's—will be silenced or activated. Normally, one of an identical pair of alleles from one parent is expressed in the same way as the other of the pair from the other parent. In imprinting, the alleles of a given pair of genes are not expressed in an equivalent manner, depending on the parent of origin. A gene is said to be maternally imprinted if the allele derived from the mother is the one that is silenced or imprinted and is paternally imprinted if the allele contributed by the father is inactivated. Thus, certain genes may be expressed from either maternal or paternal chromosomes, depending on the imprinting. This phenomenon has been observed in Angelman syndrome, a severe form of mental retardation and ataxia (Lashley, 1998).

Multifactorial Genetic Conditions. The cause of many birth defects and common adult-onset health conditions such as arthritis, diabetes, and cancer is multifactorial and complex. Multifactorial genetic conditions are thought to occur as a result of multiple gene mutations and environmental influences that combine to cause birth defects and other diseases. Multifactorial genetic conditions tend to cluster in families but do not follow the characteristic pattern of inheritance seen with mendelian disorders. Table 7-2 provides characteristics of multifactorial genetic conditions.

Neural tube defects (e.g., spina bifida, anencephaly) are an example of a multifactorial genetic condition. In most instances, neural tube defects occur as a result of both genetic and environmental influences that combine during early embryonic development and cause incomplete closure of the neural tube. Less commonly, neural tube defects are a feature of a chromosomal syndrome such as trisomy 18 or result from prenatal exposure to certain medications such as valproic acid.

It is now known that folic acid taken in the prescribed amount of 4 mg daily before conception and during the first 3 months of pregnancy reduces the recurrence of neural tube defects by 70% in women who have had a previously affected pregnancy. Daily folic acid (0.4 mg) taken in the form of a multivitamin is currently recommended for all women in childbearing years to prevent the occurrence of neural tube defects. Folic acid has been shown to be an important environmental element that plays a critical role in fetal development, which influences the outcome of genetic susceptibility to neural tube defects (Centers for Disease Control and Prevention, 1992). Examples of other multifactorial genetic conditions are listed in Table 7-2.

Complex genetic disorders such as diabetes, heart disease, common cancers, autoimmune disorders, and osteoarthritis result from the interplay of environment, lifestyle, and the small effects of many genes. For example, recent research demonstrates that genetics may influence both disease onset and progression in many clients with osteoarthritis. The candidate genes for common forms of osteoarthritis include the vitamin D receptor gene, insulin-like growth factor (IGF)-1 genes, and *COMP* genes. It is likely that that most genes related to osteoarthritis affect disease occurrence in many joints, although there may be specific genes for specific sites.

GENETIC DISORDERS CAUSED BY CHROMOSOME ABNORMALITIES

Alterations in the number or structure of chromosomes are a major cause of birth defects, mental retardation, and malignancies. Chromosomal abnormalities occur in approximately 1 in every 160 live born infants and are present in more than 50% of all spontaneous first trimester miscarriages (Lashley, 1998). Chromosomal abnormalities may involve one or more autosomes, the sex chromosomes, or both. The most common type of chromosomal abnormality, called *aneuploidy,* involves an abnormal chromosome number caused by an extra or missing chromosome. Aneuploidy is always associated with some degree of mental or physical disability or both.

Nondisjunction is the term used to describe failure of paired chromosomes to separate during meiosis. This is the most common cause of aneuploidy. Women who are 35 years of age or older have an increasing risk for aneuploid pregnancies and are therefore offered prenatal testing and counseling. Down syndrome (trisomy 21) is an example of aneuploidy in which there is an extra number 21 chromosome. Having three number 21 chromosomes causes the facial hypertelorism of Down syndrome, mental retardation, congenital heart defects, thyroid, and vision problems. Turner's syndrome is another example of aneuploidy in which girls lack a second X chromosome, which causes them to be of short stature and infertile. Table 7-3 gives examples of common abnormalities of chromosomal number.

Abnormalities may also involve structural rearrangement within or between chromosomes. Less common than aneuploidy, chromosomal rearrangements occur in 1 of every 500 newborns (Gardiner & Sutherland, 1996). A chromosomal rearrangement is said to be "balanced" when the chromosome set contains all of the correct chromosomal material but is arranged in an unusual manner. A chromosomal rearrangement is "unbalanced" when there is missing or extra chromosomal material, such as with deletions or duplication of smaller subchromosomal segments.

People who carry balanced rearrangements usually do not have associated physical or mental problem, yet balanced chromosomal rearrangements can become unbalanced with meiotic division and subsequent reproductive efforts, which may result in physical and/or mental disabilities in offspring or spontaneous pregnancy losses.

TABLE 7–3. *Examples of Chromosomal Abnormalities*

Down syndrome (trisomy 21)
Klinefelter's syndrome (47,XXY)
Turner's syndrome (45,X)

Therefore, known carriers of balanced chromosomal rearrangements are offered prenatal counseling and testing.

Chromosomal analysis requires a tissue sample (e.g., blood, skin, amniotic fluid) with special preparation and staining, which permits chromosomes to be studied under a microscope, a study called *cytogenetics*. Two common indicators for chromosome analysis are to confirm a suspected diagnosis such as Down syndrome or after two or more unexplained spontaneous abortions. Newer laboratory techniques are available that allow for very detailed chromosomal analysis. Fluorescent in situ hybridization (FISH) permits detection of microdeletions and other small abnormalities found in subtle chromosomal rearrangements. Cytogenetics is a rapidly evolving field (Lashley, 1998; Rimoin, Connor, & Pyeritz, 1996).

INCORPORATING GENETICS INTO HEALTH CARE: NURSING RESPONSIBILITIES

New information and understanding of the genetic contribution to health and disease are expanding as genetic discoveries unfold the mysteries of the human genome. Nurses need to become familiar with the basic principles of human genetics to obtain a genetic family history and to be able to explain genetic information to clients. A knowledge of human genetics enables nurses to appropriately refer individuals and families for detailed evaluation and counseling, to provide them with appropriate genetic resources, and to collaborate in client management.

Genetic Counseling and Evaluation Services and Nursing Care

Genetic services are available at local, regional, and national levels and provide genetic information, education, and support to clients and families with current and future genetic health concerns. In each location, genetic professionals (e.g., medical geneticists, genetic counselors, genetics advanced practice nurses) provide specified genetics services to clients and families referred by their primary care providers. Working as a team, genetic specialists obtain and interpret complex family history information, evaluate and diagnose genetic conditions, interpret and discuss genetic test results, and support clients and families throughout the counseling process. Individuals and their families are educated to understand the relevant aspects of genetics to their case, which enables them to make informed health decisions and helps them integrate this genetic information into their daily lives (Lea, Jenkins, & Francomano, 1998).

Nursing is a practice that encompasses all of life's stages. Blending genetics with nursing practice means adding a genetics orientation to nursing care of clients throughout the life span. Nurses and other health care professionals now become responsible for the client's

TABLE 7–4. *Sources of Genetic Information*

Ethnic background	Medical records
Family history	Medical diagnoses
Physical assessment	Client's DNA
Laboratory testing	

From Scanlon, C., & Fibison, W. (1995). *Managing genetic information.* Washington, DC: American Nurses Association.

changing genetic-related health needs over time. Nurses carry out five main activities important to genetics care: (1) help collect and interpret relevant family and medical history, (2) identify clients and families in need of further genetic evaluation and counseling for referral to appropriate services, (3) offer genetic information and resources to clients and families, (4) collaborate with genetic specialists, and (5) participate in management and coordination of care of clients with genetic conditions. A *Statement on the Scope and Standards of Genetics Clinical Nursing Practice* (International Society of Nurses in Genetics, 1998), published by the American Nurses Association, is available to guide nurses in their practice of genetic health care. These standards delineate the responsibilities for all nurses to provide genetic health care.

Genetic information is any information concerning a person's inherited health, that is, a trait, a presymptomatic predisposition, or a heritable disorder, as well as any DNA changes acquired during the person's lifetime (Scanlon & Fibison, 1995). Sources of genetic information are listed in Table 7–4. Issues surrounding genetic information make its management a major challenge. Genetic information can be the basis for social, medical, and economic prejudices and therefore can greatly affect the client and the client's family.

ETHICAL, LEGAL, AND SOCIAL IMPLICATIONS FOR NURSES

Genetic advances demand that all nurses consider their responsibilities in handling genetic information because it has many ethical, legal, and social implications. Ethical genetic issues include privacy, confidentiality, access to and justice in health care, and informed health decisions. These ethical issues are not new to nurses, but their application to genetics clinical practice now and in the future present additional and unique ethical dimensions that require nursing attention (Scanlon & Fibison, 1995). Ethical questions relating to genetics occur in various realms and in all levels of nursing practice. At the level of direct client care, nurses will be involved in offering genetic information, testing, and gene-based therapeutics. Nurses, individually and collectively, premise client care on the values of self-determination and personal autonomy. The code for nurses states "clients should be as fully involved as possible in the planning and implementation of their own health care" (American Nurses Association, 2001). To participate fully, clients need appropriate, accurate, and complete information given at such a level and in such a form that the client and family are able to make their own fully informed personal, medical, and reproductive health decisions. Nurses, as the most omnipresent health care professionals, are invaluable in the informed consent process. Nurses can help clarify clients' values and goals, assess their understanding of information, protect clients' rights, and support clients' decisions. Nurses can advocate for client autonomy in health decisions.

For all of its potential benefits, new genetic testing options also entail multiple risks. Because information is revealed about others through genetic testing, for example, both the decision to be tested and the results can have a tangible effect on the tested person's family. The fact that some family members may not want to know their risks or to have others know the risks has an impact on the tested person's decisions and reactions (Grady, 1998).

The risk of discrimination in health and life insurance, in jobs, and in other areas of life is real and pervasive. Restrictions in life choices, either self-imposed or prescribed by society, are another risk. Self-imposed restrictions may result in missed opportunities for marriage, childbearing, or career choices, which might later be regretted. Restrictions imposed by others (e.g., insurers, employers) may result in frustration, anger, isolation, and despair (Grady, 1998).

Nurses will be involved in ensuring privacy and confidentiality of genetic information derived from such sources as family history assessments, genetic tests, and other genetic interventions. Research has shown that many Americans are increasingly concerned about threats to their personal privacy. Nurses managing genetic information must be aware of the potential ethical issues related to privacy and confidentiality of genetic information and of individual privacy versus family need for genetic information. Equal access to genetic services and treatment is another ethical concern for nurses.

Having an ethical foundation will provide nurses with a framework for handling with integrity those ethical issues that arise. It supplies the basis for communicating genetic information to a client, to a family, to other care providers, to community agencies and organizations, and to society as a whole. It provides support for clinical situations presenting nurses with new moral and ethical dilemmas. Principle-based ethics offers nurses moral guidelines with which to choose and justify nursing practice. The emphasis is on ethical principles of beneficence (to do good) and nonmaleficence (to do no harm) to help solve ethical dilemmas that may arise in clinical care. Respect for persons is the ethical foundation that directs all nursing care. An ethical foundation based on these principles and one that incorporates an ethic of care helps prescribe nursing activities that support clients

and families who are facing genetics-related health and reproductive decisions and consequences (American Nurses Association, 2001; Lea, 2000; Scanlon & Fibison, 1995).

THE CHANGING FACE OF GENETIC-RELATED HEALTH CARE: FUTURE GENETIC TECHNOLOGIES

Biotechnology and genetic discoveries are increasing opportunities for clients, families, and communities to participate in the direction and design of their own health. Individual risk profiling is one example. Individual risk profiling is expected to be at the core of information-based clinical care. Identifying risk proactively opens up new opportunities for health promotion and management. Nurses with their history of providing family-centered and holistic care in all practice settings can help create new dimensions to nursing practice that incorporate theses genetic therapeutics (Lea, 2000).

Gene Chips

One discovery that offers great promise in the area of individual risk profiling is a new technology called *gene chips*. Gene chips are constructed to monitor the entire genome on a single chip so that researchers can have a better view of the interaction among thousands of genes simultaneously (Collins, 1999; DeRisi, Penland, Brown, Bittner, Meltzer, Ray, Chen, Su, & Trent, 1996). Gene chips are being designed for use as diagnostic vices. For example, gene chips are used clinically to detect human immunodeficiency virus sequence variations and to detect cancer gene mutations in breast tissue to help with diagnosis and design of treatment. Use of gene chips holds promise, along with family histories and data from large population studies, for establishing a person's risk of developing common, adult-onset disorders. Obtaining a blood sample and applying it to baseline scan using a gene chip could provide helpful information about a person's risk profile and help direct prevention strategies that could be used (Collins, 1999). Gene chips can also be used to learn more about the association of polymorphisms (genetic changes within a population) with disease, for example, arthritis or osteoporosis. Gene chips can help with understanding the mechanisms that lead to such diseases and monitoring client response to treatment (DNA Microarray [Genome Chip], www.GeneChips.com).

Pharmacogenetics

Individual genotyping will radically alter the way new drugs are developed and marketed. This growing field is called *pharmacogenetics,* a new area of genetics that combines genomics with molecular pharmacology. Pharmacogenetics is the study of how a person's genes determine his or her response to a drug; this knowledge is now being used to tailor therapeutics more effectively and to improve results for clients on clinical trials. With greater understanding of how different genotypes respond to different medications, drugs can become more customized and target those who are most likely to benefit. Testing may be performed, for example, to identify gene mutations in the cytochrome P450 gene, which codes for enzymes that play a major role in the regulation of the way a person's body metabolizes drugs. The ability to distinguish between individuals who are fast and slow drug metabolizers will allow health care providers to more precisely determine appropriate drug doses (Regaldo, 1999).

Gene Therapy

Gene therapy (i.e., the transfer of corrected or altered genes into a person's cells) is believed by many to constitute one of the next major medical advances. Gene therapy is emerging as another revolutionary development in genetic medicine that has the potential to change treatment and management of many genetic disorders. Until recently, it was not possible to correct the underlying malfunctions in protein production that can lead to the development of diseases such as cancer. New applications of gene therapy based on advances in our understanding of the human genome may permit treatment of disease directly at the level of the gene mutation itself. Gene therapy trials for a variety of conditions, including Gaucher's disease, cystic fibrosis, immune deficiencies, and many cancers, are now in progress. Further development will be necessary before gene therapies come into widespread use for a broad spectrum of disorders.

Genetic Engineering

The health benefits from biotechnology and genetic discoveries extend into the realm of genetic engineering. Researchers predict that within the next decade, tissue engineering will grow from a purely research field to applications of tissue engineering including blood products, artificial skin, bioartificial organs, vascular grafts, and cartilage. Society is already accustomed to corrective and replacement parts (e.g., hip and knee replacements, prosthetic limbs). Scientists predict that there will be wide acceptance of bionic parts that increase opportunities for replacement, correction, and enhancement (Zajtchuk, 1999).

GENETIC RESOURCES FOR NURSES AND FAMILIES

To keep pace with the rapidly expanding genetic technologies and their clinical applications, nurses will need to be responsible for their own knowledge. Nurses are expected to use genetic information wisely to mitigate suffering and improve the equality of client, family, and community life (Anderson, Monsen, Prows, Tinley, & Jenkins,

2000). The future challenges of genetic services require that all nurses have a solid understanding of ethical, legal, and social issues; informed consent; privacy; and confidentiality of genetic information—and knowledge of reliable genetic health information for their own professional development and for the clients and families they care for.

The International Society of Nurses in Genetics (ISONG) is a professional nursing society dedicated to the scientific, professional, and personal development of nurses in the management of genetic information. ISONG is developing an infrastructure to ensure that genetic education is disseminated and that this knowledge is increasingly used by nurses around the world (ISONG, www.nursing.creighton.edu/isong). The profession of nursing is responding to the call for increased genetic content in nursing education for current and future delivery of genetic services. A variety of new genetics educational and research resources and opportunities for nurses have become available to support the integration of genetics into their practice. The National Coalition for Health Professional Education in Genetics (NCHPEG) is one example. This interdisciplinary coalition has developed competencies in genetics essential for all health care professionals (NCHPEG, www.nchpeg.org).

The way in which clients communicate with health care providers and access health information is changing with the introduction of new genetic technologies and web-based innovations. One new communication pathway that is developing among clients and health care providers are the self-help groups. The Genetic Alliance is one such well-established group. The Alliance recognizes the importance of peer support and accurate, user-friendly information for those afflicted with genetic disorders. It offers an online directory of support organizations, as well as establishes support groups for conditions that have recently been discovered to have a genetic component (www.geneticalliance.org). Nurses should be aware of these and other important client and professional online resources so that they can access and provide the most up-to-date and reliable genetic information. The "Internet Resources" section in this chapter lists important and reliable web-based genetics resources for nurses and their clients.

SUMMARY

New genetic discoveries are revolutionizing medical approaches to diagnosis, management, and treatment of human disease. These new discoveries require that all nurses become familiar with basic genetic principles and apply them to clinical nursing practice. With this knowledge, nurses will be better prepared to participate in genetic family history and physical assessments, identify those individuals and families in need of further genetic information and services, provide accurate and balanced genetic information, and collaborate in the care of clients and families who are at risk for genetic disorders. New genetic technologies will also affect other important aspects of nursing care. Gene chip technology will create opportunities for individualized genetic profiling, which can identify disease predispositions and begin preventive treatment measures. Pharmacogenomics will alter the way in which new drugs are developed and prescribed. Gene therapy offers hope for a variety of genetic conditions such as autoimmune arthritis and Gaucher's disease, and genetic engineering promises to offer new opportunities for tissue replacement, correction, and enhancement. Nurses and all other health professionals must become familiar with these technologies that are creating new pathways for health promotion, prevention, and management. They must become fluent with associated ethical, legal, and social implications of these new genetic technologies and their applications. Having this knowledge will provide the ethical framework needed to effectively respond to all clients' genetic health needs over their lifetime.

INTERNET RESOURCES

Centers for Disease Control, Office of Genetics & Disease Prevention: www.cdc.gov/genetics; offers information about the effect of genetics research on public health and disease prevention

Genetic Alliance: www.geneticalliance.org; a nonprofit coalition of genetic support groups: includes list of genetic organizations

Human Genome Project Information: www.ornl.gov/hgmis; wealth of information about the Human Genome Project, including ethical, legal, and social issues; has a glossary and good information about genetics

International Society of Nurses in Genetics, Inc. (ISONG): www.nursing.creighton.edu/isong; a professional nursing society dedicated to the scientific, professional, and personal development of nurses in the management of genetic information

March of Dimes: www.modimes.org; provides educational programs for nurses in genetics, Fact Sheets on genetic conditions

National Coalition for Health Professional Education in Genetics (NCHPEG: www.nchpeg.org; offers up-to-date information on national genetics educational initiatives; promotes access and dissemination of genetics information to health care professionals

OMIM: Online Mendelian Inheritance in Man: www.ncbi.nlm.nih.gov/entrez/query.fcgi?db= OMIM

REFERENCES

American Nurses Association. (2001). *Code for nurses with interpretive statements.* Washington, DC: Author.

Anderson, G., Monsen, R. B., Prows, C. A., Tinley, S., & Jenkins, J. (2000). Preparing the nursing profession for participation in a genetic paradigm in health care. *Nursing Outlook, 48,* 23–27.

Baltimore, D. (2001). Our genome unveiled. *Nature, 409,* 814–816.

Centers for Disease Control and Prevention. (1992). Recommendations for the use of folic acid to reduce the number of cases of spina bifida and other neural tube defects. *MMWR Morbidity and Mortality Weekly Report, 41,* 1–7.

Collins, F. S. (1999). Shattuck lecture: Medical and societal consequences of the Human Genome Project. *New England Journal of Medicine, 341,* 28–37.

DiRisi, J., Penland, L., Brown, P. O., Bittner, M. L., Meltzer, P. S., Ray, M., Chen, Y., Su, Y. A., & Trent, J. M. (1996). Use of cDNA microarray to analyze gene expression patterns in human cancer. *Human Genetics, 14,* 457–460.

DNA Microarray (Genome Chip). www.Gene-Chips.com

Gardiner, R. R. M., & Sutherland, G. R. (1996). *Chromosome abnormalities and genetic counseling* (2nd ed.). New York: Oxford University Press.

Grady, C. (1998). Ethics, genetics, and nursing practice. In D. H. Lea, J. Jenkins, & C. A. Francomano (Eds.), *Genetics and clinical practice: New directions for nursing and health care* (pp. 221–246). Boston: Jones and Bartlett.

Hartl, D., & Jones, E. W. (1998). *Genetics principles and analysis* (4th ed.). Boston: Jones and Bartlett.

International Society of Nurses in Genetics, Inc. (1998). *Statement on the scope and standards of genetics clinical nursing practice.* Washington, DC: American Nurses Association.

Lashley, F. R. (1998). *Clinical genetics in nursing practice* (2nd ed.). New York: Springer.

Lea, D. H. (2000). A clinician's primer in human genetics: What nurses need to know. *Nursing Clinics of North America, 35,* 583–614.

Lea, D. H., Jenkins, J. F., & Francomano, C. A. (1998). *Genetics in clinical practice: New directions for nursing and health care.* Boston: Jones and Bartlett.

National Institutes of Health, National Cancer Institute. (1995). *Understanding gene testing.* (NIH Pub No. 96-3905). Washington, DC: U.S. Department of Health and Human Services.

Nussbaum, R. L., McInnes, R. R., & Willard, H. F. (2001). *Thompson and Thompson: Genetics in medicine* (6th ed.). Philadelphia: WB Saunders.

OMIM: Online Mendelian inheritance in man. Available at www.ncbi.nlm.nih.gov/omiim/stats/html

Regaldo, A. (1999). Inventing the pharmacogenomics business. *American Journal of Health-Systems Pharmacology, 56,* 40–50.

Rimoin, D., Connor, J. M., & Pyeritz, R. (1996). *Emery-Rimoin principles and practice of medical genetics* (3rd ed.). New York: Churchill Livingstone.

Scanlon, C., & Fibison, W. (1995). *Managing genetic information.* Washington, DC: American Nurses Association.

Williams, J. K., Prows, C., & Lea, D. H. (2000). Genetics resources for nurses. *Journal of Nursing Education, 39(1),* 45–48.

Wolpert, C. M. (2000). Human genomics in clinical practice: Bridging the gap. *Clinicians Reviews, 10(7),* 67–86.

Zajtchuk, R. (1999). New technologies in medicine: Biotechnology and nanotechnology. *Disease-a-Month, 45,* 449–495.

8

Assessment of the Musculoskeletal System

ANN BUTLER MAHER

ASSESSMENT

Systematic assessment is the basis of professional nursing practice. This chapter focuses on the subjective and objective data specific to the assessment of musculoskeletal problems.

In addition to sports preparticipation physicals and examinations for specific orthopaedic problems, nurses often participate in or perform employment-related assessments. In this context, it is essential to distinguish between a pre-employment evaluation and a preplacement evaluation. A pre-employment evaluation is an examination or inquiry performed before a job is offered. The Americans with Disabilities Act (1990) prohibits pre-employment medical evaluation but does allow physical agility tests as well as inquiries that ask applicants to describe or demonstrate how they will be able to perform essential job-related functions (Geaney, 1993). These inquiries cannot be phrased in terms of an applicant's disability.

A preplacement examination or inquiry is one performed after an offer of employment is made but before assignment to a specific job. The job offer may be conditional on the results of the preplacement evaluation as long as it is required of all potential employees and the exclusionary criteria involve essential functions of the job and do not discriminate against individuals with disabilities (McCrae & Yorker, 1993).

Current employees may be evaluated for fitness to work following an accident or illness. Such examinations evaluate the worker's capability to perform specific job functions without risk to himself or herself or others. Explicit job criteria are essential to adequately assess fitness for work. See Chapter 3 for more information on worker assessment.

INTERVIEW

The musculoskeletal assessment begins with an interview to obtain subjective data. The interview reflects the four subsystems on which comprehensive nursing care is based and asks specific questions to obtain information about the biophysical, psychological, sociologic, and cultural aspects of the patient's life.

General Biographic Data

General biographic data include information about age, gender, ethnicity, occupation, site of residence, and type of residence (all on one floor, stairs required for access).

Biophysical Subsystem

Areas of assessment related to the biophysical system include current and previous health status; the nature of the problem or complaint that prompted the individual to seek care; and the related effects or changes in the areas of mobility, strength, and activities of daily living.

For children, assessment information should include prenatal history, growth and development milestones, and gross and fine motor development (Table 8–1). Birth history data should include abnormal presentation, large for gestational age, or birth injuries. One should also ask about immunizations and history of repeated streptococcal infections.

The nurse discusses activities of daily living with the patient to determine whether changes in functional status have occurred and, if so, over what period such changes have taken place (Box 8–1).

Most commonly, the problem or chief complaint is related to pain, a change in appearance, or a change in

TABLE 8–1. *Expected Motor Development Sequence in Children, Birth to 9 Years of Age*

AGE	FINE MOTOR DEVELOPMENT	GROSS MOTOR DEVELOPMENT
1 month		Turns head to side; keeps knees tucked under abdomen; gross head lag and rounded back when pulled to sitting position
2 months		Holds head in same plane as rest of body; can raise head and hold position
3 months	When supine, puts hands together; holds hands in front of face	Raises head to 45 degrees; may turn from prone to side position; slight head lag when pulled to sitting position
4 months	Grasps rattle; hands held together	Actively lifts head, looks around; rolls from prone to supine position; no head lag when pulled to sitting position; attempts to bear weight when held standing up
5 months	Can reach and pick up object; plays with toes	Able to push up from prone position with forearms and maintain position; rolls over prone to supine to prone; back straight when sitting
6 months	Drops object to reach for another offered; holds rattle or spoon	Sits, posture shaky, uses tripod position; raises abdomen off table when prone; when standing, supports almost full weight
8 months	Transfers object between hands; holds object in each hand	Sits alone, uses hands for support; bounces in standing position; pulls feet to mouth
8 months	Begins thumb-finger grasping	Sits without support
9 months	Bangs objects together	Begins creeping, abdomen off floor; stands holding on when placed in position
10 months	Points with one finger; picks up small objects	Pulls self to standing position, unable to let self down; walks holding onto stable objects
11 months		Walks around room holding onto objects; stands securely, holding on with one hand
12 months	Feeds self with cup and spoon fairly well; offers toy and releases it	Sits from standing posture; twists and turns, maintaining posture; stands without support momentarily
15 months	Puts raisin into bottle; takes off shoes; pulls toys	Walks alone well; seats self in chair
18 months	Holds crayon, scribbles spontaneously	Walks up and down steps holding one hand; some running ability
2 years	Turns doorknob; takes off shoes and socks; builds two-block tower	Walks up stairs alone, two feet on each step; walks backward; kicks ball
30 months	Builds four-block tower; feeds self more neatly; dumps raisin from bottle	Jumps from object; throws ball overhand; walking more stable
3 years	Unbuttons front buttons; copies vertical line within 30 degrees; copies circle; builds eight-block tower	Walks up stairs alternating feet; walks down stairs two feet on each step; pedals tricycle; jumps in one place; performs broad jump
4 years	Copies cross; buttons large buttons	Walks down stairs alternating feet; balances on one foot for 5 seconds
5 years	Dresses self with minimal assistance; colors within lines; draws three-part human	Hops on one foot; catches bounced ball two of three times; heel-toe walking
6 years	Copies square; draws six-part human	Jumps, tumbles, skips, hops; walks straight line; skips rope with practice; rides bicycle; heel-toe walking backward
7 years	Prints well, begins to write script	Skips and plays hopscotch; running and climbing more coordinated
8 years	Mature handwriting skill	Movements more graceful
9 years		Eye-hand coordination developed

Adapted from Bowers, A. C., & Thompson, J. N. (1988). *Clinical manual of health assessment.* St. Louis: Mosby.

BOX 8–1.
Activities of Daily Living (ADL) Assessment

Self-care
Dressing, undressing, clothing
  Keeping clothes in good repair (mending)
  Access to clothes
  Getting into and out of underwear (bra, girdle, under-
    pants, pantyhose, stockings, garter belt)
  Putting on and removing pants
  Getting arms in sleeves
  Managing zippers, buttons, snaps (especially in back), ties
  Putting on socks, shoes, tying laces
  Applying prostheses (e.g., glasses, hearing aids)
Grooming and hygiene
  Washing, drying, brushing hair
  Brushing teeth
  Cleaning and putting in dentures
  Shaving
  Nail care (feet and hands)
  Applying makeup
  Preparing bath water and testing temperature
  Getting into and out of tub, shower
  Reaching and cleaning all body parts
Elimination
  Position altered for urination or sitting on toilet
  Ability to wipe self
  Lowering onto and rising from toilet

Mobility
Difficulty climbing or descending stairs (Is bedroom or
    bathroom on upper level? How many stairs or flights
    to apartment or house?)
Sitting up, rising from bed
Lowering to or rising from chair
Walking (short and long distances); describe necessity for
    walking
Opening doors
Reaching items in cupboards
Necessity for lifting (and any difficulty)

Communication
Dialing telephone
Reading numbers
Hearing over telephone
Answering door
Immediate access to neighbors, help

Eating
Access to market
Preparing food (opening cans, packages, using stove, reach-
    ing dishes, pots, utensils)
Handling knife, fork, spoon (cutting meat)
Getting food to mouth
Chewing, swallowing

Housekeeping, Laundry, House Upkeep
Making bed
Sweeping, mopping floors
Dusting
Cleaning dishes
Cleaning tub, bathroom
Picking up clutter (to patient's satisfaction)
Taking out trash, garbage
Use of basement (stairs, cleaning)
Laundry facilities (in home or near residence, washtub,
    clothesline)
Yard care (garden, bushes, grass)
Other home maintenance concerns (e.g., access to fuse box,
    storm windows, furnace filters, painting)

Medications
Large number of prescriptions
Difficulty remembering
Ability to see labels and directions
Medications kept in one area

Access to Community
Busline
Walking
Driving (self or service from others)
Church, dry cleaning, drugstore, bank, health care facility,
    dentist, other community agencies

Other
Caring for spouse, relative, or companion
Financial management (able to write checks, make
    payments, cash checks)
Care of pet(s)

From Bowers, A. C., & Thompson, J. N. (1988). *Clinical manual of health assessment* (p. 28). St. Louis: Mosby.

function. Questions that may help elicit information about the biophysical subsystem include the following:

1. Is there any part of your body that normally gives you trouble?
2. Tell me about what brought you to the office (clinic, outpatient center, etc.).
3. Have you ever had this problem before?
4. Have you had to make any changes in your daily work schedule (routine)?
5. Are there things that are more difficult to do or that you are unable to do now?

Generally, musculoskeletal problems give rise to a specific array of symptoms (Box 8–2), the various dimensions of which can be delineated using the series of questions outlined in Box 8–3.

The symptom of pain merits special attention in the orthopaedic patient. Has the patient's perceived site of pain moved? If the pain is associated with injury, did it occur at the time of injury or later? Does the patient reposition himself or herself frequently in an attempt to alleviate pain? Is pain affecting the patient's sleep? For a complete discussion of assessment of both acute and chronic pain, see Chapter 5.

The health history takes into account chronic conditions that may directly affect musculoskeletal integrity, such as diabetes and blood dyscrasias. Inflammatory diseases and past infections may have delayed effects on musculoskeletal integrity, often evidenced by changes in posture and movement patterns. The nurse should ask if anyone else in the family has ever had these symptoms or

---

BOX 8–3.

Interview Questions Regarding Symptoms

Chronology
When was the symptom first noted, and what course has it followed?
Was the onset slow, sudden, or insidious?
How long have you had the problem?

Recurrence
Is this the first time you have had the symptom?
If not, how many times and how often has it occurred before?
Under what circumstances does the symptom start?

Location
Where do you feel or notice the symptom?
Does it stay there, or does it (has it) spread to other parts of your body?

Quality
What is it like?
How intense or severe is it?
What makes it better or worse?

Inciting Trauma
Is the symptom related to a previous injury or accident?
If so, what was the nature of the injury or accident?
When did it occur?
Did the symptom arise from one isolated traumatic episode or from several, repeated episodes over time?

Associated Manifestations
What other symptoms are associated with this symptom or problem?

BOX 8–2.

Musculoskeletal Symptomatology

Pain
Deformity
Weakness
Limitations of movement
  Joint stiffness
  Joint locking or unlocking
Abnormally excessive joint movement
  Instability
  Giving way
Swelling
Sensory changes
  Paresthesias
  Referred pain
Vascular changes
  Chronic peripheral ischemic changes, such as white, brittle skin
  Loss of hair
  Abnormal nails on fingers or toes
  Overall color of a limb

---

similar problems. Information about past hospitalizations and surgeries may provide relevant details.

If the patient is a recent immigrant, the nurse should ask about environmental differences between the former home and the current home. For example, rickets may develop in darker-skinned individuals who move to areas with less sunlight without concomitantly increasing their dietary sources of vitamin D.

Information about travel destinations within the past year can be helpful in evaluating exposure to specific diseases (e.g., Lyme disease). Exposure to sexually transmitted diseases (through unprotected sex or by such accidents as needlesticks), as well as diagnosis or treatment for these diseases, should be ascertained because some have musculoskeletal manifestations.

Current and previous use of medications must be identified. Long-term use of steroids leads to osteoporosis and muscle weakness. Anticoagulant use and, to a lesser extent, use of nonsteroidal antiinflammatory drugs, may cause bleeding disorders that contribute to such conditions as hemarthrosis (i.e., bleeding within the joint space). Anticonvulsants are associated with osteomalacia, and phenothiazine use may cause gait disturbances. Exogenous estrogens may delay the progression of osteoporosis.

Other previous therapeutic measures that the patient may have undergone can also be identified. For example, the patient may have had physical or occupational therapy in the past. Previous diagnostic studies are also relevant. The nurse should ask the patient about previous exposure to x rays and tests or procedures specific to musculoskeletal or neurologic problems, such as myelogram, joint aspiration, computed tomography scans, or magnetic resonance imaging.

Psychological Subsystem

The psychological subsystem includes the patient's attitudes toward illness, previous experience with illness and hospitals, body image, self-concept, emotional status, coping style, and knowledge of the specific health problem and the health care system.

If the patient is a child, the parent should be reassured that the staff is reliable and caring and that their primary concern is determining the cause of the child's problem. Every attempt should be made to conduct the examination without producing pain or discomfort. Older children, particularly adolescents, may prefer to be alone with you, away from the parent. The child should be accorded such privacy when possible.

Questions that can assist data collection in this subsystem include the following:

1. Is there anything worrying you right now?
2. Have you ever been in the hospital? What was that like for you?
3. Tell me what you know or have been told about your problem. What is there about your illness or condition that you do not understand or that you find confusing?
4. What concerns you most about your current problem?
5. What is it that you expect from your visit today?

While the patient or parent is responding to your questions, note affect, positioning, and facial expressions. Are these actions consistent with the responses the patient is giving? Silences are important and may indicate that the patient or parent has something he or she wishes to discuss with or tell the nurse but is hesitant to do so. The nurse should allow the silence and not rush on to the next set of questions. It may be helpful to say, "You seem as if you wanted to tell me something more." For a more complete discussion of psychosocial issues, see Chapter 2.

Sociologic Subsystem

The sociologic subsystem primarily concerns the patient's function in roles and groups within the larger social system (family, community, work). Areas for assessment include the patient's role within the family and the patient's occupation. Are there current sources of stress (at home, at work, financially)?

If the primary language of the patient is different from that of the examiner, an interpreter may be necessary. The examiner must be careful to determine that the interpreter understands his or her meaning and that the examiner does not use words that cannot be translated or medical terminology that the interpreter does not understand. For specific guidelines on working effectively with interpreters, see Poss and Rangel (1995). The patient may be able to read and write English better than he or she can speak or understand it. In such cases, a written questionnaire can provide more accurate information.

Types of questions to ask and statements to elicit information about this subsystem include the following:

1. What is your occupation? Describe your work. Are you exposed to hazardous materials (e.g., chemicals) or unsafe conditions (e.g., poor ventilation)? Is appropriate personal protective equipment available (e.g., goggles, hard hats)?
2. Is your current problem interfering with your work responsibilities? Have you lost time from your job because of this problem?
3. Who lives with you? Do you have anyone dependent on you financially?
4. Does anyone else in your family have this problem?
5. Do you have a religious affiliation or spiritual beliefs that prescribe some guidelines for health and management of illness (e.g., dietary practices, prohibition against transfusions)?

Culture and Health

Knowledge of the patient's cultural background is essential because cultural response to disease plays a role in patient expectation and motivation. Assessment of sociologic and cultural factors is often combined. However, with a growing understanding of the integral role that culture plays in influencing behavior, a more comprehensive cultural health assessment may be helpful (Box 8–4).

All cultures have some types of home remedies or traditional healers that they may try before seeking help from nurses or physicians. In a nonjudgmental manner, the nurse should inquire whether any such remedies have been tried, what they entailed, how long they were used, and what results the patient experienced.

It is important to ascertain who makes the decisions within the family. In some cultures, the eldest man makes all decisions and his agreement for further evaluation and testing may be necessary. If the patient is a child, the mother or grandmother may be the one to make the decision.

Eye contact is viewed differently in different cultures. Some cultures view direct eye contact as a sign of

BOX 8–4.
Cultural Health Assessment Guide

Cultural Affiliations
What is your ethnic background, your ancestry?
Where were you born?
How long have you/your parents resided in this country?
What ethnic/cultural group do you identify with or belong to?
What languages do you speak, speak at home?
Are the endemic diseases, health problems, or health benefits known in this group?

Value Orientation
What do you consider important in life, in the upbringing of your family?
What are your aspirations or your dreams? If you can change the way things are, what would that be?

Cultural Practices/Taboos
Give examples of cultural expectations related to male/female, child/adult, single/married, young/old, persons in authority.
Give examples of cultural taboos: dressing, nutrition, actions/behaviors.
Describe cultural expectations related to time, distance/space (touching), communication.

Family/Home Environment
Who lives in your household? How are they related to you? Who constitutes your family?
Are there people who are not blood relatives or immediate family you consider part of your family? Why?
How do people in your household interact with each other: performance of chores, decision making (e.g., school, marriage, health), financial responsibility, conflict management, child care, parenting responsibilities, elder care, obligations to each other?
Tell me what a typical weekday/weekend is like in your household.
Who do you go to when you need something/help? Give an example.
How does patient/family define their economic status?

Communication/Interaction with Others
What is the preferred language at home?
What is the preferred language outside of home? Why?
What is the language you are most comfortable speaking? Why?
What are the differences in communication at home with communication outside (including nonverbal)?

Health Beliefs and Practices
When is one considered sick or ill versus healthy or well? Give an example.
What are some ways that parents/grandparents self-treat illnesses? Give examples.
Who is the preferred healer? Why?
Does family seek professional health care providers? When?
Who makes decisions regarding choice of care providers and when to seek one?
What specific practices/rituals do you and your family observe related to health maintenance or treatment of illnesses (e.g., food, religious, magic/superstition). Give examples.
Give examples of cultural taboos related to health and illness.

Experience with Professional Health Care
Who are the care providers you see? How often? When do you see them?
Who are your preferred professional caregivers? Why?
What are the differences between your own folk/home caregiving and that of professional caregiving?
What experiences with professional caregivers/caregiving were good, unacceptable, or bad? Why?
What accommodations or adjustments were made for your own beliefs and practices?
What adjustments were demanded from you and your family by professional caregivers?

Experience with Outsiders
What were some positive and negative aspects of your experience? Describe these experiences.
How did you learn expectations of outsiders?
What difficulties were encountered in accommodating expectations of others?
What strategies do you use or what resources are available to you to create positive changes in your life?

Courtesy Dula Pacquiao, Ed.D., R.N., Union, NJ. Adapted with permission.

disrespect, and persons from that culture lower their eyes when speaking to a person in authority. The nurse should not misinterpret this behavior.

The nurse must also be alert to the patient who may answer yes to be polite even when he or she does not understand the question. This may be a common response in Vietnamese and Japanese patients in particular.

PHYSICAL EXAMINATION

The second part of the musculoskeletal assessment involves obtaining objective data through physical examination of the patient. While this part of the assessment is being conducted, the patient should be assured privacy and provided a comfortable environment. Rapport developed during the interview further assists the nurse with the physical evaluation aspect of the assessment. The physical examination can be divided into the general overview and the local assessment. A tape measure and goniometer are tools particularly helpful in conducting the physical evaluation of the musculoskeletal system.

General Overview

The general overview focuses on an inspection of the body and includes assessment of both gait and posture. Initially, the nurse observes general appearance, body build, contours, alignment, and symmetry. The patient should sit, stand, walk, and turn around while walking, unless unable to do so. Anatomic terms used to describe specific areas and planes of the body are illustrated in Figure 8–1.

Posture. The nurse evaluates posture unless the patient cannot stand. *Posture* refers to the relative orientation of the body as defined by the composite positions of the various body joints. A posture is correct when stress applied to each joint is minimal. A faulty posture increases stress on the joints. Postural changes occur normally as a child ages (Fig. 8–2), but dorsal kyphosis is typically seen in older persons. Faulty postures are illustrated in Figure 8–3.

Lordosis refers to an excessive backward (posterior) concavity of the spine. It is commonly associated with sagging shoulders, medial rotation of the legs, and exaggerated pelvic angle. Excessive lordosis may result in swayback, in which the lumbosacral spine curves rather sharply, and the thoracolumbar spine exhibits kyphosis. *Kyphosis* refers to an excessive forward (anterior) concavity

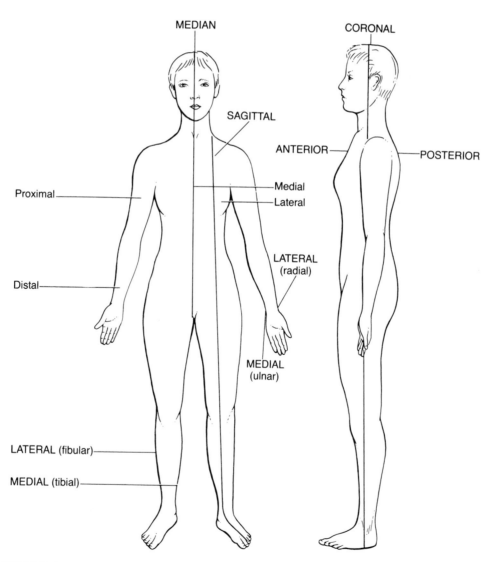

FIGURE 8–1. Anatomic terms. (From Swartz, M. H. [1998]. *Textbook of physical diagnosis* [3rd ed., p. 450]. Philadelphia: WB Saunders.)

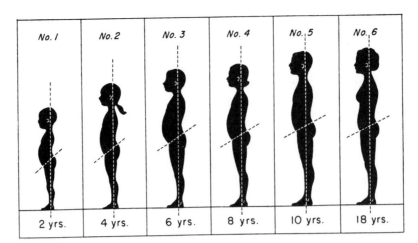

FIGURE 8–2. Postural changes with age. (From McMorris, R. O. [1961]. *Pediatric Clinics of North America, 8,* 214.)

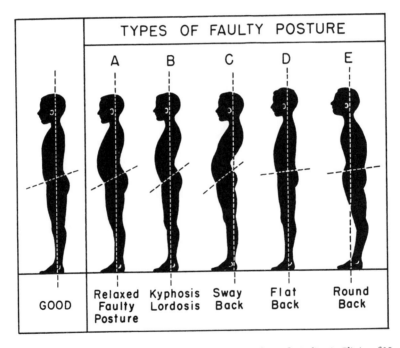

FIGURE 8–3. Types of faulty posture. (From McMorris, R. O. [1961]. *Pediatric Clinics of North America, 8,* 217.)

of the spine. It usually involves the thoracic aspect of the spine.

Scoliosis is a lateral curvature of the spine, of which there are several types. It occurs most frequently in the thoracic region, but it may also be identified in the thoracolumbar junction or the lumbar spine. Scoliosis of the cervical spine is called a *torticollis.* Scoliosis is discussed in detail in Chapter 17.

Postural problems rarely occur in isolation. They are usually accompanied by other symptoms (e.g., pain). Aside from the general orthopaedic history, other factors may provide clues to postural problems, including the following (Magee, 1997):

1. Family history of back problems
2. Age at which growth spurt occurred
3. Onset of menarche in females (the point at which two thirds of adolescent growth spurt is completed)
4. Voice change in males
5. Difficulty in fitting clothes
6. Breathing difficulties
7. Hand dominance

The nurse should observe the patient from anterior, lateral, and posterior perspectives while the individual is standing, flexing forward (at the waist), and sitting. The patient should also be observed while he or she is lying in both supine and prone positions. During these maneuvers, the nurse should note postural deviations and any abnormally protruding or sunken areas.

Gait. Normal gait involves two phases: stance and swing. The *stance* (weight-bearing) phase begins with the *heel strike,* in which the foot makes initial contact with the ground surface and weight is transferred from the contralateral foot. From there, *foot flat* and then *midstance* occur, representing the gradual redistribution of weight evenly across the foot as the body's center of gravity becomes placed directly over the foot. With continued forward movement, *pushoff* occurs and weight is gradually transferred back to the contralateral foot.

The *swing* (non–weight-bearing) phase begins with *acceleration,* during which the foot is lifted off the ground and begins an arc of movement forward. In *midswing,* the foot gradually completes its arc of movement past the opposite leg. It finally reaches *deceleration,* in which the foot is placed forward from the outstretched leg in preparation for heel strike.

There are normal age variations in gait. Toddlers may exhibit an exaggerated lumbar curve and wide-based stance as they learn to walk and run. Arms are held out for balance, and weight bearing is on the inside of the foot. After age 3, the base narrows and the arms are closer to the sides. Weight bearing shifts, with shoes wearing primarily on the outside of the heel and the inside of the toe.

Gait patterns change with aging and are more apparent after age 85. Older women have a narrower base and a waddling gait, whereas men develop a wider-based gait. The older man's walk is characterized by less arm swinging, shorter steps, and decreased steppage height. Both men and women have slower walking speed and spend more time in the stance phase than the swing phase of gait.

Abnormal gaits are the result of both musculoskeletal and neurologic problems. Table 8–2 describes common abnormal gaits.

Local Examination

The local examination is integrated with assessments of range of motion (ROM) and muscle function. Each area should be inspected for symmetry, nodules or masses, swelling (soft tissue or joint), deformities, redness, and variations in skin color. The nurse should palpate for tenderness, warmth, skin texture, bone continuity, abnormal mobility, bone or joint crepitus, and muscle weakness or hyperactivity.

Range of Motion. There are six basic types of joint motion:

1. Flexion and extension
2. Dorsiflexion and plantar flexion
3. Adduction and abduction
4. Inversion and eversion
5. Internal and external rotation
6. Pronation and supination

In addition, the shoulder can also demonstrate circumduction. Figure 8–4 illustrates these motions.

TABLE 8–2. *Abnormal Gaits*

GAIT	CAUSE	DESCRIPTION
Antalgic	Multiple disorders	Pain or discomfort in the lower extremity on weight bearing; bears weight on affected extremity as little as possible; shortened stride
Ataxic	Neurogenic (cerebellar)	Staggering, uncoordinated gait; sway may be evident
Festinating	Neurogenic (Parkinson's disease)	Body held rigidly with neck, trunk, and knees flexed; delayed start with short, quick, shuffling steps; speed may increase with distance as if individual unable to stop (festination)
Short leg	Structural (DDH, DJD, fracture)	Leg length discrepancy of 1 in. or more; walks with a limp unless corrective footwear worn
Spastic	Neurogenic (cerebral palsy, hemiplegia)	Jerky, uncoordinated movement; short steps with dragging or scraping of foot; crossed-knee (scissors) gait
Steppage	Neurogenic (peroneal nerve injury or paralyzed dorsiflexor muscles)	Increased hip and knee flexion in order for foot to clear the floor; foot slaps down and along ground; footdrop is evident
Trendelenburg	Myogenic (DDH, coxa plana)	Associated with positive Trendelenburg test—pelvis drops on normal side when patient bears weight on affected side; with bilateral weakness, there is an accentuated side-to-side movement (ducklike waddle) to keep the center of gravity over the stance

DDH, developmental dysplasia of the hip; DJD, degenerative joint disease.

Adapted from Salmond, S. W., Mooney, N. E., & Verdisco, L. A. (1991). *Core curriculum for orthopaedic nursing* (2nd ed.). Pitman, NJ: National Association of Orthopaedic Nurses. Adapted with permission.

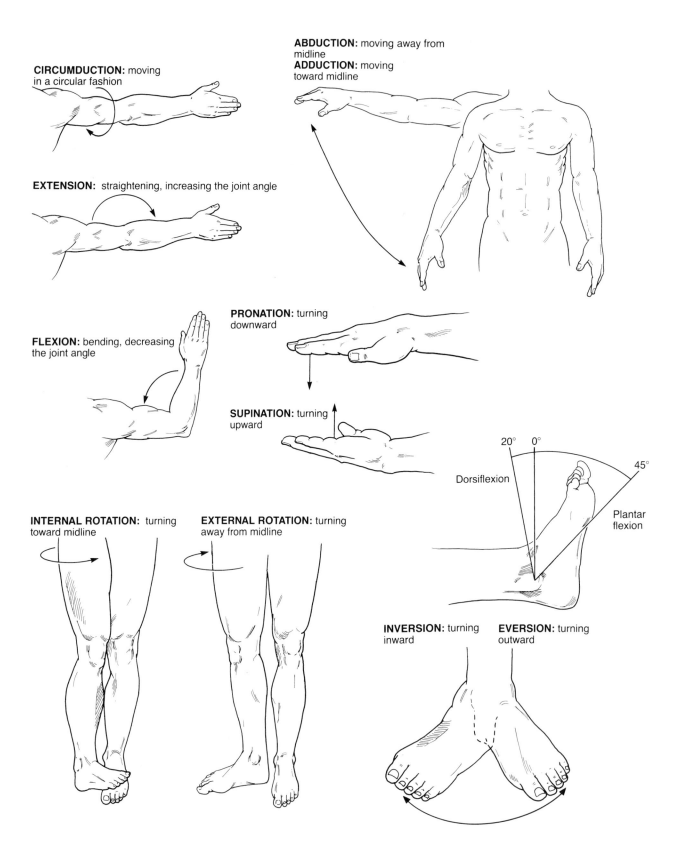

CIRCUMDUCTION: moving in a circular fashion

EXTENSION: straightening, increasing the joint angle

FLEXION: bending, decreasing the joint angle

ABDUCTION: moving away from midline
ADDUCTION: moving toward midline

PRONATION: turning downward

SUPINATION: turning upward

INTERNAL ROTATION: turning toward midline

EXTERNAL ROTATION: turning away from midline

20°   0°
Dorsiflexion
45°
Plantar flexion

INVERSION: turning inward

EVERSION: turning outward

FIGURE 8–4. Joint movements.

Both passive and active movements should be evaluated. Passive ROM requires that the patient keep the muscles relaxed while the examiner moves the joint. Active ROM requires that patients use their own muscles for movement.

Passive ROM usually equals active ROM except when there is paralysis of muscles or ruptured tendons. As the joint moves through ROM, any stiffness, clicking, or limitation of movement should be noted. Box 8–5 shows normal ROM of specific joints, measured in degrees of a circle with the joint as the center. When joint mobility is limited abnormally, the examiner should use a goniometer to measure the arc of movement, in degrees, of the affected joint (Fig. 8–5).

Muscle Function. Muscles are assessed for bulk, strength, tone, and nature of muscle contraction. This evaluation can be hampered considerably when ROM is decreased or contracture or pain is present. The nurse should inspect the muscle mass for atrophy, always comparing it with the contralateral limb. Is there any muscle hypertrophy not associated with exercise? Muscle strength is evaluated by having the patient move actively against resistance. Table 8–3 presents the Lovett scale, a commonly used grading scale.

Muscle tone is the slight residual tension in a voluntarily relaxed muscle. While putting the muscle through

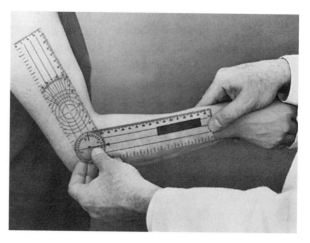

FIGURE 8–5. Use of the goniometer to measure elbow motion. (From Reider, B. [1999]. *The orthopaedic physical examination* [p. 11]. Philadelphia: WB Saunders.)

passive ROM, the nurse should evaluate for spasticity, hyperreflexia, or fasciculations, always comparing one side with the other.

Remember that decreased strength in older persons is caused by decreased muscle mass, so changes in this area should be anticipated during the physical evaluation.

BOX 8–5.
Normal Range of Motion (Shown in Degrees)

Cervical Spine
Flexion: 80–90
Extension: 70
Side flexion: 20–45
Rotation: 70

Thoracic Spine
Forward flexion: 20–45
Extension: 25–45
Side flexion: 20–40
Rotation: 35–50
Costovertebral expansion*
Rib motion*

Lumbar Spine
Forward flexion: 40–60
Extension: 20–35
Side flexion: 15–20
Rotation: 3–18

Shoulder
Elevation through abduction: 170–180
Elevation through forward flexion: 160–180
Lateral rotation: 80–90
Medial rotation: 60–100
Hyperextension: 50
Adduction: 50
Horizontal adduction and abduction: 130
Circumduction: 200

Elbow
Flexion: 140–150
Extension: 0–10
Supination (forearm): 90
Pronation (forearm): 80–90

Wrist
Abduction (radial deviation): 15
Adduction (ulnar deviation): 30–45
Flexion: 80–90
Extension: 70
Pronation (forearm): 85–90
Supination (forearm): 85–90

Hip Flexion: 110–120
Extension: 10–15
Abduction: 30–50
Adduction: 30
Lateral rotation: 40–60
Medial rotation: 30–40

Knee
Flexion: 0–135
Extension: 0–15
Medial rotation (of tibia on femur): 20–30
Lateral rotation (of tibia on femur): 30–40

Ankle
Plantar flexion: 50
Dorsiflexion: 20
Supination: 45–60
Pronation: 15–30

*Maneuvers other than measuring arcs of motion are used for assessment in these instances.

TABLE 8–3. *Grading Muscle Strength—Lovett Scale*

0	ZERO (0)	NO PALPABLE CONTRACTION OF MUSCLE
1	Trace (T)	Palpable contraction of muscle; no joint motion
2	Poor (P)	Complete ROM with gravity eliminated
3	Fair (F)	Complete ROM against gravity; no added resistance
4	Good (G)	Complete ROM against gravity; some added resistance
5	Normal (N)	Complete ROM against gravity with full resistance

ROM, range of motion.

TABLE 8–4. *Peripheral Vascular Assessment Parameters*

	NORMAL	INADEQUATE ARTERIAL SUPPLY	INADEQUATE VENOUS RETURN
Color	Pink	Pale or white	Blue (cyanotic), mottled
Temperature	Warm	Cool	Hot
Capillary refill	1–2 s	>2 s	Immediate
Tissue turgor (edema)	Full	Hollow or prunelike	Distended or tense

Adapted from Sermeus, S. M. (1984). Reconstructive microsurgery: High-tech, high-touch nursing. *Orthopaedic Nursing, 3*(2), 12. Reprinted with permission.

This decreased mass does not generally interfere with activities of daily living, however, because it occurs gradually and the individual adapts to compensate for the loss.

Neurovascular Assessment. The neurovascular assessment includes assessment of peripheral circulatory and peripheral neurologic integrity. When doing a routine physical assessment or obtaining baseline information, the nurse should always compare one side with the other for consistency. When evaluating an extremity after injury or suspected damage, the nurse should check the unaffected side first and use that as the baseline. On an injured extremity, findings distal and proximal to the site of the injury should be compared.

To evaluate peripheral vascular integrity, the color, capillary refill time, temperature, presence of peripheral pulses, and degree of swelling in the body part should be checked. The dorsum (back) of the hand can be used to evaluate temperature (Table 8–4). Pulse points that should be included are brachial, radial, ulnar, femoral, popliteal, posterior tibialis, and dorsalis pedis. To evaluate peripheral neurologic integrity, both sensation and motion must be assessed. Figure 8–6 outlines the techniques for evaluating the major nerve function in the upper extremity (radial, ulnar, and median nerves) and the lower extremity (peroneal and tibial nerve). The patient should close the eyes while sensation is being checked. Touching the digits lightly, for example, should be perceptible to the patient if sensation is normal. If the patient complains of paresthesias, or a "pins-and-needles" feeling, further evaluation is warranted.

The patient should be able to demonstrate active movement of a specific joint when requested to do so. Passive ROM of digits or toes that elicits pain or increased

pain in the arm or leg is a symptom of compartment syndrome and requires immediate targeted assessment. For a complete discussion of compartment syndrome, see Chapter 10.

When casting material does not allow for palpation of peripheral pulses, observation of edema formation, or joint movement, the nurse relies on the remaining parameters of the neurovascular assessment, such as color, temperature, sensation, and pain. These still provide adequate indication of the status of neurovascular integrity.

Once the neurovascular assessment is complete, the nurse must document the findings. When possible, as in the case of elective surgery, the nurse should identify baseline findings pertinent to the neurovascular assessment. These findings then serve as the basis for comparison for changes that may occur later in the patient's clinical course.

Head-to-Toe Assessment. In the progression from head to toe, ROM, muscle strength, and sensation are assessed. Where bilateral movement is to be evaluated, the unaffected side should be checked first if an abnormality is present or suspected. In this way, the examiner establishes the baseline for normal function between bilateral joints.

The nursing examination initially focuses on the patient's active movements to discover where function may be disrupted. If any disruption is noted, passive movements followed by resisted isometric movements are performed. If ROM is not full for any given joint (or joint complex, as in the spine), care must be taken to prevent the patient from experiencing further injury or aggravation of symptoms. Table 8–5 outlines specific tests performed, as well as their purpose, technique, and findings.

Text continued on page 210

Peroneal Nerve

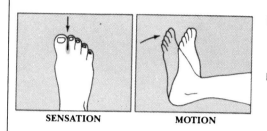

- ☐ **SENSATION**
  Prick the web space between the great toe and second toe
- ☐ **MOTION**
  Have patient dorsiflex ankle and extend toes at the metatarsal phalangeal joints

Tibial Nerve

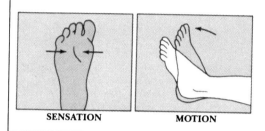

- ☐ **SENSATION**
  Prick the medial and lateral surfaces of the sole of the foot
- ☐ **MOTION**
  Have patient plantar flex ankle and toes

Radial Nerve

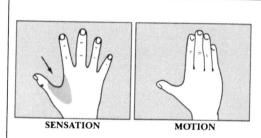

- ☐ **SENSATION**
  Prick the web space between the thumb and index finger
- ☐ **MOTION**
  Have patient hyperextend thumb then wrist and hyperextend the four fingers at the MCP joints

Ulnar Nerve

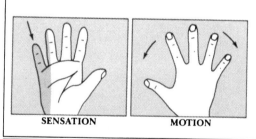

- ☐ **SENSATION**
  Prick the distal fat pad of the small finger
- ☐ **MOTION**
  Have patient Abduct all fingers

Median Nerve

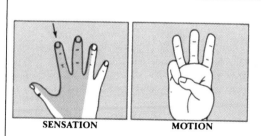

- ☐ **SENSATION**
  Prick the distal surface of the index finger
- ☐ **MOTION**
  Have patient oppose thumb and small finger; note whether patient can flex wrist

FIGURE 8–6. Neurovascular assessment of the upper and lower extremities. MCP, metacarpophalangeal. (From Stearns G. M., & Brunner, N. A. [1987]. *Operative care* [Vol. 1, p. 89]. Rutherford, NJ: Howmedica.)

TABLE 8–5. *Tests of Musculoskeletal Function*

SITE AND TEST OR SIGN	PURPOSE	TECHNIQUE	FINDINGS	COMMENTS
Shoulder				
Adson's maneuver	Evaluates blood flow in subclavian artery; tests for thoracic outlet syndrome	Palpate radial artery while abducting, extending, and externally rotating the arm; have patient take a deep breath and turn head toward arm being tested	*Negative:* Pulse remains strong *Positive:* Marked decrease or loss of radial pulse during the test	Blood flow can be compromised by cervical rib, tumor, hematoma, or infection that has tightened neck muscles Pulse may be diminished somewhat in negative test
Apley's scratch test	Evaluates shoulder ROM	1. Have the patient reach behind the head and touch the top of the opposite scapula 2. Have the patient reach behind the back and touch the bottom of the opposite scapula	Inability to perform as instructed indicates less than normal ROM for shoulder	Limited ROM decreases functional ability (e.g., combing hair, pulling up a zipper, placing something in a back pocket)
Drop arm test	Evaluates for rotator cuff tear	Examiner abducts patient's shoulder to 90 degrees; instructs the patient to slowly lower the arms to the side (see Fig. A)	*Negative:* Able to comply with instructions *Positive:* Arm drops suddenly, or severe pain is felt in shoulder as arm is lowered	Positive test indicates tear in rotator cuff

A, Drop arm test.*

SITE AND TEST OR SIGN	PURPOSE	TECHNIQUE	FINDINGS	COMMENTS
Elbow				
Tennis elbow test	Evaluates for lateral epicondylitis	Examiner holds patient's elbow (thumb on lateral epicondyle); pronates the patient's forearm, flexes the wrist fully, and extends the elbow	*Negative:* No pain *Positive:* Pain over lateral epicondyle of the humerus	Lateral epicondylitis is commonly seen in individuals who work at computers (word processing, data entry)

Wrist and Hand

Finkelstein's test	Test for de Quervain's disease (tenosynovitis of the thumb)	Patient makes a fist with the thumb inside the fingers; examiner holds the patient's forearm steady and deviates the wrist toward the ulnar side	*Negative:* No pain with maneuver *Positive:* Patient feels pain over abductor pollicis longus and extensor pollicis longus tendons	Test may cause some discomfort in normal individuals, so compare pain caused on affected side relative to normal side

Lumbar Spine

Gaenslen's test	Evaluates sacroiliac joint pathology	*Method 1:* Patient lies on side with upper leg (test leg) hyperextended at the hip; patient holds the lower leg flexed against the chest; examiner stabilizes the pelvis and extends the hip of the upper leg *Method 2:* Patient lies supine with one buttock off the edge of the examining table; patient flexes both legs to chest, then slowly extends the test leg (the leg off the table)	*Negative:* No pain in sacroiliac area with extension of test leg *Positive:* Pain in sacroiliac area when test leg hyperextended	Positive tests can be caused by an ipsilateral sacroiliac joint lesion, hip pathology, or an L4 nerve root lesion
Straight leg raising (Lasègue's test)	Evaluate for presence of HNP	*Involved leg:* Patient is supine; examiner passively raises leg with knee extended until pain is felt; leg is then extended slowly until there is no pain or tightness; examiner dorsiflexes the patient's foot *Uninvolved leg:* Patient is supine and leg is raised in manner described above (see Fig. B)	*Negative:* No pain *Positive:* Pain with dorsiflexion of foot *Positive:* Pain in opposite leg (not test leg) strongly suggests HNP	Pain in posterior thigh indicates hamstring tightness; pain down entire leg indicates sciatic nerve involvement

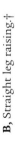

B, Straight leg raising.†

---

*From Wittert, D. D. (1986). *Orthopaedic Nursing 5*(4), 20.
†From Magee, D. J. (1992). *Orthopedic physical assessment* (2nd ed.). Philadelphia: WB Saunders.

Table continued on following page

TABLE 8–5. *Tests of Musculoskeletal Function Continued*

SITE AND TEST OR SIGN	PURPOSE	TECHNIQUE	FINDINGS	COMMENTS
Hoover's test	Helps determine whether patient has genuine weakness in one leg (due to lumbar spine pathology) or may be a malingerer	Patient lies supine; examiner cups patient's heels in his hands; patient is asked to raise the weak leg	*Negative:* When attempting to raise one leg, downward pressure is normally felt on the other *Positive:* When weak leg raising is attempted and other foot does not press downward, at least some of weakness is feigned	
Milgram's test	Evaluate for HNP	Patient lies supine and raises legs about 2 inches off the examining table	*Negative:* Patient able to hold legs off table for 30 s *Positive:* Patient unable to hold position for 30 s	
Trendelenburg test	Tests strength of gluteus medius muscle	Patient is standing with back to examiner; examiner observes the dimples over posterior iliac spines, which should be equal when the patient's weight is distributed evenly; examiner has patient lift one foot off the ground (see Fig. C)	*Negative:* Pelvis on unsupported side elevates *Positive:* Pelvis on unsupported side remains in place or drops	Patient with positive test has characteristic ducklike gait (see Table 8–2)

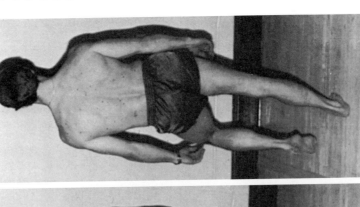

Negative   Positive

C, Trendelenburg test.†

Hip

Ortolani's maneuver	Evaluates for developmental dysplastic hip (DDH)	Infant in supine position with hips flexed; abduct and externally rotate thighs; pressure is applied against greater trochanters of femur (see Fig. D)	*Negative:* External rotation is smooth, without sound *Positive:* Feel or hear a click as the femoral head slides over the acetabular rim	Valid for only first few weeks after birth; should not be repeated too often because it can potentially cause damage to articular cartilage of femoral head

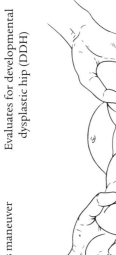

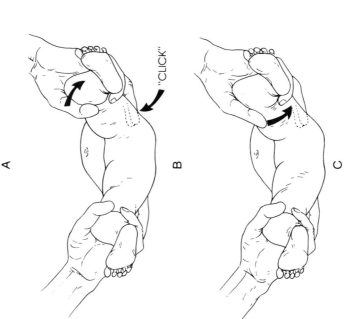

D, Ortolani's sign and Barlow's test. In the newborn, both hips can be equally flexed, abducted, and externally rotated without producing a click.† *A,* Normal. *B,* Ortolani's sign or Barlow's test, first part. *C,* Barlow's test, second part.

†From Magee, D. J. (1992). *Orthopedic physical assessment* (2nd ed.). Philadelphia: WB Saunders.

Table continued on following page

TABLE 8–5. *Tests of Musculoskeletal Function* Continued

SITE AND TEST OR SIGN	PURPOSE	TECHNIQUE	FINDINGS	COMMENTS
Barlow's test	Evaluates for DDH	Perform Ortolani's maneuver as shown in Figure D; then examiner uses the thumb to exert pressure backward and outward on inner thigh	*Positive:* If femoral head slips out over posterior rim of acetabulum and reduces when pressure is removed, hip is "unstable"; it is not dislocated, but is dislocatable	Use for infants up to 6 months; do not repeat too often as it may cause dislocated hip as well as damage to head of femur
Patrick's test	Determines whether there is limitation of ROM at hip joint	Patient lies supine with heel of test leg placed on opposite knee; examiner lowers test leg in abduction toward examining table	*Negative:* (normal result) test leg falls to table or is parallel with opposite leg *Positive:* Test leg remains higher than opposite leg; may be pain in inguinal area (hip problem) or in sacroiliac area (sacroiliac problem)	FABER; decreased ROM can be caused by problem at hip joint or iliopsoas spasm
Leg Leg length discrepancy	Determines whether one leg is shorter than the other	*True leg length:* Patient lies supine; examiner measures from a fixed point (anterior iliac spine) to medial malleolus (fixed point) (see Fig. E) *Apparent leg length:* Patient lies supine; examiner measures from a nonfixed point (umbilicus) to medial malleolus (fixed point)	*Normal:* Measurements should be equal or within 1 cm *Abnormal:* Greater than 1 cm difference equals true bone discrepancy *Positive:* True leg length equal; apparent leg length unequal	Determine whether true leg length discrepancy is above or below the knee; if apparent leg length is unequal, further evaluate for pelvic obliquity or adduction or flexion deformity of hip
Knee Drawer test	Evaluates ligament stability in knee	*Anterior test:* Patient lies on back; knee flexed to 90 degrees and hip to 45 degrees; examiner holds foot of test leg in place and draws tibia forward on femur; (examiner's hands are around the tibia with the thumbs on the medial and lateral joint lines of knee [see Fig. F])	*Negative:* Movement ≤6 mm *Positive:* Movement >6 mm indicates tear in ACL	Assure that PCL is not injured, or anterior drawer test may be false positive; if PCL injury suspected, check for posterior sag sign (gravity drawer test)

E, Measuring true leg length.‡

Knee *Continued*

Drawer test *Continued*

Posterior test: Position patient as above; tibia is pushed back on femur

Negative: Tibia does not move back

Positive: Feel and observe backward movement of tibia; indicates injury to PCL

Positive: Tibia sags back on the femur; indicates PCL is torn

Gravity test: (posterior sag sign); patient lies supine with hips flexed to 45 degrees, and knees to 90 degrees (see Fig. G)

With minimal swelling, sag is very evident; there is obvious concavity distal to the patella

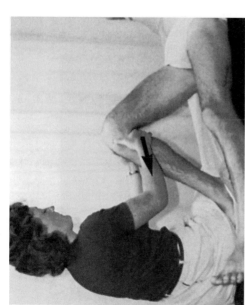

F, Position for drawer sign.†

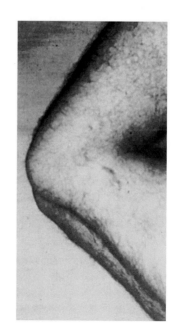

G, Posterior sag sign.§

†From Magee, D. J. (1992). *Orthopedic physical assessment* (2nd ed.). Philadelphia: WB Saunders.
‡From Jarvis, C. (1992). *Physical examination and health assessment.* Philadelphia: WB Saunders.
§From O'Donoghue, D. H. (1984). *Treatment of injuries to athletes.* Philadelphia: WB Saunders.

Table continued on following page

TABLE 8–5. *Tests of Musculoskeletal Function Continued*

SITE AND TEST OR SIGN	PURPOSE	TECHNIQUE	FINDINGS	COMMENTS
Genu valgum	Assesses for knock-knees	Measure space between medial malleoli when knees are together	*Negative:* Less than 10 cm space *Positive:* More than 10 cm space	Physiologic genu valgum most pronounced by 3-4 years old and resolves by 7 years old
Genu varus	Assesses lateral bowing of legs	Measure space between knees when medial malleoli are together; patient stands facing examiner	*Negative:* Less than 4 cm space *Positive:* More than 4 cm space persistently	Normal for child until about 18 months old
Lachman's test	Evaluates injury to ACL	Patient lies supine with knees between full extension and 30 degrees; one hand stabilizes femur and other hand moves tibia forward (see Fig. H)	*Positive:* When tibia moves forward, infrapatellar tendon slope disappears	This test is the best indicator for ACL injury

INFRAPATELLAR TENDON SLOPE

STABILIZE

H, Hand position for Lachman's test.†

208

| McMurray's test | Evaluates for medial and lateral meniscus injury | Patient lies supine with injured leg fully flexed; examiner cups heel with one hand and places other hand on the knee (fingers on medial joint line, thumb on lateral joint line) and rotates the tibia medially, changing the degrees of flexion; then rotates the tibia laterally repeatedly, changing the degrees of flexion (see Fig. I) | Positive: If a snap, or click is heard, there is probably a meniscal tear | Evaluation of meniscal injuries is difficult and requires considerable experience; because menisci have no blood or nervous supply, there may be no pain or swelling with injury |

Medial meniscus

Lateral meniscus

I, McMurray's test.†

---

†From Magee, D. J. (1992). *Orthopedic physical assessment* (2nd ed.). Philadelphia: WB Saunders.
ACL, anterior cruciate ligament; DDH, developmental dysplastic hip; FABER, flexion, abduction, and external rotation; HNP, herniated nucleus pulposus; PCL, posterior cruciate ligament; ROM, range of motion.

REFERENCES

Americans with Disabilities Act. (1990). 42 USC 12101.

Geaney, J. H. (1993). Medical examinations under the Americans with Disabilities Act. *New Jersey Medicine, 90*(1), 36–38.

Jarvis, C. (2000). *Physical examination and health assessment.* (3rd ed.). Philadelphia: WB Saunders.

Magee, D. J. (1997). *Orthopedic physical assessment* (3rd ed.). Philadelphia: WB Saunders.

McCrae, J. C., & Yorker, B. (1993). Update on the Americans with Disabilities Act for occupational health nurses. *AAOHN Journal, 41,* 250–258.

Poss, J. E., & Rangel, R. (1995). Working effectively with interpreters in the primary care setting. *Nurse Practitioner, 20*(12), 43–48.

Reider, B. (1999). *The orthopaedic physical examination.* Philadelphia: WB Saunders.

BIBLIOGRAPHY

Boyd, R. J. (1995). Evaluation of back pain. In A. M. Goroll, L. A. May, & A. G. Mulley (Eds.), *Primary care medicine* (3rd ed.). Philadelphia: Lippincott.

Hoffman, H., & Guidotti, T. L. (1994). Basic clinical skills in occupational medicine. *Primary Care, 21,* 225–236.

Matson, C. C., Holleman, W. L., Nosek, M., & Wilkinson, W. (1993). Impact of the Americans with Disabilities Act on family physicians. *Journal of Family Practice, 36,* 201–206.

Rauscher, N. A. (1996). Musculoskeletal assessment. In S. W. Salmond, N. E. Mooney, & L. A. Verdisco (Eds.), *Core curriculum for orthopaedic nursing* (3rd ed.). Pitman, NJ: National Association of Orthopaedic Nurses.

9

Diagnostic Modalities for Orthopaedic Disorders

JANE E. SMITH

Diagnosis of orthopaedic conditions is accomplished through a variety of modalities. This chapter focuses on those procedures used most frequently in the care of the orthopaedic client. Elements included in the explanation of these modalities are definition; history; equipment; specific indications; and preprocedure, intraprocedure, and postprocedure care. A summary of the nursing considerations is presented in Table 9–1.

RADIOGRAPHIC STUDIES

The use of radiographs and other radiographic studies in conjunction with the client's history and clinical presentation has greatly improved the care provided in the field of medicine and the specialty of orthopaedics. As we begin the new millennium, the costs of these diagnostic tests will come under more scrutiny. Hillman (1997) stated that diagnostic imaging has led to approximately 50% of the increases in health care costs during the past decade. Evidence-based practice and national guidelines are guiding best practice in the field of radiology. Collaboration between the health care provider and the radiologist is becoming more important because managed care is affecting reimbursements. Discussion with the radiologist can eliminate inappropriate testing, enhance information gained from the history and physical examination, and help evaluate imaging modalities.

Definition

An *x ray* is a high-energy photon beam. When an electrically produced electron beam is focused on a metal target, the atoms of the target absorb the electrons and produce an x ray. The x-ray beam can in turn be modified to provide a visual picture called a *roentgenogram*.

History

"I have discovered something interesting, but I do not know whether or not my observations are correct" (American College of Radiology, 1993). These are the words of Wilhelm Conrad Roentgen in 1895. He made the discovery that a specific ray could see through skin and the underlying tissues and project an image of bone. Since the year of his initial discovery, scientists have expanded and refined the field of radiology.

Equipment

The x-ray machine serves as the electron source, controlling amperage, voltage, and exposure time. The device that produces the fast-moving electrons is the x-ray tube. A lead-shielded window and a lead tube casing provide the housing for the x-ray tube, allowing only a small fraction of the x rays through the portal. The intricate details of the tube and the circuitry responsible for producing electrons are not within the scope of this text.

Two properties of x-rays significant to diagnostic radiology are their fluorescence and photosensitization. Accessories that make radiography possible include the various types of x-ray film, x-ray cassettes with their enclosed intensifying screen, and conventional cassettes contained within a plastic or cardboard film holder. In addition, the following improvements have made the use of x-rays more precise: the stationary and moving grids and various cones, apertures, and adjustable diaphragms for delimiting the x-ray beam. Various contrast media are employed in several radiographic examinations.

The fluoroscopic screen is commonly used by the radiologist to convert x-rays to visible light rather than to ultraviolet light. The image is immediately visualized on a television monitor. However, the image is not as clearly delineated as the photographic image on the x-ray film.

TABLE 9–1. *Overview of Nursing Considerations*

DIAGNOSTIC MODALITY	NURSING CONSIDERATIONS
Radiology	No special preparation is needed.
Computed tomography (CT)	Determine patient allergies and patient claustrophobia. Contraindicated in pregnancy. Remove jewelry and metal objects. If contrast material involved, signed consent form may be necessary.
Magnetic resonance imaging (MRI)	Patients with pacemakers, electric neurostimulators, and intracranial aneurysm clips are excluded from MRI. Determine patient claustrophobia. Convert IVs to heparin locks. Pregnant patients are usually excluded in first trimester. Remove all jewelry; a gold ring may be left on. Patient must be able to tolerate a supine position for at least 20 minutes without motion. Patient must be able to tolerate room air for at least 1 hour.
Myelography	Food and fluids withheld 4 hours before. Patient should void. *Oil:* Patient supine for 12–16 hours after myelogram. *Water:* Head of bed elevated 45 degrees 6–8 hours. Adverse reactions occur 3–8 hours after procedure and generally disappear within 24 hours, but headache may persist for several days.
Bone scan	A radioisotope is injected approximately 3 hours before the scan. Push fluids (if not contraindicated) before and after the procedure. Have patient void immediately before the examination. The radioisotope is excreted via the kidneys; wear gloves when handling urine-contaminated objects. Pregnant staff should consult their institution's policies for their recommended exposure to the patient.
Arthrography	Monitor for signs and symptoms of infection. Consent form necessary.
Electromyography (EMG)	No special preparation. Warm compresses or ice may be applied to examination site for discomfort. Analgesics may be ordered.
Arthroscopy	Monitor for signs and symptoms of infection. Observe for hematoma formation. Monitor for neuromuscular changes. Consent form necessary.
Joint aspiration	Assess for allergies to antiseptic solutions and local anesthetics, bleeding tendencies, current anticoagulant therapy, or presence of infection in area to be aspirated.
Bone marrow	Identify bleeding tendency, allergies, anxiety levels, need for premedication. Consent form necessary. Bed rest minimum of 1 hour after procedure. Application of a pressure dressing.

The fluoroscope permits better client positioning and instantaneous depiction of a particular anatomic part. In the client with a dislocated total hip prosthesis, the physician might order an anteroposterior radiograph of the pelvis to include both hips to confirm the dislocation and follow with a closed reduction under fluoroscopy to reestablish prosthetic integrity.

Image amplifiers used with radiography and fluoroscopy increase the accuracy and decrease the client's exposure. Images can be photographed or televised. A photograph of a fluoroscopic image is called a *photoroentgenogram.*

To accommodate the client's condition, portable x-ray machines are available and can be transported to the client's bedside or home.

Safety Features

A variety of shielding devices and equipment, including lead aprons, lead-lined walls, lead-lined gloves, and dosimeters (or x-ray badges), are available to protect the client and radiology personnel from exposure.

To identify an individual's radiograph, a numerical coding system and the client's name should be used. Such a system eliminates the potential for misfiling, which results in an erroneous interpretation of the client's

condition and incorrect treatment. Identification systems vary across the country; however, the following data are essential:

- Name and address of the radiologist or institution
- Name and identification number of the client
- Date of the examination
- Side of the body being examined or a clear label of one side
- Time intervals between films if obtained in sequence

Specific Indications

A radiograph can provide visual support for any number of possible diagnoses in both adults and children. Although fracture management is the primary indication, hereditary, congenital, developmental, infectious, inflammatory, neoplastic, metabolic, vascular, neurogenic, and degenerative disorders can also be evaluated with radiographs. In many cases, additional views in combination with special studies can assist in differential diagnosis of diseases or disorders.

Radiographs can reveal specifics on bone deformity, joint congruity, bone density, and calcification. Bone texture, size, shape, localized destruction, sclerosis, and fractures are also assessed with radiographs.

Radiologic capabilities can be enhanced through the use of special techniques, including computed tomography (CT), magnetic resonance imaging (MRI), myelography, and bone scan. Each of these modalities is discussed in detail. Use of these special techniques may require the client to sign a consent form. Individual hospital policies or protocols should be reviewed.

Radiographs

Preprocedure Preparation. Except in clients in whom special techniques are used in combination with x rays, client preparation is minimal. When the portable x-ray machine is used, an x-ray cassette is positioned directly under the area to be filmed. Clients seen in the radiology department are instructed to sit, stand, or lie in the appropriate position. The client is always told to "hold still" while the radiograph is being taken so that the picture will be clear. Braces, splints, or traction should remain in place unless the physician specifically requests that they be removed.

X rays are not painful in themselves, but positioning may cause discomfort. The use of pain medication or analgesics, muscle relaxants, or tranquilizers may help control any discomfort and facilitate client cooperation. Immobilization devices are available to prevent movement during radiography.

Radiologic Procedure. The client receives general instruction, usually by a radiology technician, regarding the limited exposure to radioactive materials and the proper position for the specific x ray. Most of the time needed to obtain a radiograph (15 minutes to 1 hour) is spent in client positioning. The total amount of time depends on the number and type of views ordered. The radiograph itself takes no longer than 5 to 10 seconds. Client exposure to radioactive materials is minimized. When a radiograph is ordered, the client's protection from the acute and chronic effects of overexposure must be considered.

Protecting the Client. Acute effects of overexposure are hair loss and erythema. Chronic effects are evident in the blood-forming organs. Induction of malignant tumors or cataracts, impairment of fertility, reduction of life span, and genetic changes are all possible chronic effects.

We do not actually know the limitation to impose on diagnostic procedures except to avoid untoward reaction or visible reactions of any kind. Radiation hazards to the embryo or fetus are particularly important. If a woman is known to be pregnant, radiation should be avoided completely in the first trimester and as much as possible thereafter. Because the gonads, testes, and ovaries are sensitive to radiation, lead shielding is used to reduce radiation exposure to these tissues. Whatever the type of radiograph ordered, the principal safety factor is physical

distance from the x-ray source. The energy of radiation decreases with distance.

It is possible to diminish the client's x-ray exposure in one or more of the following ways.

Maximum filtration of the primary beam. Added filtration has very little effect on the resulting quality of roentgenograms, and the necessary increase in the exposure time is relatively small.

Higher voltage. An increase in voltage intensifies the penetration of the beam, thereby relatively diminishing the total quanta of x rays that strike the skin of the client. The quality of the radiograph is not significantly altered.

Increased target-to-skin distance. Minimum standards in inches have been established for both radiography and fluoroscopy.

Small field of radiation. The smallest field of radiation necessary to achieve the desired diagnostic result can be achieved with cones in radiography and an adjustable diaphragm in fluoroscopy.

Diminished fluoroscopic exposure. Maximum and minimum levels of exposure in roentgens per minute to an irradiated area of skin have been established.

Calculation of dosage to clients in diagnostic examinations. Various tables and nomograms are available to calculate the actual dose of radiation delivered. These values differ and vary with the technique used.

Protecting Health Care Personnel. Protection against radiation hazard for the physician, nurse, or technician is also an important consideration. The most common injury sustained is to the hands. Protective measures include the following instructions:

- Any personnel near an x-ray machine should wear protective lead gloves and a lead-lined apron or its equivalent. The use of a full-length lead-lined screen is always appropriate. Dosimeters should be worn throughout the entire workday and provided for ancillary personnel assisting with radiologic procedures.
- Any unprotected body parts, such as hands, wrists, or arms, should never be exposed to the x-ray beam.
- Appropriate protective eyewear should be provided preceding fluoroscopy without image amplification.
- Kilovoltage and milliamperage settings based on national standards should be adopted for fluoroscopy.
- General principles for fluoroscopy use should be adhered to, such as avoiding the use of a fluoroscope when the client is not intercepting the beam. The examination should be concluded as quickly as possible, and an automatic timing device in the circuit can be used to automatically turn off the machine if time limits are exceeded.

Even though sufficient protection is worn, metabolic changes can occur as a result of the voltages used to energize x-ray tubes. The most effective assurance of safety is the enclosure of all high-voltage parts in a shock-proof container. If, for some reason, high-voltage conductors are exposed, operators should remain at a liberal distance. This distance is usually specified by local building codes and national safety standards.

Interpretation. The interpretation of a radiograph is a complex process, which has been outlined by Stearns and Stearns (1986) in Box 9-1. The x-ray film should be placed on a view box to give the examiner the perspective of looking at the client from the front. The exception is a spine film, which is viewed as though looking at the client from the back.

Postprocedure Care and Instructions. The client may resume diet and activity. Comfort measures (e.g., positioning, pain medication) may be necessary if the procedure has required painful positioning.

Computed Tomography/Computed Axial Tomography

Definition. A CT scanner is a high-powered computer coupled with a special x-ray system. CT uses x-ray beams that intersect and a scanner that takes sectional pictures, or cuts, of the entire body or of a particular area.

BOX 9–1.
X-Ray Interpretation

A. Note name and date.
B. Identify film type and area of body radiographed; comment on technique and the quality of film.
C. Note all views taken or attempted.
D. Describe soft tissues.
E. Describe bony contour.
F. Check for open epiphyses (estimate maturity).
G. Look for specific abnormalities.
  1. Altered density or texture
  2. Changes in size or shape
  3. Localized bone destruction or sclerosis
  4. Calcification of bone or soft tissue
  5. Fracture deformity
  6. Joint congruity
H. Scan all areas of each bone.
  1. Epiphysis
  2. Physis, zone of provisional calcification
  3. Metaphysis
  4. Diaphysis
  5. Cortex
  6. Cancellous
  7. Endosteum
  8. Periosteum
I. Draw conclusions or make diagnosis.
J. Recommend further studies as indicated.

From Stearns, H. C., & Stearns, C. M. (1986). Orthopaedic radiology. *Orthopaedic Nursing, 5*(2), 26–31.

The computer portion of the apparatus reconstructs these pictures into a useful visible image on a screen. CT may be applied to any area of the body and may use more than one axis.

CT, transverse axial tomography, computerized transverse axial tomography, computer-assisted tomography, and *reconstructive tomography* are all terms that refer to the same diagnostic technique. The advent of CT has enabled examiners to evaluate bone, soft tissue tumors, nerves, vessels, and bone mineral density in a variety of clients using a noninvasive procedure.

History. Hounsfield and Cormack are credited with the invention of CT in the late 1960s. Early scanners were extremely slow. The first clinical application of CT was for head images. This occurred in the 1970s, and a single slice took approximately 8 minutes (Galen, 1999). Currently, CT scanners can scan the entire body in a matter of minutes.

Equipment. The scanner consists of a large, vertically oriented ring containing an x-ray source that encircles or rotates around the client. Sensors detect the x rays and send the information to a computer, which reconstructs the image on a video screen. Film copies are also generated for interpretation by the radiologist. Three-dimensional images can be constructed.

Specific Indications. CT is used to evaluate bone structure. When plain radiographs prove to be inconclusive or show the treatment plan has not resulted in improvement, CT may identify fractures or loose bodies within a joint (Hines, 1999).

CT is useful in several musculoskeletal conditions. First is back and leg pain. Although conservative treatment should be used initially, CT can identify herniated discs, compression fractures, spinal stenosis, and spinal tumors. When combined with myelography, CT has high sensitivity and specificity for herniated discs and spinal stenosis. The combination of these two modalities provides additional information about nerve compression (Hines, 1999).

Other indications for the use of CT specific to orthopaedics include the evaluation of skeletal metastasis in a variety of cancers, osteosarcoma, sacroiliac joint disease, pseudoarthrosis, and neurologic deficits (Moye, 1996). CT also has the advantage of being noninvasive and painless.

There are several very serious disadvantages of CT. It is an expensive procedure when compared with ordinary radiography. CT is contraindicated in pregnancy because of the radiation exposure. Finally, there is a possibility of not obtaining a definitive result because of client motion during the examination.

Preprocedure Preparation. Before CT, the client should receive an explanation of the procedure and its purpose. One must ascertain whether the client is claustrophobic. A sedative may be administered for claustrophobia. One must also determine whether the client has any iodine allergies if contrast medium is to be used. Diphenhydramine (Benadryl) or cortisone must be available for administration during the procedure if needed.

The client must remain still during this procedure. The client should be told that he or she may hear clicking or whirling noises from the movement of the scanner during the examination. The client may be restricted to nothing by mouth before the scan. Jewelry and metal objects are removed.

The contrast material may be injected or orally ingested and may cause a warm, flushed feeling. Because a contrast material is used, a consent form may be necessary. Nurses should consult their institution's policy and procedure manual.

Computed Tomography Procedure. The client is usually supine on a horizontal table and is instructed to lie still during the examination. The scanner is positioned and makes a 180-degree scan of the area, 1 degree at a time. The computer processes information as it is received, and images begin to appear on the screen almost immediately. The length of the procedure varies depending on the number of areas to be scanned.

The procedure for CT is simple and straightforward, although the equipment is complicated. The only risk to the client having CT is the radiation exposure.

In CT, air appears black, bone appears white, and soft tissue appears in shades of gray. The relationship between these colors and shades provides the examiner with the information to interpret the scan. Figure 9–1 shows a representative CT scan of the pelvis.

Postprocedure Care and Instructions. Minimal postprocedure care is required after CT. The nurse must be aware of and observe for an allergic reaction if a contrast material is used. Should an allergic reaction occur, antihistamines (Benadryl) or steroids (cortisone) might be administered per protocol. In the case of anaphylaxis, resuscitation measures must be instituted.

The client may experience discomfort from lying still for an extended time. Comfort measures include assisting the client to assume a comfortable position and providing medication for pain as ordered and indicated.

Magnetic Resonance Imaging

Definition. MRI shows the hydrogen density of tissue within the body. The hydrogen atom is the basis for MRI because the body is composed primarily of hydrogen atoms and because of the magnetic qualities of the hydrogen atom itself.

In general, the magnetic field in the scanner causes the hydrogen atom to align along an axis with the poles of the magnet. Radio waves produced by the scanner act on the protons in the nucleus, pulling the atom out of

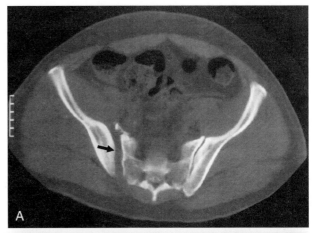

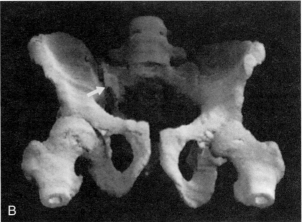

FIGURE 9–1. *A,* A representative computed tomography (CT) scan of the pelvis, demonstrating displacement of the sacroiliac joint *(arrow)*. *B,* A three-dimensional CT scan of the pelvis with widening of the sacroiliac joint *(white arrow)*. (From Engle, C., & Gruen, G. S. [1993]. Vertical shear fractures of the pelvis. *Orthopaedic Nursing, 12*[5], 58–59.)

alignment and causing a random configuration. Realignment of the hydrogen atom occurs when the radio waves are discontinued. During realignment, the hydrogen atoms give off an electric signal. These signals are translated into an image through the computer component of the MRI. Tissues with minimal hydrogen density are not visualized, and conversely, the areas with highest hydrogen density are clearly visualized.

History. Conceived in 1946, applications of MRI were anticipated in the basic science fields of physical and organic chemistry as well as in solid-state physics, biophysics, and biochemistry.

Early pioneers in MRI used themselves in biologic experiments. In the 1950s, Edward Purcell reputedly placed his head in an MRI coil and magnet in an attempt to observe the differences in the MRI signal or the line shape stimulated by thinking profoundly or focusing on a specific task versus having a blank mind. Although this type of experimentation cannot be interpreted as an imaging experiment, it does point out that the early practitioners recognized the possibility of applying this process to biologic systems. Damadian published data on MRI and applied for a patent in 1972 and clinical trials began in 1980.

Equipment.   The principal equipment for MRI is the imaging suite, which houses the MRI scanner and the imaging table. An intercom system or similar device for verbal communication between the client in the imaging room and either the physician or technologist in the monitoring room is of primary importance. Visual observation of the client is conducted through a closed-circuit television system. Nonferromagnetic stretchers should be used to transport clients. A well-stocked crash cart is available for emergencies, and the magnet's power-down switch is located in a prominently accessible area. The computer component is also located outside the scanning room.

Safety Issues.   General precautions to ensure the safety of personnel include the following:

- Access to the imaging area should be limited.
- Signs should be prominently displayed to warn persons with cardiac pacemakers or neurostimulators *not* to enter the room.
- All metal objects should be removed from personnel before entering the imaging room. Ferromagnetic objects can be drawn into the center of the magnetic field with a force that turns a minor metal object (e.g., a safety pin) into a dangerous high-velocity missile.
- Credit cards and wristwatches with mechanical parts should be removed to prevent magnetic tape erasure and watch malfunction.
- All personnel must know where the magnet's power-down switch is located to initiate immediate action in the event of a fire emergency.

If safety standards are maintained, accidents can be prevented. The activities within the MRI area should be organized and efficient, and common sense should be the basic guideline for all personnel in avoiding injury to themselves or to a client.

Specific Indications.   MRI is considered more sensitive than CT, particularly when used in diseases involving a change in tissue water content, such as disc disease, strokes, and tumors. Specific applications of MRI for the musculoskeletal system include evaluating the spine, bone, and joint structure and diagnosing diseases such as arthritis, avascular necrosis, soft tissue tumors, multiple sclerosis, and infection. MRI has been found effective in differentiating cellulitis from osteomyelitis (Hines, 1999).

MRI may be the preferred method of examination for intraspinal contents. Both myelography and CT reflect bone artifacts that obscure the spinal canal, but MRI does not. MRI can indicate the presence of a degenerated disc or a herniation by evaluating asymmetry of the epidural fat. It also can evaluate disc space and the height of the vertebral body.

Because of the absence of hydrogen atoms in the cortical bone, it is possible to distinguish cortical bone from soft tissue and bone marrow. Therefore, diseases affecting the marrow cavity, such as tumors and osteomyelitis, are readily visualized with MRI.

MRI effectively differentiates among muscle, tendon, and ligaments, providing a clear anatomic delineation of joint structures, particularly the anterior and posterior cruciate ligaments. MRI can be used to guide arthroscopic surgery (Galen, 1999).

Early diagnosis and staging of avascular necrosis can be made using MRI. As soon as fibrovascular tissue replaces bone marrow, osteonecrosis can be detected. The diseased hip usually shows an MRI of decreased intensity compared with the normal hip. This modality is more sensitive than CT or radiography in the early detection of avascular necrosis (Galen, 1999).

Evaluation of multiple sclerosis was the earliest application of MRI to the musculoskeletal system. The sclerotic lesions in the brainstem, cerebellum, and spinal cord characteristic of multiple sclerosis are readily apparent on an MRI. Because of its sensitivity to these lesions, MRI is the most commonly used technique today in the diagnosis of multiple sclerosis.

Preprocedure.   A number of practical considerations or general precautions must be taken to ensure client safety with the use of MRI. It is currently recommended that clients with cardiac pacemakers, electric neurostimulators, and intracranial aneurysm clips be excluded from MRI examination. Iron, nickel, and cobalt, referred to as *ferromagnetic elements,* are affected by the magnetic field and place the client at risk for displacement or dislocation. Metal plates, pins, screws, or surgical staples within the body pose no risk during MRI if they have been in place for more than 4 to 6 weeks. The presence of a metal body can distort the magnetic resonance image. Metals without measurable ferromagnetic properties can also produce image distortion.

Any client requiring life support equipment should also be excluded from MRI examination. Client care items, such as an oxygen tank or intravenous pole, can become airborne projectiles if pulled into the magnetic system.

In the event of a medical emergency during MRI, such as a grand mal seizure or cardiopulmonary arrest, it is of paramount importance that MRI personnel be prepared and able to gain easy access to the client in the imaging room. Resuscitative measures can be initiated in the imaging room, but the client should be transferred as quickly as possible to an adjacent room to minimize any potential hazards to members of the staff and to the MRI equipment from the inadvertent presence of scissors or metal instruments carried into the room.

There is limited data on the effects of MRI on the developing fetus. Pregnant clients are usually not scanned, especially during the first trimester. However, when the use of ionizing radiation in an examination is required, it is preferable to consider MRI.

The client's weight and abdominal girth must be within appropriate parameters to accommodate the scanner. Clients exceeding the approximate measurements for the scanner are not eligible for MRI examination. Machines to accommodate larger clients exist but may not be conveniently available.

Potential candidates for MRI must be able to tolerate a supine position for at least 20 minutes without motion. During this time, only verbal communication is maintained and the client is actually out of visual range.

In preparing a client for MRI examination, these four steps should be followed:

1. Screen for contraindications.
2. Explain to the client what the study encompasses.
3. Remove all external metal devices or objects.
4. Make the client as comfortable as possible.

Hospitals or imaging centers offering MRI should have a formalized eligibility questionnaire to ensure that all pertinent information is gathered about medical illnesses, previous surgical procedures, and the possibility of pregnancy. Special inquiry should be made about cardiac pacemakers, neurostimulators, prosthetic heart valves, joint prostheses, ocular foreign bodies (contact lenses), and cerebral aneurysm surgery.

Any intravenous lines should be converted to a heparin lock. The client should be able to tolerate at least 1 hour on room air without the need for supplemental oxygen therapy. For individuals who have a tendency toward claustrophobia, a tranquilizer may be prescribed.

If there is a possibility that a metal fragment might be lodged in a client's body, a radiograph should be obtained for verification. Metal detectors may be used before scanning a client as a routine part of the screening process.

If there are no contraindications to the examination, the client should be given a detailed explanation of the procedure to ensure cooperation and to allay apprehension. This instruction should mention the estimated duration of the study (30 to 90 minutes for completion of the entire examination), the noise of the gradient coils (constant drumming sound), and the confinement within the magnet because of the small size of the MRI inner chamber. Earplugs or headphones for music may help with the noise. The newer, more open MRI scanners may help alleviate the claustrophobia, but the images may not be as precise.

The client is allowed to stretch between scans but must remain absolutely still while inside the MRI scanning chamber. As mentioned previously, communication is maintained throughout the entire procedure using an intercom system. After orienting the client to the procedural process, the nurse should provide suitable attire, eliminating snaps, zippers, and metal fasteners. All miscellaneous metal items should be removed from the client's body, including hairpins, safety pins, jewelry, eyeglasses, wristwatches, dentures, hearing aids, brassieres, and boxer shorts with snaps. A wedding band made from gold may be allowed, but this is at the discretion of MRI department personnel. It may not be necessary to remove dentures or bridgework if the scan is for the trunk or lower body. The MRI department should be consulted for specific instructions. Client valuables should be secured.

Before the examination, the client is asked to void, unless the pelvis is the area to be scanned. In this case, the bladder should be at least half full when the study is initiated.

Young children tolerate MRI poorly. They are unable to remain still during the examination, and sedation may be required. Older children tend to cooperate if the procedure is adequately explained and verbal reassurance is given. In the case of newborns or infants younger than 2 months of age, sedation is not usually required as long as they are secured in blankets and a restraining board is used.

Procedure

Client Positioning. The client undergoing MRI is placed on an imaging table with pillows positioned beneath the head and knees to prevent back pain and possible early termination of the examination. The imaging room is usually kept cool, and therefore sheets are provided for the client's comfort. The client should be able to communicate immediately—a fact that should be verified before the beginning of the examination. The client is instructed to breathe normally and remain still for as long as possible throughout the course of the examination. If for some reason the client cannot tolerate the procedure, it is discontinued.

Interpretation. There are three basic *imaging planes:* transaxial, sagittal, and coronal. The zero reference for these planes is matched to the anatomic part to be examined. Adjustments to the imaging planes are completed by positioning the client as follows:

- Cephalad or caudad in the transaxial plane
- Left to right in the sagittal plane
- Elevating the client or the involved extremity for the coronal plane

The majority of techniques use a multisection protocol providing a set of images that can be described by the number, thickness, and distance between sections and by the position of the center section relative to the zero reference of the imaging plane.

Multisection imaging, which uses the maximum number of sections that can be obtained, is determined by the different pulse sequences. Generation of a series of contiguous section images is not always available. When not available, a maneuver called *interleaving* can be used.

When using low or intermediate field-strength magnets, data are collected many times during the imaging sequence. The average of the signal intensity values is entered into image processing, and the collected data are described (Fig. 9–2). A form of geometric magnification called *zoom imaging* can also be used to evaluate small anatomic areas.

Postprocedure Care and Instructions. Normal diet and activity may be resumed. The client may experience discomfort from lying still for an extended time. Comfort measures include assisting the client to assume a comfortable position and providing medication for pain as ordered and indicated.

Myelography

Definition. Myelography is the evaluation of the spinal canal and its contents by the introduction of a contrast medium into the sac (dura) surrounding the

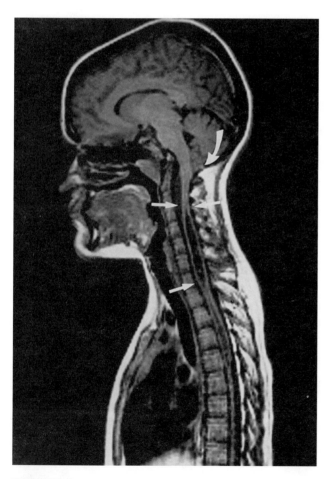

FIGURE 9–2. T_1-weighted sagittal magnetic resonance image of a large syrinx cavity *(small white arrows)* that extends from C2 to T5 and expands the cervical cord. (From Michals, E. A., & Ransey, R. G. [1996]. Syringomyelia. *Orthopaedic Nursing, 15*[5], 34.)

spinal cord and nerves. Fluoroscopy is used to guide the introduction of the contrast medium and to record the radiograph. CT and MRI can also be used as a component of the procedure. A myelogram can indicate a block in the flow of cerebrospinal fluid (CSF) and reveal distortion of the epidural, dural, and subarachnoid spaces.

History. Walter Edward Dandy, an American neurosurgeon, using gas as the contrast agent, performed the first myelogram in 1919. The procedure was taken one step farther by the Swedish neuroradiologist Erik Lindergrin, who injected air into the spinal canal while removing large amounts of CSF. Tomograms of the area were then obtained. This procedure detected only gross abnormalities, such as tumors or cysts. Because of the use of negative contrast medium (gas or air) and the loss of spinal fluid, these procedures were very painful and time-consuming and required special training and equipment that were not easily accessible in small towns and rural communities.

During the 1920s and 1930s, the search for a better contrast medium continued. Agents such as iodized oil (Lipiodol) and thorium oxide (Thorotrast) were tried and discarded because of such side effects as meningeal reactions, adhesive arachnoiditis, neck stiffness, and severe cramping. In the early 1970s, a contrast medium called *Demer X* was thought to be acceptable but was found to cause excessive meningeal irritation and hyperexcitability of the central nervous system (CNS). The development of metrizamide effectively resolved these problems.

Equipment. Myelograms are performed in a radiology department using a fluoroscope and an x-ray table that tilts. In addition to the lumbar puncture tray, gloves, and syringes used by the radiologist, a contrast medium is needed.

Myelograms can be performed using a water-soluble or oil-based contrast medium. Metrizamide, a nonionic, water-soluble contrast medium, is the agent of choice because it does not need to be removed from the subarachnoid space and it provides a clear and detailed visualization of the nerve roots. In combination with a CT scan or MRI, a myelogram allows soft tissue structures and the spinal canal to be distinguished.

Iophendylate (Pantopaque) is an oil-based contrast medium that does not mix with CSF and tends to form globules in the spinal canal. Because of the viscosity of iophendylate, visualization of the nerve roots can be cloudy. This oil-based medium must be removed from the spinal canal at the completion of the procedure. Iophendylate, however, is non-neurotoxic.

Specific Indications. Myelography has contributed significantly to the overall diagnostic evaluation of the spine. This procedure provides information specific to a selected group of spinal disorders, such as disc herniation, tumors, degenerative arthritis, spinal stenosis, congenital anomalies, and root cysts of the spine. With the sophistication of less invasive techniques, such as CT and MRI, myelography may no longer be the diagnostic tool of choice. However, when used in combination with a CT scan or MRI, an extremely detailed evaluation of the spinal column can be made, including soft tissue structures inside the spinal canal, as well as the bones and paraspinal tissue.

The disadvantages of myelography are the multiple side effects associated with it. The most common client complaints are headache, nausea, and vomiting. Other possible side effects are mental confusion, difficulty in voiding, and allergic reactions.

Preprocedure Preparation. Myelograms have become an ambulatory test during the past decade. On the day before the examination, the client should be instructed to drink extra fluids. This increases the fluids in the body and decreases the risk of developing a spinal headache. The client is instructed to refrain from eating or drinking after midnight the day before the test. Arrangements should be made for a family member or friend to be available to bring the client home after the procedure.

If the client takes daily medications, he or she should consult the nurse about taking them before arriving for the test. Warfarin (Coumadin), heparin, and some diabetic medications are withheld or the dosages altered. Metformin hydrochloride (Glucophage) may be withheld 48 hours after the procedure because of the effects of the contrast medium on renal function. Once renal function has been reevaluated and found to be normal, metformin hydrochloride may be resumed. Phenothiazines, tricyclic antidepressants, monoamine oxidase (MAO) inhibitors, and CNS stimulants should be discontinued before the myelogram and held for at least 24 hours after the procedure because they lower the seizure threshold.

Before the myelogram, the procedure is explained to the client and a consent form is obtained. Preexisting allergies to iodine should be documented. Adverse reactions to iodine-based dye include hives, swelling, and difficulty breathing. If it is anticipated that an MRI will be part of the procedure, the client must be screened for a pacemaker, aneurysm clips, or other metal implants that would preclude this type of imaging. The client should void before the procedure.

Myelogram Procedure. The client is placed on the x-ray table in the prone position with his or her feet against a footrest. This prevents the client from slipping off the table when it is in the upright position. The client's back is prepared with povidone-iodine unless the client is allergic. A lumbar puncture is performed by the radiologist. After removing the stylet from the spinal needle, approximately 10 mL of CSF is removed for chemical and cytologic studies. The stylet is replaced while the physician draws the contrast medium into a syringe. The stylet is then removed and the radiologist slowly injects 1 mL of contrast material into the lumbar puncture needle. The client then undergoes fluoroscopy on the tilt table to determine the presence of the contrast material in the subarachnoid space. Once placement is confirmed, the remaining contrast medium is injected. The stylet is replaced, and the needle is left in the subarachnoid space.

The lights are dimmed, the tilt table is moved to various degrees, and the spinal subarachnoid space is fluoroscoped to visualize the surrounding structures. Spot films are completed as necessary.

If an oil-based contrast medium is used, it is removed at this time. This procedure is done aseptically. The stylet of the spinal needle is removed, syringe is attached, and contrast medium is aspirated. The stylet is replaced, and the needle is removed in the same manner as when a nonionic, water-soluble dye is used. The client's skin is cleaned, and a small dressing or Band-Aid is applied. The client is returned to bed via a stretcher. If CT or MRI scans are planned, the client will be taken to that area at the appropriate time. CSF is sent for laboratory analysis immediately after the completion of the procedure. Total examination time is 30 to 90 minutes. Additional scans increase the examination time.

Interpretation. It is the physician's responsibility to document the procedure performed, date and time, amount and character of fluid removed, CSF pressures, preliminary x-ray findings, amount of contrast medium removed (if applicable), any significant reactions, and comments.

Postprocedure Care and Instructions. If an oil-based dye (Pantopaque) is used and removed, the client is maintained in the supine position for 12 to 16 hours. If a nonionic, water-soluble dye (metrizamide) is used, the client may have the head of the bed elevated about 45 degrees for 6 to 8 hours, depending on the physician's preference.

The client should be observed for meningeal irritation. Complaints of headache, fever, nausea and vomiting, or convulsions should be reported and treated as per prescribed protocol. Adverse reactions occur within 3 to 8 hours after injection and generally disappear within 24 hours. Administration of phenothiazines (Compazine) and psychotropic drugs should be suspended for 48 hours before the procedure and for at least 24 hours after the procedure because they lower the seizure threshold.

Some headaches may persist for several days. Authorities believe that fluid intake should be encouraged to increase the excretion of the dye and to replace any lost

CSF. Recommendations are not specific with respect to amount of fluids required. A blood patch may be necessary for a persistent headache. This procedure is performed by an anesthesiologist to seal the small hole created in the dura during the myelogram. A small amount of blood is taken from the client's arm and injected into the dural sac preventing further leakage of CSF (Spinasanta, 2001).

Bone Scan

Definition. A bone scan is a nuclear medicine study involving the use of radionuclides that have an affinity for bone. A *radionuclide* is an unstable nucleus and its orbital electrons. The radionuclide most commonly used for bone scans today is technetium tagged to phosphate or diphosphate. Its chemical symbol is ^{99m}Tc. Radionuclides and sophisticated scanning equipment provide information valuable in the diagnosis of metastatic and metabolic bone diseases, degenerative bone and joint diseases, fractures, and osteomyelitis.

History. The field of nuclear medicine had its origin in 1896 when Becquerel discovered radioactivity (Galen, 1999). More recent developments in nuclear medicine date from 1935, when Chiewitz and von Hevesy first reported that "an artificially produced radionuclide used as a tracer or indicator for metabolic studies coincidentally involved a radionuclide that localized in the skeleton" (Freeman, 1984, p. 182). Further advances in radionuclide development include the discovery and use of isotopes of strontium, calcium fluoride, and gallium. Until the 1970s, strontium was considered the radionuclide of choice for skeletal imaging. In 1971, technetium-tagged phosphates were introduced and were shown to selectively and rapidly localize in the skeleton.

Equipment. To project a meaningful image, the following equipment is necessary: the radionuclide, a gamma camera, and a scanning table. A gamma camera consists of a collimator, a scintillation crystal, photomultiplier tubes, a pulse height analyzer, and a control console. Further description of these components can be found in the section on procedure.

Specific Indications. One of the primary indications for a bone scan is the presence of various primary malignancies that metastasize to the bone. These metastatic lesions arise from breast, prostate, lung, lymph, thyroid, brain, and renal cancers. Bone scans are used to detect metastatic bone involvement at early stages because they can provide definitive information much earlier (months) than traditional radiographs. When tumors metastasize to bone, abnormal bone growth is stimulated. The bone scan visualizes increased energy that is emitted by the collection of radionuclide in the area (American College of Radiology, 1993). The major

disadvantage of bone scanning under these circumstances is that skeletal imaging cannot separate malignant from benign bone tumors.

Other indications for skeletal imaging include suspected osteomyelitis, fractures, avascular necrosis, rheumatoid arthritis, osteoarthritis, and various metabolic diseases (e.g., Paget's disease). Skeletal imaging is useful in the differential diagnosis of osteomyelitis, which can often be distinguished from cellulitis. A disadvantage in this case is the need to take multiple projections and magnified views to adequately assess the areas of suspected osteomyelitis. Skeletal imaging may also be extremely useful for delineating some fractures that are difficult to see on radiographs, as well as detecting a loose or infected prosthesis.

Preprocedure Preparation. Before a bone scan, the client should receive a thorough explanation of the procedure. The client's level of knowledge must be assessed and the explanation gauged accordingly. All of the client's questions should be answered. The procedure is not painful, although the client must lie still for the examination and therefore may experience some discomfort. Medication should be provided before the scan is obtained if necessary. A consent may be required depending on institutional policy.

The duration of the procedure varies from 10 minutes to 1 hour. Approximately 3 hours before the scan, the client is given an intravenous injection of technetium phosphate. The client metabolizes the radiopharmaceutical and excretes it rapidly through the urinary system. Therefore, the client should be instructed, encouraged, and assisted to drink large quantities of fluids (if fluid intake is not otherwise contraindicated). The fluids help hydrate the client and cause frequent voiding, reducing the radiation dose to the bladder. The client's bladder should be emptied immediately before the bone scan because a full bladder can obscure the pelvic area (Moye, 1996). A client who is incontinent should be cleansed and given a clean gown because radionuclide-contaminated clothing or skin may yield an inaccurate scan.

Bone Scan Procedure. A bone scan is a relatively simple procedure, which may be performed on either an inpatient or on an ambulatory basis. Skeletal imaging is done 2 to 3 hours after the radionuclide injection. The client is transferred to a scanning table, and the pictures are taken. The scanning table is a hard, flat surface that clients may have difficulty tolerating because the procedure takes 30 to 60 minutes. The client should be reminded to remain as still as possible because any movement during the scan could produce an unacceptable result. Bone scans produce skeletal images in the following manner. Technetium phosphate localizes in bone and emits gamma radiation, or x rays. As the client lies on the scanning table, these gamma rays pass through the collimator, a device that limits the access of gamma rays to the gamma camera. The photomultiplier tubes then detect and amplify those scintillations produced by the interactions of the gamma rays and the crystal. The pulse height analyzer discards signals from the background and scattered radiation. The image is produced when the scintillations reach the cathode-ray tube, a process that takes a matter of seconds.

Interpretation. A bone scan is read by the radiologist. A normal scan should be symmetrical. Uniformity and symmetry of distribution of the radiopharmaceutical in the skeleton is the most important determinant of a normal scan. Bone scans have areas of increased uptake, referred to as *hot spots,* and areas of decreased uptake, referred to as *cold spots.* Areas of abnormally increased or decreased activity in any bone should be examined carefully (Fig. 9–3).

Postprocedure Care and Instructions. Following this procedure, the client is once again instructed to drink large quantities of fluids and to void frequently for the next 24 to 48 hours. If the procedure is performed on an inpatient basis, the client should be positioned comfortably in bed and given medication for pain as ordered and

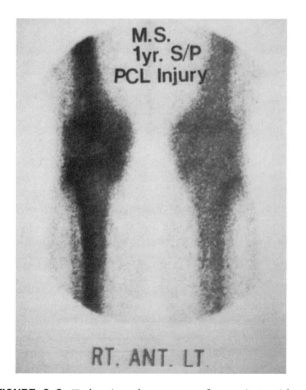

FIGURE 9–3. Technetium bone scan of a patient with a chronic posterior cruciate ligament (PCL) injury. Note the diffuse uptake in the affected right knee. The association of chondral injury with chronic PCL injuries is well documented with bone scan images. (From Miller, M. D., Cooper, D. E., & Warner, J. J. P. [1995]. *Review of sports medicine and arthroscopy* [p. 17]. Philadelphia: WB Saunders.)

indicated. The scan itself is not painful, but lying still may produce extreme discomfort.

It is important to remember that ^{99m}Tc is eliminated from the body via the kidneys. Therefore, the client's urine is radioactive and should be handled only while wearing latex gloves. Pregnant staff members and visitors should use discretion in the length of time they spend with the client. Institutional policies on exposure to radioactive materials should be consulted.

ELECTROMYOGRAPHY AND NERVE CONDUCTION TESTS

Definition

Electromyography (EMG) is the examination of the electric potentials of muscles. EMG is used in the detection and diagnosis of primary muscle disease and of disruptions in the transmission of electric impulses at neuromuscular junctions and in the differentiation between motor symptoms that are secondary to neurologic disturbance. Nerve conduction tests measure the time needed to transmit an electrical stimulus along the course of the nerve. A healthy nerve transmits the signal faster and stronger than a nerve that is pinched or damaged.

History

EMG enjoys a distinguished history. Contributors to its development include Leonardo da Vinci, who studied muscles and their functions, and Francisco Redi, who in 1666 first deducted the principle of muscle-generated electricity. Luigi Galvani further advanced this study when he observed a relationship between muscle contraction and electricity (Basmajian & DeLuca, 1985). In the late 1800s, Guillaume Duchenne began the science of EMG when he became the first to use electricity to systematically assess the dynamics of intact skeletal muscle (Basmajian, 1962).

Equipment

The equipment used during EMG is similar to that used for electroencephalography or electrocardiography. The electromyograph consists of three electrodes, an amplifier, a strip-chart recorder, and an oscilloscope. Of the electrodes, one adheres to the surface and is actually a modified electroencephalograph electrode. The electrodes can be made of metal, rubber, or synthetic materials; the choice of material depends on the practitioner's preference. There are two types of inserted electrodes, which are referred to as *needle* and *wire electrodes.* The needle electrode, the first to be used, is still used today. It is basically a hollow needle, 24 to 28 gauge, from 0.5 to several inches long, and insulated on the outside with Teflon or another similar material. Wire electrodes may be constructed from a variety of metals and are often inserted using a hypodermic needle. The type of electrode is highly individualized and extremely important because

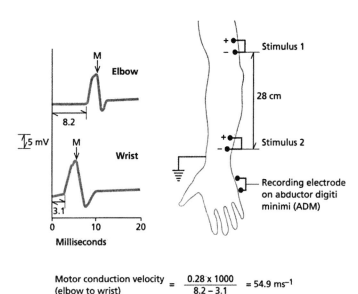

FIGURE 9–4. Measurement of motor conduction velocity of the ulnar nerve. A recording electrode on the abductor digiti minimi records the muscle action potential (M) from the ulnar nerve at the elbow (Stimulus 1) and at the wrist (Stimulus 2). From these values, the motor conduction velocity can be calculated. (From Kumar, P., & Clark, M. [1994]. *Clinical medicine* [p. 878]. London: Bailliere Tindall.)

$$\text{Motor conduction velocity (elbow to wrist)} = \frac{0.28 \times 1000}{8.2 - 3.1} = 54.9 \text{ ms}^{-1}$$

the material chosen affects the transmission of electric impulses. Figure 9-4 provides a representation of the measurement of nerve conduction.

Specific Indications

EMG is used to evaluate a wide variety of client complaints, including skeletal muscle weakness, general muscle weakness, pain, alterations in gait, and various types of deformity and disability. EMG can also be used to differentiate between myopathic and neuropathic conditions that demonstrate specific patterns of activity. This technique is also helpful in the detection of lower motor neuron lesions, in the assessment of degenerative disc disease, and in the evaluation of suspected defects in electric signal transmission at neuromuscular junctions. Nerve conduction velocity, which can be measured during EMG, is useful in the diagnosis of neuropathies and nerve entrapment syndromes (e.g., carpal tunnel syndrome).

Relative contraindications to EMG are suspected bleeding disorders, postmastectomy edema on the extremity to be tested, and contagious skin infections. There are no absolute contraindications.

Preprocedure Preparation

There is no special preparation necessary before an EMG. The client should be given an explanation of the procedure and some idea of what to expect during it. The client must understand that it is a diagnostic procedure. A physician generally performs this procedure.

EMG Procedure

The client is asked to sit or lie down (either supine or prone). The skin is then cleansed, and the electrodes are applied. Normal muscles at rest have no action potentials. Action potentials are tested by asking the client to alternately constrict and relax various muscles. At differ-

ent intervals and varying sites, the needle or wire electrode is inserted into the muscle. The signal is then transmitted to the amplifier, and an auditory representation of the action potentials is achieved. At the same time, the signal is transmitted to the oscilloscope and strip-chart recorder. The oscilloscope provides an immediate visual representation. The strip-chart recording provides a permanent hard-copy record. With the assistance of computers, much of this information can be stored on disks. The procedure can last from 30 minutes to 2 hours. Results can be interpreted immediately.

Postprocedure Care and Instructions

Following an EMG, the client should be assisted into a comfortable position. Warm compresses or ice may be applied if the client reports extended discomfort. Analgesics should be administered as ordered. If the procedure has been completed on a client with a known or suspected bleeding disorder, close observation and assessment of electrode insertion sites are necessary. Complications from this procedure are uncommon.

ARTHOGRAPHY

Definition

Arthrography is a radiologic procedure using radiographs, CT, or MRI to view a joint after a contrast medium has been injected into the joint. Arthrography is considered an invasive procedure because it involves injection into a joint (sterile cavity). Arthrography may be performed on the hip, knee, shoulder, elbow, ankle, or wrist.

History

Arthrographic examination of specific joints has been performed since 1905 (Ricklin, Ruttiman, & DeBuono,

1971). The first contrast medium used was room air. Oxygen was also used as a contrast medium in the early development of arthrography. Further developments in arthrography did not occur until the early 1930s (Goldman, 1982; Grech, 1977), when shoulder and hip arthrography were reported. Room air was the contrast medium in these studies also.

Radiologists currently use saline, iodinated, or gadolinium-based contrast medium when performing arthrograms. The selection of contrast material and techniques used varies with the joint being studied. Meniscal retears have been visualized best when magnetic resonance (MR) arthrography with gadolinium-based contrast material was used (Sciulli, Boutin, Brown, Nguyen, Muhle, Lektrakul, Pathria, Pedowitz, & Resnick, 1999). MR arthrography is also an appropriate diagnostic procedure for persistent shoulder pain. CT arthrography has been used in diagnosing elbow injuries (Baker & Jones, 1999).

Equipment

The equipment needed to perform an arthrographic examination is minimal and includes needles (25 gauge and 18 to 22 gauge), syringes (5, 10, and 20 mL, preferably of the Luer-Lok type), local anesthetic, antiseptic or antimicrobial solution, sterile drapes, sterile gloves, and contrast material. Epinephrine is optional. Other equipment includes fluoroscopic, x-ray, CT or MR equipment; specialized frames or bolsters to sufficiently relax the joint capsule; and elastic bandages.

Specific Indications

Arthrography is a valuable diagnostic tool when combined with client history and physical examination. Arthrography may be used to evaluate the integrity of structures within the joint (ligaments, tendons, and the menisci). The indications for arthrography vary depending on the joint to be examined and generally include unexplained joint discomfort or pain, arthritis, dislocations, and synovial abnormalities (Moye, 1996).

The advantages of arthrography over other diagnostic modalities are simplicity, low risk, and accuracy. The primary advantage of arthrography, however, is that it enables the examiner to directly view the encapsulated joint.

Preprocedure Preparation

Arthrography should be thoroughly described to the client before the examination. The procedure usually takes place in the radiology department and is performed by either a radiologist or an orthopaedist. The physician should obtain an informed consent from the client.

Before the examination, a thorough client history must be obtained, including any allergies to iodine or the specific contrast substance. The explanation should include what the procedure entails; what, if any, discomfort is to be expected; the length of the procedure; and the aftercare and follow-up.

Arthrography Procedure

During arthrography, the client is positioned in a manner that facilitates easy access to the joint. For most arthrographies, this position is initially supine. Frames, bolsters, and pillows are used to fully extend the joint capsule. Once the client is positioned, the area to be examined is scrubbed with an antiseptic or antimicrobial agent and draped using aseptic technique. The area is then anesthetized using a 25-gauge needle and a local anesthetic agent, such as lidocaine.

Any joint effusion should be aspirated to prevent the contrast material from becoming overly dilute. Any fluid obtained should be sent for culture and sensitivity if infection is suspected. An 18- to 22-gauge needle is inserted into the joint space, using landmarks as a guide and possibly under fluoroscopic control (Fig. 9–5). Depending on physician preference, air may be injected into the joint space to distend it. Following this, the contrast medium is injected. The quantity of contrast medium varies depending on the joint being examined as well as physician preference and experience. After injection of the contrast medium, the joint is put through its range of motion, either actively or passively, to allow the contrast medium to fully cover the joint surfaces. Films are then taken. Radiographs, fluoroscopy, or tomograms may be used.

Risks of the procedure include the possibility of extracapsular as opposed to intracapsular injection of the contrast material, infection, and injection of the contrast medium into the bone. There is also the risk of allergic reactions or of anaphylaxis when a contrast medium is used. Other than infection, few complications are associated with arthrography. Other complications include exacerbation of existing joint pain, inadvertent axillary blocks with shoulder arthrography, persistent crackling noises within the joint, and sterile synovitis (Moye, 1996).

Postprocedure Care and Instructions

Following arthrography, the client should be instructed to rest the joint for 6 to 12 hours. This rest may include immobilization. A mild pain reliever may be prescribed, and ice and an elastic bandage may be applied to the joint. In addition, the client should be instructed that crackling or squishing sounds might be heard in the joint for a few days after the procedure. This is to be expected but should be reported to the physician if it persists longer than a few days. The client should be instructed about the signs and symptoms of infection and told to report any that occur to the physician, although infection after arthrography is rare if aseptic technique is used.

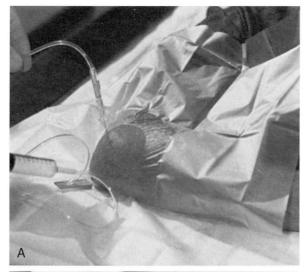

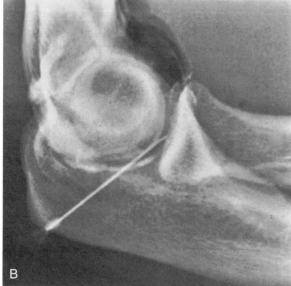

FIGURE 9–5. *A,* Needle in position with attached extension tube for contrast injection with fluoroscopic visualization. *B,* Spot film of elbow with the needle in place during injection for arthrography. (From Sauser, D. D., Thordarson, S. H., & Fahr, L. M. [1990]. Imaging of the elbow. *Radiology Clinics of North America, 28,* 930.)

ARTHROSCOPY

Definition

Arthroscopy is the examination of the interior of a joint with a small fiberoptic tube called an *arthroscope.* Arthroscopic procedures are most commonly performed on the knee. Advances in technology have lead to the ability to perform arthroscopic procedures on the ankle, hip, wrist, elbow, shoulder, temporomandibular joint, and spine.

Arthroscopy allows for extensive and accurate visualization of a joint cavity. It has become a highly cost-effective procedure, which, in most cases, can be done as an ambulatory procedure. However, the major advantage of arthroscopy is the immediately improved joint mobility the procedure affords.

History

Kenji Takagi is credited with the development of arthroscopy in 1918. Fiber light was first used in the late 1950s and Watanabe and associates performed the first meniscectomy in 1962.

In 1973, changes in the original arthroscopic technique reduced examination time, allowed the use of local anesthesia, and eliminated the cumbersome irrigation system, thereby reducing the need for extensive incision and suturing.

Today, technical and optical improvements, such as miniature hand and motorized instruments, lens systems, and fiberoptic light transmission devices, have contributed to the tremendous growth of interest in the field of diagnostic arthroscopy.

Equipment

Arthroscopic procedures are extremely dependent on the use of precise and intricate instrumentation and equipment. Failure of the equipment prevents proper examination of the joint space. Therefore, familiarity with the use and repair of the arthroscopic equipment is important for the staff in the operating room.

The typical arthroscope is constructed of a small-diameter outer metallic casing through which fiberoptic light bundles are passed. No single arthroscope is ideal for use in every client or in every procedure. However, the need for larger arthroscopes is determined by the orthopaedic surgeon, who may prefer them for surgical procedures when television monitoring is used and when the client is under general anesthesia.

Because of the small diameter of the arthroscope, a high-intensity light source is necessary to provide illumination of the joint space. The high-intensity light is attached to a fiberoptic cable, which in turn is attached to the arthroscope. Every dimension of the light transmission system must be optimal to provide the best imaging.

Sharp and blunt trocars are used to make a path through which to insert the arthroscope. The sharp trocar penetrates the skin and joint capsule, and the blunt trocar is inserted into the sheath and pushed through the synovium of the joint. The arthroscope itself is extremely fragile and is therefore housed in a metal sheath that is slightly larger in diameter than the arthroscope. It serves to protect the arthroscope, preventing damage during the procedure. Irrigation valves attached to the metal sheath are used for fluid inflow or for suctioning blood and tissue. Irrigation and distention are essential parts of the surgery. Because the normal joint fluid is oily in consistency, it is difficult to see through and must be drained and replaced with a medium (saline) that provides better visualization. Light can also be obscured within the joint itself because of the presence of blood and tissue debris and because of the joint's configuration. Therefore, it is important to maintain a flow of clear saline solution into the joint.

A suction device enables a constant flow of saline through the joint, removing debris produced with cutting or trimming. Carbon dioxide gas may also provide a clear medium for distention of the joint during the procedure.

Probes and grabbers are commonly used to manipulate the cartilage and ligaments in the joint space during the procedure. Simultaneous television viewing and recording of the examination are becoming a standard practice, providing an educational tool for physician and client as well as accurate documentation of the procedure.

Specific Indications

The advantage of arthroscopic examination as a diagnostic modality is that the diagnosis of pathologic abnormalities is based on direct observation rather than presumptive evidence obtained through client history, physical examination, laboratory tests, or radiographs.

Clients who are candidates for arthroscopy generally fall into one of three categories:

1. Clients who injure themselves in an accident or through trauma, such as twisting or falling
2. Clients who are experiencing a disease process, such as exacerbations of degenerative or rheumatic disease
3. Clients who are having unexplained symptomatic joint complaints

Many times, the client complains that the affected joint "locks," "gives way," or swells. With arthroscopy, an orthopaedic surgeon can visualize the joint and determine which area is responsible for the client's complaint.

From the client's point of view, arthroscopy has the advantage that it can be performed on an ambulatory basis, thus reducing the cost.

Some complications are associated with arthroscopic procedures. In addition to hematoma formation and infection, reactions to anesthesia may occur. Because arthroscopic procedures may be performed with local or regional blocks, these complications are rare.

Equipment breakage is one of the most common complications in knee arthroscopy. Additional surgery is needed to retrieve the free piece from the joint cavity.

Damage to adjacent blood vessels and nerves are complications in arthroscopic examination of the knee, hip, ankle, and elbow.

Spinal thoracoscopic procedures have additional potential complications. Atelectasis and lung collapse may occur postoperatively as a result of the procedural approach. Lymphatic injuries, sympathectomy, and dural

tears are also possible complications (Kuklo & Lenke, 2000).

Preprocedure Preparation

Before an arthroscopic procedure, the client should be asked to report any illness or infection and to list any medications. It may be necessary to discontinue some medications, especially aspirin or warfarin, before the procedure. Preadmission laboratory samples or tests (e.g., radiographs, hematocrit, hemoglobin, urinalysis) should be completed as ordered. Preoperative pulmonary function tests may be ordered before spinal thoracoscopic procedures (Kuklo & Lenke, 2000).

It must be reinforced to the client that he or she should not eat or drink anything after midnight the night before surgery; this includes drinking water and chewing gum. A consent form is needed for this surgery. The anesthesiologist usually visits with the client before surgery to discuss and obtain permission for anesthesia. Medication may be ordered to relax the client, and an intravenous line is generally started.

Arthroscopic Procedure

Arthroscopy can take from 15 minutes to several hours, depending on the client's pathologic condition and on the surgeon's technique. The procedure begins with draping the client's joint and positioning the extremity. The joint may or may not be placed in a stabilizing mechanism, depending on physician preference.

Some physicians prefer to use a tourniquet and a blood evacuation system. Some believe that visualization is increased if blood is evacuated from the joint, but others believe that the danger of ischemia is too great for the minimal improvement obtained from use of the tourniquet.

The irrigation system is then set up, usually controlled with foot pedals by the physician. A portable or a wall suction unit is used for evacuating the joint cavity and irrigation fluids.

The actual procedure begins with a small stab wound into the joint area. Next, the sharp and then the blunt trocars are inserted into the joint. The trocars are pulled through a cannula, which is left in place to keep the wound open. This wound is first used for irrigation and distention. The arthroscope is placed through the cannula, and the light source is attached.

Additional portals are made for passage of instruments. The joint space is evaluated using various probes to manipulate the soft tissues and cartilage.

The entire operating room staff can view the procedure on a television monitor while the physician views the joint directly through the arthroscope. The procedure may be videotaped. After the diagnostic arthroscopy has been completed, the orthopaedic surgeon may choose to proceed with arthroscopic surgery or to open the joint for arthrotomy.

Before removing the arthroscopic equipment, the fluid within the joint space must be drained. The stab wounds are generally not sutured unless they are gaping. Because most arthroscopies are performed as ambulatory surgery, clients are allowed to return home the same day provided they are alert, have voided, and are taking postoperative food and fluids without nausea or vomiting. Lower extremity arthroscopies may require the ability to ambulate with crutches. Bulky dressings with elastic wraps are usually applied, and occasionally, an immobilizer splint may also be applied. Spinal thoracoscopy clients are admitted for monitoring because of potential complications.

Postprocedure Care and Instructions

Initially, the client should be instructed to keep the extremity elevated as much as possible for the first 48 hours to reduce edema. Ice should be applied for at least 24 hours after the surgery.

The client is usually allowed partial weight bearing immediately, although crutches may be used for 24 to 48 hours. A mild analgesic, such as acetaminophen, is usually prescribed for pain control, although clients may remain in the hospital until pain is under control. Postoperative physical therapy is beneficial for muscle strengthening.

A visit to the orthopaedic surgeon is recommended approximately 7 days postoperatively for evaluation of the puncture wounds and muscle strength. It is important to stress to clients that they should call the surgeon if they notice increased swelling, elevated temperature, or increased pain in the joint. A small effusion in the joint is common.

The client can usually shower 48 hours after the surgery, although soaking in a tub is not generally recommended for at least 4 days after arthroscopy. Return to work and other activities are determined by the surgeon based on the procedure performed.

JOINT ASPIRATION

Definition

Joint aspiration, or *arthrocentesis,* is a procedure carried out to obtain synovial fluid for examination. In addition to serving as a diagnostic tool, joint aspiration may also serve as a treatment for septic arthritis. Any synovial joint may be the target of aspiration, including the ankles, knees, hips, wrists, elbows, and shoulders.

History

Documented literature on the history of joint aspiration is markedly limited. The procedure seems to have been accepted in various forms since the earliest of times, but there is no definitive mention of its inception.

Equipment

The instruments and equipment for an arthrocentesis should be sterile. Aseptic technique is essential. Equipment includes antiseptic solution, topical and/or local anesthetic, sterile needles (one 25 gauge and a few that are 20 gauge or larger), syringes, drapes, gloves, dressings or Band-Aids, and culture or test tubes. The procedure may be performed without x-ray visualization (blind) or be performed with fluoroscopic control.

Specific Indications

This procedure is recommended to establish the presence of infection in a joint or joint cavity, such as septic arthritis and acute hematogenous osteomyelitis (Jaffe, Greco, & Wade, 1996). Joint aspiration may also be performed to evaluate inflammatory disorders before arthrography, to relieve pain when joint effusion is present, and to instill anti-inflammatory medications into the joint. The advantages of joint aspiration include safety, simplicity, and quantity of information revealed, as well as prevention of complications associated with joint swelling and effusion. These complications include stretching of the ligaments surrounding the joint, pressure on the joint capsule, interference with circulation, and irritation of nerve endings resulting in muscle spasms. The disadvantage of this procedure is the potential risk of infection.

Preprocedure Preparation

Before joint aspiration, the client should be assessed for allergies to the antiseptic solutions and local anesthetics. Assessment should also determine the presence of any bleeding tendencies or infection in the area to be aspirated and the current use of any anticoagulants. The client's anxiety level and knowledge level should be assessed because some teaching is necessary. The process of joint aspiration is explained to the client, as is the need for the procedure, its duration, expected results, and possible complications.

Joint aspiration is usually considered invasive, and informed consent is usually obtained before initiating the procedure. Nurses should check their institution's policy and procedure manual to determine whether such consent is required.

Joint Aspiration Procedure

The aspiration procedure is relatively simple. If the procedure is performed blind, it may be done in the client's room or physician's office. The procedure may be performed in the operating room (rarely) or in the radiology department if fluoroscopic control is desired.

Client Positioning. Client positioning varies, the deciding factor being the joint to be aspirated. A position of comfort with the area of the joint to be aspirated exposed is desirable. The client may need premedication for pain or anxiety before the procedure, although this is unlikely. The affected joint is prepared with an antiseptic solution, and a local anesthetic is injected into the skin and surrounding soft tissues. The area is then draped, sterile gloves are donned, and a 20-gauge or large-bore needle is inserted into the joint space. Synovial fluid is then aspirated. If the effusion is large, several large syringes may be needed to reduce the swelling. In clients with inflammatory disorders, a steroid with or without local anesthetic may be injected after aspiration. The aspiration site is dressed with a Band-Aid or sterile dressing, and the client is assisted to a comfortable position. The procedure lasts approximately 15 to 30 minutes.

Evaluation. The synovial fluid aspirated from the joint is examined in a variety of ways. According to D'Ambrosia (1986), five factors are studied grossly: volume, color, clarity, viscosity, and mucin clot formation. Synovial fluid should be colorless or straw colored, transparent, present in small amounts, and of low viscosity (D'Ambrosia, 1986). Mucin clot formation is to be expected. The characteristics of the clot determine the presence or absence of an inflammatory or infectious condition. Blood may be present in the specimen if the client has a bleeding disorder or has sustained a traumatic injury to the joint.

Microscopic examination of the synovial fluid is also performed, including cell counts, Gram stains, and inspection for formed elements. Infection is suspected when the cell count reveals greater than 25,000 leukocytes per milliliter and more than 25% polymorphonuclear cells (Salvati & Brause, 1988). Formed elements include urate, calcium, pyrophosphate, and cholesterol crystals, along with cartilage debris. Glucose and total protein content are evaluated and compared with levels in blood. In septic arthritis, the glucose content of synovial fluid is considerably lower than that in the blood, and the protein content is elevated. In addition to microscopic examination, aerobic and anaerobic cultures should be done. Specimens should be transported to the laboratory immediately or placed in an appropriate medium.

Postprocedure Care and Instructions

Joint aspiration may be performed in an inpatient or an ambulatory setting or in a physician's office or clinic. If the procedure is performed in the hospital, the nurse is responsible for assessing the client for signs and symptoms of infection and bleeding and for reporting them to the physician. The nurse is also responsible for teaching the client the signs and symptoms of infection to watch for at home. Continued or additional joint swelling, elevated temperature, purulent drainage, redness, and increased pain or tenderness at the site of aspiration must be reported to the physician.

BONE MARROW EXAMINATION

Definition

Bone marrow, located within cancellous bone and in cavities of long bone, functions primarily to manufacture erythrocytes, leukocytes, and platelets. There are two types of bone marrow: red, which produces the blood cells, and yellow, which produces blood cells only in times of shock and severe hemorrhage. Bone marrow examination includes aspiration, biopsy, and microscopic evaluation of the red marrow, primarily for diagnostic purposes.

History

The earliest date noted for bone marrow examination is 1903. Improvements in the design of the needles, the aspiration technique itself, and the techniques used to mount and examine the tissue samples have made this a valuable procedure in the diagnosis, evaluation, and treatment of many orthopaedic and oncologic disorders.

Equipment

The equipment used to perform bone marrow aspiration and biopsy includes needles and syringes, sterile setup, local anesthetic, skin antiseptic, and laboratory supplies. Bone marrow aspiration requires aspiration needles with stylets, bone marrow (biopsy) needles with stylets, and 22- and 25-gauge needles. Two syringes, 5 to 20 mL, are also necessary. A sterile setup should include gloves, drapes, dressing, and scalpel. The necessary laboratory supplies are test tubes, culture tubes, slides, and fixatives.

The types of equipment used may vary with physician preference, actual procedure performed, and the diagnosis being considered. There are a variety of needles available for aspiration and biopsy, including Rosenthal (aspiration), Craig, Westerman-Jensen, Johannah, and Jamshidi (biopsy). These needles vary in lumen size, shape, and length. All equipment must be sterile because this procedure is invasive and therefore has the potential for introducing bacteria into the marrow cavity.

Specific Indications

Bone marrow is examined to confirm or rule out a suspected diagnosis, to direct the course of treatment, or to follow responses to treatment. Hematologic disorders as well as primary and metastatic tumors are diagnosed with bone marrow aspiration and biopsy. Metabolic bone disease, multiple myeloma, and infectious diseases are among the orthopaedic indications for bone marrow examination.

Bone marrow examination can be diagnostic for certain disorders, although it does not always provide specific or even relevant information. Bone marrow aspiration and biopsy is a relatively quick and simple procedure, which entails no great risk to the client. Contraindications to this procedure are few. The only absolute contraindication is hemophilia and related bleeding disorders.

Preprocedure Preparation

Before bone marrow examination, thorough client assessment and instructions are necessary. Client assessment includes questions designed to identify any bleeding tendencies or disorders, any allergies (especially to local anesthetics), level of anxiety, and need for premedication. Should the client need premedication, obtain a physician's order for a pain reliever or tranquilizer or both.

Client teaching includes a brief description of the procedure, the need for a small incision, the use of a pressure dressing, the need for at least 1 hour of bed rest, and the possibility of discomfort or pain. The type of skin preparation needed for the procedure, such as povidone-iodine scrubs, should be described. In addition to client teaching, the client may need psychosocial support because not only will there be anxiety about the procedure but there also may be anxiety associated with the impending diagnosis.

Informed consent and a description of the benefits and risks of the procedure are the physician's responsibility. Bone marrow examination is an invasive procedure, and most institutions require a signed permission from the client. Nurses should consult their institution's policy and procedure manual.

Bone Marrow Aspiration Procedure

The client may be premedicated with a pain reliever or tranquilizer 30 minutes before the procedure. Client positioning varies depending on which site is chosen for aspiration or biopsy. The client is placed on his or her abdomen (prone) or on his or her side with the top knee flexed. The posterior superior iliac crest is the preferred site. The anterior iliac crest may be used if the client is very obese (Nettina, 1996). In adults, other sites that may be used are sternum and spinous process of the vertebrae. In children younger than 18 months, the tibia is used but for aspiration only.

The area of aspiration is scrubbed with an antiseptic solution. This area is then draped and marked, and a local anesthetic is injected. If a biopsy is to be performed, the physician makes a small incision to facilitate needle access. The needle with stylet is inserted into the bone until the physician feels a give, or pop, indicating that the needle is in the marrow cavity. After the stylet is removed, a syringe is attached and a small amount of marrow is aspirated. More than one specimen may be aspirated. Once the specimens have been obtained, the stylet is replaced and the entire apparatus is quickly removed.

Postprocedure Care and Instructions

A dry sterile dressing is applied along with pressure at the puncture site. This pressure should be firm but gentle. If a biopsy has been performed, the client is kept on bed rest for approximately 1 hour. It is important to assess the client for signs and symptoms of hemorrhage. Also, the nurse should check vital signs frequently, assess level of consciousness, and monitor the quantity and character of any drainage.

There should be little, if any, pain associated with this procedure, although a mild analgesic may be indicated. Severe or unrelenting pain may indicate a fracture. The biopsy site may be sore for 2 to 3 days.

Complications of bone marrow examination include osteomyelitis, bleeding, and hematoma formation, as well as perforation of the sternum and iliac bone. The client should be monitored for signs and symptoms of cardiac tamponade (for sternal bone marrow aspirations) and retroperitoneal hemorrhage (for iliac crest aspirations). Signs and symptoms of osteomyelitis include redness and swelling at the site, severe pain and tenderness, anorexia, malaise, and fever.

NURSING CONSIDERATIONS

The pertinent nursing considerations for each diagnostic modality are provided in Table 9-1.

INTERNET RESOURCES

Radiological Society of North America: www. radiologyinfo.org/content/mr_musculoskeletal.htm
Spine Universe: www.spineuniverse.com

REFERENCES

American College of Radiology. (1993). *Radiology: An inside look.* Reston, VA: Author. [On-line]. Available at www.acr.org

Baker, Jr., C. L., & Jones, G. L. (1999). Arthroscopy of the elbow. *The American Journal of Sports Medicine, 27*(2), 251–264.

Basmajian, J. V. (1962). *Muscles alive: Their function revealed by electromyography.* Baltimore: Williams & Wilkins.

Basmajian, J. V., & DeLuca, C. J. (1985). *Muscles alive: Their function revealed by electromyography* (5th ed.). Baltimore: Williams & Wilkins.

D'Ambrosia, R. D. (1986). *Musculoskeletal disorder, regional examination and differential diagnosis* (2nd ed.). Philadelphia: Lippincott.

Freeman, M. (1984). *Freeman & Johnson's clinical radionuclide imaging.* New York: Grune & Stratton.

Galen, B. A. (1999). Diagnostic imaging: An overview. *Primary care practice: A peer-reviewed series.* [On-line]. Available at www.nursing-center.com

Goldman, A. B. (1982). *Shoulder arthrography technique, diagnosis, and clinical correlation.* Boston: Little, Brown.

Grech, P. (1977). *Hip arthrography.* Philadelphia: Lippincott.

Hillman, B. J. (1997). Diagnostic imaging in 2001: A health economics perspective. *European Journal of Radiology, 7*(14), S251–S252.

Hines, S. E. (1999). How to choose between CT and MRI for musculoskeletal pain. *Patient Care, 33*(17), 54–70.

Jaffe, K., Greco, C., & Wade, J. (1996). Orthopaedic emergencies and infections. In V. A. Masear (Ed.), *Primary care orthopaedics.* Philadelphia: WB Saunders.

Kuklo, T. R. & Lenke, L. G. (2000). Thoracoscopic spine surgery: Current indications and techniques. *Orthopaedic Nursing, 19*(6), 15–22.

Moye, C. E. (1996). Diagnostic studies. In S. W. Salmond, N. E. Mooney, & L. A. Verdisco (Eds.), *Core curriculum for orthopaedic nursing* (3rd ed.). Pitman, NJ: National Association of Orthopaedic Nurses.

Nettina, S. M. (Ed.). (1996). *Lippincott manual of nursing practice* (6th ed.). Philadelphia: Lippincott-Raven.

Ricklin, P. Ruttiman, A., & DeBuono, M. D. (1971). *Meniscus lesions: Practical problems of clinical diagnosis arthrography and therapy.* New York: Grune & Stratton.

Salvati, E. A., & Brause, B. D. (1988). The examination of the case. In D. Schlossberg (Ed.), *Orthopaedic infection.* New York: Springer-Verlag.

Sciulli, R. L., Boutin, R. D., Brown, R. R., Nguyen, K. D., Muhle, C., Lektrakul, N., Pathria, M. N., Pedowitz, R., & Resnick, D. (1999). Evaluation of the postoperative meniscus of the knee: A study comparing conventional arthrography, conventional MR imaging, MR arthrography with iodinated contrast material, and MR arthrography with gadolinium-based contrast material. *Skeletal Radiology, 28*(9), 508–514.

Spinasanta, S. (2001). *Myelogram (myelography).* [On-line]. Available at www.spineuniverse.com

Stearns, H. C., & Stearns, C. M. (1986). Orthopaedic radiology. *Orthopaedic Nursing, 5*(2), 26–31.

Complications of Orthopaedic Disorders and Orthopaedic Surgery

TERESA A. PELLINO, MARY ANN S. PRESTON, NANCY BELL, MONICA J. NEWTON, and KATHLEEN HANSEN

COMPARTMENT SYNDROME

Definition

A *compartment* is an area in the body where muscles, nerves, and blood vessels are encompassed within tissue such as bone or fascia. There are 46 anatomic compartments within the body, 36 of which are located in the extremities. Compartment syndrome is high pressure in the muscle compartment in the closed fascial space. Compartment syndrome causes capillary blood perfusion to be reduced below a level necessary for tissue viability and is classified as acute, chronic, or crush.

Incidence

The most frequently involved muscle compartments are the four of the lower leg: the anterior, superficial posterior, deep posterior, and lateral (Fig. 10–1). Compartment syndrome can also involve the hand, forearm, upper arm, shoulder, thigh, foot, lumbar paraspinal, extraocular, and gluteal muscles (Gellman & Buch, 1998; McQueen, Gaston, & Court-Brown, 2000; Yamaguchi & Viegas, 1998).

The space for the compartment's contents must be limited, and tissue pressure must be increased for compartment syndrome to occur. Space limitations can result from external compression (e.g., from a cast or splint) or from restrictions inherent in the client's skin, fascia, or epimysium. Increased tissue pressure can result from increased compartmental contents (e.g., edema or blood) or a combination of external and internal sources. Box 10–1 lists common causes of acute compartment syndrome.

Acute Compartment Syndrome. Acute compartment syndrome is the most severe form, often requiring surgical intervention. The acute form may also be called anterior tibial syndrome, calf hypertension, Volkmann's ischemic paralysis, and march gangrene.

Volkmann's contracture, limb deformity resulting from unrelieved compartment syndrome (Fig. 10–2), may require reconstructive surgery.

Acute compartment syndrome occurs as frequently in children as in adults. Fractures, particularly supracondylar fractures of the humerus are common causes of compartment syndrome in children. Additional causes of compartment syndrome in children include high-velocity injuries, infiltrated arterial or intravenous (IV) infusions, and in utero limb compression in neonates (Blakemore, Cooperman, Thompson, Wathey, & Ballock, 2000).

Chronic Compartment Syndrome. Chronic, or exertional, compartment syndrome results from increasing pressure in the compartment from exercise. Exercise increases capillary surface area and capillary pressure, leading to increased transcapillary filtration without increased reabsorption. Muscle volume can increase as much as 20%. Fascial compliance is decreased in some individuals, prohibiting expansion of the muscle compartment. Increased pressure leads to ischemia and pain. Neurologic deficits are rare with chronic compartment syndrome, and they generally resolve with rest. If exercise is continued despite pain and neuromuscular deficit, the acute form of compartment syndrome may develop and require decompression. Chronic compartment syndrome is also called *exercise ischemia, exercise myopathy,* and *recurrent compartment syndrome.* The exact prevalence of chronic compartment syndrome is not known.

Crush Syndrome. Crush syndrome comprises the multicompartment, systemic effects of severe muscle necrosis resulting from crush injuries that externally

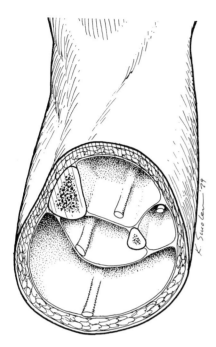

FIGURE 10–1. Four compartments of the leg. (From Mubarak, S. J., & Hargens, A. R. [1981]. *Compartment syndromes and Volkmann's contracture* [p. 38]. Philadelphia: WB Saunders.)

compress the compartment. Bleeding and edema from fracture or fluid shifts contribute to the injury. Muscle infarction within the compartment leads to myoglobinemia, extracellular fluid loss, acidosis, hyperkalemia, renal failure, shock, and cardiac arrhythmias. Individuals who were trapped under a fallen object or under equipment or those who overdosed on a drug and fell asleep with a limb beneath their body are at risk for crush syndrome. Persons treated with a pneumatic antishock garment or military antishock trousers and those who suffered a wringer-type injury may also develop crush syndrome. The compartments of the lower extremities are the most commonly affected muscle compartments.

Pathophysiology

A muscle compartment contains muscles, arteries, veins, and nerves enclosed in the space between the fascia and the bone (Fig. 10–3). Fascia is a dense, regular, connective tissue. The biomechanics and function of fascia are poorly understood, but it is thought to enhance the power of underlying muscle. If fascia is removed, the muscle can balloon out, decreasing the contractile efficiency of the muscle. Removal of the fascia can decrease muscle strength by 15%.

Interstitial fluid is formed by the filtration of water and dissolved crystalloids because of hydrostatic pressure of the blood within the capillary (Starling's law). The colloids of plasma are retained by the capillary wall and exert contrary force by the action of osmotic pressure. Fluid tissue pressure, capillary fluid pressure, and the effective osmotic pressures of tissue fluid and plasma determine the exchange of fluid across the vessel wall. These pressures determine the fluid balance between the intravascular and the extravascular spaces of the compartment. At the arterial end of the capillary, the hydrostatic pressure in the vessel is greater than the osmotic pressure, promoting fluid movement out of the capillary. In contrast, fluid is reabsorbed into the capillary at the venous end because the osmotic pressure in the capillary is greater than the hydrostatic pressure.

There are two basic causes of compartment syndrome: decreased compartment size and increased contents in the compartment. Specific causes for each category are listed in Box 10–1.

Acute Compartment Syndrome. The initial injury may be proximal to the compartment, resulting in decreased blood flow below the level of the injury. The decrease in blood flow causes hypoxia in the cells of the capillary wall, and the capillary begins to lose its integrity. The colloid proteins escape into the soft tissue, drawing fluid with them. Swelling results, exacerbating the problem. If the initial damage is to the muscles, the swelling begins in the muscle as a result of hemorrhage and damage to the capillaries (Fig. 10–4).

The pressure relationships within the compartment change. The compartment can distend only so far (because the fascia and bone restrict it), so the pressure

---

BOX 10–1.
Common Causes of Acute Compartment Syndrome

External Compression
Tight dressings, casts, braces, or traction
Closure of fascial defects
Pneumatic antishock garments
Surgical positions, particularly the lithotomy or hemilithotomy position
Automatic blood pressure monitoring devices
Eschar from burns

Increased Compartment Content
Trauma (especially fractures)
Contusions
Bleeding disorders or anticoagulation
Burns
Vascular repair
Exercise
Immobility following drug or alcohol overdose or falls
Venous obstruction
Ischemia
Infiltrated IV sites
Frostbite
Venomous bites

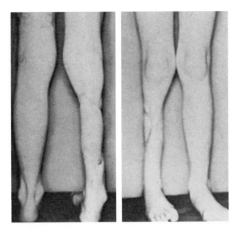

FIGURE 10–2. Posterior and frontal views of the legs of a 14-year-old girl who 10 years previously had sustained a fracture of the right femur. She had been treated in Bryant's traction and developed a deep posterior compartment syndrome and a skin lesion that required grafting. Note the cavus of the foot, equinus and adduction of the forefoot, and varus of the hindfoot. (From Mubarak, S. J., & Hargens, A. R. [1981]. *Compartment syndromes and Volkmann's contracture* [p. 199]. Philadelphia: WB Saunders.)

inside the compartment begins to rise. The critical factor in compartment syndrome is an elevated intracompartmental pressure sufficiently high to compromise the intracompartmental microcirculation. If the soft tissue pressure is greater than the intravascular pressure, the vessels begin to collapse. One might expect that low tissue pressure arrests circulation, but an increased tissue pressure applied to the walls of collapsible vessels produces a corresponding increase in the pressure within those vessels. This increased venous pressure lowers the local arteriovenous pressure gradient. Blood continues to flow down the pressure gradient from the arteries to the veins. Changes in the local arteriovenous gradient affect local blood flow, which, in turn, is determined by the local arteriovenous gradient. Intracompartmental pressures of 30 to 40 mm Hg are high enough to compromise muscle microcirculation. As venous structures begin to collapse, the blood outflow is obstructed, resulting in further leakage of proteins and fluid into the soft tissues. When the pressure is high enough to decrease flow of the arterioles, blood supply is cut off, and the muscle becomes necrotic. Pressures of 65 mm Hg in the forearm and 55 mm Hg in the calf can produce complete cessation of tissue circulation in normovolemic clients.

As tissue fluid pressure increases, capillary blood flow decreases. If there is a prolonged period of microcirculatory ischemia, necrosis of the intracompartmental tissues, including muscle and nerve tissue, results.

Pressure tolerance varies among clients, depending on the duration of the pressure increase and changes in arterial pressure. The metabolic demands of the tissue also play a role in the tolerance of increased tissue pressure. Higher tissue pressures can be tolerated for less time than lower tissue pressures. Decreased local arterial pressure lowers local blood flow to the area by reducing the local arteriovenous gradient, as described previously. Local arterial pressure may be decreased in the presence of shock or peripheral vascular disease or when the limb has been elevated above heart level. Traumatized tissue may have a higher metabolic demand, thus requiring more blood flow for viability than resting, uninjured muscle.

Chronic Compartment Syndrome. Although the pathophysiology of chronic compartment syndrome is not as well understood as that of the acute form, many of the same principles apply. Repeated muscle contractions during exercise can increase muscle bulk by 20%. Because the envelope surrounding the muscle is unyielding, tissue pressures rise. Transudation of fluid into the interstitial space because of arteriovenous gradient changes occurs if the tissue pressure does not return to normal with muscle relaxation. In addition, with each stretching trauma, the fascia can become inflamed and injured, resulting in fascial scarring, which further decreases the size of the compartment and decreases the minimal elasticity of the fascia itself. It is also hypothesized that chronic compartment syndrome may be the result of the accumulation of metabolic wastes within the compartment that occurs during exercise. During exercise, the compartmental pressures alter the arteriovenous pressure gradients, which

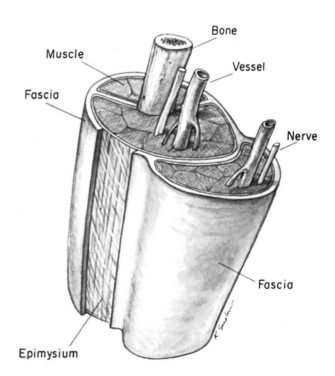

FIGURE 10–3. Components of a generalized muscle compartment. (From Mubarak, S. J., & Hargens, A. R. [1981]. *Compartment syndromes and Volkmann's contracture* [p. 18]. Philadelphia: WB Saunders.)

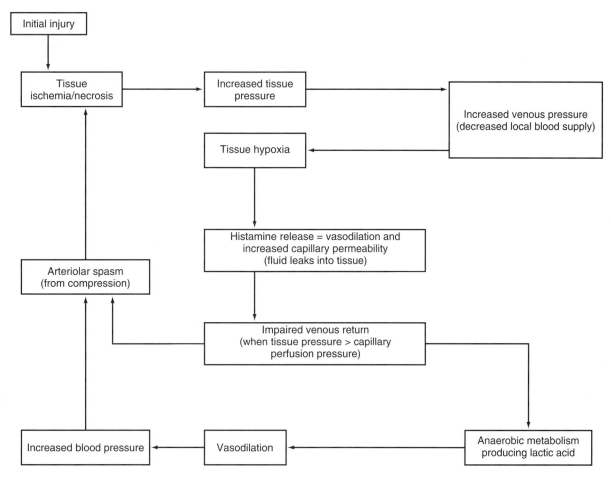

FIGURE 10–4. Pathophysiology of acute compartment syndrome. (From Ross, D., & Evans, R. [1994]. A patient with acute compartment syndrome. *Clinical simulations in medical-surgical nursing III, Medi-Sim computer assisted instruction.* Baltimore: Williams & Wilkins.)

causes the metabolic wastes to accumulate in the muscle tissues, creating pain. When the client rests, the pressures decrease, allowing the wastes to be removed and thus decreasing the pain (Ross, 1996).

Crush Syndrome. Myoglobinuric renal failure is the hallmark of crush syndrome. Myoglobin is released from muscle tissue that has become ischemic because of compression, and myoglobinuria results. The presence of the systemic symptoms of crush syndrome seems to depend on the amount of muscle that is necrotic. In other words, the more muscle compartments involved, the greater the likelihood of systemic manifestations. When a large amount of muscle is infarcted, the sarcolemma loses its functional integrity, creating intracellular edema. Intracellular edema, along with the interstitial edema from capillary ischemic damage, produces third-space loss. Hypovolemia with hypotension or shock may result. Myoglobin is released into the circulation, where it can occlude the distal convoluted tubule and precipitate renal failure. It is also thought that myoglobin may have a toxic effect on the kidney.

Potassium is also released from the damaged muscle cells. Because of renal failure, this excess potassium is not excreted, and the resulting hyperkalemia may cause cardiac arrhythmias.

Assessment

A nursing history should contain information about potential causes of compartment syndrome. Information should be obtained about causes of injury; position of the arms and legs during and after injury, surgery, or immobilization (to assess for potential areas of compression); type of surgery performed; exercise patterns; and other risk factors. Box 10-2 summarizes the signs and symptoms of compartment syndrome.

Acute Compartment Syndrome. The assessment of acute compartment syndrome can best be accomplished by assessing for the "6 Ps": pain, paresthesias, paresis, pressure, pink skin color, and pulse (distal pulse present) (Hargens & Mubarak, 1998). The primary symptom of compartment syndrome is increasing pain or pain that is out of proportion to the injury. Attention should be paid

---

BOX 10–2.
Assessment for Compartment Syndrome

Acute Compartment Syndrome
Cause of injury
Position of body during and after injury, surgery, or
     immobilization
Increasing pain
Deep, throbbing, unrelenting, localized pain
Pain on passive stretch of compartment
Paresthesias
Skin tense, shiny
Sensory deficits
Motor weakness
Pulse is almost always present

Chronic Compartment Syndrome
Aching, tightness, or squeezing in limb
Associated with exercise
Muscle tenderness
Numbness, paresthesias
Exercise patterns

Crush Syndrome
Cause and length of limb compression
Possible sources of compression
Position in which found
Use of pneumatic antishock garment (how long?)
Deep, unremitting, poorly localized pain
Tense, swollen extremity
Hypovolemia
Urine output decreased initially, then increased

---

to the client who continues to complain of pain after receiving analgesics or who states that the pain is continually worsening. Clients generally complain of a deep, throbbing feeling of pressure that is unrelenting and localized. The hallmark sign of compartment syndrome is pain on passive stretch. For example, in anterior compartment syndrome, leg pain increases on plantar flexion.

Clients may also report paresthesias, that is, a feeling of "pins and needles," or they say the extremity feels like it is "asleep." Sensory deficits associated with the nerve in the affected compartment are among the first signs of acute compartment syndrome. Table 10–1 details the nerve assessment for various compartments. In addition to assessing the client for paresthesias, it is important to assess the client's two-point discrimination to determine whether he or she can differentiate between sharp and dull. The client may be able to feel pressure or touch but may not be able to discriminate, which is a sign of decreasing neurovascular function.

Clients with compartment syndrome may have weakness, that is, paresis, in the extremity distal to the injury because of the compression on the nerves. If trauma has occurred, the site of injury as well as areas that may have incurred bruising or compression should be examined. The area over the compartment may feel tense, and the skin may be shiny and warm.

Arterial flow to the extremity is generally present until compartment pressures are elevated to a level above systolic pressure. Therefore, unlike arterial injury, the skin is usually still pink and the distal pulse is present. If the client develops pulselessness where there previously was a pulse or develops pallor of the extremity, action must be taken quickly. The client's contralateral extremity should also be assessed because this can provide a baseline, as well as serve as a control, of the client's normal neurovascular status.

Acute compartment syndrome generally occurs within 6 to 8 hours after injury, but it may take as long as 2 days to manifest.

Chronic Compartment Syndrome. Young, active individuals are most commonly affected by chronic compartment syndrome. It can occur in males and females. The lower leg is most commonly affected, but the syndrome also occurs in the thigh, hand, and forearm. The primary complaint is aching, tightness, squeezing, or cramping in the affected limb. Symptoms are associated with activity and may disappear immediately after exercise is stopped or continue for a few minutes or a day.

Pain is usually localized to the specific compartment. Bilateral pain is present in 90% of clients. A history of previous fracture, knee surgery, or casting should be obtained.

Generally, no notable swelling occurs in chronic compartment syndrome, but mild muscle tenderness of the compartment may be present. Muscle hernias may or may not be palpable. Skin condition, pulses, capillary filling, range of motion, and deep tendon reflexes are usually normal. In severe cases, numbness and paresthesias may be present and correlate with the involved muscle compartment (see Table 10–1).

Crush Syndrome. Information about the cause and duration of limb compression should be obtained. The type of accident and possible sources of external compression, such as debris, need to be examined. In drug overdose cases or cases in which clients have fallen and not been able to move, it is important to learn the position in which the client was found to determine which compartments were compressed. The amount of pressure used and the amount of time a client has been in a pneumatic antishock garment or military antishock trousers should be noted.

If the client is conscious, he or she may report deep, unremitting, and poorly localized pain. In many cases, however, the client may not be able to give an adequate history or verbalize the pain status.

Examination often reveals a tense and swollen extremity. Minimal swelling may be due to dehydration and peripheral vasoconstriction from shock. Localized skin pressure changes accompanied by erythema, bullae, or vesicles may occur.

Signs of hypovolemia may be present, including such hemodynamic changes as decreased blood pressure, increased heart rate, and altered cardiac output and central venous pressure. The client may have cool, clammy skin.

Urine output initially decreases in the oliguric stage of acute tubular necrosis. An output below 400 mL per 24 hours can be expected. During the diuretic phase, increased urine output occurs. The urine may be red-brown because of myoglobinuria.

TABLE 10–1. *Nerve Assessment*

COMPARTMENT	NERVES INVOLVED	SIGNS AND SYMPTOMS
Anterior leg	Deep peroneal	Decreased dorsiflexion of foot and toes
		Tense and tender lateral to tibial crest
		Anterior pain with toe, foot, or ankle plantar flexion
Lateral leg	Superficial peroneal	Decreased foot and ankle eversion
	Deep peroneal	Sensory deficit over dorsum of foot and perhaps first web space
Superficial posterior leg	Tibial	Decreased plantar flexion of ankle
	Sural	Posterior calf pain with active plantar flexion and passive ankle dorsiflexion
		Sensory deficit over lateral aspect of foot
Deep posterior leg	Tibial	Tenseness hard to detect
	Saphenous	Passive pain with dorsiflexion of toes or foot, everting foot
		Paresis in toe flexors and foot invertors
Foot (medial, lateral, central, interosseous)	Digital	Difficult to separate four compartments
		Tense and swollen
		Decreased motions
		Passive stretch pain
Gluteal (3) (tensor, medius/ minimus, maximus)	Sciatic	Buttock tenderness and tenseness
		Decreased extension and abduction of hip
		Gluteal stretch pain with hip adduction or flexion
		Paresthesias along distal sciatic
Iliacus (inner wall of pelvis)	Femoral	Very rare, occurs with hemorrhage in pelvis
		Hip held in flexion
		Pain with hip extension
		Tenderness along inguinal ligament
		Dysesthesia around knee and distally in saphenous nerve
Thigh		
Anterior	Femoral	Decreased knee extension
		Keeps knee in extended position
		Passive flexion of knee leads to pain in anterior thigh
		Active quadriceps contraction leads to pain
		Paresthesia over knee and medial aspect of leg and foot
		Tense and tender over anterior thigh
Posterior	Obturator	Decreased knee flexion
	Sciatic	Passive knee extension leads to posterior thigh pain
		Sensory and motor deficits of distal sciatic if significant pressure elevation
		Tender and tense over medial thigh
		Paresthesia and paresis along obturator
Forearm		
Volar	Median	Sensation and motor function on flexor or palmar surface of the hand
	Ulnar	Decreased strength in finger and thumb flexors
	Anterior interosseous	Passive extension of the fingers causes pain in volar forearm
		Paresis of intrinsic muscles
		Tenseness and tenderness over volar forearm
Dorsal	Posterior interosseous	Decreased wrist and finger extension
		Hand may assume extended position
		Passive finger or wrist flexion leads to pain in dorsal forearm
		Sensory deficit usually minimal

Assessment in obtunded clients is challenging because they cannot report the classic symptoms of compartment syndrome. A high degree of suspicion in high-risk clients is warranted. Physical examination should include palpation of the suspected compartments for tenseness. In the hand, a classic symptom of compartment syndrome is the intrinsic-minus position in which the metacarpophalangeal joints are in extension and the interphalangeal joints are in flexion (Ouellette, 1998). Ortiz and Berger (1998) recommend carefully observing the obtunded client for signs of pain, such as increased heart rate or blood pressure and withdrawal of the extremity, with passive stretch of the compartments.

Diagnostic Evaluation

The definitive sign for any type of compartment syndrome is increased pressure. In alert and cooperative clients, signs and symptoms of compartment syndrome should suggest the need for tissue pressure measurement. In uncooperative or comatose clients, tissue pressure may need to be monitored continually.

Acute Compartment Syndrome. Intracompartmental pressure can be measured by threading an indwelling catheter with nonabsorbable sutures; a side-ported, slit-tip, or transducer-tipped catheter; or a large-bore needle into the compartment and reading the pressure on a manometer or specially designed pressure monitor. Continuous monitoring can be accomplished using a wick, slit-tip, or transducer-tipped catheter connected to a pressure monitor. The needle or catheter is inserted through the fascia of the involved muscle at the junction of the compartment. Pressure is measured in millimeters of mercury. Needle measurements of intramuscular pressure can be erroneous because of occlusion of the needle tip by tissue and changes in pressure may not be detected. The wick or slit-tip catheters avoid some problems but are dependent upon client position and require equilibration and injection of saline. The electronic transducer-tipped catheter may provide the best technology in the future because these concerns are avoided with this method (Hargens & Mubarak, 1998; Willy, Gerngross, & Sterk, 1999). Normal compartment pressure is between 0 and 8 mm Hg. Nerve tissue seems to be more sensitive than muscle tissue to the effects of increased pressure. If the compartment pressure is greater than 30 mm Hg for 8 hours, nerve damage can occur. Permanent muscle damage can begin after 4 to 12 hours of ischemia.

Continuous compartment monitoring should be used in comatose, unresponsive, or uncooperative clients when compartment syndrome is suspected. Continuous or one-time pressure monitoring should be done to confirm the diagnosis of compartment syndrome, to rule out peripheral nerve injury, to assess decompression, and to monitor skin closure during surgery. Monitoring can rule out ischemic neurologic damage and arterial injury.

Efforts to find a noninvasive technique for compartment pressure monitoring are under way. The use of near-infrared spectroscopy for monitoring pressure in trauma clients with a clinical diagnosis of compartment syndrome compared with control clients has been reported by Giannotti, Cohn, Brown, Varela, McKenney, and Wiseberg (2000). This method uses light transmission and absorption to measure oxygen saturation. A probe is placed on the skin over the suspected compartment. Oxygenation of the compartments was found to be significantly lower in clients with known compartment syndrome before fasciotomy than in the corresponding unaffected extremity compartments or in the affected compartments postfasciotomy or in clients who did not have clinical symptoms. There was some variability among clients, however, and this method cannot evaluate the deep posterior compartment. The authors advise further investigation of the method to determine its application in clinical settings (Giannotti et al., 2000).

Measurement of skin surface pressure (SSP) under a cast has been compared with intracompartmental pressures in an inflatable forearm model and an animal model (Uslu & Apan, 2000). SSP measurements were highly correlated with intracompartmental pressures. This technique may hold promise for monitoring clients who are casted; however, clinical studies are lacking at this point.

Most laboratory tests are not helpful in diagnosing compartment syndrome. Creatine kinase (CK, formerly creatine phosphokinase [CPK]) levels may be elevated and myoglobinuria may be present, but these indicate that muscle damage has already occurred and may be due primarily to other injuries.

Chronic Compartment Syndrome. Diagnosis is made by identifying a positive clinical pattern of pain with exercise, establishing that the pain corresponds to a muscle compartment, and measuring compartment pressures. Compartment pressures are usually chronically elevated, but some practitioners advise measuring the pressure after exercise. Resting pressures are usually 15 to 30 mm Hg in these clients. Postexercise pressures above 30 mm Hg are considered abnormal. Pedowitz, Hargens, Mubarak, and Gershuni (1990) suggest the criteria of a resting pressure higher than 15 mm Hg and a 1-minute postexercise pressure higher than 30 mm Hg or a 5-minute postexercise pressure higher than 20 mm Hg as indicative of a chronic compartment syndrome.

Magnetic resonance imaging (MRI), which is being studied as an adjunct to diagnosis of chronic compartment syndrome, assesses muscle density changes or changes in cross-sectional areas of muscle. MRI has the advantages of being noninvasive and allowing evaluation of several compartments. MRI may also help clarify the pathophysiologic changes occurring in chronic compartment syndrome.

Crush Syndrome. In addition to increased compartment pressures, clients with crush syndrome manifest systemic symptoms. Changes in hemodynamics, such as decreased central venous pressure, decreased wedge pressures, and decreased cardiac output, result from hypovolemia. Hemoglobin and hematocrit values may increase because of hemoconcentration.

Signs of rhabdomyolysis (a synonym for crush syndrome) include an increase in serum myoglobin level to greater than 1.5 mg/dL; myoglobinuria; positive *O*-toluidine test; positive spun plasma test; and increased serum potassium and muscle enzyme levels, such as aldolase, aspartate transaminase (AST; formerly serum glutamic oxaloacetic transaminase [SGOT]), lactate dehydrogenase (LDH), and CK. The CK usually shows an elevation greater than 10,000 IU.

Increased blood urea nitrogen (BUN) and creatinine and altered serum potassium, phosphorous, calcium, and sodium levels accompany the renal failure with crush syndrome. During the oliguric phase, phosphorous, potassium, BUN, and creatinine levels are elevated, and the calcium level is decreased. Decreased sodium and potassium levels and elevated BUN and creatinine levels are typical of the diuretic phase. Creatinine and BUN return to normal levels, the phosphorous level decreases, and the calcium level increases during the recovery phase. The urine sodium level increases, and urine specific gravity decreases.

High, peaked T waves, ST-segment depression, increased QRS duration and PR intervals, and premature ventricular complexes are characteristic of the cardiac changes that accompany the hyperkalemia from muscle damage.

Treatment Modalities and Related Nursing Management

Acute Compartment Syndrome. The primary treatment for compartment syndrome is to relieve the source of pressure. This may involve loosening external constriction (e.g., bivalving a cast and Webril), loosening dressings, or removing tight stockings. For clients with thermal burns, this may be accomplished by debridement of eschar. If the relief of external pressure is not effective and the compartment pressure rises, a fasciotomy may be necessary.

Treatment for an increase in the contents of the compartment initially involves keeping the limb at heart level. Limb elevation above heart level decreases local arterial perfusion and further compromises local blood flow. Adequate hydration should be maintained to preserve mean arterial blood pressure. If compartmental pressure is not relieved and the signs and symptoms progress, a fasciotomy may be required.

Other treatment modalities have been tried, with varying degrees of success. Vasodilators and sympathetic nerve blocks do not seem to increase tissue perfusion in compartment syndrome. Hypertonic mannitol has not been proven effective in clinical studies. Hyperbaric oxygen can be used as a treatment adjunct to decrease postischemic swelling and improve peripheral ischemia after fasciotomy (Fitzpatrick, Murphy, & Bryce, 1998).

There is some controversy about what tissue pressure measurements are indications for a fasciotomy. Although authors disagree on a definitive pressure measurement recommendation, pressures of 30 to 45 mm Hg in conjunction with a positive clinical examination are generally accepted criteria. A critical factor is the difference between the mean arterial pressure and compartment pressure, called the *delta pressure*. Delta pressures at or above 30 mm Hg warrant consideration for fasciotomy. If the blood pressure falls, the client may not be able to tolerate as high an increase in compartment pressure. Thus, absolute values of pressure are not as important as individual consideration of the client's hemodynamic status and pressure measurements.

In children, physiologic differences make it even more difficult to determine pressures indicative for fasciotomy. It is not known if tissue pressures in children are different from those in adults. Future growth must be considered in treating the child with compartment syndrome. Fasciotomy-fibulectomy, which may be used in adults, should not be in children because it may impair growth.

The purpose of a fasciotomy is to relieve tissue pressure and reestablish tissue perfusion. At least one skin incision is made, and the fascia is relaxed with dissecting scissors. The skin itself may contribute to increasing the tissue pressure when swelling occurs, so the incisions are left open for several days, and bulky, wet dressings are applied. The extremity is re-evaluated, and the compartment is closed usually in 3 days for the upper extremities and 5 days for the lower extremities. Complications as a result of fasciotomy, such as loss of fracture stabilization, necrosis of the bone, delayed union or nonunion of fractures, and infection, can occur. The compartment syndrome may recur after closure.

Chronic Compartment Syndrome. Some advocate nonsurgical treatment for chronic compartment syndrome, but others believe that nonsurgical treatment, except for cessation of activity, is of limited use. Physical therapy, stretching, footwear changes, anti-inflammatory drugs, orthotic devices, and diuretics may be prescribed for the client with chronic compartment syndrome.

Fasciotomy or partial fasciectomy is the definitive treatment for chronic compartment syndrome. Generally, the procedure can be performed on an outpatient basis with local anesthesia. Dressings are removed after 48 hours. Full weight bearing can be expected on the third postoperative day, and clients often return to stretching exercises of the involved compartment about 2 weeks after surgery. Most clients return to their normal activity levels within 3 months.

Crush Syndrome. Treatment for crush syndrome is aimed not only at resolving increased muscle tissue pressure through the use of fasciotomy but also at managing the potentially life-threatening systemic effects of the syndrome. Rapid crystalloid fluid replacement must be instituted to offset the hypovolemia from third-space loss. Monitoring of hemodynamic parameters is essential.

The treatment of acute tubular necrosis varies with the stage of the disease. During the oliguric phase, maintaining fluid and electrolyte balance is the prime consideration. Hyperalimentation and dialysis may be necessary to handle the hypercatabolism experienced during this stage. Furosemide and mannitol may be given to expand circulating volume, increase renal perfusion, increase pressure in the renal tubule to overcome obstruction, and dilate the renal artery. A urine output of 100 to 200 mL/hr is the goal once myoglobinuria is present.

Treatment for hyperkalemia may include IV calcium to stabilize the myocardium, sodium bicarbonate to improve acidosis and displace potassium, and insulin and glucose IV to move potassium into the cell. Sodium polystyrene sulfonate (Kayexalate) taken orally or given as an enema may be needed to reduce serum potassium levels.

Nursing Management

Nursing diagnoses that may apply to the client with a suspected or confirmed compartment syndrome include high risk of peripheral neurovascular dysfunction and pain related to increased tissue pressure, anxiety related to pain and potential surgery or knowledge deficit related to compartment syndrome and its treatment, kinesthetic sensory alternations related to nerve damage, and body image disturbance related to decreased limb function and surgical scars. In addition, clients undergoing fasciotomy may also be at risk for infection related to open surgical wounds. Individuals with crush syndrome are also at risk for alteration in renal tissue perfusion.

High Risk for Peripheral Neurovascular Dysfunction

Circulatory Care. The nurse is responsible for monitoring the client for compartment syndrome. Neurovascular and pain assessment must be done at least every 4 to 8 hours for all orthopaedic clients and even more often (every 1 to 2 hours) in the immediate postoperative period and for clients who are at greatest risk for or who have shown signs of developing compartment syndrome. Those at risk include clients who have had upper or lower extremity surgery or sustained fractures in the past 8 hours; clients who have been in one position for an extended period (e.g., clients who were in a lithotomy position for surgery for several hours) (Heppenstall &

Tan, 1999); clients receiving anticoagulation therapy (McLaughlin, Paulson, & Rosenthall, 1998); and clients who have recently had a cast, splint, brace, traction, or pneumatic antishock garment applied. The physician should be notified immediately if any signs of compartment syndrome occur.

Special attention should be paid to the client who is not able to communicate pain or who has altered sensation. As described previously, palpation of the suspected compartments and careful assessment of signs of pain (elevated heart rate or blood pressure or withdrawal of the extremity) should be implemented for the client unable to communicate. There have been some reports of epidural analgesia or nerve blocks masking symptoms of compartment syndrome (Hyder, Kessler, Jennings, & De Boer, 1996; Tang & Chiu, 2000), or delaying treatment of compartment syndrome (Dunwoody, Reichert, & Brown, 1997). There are no randomized trials that support these findings, and other authors raise questions about these reports (Mubarak & Wilton, 1997; Politis, 1998; Schmitz, Brown, Stoner, & Vollers, 1997). Mubarak and Wilton (1997) stated that whatever mode of analgesia is used, a high index of clinical suspicion, detailed examination, and compartment pressure measurements are the cornerstones for diagnosis and treatment of compartment syndrome.

The affected limb should be maintained at heart level. The nurse may need to bivalve the cast and split the underlying soft dressings (at physician instruction) and remove dressings to relieve external pressure.

The use of ice should be avoided in clients suspected of developing compartment syndrome. Intake and output should be carefully monitored and recorded. Volume replacement should be adequate to prevent any decrease in mean arterial pressure.

Caution must be taken in deflating antishock garments because blood pressure may drop rapidly. The duration and degree of use of these garments should be limited as much as possible and noted on the chart.

Pain

Pain Management. Alleviating the source of increased tissue pressure is the ultimate intervention for pain. Administering analgesics and comfort measures may aid in making the pain more tolerable for the client until the pressure is reduced (see Chapter 5). Measures to reduce anxiety also should be used.

Anxiety/Knowledge Deficit

Anxiety Reduction, Teaching: Disease Process and Procedure/Treatment. The development of compartment syndrome is an unexpected event for clients. The nurse should observe clients for signs and symptoms of anxiety, such as elevated heart rate and blood pressure;

frequent, repeated questions about their condition and treatment; and an inability to focus on instructions and explanation. The cause of client anxiety should be determined through careful listening and questioning. Nursing interventions should focus on relieving client anxiety by the use of pain-relieving measures (medications and comfort measures) and by simple explanations of what compartment syndrome is and its monitoring and treatment. The client's family or significant others should be included in these explanations. Continued support and explanations should be given throughout hospitalization and follow-up care.

Sensory Alterations

Circulatory Precautions. If residual sensory alterations are anticipated, the client should be counseled about care of insensate skin, including checking water temperature before immersing the extremity, avoiding the use of sharp objects (e.g., nail clippers, razor blades) around the insensate area, and closely inspecting the skin to detect abrasions.

Body Image Disturbance

Body Image Enhancement. Efforts should be made to establish a trusting nurse/client relationship to allow the client to describe feelings about concerns with body image. Realistic expectations about recovery of function and skin appearance should be discussed with the client and significant others. Appropriate referrals should be made. Occupational therapy may be needed for alterations in self-care and home care. A social worker may need to become involved if the client anticipates changes in employment. A plastic or reconstructive surgeon may become involved for wound closure or coverage.

Potential for Infection

Infection Protection and Control. Vital signs should be monitored closely for increases in temperature and heart rate. The client's skin and wound should be monitored for evidence of infection, such as foul drainage, redness, and increased swelling. Blood and wound cultures need to be obtained as indicated. Sterile technique is used for dressing changes every 8 hours. White blood cell counts and sedimentation rates need to be evaluated, and abnormalities must be reported. Prophylactic antibiotics should be given as prescribed.

Alteration in Renal Tissue Perfusion

Fluid/Electrolyte Management. In crush syndrome, adequate fluid is needed to dilute the myoglobin in the blood and renal tubules. Alkaline crystalloids at a rate of 500 mL/hr may be needed to maintain the urine

pH above 6.5. With hydration, the nurse must be alert for symptoms of pulmonary edema, congestive heart failure, and hypertension. Diuretics should be monitored, with a goal of maintaining urine output above 300 mL/hr. Urine should be tested for red blood cells (myoglobin is carried in this manner). Muscle enzyme, potassium, and serum pH levels also should be monitored.

Summary

Compartment syndrome can occur after trauma, immobilization, and surgery. Astute nursing assessment and early intervention to relieve compartment pressure is essential in preventing long-term consequences.

DEEP VENOUS THROMBOSIS

Definition

Various thromboembolic conditions may occur in orthopaedic clients, including thrombophlebitis, deep venous thrombosis (DVT), and pulmonary embolism (PE). *Thrombosis* is the formation of a blood clot (thrombus) in a vessel, and *phlebitis* is the inflammation of a vein. *Thrombophlebitis* occurs when both of these conditions are present. A thrombus is considered a *DVT* when a clot occurs in a deep vein of the lower extremity. A clot that travels to the pulmonary circulation is termed a *PE*. This section of the chapter deals with thrombophlebitis and DVT. PE is covered in another section of this chapter.

Incidence and Risk Factors

Clients who sustain orthopaedic trauma or undergo orthopaedic surgery are at high risk for developing DVT. Venous thromboembolism is responsible for 500,000 deaths annually in industrialized countries, yet it is probably the most preventable cause of death in elective orthopaedic surgery. Rates of DVT and fatal PE in unprotected orthopaedic clients is high, reaching greater than 40% in clients undergoing knee and hip arthroplasty or sustaining multiple trauma. For these clients, the proximal DVT rate is 15% or greater, and the fatal PE rate is 15% or greater (Paiement & Mendelsohn, 1997). The pooled rate of DVT reported from a review of studies involving trauma clients was 11.8% (Velmahos, Kern, Chan, Oder, Murray, & Shekelle, 2000a). Individuals who sustain a spine fracture and those who have a spinal cord injury have a twofold and threefold increase in the odds of developing DVT compared with other trauma clients (Velmahos, Kern, Chan, Oder, Murray, & Shekelle, 2000b). Risk factors related to blood coagulation, vascular injury, and venous stasis may also be present (Box 10-3). A systematic assessment of this risk should be performed in every client and an appropriate plan of care implemented.

DVT rarely occurs in children, possibly because of their short veins and frequent movement compared with that of adults who are in bed when ill or in traction.

BOX 10–3.
Risk Factors and Contributing Diseases for Deep Vein Thrombosis

---

The development of venous thrombosis is based on three factors known as *Virchow's triad:*

1. Trauma to the vessel
2. Venous stasis
   Bed rest or immobility
   Myocardial infarction
   Congestive heart failure
   Hypotension
   Chronic obstructive pulmonary disease
   Obesity
   Pregnancy
   Estrogen intake
   Previous deep venous thrombosis
   Extrinsic compression
   Surgery
   Paraplegia
3. Hypercoagulability
   Pregnancy
   Cancer
   Estrogen intake
   Myeloproliferative disorders

Pathophysiology

Venous stasis, vessel damage, and altered clotting mechanisms all contribute to thrombus formation. These three risk factors were identified by Rudolf Virchow in 1846 and are termed *Virchow's triad*. Thrombosis occurs because of an imbalance between the thrombogenic factors and protective mechanisms. Thrombogenic factors include damage to the vessel wall, platelet aggregation, blood coagulation, and stasis. The protective mechanisms include an intact endothelium, adequate blood flow to dilute clotting factors or disrupt platelet aggregates, inactivation of coagulation factors by the liver, and a functioning fibrinolytic system.

An injury to a vessel triggers the hemostatic process. The intrinsic and extrinsic pathways of blood coagulation are involved (Fig. 10–5). Platelets adhere to the damaged endothelium or exposed subendothelium. If the blood flow in the area is diminished, the platelets aggregate. When the platelets begin to aggregate, adenosine diphosphate is released and further aggregation occurs. The release of platelet factors activates thrombin, which induces formation of a platelet plug and forms fibrin from fibrinogen (factor I). At the same time, plasma proteins react with the subendothelium. Exposed tissues or macrophages present tissue factor (factor III, or thromboplastin) to the blood at the injured site, triggering the extrinsic phase of blood coagulation. Platelets are stimulated to expose or assemble membrane glycoproteins IIb and IIa, which bind fibrinogen and von Willebrand factor and support platelet recruitment and aggregation. Enzyme-cofactor complexes assemble on the platelet surface, accelerating factor X and prothrombin (factor II) activation. This leads to thrombin formation and the subsequent conversion of factors V and VIII into activated cofactors and stimulates platelet secretion. The intrinsic pathway is initiated when factor XII is activated by exposure of the blood to the damaged vessel wall. The intrinsic and extrinsic pathways both activate factor X, which converts prothrombin to thrombin. Protective factors that generally inhibit clot formation or break down fibrin may not be able to reach the forming thrombus because of venous stasis.

Once a thrombus is formed, it may undergo lysis (partial or complete), become organized, persist as unorganized or partially organized fibrin, or become dislodged and carried in the circulation as an embolus.

Assessment

Clinical diagnosis of DVT is fairly nonspecific and often inaccurate. Many individuals may have a DVT without any symptoms of the disorder. In addition, symptoms of a DVT may be present, but objective signs may not. If signs and symptoms of a DVT are present, other conditions of muscle, subcutaneous tissues, joints, and other structures need to be ruled out because clinical manifestations of DVT are nonspecific.

Subjective Assessment: Nursing History. Inflammation and obstruction are the key causes of DVT symptoms. The most common symptoms are pain and tenderness at or below the site of thrombosis. The amount of pain and tenderness present is not indicative of the size or extent of thrombosis. The pain may be described as aching, cramping, sharp, dull, severe, or mild. The discomfort may be constant or intermittent and often increases with movement and weight bearing.

Objective Assessment: Physical Examination. Swelling at or below the site of thrombosis is caused by edema as a result of venous obstruction or inflammation. Swelling resulting from inflammation is generally localized to the site of thrombosis, and the client usually complains of pain and tenderness at the site. Swelling resulting from venous obstruction is distal to the obstruction and not associated with pain. Mild to severe pitting edema may be seen. Elevating the leg often lessens the swelling, but swelling may recur with ambulation. The site may be red. Homans' sign (forced dorsiflexion of the foot causing discomfort in the upper calf) is not specific to or sensitive for DVT. It is present in less than one third of symptomatic clients with DVT and in more than 50% of symptomatic clients who do not have DVT.

Diagnostic Evaluation

Various diagnostic studies can detect DVT. The use of specific tests varies depending on the suspected location of the thrombus and whether the test is for clinical or research purposes. Venography is considered the standard for clinical diagnosis, but it is an invasive procedure with a number of side effects.

At present, blood tests are not recommended for detecting clients at risk for postoperative thrombosis because these clients can be recognized by clinical risk factors alone. Fibrinolytic activity measurement may improve the predictive power, but the improvement is marginal and involves expensive tests. Fibrinopeptide-A assay and the fibrin/fibrinogen fragment-E assay are sensitive to venous thromboembolism in symptomatic clients. They are not specific to DVT, however, and must be performed by radioimmunoassay, making them complicated for clinical use.

Venous Ultrasound Imaging. In the past years, venous ultrasound imaging has grown tremendously popular in the use of diagnosing venous thrombosis. It is both a sensitive and accurate noninvasive examination for locating thrombus within the deep and superficial venous systems. This technique has almost completely replaced contrast studies as the standard evaluation for the diagnosis of lower and upper DVT.

Noninvasive venous imaging is the use of an ultrasound scanning probe and gel that is placed on the skin to aid in the ultrasound transmission from the transducer into the tissue. Sound waves hit the moving red blood cells and return the sound waves to be converted and displayed as images on a monitor. Some technologists use only grayscale (tissue) interrogation, whereas others use color imaging (direction of flow) in conjunction with grayscale. Duplex scanners combine real-time imaging and pulsed Doppler capabilities to provide both anatomic and physiologic information of the blood vessels.

Ultrasound examinations use important criteria to diagnose a thrombus in a vein: direct visualization of the thrombus lying in the vein; loss of compressibility of the vein; dilation of the lumen of the vein; and changes in the flow dynamics within the vein, such as loss of spontaneity and phasicity with poor or no augmentation

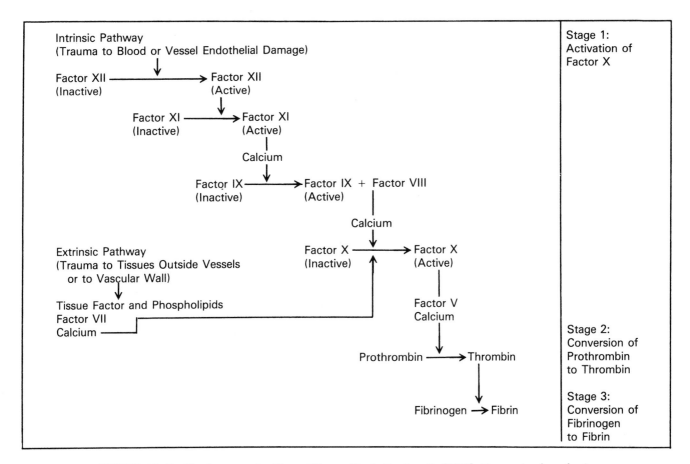

FIGURE 10–5. Clotting cascade. (From Wittert, D., & Barden, R. [1985]. Deep vein thrombosis, pulmonary embolism, and prophylaxis in the orthopedic patient. *Orthopedic Nursing, 4,* 28.)

to distal compression or Valsalva's maneuvers. There may be total absence of flow in obstructive thrombus or disturbed flow around a partial or nonocclusive thrombus. Determining the age of a thrombus is rather difficult. Within a day or two, the thrombus becomes echogenic as the red blood cells begin to organize. In clients with a history of DVT or chronic venous changes, the vessel lumen tends to become narrowed and echogenic as the overall diameter of the vessel decreases. Valvular incompetence can easily be determined by seeing and hearing reflux or abnormal reversal of flow following an augmentation (Zwiebel, 2000).

The extent of the thrombus and which vessels are involved can be immediately determined. Follow-up examinations for propagation or recanalization of the thrombus can be done comfortably. The reported accuracy of ultrasound imaging for the diagnosis of acute DVT from the popliteal (knee) vein and proximal is approximately 90% to 95%, whereas the sensitivity in clients with calf symptoms is 80% (Polak, 1992). Imaging examinations of the calf are more difficult because of their small size and the large number of deep calf veins—paired posterior tibial, peroneal, and anterior tibial veins. Serial ultrasound scans can be used to follow clients with thrombi of the calf for propagation into the popliteal vein.

A few limiting factors of ultrasound scanning of the deep veins are in areas of ligaments, such as at the adductor canal level and the proximal calf, which hamper compression of vessels. Vessels in obese clients and in those with large amounts of swelling may not be well visualized (Zwiebel, 2000). The positioning of the orthopaedic client may be difficult secondary to traction, splints, and immobility of the surgical limb, making the examination difficult. Complications of diagnostic ultrasound are essentially nonexistent.

Venous Doppler. Continuous-wave Doppler is used to evaluate venous flow patterns of the leg or arm. For this examination, the client should lie supine on a cart or bed, head up at least 30 degrees, the leg externally rotated, and the knee flexed outward. The Doppler is placed at four sites on each leg: over the common femoral vein, superficial vein, popliteal vein, and the posterior tibial vein. The corresponding arteries are used as landmarks to identify the deep vessels. When the probe is positioned over the vessel, normal venous signals are heard spontaneously and are phasic, changing with respirations. When the extremity is compressed distal to the probe, an augmentation of the signal is heard as the venous blood passes by the Doppler probe. With Valsalva's maneuvers or compression proximal to the Doppler, the signal ceases and then augments with release of compression.

This technique requires an experienced examiner and has several limitations. Nonocclusive thrombi may not

alter flow hemodynamics. Normal signals may be heard in clients who have double femoral or popliteal veins in which one is patent and the other is thrombosed. Extrinsic compression of a vein by tumor, hematoma, or poor positioning may cause abnormal signals that cannot be differentiated from thrombus.

Venous Doppler is sensitive to proximal vein thrombosis but less sensitive to calf vein thrombosis because of the large number of calf veins. Venous Doppler examination is still used, but mainly as a screening examination because it is portable and inexpensive, provides quick bilateral evaluation, and has high client acceptance. If a thrombus is suspected, impedance plethysmography (IPG) or ultrasound scanning also should be done to the abnormal extremity.

Impedance Plethysmography. Before ultrasound scanning was available, IPG was done routinely with venous Doppler examinations to determine the presence of thrombus. IPG is a noninvasive examination that measures changes in electrical resistance (impedance) that reflect volume changes in limb blood content.

As with the Doppler examination, the IPG relies on good positioning of the client and may be difficult in the orthopaedic client. Limitations to this testing are similar to those of the venous Doppler in that it may not detect a nonocclusive thrombus. IPG is diagnostic only from above the top electrode (proximal calf) upward. Thrombi of the calf may not be detected by this technique. An abnormal test result is positive for thrombus in the leg but does not identify the exact location or extent of occlusion. A false-positive result may occur in clients with unrecognized muscle contractions that stop venous filling; in clients with right-sided heart failure, on mechanical ventilation, or with severe arterial disease in the leg; or in clients who cannot be positioned properly, such as those with orthopaedic traction.

Venography. Venography remains the gold standard for venous testing. However, a small number of these examinations are performed as compared with noninvasive techniques. Ascending venography is the most common technique used for definition of DVT. The client is in a 45-degree upright position and non–weight bearing on the leg to be examined. A tilt-table can be used for positioning. Tourniquets may be used at the calf and thigh level. A needle is inserted into the dorsal foot vein, and contrast medium is injected. Films are taken as the contrast medium fills the veins and the tourniquets are removed. Filling defects of the veins are diagnosed as thrombus. If only the iliac veins and vena cava need to be assessed, a venacavogram is performed by inserting a needle into the femoral vein and injecting contrast material. Venograms are performed when noninvasive tests are unavailable, equivocal, or negative in the face of a strong clinical suspicion of thrombotic occlusion. Venography allows differentiation between acute and chronic disease and can accurately define anatomy before surgical procedures. Venography also can distinguish between intrinsic thrombus and extrinsic venous compression. Descending venography is used to assess venous valvular incompetence.

Venography is a difficult technique that requires experience to execute and interpret adequately. Potential problems with venography are false-positive or false-negative results because of failure to inject the dye into the dorsal foot vein or to adequately fill the femoral and iliac veins. Generally, errors on the false-positive side are due to inadequate venography techniques. Side effects of venography include pain in the foot during dye injection. Pain is probably related to direct damage to the venous endothelium by the contrast medium. This may produce phlebitis and even DVT in a small percentage of clients (1 in 30 clients who have normal venograms). Hypersensitivity to the dye and local skin and tissue necrosis because of extravasation of contrast material at the site of injection are less common side effects.

Treatment Modalities and Related Nursing Management

Prevention of DVT is a primary goal for the care of clients who have sustained orthopaedic trauma or surgery. Identification of high-risk groups is the first step in prevention (see Box 10–3). The incidence of DVT in clients following total hip and knee arthroplasty is so high, however, that prophylaxis should be provided regardless of other risk factors.

Research into the best and safest means of prophylaxis is ongoing and ever changing. Pharmacologic agents and physical-mechanical measures have been tested with varying results. A brief review of the information from the American College of Chest Surgeons' Fifth Consensus Conference on Antithrombotic Therapy (1998), an expert trauma panel funded by the Agency for Healthcare Research and Quality (Velmahos et al., 2000a, 2000b), and other guidelines established from summarized research by the National Guideline Clearinghouse is presented here under the specific pharmacologic or mechanical measure. Because of limited studies in terms of methods and numbers of clients, Velmahos and colleagues (2000a) stated that currently there is no evidence that any existing method of venous thromboembolism prophylaxis is clearly superior to other methods or even to no prophylaxis in trauma clients. At present, subcutaneous fixed-dose low-molecular-weight heparin (LMWH), adjusted-dose oral anticoagulation, or adjusted-dose unfractionated heparin (UH) is recommended for prophylaxis following various lower extremity procedures. Intermittent pneumatic compression and elastic stockings also have roles in DVT prevention. In addition, epidural

anesthesia and noncemented prostheses may decrease the incidence of DVT in appropriately selected clients. When anticoagulant-based prophylaxis is not feasible because of active bleeding, high-risk clients may be candidates for inferior vena caval filter placement.

Physical Measures. Early ambulation, elevation of the foot of the bed, ankle exercises, graded compression elastic stockings, and intermittent external pneumatic compression (IPC) can reduce the incidence of DVT. Elevation of the foot of the bed (without bending the knee) promotes venous return. Rhythmic dorsal and plantar flexion can increase the blood flow in the lower extremities and increase maximum flow in the femoral vein.

For elastic stockings to be effective in increasing venous return, and thereby decreasing the incidence of DVT, a graded pressure must be present in the stocking. Compression is applied to the ankle and calf, with greater pressure applied distally. Knee-high stockings are effective and also prevent the undesirable "garter effect" of thigh-high stockings. In addition, proper fit, preoperative placement (before induction of anesthesia), and consistent use are key components in the effectiveness of the stockings.

IPC involves the application of leggings that intermittently inflate in an ankle-to-thigh pattern to promote venous return. IPC has been shown to be extremely effective in DVT prophylaxis following total knee replacement and is thought to provide benefit in DVT prophylaxis in all orthopaedic cases (Wood, Kos, Abnet, & Ista, 1997). It is believed that IPC prevents DVT by mechanically decreasing blood pooling in the legs and increasing the rate and velocity of venous flow in the lower extremities, thus promoting clearance and mixing (with inhibitory factors) of activated coagulation factors. Pneumatic compression is also thought to have a fibrinolytic effect that counteracts hypercoagulability caused by surgery. This technique should be started before the induction of anesthesia or as soon as possible postoperatively and continued as long as the client is on bed rest.

Complications such as constriction and increased muscle compartment pressure and skin pressure may accompany the use of mechanical measures. In addition, compression stockings may not be usable because of such devices as casts, traction, and braces, particularly in trauma clients.

When compression stockings and IPC cannot be used, impulse technology can be employed. This technique uses a foot pad that applies pressure from a puff of air on the sole of the foot. The venous plexus of the foot is compressed, just as it is by the pressure occurring in normal ambulation. The resulting blood flow is highly pulsatile, sending a column of blood back to the heart by increasing venous velocity in the post-tibial, popliteal, and femoral veins. With each impulse, the plexus empties in milliseconds.

The foot pump is effective in reducing proximal thrombosis after hip or knee replacements, spine surgery, and hip fracture reduction. It also reduces swelling, pain, and compartment pressures after trauma and surgery.

Pharmacologic Agents

Warfarin. Adjusted-dose warfarin therapy has been found to be safe and effective in reducing the incidence of DVT after total hip replacement and hip fracture repair, but it is less effective after total knee replacement. Warfarin affects prothrombin time (PT) and international normalized ratios (INR) by competing with vitamin K. Generally, clients receive warfarin the evening before surgery and immediately after surgery. The dosage is then adjusted to maintain the INR within a 2.0 to 3.0 target range.

Unfractionated Heparin. Adjusted-dose UH has been found to be effective for DVT prophylaxis after total hip replacement. Heparin binds with antithrombin III to prolong the partial thromboplastin time (PTT). Adjusting the preoperative low-dose UH with postoperative heparin dosage to keep the PTT at approximately 1.5 times normal is more effective than the traditional, fixed, low-dose heparin regimen.

Side effects of warfarin and unfractionated heparin. Hematomas and gastrointestinal bleeding have been reported side effects with both heparin and warfarin. The anticoagulant effects of warfarin are reversed by the administration of fresh frozen plasma, blood, and vitamin K. Although warfarin is contraindicated in pregnancy, heparin products are safe to use.

Low-Molecular-Weight Heparin. Several studies in the orthopaedic literature note that LMWH outperforms UH for venous thromboembolism and prophylaxis and is more efficacious than oral anticoagulants in knee replacement, with few hemorrhagic side effects. There are now data to suggest that LMWH is superior to UH for prophylaxis in moderate- to high-risk trauma clients (Eastern Association for the Surgery of Trauma, 1998).

A fixed dose is given subcutaneously once or twice per day. Monitoring PTT is not necessary with this regimen. It is more effective than low-dose UH and is equally effective as or superior to adjusted-dose heparin and low-intensity warfarin. All heparins reverse with protamine sulfate.

Aspirin. Aspirin has had conflicting results in preventing DVT. It can reduce the incidence of DVT after total hip replacement, but it is inadequate when compared with other regimens.

Other Therapies. Other common historical prophylaxes now used only in special circumstances include dextran and antithrombin III therapies. This is due primarily to their lack of cost-effectiveness and improved results with newer therapies.

Anesthetic and Surgical Techniques. Regional anesthetics (e.g., epidural and spinal anesthesia) and analgesics have been found to reduce the incidence of DVT following total hip and total knee arthroplasty. There is evidence that a regional lumbar block of the L1 and L2 spinal nerves increases blood flow to the legs, thereby reducing platelet aggregation and blood viscosity.

The incidence of DVT has been reported to be minimal in clients receiving noncemented hip prostheses compared with those in whom methyl methacrylate was used for prosthesis insertion. Potential factors in reducing DVT were younger age, shorter operating room time (clients with noncemented hip prostheses were younger and had less time in surgery), and avoidance of intramedullary injection of methyl methacrylate. It was hypothesized that cement injection might affect coagulation and that the heat generated from injection might damage endothelial cells.

Treatment of Deep Venous Thrombosis. There is some controversy regarding which of the clients who develop DVT should be treated. It is generally accepted that clients who develop a large proximal DVT need to be treated. The controversy primarily concerns the likelihood of a calf thrombus extending or embolizing. Based on the most current evidence, clients with calf DVT have two options: (1) to undergo anticoagulation for 3 months or (2) to be followed with several noninvasive tests for 10 to 14 days to identify proximal extension of thrombus (Clagett, Anderson, Heit, Levine, & Wheeler, 1995).

Reasons to treat calf vein DVT include prevention of significant problems with valvular incompetence and venous stasis conditions. It is estimated that only about 3% of pulmonary emboli arise from isolated calf vein thrombi. Calf vein thrombus is known to propagate into the popliteal vein in up to 28% of cases, posing further risk of pulmonary embolization (Zweibel, 2000).

Heparin has been the mainstay of thrombotic therapy for hospitalized clients with DVT. An initial IV bolus is given (5000 U). After the DVT is confirmed, another bolus of 5000 to 10,000 U is given. A continuous IV drip at 1300 U/hr is then started and titrated to maintain the PTT at 0.5 to 2.5 times the control or baseline (blood heparin level 0.2 to 0.4 U/mL). Therapy is continued for 5 to 10 days. On the second or third day of treatment, warfarin is started. Warfarin should be overlapped with heparin for 4 to 5 days and until the INR target range has been attained (2.0 to 3.0). In some clients, heparin and warfarin can be started on the same day. Warfarin is continued for 3 to 6 months. A side effect of heparin is thrombocytopenia. Platelet counts should be checked daily. In addition, the client should be monitored for bleeding. In some cases, IV heparin is used for a short hospitalization, during which time the client is stabilized and is taught about discharge issues with LMWH.

LMWH is now being used for both inpatient and outpatient DVT treatment. Warfarin is started conjunctively on day 1. The INR is monitored to determine the efficacy of warfarin therapy. Platelets are checked between day 3 and 5. LMWH is stopped between day 5 and 7 and when the INR is between 2.0 and 3.0.

Fibrinolytic therapy is rarely used in orthopaedic clients because it is relatively contraindicated in those who have undergone surgery in the past 10 days and those who have had severe trauma.

Surgery is performed only rarely to treat DVT. Venous interruption (ligation of a proximal vein to prevent embolization from more distal veins) is used only if hemorrhagic complications occur or are anticipated from anticoagulant therapy or if anticoagulant therapy fails. The potential problems of the procedure are permanent obstruction of venous drainage, venous hypertension, edema, ulceration, and the possibility of thrombosis above the ligation. Venous thrombectomy is used to treat phlegmasia cerulea dolens (venous obstruction in which limb viability is jeopardized), but it provides relief of only the acute symptoms of venous obstruction. In many cases, thrombosis occurs again after the procedure.

Nursing Management

The nursing concerns that may be present in clients at risk for developing DVT or those who have developed DVT include possible alteration in peripheral circulation, pain, possible bleeding complications, and anxiety related to inadequate knowledge about DVT and its treatment.

Alteration in Peripheral Circulation

Respiratory Care, Embolus Precautions. Nursing care of the postoperative or post-trauma orthopaedic client includes assessment of risk factors and intervention to reduce the incidence of DVT. Frequent position changes, early and frequent ambulation, and elevation of the foot of the bed (not bending the knee) help promote venous return. The client should be taught and encouraged to perform ankle exercises. Gradient elastic or pneumatic compression stockings (or both) should be worn by clients who are at risk for DVT. The legs should always be measured before the application of stockings. Knee-high stockings should be used when thigh-highs roll and produce a "garter effect." Encouragement and response to client complaints about the devices may increase usage. Clients may complain about being too warm in the pneumatic compression stockings. Adjustment of the room temperature, use of the cooling option

if available, or fewer blankets on the lower extremities may alleviate this complaint.

Pain

Physical Comfort Promotion, Pain Management. Clients who develop DVT may complain of discomfort in the affected extremity. Warm, moist heat to the affected area, elevation of the extremity, analgesics, and relaxation techniques may alleviate this discomfort. Aspirin and nonsteroidal anti-inflammatory drugs (NSAIDs) are contraindicated in clients who are receiving anticoagulants.

Bleeding Complications

Tissue Perfusion Management: Bleeding Precautions. Clients receiving anticoagulants, whether prophylactic or therapeutic for DVT, need to be monitored for signs and symptoms of bleeding. Urine, stool, and sputum should be monitored closely. Increased blood output in drains should be noted and reported to the physician. Laboratory results (hematocrit, PTT, PT, INR) should be checked and reported to the physician. Complete blood counts and platelet results should also be monitored as appropriate. Complaints about light-headedness, fatigue, and similar symptoms should be followed closely. Vital signs need to be monitored. Care must be taken to avoid medications that interact with the anticoagulants (Box 10–4), particularly aspirin and NSAIDs.

Anxiety

Client Education, Teaching, Individual Psychological Comfort Promotion, Anxiety Reduction. The client should be educated about prophylactic and therapeutic measures for DVT. Risk factors should be discussed. The client's role in prevention, through means such as ankle exercise, increased ambulation, and adherence to the medication regimen, should be stressed. Clients being prescribed anticoagulants when discharged home need to understand their effects and what signs and symptoms signal potential problems.

Summary

DVT is a common occurrence in the orthopaedic client population. Careful assessment, client specific prophylactic measures, prompt treatment, and diligent nursing care can significantly decrease morbidity and mortality from this complication.

PULMONARY EMBOLISM

PE is estimated to cause as many as 50,000 deaths in the United States each year. Untreated PE mortality is as high as 30%, and mortality rates for treated clients range from 2% to 3% (Tai, Atwal, & Hamilton, 1999). Unfortunately, signs and symptoms are often nonspecific, and diagnosis may be delayed or missed. More than 70% of clients who die from PE do not have the diagnosis considered before death. However, less than 35% of all clients suspected of having PE actually have it. Clinicians need to have a high degree of suspicion, especially in high-risk clients (Rosenow, l995). PE can be considered a major complication of DVT, which is a common complication of orthopaedic injuries, multiple trauma, and surgical procedures. Knowledge of the pathophysiology, diagnosis, treatment, and prevention of PE is critical for the orthopaedic nurse.

Definition

A PE is a clot or other foreign matter (air, fat, tissue, or amniotic fluid) that becomes lodged in a pulmonary arterial vessel. This section of the chapter deals with PE

BOX 10–4.
Drugs That Affect Anticoagulant Therapy (Partial Listing)

Drugs That Prolong Prothrombin Time (PT)
Allopurinol (Zyloprim)
Amiodarone (Cordarone)
Anabolic steroids
Antibiotics (broad-spectrum)
Chloral hydrate
Chloramphenicol
Cimetidine (Tagamet)
Clofibrate
Danazol (Danocrine)
Disulfiram (Antabuse)
Estrogen
Gemfibrozil (Lopid)
Glucagon
Heparin
Influenza virus vaccine
Metronidazole (Flagyl)
Miconazole (Monistat)
Nalidixic acid (NegGram)
Nonsteroidal anti-inflammatory drugs (NSAIDs)
Phenytoin (Dilantin) when first started
Salicylates
Sulfinpyrazone (Anturane)
Sulfonamides
Sulfonylureas
Thyroid preparations

Drugs That Shorten PT
Antacids
Barbiturates
Cholestyramine resin (Questran)
Glutethimide (Doriden)
Griseofulvin (Fulvicin, Grisactin)
Phenytoin (Dilantin) with long-term use
Rifampin (Rifadin, Rimactane)

---

resulting from dislodged thrombi. Decreased or absent blood flow distal to the embolus results when a thromboembolism lodges in the pulmonary circulation.

Incidence and Risk Factors

As many as 300,000 to 600,000 hospitalizations per year are associated with DVT or PE (Velmahos, Kern, Chan, Oder, Murray, & Shekelle, 2000a). Clinically significant PE has been reported to be as high as 20% in clients undergoing hip surgery, with a 1% to 3% incidence of fatal PE. Trauma clients have a reported 10% to 90% incidence of DVT and a 1% to 22% incidence of PE (Knudson, Morabito, Paiement, & Shackelford, 1996).

Because DVT is a major cause of PE, many risk factors for DVT and PE are similar. First described in 1846, Virchow's triad (as reviewed in the DVT section of this chapter) still provides a good framework for examining DVT risk factors. Inherited risk factors affect coagulability and include antithrombin III deficiency, disorders of plasminogen and plasminogen activation, proteins C and S deficiency, and dysfibrinogenemia. Acquired risk factors include surgical procedures that cause trauma to the vessel; immobilization; cancer; estrogen use; venous insufficiency; chronic diseases, such as CHF and chronic obstructive pulmonary disease (COPD); obesity; changes in the clotting cascade (because of injury or shock); and age (increased risk for clients older than 40). A previous history of DVT and PE is also a significant risk factor. Additional risk factors present in the multiple-trauma population include pelvic and long-bone fractures, head injury, and spine injury, although one meta-analysis found only increased age, spine fracture, and spinal cord injury to be predictive factors for development of DVT (Velmahos et al., 2000b).

Pathophysiology

Most pulmonary emboli occur as a result of DVT (refer to the DVT section of this chapter for a review of the clotting process and thrombus formation). When a venous thrombus or a part of a thrombus dislodges from its primary site, it becomes an embolus. The embolus then travels the venous circulation to the right side of the heart and can be ejected into the pulmonary circulation. A major pulmonary artery or one of its branches is affected, depending on the size of the clot and location of the adherence. Perfusion distal to the embolus is then partially or completely occluded.

To understand the effect of PE, it is important to understand the relationship between ventilation and perfusion. For optimal gas exchange to occur within the lungs, ventilation (the movement of air in and out of the lung) must match perfusion (blood flow through the pulmonary vascular system) (Fig. 10–6). The pulmonary circulation normally is a low-pressure (approximately 25/10 mm Hg) system, so pulmonary blood flow is gravity dependent. In an upright person, the preponderance of

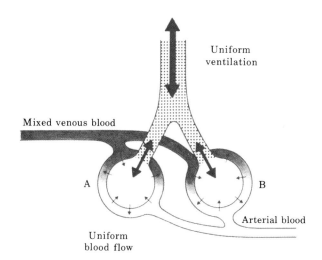

FIGURE 10–6. Schematic representation of gas exchange in an idealized two-compartment model of the lung in which there is uniform distribution of ventilation and blood flow. (Adapted from Comroe, J. H., Jr., Forster, R. E., II, Dubois, A. B., Briscoe, W. A., & Carlsen, E. [1962]. The lung. *Clinical physiology and pulmonary function tests* [2nd ed.]. Chicago: Year Book.)

blood flows to the dependent area or the bases of the lungs. In a supine person, the major quantity of blood flows to the posterior fields and bases. Ventilation is higher at the apices of the lungs than at the bases. However, the bases have a greater capacity for expansion than the already expanded apices. With normal or deep breathing, ventilation increases at the bases and air comes in contact with the bloodstream, allowing for optimal matching of ventilation and perfusion (see Fig. 10-6). This matching allows for optimal gas exchange and oxygenation of pulmonary blood.

Gas exchange occurs at the membrane interface between the alveoli and pulmonary capillaries. Diffusion (movement of gas across the membrane) is dependent on a pressure gradient. Oxygen partial pressure is greater in the alveoli than in the pulmonary capillaries, so oxygen diffuses into the capillaries, where it is disseminated to the tissues via the arterial circulation. Because carbon dioxide has a higher partial pressure in the pulmonary capillaries than in the alveoli, it diffuses into the alveoli, where it can be removed through exhalation.

When an embolus blocks a pulmonary artery or branch, flow distal to the embolus is either partially or totally occluded, depending on the size of the embolus. Initially, ventilation is not affected, and the result is an area of ventilation without perfusion (occlusion assumed). If the involved area is small, the effect is minimal. Other lung units supply sufficient oxygen to meet current needs. However, if the involved area is large, a significant area of gas exchange is obliterated and the systemic effects of decreased oxygen content and increased carbon dioxide become evident.

Ventilation continues in the alveoli that are not receiving perfusion, resulting in alveolar dead spaces, which continue to be ventilated but are unable to contribute to gas exchange (Fig. 10-7). This results in fewer alveoli participating in gas exchange, which can lower arterial oxygenation (Pao_2). The dead spaces (wasted ventilation) require an energy cost without providing benefit. The greater the area of dead space ventilation, the more gas exchange area lost and the more energy used to ventilate areas that are not contributing to oxygenation.

The lungs compensate for the dead space ventilation by pneumoconstriction, that is, by increasing airway resistance and diverting more ventilation to the well-perfused lung areas, thereby decreasing dead space ventilation. This pneumoconstriction is thought to be related to bronchoalveolar hypocarbia, hypoxia, humoral agents such as serotonin and histamine, and thrombin activation caused by the presence of the clot(s).

This insult to the lungs also causes a loss of surfactant. Surfactant (the lipoprotein produced by type II alveolar cells) reduces surface tension and prevents collapse of alveoli. The loss of surfactant predisposes the client to collapse of alveoli and allows transudation of capillary fluid into the alveoli, thereby adding atelectasis to the signs of ventilation/perfusion mismatching. Some lung units are poorly ventilated because of the atelectasis, but they continue to receive good perfusion. Because they

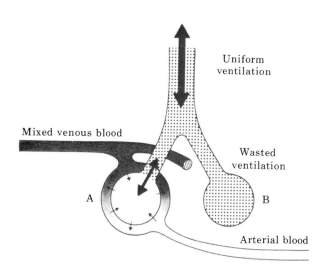

FIGURE 10–7. A schematic representation of a two-compartment model of the lung showing the effect of pulmonary arterial obstruction on wasted ventilation. When blood flow to unit B ceases, any ventilation to the unit is wasted because it cannot contribute to gas exchange. Gas exchange in unit A depends on the amount of ventilation and blood flow to the unit. (Adapted from Comroe, J. H., Jr., Forster, R. E., II, Dubois, A. B., Briscoe, W. A., & Carlsen, E. [1962]. The lung. *Clinical physiology and pulmonary function tests* [2nd ed.]. Chicago: Year Book.)

are poorly ventilated, the blood flowing past them is unable to pick up sufficient oxygen and returns to the heart poorly oxygenated, further lowering the Pao_2.

Hemodynamic consequences of PE include pulmonary artery hypertension resulting from the increased pulmonary artery resistance and pressure. The increased resistance and pressure may be limited to a small area distal to the embolus or, in the case of a large embolus, may result in significantly increased pulmonary artery pressure (as when more than 50% of the pulmonary vascular bed is occluded). Increased right ventricular work results from the increased pressure against which the right ventricle must pump. Decreased blood flow to an area of lung parenchyma eventually causes atelectasis or collapse of alveoli. Now ventilation is also affected. If the atelectatic area extends beyond the nonperfused area, the result is an intrapulmonary shunting or an area of decreased or absent ventilation with perfusion present. Blood flowing past this nonventilated unit has little or no oxygen to pick up and thus returns to the left side of the heart with nearly the same oxygen supply as on the venous side.

The combination of dead spaces and shunt units can severely hamper oxygenation, leaving the client hypoxemic (decreased Pao_2).

Assessment

Pulmonary emboli are often undetected or misdiagnosed because of the nonspecificity of PE symptoms. The symptoms also vary depending on size, location, number of emboli, degree of occlusion, area of involvement, and occurrence of infarction.

Approximately one third of deaths caused by PE occur within 1 hour of onset. These may be the cases in which the client complains of severe dyspnea, chest pain, and a sense of impending doom and suffers rapid circulatory failure. In the case of a massive PE, diagnosis and successful treatment may be next to impossible because of the extensive loss of gas exchange area and the intense strain on the right side of the heart because of pulmonary hypertension. Some clinicians are reporting successful resuscitation with the use of thrombolytics in these cases.

The most common symptoms of PE are unexplained dyspnea and chest pain, with sudden-onset dyspnea and pleuritic-type chest pain most typical (Manganelli, Palla, Donnamaria, & Giuntini, 1995). In addition, symptoms of hypoxia, such as apprehension, confusion, and anxiety, are present. Many clients with PE go undiagnosed, so a high degree of suspicion is appropriate in clients at risk when chest pain and dyspnea occur acutely.

Hypoxia from PE is manifested by tachypnea, tachycardia, and dyspnea. Breath sounds may be diminished, and crackles (rales) and wheezes may be evident, especially after the advent of atelectasis. Cough may accompany the symptoms as well as less common findings, such as fever,

diaphoresis, hemoptysis, and pleuritic chest pain. A split S_2 may be heard. Clients may become anxious or complain of a sense of dread. Because many of these findings can occur with other conditions causing hypoxia, diagnostic tests are crucial.

Ongoing assessments after PE is diagnosed are important for evaluating the impact of the disorder and the effectiveness of the treatment. The nurse must monitor blood pressure, heart rate, and urine output and to assess skin temperature and color, which can warn of impending shock manifested by hypotension. If the client is suspected of having a massive PE or is hemodynamically unstable, an immediate transfer to the intensive care unit is indicated. Assessment of respiratory rate, depth, and effort, as well as quality of breath sounds and oxygenation using oximetry or arterial blood gases (ABG), is pertinent to determining what interventions may be needed to maintain respiratory stability. The nurse should be alert to increasing crackles or decreased breath sounds as well as deteriorating mental status or subjective reports of dyspnea, anxiety, and pain.

Diagnostic Evaluation

Ventilation/Perfusion Scan. The ventilation/perfusion ($\dot{V}/\dot{Q}$) scan is often the first test ordered for evaluation of the client with suspected PE. It is less invasive than pulmonary angiography, and in many centers, it may be more readily available. It is actually two tests: one of ventilation and the other of pulmonary perfusion. The client inhales a radiolabeled gas for the ventilation scan. X-ray images are taken during breath-holding to demonstrate distribution of the gas. Poorly ventilated areas appear lighter on the images. The ventilation scan in PE should be normal early in the course of the disorder (because PE is a vascular disease) unless there is an underlying pathologic condition, such as COPD, pleural effusion, or pneumothorax.

The perfusion scan involves injecting the client with radiolabeled albumin. The particles become distributed in proportion to pulmonary blood flow and are trapped in the capillaries. Radiographs in several different positions demonstrate the distribution of flow. The embolized area does not allow radioisotope access and appears as a lighter patch, or cold spot.

The two scans are considered together. A PE should show as a vascular or perfusion defect without a defect in ventilation (Fig. 10-8). Many conditions can cause abnormal $\dot{V}/\dot{Q}$ scans, including COPD, vasculitis, pulmonary edema, tumors, tuberculosis, and sarcoidosis. Often, a chest x-ray film corroborates findings.

A normal $\dot{V}/\dot{Q}$ scan without a perfusion defect may effectively rule out PE. Large perfusion defects that do not appear on the ventilation scan are associated with a high probability for PE. Defects present on both perfusion and ventilation scans cannot rule out the presence of PE and are considered indeterminate. Even a so-called low-

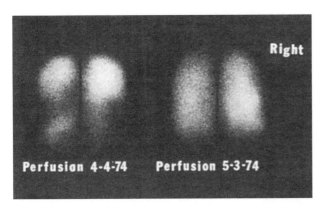

FIGURE 10–8. *(Left)* Perfusion scan in client with major, bilateral emboli. *(Right)* One month later, essentially complete resolution has occurred. (From Moser, K. [1988]. Pulmonary embolism. In J. F. Murray & J. A. Nadel [Eds.], *Textbook of respiratory medicine* [p. 1304]. Philadelphia: WB Saunders.)

probability scan has been associated with a positive angiogram in 15% to 30% of clients, with a 30% prevalence of PE. The Prospective Investigation of Pulmonary Embolism Diagnosis, a multimillion-dollar trial sponsored by the National Heart, Lung, and Blood Institute, found that indeterminate or low-probability results on $\dot{V}/\dot{Q}$ scans are not accurate predictors of the presence of PE. Angiography should be used to confirm the diagnosis in clients with indeterminate results (Tai, Atwal, & Hamilton, 1999).

Pulmonary Angiography. Angiography is still considered the reference standard for the diagnosis of PE. However, it is an invasive procedure and has some risk. The mortality rate is 0.24% to 0.60%, but morbidity can be significant in clients with diabetes mellitus, uremia, congestive heart failure, and some chronic lung diseases. The procedure entails placement of a catheter into the pulmonary artery (as in a catheterization of the right side of the heart). The preferred approach is percutaneous cannulation of the right femoral vein. Contrast material is then injected under pressure to image the pulmonary arterial vasculature. A pulmonary thromboembolus shows as a vascular cutoff or filling defect (Fig. 10–9). Specialized skill is required to perform and interpret the test, and it may not be available in all centers.

Spiral Chest Computed Tomography. Newer, high-speed spiral computed tomography (CT) modalities may be useful to confirm the diagnosis of PE in the client with an indeterminate $\dot{V}/\dot{Q}$ scan. Recent studies have shown spiral CT to be very reliable in the diagnosis of PE, with specificity and sensitivity equivalent to that of pulmonary angiogram and greater than that of $\dot{V}/\dot{Q}$ scan (Tai, Atwal, & Hamilton, 1999). It is noninvasive and capable of providing multiplanar images of the pulmonary vasculature and parenchyma.

Arterial Blood Gases. Although not specific to PE, ABG can be helpful in identifying the hypoxemia that often accompanies PE. Often, early ABG analysis associated with small emboli shows only a mild or moderate fall in Pao_2. The number of alveolar units affected and the client's underlying lung condition determine how effectively the rest of the lung can carry on the process of gas exchange. (See the pathophysiology section for a discussion of shunting and dead space.) This mild hypoxemia may be associated with respiratory alkalosis (low $Paco_2$) as the client increases respiratory rate and perhaps respiratory depth to increase oxygenation, thereby exhaling more CO_2. As the condition worsens or as the client tires from the increased respiratory effort, the ABG may deteriorate, resulting in a further fall in Pao_2 and a rise in $Paco_2$.

Chest X-ray Film. The chest x-ray film is not conclusive in diagnosing PE. It may be normal or show signs of effusions, infiltrates, atelectasis, or an elevated hemidiaphragm. However, the chest x-ray film may help rule out other conditions and is useful to compare with scans.

Electrocardiogram. The electrocardiogram may show nonspecific ST and T-wave changes but is not particularly helpful in making the diagnosis of PE. In the case of a massive PE, signs of right-sided heart strain may be evident. However, the electrocardiogram may be

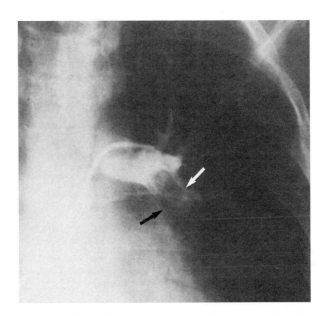

FIGURE 10–9. Selective pulmonary angiogram showing large filling defect *(arrows)* at distal end of left main pulmonary artery. The embolus is totally occluding the lingular and left lower lobe arteries. (From Moser, K. [1988]. Pulmonary embolism. In J. F. Murray & J. A. Nadel [Eds.], *Textbook of respiratory medicine* [p. 1311]. Philadelphia: WB Saunders.)

helpful in ruling out other problems, such as myocardial infarction.

Echocardiogram. The cardiac echocardiogram may demonstrate the presence of intracardiac clot or signs consistent with right ventricular dysfunction.

Tests for Deep Venous Thrombosis. Because most pulmonary emboli are the result of a dislodged DVT, diagnostic tests for DVT are performed to identify a possible source for the PE and risk for dislodgment of additional emboli. Refer to the section on DVT in this chapter for further discussion on its diagnosis.

Treatment Modalities and Related Nursing Management

Treatment focuses on preventing further thrombosis or limiting the size of the current thrombus and providing cardiopulmonary support.

Anticoagulation. Currently, heparin remains the drug of choice for anticoagulation. It does not have the ability to dissolve clots, but it can prevent formation of new thrombi or propagation of existing ones. It enhances the inhibitory actions of antithrombin III, thereby blocking the conversion of prothrombin to thrombin and fibrinogen to fibrin. Uncommon but very serious adverse effects of heparin therapy include thrombocytopenia and arterial thrombosis (Box 10–5).

For treatment of diagnosed PE, heparin is given as a loading bolus of 5000 to 15,000 U intravenously, followed by a continuous infusion regulated by clotting time. The use of weight-based dosing nomograms, which specify heparin dosage adjustments based on body

---

BOX 10–5.
Adverse Effects of Heparin Therapy

Hemorrhage
Urticaria
Anaphylactic shock
Alopecia
Osteoporosis (with long-term use)
Thrombocytopenia (low platelet count)*
Arterial thrombosis (white clot syndrome)
Skin necrosis with subcutaneous injection (may herald more serious heparin-induced thrombosis)

*Heparin-induced thrombocytopenia can be (1) acute reversible form seen immediately after an IV bolus, (2) mild thrombocytopenia developing 2–4 day after heparin therapy and resolving in 1–5 day even if heparin is continued, or (3) delayed onset (day 6–14) persistent thrombocytopenia resulting from formation of heparin-dependent antibodies (may be associated with heparin resistance and arterial thrombosis). Heparin must be discontinued immediately.
Data from Cola, C., & Ansell, J. (1990). Heparin-induced thrombocytopenia and arterial thrombosis: Alternative therapies. *American Heart Journal, 119,* 368–370.

---

weight and in response to any given activated partial thromboplastin time (aPTT), is showing promising results (Raschke, Reilly, Guidry, Fontana, & Srinivas, 1993). Heparin therapy is usually continued for 7 to 10 days, depending on the client's risk factors and activity.

LMWHs appear to have a more predictable anticoagulant response with a lower risk of bleeding complications and a longer half-life than UHs. Their safety and effectiveness in treating DVT is well established (Simonneau, Sors, Charbonnier, Page, Laaban, Azarian, Laurent, Hirsch, Ferrari, Bosson, Mottier, & Beau, 1997). LMWHs are increasingly being advocated as an alternative to IV heparin therapy for PE. They offer the benefit of simple, subcutaneous administration without the need for monitoring of clotting times but are more expensive than UH. Simonneau and colleagues (1997) randomized a group of 612 stable clients with symptomatic PE to either fixed-dose subcutaneous LMWH or adjusted-dose IV fractionated heparin regimens. Both groups received concurrent warfarin therapy. No differences were found between the groups with respect to recurrence of thromboembolism, bleeding episodes, and mortality rates.

Oral anticoagulants (warfarin) are started within 3 days of initiation of heparin therapy to achieve the peak effect of the anticoagulant on prothrombin activity. The PT/INR is measured to regulate the warfarin dosage. The PT and aPTT have been found to vary depending on the activity of the thromboplastin used. To standardize results, an INR is used, thus avoiding differences in PT ratio that can occur from batch to batch of thromboplastin reagents. The INR is now considered the reference standard in monitoring coagulation. PTT/INR is determined before initiation of the drug and periodically until the maintenance dose is determined and stabilized. During the overlap of therapy, PTT and PT/INR levels are monitored, the heparin dosage is decreased, and the warfarin dosage is adjusted. Debate continues regarding the optimal duration of warfarin therapy. It is usually continued for 3 to 6 months after discharge, although some researchers suggest that as few as 4 weeks of anticoagulation may be adequate to prevent recurrence in certain subgroups of clients (Schulman, Rhedin, Lindmarker, Carlson, Larfars, Nicol, Loogan, Svensson, Ljungberg, & Walter, 1995). Client education about the effects and potential hazards associated with anticoagulant therapy is important and should be started with the initiation of treatment. Arrangements may need to be made for scheduled monitoring of INR and dosage changes before discharge. Discharge instructions should be provided in writing (Table 10–2).

Thrombolytic Therapy. Thrombolytic therapy in myocardial infarction has been proved effective and has gained widespread use. Thrombolytic therapy in combination with heparin seems to be indicated in massive PE associated with hypotension or severe hypoxemia. Significant risk of stroke or major hemorrhage (especially in the

TABLE 10–2. *Client Education: Warfarin*

FOCUS	TEACHING POINTS
Diet	Avoid foods high in vitamin K (affects clotting factors): 　Mayonnaise 　Oils (canola, salad, soybean) 　Vegetables (broccoli, brussels sprouts, cabbage, collard greens, raw turnip or mustard greens, watercress lettuces, cucumber peel, green scallions, parsley) 　Beef liver 　Green tea or herbal teas containing tonka beans, sweet clover, or sweet woodruff
Activity	Talk with your health care provider before you take a trip or participate in a physical activity. Strenuous activity may require dosage adjustment or extra precautions to prevent bleeding. Travel may result in sitting for long periods—precautions such as frequent moving about may be necessary. If you are gone for a long time, another health care provider may need to follow your therapy.
Tests	Have your blood checked as ordered by your health care provider. Your warfarin dosage is based on clotting studies (PT or INR). Your health care provider will adjust the dosage based on these studies. Too much can cause bleeding; too little may not prevent venous clots from forming again. Your target PT is _____ . Your target INR is _____ .
Treatments	Notify physicians, dentists, and other health care providers before any procedures. Certain procedures may cause bleeding and should be avoided or delayed or precautions should be taken to control or prevent prolonged bleeding.
Teaching	Avoid the following: 　Smoking (or greatly reduce) 　Aspirin 　Alcohol 　These substances can affect clotting factors and may require a warfarin dosage adjustment. Wear a Medic Alert bracelet. Health care providers can be alerted to watch for bleeding or avoid the risk of certain procedures even when you may be unable to communicate during an emergency. Report symptoms of internal bleeding: 　Headache (continuous) 　Dizziness 　Faintness 　Chest pain 　Pelvic pain 　Lumbar pain Observe for and report signs of bleeding: 　Blood in urine 　Bright red or black tarry stools 　Vomiting blood 　Bleeding gums or pink toothbrush 　Nosebleeds 　Bloody sputum 　Oozing from shaving or minor cut 　Unusually heavy menstrual flow 　Purplish skin spots 　Easy bruising
Medications	Take the pill at the same time every day to help ensure steady clotting levels. Do not take an extra pill if you forget a dose—instead notify your health care provider for advice. Do not take any other medications without first checking with your health care provider. Other medications can change warfarin's effect (see Box 10–4).

postoperative period and in older clients with diastolic hypertension) may limit the benefits of this therapy in clients with major emboli but no hemodynamic compromise.

Currently available therapeutic agents include streptokinase, urokinase, and recombinant tissue–type plasminogen activator (rt-PA), which was approved for use in the treatment of PE in June 1990 by the U.S. Food and Drug Administration. Thrombolytic therapy accelerates clot lysis, hastens pulmonary tissue reperfusion, reverses right-sided heart failure, and improves pulmonary capillary blood volume. Local pulmonary arterial infusion of rt-PA appears to have no advantage over peripheral administration of the drug. Clinical trials are being conducted to determine the most effective dose, time window, and duration of therapy with the fewest adverse effects.

Surgical and Invasive Procedures. In clients for whom anticoagulant therapy is contraindicated or whose cardiopulmonary status is tenuous, more aggressive approaches are taken.

Inferior Vena Caval Filter. The inferior vena caval (IVC) filter is inserted under fluoroscopy via the femoral vein. Once deployed and anchored, it traps emboli and prevents their travel to the pulmonary circulation. Placement of a filter does not alter the potential for recurrent venous thrombosis, but the danger of PE resulting is minimized. Indications for IVC filter placement in the client with PE include strong contraindication for anticoagulant therapy (acute brain injury, major surgery), complications requiring cessation of anticoagulant therapy, and recurrent embolism despite adequate anticoagulation. IVC filters are usually placed percutaneously by interventional radiologists. Inferior venacavograms are done before filter placement to determine the caval diameter, location of the renal veins, and presence of thrombus within the cava. Many different types of filter have been used, but no large-scale prospective comparative studies exist to demonstrate superiority of any one type of device (Tai, Atwal, & Hamilton, 1999). Complications associated with IVC filters include migration of the filter, embolism to the pulmonary artery, and caval perforation or occlusion. IVC filters are usually left in place permanently; several authors have asserted that they have acceptable long-term safety and low complication rates (Langan, Miller, Casey, Carsten, Graham, & Taylor, 1999; Rogers, Strindberg, Shackford, Osler, Morris, Ricci, Najarian, D'Agostino, & Pilcher, 1998). Once the filter has been inserted, the nurse should assess for complications, such as bleeding at the venipuncture site. Anticoagulation may be resumed after filter placement if indicated.

Prophylactic IVC Filters. Certain high-risk clients may benefit from prophylactic placement of IVC filters (Rogers, Shackford, Ricci, Huber, & Atkins, 1997). Existing studies of the effect of prophylactic IVC filters on the incidence of PE in the trauma population are observational and use comparisons to historical controls. Nonetheless, some do suggest that prophylactic IVC filters may reduce the risk of both PE and fatal PE in some groups of trauma clients (Velmahos et al., 2000b). Commonly cited indications for prophylactic IVC filter insertion in the trauma population include prolonged immobilization with multiple injuries, closed head injury, pelvic fracture, multiple long-bone fracture, spine fracture (Langan et al., 1999), infrarenal venous injury (Spain, Richardson, Polk, Bergamini, Wilson, & Miller, 1997), and contraindication

of other modalities such as anticoagulation and sequential compression. Debate continues as to which clients are at highest risk for PE and would therefore be most likely to benefit from prophylactic filter placement (Brasel, Borgstrom, & Weigelt, 1997; McMurtry, Owings, Anderson, Battistella, & Gosselin, 1999; Spain et al., 1997; Velmahos et al., 2000b).

Pulmonary Embolectomy. Pulmonary embolectomy is an invasive procedure reserved for clients who are hemodynamically compromised and for whom conservative treatment is ineffective. This procedure involves extraction of the embolus from the pulmonary artery. Embolectomy was traditionally performed using general anesthesia and extracorporeal circulation but currently can be performed in some cases using local anesthesia and a special IV suction catheter. Data on outcomes from surgical embolectomy largely predate the use of thrombolytic therapy. Catheter embolectomy is still an evolving technology.

Supplemental Oxygen. Oxygen may be administered by nasal cannula or mask to prevent the effects of hypoxia. ABG or oximetry can be used to assess the need for and the response to oxygen therapy. In the case of a large PE or pulmonary infarction in which there is significant pulmonary dead space or intrapulmonary shunting, intubation and mechanical ventilation may be indicated.

Nursing Management

The major goals of nursing intervention are to prevent PE (through interventions to prevent DVT) and to minimize complications if PE does occur.

Altered Tissue Perfusion: Cardiopulmonary

Embolus Precautions/Embolus Care: Pulmonary. Pulmonary tissue perfusion may be compromised as a result of blockage of a portion of the pulmonary circulation by an embolus. Although the nurse may not be able to directly affect the outcome of this physiologic event, he or she must continue to assess the client for improvement or deterioration in response to the insult. Blood pressure, heart rate, urine output, and skin temperature and color can warn of hemodynamic compromise.

The nurse is also responsible for the administration and monitoring of anticoagulants and thrombolytics. Knowing the expected therapeutic response and potential adverse effects of these agents and monitoring laboratory results are important because the nurse collaborates with the physician for optimal client care.

Impaired Gas Exchange

Respiratory Monitoring, Embolus Care: Pulmonary. Gas exchange is impaired in the client with PE because of the ventilation/perfusion mismatch and intrapulmonary shunting. This impairment is manifested by decreased PaO$_2$, tachycardia, and tachypnea, and often by neurologic manifestations of hypoxemia.

Oximetry, a noninvasive test, or ABG analysis can yield valuable information on how well the client is oxygenating. Arterial oxygen pressure should be greater than 60 mm Hg (80 to 100 mm Hg is desirable), and the O$_2$ saturation should be greater than 90% (95% and above is desirable).

The client should be monitored for increased respiratory distress: dyspnea, tachypnea, and anxiety. Supplemental oxygen is given to augment the diffusion at the alveolar capillary membrane. The nurse should monitor the effect of oxygen on respiratory rate, dyspnea, and anxiety, especially if the oxygen is removed for any reason.

Because gas exchange is impaired, limiting the client's oxygen demand is important. Limiting and spacing activity, providing rest periods, controlling anxiety and pain, and augmenting ventilation by ensuring deep breathing and proper positioning are important.

The impaired gas exchange caused by PE may lead to activity intolerance because of hypoxemia. The client may respond with tachypnea and shallow breathing. Anxiety and fear may exaggerate this response. The nurse must ensure that clients maximize ventilation by instructing them to take deeper breaths at a slower rate. An increased respiratory rate is to be expected as a compensatory mechanism to increase ventilation, but the client should be coached to avoid shallow breathing. Nursing measures that reduce fear and anxiety also assist clients to achieve an optimal breathing pattern.

Anxiety

Anxiety Reduction. Anxiety related to hypoxemia, dyspnea, and fear is manifested by tachypnea, tachycardia, subjective responses, and lack of concentration. Dyspnea can cause anxiety. However, anxiety worsens dyspnea, and the client can be caught in a vicious cycle. Anxious states also cause an increased oxygen demand, which must be avoided in this client population.

Clear explanations of the problem and treatment as well as discussion of how clients can participate in their recovery can be helpful. Listening to the client's fears and offering support and explanations may help alleviate the fears.

Knowledge Deficit

Teaching: Disease Process and Procedure/ Treatment. Knowledge deficits related to diagnosis, treatment, risk factors, and care at home can be manifested by questions, uncertainty, anxiety, and lack of participation in self-care. Client education about the diagnosis and treatment plan should be based on the client's educational level, readiness to learn, and physical

stability. Instruction on anticoagulant therapy should be started when the anticoagulants are administered and enhanced when warfarin therapy is initiated (see Table 10–2). Risk factors and situations to avoid (e.g., prolonged sitting, crossing legs, wearing tight stockings) should be included. Written instructions augment oral instructions and should be given before the day of discharge for optimal learning and discussion.

Summary

PE remains a significant complication after multiple trauma and orthopaedic injury and surgery. PE typically is a consequence of DVT. Diagnosis of both PE and DVT can be difficult and requires specialized tests (V̇/Q̇ scanning and angiography) for confirmation. The size of the embolus and extent of lung involvement determine the seriousness and outcome of PE. Nurses can play a key role in the prevention and early detection of PE, thereby reducing client morbidity and mortality. Heparin therapy has been a primary treatment modality, but other modalities such as LMWH and thrombolytic therapy are emerging and currently being studied to determine their role in the treatment of PE.

FAT EMBOLISM SYNDROME

Fat embolism following trauma and long-bone fracture is a major cause of morbidity and mortality. The exact mechanism of the pathophysiologic process that produces fat embolism still has not been completely identified. Mortality rates from fat embolism syndrome have significantly decreased over the past decade, although prevention and treatment modalities continue to be explored.

Definition

Fat embolism is the presence of fat globules in lung parenchyma and peripheral circulation, typically after a long-bone fracture, major trauma, or orthopaedic surgical procedure. *Fat embolism syndrome* (FES) is a serious manifestation of fat embolism that may present as an acute respiratory insufficiency because of decreased alveolar diffusion of oxygen, thrombocytopenia, or deteriorating mental status.

Incidence

Fat embolism occurs most frequently after long-bone fracture, particularly in clients with multiple long-bone fractures or concomitant pelvic fractures. Embolic fat in the blood has been found in at least 90% of clients with major trauma to soft tissue or bone. In a group of fatally injured blunt force trauma victims, 68% had pulmonary fat emboli present on autopsy (Mudd, Hunt, Matherly, Goldsmith, Campbell, Nichols, & Rink, 2000).

Subclinical FES has been speculated to occur in at least 50% to 100% of clients with a fracture of a long bone or the pelvis. However, the incidence of post-traumatic episodes that develop into overt FES requiring intervention is approximately 0.5% to 2.2% for single long-bone fractures and 5% to 10% with multiple fractures (Johnson & Lucas, 1996). Clients with multiple fractures may also have other severe associated injures that mask FES or account for its clinical signs and symptoms.

The development of FES in clients at risk varies with the number and type of fracture (open vs. closed). The overall incidence of FES is 1% to 2% with tibia or femoral shaft fractures and 5% to 10% with fractures of both bones or multiple bone fractures, particularly those associated with pelvic injuries. FES may occur more often after a closed fracture than after an open one treated by external decompression. It is widely accepted that clients with delayed open reduction and internal fixation (ORIF) have a higher incidence of clinical FES than clients treated with ORIF within 24 to 48 hours of injury.

Debate remains as to the contribution of method of fracture fixation to risk of FES. Some researchers contend that surgical techniques in which high pressures are applied to the intramedullary canal, such as intramedullary nailing of long-bone fractures or insertion of prosthetic components in total joint replacement procedures, increases the risk of pulmonary complications (Muller, Rahn, Pfister, & Meinig, 1994; Pitto, Koessler, & Kuehle, 1999). FES has been reported after many orthopaedic procedures, most commonly total joint replacement and hemiarthroplasty of the hip and knee and intramedullary nailing of the femoral shaft. Rare cases of FES have been reported after spinal fusion, femoral elongation, and closed femoral osteotomy. FES has also been reported in association with osteomyelitis, contusions, lacerations or incision of adipose tissue, and septicemia. An increased risk of FES has been reported with myelodysplasia disorders, collagen vascular disorders, osteoporosis, increased liquid marrow fat content, liposuction, and external immobilization causing medullary cavity enlargement.

Children have a much lower incidence of FES than adults; children develop the clinical syndrome 100 times less frequently than adults with comparable injuries. It has been postulated that the marrow fat content of children differs significantly from that of adults; marrow fat in children has smaller amounts of liquid triolein.

The mortality rate following FES ranges from 5% to 15% (Bulger, Smith, Maier, & Jurkovich, 1997; Johnson & Lucas, 1996), with higher death rates related to the severity of the FES and number and severity of associated injuries. Death usually occurs from respiratory complications. Coma, severe adult respiratory distress syndrome (ARDS), pneumonia, and congestive cardiac failure are grave prognostic signs. Long-term morbidity is associated with focal cerebral neurologic deficits.

Pathophysiology

Two theories exist regarding the source of fat globules that migrate to the lungs. The first postulates that direct trauma disrupts fat cells in the marrow of fractured bones or contused soft tissues. Fat droplets enter the venous system through torn veins at the injury site. The droplets travel to the pulmonary vascular bed and become trapped as emboli in lung capillaries. Fat droplets reach the lung within moments after injury or during the course of surgery. Some droplets go through the lungs to the systemic circulation and embolize to other body parts, such as the brain, kidneys, retina, or skin.

The second theory asserts that embolic fat is derived from circulating blood lipids. The metabolic response to the stress of injury alters the physiologic emulsion of fat in plasma. The release of catecholamines after trauma mobilizes free fatty acids from the body's fat deposits (Muller et al., 1994). Normal chylomicrons (less than 1 μm) coalesce and form fat globules 10 to 40 μm in diameter. This theory is supported by the occurrence of fat emboli in nontraumatic but stressful conditions.

The initial effects of pulmonary fat microembolism (regardless of the source) are mechanical. Pulmonary perfusion pressure increases, vessels become engorged, and the lung becomes more rigid and less compliant. This increases the workload of the right side of the heart. As breathing becomes more difficult, the right side of the heart dilates in an effort to increase cardiac output, thereby requiring increased venous return. At this point, the individual is especially susceptible to the effects of hypovolemic shock with decreased central venous return. Death at this stage results from acute right-sided heart failure. (Further information about the effects of embolism on the lungs can be found in the section on PE.)

The next phase of FES involves the effects of free fatty acids on the lungs. Neutral fat globules released from the body's fat deposits occlude small pulmonary vessels (less than 20 μm) and become trapped in the pulmonary circulation, where they are hydrolyzed by the enzyme lipoprotein lipase into free fatty acids. The alveolocapillary membrane reaction in FES is the same as that in ARDS. Fat embolism is considered an etiologic factor in ARDS and, by some investigators, only a variant of ARDS. Free fatty acids produce endothelial damage, increase capillary permeability, and inactivate lung surfactant by damaging type II pneumocytes. Increased capillary permeability leads to hemorrhagic pulmonary edema because of protein-containing fluid leaking into interstitial spaces and alveoli. Loss of surfactant activity causes patchy alveolar collapse, and formation of a protein-rich hyaline membrane decreases the alveolocapillary exchange surface. Decreased oxygen diffusion from alveoli to lung capillaries from the thickened membrane results in severe hypoxia. Concurrent release of thromboplastin from the fat hydrolysis may initiate intravascular

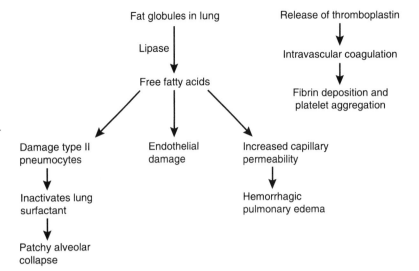

FIGURE 10–10. Pathophysiology of fat embolism syndrome.

coagulation, leading to fibrin deposition and platelet aggregation (Fig. 10-10).

Inflammatory mediators (cytokines) also play a role in the pathologic changes seen in FES. Pulmonary vasospasm and bronchospasm are caused by the release of amines from the breakdown of platelets and mast cells and from the fracture site, as well as histamine from the lung parenchyma. This vasospasm causes venous constriction and congestion of the pulmonary capillary bed. Catecholamine release causes platelet aggregation and contributes to microemboli in the lungs, brain, and other tissues. Platelets aggregate on fat particles and may cause disseminated intravascular coagulation (DIC). Platelets break down, causing thrombocytopenia and decreasing plasma fibrinogen. Petechiae may occur from the thrombocytopenia. Free fatty acids can cause red cell hemolysis, resulting in decreased hemoglobin.

The severity of reaction in FES depends on the amount of fat released and the general condition of the client. Hypovolemia and shock are especially dangerous because of the association between hypoperfusion and release of catecholamines and other cytokines and increased adhesion and aggregation of platelets. About 50% of clients with major fat embolism involving systemic symptoms have residual damage of the brain, lungs, heart, kidneys, and eyes. Findings on autopsy of cases of FES show fat globules, alveolar macrophage proliferation, interstitial edema, intra-alveolar edema, and hemorrhage in the lungs. The lung tissue resembles that seen in ARDS. Brain capillaries are plugged by fat, and surrounding hemorrhage is present. Kidneys demonstrate glomerular fat plugs. Cutaneous petechiae are present, showing capillaries plugged by fat with surrounding hemorrhage.

Assessment

Fat embolism syndrome can be viewed as a continuum from a subclinical form (usually undetected and untreated) through a fulminant form. FES is identified by evaluating a collection of possible signs and symptoms in the client at risk and remains a diagnosis of exclusion.

The clinically apparent form of FES generally occurs within 24 to 48 hours of injury. This form usually presents with respiratory insufficiency, mental status changes, and in some cases, petechiae. A 100% survival rate for this form has been reported in a number of studies.

The severe, fulminant form develops up to 12 hours after injury, with massive embolization, prominent neurologic involvement, and cardiovascular collapse. Symptoms may be masked intraoperatively by general anesthesia. This form may progress rapidly to death.

Clients with FES generally have a history of traumatic injury, long-bone fracture, or an orthopaedic procedure (e.g., total joint arthroplasty). The most common presenting symptoms are those of acute respiratory insufficiency (e.g., tachypnea, dyspnea, use of accessory muscles) and hypoxemia (i.e., cerebral symptoms, such as restlessness, apprehension, anxiety, agitation, confusion, stupor, or coma). Cerebral symptoms may result from hypoxia or embolic fat to the brain.

Hypoxemia, tachycardia, tachypnea, and pyrexia are consistently seen in clients with FES. Rales and rhonchi may be heard on auscultation of the lungs. Cutaneous petechiae, primarily on the upper chest, axilla, oral mucosa, conjunctivae, and neck, are seen in 50% to 60% of clients. Approximately 10% of clients develop respiratory failure requiring intubation and mechanical ventilation.

Diagnostic Evaluation

Several changes occur in laboratory studies in FES, the most indicative of which are the changes in ABG. Severe hypoxemia is the hallmark sign. Initially, the $Paco_2$ drops as a result of hyperventilation. As the respiratory insufficiency continues, however, $Paco_2$ can be expected to rise as a result of impaired oxygen delivery and metabolic acidosis.

Chest x-ray films may be normal initially and may progress to show a diffuse, fluffy, bilateral infiltrate. In more severe cases, diffuse opacities may be seen. MRI can be used to detect cerebral lesions (Takahashi, Suzuki, Osakabe, Asai, Miyo, Nagashima, Fujimoto, & Takahasi, 1999).

V̇/Q̇ scans may be useful in excluding PE as a cause of acute hypoxemia but are not generally helpful in the diagnosis of FES. Nonspecific peripheral defects may be seen, but on the whole, the emboli tend to be too small to be detected (Bulger et al., 1997).

FES is associated with a sudden fall in hematocrit value with the onset of symptoms. The anemia has been associated with hemorrhage into the lungs because of microangiopathy and with blood loss at injury. Thrombocytopenia (platelet count less than 150,000/mL) is considered diagnostic for FES.

Fat globules are found in the urine of less than 50% of clients, but this is not a diagnostic finding because lipiduria may be seen in trauma clients who do not show symptoms of FES (Bulger et al., 1997).

Examination of fluid from bronchoalveolar lavage for fat cells in intubated clients has been suggested as a method of confirming the diagnosis of FES (Mimoz, Eduoard, Beydon, Quillard, Verra, Fleury, Bonnet, & Samii, 1995). Some authors have suggested that this is not specific for FES (Stanley, Hanson, Hicklin, Galzier, Ervanian, & Jadali, 1994), and the exact cutoff criterion has not been determined.

Criteria for Diagnosis of Fat Embolism Syndrome.
Widely used in the past, Gurd's criteria for diagnosis of FES include respiratory insufficiency (hypoxemia, pulmonary edema), cerebral involvement, and petechial rash as major features. The minor features include pyrexia, tachycardia, thrombocytopenia, retinal emboli, drop in hematocrit value that cannot be accounted for by other sources of blood loss or IV fluid dilution, and fat in the urine and sputum. At least one major and three minor features should be present for a positive diagnosis. Other investigators have focused on more refined indicators of respiratory insufficiency for diagnosis. When acute respiratory insufficiency is the major presenting symptom, it is important to exclude other treatable causes, such as pneumothorax, volume overload, and PE, before making the diagnosis of FES.

Treatment Modalities and Related Nursing Management

The first aim of treatment is prevention of FES. Accepted principles in treating long-bone fracture are careful handling, adequate splinting, and elimination of unnecessary manipulation of the affected extremity or pelvis. ORIF within 24 to 48 hours after the injury is recommended. Early aggressive resuscitation to prevent hypovolemic shock, adequate analgesia, administration of blood through a 20-μm filter, and prevention of sepsis are also standard in the care of fracture clients.

Surgeons continue to explore new operative techniques designed to decrease the incidence of FES during orthopaedic procedures. Intraoperative precautions in joint replacement surgery include removing the products of medullary reaming by lavage or aspiration and venting the shaft to lower intramedullary pressure. Aspiration of the intramedullary canal marrow before placement of the alignment guide pin in total knee arthroplasty has been recommended. Venting can be done by placing a catheter down the canal or drilling a hole in the shaft. Increasing the inspired oxygen concentration when the cement and prosthesis are inserted, monitoring cardiopulmonary parameters, and maintaining the intravascular volume are additional recommendations. Pitto, Blunk, and Kossler (2000) recommend use of a bone vacuum technique during cementing of the femoral component during total hip arthroplasty.

Use of corticosteroids to prevent FES has been advocated but remains controversial. Methylprednisolone is hypothesized to prevent FES by several mechanisms, including maintaining vascular integrity by protecting the capillary endothelium, stabilizing the lysosomal membrane of granulocytes, stabilizing the complement system activation, and slowing the platelet aggregation. Although early studies suggest a potential benefit from prophylactic treatment with corticosteroids in clients at risk for FES, the lack of a consensus on predictive markers for clients in whom FES will develop could lead to unnecessary steroid treatment in some clients. Human trials of corticosteroids for *treatment* of FES have been poorly controlled, and concerns about increased risk of infection in multiple-injured or postoperative clients have limited their use (Bulger et al., 1997).

If FES develops, therapy is largely supportive and aimed at preserving respiratory integrity. Oxygen is administered by mask or nasal cannula. Intubation and continuous positive airway pressure may be necessary. Frequent ABG measurement may be required. Arterial oxygen pressure should be maintained at a minimum of 60 to 70 mm Hg.

Clients with the subclinical and overt forms of FES often respond well to oxygen therapy. Clients who develop the fulminant form are more likely to require long-term mechanical ventilation and positive end-expiratory pressure to maintain oxygenation. Supportive therapy for these clients is similar to that required for clients with ARDS.

Maintenance of adequate intravascular volume is also of primary importance. Adequate fluid and blood replacement is essential in the prevention of shock and maintenance of adequate oxygen delivery. Hypotension must be treated aggressively. Some clients may require pulmonary artery catheters for accurate measurement of cardiac output and vasoactive medications for optimization of hemodynamic parameters. Low-dose dopamine may improve urinary output, prevent interstitial pulmonary edema, and increase cardiac output. A continuous infusion of nitroglycerin may be needed to decrease mean pulmonary arterial pressure and right ventricular afterload.

Some treatments used in the past, such as 5% ethyl alcohol, heparin, and low-molecular-weight dextran, have been shown to be ineffective or may be detrimental to the client with FES. The use of heparin to decrease lipemia is contraindicated. One of the endproducts of the reaction of the lipoprotein lipase and fat is free fatty acid, which may further aggravate lung damage.

Nursing Management

Nursing care, like medical care, is aimed at prevention and early recognition of FES, and minimization of injury if it does occur. Nursing diagnoses for the client at risk for FES include potential for injury from fat emboli. Nursing diagnoses for the client who develops FES include ineffective breathing pattern, impaired gas exchange, ineffective airway clearance, fear and anxiety, and compromised or ineffective individual or family coping.

Risk for Injury from Fat Emboli

Positioning/Respiratory Monitoring. The cautious handling of fractured extremities and the avoidance of unnecessary manipulation of the fracture site are interventions aimed at preventing additional fat release. Clients at high risk for FES should be carefully assessed and monitored for symptoms of hypoxemia. Lung auscultation and observation for dyspnea, shallow respirations, restlessness, and agitation should be carried out routinely. ABG should be analyzed if there is a suspicion of oxygen deficit.

Fluid Monitoring and Resuscitation. Intake and output should be recorded accurately, and the client should be monitored for signs of shock. Adequate fluid replacement is important in influencing the outcome of FES.

Ineffective Breathing Pattern/Impaired Gas Exchange/Ineffective Airway Clearance

Airway Management/Oxygen Therapy/Respiratory Monitoring/Mechanical Ventilation. Elevating the head of the client's bed, if not contraindicated, will promote easier breathing. The client should be assisted in deep breathing and coughing. Changing the client's position frequently will prevent pooling of secretions. Results of blood gas analysis should be monitored and reported. Oxygen should be delivered by cannula or mask. If the client is unable to achieve adequate oxygenation, intubation and mechanical ventilation may be necessary.

The nurse should provide support and reassurance at all times. Monitoring of hemoglobin and hematocrit values and replacement of blood are critical in promoting adequate oxygen delivery.

Fear and Anxiety

Anxiety Reduction/Teaching: Procedure/Treatment. Fat embolism syndrome and its treatment should be explained to the client at the appropriate time. The nurse should stay with the client until fear is alleviated. The client should be reassured that he or she is being monitored and that appropriate treatment will be given.

Compromised or Ineffective Individual or Family Coping

Coping Enhancement/Family Support. All procedures and treatments should be explained. The client and family should be encouraged to ask questions and communicate their concerns. If the client must be transferred to the intensive care unit, adequate explanation should be given and the client should be accompanied by familiar personnel. Means of communication, such as writing, pointing, or using an alphabet board, should be provided to the client who needs intubation and mechanical ventilation.

Summary

FES can be a devastating complication of orthopaedic injuries and surgery. With cautious handling, prompt recognition of symptoms, and adequate treatment of the syndrome, morbidity and mortality can be dramatically decreased. The orthopaedic nurse is instrumental in assessing clients at risk and initiating treatment measures. Prompt recognition of respiratory compromise, calm reassurance, and education are key interventions in caring for the client with FES.

BLOOD LOSS AND HEMORRHAGE

Blood loss is a common occurrence in orthopaedic surgery, particularly with trauma, fractures, joint replacements, and extensive spinal procedures. Surgical clients are the recipients of most of the blood transfusions today in the United States (Fiebig, 1998). The future is promising for the continued development and evaluation of methods to decrease blood loss, as well as for changes in practice of blood administration and for the development of alternatives to blood replacement.

Etiology

Blood loss may occur as a result of trauma, surgery, blood clotting disorders, and abnormalities or erosion of blood vessel walls. In addition, slipped ligatures during or after surgery, infection, soft tissue damage, ulcers, and medications (e.g., NSAIDs, anticoagulants) may induce blood loss.

Incidence

Orthopaedic Surgical Procedures. Significant blood loss may occur with various orthopaedic surgical procedures, both during the procedures and in the postoperative period. Some variables have been associated with increased blood loss during orthopaedic procedures. Clients undergoing bilateral joint replacements and those with revision arthroplasty surgery have higher blood losses and a higher need for blood replacement than clients undergoing single, primary arthroplasty, especially total knee arthroplasty (Bierbaum, Callaghan, Galante, Rubash, Tooms, & Welch, 1999; Larocque, Gilbert, & Brien, 1997). Although some authors have reported that noncemented total hip and knee arthroplasty components have been associated with increased blood loss compared with cemented prostheses (An, Mikhail, Jackson, Tolin, & Dodd, 1991), recent authors have not found this difference (Anders, Lifeso, Landis, Mikulsky, Meinking, & McCracken, 1996; Nuttall, Santrach, Oliver, Horlocker, Shaughnessy, Cabanela, & Bryant, 1996). An and colleagues (1991) postulated that the cement may plug bleeding sites from the bone. The incidence of blood transfusion in total joint arthroplasty has been reported to be higher for clients with lower preoperative hemoglobin, older clients, and those with lower body weights (Larocque, Gilbert, & Brien, 1997; Nuttall et al., 1996). NSAIDs, including aspirin, also increase the loss of blood in the postoperative period because of their interference with platelet aggregation. Swain, Nightingale, and Patel (2000) found increased blood transfusion with intertrochanteric fractures as compared with intracapsular fractures, and variance was also effected by the surgical repair approach.

Blood Clotting Abnormalities. The most common inherited blood clotting abnormality is hemophilia, an X-linked disorder characterized by a deficiency of clotting factor VIII. Hemophilia B is a deficiency of factor IX. Von Willebrand's disease is the second most common inherited hemorrhagic disorder. It is associated with prolongation of normal bleeding time because of a deficiency of von Willebrand's factor.

Blood clotting disorders may also be acquired. Malabsorption syndromes, liver disease, and biliary atresia may all result in vitamin K deficiency and lengthened clotting times. Medications (e.g., warfarin) may also effect the prothrombin time.

Pathophysiology

For hemostasis to occur, the clotting system must be intact. Figure 10-5 shows the clotting cascade. Any deficiency in the factors or medications interfering with the clotting cascade can precipitate blood loss. There are also instances during surgery or with a postoperative drain in place, for example, when even an intact clotting system is not sufficient to stop blood loss as quickly as it occurs. Other measures, such as pressure at the site of bleeding, must be taken to decrease blood loss until a clot is able to form at the site of bleeding.

An adequate amount of red blood cells in the blood is needed to transport oxygen for cell survival. The vital organs—the brain, heart, kidneys, and liver—are particularly susceptible to damage from hypoxia resulting from blood loss.

Assessment

Subjective Assessment: Nursing History. Increased anxiety and dizziness may characterize blood loss in the conscious client. The client may complain of restlessness, feelings of increased heart rate, and a "clammy" feeling, especially with rapid blood loss. Fatigue, drowsiness, and weakness may be more common complaints with slower blood loss. The client may report increased pain, tenderness, and decreased joint mobility.

Objective Assessment: Physical Examination. Blood loss is manifested by drainage from any part of the body, wounds, or drains; hypotension; rapid respiration; tachycardia; and irregular pulse. There may be swelling at the site. The client may appear restless and have a grayish pallor and cool, moist skin. A decrease in urine output often is noted. Clients with anemia demonstrate signs of hypoxia such as light-headedness, weakness, angina, and dyspnea. A younger healthy client tolerates a lower hemoglobin level than an older client with chronic cardiorespiratory disease process.

Diagnostic Evaluation. A complete blood count shows a decrease in red blood cells, hemoglobin, and hematocrit values. It should be noted, however, that if the client is hypovolemic, the hematocrit may not be decreased because it is a ratio of blood cells to serum. Coagulation studies may be done to determine whether a clotting abnormality is present. Tests for blood in the stool (guaiac) and urine can be carried out to facilitate determination of the site of blood loss if it is not readily apparent. Use of angiography may facilitate assessment of bleeding vessels and the need to return to the operating room for control.

Treatment Modalities and Related Nursing Management

The first goal in treating a client losing blood is to stop or minimize the blood loss. Pressure to the area of bleeding (manual or dressings), electrocautery, tourniquets, or pneumatic antishock garments may be used to decrease blood loss. Chemical means may also suppress blood loss.

Blood and fluid replacement are the major treatments for minimizing the damaging effects of blood loss.

The American Society of Anesthesiologists (1996) published their findings of a review of 1417 articles and expert opinion consultation in an attempt to establish evidence-based guidelines for indications for blood transfusions. Blood is rarely required for hemoglobin levels greater than 10 g/dL and almost always indicated for hemoglobin levels less than 6 g/dL. The client's hemoglobin level combined with the individual client's risk to develop complications from hypoxia are the recommended transfusion triggers. Thus, the singe rule of "10/30" (hemoglobin of 10 g/dL and a hematocrit of 30%) is outdated.

Transfusion therapy includes administration of components of blood:

- *Erythrocyte:* Red blood cells carry oxygen to tissues and organs. Hemoglobin binds with oxygen for use in cellular metabolism. Administration of packed red blood cells is used to restore the oxygen carrying capacity of blood.
- *Platelets:* Platelets provide hemostasis by adhering to the damaged endothelium to form a platelet plug.
- *Fresh frozen plasma:* This is transfused for multiple factor deficiencies because it provides enzymes of the thrombotic and fibrinolytic systems of coagulation. Clinical situations include liver disease and massive transfusion (following 6 to 10 U red blood cell transfusion).
- *Cryoprecipitate:* Cryoprecipitate contains coagulation proteins (factor VIII, fibrinogen, fibronectin, and factor XIII) and should be given to clients deficient in these coagulation proteins who are at risk of hemorrhage and to clients who have undergone massive transfusion therapy.
- *Definitions:*
  Allogeneic blood—blood obtained for transfusion from an individual other than the client.
  Autologous blood—blood donated from the client in anticipation of transfusion that is given back to the same client if the need for transfusion occurs.

Allogeneic Blood Transfusions. Fear of transmission of viral agents from blood transfusions has led to the implementation of intense measures to ensure that the blood supply is safe and to the development of alternatives to transfusion therapy (Ness, 1999). Although safer than before, allogeneic blood transfusions still have potential risks. Because of these risks, clients should provide consent before allogeneic blood transfusion, unless they are involved in a life-threatening emergency situation. The Joint Commission on Accreditation of Healthcare Organizations' standard includes the requirement for obtaining client consent before transfusion (Belanger, 1999). The estimated risks associated with blood and blood product transfusions are listed in Box 10-6.

BOX 10-6.
Estimated Risks Associated with Blood and Blood Product Transfusions

Hepatitis B	(1/30,000–1/250,000) per unit transfused
Hepatitis C	(1/30,000–1/150,000) per unit transfused
HTLV	(1/250,000–1/2,000,000) per unit transfused
HIV/AIDS	(1/200,000–1/2,000,000) per unit transfused
Bacterial contamination	
RBCs	1/500,000 per unit transfused
Platelets	1/12,000 per unit transfused
Acute hemolytic reaction	1/250,000–1/1,000,000 per unit transfused

HTLV, human T-cell lymphotropic virus; HIV/AIDS, human immunodeficiency virus/acquired immunodeficiency syndrome.
From Goodnough, L. T., Brecher, M. E., Kanter, M. H., & Aubuchon, J. P. (1999). Transfusion medicine. *New England Journal of Medicine, 340*(6), 438–447.

The clinical significance of the immunosuppression following allogeneic blood transfusions is widely debated and clinical outcomes are conflicting (Aubuchon, 1997). The potential of an increased risk of infection from immunosuppression to the orthopaedic client must be considered against the benefit of transfusion therapy. Use of leukocyte reduction by filtration decreases the client's exposure to the allogeneic leukocytes. Clients may experience decreased febrile reactions, alloimmunization, and platelet refractoriness.

Massive transfusion protocols for the exsanguinating client usually require uncrossmatched type O negative blood for first-line transfusion. In such a life-threatening situation, the risks are secondary to sustaining life.

Directed Donation. This is blood donated by friends, family, or co-workers specifically for an identified client's use. Understanding that the blood came from a known person may decrease the client's anxiety, but this may be misleading. In fact, studies point to no reduction in infectious disease transmission. Directed donation is therefore offered but not usually encouraged. This practice may lead to a direct charge of $100 to $300 per unit to the client.

Autologous Blood Transfusions. Autologous blood may be collected either in the preoperative period (via predonated autologous deposits), intraoperatively (via salvage by cell saver), or in the postoperative period (via salvage by an autotransfusion system). Autologous blood may then be transfused to the client without the majority of the risks involved in allogeneic transfusion, although autologous transfusion is not risk free (Fiebig, 1998). During the intraoperative phase, the majority of red blood cells transfused for total hip and knee arthroplasty at the Mayo Foundation were autologous (Warner, Warner, Schroeder, Offord, Maxson, & Santrach, 1998).

Preoperative Autologous Blood Donation. The National Heart, Lung, and Blood Institute Panel (NHLBIP, 1995) has recommended reserving use of preoperative autologous blood donation (PABD) for use in elective procedures in which there is at least a 10% likelihood for the need for transfusion. This includes total hip and knee arthroplasty and major spine procedures with instrumentation (NHLBIP, 1995). In an analysis of 9482 clients having total hip or knee arthroplasty, Bierbaum and colleagues (1999) reported that 57% of the total hip arthroplasty clients and 39% of the total knee arthroplasty clients received a blood transfusion. This included primary, bilateral, and revision surgeries. Of the clients receiving blood, 66% received PABD.

The recommended amount of blood that should be predeposited varies depending on the ability of the client to donate and the complexity of the procedure. Clients scheduled for surgery may donate a unit of blood (or less if the client weighs less than 110 pounds) every 4 to 7 days. Predeposit donation should be completed at least 72 hours before the scheduled procedure. The client must have a hematocrit level of 33% and a hemoglobin level of 11 g/dL for donation (NHLBIP, 1995). The only true contraindication to autologous donation is the presence of bacteremia. If the client has other comorbidities in which a decrease in the oxygen-carrying capacity of the blood may be detrimental, such as severe angina, aortic stenosis, anemia, pulmonary disease, hemodynamic instability, or pregnancy, autologous donation may be contraindicated (Testa & Tobias, 1996). However, when these conditions are present, each case is reviewed individually to determine the risk/benefit ratio of autologous donation. Table 10–3 outlines general information about and advantages and disadvantages of PABD.

Client information on dietary habits and methods for increasing iron intake should be presented before the predeposit is done. Iron supplements to stimulate red blood cell production are required. Clients need to be informed they may require allogeneic blood transfusion if additional units of blood are required (beyond the amount predeposited). If the client does not need the autologous blood, the unused blood is destroyed because it does not meet requirements for allogeneic donation. If the surgical date is changed, the blood that has been collected may be frozen or reinfused before surgery.

In recent years, there has been some controversy about the advantages and need for PABD and the national overall use of PABD has decreased 41.8% from 1992 to 1997 (National Blood Data Resource Center, 1999). Data about costs of PABD versus allogeneic blood are conflicting and confusing because researchers consider different variables in their analyses. Sonnenberg, Gregory, Yomtovian, Russell, Tierney, Kosmin, and Carson (1999), for example, raised the issue of cost of treating infection if there is an increased risk of bacterial transmission in allogeneic transfusions compared with autologous blood as some authors have proposed. There are also the issues of the discard rate of PABD, reported to be in the range of 15% to 45%, and the need for allogeneic transfusion in clients who have predonated blood, reported at 9% to 15% (Bierbaum et al., 1999; Billote, Glisson, Green, & Wixson, 2000; National Blood Data Resource Center, 1999). An issue not discussed in the literature is the impact of reducing PABD on the national blood supply. Although there appear to be some disadvantages, PABD remains a good alternative for blood replacement, particularly for clients undergoing revision total hip arthroplasty, bilateral total knee or total hip arthroplasty, and major spine surgery with instrumentation.

Intraoperative Blood Salvage and Autotransfusion. Intraoperative blood salvage and reinfusion involves collecting shed blood by aspiration from the surgical site, concentrating the aspirate, and washing the red cells before reinfusion. This technique is used primarily for clients for whom large blood losses without contamination are anticipated during surgery (e.g., spine fusions and bilateral or revision joint replacements). Because a flat fee generally is charged for setup and use, this method of autotransfusion is expensive relative to other methods unless large volumes of blood are lost. Intraoperative blood salvage can be used in emergency and trauma situations. Intraoperative blood salvage and reinfusion is contraindicated for clients with infection or malignancy.

From 50% to 60% of the red blood cells from the shed blood are salvageable for reinfusion. Several techniques have been advocated to increase the viability of salvaged cells and to increase the recovery of drainage. Open-tipped plastic suction hoses with pressures less than 100 mm Hg decrease cell destruction. Pooling or clotting of blood in the wound should be avoided, and sponge use should be limited.

Devices for collection of blood intraoperatively that return unwashed blood to the client are also available. These devices work similarly to the postoperative collection devices (described in the next section), and blood can be returned to the client either intraoperatively or postoperatively.

Postoperative Blood Salvage and Autotransfusion. Postoperative blood salvage involves collection of shed blood through suction into a reservoir, filtration (and, in some cases, washing) of the drainage, and reinfusion of blood through the client's venous line (Fig. 10-11). Reinfusion can be continuous or intermittent in the postoperative period. Postoperative autotransfusion is used in total joint replacement surgery, spinal procedures, and in some cases of trauma; it can significantly decrease the amount of allogeneic blood transfusions needed (Grosvenor, Goyal, & Goodman, 2000).

In some instances, the intraoperative cell washing device stays with the client in the postanesthesia care unit, pulling the blood from the postoperative drain. However, this method of postoperative salvage is labor intensive and generally not cost-effective.

Postoperative autotransfusion is not used for clients with a malignant lesion or an infection near the operative site. It is also contraindicated in clients with severe coagulation disorders, renal failure, or trauma with fecal or urinary contamination or if the wound is more than 4 hours old. Other contraindications include the use of irrigants that are not injectable (e.g., povidone-iodine, bacitracin), hemostatic agents, or agents that may cause clotting in the device (e.g., thrombin gelatin foam, microcrystalline collagen).

According to the American Association of Blood Banks, blood collection in the reservoir can last up to 6

TABLE 10–3. *Blood Replacement Alternatives: Advantages and Disadvantages*

ALTERNATIVE	ADVANTAGES	DISADVANTAGES
Predeposit Autologous Donation 1 unit of blood can be donated every 4–7 days, providing hematocrit is >34%. Blood may be stored for 35–42 days without freezing. The last unit of blood should be donated at least 72 hr before surgery. Criteria for predeposit autologous blood donation are less stringent than those for homologous blood donation; therefore, the blood is destroyed if not used by the client. Criteria for autologous blood donation include (1) no history of cardiovascular disease, severe respiratory disease, recent severe asthma attacks, or seizures since infancy; (2) age 12–75 yr (may be waived); (3) adequate red blood cells (RBCs) (hemoglobin >11 g and hematocrit >34%); (4) if client weighs <110 pounds, blood is drawn per body weight; and (5) no active infection. Women of childbearing age may benefit from autologous blood because homologous blood may cause formation of antibodies that might interfere with future pregnancies.	Decreases possibility of blood reactions, alloimmunization, and transmission of infectious agents. Has a high client acceptance level. Is cost-effective compared with other forms of autotransfusion. Does not prolong operative or anesthesia time or require additional equipment. Involves client in care. Clients may be more likely to donate blood in the future for own or homologous use.	Hematocrit must be >34%. Storage may be a concern. Change in operative dates may cause blood to become outdated. Donation is time-consuming and involves travel for client. Cost may increase because of tracking. Client must have veins that are adequate for venipuncture with large-bore needles. Can be used only for elective procedures. Client often has a decreased hemoglobin and hematocrit level at the time of operation. Unused blood will be discarded.
Intraoperative Blood Salvage Uses portable centrifuges and cell washers. Blood and debris from surgical field aspirated and mixed with dilute solution of heparin or citrated dextrose. Mixture passed through 140-μm filter, then roller-pumped to bowl in centrifuge. The RBCs are washed with normal saline. Centrifugal force separates RBCs from waste products. Suspension of RBCs (approximately 50% of shed RBCs are saved) in saline is pumped into blood bag and transfused through 20- to 40-μm filter.	Decreases risks of transfusion reactions, alloimmunization, transmission of infectious agents. Is cost-effective in clients with large intraoperative blood loss. Can be used for emergency and trauma situations. May have better oxygen-transport capacity than banked blood. No long-term prior arrangements are necessary.	Additional costs, particularly if small intraoperative blood loss. Potential complications of infection, microembolization, hemoglobinopathy, nephrotoxicity, disseminated intravascular coagulation, and thrombocytopenia. Contraindicated with infection and malignancy. Potential deficiency of clotting factors and platelets.

Table continued on following page

TABLE 10–3. *Blood Replacement Alternatives: Advantages and Disadvantages* Continued

ALTERNATIVE	ADVANTAGES	DISADVANTAGES
Postoperative Blood Salvage Cell saver may be continued postoperatively. Closed system may be used with continuous or intermittent infusion. With continuous autotransfusion, the blood is collected in a reservoir (with a source of suction), and the tubing from the outflow port is threaded through an infusion pump to the client's peripheral or central venous line. The rate of reinfusion is adjusted every 0.5–1 hr according to the amount of bleeding and need for volume replacement. For intermittent infusion, the blood is collected in the device's reservoir and reinfused after the collection period. As the rate of bleeding decreases (or at a predetermined time according to institutional policy), the reinfusion is stopped and the system is converted to a standard wound drain to collect further drainage. All blood for autotransfusion is filtered through a gross clot prefilter and a standard 20- to 40-μm aggregate filter before reinfusion. After collecting blood for 6 hr, blood must be reinfused, generally over 2–4 hr.	Decreases risks of transfusion reactions, alloimmunization, transmission of infectious agents. Normal potassium level. Acceptable to most biblical and religious convictions. Temperature closer to body temperature. Costs not significantly higher than homologous blood transfusions in most institutions. RBCs are able to survive the salvage process.	Potential of reinfusion of bone, metal, methyl methacrylate debris, and fat that has been collected. Requires additional training of nursing personnel. Potential for microemboli. Contraindicated with infection or malignancy. May increase risk of hemorrhage if preexisting blood dyscrasia or clotting anomaly is present. Increased levels of free plasma hemoglobin may cause renal damage. Contraindicated in trauma with fecal or urinary contamination and in wounds >4 hr old. Cannot reinfuse blood that has been exposed to noninjectable irrigants or hemostatic agents.

hours. Following the collection period, blood should be reinfused over 2 to 4 hours. It is possible to have multiple transfusions from use of postoperative devices.

The blood salvaged in these collection devices has been proven to be safe and of good quality. The average hematocrit is 24% to 34%, and the average hemoglobin is 8.9 to 11.5 g/dL. These numbers decrease with each successive device used. It has also been found the erythrocytes collected in the autotransfusion unit have a normal survival rate.

The prefilters within the devices remove the large particles that may come through the drainage tubing, including bone and cement fragments, blood clots, and large fat particles. Although it is recognized that the

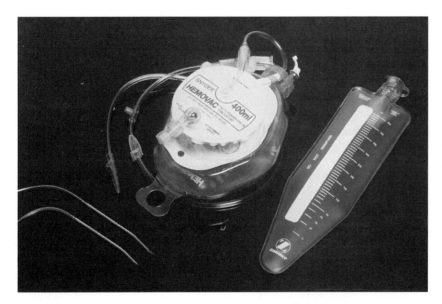

FIGURE 10–11. A postoperative orthopaedic autotransfusion device. (Courtesy of Zimmer, Inc., Warsaw, IN.)

amount of fat particles in the salvaged blood is high, studies have been inconclusive about the significance of reinfusing these particles back to the client because most of the fat particles in the salvaged blood are less than 9 µm in size. Because the pulmonary literature indicates anything less than 40 µm does not cause pulmonary complications, it is thought that these particles cause no harm to the client. Some of the commercially available devices have incorporated methods to help remove the fat from the salvaged blood before reinfusion. The use of a leukocyte depletion filter also reduces the number of fat particles when compared with a 40-µm microaggregate filter. This is an area that requires much more research.

Another concern is the possible reinfusion of polymethyl methacrylate (PMMA) monomer to the client when the salvaged blood was reinfused. In cases in which cemented prostheses are used, at the time the cement is introduced, the possibility exists for the client to become hypotensive as the monomer reaches the vasculature. The highest levels of PMMA monomer have been detected at 5 minutes after insertion of the wound drain. These were below toxic level, however, and did not cause hypotension. After storage of the blood at room temperature for 6 hours—the average collection time—the PMMA monomer was no longer detectable. Therefore, the PMMA monomer has been found not to cause problems for clients.

To date, few complications have been reported in the literature for clients who have received salvaged blood. The majority of reported complications have been febrile reactions, particularly when the recommended collection time was exceeded. Evans, Rubash, and Albrecht (1993) found no increase in febrile reactions when comparing clients who had been reinfused with those who had not. Rare complications include hypotension, airway edema, and transfusion reaction symptoms.

Preoperative Hemodilution. Preoperative hemodilution is a technique used to decrease the amount of blood lost during an operative procedure, although its use in orthopaedic surgery is limited (Sculco, 1995). Preoperative hemodilution is generally carried out by the anesthesia care provider immediately before beginning the operative case but after anesthesia has been induced. Units of blood are withdrawn from the client through a large IV line, replaced with colloid or crystalloid, and reinfused as needed either during or after the procedure. The hematocrit is generally decreased to 24% to 28% using a calculation formula so as not to compromise the oxygen-carrying capacity to the tissues. If preoperative hemodilution is to be used, the client must have an initial hematocrit level of at least 38%. The advantages of this procedure are there is blood readily available as needed during and after the procedure and the intraoperative blood lost is very dilute. The obvious disadvantage is the decrease in the oxygen-carrying capacity of the remaining blood. In addition, coagulation factors and platelets are

diluted (Goodnough, Despotis, Merkel, & Monk, 2000). Clients generally must be in good health to tolerate preoperative hemodilution.

Hypotensive Anesthesia. Controlled hypotensive anesthesia has been used to decrease intraoperative blood loss during total hip arthroplasty and spinal surgery. Hypotensive anesthesia involves administering agents to maintain the client's mean arterial blood pressure approximately 20 mm Hg below the average preoperative blood pressure. Arrhythmia, cerebrovascular accident, myocardial infarction, and renal or hepatic damage are potential complications of controlled hypotensive anesthesia. Maintenance of the systolic blood pressure above 70 mm Hg perfuses vital organs and minimizes complications. Carotid stenosis, coronary artery disease, and renal impairment are contraindications to this anesthetic technique. A decreased urine output is often noted after hypotensive anesthesia.

Hypothermia. Cooling of the client to temperatures of 30°C and lower decreases metabolic and oxygenation demands of tissue. This is commonly achieved in cardiovascular surgery with use of the heart/lung bypass machine. Induced hypothermia is not a common practice in orthopaedic surgery (Cooley, 1995).

Surgical Techniques. The surgical technique plays an important role in determining the amount of surgical blood loss. Surgeons can use several methods to minimize blood loss (Nelson & Fontenot, 1995). Preoperative planning allows the surgeon to determine the technique that will be used before the actual case and allows the surgical team to have the necessary equipment available and prepare for possible complications that may arise. Adequate preoperative planning and skill of the individual surgeon may also decrease the surgical time, which also limits the amount of blood lost.

Surgeons may use several methods to decrease the amount of blood lost intraoperatively. Techniques used directly in the surgical wound include sponge packing, use of electrocautery and suture ligatures, and the application of hemostatic agents to the bleeding tissue. Intraoperative use of a pneumatic tourniquet placed on an extremity for surgical procedures on the arm or leg can create an essentially bloodless field. As described previously, there is conflicting evidence that cemented prostheses may have decreased blood loss as compared with uncemented prostheses in total joint arthroplasty.

Crystalloid and Colloid Volume Replacement. Hypovolemia is the primary concern in acute blood loss, which should be treated with administration of crystalloids or colloids to maintain an adequate blood pressure. Appropriate crystalloid volume replacement for blood loss is a physiologic, isotonic salt solution (with or without dextrose) such as normal saline and lactated Ringer's solution. Electrolytes, such as potassium, are added based on clinical and laboratory assessment. Examples of colloid solutions are 6% hetastarch (Hespan), albumin, and dextran. Colloids remain in the intravascular space longer than crystalloids but may cause dilutional coagulopathy.

Generally, a larger volume of crystalloid than colloid solution is needed for fluid volume expansion (approximately 3 mL of crystalloid is needed for each milliliter of blood lost). Systemic tissue edema is one consequence of large infusions of crystalloid solutions. Colloid infusion has been associated with an increase in the development of pulmonary edema, particularly in trauma clients.

Pharmacologic Therapy: Recombinant Erythropoietin. Erythropoietin is a glycoprotein growth factor that stimulates red blood cell production and is produced by healthy kidneys. Use of recombinant erythropoietin, which is manufactured by recombinant DNA technology and has the same biologic effects of endogenous erythropoietin, has been approved in the United States for several uses, including treatment of anemic clients scheduled for elective surgical procedures (Geier, 1998). In two large studies (105 and 208 sample size) of clients undergoing unilateral total hip replacement, use of erythropoietin decreased the need for intraoperative and postoperative blood transfusions (Biesma, Marx, Kraaijenhagen, Franke, Messinger, & van de Wiel, 1994; Canadian Orthopedic Perioperative Erythropoietin Study Group, 1993).

Use is contraindicated with uncontrolled hypertension and with known hypersensitivity to human albumin and mammalian cell-derived products. Erythropoietin may be associated with an increased risk of thrombotic and vascular events. All clients should receive oral supplemental iron with the initiation of erythropoietin therapy, and supplemental iron should continue until therapy is stopped. A baseline hemoglobin level should be evaluated to ascertain that the client's hemoglobin is between 10 and 13 g/dL. Erythropoietin may be administered subcutaneously or intravenously. Medication storage requires refrigeration.

The cost of erythropoietin is considered quite high. Dosing for preoperative autologous blood donation is about 600 U/kg, administered twice a week. However, use of erythropoietin preoperatively for clients with a satisfactory hemoglobin level who are donating blood could lead to a decreased dependence on allogeneic blood use and more effective use of autologous donation.

Withholding of Nonsteroidal Anti-inflammatory Drugs. The use of preoperative NSAIDs, including aspirin, has been associated with an increase in postoperative blood loss and bleeding complications following total hip arthroplasty. The incidence of postoperative bleeding complications greatly increases with the use of NSAIDs that have a half-life of more than 6 hours. These NSAIDs include diflunisal, naproxen, sulindac, aspirin, and piroxicam.

NSAIDs inhibit cyclooxygenase (COX; an enzyme that catalyzes the formation of prostaglandin from arachidonic acid) and therefore interfere with platelet aggregation. It is preferable to eliminate as much of the drug from the blood as possible. The time of discontinuation of an NSAID preoperatively should be determined by the half-life of the drug. Withholding the drug for five times the length of its half-life allows it to be completely eliminated before surgery. If NSAIDs must be used preoperatively, it is recommended that drugs with a half-life of less than 6 hours be used. The use of COX-2 inhibitors preoperatively is under investigation.

Combined Modalities. It is important to note that many surgeons use a combination of the techniques discussed to decrease the amount of blood lost during surgery and to decrease the amount of allogeneic blood used. It is important that an autologous blood/blood conservation approach be used, when possible, to minimize blood loss and decrease the client's risk of receiving allogeneic blood. The Blood Management Practice Conference has developed an algorithm (Fig. 10–12) that aids in the decision-making process of which donation/blood conservations should be used in clients who will be undergoing elective surgery (Spence, 1995).

Nursing Management

Nursing diagnoses associated with blood loss and fluid or blood replacement include activity intolerance/fatigue, anxiety, fluid volume deficit, altered nutrition (less than body requirements), potential fluid volume excess, and potential for injury from transfusion reaction.

Activity Intolerance/Fatigue

Energy Management. Cell oxygenation decreases as red blood cell levels decrease, possibly causing reduced activity tolerance and fatigue from even simple tasks. In addition to measures to increase red blood cell levels, interventions to decrease fatigue should be instituted. Activities should be paced, and assistance should be provided as needed until the client regains strength. Physical therapists should be notified of decreased blood counts so that they can assess clients more closely for fatigue and modify activity as needed. In some instances, it may be necessary to withhold or reschedule therapy until blood replacement is completed.

Anxiety

Anxiety Reduction. Anxiety may be related to unanticipated blood loss, need for transfusions, and fear of viral transmission. Anticipated blood loss should be discussed before elective surgeries, and the various options should be explained to the client. The client should

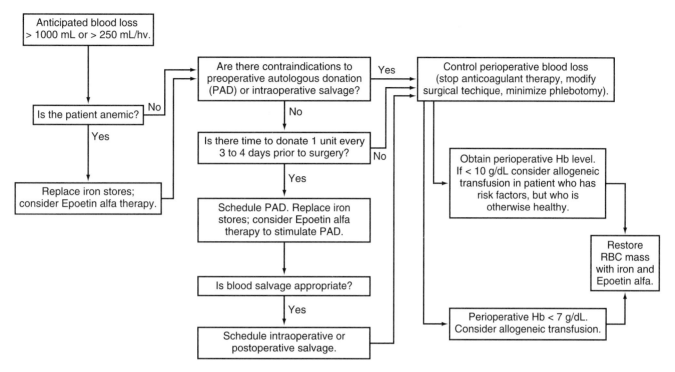

FIGURE 10–12. Blood management algorithm for elective surgery. (From Spence, R. K. [1995]. Surgical red blood cell transfusion practice policies. *American Journal of Surgery, 170,* 5S. Copyright 1995 by Excerpta Medica Inc. Reprinted by permission of publisher.)

be an active participant in making decisions about blood transfusion options. Risks, benefits, and alternatives to transfusion therapy should be discussed with the client. Clients with religious beliefs that forbid the acceptance of blood products should be provided with client advocacy support.

Fluid Volume Deficit

Fluid Management and Blood Products Administration. Fluid volume deficit may be related to blood loss from hypovolemia or hemorrhage. The client's vital signs, clinical status, and laboratory values (hemoglobin, hematocrit, PT—commonly expressed as the INR, PTT, and electrolytes) should be assessed after any procedure or trauma. Blood loss from drains, incisions, and wounds should be monitored closely. Urine, sputum, nasogastric drainage, and stool should be checked for obvious or occult blood if there is concern about possible blood loss from these sites (e.g., with clients using anticoagulants).

Risk factors for increased blood loss should be assessed, and measures should be taken to decrease risks when possible. NSAIDs use should be stopped preoperatively, especially those drugs that have a half-life of more than 6 hours. The effects of anticoagulants may need to be reversed if there is excessive bleeding or if clotting times are prolonged above therapeutic levels. Vitamin K is given to reverse the effects of warfarin, and protamine sulfate is given to reverse the effects of heparin.

The nurse is responsible for assessing the client's need for blood and fluid replacement, for providing safe and appropriate replacement, and for assessing the client's response to therapy. Safe administration of blood products includes ensuring accurate client and blood product identification before administration, monitoring of the blood product infusion and client response, and prompt identification and intervention when adverse reactions occur.

Altered Nutrition

Nutrition Management. An alteration in nutrition (less than body requirements) can occur after blood loss or blood donation. Iron supplements may be required (and are recommended during and after PABD). The client may take ferrous gluconate or ferrous sulfate. Both are available without a prescription. Ferrous gluconate is not as well absorbed as ferrous sulfate, but many clients find it less irritating to the gastrointestinal system. The client should be told that the stool may appear black or tarry while taking iron supplements. Clients also should be advised to increase dietary iron when they are able to tolerate a general diet.

Potential Fluid Volume Excess

Fluid Management. During fluid or blood administration, the client should be monitored closely for fluid volume overload or excess. Signs and symptoms include shortness of breath, edema, rales on lung auscultation, and increased blood pressure. If there are concerns about fluid overload, additional measures during transfusion therapy should be taken. The rate of transfusions should be closely monitored and adjusted based on client reaction. Drainage collected by postoperative salvaging techniques may be washed and centrifuged to decrease the volume that is reinfused.

High Risk for Injury from Transfusion Reaction

The client's vital signs and clinical status should be monitored closely during any type of administration of blood or blood products. Symptoms of a transfusion reaction include chills, a burning sensation at the IV site, chest or back pain, and dyspnea. Fever, hypotension, flushing, hemoglobinuria, oliguria, shock, and bleeding are objective signs of a reaction.

If a reaction is suspected, the blood transfusion should be stopped immediately and the physician should be notified of pertinent signs and symptoms. Antipyretics may be ordered. The client's cardiovascular and renal status should be monitored closely.

Interventions to minimize reactions include scrupulous checking of client and blood identity when administering allogeneic or autologous blood, changing the 20- to 40-μm filter with each unit transfused, and labeling collected blood if cells are to be washed (per institution policy). With administration of large amounts of blood containing citrate dextrose solution (an anticoagulant agent) or fresh frozen plasma, calcium chloride may be needed to prevent citrate toxicity and cardiac failure.

Innovations and Future Trends

Blood Substitutes. Because of the unique properties of blood, the development of a substitute has been difficult (Robb, 1999). Research continues to search for a substitute for red blood cell replacement. The advantages of such a substitute include no risk of transmissible disease, no need to crossmatch, a long shelf life, and a larger supply than with allogeneic blood transfusions. Synthetic oxygen-carrying compounds and solutions of hemoglobin are the main avenues of current research. Toxicity and a short intravascular half-life have been the biggest limitations in their development.

Use of perfluorochemical has been one approach. Perfluorochemicals contain fluorine, which is highly soluble to oxygen and carbon dioxide. Passive transport of oxygen from the lungs to the tissue occurs. Storage, undesirable side effects, and limited efficacy have prevented its widespread use.

Hemoglobin-based oxygen carrier solutions offer a more promising future (Robb, 1999). Researchers modify the hemoglobin molecule obtained from human and animal resources. Clinical trials are under way. Long-term effects of blood substitute products include hyperten-

sion, renal dysfunction, tachycardia, and gastrointestinal distress. The cost of these substitutes is significant to cover the extensive expenses of research and development.

Cryopreservation of red blood cells is an expensive but viable option (Sacher & Sandler, 1999). Storage is successful at −80°C for years. Use may include storage of rare and specific red blood cell phenotypes and universal type O for emergency use.

Summary

Blood is a limited resource that saves lives. Blood loss can be anticipated or unanticipated during orthopaedic surgery and trauma. With increasing concern about the transmission of infectious agents through allogeneic blood transfusion, a great deal of research is being conducted on alternatives for oxygen transport and red blood cell replacement; this research has lead to a decline in the transfusion trigger for blood transfusion. At the same time, the rapid aging of Americans may effect the amount of allogeneic blood supply available, yet place a simultaneous increase demand for it. The treatment of client hemorrhage will continue to evolve.

INTERNET RESOURCES

Blood Transfusions: Knowing Your Options; Pall Corporation: www.bloodtransfusion.com
National Guideline Clearinghouse (search for deep venous thrombosis): www.guideline.gov

REFERENCES

Compartment Syndrome

Blakemore, L. C., Cooperman, D. R., Thompson, G. H., Wathey, C., & Ballock, R. J. (2000). Compartment syndrome in ipsilateral humerus and forearm fractures in children. *Clinical Orthopaedics and Related Research, 376,* 32–38.

Dunwoody, J. M., Reichert, C. C., & Brown, K. L. B. (1997). Compartment syndrome associated with bupivacaine and fentanyl epidural analgesia. *Journal of Pediatric Orthopaedics, 17,* 285–288.

Fitzpatrick, D. T., Murphy, P. T., & Bryce, M. (1998). Adjunctive treatment of compartment syndrome with hyperbaric oxygen. *Military Medicine, 163,* 577–579.

Gellman, H., & Buch, K. (1998). Acute compartment syndrome of the arm. *Hand Clinics, 14,* 385–389.

Giannotti, G., Cohn, S. M., Brown, M., Varela, J. E., McKenney, M. G., & Wiseberg, J. A. (2000). Utility of near-infrared spectroscopy in the diagnosis of lower extremity compartment syndrome. *The Journal of Trauma, 48,* 396–401.

Hargens, A. R., & Mubarak, S. J. (1998). Current concepts in the pathophysiology, evaluation, and diagnosis of compartment syndrome. *Hand Clinics, 14,* 371–383.

Heppenstall, B., & Tan, V. (1999). Well-leg compartment syndrome. *Lancet, 354,* 970.

Hyder, N., Kessler, S., Jennings, A. G., & De Boer, P. G. (1996). Compartment syndrome in tibial shaft fracture missed because of a local nerve block. *Journal of Bone and Joint Surgery, 78B*(3), 499–500.

McLaughlin, J. A., Paulson, M. M., & Rosenthall, R. E. (1998). Delayed onset of anterior tibial compartment syndrome in a patient receiving low-molecular-weight heparin: A case report. *Journal of Bone and Joint Surgery, 80A,* 1789–1790.

McQueen, M. M., Gaston, P., & Court-Brown, C. M. (2000). Acute compartment syndrome: Who is at risk? *Journal of Bone and Joint Surgery, 82B,* 200–203.

Mubarak, S. J., & Wilton, N. C. T. (1997). Compartment syndromes and epidural analgesia. *Journal of Pediatric Orthopaedics, 17,* 282–284.

Ortiz, J. A., & Berger, R. A. (1998). Compartment syndrome of the hand and wrist. *Hand Clinics, 14,* 405–418.

Ouellette, E. A. (1998). Compartment syndrome in obtunded patients. *Hand Clinics, 14,* 431–450.

Pedowitz, R. A., Hargens, A. R., Mubarak, S. J., & Gershuni, D. H. (1990). Modified criteria for the objective diagnosis of chronic compartment syndrome of the leg. *American Journal of Sports Medicine, 18,* 35–40.

Politis, G. D. (1998). Postoperative epidural analgesia and neurologic complications. *American Journal of Orthopedics, 27,* 757–758.

Ross, D. G. (1996). Chronic compartment syndrome. *Orthopaedic Nursing, 15,* 23–27.

Ross, D., & Evans, R. (1994). A patient with acute compartment syndrome. *Clinical simulations in medical-surgical nursing III, Medi-Sim computer assisted instruction.* Baltimore: Williams & Wilkins.

Schmitz, M. L., Brown, R. E., Stoner, J. M., & Vollers, J. M. (1997). Compartment syndromes associated with postoperative epidural analgesia, Commentary. *Journal of Bone and Joint Surgery, 79A,* 1271–1272.

Tang, W. M., & Chiu, K. Y. (2000). Silent compartment syndrome complicating total knee arthroplasty: Continuous epidural anesthesia masked the pain. *Journal of Arthroplasty, 15*(2), 241–243.

Uslu, M. M., & Apan, A. (2000). Can skin surface pressure under a cast reveal intracompartmental pressure? *Archives of Orthopaedic & Trauma Surgery, 120,* 319–322.

Willy, C., Gerngross, H., & Sterk, J. (1999). Measurement of intracompartmental pressure with use of a new electronic transducer-tipped catheter system. *Journal of Bone and Joint Surgery, 81A,* 158–168.

Yamaguchi, S., & Viegas, S. F. (1998). Causes of upper extremity compartment syndrome. *Hand Clinics, 14,* 365–370.

Deep Venous Thrombosis

American College of Chest Physicians. (1998). Fifth ACCP consensus conference on antithrombotic therapy. *Chest, 114,* 611S–633S.

Clagett, G. P., Anderson, F. A., Heit, J., Levine, M. N., & Wheeler, H. B. (1995). Prevention of venous thromboembolism. *Chest, 108*(Suppl), 312S–334S.

Cola, C., & Ansell, J. (1990). Heparin-induced thrombocytopenia and arterial thrombosis: Alternative therapies. *American Heart Journal, 119,* 368–370.

Eastern Association for the Surgery of Trauma. (1998). Practice management guidelines for the management of venous thromboembolism in trauma patients. *Journal of Trauma, 44,* 941–956.

Paiement, G. D., & Mendelsohn C. (1997). The risk of venous thromboembolism in the orthopedic patient, epidemiological and psychological data. *Orthopedics, 20*(Suppl), 7–9.

Polak, J. F. (1992). *Peripheral vascular sonography.* Baltimore: Williams & Wilkins.

Velmahos, G. C., Kern, J., Chan, L. S., Oder, D., Murray, J. A., & Shekelle, P. (2000a). Prevention of venous thromboembolism after injury: An evidence-based report. Part I: Analysis of risk factors and evaluation of the role of vena caval filters. *Journal of Trauma-Injury, Infection & Critical Care, 49,* 132–139.

Velmahos, G. C., Kern, J., Chan, L. S., Oder, D., Murray, J. A., & Shekelle, P. (2000b). Prevention of venous thromboembolism after injury: An evidence-based report. Part II: Analysis of risk factors and evaluation of the role of vena caval filters. *Journal of Trauma-Injury, Infection & Critical Care, 49,* 140–144.

Wittert, D., & Barden, R. (1985). Deep vein thrombosis, pulmonary embolism, and prophylaxis in the orthopaedic patient. *Orthopaedic Nursing, 4*(4), 27–32.

Wood, K. B., Kos, P. B., Abnet, J. K., & Ista, C. (1997). Prevention of deep-vein thrombosis after major spinal surgery: A comparison study of external devices. *Journal of Spinal Disorders, 10,* 209–214.

Zwiebel, W. J. (2000). *Introduction to vascular ultrasonography* (4th ed.). Philadelphia: WB Saunders.

Pulmonary Embolism

Brasel, K. J., Borgstrom, D. C., & Weigelt, J. A. (1997). Cost-effective prevention of pulmonary embolus in high-risk trauma patients. *Journal of Trauma-Injury Infection and Critical Care, 42,* 456–460.

Knudson, M. M., Morabito, D., Paiement, G. D., & Shackelford, S. (1996). Use of low molecular weight heparin in preventing thromboembolism in trauma patients. *Journal of Trauma-Injury, Infection & Critical Care, 41,* 446–459.

Langan, E. M., Miller, R. S., Casey, W. J., Carsten, C. G., III, Graham, R. M., & Taylor, S. M. (1999). Prophylactic inferior vena cava filters in trauma patients at high risk: Follow-up examination and risk/benefit assessment. *Journal of Vascular Surgery, 30,* 484–488.

Manganelli, D., Palla, A., Donnamaria, V., & Giuntini, C. (1995). Clinical features of pulmonary embolism. *Chest, 107* (Suppl 1), 25S–31S.

McMurtry, A. L., Owings, J. T., Anderson, J. T., Battistella, F. D., & Gosselin, R. (1999). Increased use of prophylactic vena cava filters in trauma patients failed to decrease overall incidence of pulmonary embolism. *Journal of the American College of Surgeons, 189,* 314–320.

Raschke, R., Reilly, B., Guidry, J., Fontana, J. R., & Srinivas, S. (1993). The weight-based heparin dosing nomogram compared with a "standard care" nomogram. A randomized controlled trial. *Annals of Internal Medicine, 119,* 874–881.

Rogers, F. B., Shackford, S. R., Ricci, M. A., Huber, B. M., & Atkins, T. (1997). Prophylactic vena cava filter insertion in selected high-risk orthopaedic trauma patients. *Journal of Orthopaedic Trauma, 11,* 267–272.

Rogers, F. B., Strindberg, G., Shackford, S. R., Osler, T. M., Morris, C. S., Ricci, M. A., Najarian, K. E., D'Agostino, R., & Pilcher, D. B. (1998). Five-year follow-up of prophylactic vena cava filters in high-risk trauma patients. *Archives of Surgery, 133,* 406–412.

Rosenow, E. (1995). Venous and pulmonary thromboembolism: An algorithmic approach to diagnosis and management. *Mayo Clinic Proceedings, 70,* 45–49.

Schulman, S., Rhedin, A. S., Lindmarker, P., Carlson, A., Larfars, G., Nicol, P., Loogan, E., Svensson, E., Ljungberg, B., & Walter, H. (1995). A comparison of six weeks with six months of oral anticoagulant therapy after a first episode of venous thromboembolism. Duration of anticoagulation trial study group. *New England Journal of Medicine, 332,* 1661–1665.

Simonneau, G., Sors, H., Charbonnier, B., Page, Y., Laaban, J. P., Azarian, R., Laurent, M., Hirsch, J. L., Ferrari, E., Bosson, J. L., Mottier, D., & Beau, B. (1997). A comparison of low-molecular-weight heparin with unfractionated heparin for acute pulmonary embolism. *New England Journal of Medicine, 337,* 663–669.

Spain, D. A., Richardson, J. D., Polk, J. C., Bergamini, T. M., Wilson, M. A., & Miller, F. B. (1997). Venous thromboembolism in the high-risk trauma patient: do the risks justify aggressive screening and prophylaxis? *Journal of Trauma-Injury, Infection & Critical Care, 42,* 463–467.

Tai, N. F. M., Atwal, A. S., & Hamilton, G. (1999). Modern management of pulmonary embolism. *British Journal of Surgery, 86,* 853–868.

Velmahos, G. C., Kern, J., Chan, L. S., Oder, D., Murray, J. A., & Shekelle, P. (2000a). Prevention of venous thromboembolism after injury: An evidence-based report. Part I: Analysis of risk factors and evaluation of the role of vena caval filters. *Journal of Trauma-Injury, Infection & Critical Care, 49,* 132–139.

Velmahos, G. C., Kern, J., Chan, L. S., Oder, D., Murray, J. A., & Shekelle, P. (2000b). Prevention of venous thromboembolism after injury: An evidence-based report. Part II: Analysis of risk factors and evaluation of the role of vena caval filters. *Journal of Trauma-Injury, Infection & Critical Care, 49,* 140–144.

Fat Embolism Syndrome

Bulger, E. M., Smith, D. G., Maier, R. V., & Jurkovich, G. J. (1997). Fat embolism syndrome: A 10-year review. *Archives of Surgery, 132,* 435–439.

Johnson, M. J., & Lucas, G. L. (1996). Fat embolism syndrome. *Orthopedics, 19,* 41–49.

Mimoz, O., Edouard, A., Beydon, L., Quillard, J., Verra, F., Fleury, J., Bonnet, F., & Samii, K. (1995). Contribution of bronchoalveolar lavage to the diagnosis of posttraumatic pulmonary fat embolism. *Intensive Care Medicine, 21,* 973–980.

Mudd, K. L., Hunt, A., Matherly, R. C., Goldsmith, L. J., Campbell, F. R., Nichols, G. R., II, & Rink, R. D. (2000). Analysis of pulmonary fat embolism in blunt force fatalities. *Journal of Trauma, 48,* 711–715.

Muller, C., Rahn, B. A., Pfister, U., & Meinig, R. P. (1994). The incidence, pathogenesis, diagnosis, and treatment of fat embolism. *Orthopaedic Review, 23,* 107–117.

Pitto, R. P., Blunk, J., & Kossler, M. (2000). Transesophageal echocardiography and clinical features of fat embolism during cemented total hip arthroplasty. A randomized study in patients with a femoral neck fracture. *Archives of Orthopaedic & Trauma Surgery, 120,* 53–58.

Pitto, R. P., Koessler, M., & Kuehle, J. W. (1999). Comparison of fixation of the femoral component without cement and fixation with use of a bone-vacuum cementing technique for the prevention of fat embolism during total hip arthroplasty. A prospective, randomized clinical trial. *Journal of Bone & Joint Surgery, 81,* 831–843.

Stanley, J. D., Hanson, R. R., Hicklin, G. A., Glazier, A. J., Jr., Ervanian, A., & Jadali, M. (1994). Specificity of bronchoalveolar lavage for the diagnosis of fat embolism syndrome. *American Surgeon, 60,* 537–541.

Takahashi, M., Suzuki, R., Osakabe, Y., Asai, J. I., Miyo, T., Nagashima, G., Fujimoto, T., & Takahashi, Y. (1999). Magnetic resonance imaging findings in cerebral fat embolism: correlation with clinical manifestations. *Journal of Trauma, 46,* 324–327.

Blood Loss

American Society of Anesthesiologists Task Force on Blood Component Therapy. (1996). Practice guidelines for blood component therapy. *Anesthesiology 84,* 732–747.

An, H. S., Mikhail, W. E., Jackson, W. T., Tolin, B., & Dodd, G. A. (1991). Effects of hypotensive anesthesia, nonsteroidal antiinflammatory drugs, and polymethyl methacrylate on bleeding in total hip arthroplasty patients. *Journal of Arthroplasty, 6,* 245–250.

Anders, M. J., Lifeso, R. M., Landis, M., Mikulsky, J., Meinking, C., & McCracken, K. S. (1996). Effect of preoperative donation of autologous blood on deep-vein thrombosis following total joint arthroplasty of the hip or knee. *Journal of Bone and Joint Surgery, 78A,* 574–580.

Aubuchon, J. (1997). Transfusion options. *Archives of Pathology & Laboratory Medicine, 121,* 40–47.

Belanger, A. C. (1999). Joint Commission on Accreditation of Healthcare Organizations' expectations for transfusion medicine in health care organizations. *Archives of Pathology & Laboratory Medicine, 123,* 472–474.

Bierbaum, B. E., Callaghan, J. J., Galante, J. O., Rubash, H. E., Tooms, R. E., & Welch, R. B. (1999). An analysis of blood management in patients having total hip or knee arthroplasty. *Journal of Bone and Joint Surgery, 81A,* 2–10.

Biesma, D. H., Marx, J. J., Kraaijenhagen, R. J., Franke, W., Messinger, D., & van de Wiel, A. (1994). Lower homologous blood requirement in autologous blood donors after treatment with recombinant human erythropoietin. *Lancet, 344,* 267–270.

Billote, D. B., Glisson, S. N., Green, D., & Wixson, R. L. (2000). Efficacy of preoperative autologous blood donation: Analysis of blood loss and transfusion practice in total hip replacement. *Journal of Clinical Anesthesia, 12,* 537–542.

Canadian Orthopaedic Perioperative Erythropoietin Study Group. (1993). Effectiveness of perioperative recombinant human erythropoietin in elective hip replacement. *Lancet, 341,* 1227–1232.

Cooley, D. A. (1995). Conservation of blood during cardiovascular surgery. *American Journal of Surgery, 170*(6A Suppl), 53S–59S.

Evans, R. L., Rubash, H. E., & Albrecht, S. A. (1993). The efficacy of postoperative autotransfusion in total joint arthroplasty. *Orthopaedic Nursing, 12,* 11–18.

Fiebig, E. (1998). Safety of the blood supply. *Clinical Orthopedics and Related Research, 357,* 6–18.

Geier, K. (1998). Perioperative blood management. *Orthopaedic Nursing, 17*(Suppl), 6–36.

Goodnough, L. T., Brecher, M. E., Kanter, M. T., & Aubuchon, J. P. (1991). Estimated risks associated with blood and blood transfusions. *New England Journal of Medicine, 340,* 438–447.

Goodnough, L. T., Despotis, G. J., Merkel, K., & Monk, T. G. (2000). A randomized trial comparing acute normovolemic hemodilution and preoperative autologous blood donation in total hip arthroplasty. *Transfusion, 40,* 1054–1057.

Grosvenor, D., Goyal, V., & Goodman, S. (2000). Efficacy of postoperative blood salvage following total hip arthroplasty in patients with and without deposited autologous units. *Journal of Bone and Joint Surgery, 82A,* 951–954.

Larocque, B. J., Gilbert, K., & Brien, W. F. (1997). A point score system for predicting the likelihood of blood transfusion after hip or knee arthroplasty. *Transfusion, 37,* 463–467.

National Blood Data Resource Center. (1999). *Comprehensive report on blood collection and transfusion in the United States.* Bethesda, MD: Author.

National Heart, Lung, and Blood Institute Panel on the Use of Autologous Blood. (1995). Transfusion alert: Use of autologous blood. *Transfusion, 35,* 703–711.

Nelson, C. L., & Fontenot, H. J. (1995). Ten strategies to reduce blood loss in orthopedic surgery. *American Journal of Surgery, 170,* 64S–68S.

Ness, P. M. (1999). Integrating the new generation of blood components into transfusion practice. *Transfusion, 39,* 1027–1030.

Nuttall, G. A., Santrach, P. J., Oliver, W. C., Jr., Horlocker, T. T., Shaughnessy, W. J., Cabanela, M. E., & Bryant, S. (1996). The predictors of red cell transfusion in total hip arthroplasty. *Transfusion, 36,* 144–149.

Robb, W. J. (1999). Massive transfusion in trauma. *AACN Clinical Issues, 10*(1), 69–84.

Sacher, R. A., & Sandler, S. G. (1999). Impact of innovations on transfusion medicine. *Archives of Pathology & Laboratory Medicine, 123,* 672–676.

Sculco, T. P. (1995). Blood management in orthopedic surgery. *American Journal of Surgery, 170,* 60S–63S.

Sonnenberg, F. A., Gregory, P., Yomtovian, R., Russell, L. B., Tierney, W., Kosmin, M., & Carson, J. L. (1999). The cost-effectiveness of autotransfusion revisited: implications of an increased risk of bacterial infection with allogeneic transfusion. *Transfusion, 39,* 808–817.

Spence, R. K. (1995). Surgical red blood cell transfusion practice policies. *American Journal of Surgery, 170,* 3S–12S.

Swain, D. G., Nightingale, P. G., & Patel, J. V. (2000). Blood transfusion requirements in femoral neck fracture. *Injury, 31,* 7–10.

Testa, L. D., & Tobias, J. D. (1996). Techniques of blood conservation. *American Journal of Anesthesiology, 23,* 63–72.

Warner, D. O., Warner, M. A., Schroeder, D. R., Offord, K. P., Maxson, P., & Santrach, P. (1998). Changing transfusion practices in hip and knee arthroscopy, *Transfusion, 38,* 738–744.

11

Perioperative Considerations for the Orthopaedic Client

TINA KURKOWSKI

Orthopaedic surgery places the client in a uniquely vulnerable situation, and the perioperative nurse plays a vital role as client advocate within the continuum of care. Perioperative nursing practice is defined as activities performed by the professional registered nurse in the preoperative, intraoperative, and postoperative phases of the client's surgical experience. Perioperative nurses must be responsible and accountable in ensuring high-quality nursing care for clients who undergo surgery and other invasive procedures. Perioperative nurses are registered nurses (RN) who work in hospital surgical departments, day-surgery units (also called *ambulatory surgery*), clinics, and physician's offices. Perioperative nurses may work closely with the surgical client, family members, and other health care professionals. They help plan, implement, and evaluate treatment of the client. In the operating room (OR), the orthopaedic perioperative nurse may serve as any of the following:

Scrub nurse—selecting and handling instruments and supplies used for the operation

Circulating nurse—managing the overall nursing care in the OR and helping to maintain a safe, comfortable environment

RN first assistant (RNFA)—delivering direct surgical care by assisting the surgeon in controlling bleeding, providing wound exposure, and suturing during the actual procedure

Certified registered nurse anesthetist—delivering care to clients before, during, and after surgical procedures; staying with clients for the entire procedure, constantly monitoring every important body function, and individually modifying the anesthetic to ensure maximum safety and comfort

Standards of care and practice have been established by the Association of periOperative Registered Nurses

(AORN), the American Society of PeriAnesthesia Nurses (ASPAN), and the National Association of Orthopaedic Nurses (NAON).

PREOPERATIVE COORDINATION AND SURGICAL PREPARATION

Coordination and preparation of the client for the procedure refers to activities done by the RN/RNFA before the operative or invasive procedure to make the client physically, psychologically, and emotionally ready for the procedure. The preoperative period is divided into two phases: Phase 1 lasts from when the decision to have surgery is made until the client's arrival in the holding area or same-day surgery unit; Phase 2 lasts from the client's arrival before surgery through admission to the OR. Responsibilities in these phases may include one or more of the following: admitting the client, collecting laboratory specimens, obtaining the consent to treatment, and providing any ordered preprocedure treatment or care. Nurses providing these services may also provide client care during and after the procedure.

Phase 1: Assessment and Preparation

This component of the preoperative phase revolves around assessing, planning, implementing, and evaluating the client's decision to undergo surgery. This process may be completed on a hospital inpatient; however, it is more commonly performed on an outpatient basis for elective surgical procedures.

History. It is imperative to obtain a complete and accurate health history because systemic disease can affect many aspects of client care. For example, liver or kidney impairment may adversely affect medication clearance. Many anesthetics depress the myocardium and affect the vasculature. Therefore, knowledge of existing cardiovascular disease and hydration status is important. Neuromuscular disease can exaggerate responses to the neuromuscular blocking agents used to achieve muscle relaxation during surgery and, depending on the type and severity of disease, may also affect respiratory function. Pulmonary disease may affect gas exchange and lead to postoperative complications. Any anesthetic history involving difficulty with airway management requires further investigation.

Allergy Management and Latex Precautions. Knowledge of client allergies is vital. For example, iodine is an agent found in many radiographic dyes and antimicrobial skin preparation, and clients allergic to iodine may mention an allergy to shellfish. Nurses must also recognize those clients who require latex precautions and then implement appropriate nursing interventions to protect them from harm. Appropriate questions need to be asked, with terminology adapted to language the client can understand. Clients with certain food allergies, including banana, avocado, chestnut, apricot, kiwi, papaya, passion fruit, pineapple, peach, nectarine, plum, cherry, melon, fig, grape, potato, tomato, and celery, may also have a coexisting latex allergy (Kurup, Kelly, Elms, Kelly, & Fink, 1994).

Lists of nonlatex substitutes for medical supplies and devices should also be accessible. A list has been developed by Allergy to Latex Education and Resource Team (A.L.E.R.T., Inc., Milwaukee, Wisconsin, website: www.latexallergyresources.org). Because manufacturers are continuously developing nonlatex alternatives, a regular review and updating of these lists is recommended.

Medications Management. A thorough medication history is important for a total assessment. Long-term use of medications may be a factor in interaction with anesthetic agents. Noncompliance with long-term drug therapy may indicate that a chronic condition is not well controlled. Determining whether the client has taken any over-the-counter medications, such as aspirin, nonsteroidal anti-inflammatory drugs (NSAIDs), or any street drugs, is important information for the anesthesiologist. Table 11–1 highlights some common medications and their implications for anesthesia.

Medications required for the control of chronic illness may be continued until surgery. If the client is admitted the morning of surgery, the nurse must be certain to inquire about which morning doses of medications were taken. The anesthesiologist should be consulted about the unique needs of each client.

The American Society of Anesthesiologists (ASA) recommends that people stop taking herbal remedies several weeks before surgery because of potential untoward events (Reuters Health, 1999). Perioperative nurses should screen all clients for herbal medicine use. Often,

clients reveal herbal use to a nurse when they have failed to do so with their surgeon or anesthesia care provider. After ascertaining the daily dose, strength, frequency, and duration of use, a nursing diagnosis can be made and nursing interventions can be planned. For example, if a total knee arthroplasty client has been taking Gingko biloba, the client is at risk for fluid volume deficit and it would be appropriate to institute bleeding precautions (Brumley, 2000).

Family History. A family history of adverse reactions to anesthesia can signal an inherited tendency toward the same disorder. Two notable anesthetic disorders that are genetically inherited include malignant hyperthermia (MH) and atypical pseudocholinesterase levels; they are discussed later.

Social History. An evaluation of the client's home situation is especially important for discharge planning. Many orthopaedic clients have postoperative mobility restrictions that affect their functioning. Therefore, it is crucial to discover with whom the client lives, if significant others are dependent on the client for care, or if significant others are available to support the client and what environmental barriers exist in the home.

Physical Examination. The physical examination follows completion of the history. Careful evaluation and examination of major systems gives the RNFA or perioperative nurse a good idea of the client's physical status. The RNFA or perioperative nurse uses the assessment data to diagnose actual or potential health problems that may affect the client during the operative procedure period. Abnormal vital signs (pulse, temperature, blood pressure [BP], and respirations) must be communicated to the physician and anesthesia provider because they may be indicators of possible postprocedure complications. Postponement of the procedure may be necessary to treat the underlying problem associated with abnormal vital signs. Height and weight are critical for computing medication dosages, especially in pediatric clients. The skin inspection should be performed in a well-lit room. A skin infection may be cause to cancel an orthopaedic surgical procedure. For example, a client scheduled for a total joint replacement may have surgery postponed if a cellulitis was discovered. A thorough assessment of the client's peripheral pulses provides a baseline for comparison postoperatively. Gastrointestinal assessment data may provide clues for identifying constipation, diarrhea, and bowel incontinence. Urinary assessment data provide clues for identifying clients at risk for fluid volume deficit and fluid volume excess intraoperatively.

The anesthesia provider examines the client with a major emphasis on airway assessment. Issues of major concern include (1) the condition of the teeth (dentures and plates need to be removed for intubation, and loose

TABLE 11–1. *Medication History and Implications for Anesthesia*

DRUG CATEGORY	RELEVANCE TO ANESTHESIA

Cardiovascular medications
  Antiarrhythmics
  Antihypertensives
  Calcium channel blockers
  Beta blockers
  Nitrates
  Cardiac glycosides
	Crucial to cardiovascular function. In addition, many cardiovascular medications interact with anesthetic agents, augmenting response to myocardial depressant effects and other side effects.

Diuretics	Can alter fluid and electrolyte balance and may cause significant hypokalemia.

Bronchodilators
  Theophylline preparations
  Aerosol sympathomimetics
  Steroid preparations
	Crucial for optimizing pulmonary function and preventing bronchospasm.

Oral hypoglycemics and insulin	Important because of their effect on blood sugar. The anesthesia provider should determine how to avoid both hyperglycemia and hypoglycemia.
Over-the-counter medications Aspirin and nonsteroidal anti-inflammatory drugs (NSAIDs)	Many potential interactions with anesthetic agents, depending on category. Aspirin and NSAIDs can affect platelet function and increase the tendency for bleeding.

Anticoagulants
  Warfarin (Coumadin)
  Heparin
	Affect coagulation and can cause severe bleeding. Reversal agent for warfarin is vitamin K. Reversal agent for heparin is protamine sulfate.

Steroids	Exogenous administration suppresses adrenal function and may indicate the need for perioperative stress dose coverage.
Anticonvulsants	Important because of their role in seizure control.

Gastrointestinal medications
  Cimetidine
  Zantac
  Pepcid
  Prilosec
	Decrease hepatic blood flow and can prolong the metabolism of certain drugs (i.e., lidocaine, theophylline, opioids, benzodiazepines, and succinylcholine).

Monoamine oxidase inhibitors (MAOIs)
  Isocarboxazid (Marplan)
  Phenelzine sulfate (Nardil)
  Tranylcypromine sulfate (Parnate)
	Given for the treatment of depression. Meperidine (Demerol) is absolutely contraindicated in clients receiving such drugs because of catastrophic reactions ranging from severe hypertension, hyperpyrexia, and seizures to coma, severe respiratory depression, and cardiovascular collapse. This warning may apply to other opioids as well. Alert anesthesia provider that client is taking this type of medication. MAOIs are usually discontinued 10 days before elective surgery.

Lithium and tricyclic antidepressants	May interact with anesthetic agents.
Chronic use of sedatives, hypnotics, or narcotics, including illicit drugs, alcohol, and tobacco	May influence response to anesthetic agents. Can affect liver function and gas exchange.

or capped teeth must be noted because of the potential for injury and subsequent aspiration), (2) the degree to which the client can open his or her mouth, and (3) the degree to which the client can hyperextend the neck (Miller, 2000a). On completion of the physical examination, the anesthesia care provider assigns a classification status to the client that reflects the degree of illness and risk for anesthesia.

Laboratory Studies. Preoperative laboratory tests serve to confirm surgical risk factors identified during the history taking and physical examination. Laboratory testing can, when used selectively, identify additional problems as well as establish a baseline to allow assess-

ment of abnormalities discovered in the postoperative period. It is generally recognized that using preoperative tests in a low-risk population is expensive and may, in selected cases, be counterproductive (Miller, 2000a). Generally, the history and physical examination should be used to direct the ordering of tests.

Aspiration Precautions. A more tolerant approach to preoperative fasting guidelines for healthy adults undergoing elective surgery was recently recommended by a task force appointed by the ASA. The recommendations of this task force were accepted by the ASA in October 1998. The recommendation liberalizes the intake of clear liquids and specifically allows a light breakfast (e.g., toast and tea or coffee) up to 6 hours before elective surgery in the healthy client (Pandit, Loberg, & Pandit, 2000). The task force noted that intake of fried or fatty foods or meat may prolong gastric emptying time. Both the amount and type of foods ingested must be considered when determining an appropriate fasting period. Because nonhuman milk is similar to solids in gastric emptying time, the amount ingested must be considered when determining an appropriate fasting period. The guidelines suggest that it is appropriate to fast from intake of clear liquids for 2 hours or more before procedures requiring general anesthesia, regional anesthesia, or sedation/analgesia. Examples of clear liquids include water, fruit juices without pulp, carbonated beverages, clear tea, and black coffee. These liquids should not include alcohol. The volume of liquid ingested is less important than the type of liquid ingested. For children, it is appropriate to fast from intake of breast milk for 4 hours or more and infant formula for 6 hours or more before undergoing procedures that require general anesthesia, regional anesthesia, or sedation/analgesia. Older clients' gastric emptying is delayed because of decreased peristalsis and gastric motility. As a result of delayed gastric emptying, clients have increased risks for aspiration (Hazen, Larsen, & Hoot Martin, 1997). Other factors that delay gastric emptying and place the client at higher risk for aspiration include obesity, diabetes mellitus, peptic ulcer disease, stress or pain, trauma, and pregnancy (ASA, 1999).

Informed Consent. Informed consent is a legal requirement for the surgeon and anesthesia provider to disclose information to the client that enables that client to understand the procedure, its risks, and its potential outcomes before consenting to it (Pape, 1997). Implicit in such discussion is that information is presented in consideration of the client's ability to understand it; thus, consideration must be given to the client's age, education, and competence (Brazell, 1997). If the perioperative nurse/RNFA becomes aware that the client has changed his or her mind, has had a change in health status since the consent was signed, or misunderstands the procedure, or if the client's mental capacity is in doubt, the nurse/ RNFA, according to nursing standards of care, must advise a superior or the physician (Pryor, 1997). No preoperative medications should be given before obtaining proper consent.

Teaching: Preoperative, Anxiety Reduction. The trend toward ambulatory surgery decreases the time nurses spend with preoperative clients and challenges the perioperative nurse to provide effective comprehensive support in a limited amount of time. Given the time constraints in the ambulatory surgical setting, assessing and teaching the client on the day of surgery is not feasible or appropriate. Reaching out to the client a few

days before surgery either in the client's home, in the ambulatory surgery center, or by telephone is the current practice. Table 11-2 identifies specific client education. Perioperative nurses must provide adequate time for older clients to make decisions and allow sufficient time for client education. Using both verbal and written instructions and including clients' family members in preoperative teaching and discharge planning are imperative if older clients have difficulty with decision making and have evidence of memory decline.

Many orthopaedic surgical clients need assistant devices for postoperative ambulating. Instruction and return demonstration of crutch walking and walker use should definitely be completed before surgery. It is extremely difficult to learn these skills when dizziness, pain, maneuvering with bulky casts and dressings, and non–weight-bearing status predominate over the ability to use crutches or a walker.

Psychological preparation and client education are important aspects of the client's surgical experience. Client and family/significant other education can occur through discussion, printed materials, video, or computer program; it may be planned or spontaneous; or it may be formal or informal. The perioperative RN/RNFA should not rely on these materials as a substitute for nurse-facilitated client education (Rothrock, 2000). It is critical to actively listen to a client and redesign material to incorporate any concerns or fears. In a practice setting providing optimal continuity of care, the RNFA would begin identifying what the client must know and wants to know at the time the decision for surgical intervention is made. As the RNFA follows the client across the care continuum, education and interventions to decrease fear can be implemented. This continued assessment and education may prevent overwhelming of the client and family/significant others with information.

Sending the Client to the Operating Room. The client should be identified before transport to the operative suite. This is done to ensure that the correct client is transported to the operative suite at the appropriate time with all the necessary paperwork completed and in the chart. When identifying a child, the nurse should ask the parents or legal guardian what the child's name is and what procedure is being done. If the child is old enough to respond, he or she should also be asked these questions. During phase 1 care, all clients should remove dentures, prostheses, contact lenses, glasses, hearing aides, and jewelry. Some health care facilities allow the client to wear prostheses to the operative and invasive procedure suite. In such cases, the perioperative RN must secure the prostheses during the procedure. Nail polish and artificial nails may need to be removed. In some instances, clients should be asked to void on call, and any preoperative medication is administered as prescribed.

TABLE 11–2. *Preoperative Client Teaching*

FOCUS	TEACHING POINTS
Preoperative fast	Nothing by mouth (NPO) after midnight, including candy or gum because they stimulate gastric acid secretion.
	Late-day surgery: Clear liquid breakfast *may* be allowed 6–8 hr preoperatively. Pediatric clients may have clear liquids up to 2–3 hr before surgery.
Avoidance of smoking	Smoking interferes with pulmonary function.
	Avoid smoking as long as possible before surgery, at least as long as NPO status is in effect.
Preoperative preparations	Perform antimicrobial skin cleansing if ordered.
	Remove dentures, contacts, glasses, prostheses, hairpins or wigs, nail polish, artificial nails, and makeup.
	Wear OR gown and cap.
	Void on call to OR.
Safety	Place side rails up after premedication.
	Client should use call light if assistance is needed; no attempt should be made to get out of bed because of possibility of falling and consequent injury.
Preadmission interview, visit and education related to preoperative, intraoperative, and postoperative periods	Explain expectations after leaving client care unit.
	Starting of IV lines and placement of monitoring devices
	Characteristics of OR environment
	Application of oxygen
	Close monitoring of vital signs and placement on cardiac monitor
	Presence of urinary catheter, if applicable
	Review type of dressing, casts, and other devices based on type of surgery.
	Address length of PACU stay.
	Discuss waiting facilities for family and how client information can be obtained.
Postoperative pain	Discuss availability of pain medication and encourage client to request it before pain becomes severe.
Early postoperative mobilization, activity, and exercises	Discuss benefits of early activity as it relates to prevention of complications.
	Teach and have client return demonstrate coughing, deep breathing, use of incentive inspirometer, leg exercises, turning, positioning, and ambulation with assistive devices.

IV, intravenous; OR, operating room; PACU, postanesthesia care unit.

Phase 2: Presurgical Clearance

This phase of the preoperative period takes place adjacent to the OR. Names for this area are the preoperative room prep and holding area, client receiving, or preanesthesia area.

In phase 2, careful review of the consent form for accuracy and completeness is done according to facility policy. Every effort should be made to ensure that the client gave legal and informed consent. Wrong-site surgery is a devastating problem for the client and results from poor preoperative planning, lack of institutional controls, failure of the operative team to exercise due care, or a simple mistake in communication between the client and the surgeon. The American Academy of Orthopaedic Surgeons (AAOS) has an advisory statement on wrong-site surgery. This statement suggests that wrong-site surgery is preventable by having the surgeon's initials placed on the operative site using a permanent marking pen and then operating through or adjacent to his or her initials. Spinal surgery done at the wrong level can be prevented with an intraoperative x-ray film that marks the exact vertebral level (site) of surgery (AAOS, 2000).

The client's chart is reviewed for completeness: Prescribed test results and the history and physical examination must be present. Review of the preprocedure checklist is completed to determine that the client has voided, removed jewelry and prostheses, and received prescribed preprocedure medications. The nurse should validate the last time that the client had anything to eat or drink. The nurse should also investigate items on the checklist that have not been completed and take appropriate corrective action before transferring the client to the operating suite.

INTRAOPERATIVE PHASE

Transport

The preoperative phase of care ends as the client is escorted into the OR suite. The perioperative nurse completes the client interview and chart check begun in phase 2: verbal identification and bracelet checks of the client's name, surgical procedure and operative site, and surgeon's name. The nurse again validates the last time the client had anything to eat or drink and validates whether the client has any allergies to food or medications. Once the process has been successfully completed, the perioperative RN/RNFA supervises and assists in safe transfer of the client to the OR bed. Once the OR doors close, the unique nature of surgery requires the perioperative RN to be aware of and respond with compassion to the client's physical and emotional needs. The perioperative RN ensures sterile technique and anticipates the surgical team's needs to make sure it has everything required to complete the surgery successfully.

Anesthesia Administration

Assisting the anesthesia care provider is an important role of the perioperative RN/RNFA, and thus the perioperative RN/RNFA must be familiar with the various types of anesthesia and the supplies and needs involved for each. Table 11–3 reviews the various anesthetic techniques and corresponding nursing implications. General anesthesia and regional nerve blockage are the two broad anesthesia categories. Unconsciousness is integral to general anesthesia, whereas varying levels of consciousness accompany regional nerve blockade. The uninformed client may fear "being awake" during regional blockage, equating it with pain. If a regional technique is a viable option, the perioperative RN/RNFA may reinforce its value by making the client aware of the intraoperative and postoperative pain management benefits, decreased incidence of such postoperative complications as nausea and vomiting, and the availability of sedatives and amnestics during the intraoperative period (Hoshowsky, 1995).

Intraoperative Anesthesia Complications

Pulmonary Complications. Aspiration may be a significant intraoperative complication. It may occur when gag reflexes are abolished and the client is unconscious. Residual effects impede lung function and gas exchange. Aspiration of solid food or broken teeth may cause respiratory obstruction. The treatment of aspirations should be immediate and should focus on removing as much aspirate as possible by lowering the head of the table and suctioning the oropharynx and tracheobronchial tree. Oxygenation of the client must occur frequently between suctionings. Overall, it is most important to maintain the client's airway. Other common pulmonary complications may be found in the postoperative section of this chapter.

Cardiovascular Complications. Perioperative myocardial infarction carries a high mortality rate. Therefore, through the client's history, physical examination, and medication regimen preoperatively, high-risk surgical clients can be identified. Identified risk factors that can be corrected before surgery will help decrease the cardiovascular morbidity and mortality associated with surgery. Intraoperative ischemic episodes must be prevented, if possible, and treated promptly should they occur. Treatment should be directed toward optimizing myocardial oxygen consumption while minimizing oxygen demands. This can be achieved through the administration of opioids, supplemented with volatile inhalation agents, and 100% oxygen (Miller, 2000b).

Hypovolemia. Hypovolemia is a loss of circulating blood volume or deficit of extracellular fluid stemming from reduced fluid intake and hemorrhage. Surgical intervention should be aimed at locating and controlling the bleeding. The anesthesia provider has the responsibility to transfuse the client when other measures such as fluid and plasma expanders no longer help the client cope with blood loss. To make a sound decision about transfusing, knowledge of blood loss is critical. Communication about measured loss on sponges and in suction canisters should be ongoing, as should estimates when a circumstance such as the use of irrigation and blood on the drapes prevents a more accurate accounting. The client may need to be placed in the Trendelenburg position, and medication may be needed to stabilize the client's vital signs. Fluid and electrolyte imbalances may result from treatment of hypovolemia and should be managed appropriately. Options for blood replacement are discussed in Chapter 10.

Temperature Regulation. Hypothermia and MH are two potential alterations in temperature that surgical clients are at risk for. Blackburn (1994) suggested that as many as 70% of all clients undergoing surgical procedures develop inadvertent hypothermia. The incidence of MH reaction in North America and Europe is about 1 in 15,000 anesthesia procedures in children and ranges from 1 in 50,000 to 1 in 150,000 anesthesia procedures in middle-aged adults (Bell & Merli, 1998).

Unintentional perioperative hypothermia has many potentially serious consequences during and after surgery. Based on recent studies and research, clients whose core temperatures are below 36°C (96.8°F) have an increased incidence of wound infection, longer hospital stays, increased surgical bleeding, and increased risk of cardiac events (Kurz, Sessler, & Lenhardt, 1998). Mild hypothermia appears to increase incisional surgical site infection (SSI) risk by causing vasoconstriction, decreased delivery of oxygen to the wound space, and subsequent impairment of function of phagocytic leukocytes (i.e., neutrophils). Clients at greater risk of developing hypothermia include the very young, the very old, clients having procedures in which a major body cavity is opened (i.e., thoracic, abdominal, pelvic cavities), and clients having procedures lasting greater than 1 hour. Intraoperative nursing activities to prevent hypothermia should focus on increasing the ambient room air to 70°F for adults and 75°F for children, limiting body exposure, warming intravenous (IV) and irrigation solutions, applying head covering, and using forced warm air blankets. The client's temperature should be monitored intraoperatively and communicated to

TABLE 11–3. *Anesthesia and Nursing Implications*

TYPE OF ANESTHESIA*	NURSING IMPLICATIONS
I. General Anesthesia Reversible state of unconsciousness with amnesia, analgesia, reflex suppression, and muscle relaxation. Components include induction, maintenance, and emergence. Wide variety of agents and techniques are used.	Induction and emergence are critical times. During induction, the circulating nurse may need to apply cricoid pressure to displace the cricoid cartilage and close the esophagus when passing an endotracheal tube to decrease the risk of aspiration. Assess client for bilateral breath sounds after passage of endotracheal tube. Warm blankets are applied before and after surgery to attenuate shivering and warm the client. Emergence assessments include airway patency, return of reflexes and muscle strength, and ability to follow commands. Postoperative assessments include level of consciousness, airway patency, cardiovascular status, temperature, fluid balance, and return of neuromuscular function. Assess for nausea and vomiting. Determine need for postoperative analgesia based on client comfort. Perform operative site assessments as appropriate.
II. Regional Anesthesia Local anesthetics act on cell membrane, interrupting sensory pathways between the surgical site and the brain. All local anesthetics have the potential to produce side effects (influenced by maximal safe dose, vascularity, absorption, and other client variables) and allergic reactions (rare). Toxic reactions are usually seen intraoperatively. Duration of block depends on potency of drug, its duration of action, dose, technique, and client variables. Lidocaine hydrochloride (Xylocaine) acts for 1–3 hr and is commonly used for infiltration, regional IV anesthesia, peripheral nerve block, epidurals, and spinals. Bupivacaine (Marcaine) acts for 3–10 hr and may be used for the same techniques as discussed previously. The addition of epinephrine to either of the local anesthetics may prolong the anesthetic action of the medications and cause vasoconstriction, which decreases bleeding at the infiltration site.	Following administration, monitor for signs and symptoms of allergic reaction. Signs and symptoms of toxicity primarily affect the central nervous system first and then the cardiovascular system. Check for drowsiness, numbness of tongue, blurred vision, tinnitus, dizziness, restlessness, slurred speech, and muscular twitching followed by convulsions. Hypotension, bradycardia, heart block, and arrest can occur as well. Management includes stopping administration of local anesthetic, and resuscitation as appropriate with epinephrine, oxygen, intravenous fluids, aminophylline, and hydrocortisone. Good for postoperative pain control.
A. Infiltration Techniques 1. Local infiltration: subcutaneous injection at operative site. Provides sensory blockade of the skin and subcutaneous tissue of the operative area. 2. Intravascular infiltration, or Bier block, used for surgeries below elbow or knee. Double bladder tourniquet applied to operative extremity and inflated. Then local anesthetic injected into distal peripheral vein to provide anesthesia in operative extremity.	Assess need for postoperative analgesia as sensation returns (applies to all regional techniques). Helpful to get oral or intravenous analgesia on board *before* block wears off. Tourniquet time is crucial. Cannot be less than 30 min (inadequate for sufficient metabolism before release into systemic circulation) or greater than 90 min in upper extremity or 2 hr in lower extremity because of ischemia. Tourniquet must be deflated slowly and intermittently to avoid systemic bolus. Assessment of circulatory status critical postoperatively: Monitor for return of normal sensation, color, and capillary refill.
B. Peripheral Nerve Blockade Local anesthetic injected around major nerve trunk supplying surgical site, producing both sensory and motor blockade. 1. Brachial plexus block: for procedures involving the upper extremity. Accomplished via axillary, interscalene, or supraclavicular approach. Interscalene or supraclavicular approach useful for procedures of the shoulder; however, a more extensive block and pneumothorax are possible complications. Axillary technique often used for hand surgery. 2. Femoral block: used for procedures involving the knee. 3. Ankle block: used for procedures on foot and toes.	Assess for sensory and motor blockade before incision. Postoperatively, assess for return of sensory and motor function. Important to differentiate between paresthesias related to dissipation of anesthesia versus neurovascular compromise. Proper positioning and support of extremity (sling or shoulder immobilizer) are essential to protect from injury. If able to ambulate, support lower extremity until recovery complete. Use assistive devices for ambulation.

Table continued on following page

TABLE 11–3. *Anesthesia and Nursing Implications* Continued

TYPE OF ANESTHESIA*	NURSING IMPLICATIONS
II. Regional Anesthesia *Continued* **C. Central Nerve Blockade** Local anesthetic injected into spinal canal with resultant sensory motor and autonomic blockade 1. Spinal: injection made into subarachnoid space (dura is punctured). 2. Epidural: injection into epidural space. Indwelling catheter may be left in place for postoperative pain management.	Intraoperatively, assess client's level of sensory and motor blockade using dermatomal landmarks. Common dermatomal landmarks include L1–L2 (groin), T10 (umbilicus), and T4 (nipple line). Assess for high spinal (anesthetic may travel as high as C4) with respiratory impairment. Check for symmetric excursions with breath sounds: equal bilaterally. Postoperatively, monitor for return of sensory and motor function. Return of sensation can vary, with one leg regaining sensation before the other. Return of sensation to both extremities and the rectal area (which represents the lower sacral segments) is a good indication that recovery is complete. Assess motor functioning by having client wiggle toes, dorsiflex ankles, and raise and flex legs as allowed by surgery. Check for hypotension resulting from residual autonomic blockade. Management includes elevation of legs, intravenous fluids, O_2, and pharmacologic intervention as necessary. Check for urinary retention because nerves supplying bladder are affected. Check for complaints of spinal headache on second postoperative day (due to dural puncture with cerebrospinal fluid leak). Incidence decreased with 25-gauge needle for spinal injection and adequate hydration. Early ambulation does not affect incidence of headache. Symptoms include severe frontal or occipital pain that worsens in the upright position and possibly nausea, vomiting, double vision, tinnitus, and dizziness. Conservative treatment includes bed rest, hydration, and analgesics. If no response to conservative therapy, an epidural blood patch can be done: 10 mL of the client's own venous blood is injected using sterile technique into the spinal puncture site to seal the leak. Relief is usually instantaneous. Other possible but very rare complications include symptoms of meningeal irritation and cord compromise. Report complaints of fever, pain, tenderness, weakness, or paralysis to appropriate physician immediately for prompt investigation and treatment to prevent permanent neurologic impairment.
III. Intravenous Conscious Sedation to Accompany Local Anesthetics for Regional Techniques **A. Benzodiazepines** 1. Diazepam (Valium) 2. Midazolam (Versed)	Intravenous conscious sedation is used to produce a depressed level of consciousness but allows the client to maintain a patent airway and respond appropriately to verbal instruction or physical stimuli. The goals of conscious sedation are relaxation, sedation, amnesia, and analgesia, usually achieved with a balance of the two classes of medications. Intraoperative monitoring with pulse oximeter and frequent vital sign checks as per institution policy essential. Assess level of consciousness and emotional comfort. Antianxiety agents: not for control of pain. Often given with local anesthetics for relaxation and amnesia. Effects reversible with flumazenil (Romazicon). Written discharge instructions essential in ambulatory setting.
B. Opioids 1. Morphine 2. Fentanyl (Sublimaze) 3. Hydromorphone	Analgesics control pain. Assess for changes in level of consciousness, vital signs, and respiratory status. Effects reversible with naloxone (Narcan). Frequently cause nausea and vomiting and urinary retention as side effects

*Type of anesthesia depends on type and length of surgery, surgeon's and anesthesiologist's preference, and client's condition and preference.

From Mattocks-Whisman, F., & Rivellini, D. (1991). Perioperative patient care. In S. W. Salmond, N. E. Mooney, & L. A. Verdisco (Eds.), *Core curriculum for orthopaedic nursing* (pp. 154–155). Pitman, NJ: National Association of Orthopaedic Nurses.

postanesthesia care unit (PACU) nurses on discharge from the OR.

Malignant Hyperthermia Precautions. MH is a medical emergency that all perioperative nurses should be prepared to handle. Clients with the inherited MH trait have a rare skeletal muscle disease that causes them to develop life-threatening hyperthermia (i.e., body temperatures of 43.3°C [110.0°F] or higher) at the time MH-triggering agents (i.e., succinylcholine, halothane, enflurane, and isoflurane) are administered to induce general anesthesia or shortly thereafter. Continuous skeletal muscle rigidity, hypermetabolism, hypercapnia, tachypnea, and tachycardia that result in cardiac arrest and death if left untreated also characterize the MH syndrome (Donnelly, 1994). Knowledge of MH and the care of MH-susceptible clients and adequate preparation for MH crises are the cornerstones of successful client outcomes to this life-threatening syndrome.

Dunn (1997) described the circulating nurse's major role in responding to an MH crisis. The anesthesia care provider discontinues administration of all triggering agents and hyperventilates the client with 100% oxygen at a high flow rate. The nurse prepares an initial dose of dantrolene 2.5 mg/kg, which may be repeated at 20-minute intervals up to a maximum dose of 10 mg/kg until symptoms subside. The nurse and anesthesia care provider use iced IV saline solutions, a temperature-regulating blanket, and gastric and rectal ice lavage and place bags of ice around the client to cool him or her. They also obtain multiple, sequential determinations of the client's arterial and venous blood gases, central venous pressure, urine output, temperature, $ETCO_2$, serum potassium, serum calcium, serum lactate dehydrogenase, serum creatine phosphokinase, urine myoglobin, and serum clotting mechanisms. If the client continues to have cardiac arrhythmias after the acidosis and hyperkalemia are corrected, the anesthesia care provider gives procainamide or other appropriate antiarrhythmic agents. To maintain the client's urine output at more than 2 mL/kg per hour, the nurse and anesthesia care provider administer furosemide and extra IV fluids. As soon as the client is stable, he or she is transferred to the intensive care unit (ICU).

Pseudocholinesterase Deficiency. The diagnosis of atypical pseudocholinesterase deficiency is made only after a healthy client experiences prolonged neuromuscular blockade following a conventional dose of the depolarizing neuromuscular blocking agent succinylcholine. Succinylcholine has a rapid onset (30 to 60 seconds) and a short duration of action (3 to 5 minutes), making it an ideal agent for intubation. It is metabolized by pseudocholinesterase, a plasma enzyme, which has no other antagonist. Alterations in the efficacy or amount of any given client's pseudocholinesterase may cause an extended duration of neuromuscular blockade, resulting in

the client being admitted to the PACU on a ventilator. These alterations are related to genetic defects and make it important for the anesthesia provider to establish any familial history of problems with anesthesia.

Intraoperative Nursing Care

Perioperative nurses are continually involved in various forms of assessment related to client care and are skilled in identifying nursing diagnoses that are applicable to the intraoperative phase of nursing care. Appropriate assessment, planning, and implementation can lead to attaining positive, measurable outcomes for the surgical client. The most common, high-risk, and problem-prone areas are discussed here.

Fear. The surgical client frequently encounters anxiety caused by consciously recognized danger (i.e., invasive surgical procedure); this is defined as *fear*. Intraoperative nurses are at a unique advantage to choose from many appropriate interventions that will assist the client in meeting the outcome of fear control. The ratio of one RN to one client allows the RN to individualize interventions. For example, a child faced with an orthopaedic surgical procedure benefits from the nurse engaging in security enhancement, distraction, and therapeutic play. An older client with underlying dementia benefits from calming technique, touch, and security enhancement. A healthy young client undergoing an elective carpal tunnel release may benefit from anxiety reduction, emotional support, and humor.

Risk for Infection: Intraoperative. Inherent in the surgical setting is the effort to minimize the risk of nosocomial infection to the client. A deep infection after a hip or knee arthroplasty has a mortality rate of 2% to 6% and the risk of lifelong physical disability of approximately 60% (Wymenga, Van Dijke, Van Horn, & Slooff, 1990). Although unproven, the greatest risk for postoperative infection appears to be the clients themselves. Factors that may increase the risk of SSI include those related to the client's age, nutritional status, and smoking status; whether the client has diabetes, obesity, coexisting infections at a remote site, colonization with microorganisms, or altered immune response; whether the client is taking any systemic steroids; and the length of preoperative stay (Mangram, Horan, Pearson, Silver, & Jarvis, 1999).

Wound Classification. The risk of SSI also depends on whether the surgical procedure is a clean, clean-contaminated, contaminated, or dirty-infected procedure based on standard definitions of these terms. The Centers for Disease Control and Prevention (CDC) defines the four wound classes as follows (Garner, 1982):

Class I—Clean: The respiratory, gastrointestinal, or genitourinary system is not entered; primarily closed wounds; closed wound drainage system may be present; no evidence of infection; carries a 1% to 5% risk of infection

Class II—Clean-contaminated: The respiratory, gastrointestinal, or genitourinary system is entered under controlled conditions; no breaks in aseptic technique; no infection is noted; carries a 3% to 11% risk of infection

Class III—Contaminated: Open, fresh, or traumatic wounds; a major break in aseptic technique; incisional infection present; carries a 10% to 17% risk of infection

Class IV—Dirty or infected: Old traumatic wound; retained devitalized tissue present; existing clinical infection noted; carries a greater than 27% risk of infection

AORN (1996) endorsed the documentation of wound class to enable the prediction of outcomes and appropriate interventions.

Medication Administration. To prevent SSI, perioperative antimicrobial prophylaxis is recommended for various surgical procedures. Based on published data, implications for perioperative nurses involved in antibiotic administration for surgical prophylaxis are fairly straightforward. Optimal antimicrobial agents for prophylaxis are bactericidal, nontoxic, inexpensive, and active against the typical pathogens that cause SSI postoperatively. To maximize its effectiveness, IV perioperative prophylaxis should be given within 30 to 60 minutes before the time of surgical incision (Osmon, 2000). Antibiotic prophylaxis should be of short duration to decrease toxicity, antimicrobial resistance, and excess cost. Additional doses are generally recommended only when the operative procedure extends beyond 2 to 3 hours (Nichols, 1996).

Intraoperative Infection Control. Skin is the client's first line of defense against infection. Disruption of the skin from an operative incision or trauma (i.e., open fracture) compromises that line of defense by providing an entry for microorganisms. Perioperative nurses must consider the multiple factors that influence infection outcomes and risks in the surgical setting. For most SSIs, the source of pathogens is the endogenous flora of the client's skin, mucous membranes, or hollow viscera (Mangram et al., 1999). Exogenous sources of SSI pathogens include surgical personnel; the operating room environment (including air); and all tools, instruments, and materials brought to the sterile field during an operation. Duration of surgical scrub, skin antisepsis, preoperative shaving, preoperative skin preparation, duration of operation, antimicrobial prophylaxis, operating room ventilation, foreign material at the surgical site, surgical drains, and surgical technique also affect the client's risk for infection (Mangram et al., 1999).

The controversial findings regarding the mode of transmission of microorganisms causing SSIs and the influence of the OR environment on such infections continue to be topics of debate. However, it is known that airborne contamination with bacteria-carrying particles is one of the dominating causes of postoperative infection in clean surgery. The bacteria-carrying particles are generated almost exclusively by the OR staff members. During moderate physical activity, every person sheds skin scales, generating approximately 1000 bacteria-carrying particles (Friberg, 1998). The shedding rate is influenced greatly by the activity's intensity. The origin of most particle-carrying bacteria are the axilla, perineum, and the inside of the thighs; therefore, more pronounced arm movements and walking dramatically increase the shedding. The air contaminates clothing, instruments, and the wound by direct contact. In turn, the clothing and instruments indirectly transfer bacteria to the wound. Therefore, one of the OR team members' major goals is to reduce or minimize the counts of bacteria-carrying particles in the air. Efforts should be made to minimize personnel traffic during operations.

Traffic Patterns. Perioperative nurses are uniquely situated to promote good traffic control practices in the OR. AORN gives guidance in *Recommended Practices for Traffic Patterns in the Surgical Suite* (AORN, 2000) to reduce the amount of airborne contamination during surgery. Specifically, AORN recommends that movement of staff members be kept to a minimum while a surgical procedure is in progress. This includes minimizing the number of people in the OR and movement, limiting the amount of talking during surgery, and keeping the OR doors closed except during movement of staff members or equipment. In addition to AORN recommendations, the CDC guidelines for infection control (Mangram et al., 1999) emphasize the importance of traffic patterns in the surgical suite and the limitation in the number of personnel involved in the procedure. The CDC guideline also states that airborne contamination decreases with increased ventilation, which dilutes contaminated air with relatively clean filtered or outdoor air and with decreased numbers and activity of personnel.

Airflow and Filtration. Control of the air within the surgical suite is an important issue but remains controversial. The purpose of OR ventilation is to dilute and remove airborne bacteria-carrying particles. A reduction in the number of these particles is definitely beneficial; however, there is a threshold below which further reduction in colony-forming units (CFUs) fails to yield a corresponding reduction in wound infection rates. An ordinary conventional air handling system normally provides 16 to 20 air changes per hour. High-efficiency particulate air (HEPA) filters with air entering at the ceiling and slightly less air exiting at the floor creates a positive pressure in the room. This pressure prevents potentially contaminated air from entering the OR from adjacent areas. The air counts of bacteria are expected to be 50 to 150 CFU/m^3 and sometimes even more, depending on the number of people present and their level of physical activity. This degree of air contamination can be expected to yield a postoperative infection rate of 3% to 5% in clean, infection-prone surgery.

Orthopaedic rooms equipped for total joint arthroplasty procedures may have a laminar-flow air handling system. The 1999 CDC guidelines suggest consideration of performing orthopaedic implant operations in ORs supplied with ultraclean air. Laminar airflow units recirculate excessive volumes of HEPA-filtered sterile air and usually have up to 400 to 500 air changes per hour. If used correctly, they should provide less than 10 CFU/m^3 during surgical procedures. This usually results in an infection rate of less than 1%, even after infection-prone, clean surgery.

Surgical Attire. For many years, body exhaust suits were the gold standard for clothing in rooms equipped with laminar airflow units. However, they are relatively expensive and impractical (e.g., difficult to put on, warm to work in, often did not provide enough fresh air for breathing, made communication between surgical team members difficult, sudden and arterial bleeding or splashing hitting the helmet's front could obscure surgeon's vision). Therefore, not all orthopaedic surgeons accepted the body exhaust suits. Instead, disposable clothing, in combination with modern face masks and wide surgical hoods that reach out over the shoulders to prevent skin bacteria emission spread from the neck, have been found to be as efficient as body exhaust suits in suites equipped with laminar airflow units (Friberg et al., 1980). Nonwoven disposable clothing with plastic arm and front shielding combined with disposable hoods and modern face masks seem to be a bacteriologic safe clothing alternative to a body exhaust suit. The surgical hood must cover the hair and must be long enough to be tucked well underneath the sterile gown to prevent contamination emanating from the neck area (Mangram et al., 1999). Shoe covers are no longer recommended for the prevention of SSIs. There are no recommendations on how or where to launder scrub suits, on the restricted use of scrub suits to the operating suite, or for the covering of scrub suits when out of the operating suite. The CDC report considers these unresolved issues (Mangram et al., 1999).

Surveillance: Aseptic Technique. Excellent surgical technique is widely believed to reduce the risk of SSI. Principles of aseptic technique are used in establishing and maintaining a sterile field. Application of these principles requires that all team members develop and maintain a surgical conscience. Surgical conscience involves both scientific and intellectual honesty; it is a self-regulation of practice according to a deep personal commitment to the highest values. The goal of the surgical conscience is not to excuse error but to admit readily and rectify any break in technique to better serve the client. According to AORN (2000), the recommended practices of aseptic technique include the following:

- Scrubbed persons function within a sterile field.
- Use sterile items within a sterile field.
- Open, dispense, and transfer all items onto a sterile field by methods that maintain sterility and integrity.
- Constantly maintain and monitor the sterile field.
- Move within or around the sterile field in a manner that maintains sterility of the field.

Ensuring the sterility of all items used during surgery is a core competency for the perioperative nurse. The nurse should check all sterile items for signs of pinholes, tears, moisture, and lack of seal integrity (AORN, 2000). Compromise of the package compromises sterility. The item should not be used if a defect in packaging is found. Some commercially prepared items degrade over time and thus are stamped with an expiration date. If the item is outdated, it should not be used.

Sterilization. Various methods are used to sterilize items used during surgery. Manufacturer-supplied prepackaged sterile items are usually sterilized in bulk by gamma irradiation. Surgical instruments can be sterilized by steam under pressure, dry heat, ethylene oxide, hydrogen peroxide gas plasma sterilization, or peracetic acid. Flash sterilization should be performed only for client care items that will be used immediately (e.g., to reprocess an inadvertently dropped instrument). Flash sterilization should not be used for reasons of convenience, as an alternative to purchasing additional instrument sets, or to save time. Inadequate sterilization of surgical instruments has resulted in SSI outbreaks. When possible, instrument sets used to implant medical devices and the implant itself should be processed by conventional methods according to manufacturer recommendations. The importance of routinely monitoring the quality of sterilization procedures has been established.

Skin Preparation. AORN (1996) recommends preoperative cleaning, hair removal, and antimicrobial skin preparation to reduce bacterial colony count of the incision site. The 1999 CDC Guidelines (Mangram et al., 1999) recommend no hair removal preoperatively unless the hair at or around the incision site will interfere with the operation. If hair is removed, it should be removed immediately before the operation, preferably with electric clippers. Shaving is no longer recommended. The CDC also suggests that clients be required to shower or bathe with an antiseptic agent on at least the night before the operative day. An appropriate antiseptic agent, such as chlorhexidine or iodine preparations, should be used for skin preparation. A preoperative antiseptic skin preparation should be applied in concentric circles moving toward the periphery. If the area being prepared is known to be contaminated or infected, cleansing should begin at the periphery and proceed inward to the most contaminated portion. The prepared area must be large enough to extend the incision and to create new incisions or drain sites, if necessary. Orthopaedic procedures usually require scrubbing of the area for at least 5 minutes, painting the incision with antimicrobial solution, and if desired, applying alcohol solution. To prevent a chemical burn of the skin, nursing actions should be taken to avoid pooling of solutions under the client or tourniquet cuff.

In addition to preparing the client's skin, the surgical hand scrub is performed by all team members who will be at the sterile field. Before donning sterile gown and gloves, team members use antimicrobial soap and mechanical friction to remove dirt, oil, and the transient bacteria on the skin of the hands and forearms up to the elbows. The surgical hand scrub reduces the skin's residential microbial count and inhibits rebound growth of microorganisms. The CDC guidelines (Mangram et al., 1999) recommend that nails be kept short and that artificial nails not be worn. The issue of wearing nail polish remains unresolved.

Wound Care: Closed or Open Drainage. Philosophies vary greatly regarding the use of drains. Some surgeons believe that drains are more likely to cause infections than to prevent them. The CDC guidelines (Mangram et al., 1999) suggest that if drainage is necessary, one should use a closed-suction drain, place a drain through a separate incision distant from the operative incision, and remove the drain as soon as possible. The RNFA should have a working knowledge of the types of systems available and knowledge in proper assembly, insertion, activation, and removal of each system used.

Implants/Explants. Implants are commonly used in orthopaedic fixation and reconstructive surgery. They may be bioresorbable, metallic, plastic, ceramic, chemical, or biologic, such as allograft tissue and bone. To prevent stress and possible implant fracture, care should be taken to avoid damaging the surface of any implant. Bioresorbable, metallic, plastic, and ceramic implants should never be altered. The correct size and configuration should be chosen and used. Documentation of implants provides a permanent record of the device implanted for use later. For example, the surgeon may need to know the type and size of a previous implanted device for easy and efficient removal or to decide what should be placed in the client's contralateral side. Legally, documentation provides a way to identify recipients of a

particular implant should the manufacturer recall the product in the future. Documentation requirements include manufacturer name, catalog, model, lot and serial numbers, implant size and amount, sterilization load control number if the implant was institutionally sterilized, and the anatomic location of the implant(s). If the implant requires tracking by the U.S. Food and Drug Administration (FDA), that number should also be included in the documentation. In addition, any implant removed from the client should be documented as an explant. Explant documentation requires that all accessible information as noted for implants be recorded on the client's record.

Allograft tissues are being used for an increasing variety of purposes, most commonly stabilizing painful joints; promoting healing of nonunion fractures; and restoring structure, function, and cosmesis. Many types of allograft tissues are available for use: fresh frozen, freeze-dried, and decalcified. All tissues should be obtained by an agency that subscribes to the national guidelines and standards of the American Association of Tissue Banks. Adherence to these guidelines may minimize the risk of acquiring blood-borne diseases, such as hepatitis and human immunodeficiency virus (HIV) infection.

The handling of all allograft tissue begins with checking the surgical permit for consent and verification of the type and size of tissue to be used. Frozen allografts need to be thawed in sterile, isotonic, warm solution for at least 30 minutes before cutting, contouring, or implanting bone. Freeze-dried allografts also require reconstitution by instilling in sterile isotonic solution for about 30 minutes. Aerobic and anaerobic cultures of the allograft are taken to ensure sterility of the implant.

Documentation of the allograft in the intraoperative nursing care record should include the type of allograft, name of implanting surgeon, name of the tissue bank, identification or access number of the graft, and the implant location. Institutional implant logs should be completed according to the hospital's policy and procedures. Many tissue banks also require that a transplant record be completed and returned to them. The record usually includes the recipient name, surgeon name, institution name and address, the procedure performed, the type of allograft used, the ID number of the allograft, and the date of transplant.

Risk for Injury

Perioperative Positioning: Intraoperative. Probably no other specialty uses as many varied surgical positions as orthopaedics. Positions for orthopaedic surgery are usually variation of the supine, lateral, and prone positions. For procedures involving the extremities, such as knee arthroscopy or carpal tunnel release, the client is placed in a supine position. For procedure involving the shoulder, a semi-sitting position is preferred. Surgery involving the hip joint requires the client to be in a lateral position. Each position creates a challenge for the OR team. Table 11-4 depicts the various surgical positions, devices used, and nursing actions to implement the position safely. Complications from improper positioning can result in nerve compression, interference with venous return and cardiac output, compression of the eye or corneal abrasions, accidental removal of the endotracheal tube, or joint strain.

The neurologic and musculoskeletal systems are most vulnerable to injury from positioning. Significant age-related changes such as cervical arthritis, lung elastin loss, and thoracic cage rigidity must be taken into consideration when positioning the older client. Elevating the head of bed, when possible, assists in chest expansion (Hazen, Larsen, & Hoot Martin, 1997). Brachial plexus injury may occur when the arm is abducted greater than 90 degrees or when pressure is applied to the client's axilla, clavicle, or elbow. Symptoms include numbness; paresthesias; and paralysis of the arm, shoulder, or torso. To prevent injury, arms should never be abducted past 90 degrees and palms should face upward when positioned out on armboards and should face inward when the arm is to be tucked at the client's side. When using a sheet to tuck arms at sides, the entire elbow regions should be covered.

The sciatic, saphenous, peroneal, tibial, and sural nerves are the most vulnerable to injury in the lower extremity (Fig. 11-1). Sciatic nerve injury is relatively uncommon but may cause back and leg pain, weakness, or numbness. Severe abduction or flexion of the leg may cause sciatic nerve stretching. The saphenous nerve runs superficially at the medial thigh and may be impaired by direct compression from a tourniquet or arthroscopic leg holder. Peroneal nerve injury is caused by compression over the lateral aspect of the fibular head or from prolonged plantar flexion of the foot, which may cause foot-drop. The tibial nerve may be injured as it diverges at the popliteal fossa and travels down the leg to the medial aspect of the ankle. Injury may produce sensory and motor loss to the calf or sensory loss to the sole of the foot or both. The sural nerve is found laterally at the ankle and foot; injury causes a loss of sensation to the lateral aspect of the foot. Direct pressure on the ankle structures may cause injury to the Achilles tendon. Ensuring that the client's legs are uncrossed, avoiding pressure behind the knees, and providing extra padding around bony prominences of the knees and ankles helps prevent nerve injury. Additional nerves that may be injured include the pudendal and lateral femoral cutaneous nerves. Traction on the legs and pressure on the perineum from an inadequately padded perineal post on the fracture table can cause loss of perineal sensation and fecal incontinence. In the prone position, thigh pressure against a hard support bolster can lead to anesthesia on the lower lateral, anterior aspect of the thigh (McEwen, 1996).

Pressure Management. Pressure sore formation has been identified as a complication of surgery. A thinner layer of subcutaneous fat predisposes older clients to the potential for pressure sores. Decreased skin elasticity and turgor increase the risk for pressure injury and injury related to the use of adhesives (Hazen, Larsen, & Hoot Martin, 1997). A complete discussion of factors contributing to pressure sore formation can be found in Chapter 4. Health care professionals attempt to reduce the incidence of severe pressure sores by identifying people at high risk and by using prevention strategies, such as pressure-relieving equipment. It is essential that initiatives be based on the best available evidence of clinical and cost-effectiveness and that a systematic review of the evidence for the effectiveness of pressure-relieving support surfaces such as beds, mattresses, cushions, and repositioning interventions be undertaken.

At present, the most effective means of pressure relief on the operating table is unclear. Two randomized, controlled studies have evaluated different methods of pressure relief on the operating table. The first compared a viscoelastic polymer pad with a standard table and found a relative reduction in the incidence of postoperative pressure sores of 47% with use of the polymer pad for clients undergoing elective major general, gynecologic, or vascular surgery in the supine or lithotomy position (relative risk of 0.53; confidence interval 0.33 to 0.85; Nixon, McElvenny, Mason, Brown, & Bond, 1998). Aronovitch (1998) compared the MicroPulse alternating system (applied both during surgery and postoperatively) with a gel pad during surgery and standard mattress postoperatively and report a pooled relative risk of 0.21, confidence interval of 0.06 to 0.7 in favor of the MicroPulse system. Organizations should consider the use of pressure relief for high-risk clients in the OR because this is associated with a reduction in postoperative incidence of pressure sores. The relative merits of higher-tech constant low pressure and alternating pressure are unclear. Independent, well-designed, multicenter, randomized, controlled trials are needed to compare the clinical and cost-effectiveness of different types of pressure-relieving devices for individuals at different levels of risk in a variety of settings.

At the completion of surgery, it is important for the RNFA and perioperative nurse to reexamine the client's skin and neurovascular function. Any alteration of skin integrity or function must be reported to the surgeon immediately. Documentation of positioning must appear on the intraoperative nursing care record and should include aspects such as the surgical position used, devices used to position the client, personnel involved with the act of positioning, and preoperative and postoperative skin integrity and neurovascular assessments.

Text continued on page 287

TABLE 11–4. *Common Surgical Positions*

POSITION	SURGICAL PROCEDURE	DEVICES USED, NURSING ACTIONS TO POSITION CLIENT	POSTOPERATIVE ASSESSMENT AND CONSIDERATIONS
Supine	Anesthesia induction Most extremity procedures Anterior cervical spine procedures Closed reduction and nailing of femur and tibia Open reduction and internal fixation of hip	Headrest to relax neck muscles Safety strap placed 2 inches above knees Arms on armboards or tucked at sides Legs uncrossed, no part of body touching metal Lumbar roll or small pillow under knees to alleviate back pain Hand table: secured under mattress or to table frame Ensure that hand table is the same height as the OR bed Lateral stress post: secured at thigh level to bed for knee arthroscopy Footrest: secured to table to prop leg in flexed position during total knee arthroplasty Stryker frame: see reference noted later Fracture table: operative leg in traction boot or with skeletal pin to traction. Unaffected leg is in padded stirrup or over padded sling. Pad perineal post, sacral rest, and traction boot well Arms: out on armboards or in a sling across chest. Many attachments. Refer to operator's manual for directions on use	Assess for brachial plexus injury Radial nerve: Sensation tested by pricking web space between thumb and index fingers. Motion tested by having client hyperextend the thumb, wrist, and fingers at the MCP joint Ulnar nerve: Sensation tested by pricking the distal end of small fingers. Motion tested by asking client to abduct all fingers with fingers flexed Median nerve: Sensation tested by pricking distal portion of index finger. Motion tested by having client oppose thumb and little finger and flex wrist Assess client for injury to popliteal space. Too large a pillow under knees may cause venous thrombosis Assess for peroneal nerve injury caused by improper positioning of stress post Assess skin for pressure sore formation over bony prominences (i.e., sacrum, heels, occiput) Assess for alopecia Assess perineum from pressure of perineal post, foot from pressure of traction boot(s), and sacrum from pressure of sacral rest on fracture table

Supine position. (From Gruendemann, B. J. [1987]. *Positioning plus* [p. 36]. Buffalo, NY: Devon Industries.)

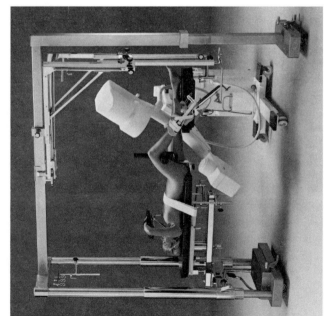

Chick Langrene fracture table. (Courtesy of Midmark Corporation, Versaille, Ohio.)

Modifications to Supine

Beach chair or semi-Fowler's

Shoulder procedures

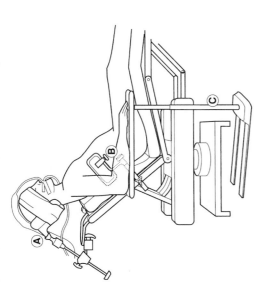

Modified beach chair position. (Courtesy of Zimmer, Inc., Warsaw, Indiana.)

Head secured to neurosurgical or orthopaedic headrest with tape to stabilize head and neck. Protect skin with gauze or towel before using tape.
Side brace: attached to bed to keep client's torso on table
Operative arm: draped free on field supported by armboard or padded Mayo stand or placed across chest
Legs uncrossed

Assessments as discussed previously.

Lowered foot of OR table

Knee arthroscopy

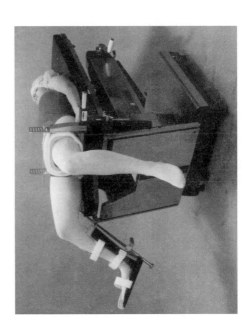

The foot of the OR table is lowered, and the leg not operated on is supported with a well-padded Allen stirrup. (Courtesy of Allen Medical Systems, Bedford Heights, Ohio.)

Leg holder surrounds operative leg on thigh
Operative leg draped free on field
Nonoperative leg held in padded Allen stirrup

Assess lower extremities for nerve injuries
Peroneal nerve: Sensation tested by pricking web space between great and second toes. Motion tested by having client dorsiflex ankle and extend toes at metatarsal phalangeal joints
Tibial nerve: Sensation tested by pricking medial lateral surface of sole of foot. Motion tested by having client plantar flex ankle and flex toes

Table continued on following page

TABLE 11–4. *Common Surgical Positions* Continued

POSITION	SURGICAL PROCEDURE	DEVICES USED, NURSING ACTIONS TO POSITION CLIENT	POSTOPERATIVE ASSESSMENT AND CONSIDERATIONS
Modifications to Supine *Continued*			
Application of cervical traction	Cervical spine procedures	Remove head section of OR table, insert neuro-surgical headrest, and tighten securely Cervical head halter traction: Apply halter as usual, add traction cording and weights as physician directs Gardner-Wells tongs: Pins are inserted into skull by surgeon. Add traction cording and weights as physician directs Stryker frame: Use to access anterior and posterior cervical spine*	Assess client for skin irritation around ears and chin
Application of finger traps	Closed reduction and pinning of wrist fractures Wrist arthroscopy	Application of finger traps is done by compressing the netting to form an opening, inserting digit, then pulling down to close Hang traps from IV pole, apply felt sling over upper arm, and affix weights for fracture reduction or distraction of joint space Commercial distraction devices (tower) for wrist arthroscopy: Follow manufacturer directions	Assess fingers of operative extremity for injury caused by finger traps. Assess client for traction injury to brachial plexus as discussed previously.

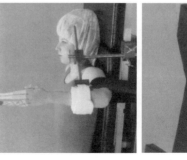 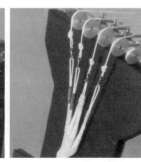

Finger traps in use via the Schlein hand positioner. (Courtesy of Allen Medical Systems, Bedford Heights, Ohio.)

Lateral

Hip and femur procedures
Selected elbow procedures
Shoulder arthroscopy

Anesthetize the client supine, then turn lateral

Hips and shoulders are simultaneously turned to avoid twisting spine

Lower shoulder is brought forward slightly

Axillary roll is placed under lower arm to protect brachial plexus

Place pillows between arms for support, or use double armboard or padded Mayo stand to support upper arm

Pillows are placed between legs. Lower leg is flexed at hip and knee, upper leg is straight

Padding is placed at knee and ankle level to protect bony prominences

Vac Pac: Cover with viscoelastic overlay, place on bed with U toward client's head, mold around client and apply suction to make firm

Hip positioning frame (McQuire, Montreal): Cover with padding, following manufacturer directions for use

Shoulder traction device: Pad hand and wrist to protect from damage, apply weights to distract humeral head from glenoid fossa, follow manufacturer directions for use

---

Assess client for skin impairment on the down side of the client. Areas of inspection should include the ear, eye, and nose, acromion process, greater trochanter, lateral condyle of the femur and tibia, lateral malleolus of the ankle. Assessment of nerve impairment to the brachial plexus, the peroneal and sural nerves should be completed as noted. The radial pulse should be checked after placement of the axillary roll and postoperatively to determine the presence or absence of circulatory injury

Hip positioning frames require examination of the skin over the ischial tuberosities

Use of shoulder traction device warrants examination of the hand, wrist, fingers, and brachial plexus. Circulatory and nerve checks should be completed once the traction apparatus is removed

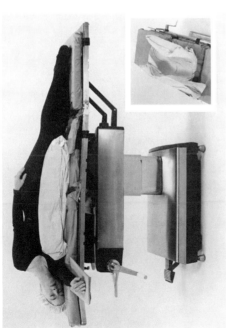

Vac Pac. (Courtesy of Olympic Medical Corporation, Seattle, Washington.)

McQuire frame and action pad set. (Courtesy of Action Products, Inc., Hagerstown, Maryland.)

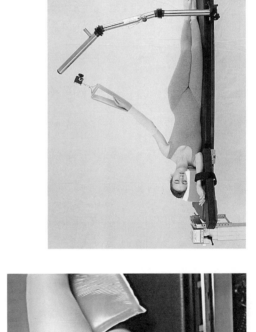

Bazooka lateral positioner. (Courtesy of Orthopedic Systems, Inc., Hayward, California.)

Table continued on following page

*See Hoshowsky, V. M. (Ed.). (1995). *Orientation to the orthopaedic operating room* (pp. 44–46). Pitman, NJ: National Association of Orthopaedic Nurses.

TABLE 11–4. *Common Surgical Positions* Continued

POSITION	SURGICAL PROCEDURE	DEVICES USED, NURSING ACTIONS TO POSITION CLIENT	POSTOPERATIVE ASSESSMENT AND CONSIDERATIONS
Prone	Thoracic and lumbar spine procedures Selected elbow procedures Posterior cervical and lower extremity procedures	Anesthetize the client supine, then turn prone by log-rolling client. Have bed immediately available to turn client supine in case of an emergency Chest rolls: Measure client from acromioclavicular joint to iliac crest for correct length chest rolls Four poster frame (Relton-Hall, CHOP), convex frame (Wilson, Kambin): Place frame on bed without x-ray parts or table pads, cover with padding Knee-chest frame (Andrews): Place frame onto foot of bed, lower foot of bed, apply viscoelastic overlay to knee area. Apply compression stockings to client's lower extremities. Position client on bed kneeling, apply buttock rest and hip guards, apply foam boots to feet and clip to underside of frame. Place foam strap around client's thighs and buttock post Be sure abdomen, genitals, and breasts hang free. Place bump under torso for chest elevation and ventilation Arms: Should be flexed at elbows. On armboards, palms down Head: Should be turned to side, no pressure on nose, eyes, or ears. Spine is straight	Assess client for skin irritation of the eyes, ears, and face Assess skin over chest, iliac crests, knees, feet, toes, and ankles. Assess for brachial nerve injury from incorrect chest roll length Assess brachial nerve for injury and shoulder for dislocation secondary to incorrect arm movement during positioning Assess genitals and breasts for pressure areas

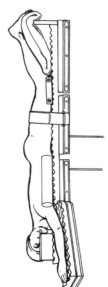

Chest rolls. (From Gruendemann, B. J. [1987]. *Positioning plus* [p. 59]. Buffalo, NY: Devon Industries.)

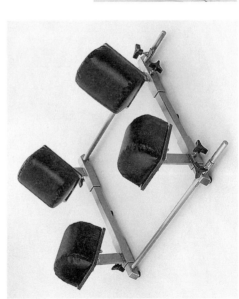

Relton-Hall surgical frame. (Courtesy of Imperial Surgical Ltd., Markham, Ontario, Canada.)

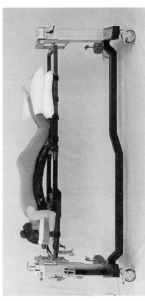

Wilson frame. (Courtesy of Orthopedic Systems, Inc., Hayward, California.)

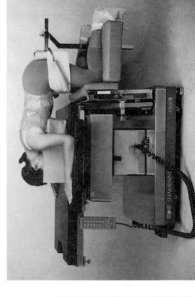 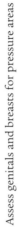

Andrews spinal frame. (Courtesy of Orthopedic Systems, Inc., Hayward, California.)

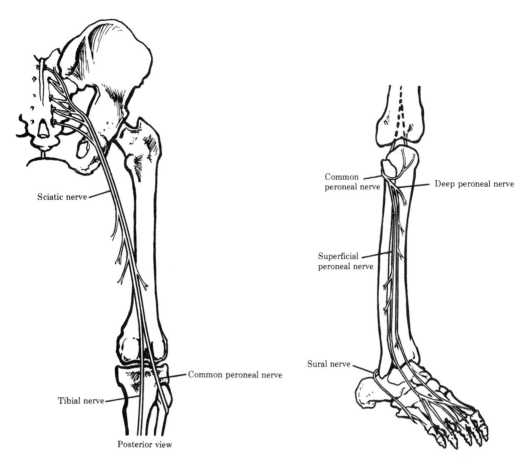

FIGURE 11–1. Nerves of the lower extremity. (From Gruendemann, B. J. [1987]. *Positioning plus* [pp. 75-76]. Buffalo, NY: Devon Industries.)

Embolus Precautions. Deep venous thrombosis (DVT) is a potentially serious complication after total hip or knee replacement. The pathophysiology of venous thrombosis involves three interrelated factors, known as *Virchow's triad:* damage to the vessel wall, slowing of the blood flow, and an increase in blood coagulability. Risk factors for DVT include age, cancer, surgery, immobilization, fractures, paralysis, smoking, use of oral contraceptives, and the antiphospholipid syndrome (Lensing, Prandoni, Prins, & Buller, 1999). In a prone position, circulation is affected by pressure on the inferior vena cava. This leads to decreased cardiac output and decreased circulating blood volume, which can result in hypotension; this hypotension may then contribute to DVT. A pillow placed under the client's pelvis may decrease pressure. DVT risk may also be increased because of intraoperative positioning for optimal access, direct vascular injury from intraoperative limb manipulation, and the use of thigh tourniquets. Use of a thigh tourniquet impairs venous drainage, damages the endothelium, confines coagulation reactants from surgical trauma below the tourniquet, and may increase the risk of venous thrombosis and large emboli. Without prophylaxis, the risk of DVT ranges from 30% to 70% following some

orthopaedic procedures. Prophylaxis, often consisting of a combination of pharmacologic and mechanical agents, reduces the risk of DVT by 50% to 64% in orthopaedic clients (Agu, Hamilton, & Baker, 1999). Pharmacologic prophylaxis should be administered per the surgeon's preference. Unlike pharmacologic agents, mechanical methods do not interfere with hemostasis and are unlikely to cause bleeding complications; consequently, they are popular with orthopaedic surgeons, and the placement of pneumatic stockings intraoperatively is common. The risk of late-onset venous thrombosis persists for at least 5 weeks after joint replacement.

Surgical Precautions. Surgical precautions involve minimizing the potential for iatrogenic injury to the client related to a surgical procedure. Electrical safety and surgical counts are discussed here. Electrosurgery is used routinely to cut and coagulate body tissue with high radiofrequency electrical current. Electrosurgical units (ESUs) may be of a monopolar or bipolar type. Monopolar units involve the use of an active electrode, usually a pencil, a generator, and a dispersive pad. Current flows from the generator through the client and back into the generator through the dispersive pad. The circulating nurse is responsible for selecting an adequate site for the dispersive pad. The site should be a smooth muscular surface close to the operative site. The pad must be in constant contact with the skin and should never be cut or altered. According to AORN's (1998a) recommended practices for electrosurgery, the dispersive electrode should not be placed over bony prominences, scar tissue, skin over an implanted metal prosthesis, hairy surfaces, or areas distal to tourniquets and pressure points. Fatty tissues or tissue directly over bone can impede electrosurgical return current flow, and there is potential for superheating if a dispersive electrode is placed on the skin over the site of an implanted metal prosthesis. Adequate tissue perfusion, which promotes electrical conductivity and dissipates heat, cannot be ensured if the dispersive electrode is placed distal to tourniquets or over scar tissue. To prevent burns from electrical current being dispersed anywhere but to the grounding pad, it is important that the client's body does not touch the metal portion of the OR bed or metallic jewelry and that electrocardiogram leads not be placed between the operative site and the dispersive pad. In addition, the pad should not be exposed to prep solution or irrigation fluid. The scrub person should keep the active electrode in its safety holster to prevent inadvertent activation, and the ESU should not be activated in the presence of flammable liquids (e.g., alcohol, tincture of benzoin). The client's skin integrity should be evaluated and documented before and after ESU use to evaluate the client's skin condition for possible injuries.

Bipolar electrocautery current flows between two tips of a bipolar forceps that is positioned around tissue. It is often used on delicate tissues. A dispersive electrode is not needed because current flows between the two tips of the bipolar forceps rather than through the client.

Special precautions should be taken when using monopolar ESU with clients who have pacemakers and automatic defibrillators (El-Gamal, Dufresne, & Saddler, 2001). Most modern pacemakers are designed to be shielded from radiofrequency current during monopolar ESU use. The circulating nurse should ensure that the current path from the surgical site to the dispersive electrode does not pass through the vicinity of the client's heart or the implanted pacemaker device. The client's pacemaker may interpret electrocautery as cardiac activity and inhibit the pacemaker from initiating a heartbeat. A client with an automatic implantable cardioverter/defibrillator (AICD) should have the AICD device deactivated before monopolar ESU is activated because using electrosurgery on a client with an activated AICD may trigger an electrical shock to the client.

The smoke plume generated from electrocautery contains chemical byproducts, and exposure to this smoke plume should be reduced. When a smoke evacuation system is used, the capture device should be placed as close to the source of the smoke plume as possible. This maximizes smoke capture and enhances visibility at the surgical site. The Occupational Safety and Health Administration (OSHA) recommends that smoke evacuation systems be used to reduce potential acute and chronic health risks to clients and personnel.

Surgical counts are a critical component in the delivery of safe perioperative nursing care. Prevention of retaining a foreign object postoperatively is of paramount importance. The legal precept of *res ipsa loquitur,* or the evidence stands for itself, is the basis on which defendants are considered guilty of leaving a foreign object in a client. The surgical team is responsible to account for all sponges, sharps, instruments, and accessory items used during the procedure. AORN's (1999) *Recommended Practices* provides guidelines for performing counts. The general guidelines include the following:

- Counts should be done by two individuals, one of whom should be a RN.
- Sponges and instruments should be counted on all procedures in which a possibility exists that a sponge or instrument could be retained.
- Sharps should be counted on all procedures.
- Do not remove counted items from the room.
- Broken items should be accounted for in their entirety.
- Closing counts should occur when closure of a body cavity begins and immediately before case completion.
- Documentation should include names and titles of personnel performing the counts, results of the counts, actions taken if count discrepancies occur, and rationale for not performing a count.

In case of an incorrect count, it is the responsibility of the RN to inform the surgeon. The surgeon should search the operative field and wound while nursing personnel perform a recount of the missing item. A search of the OR (floor, trash, linen) should be conducted if the item is not found on the field. If the search is not successful, an x-ray film is usually taken to determine whether the missing item has been retained in the client. Personnel are encouraged to fully understand and follow institutional polices regarding counts to legally protect clients and themselves.

Pneumatic Tourniquet Precautions. The pneumatic tourniquet includes an inflatable cuff, pressure source, pressure regulator, connective tubing, and a pressure display. They may be disposable or reusable. Pneumatic tourniquets primarily are used to occlude blood flow and to obtain a near-bloodless operative field, but they may also be used to confine a bolus of local anesthetic in a distal extremity during IV regional anesthesia (i.e., Bier block). Use of a tourniquet is contraindicated in clients with vascular insufficiency or neurologic impairment.

Before each use, pneumatic tourniquets should be inspected and tested because unintentional pressure loss can result from loose tubing connectors, deteriorated tubing, stopcock leaks, cuff bladder leaks, or worn cuff closures. Newer systems offer an automated, computerized microprocessor that performs self-calibration, displays elapsed inflation time, and sounds alarms. Refer to individual manufacturer's guidelines for testing and maintenance of tourniquets.

The client's extremity and skin should be assessed before application of a tourniquet. The cuff selected should be of the widest possible for the extremity and of an appropriate length. A 3- to 6-inch overlap is recommended. Based on manufacturers' instructions, application of cotton cast padding placed circumferentially without wrinkles may be suggested. If the tourniquet is applied before the surgical prep, care must be taken to avoid pooling of the prep solutions underneath the cuff to prevent a chemical burn. Pressure settings should be selected based on surgeon directions. The usual pressures for an upper extremity range from 135 to 255 mm Hg or 70 mm Hg above the client's systolic BP. Lower extremity pressures range from 250 to 450 mm Hg or two times the client's systolic BP.

Before inflation of the tourniquet, the surgeon or RNFA usually exsanguinates the limb using either an Esmarch (rubber) bandage or gravity. The tourniquet should always be inflated with the limb elevated. Once inflated, the cuff should not be readjusted. Inflation time should be kept to a minimum. It is common to notify the surgeon at 1 hour and each subsequent 15 to 30 minutes of the tourniquet inflation time. Ninety minutes is the recommended time limit for either upper or lower extremity tourniquet inflation. In addition, after a period of reperfusion (i.e., 5 minutes or more), the tourniquet may be reinflated for another 90 minutes. Tourniquets carry with them a risk of paresthesias and possible paralysis secondary to ischemia of tissues while the tourniquet is inflated.

Documentation related to tourniquet use should include cuff location; cuff pressure; time of inflation and deflation; skin and tissue integrity under the cuff before and after the use of the pneumatic tourniquet; identification, serial number, and model of the specific tourniquet; and the name of the person applying the cuff. All cuffs and equipment should be decontaminated and stored in accordance with the manufacturers' recommendations (AORN, 1999).

Medication Administration. The most common types of medications used during orthopaedic procedures are antibiotics, local anesthetics, hemostatic agents, and vasoactive drugs. Broad-spectrum antibiotics such as cefazolin sodium (Ancef) and bacitracin, or occasionally tobramycin sulfate (Nebcin), vancomycin hydrochloride (Vancocin), or gentamicin sulfate (Garamycin), are used

as prophylactic antibiotics and in irrigation fluids. Irrigation fluids are usually warm isotonic solutions (e.g., normal saline, lactated Ringer's). Irrigation may be administered into client's wound via a syringe, bulb irrigator, or pulse lavage. Pulse lavage delivers fluids at a high speed and force for debridement of tissues or irrigation alone.

Additional types of medications used in orthopaedic surgery include local anesthetics (i.e., lidocaine, bupivacaine [Marcaine], ropivacaine) used to anesthetize the area injected. Epinephrine may be added to local anesthetics to cause vasoconstriction and control bleeding. It may also be added to irrigation bags during arthroscopic surgery for the same effect. Hemostatic agents commonly used during surgery to control bleeding include thrombin, Avitene, Gelfoam, Surgicel, and bone wax. Thrombin assists in hemostasis by catalyzing the conversion of fibrinogen to fibrin for clot formation. Avitene is a microfibrillar collagen agent that acts to aggregate platelets during the conversion of prothrombin to thrombin. Gelfoam is an absorbable gelatin sponge that can absorb up to 45 times its weight in blood. It provides a physical matrix around which clot formation occurs. Surgicel is an oxidized cellulose product that can absorb up to 10 times its weight in blood. It is deactivated in the presence of thrombin. Bone wax is processed bees' wax that may be applied to the ends of cut bone to control bleeding and prevent bony regrowth. Antispasmodics (i.e., chlorpromazine [Thorazine], papaverine) are used topically to control vessel spasm during microsurgical procedures; steroidal preparations (i.e., triamcinolone [Aristicort]) can be injected to control edema.

Bone Cement. Polymethylmethacrylate (PMMA), medical bone cement, is considered a hazardous substance by OSHA. It is an acrylic substance used to secure implants to bone or to fill a joint cavity with "beads" of antibiotic-loaded cement after an infected implant is removed. The monomer (liquid) and polymer (powder) are combined on the sterile field to form the PMMA compound. The monomer is flammable and care should be taken not to spill any of the product. It may be mixed by hand, in a centrifuge, or in a vacuum that removes excess air bubbles, which may cause premature cracking of the cement structure. Environmental conditions are very important for preparation. Warm PMMA, implants, or room dramatically decrease setting time. PMMA may be refrigerated to extend setting time. As PMMA vapor is released during the mixing process, OR personnel face potential side effects from exposure. Exposure of OR personnel can be reduced significantly by using a forced-exhaust mixing stand that removes the vapor fumes from around the bowl or a vacuum pump that contains the fumes. Pregnant personnel are discouraged from being present when PMMA is to be used because of fume emission. Personnel using PMMA should not wear soft contact lenses because they are permeable to the fume emission. When bone cement is to be injected into a canal, the anesthesia care provider should be notified because reports have linked the use of PMMA to acute hypotensive episodes, creation of air and fat emboli, and cardiac arrests in surgical clients soon after implantation. Setting of cement causes an exothermic reaction, and care should be taken to prevent burns to the client's tissues. Bone cement is considered an implantable and should be documented as such on the intraoperative record.

Prosthesis of antibiotic-loaded acrylic cement (PROSTALAC) hip and knee joints were developed over the past decade by Dr. Clive Duncan, Head of the Department of Orthopedics at Vancouver Hospital; Dr. Bas Masri; Dr. Chris Beauchamp; Nancy Paris-Sceley, a biomedical engineer at the British Columbia Institute of Technology; and their colleagues (Kent, 1999). Previously, clients needed bed rest and a course of antibiotics for several weeks. The only other option for in situ antibiotics has been "beads" of antibiotic-loaded cement, but the researchers wanted to give clients a functioning joint along with the medication. The joints are made in the operating room, where the surgeon combines the antibiotic with the polymer, combines this with the monomer, and then sets it in the appropriate mold. Stainless steel is used for the stem parts of the joints and the cement coating interfaces with the bone surfaces. Research is continuing, and FDA approval is being sought.

Documentation. Documentation of perioperative nursing care is important to give an accurate accounting of the events during surgery. As more operating rooms automate processes, computerized documentation is increasing. Computerization of the perioperative record allows for easy utilization of standardized nursing languages, and many systems are equipped with case record defaults that can greatly decrease the time involved in documentation. Assessment, planning, implementation, and evaluation are critical elements of any documentation form or system. Identification of personnel providing care is integral to professional accountability. Assessment components should include pertinent history, allergies, level of consciousness, psychological readiness for surgery, sensory/communication impairments, skin appearance, and musculoskeletal and cardiopulmonary status. Preoperative admission criteria must be met and recorded. Infection control interventions, such as prep solution and location, insertion of drains, and dressing placement, must be noted. Injury prevention interventions (e.g., ESU settings, tourniquet documentation, surgical counts, positioning details, medications administered) need to be documented. Fluid volume deficit preventive measures, such as autotransfusions, urine output, and irrigation fluids, and estimated blood loss should be noted. Communication of important intraoperative events and clear description of the surgical procedure to personnel receiving the client should occur before relief to ensure positive outcomes and continuity of care.

Surgical Assistance. Assisting the surgeon with operative procedures and care of the surgical client is the focus of the RNFA during the intraoperative phase of care. The decision by a RN to practice as a first assistant must be made voluntarily and deliberately, with an understanding of the professional accountability that the role entails. The AORN's *Registered Nurse First Assistant Consumer Fact Sheet* (www.aorn.org/patient/rnfafact.htm) delineates that the intraoperative responsibilities of the RNFA include the following:

- Collaborating with the surgeon and other health care professionals for an optimal surgical outcome
- Assisting the anesthesiologist when applicable
- Assisting with client positioning, skin preparation, and draping
- Providing wound exposure
- Handling tissue appropriately to reduce the potential for injury
- Using and manipulating surgical instruments skillfully
- Controlling blood loss
- Suturing tissue

POSTOPERATIVE PHASE

Most ambulatory surgery centers have designated two separate phases of recovery of a surgical client. Phase 1 is the acute phase of recovery. The level of care and the attention paid to the client immediately on exiting the OR are consistent with that of the PACU. Established criteria must be met before clients are permitted to progress to phase 2 of recovery. Phase 2 is the surveillance phase of recovery during which the client progresses further and is readied for discharge to home in the ambulatory setting. This can be equated to the first 24 hours of a hospitalized client's stay.

Some institutions are beginning to practice fast tracking (bypassing phase 1 PACU and proceeding directly to phase 2). Currently, no agreed-upon definition of what factors are involved in fast tracking have been identified. According to ASPAN's *Position Statement on Fast Tracking* (www.aspan.org/PosStmts2.htm), institutional guidelines should include the following:

- Appropriate client selection
- Preoperative education of the client and family
- Appropriate selection and management of anesthetic agents
- Assessment criteria used to evaluate client readiness in bypassing phase 1 at the end of the surgical procedure
- Discharge criteria
- Monitoring and reporting client outcomes

Phase 1: Assessment

Orthopaedic nursing in the PACU is challenging and rigorous. In this high-tech era, the care demanded by the orthopaedic care requires vigilant general PACU knowledge and sound knowledge of orthopaedic procedures. Along with astute nursing assessment skills, skills in psychosocial nursing interventions is needed more frequently with this group because the goal of surgery is focused on restoring mobility and relieving pain and disability. The nurse must be sensitive to heightened anxieties and be empathic to individual needs.

Immediately after surgery under general, spinal, or epidural anesthesia, the client is transported to the PACU by the anesthesia care provider. Initial and ongoing assessments are necessary to evaluate the client's condition during the emergence and recovery stages.

The anesthesia care provider's report includes pertinent history and laboratory values and type of anesthesia, including preoperative and intraoperative medication and the times of administration. Communication of the type of surgery performed, along with significant OR events, including estimated blood loss and fluids administered, is shared. The anesthesia care provider remains present during this period in a collaborative manner until a thorough assessment has been made and the PACU nurse completes evaluation of the client.

In keeping with ASPAN (2000) standards, subsequent nursing actions are directed toward optimizing recovery from anesthesia, detecting and managing postanesthesia complications, providing ongoing assessments and interventions appropriate to the surgical procedure, and supporting the client emotionally. The anesthetized client is often described as "vulnerable" and "dependent" because many anesthetic agents and techniques temporarily suppress protective reflexes and vital organ function. Specific nursing care related to the orthopaedic client that begins in the PACU includes positioning, neurovascular assessment, care of immobilization devices, wound care, range-of-motion exercise, and observation for complications. Anesthesia time may be extensive for clients undergoing spinal or major reconstructive surgery; therefore, the potential for complications increases. Table 11–5 describes the general postanesthesia assessment.

Ineffective Airway Clearance and Ineffective Breathing Pattern

Airway Management. Airway problems are the most common complication in the PACU and include upper airway obstruction, respiratory depression, airway spasm, and aspiration. The vigilance of the PACU nurse is

---

TABLE 11–5. *Postanesthesia Assessment*

PARAMETER	ASSESSMENT
Patency of airway	Respiratory rate and pattern. Auscultate breath sounds.
	Presence of artificial airways (i.e., oropharyngeal or nasopharyngeal) or adjuncts (i.e., endotracheal tube) and presence and type of mechanical ventilation.
	Application of oxygen and pulse oximetry probe.
Vital sign stability	Heart rate and rhythm (with electrocardiogram as applicable), blood pressure, O_2 saturation, temperature.
	Assess any invasive hemodynamic monitoring lines, values, and waveforms (i.e., central venous pressure, pulmonary artery catheter).
Fluid status	Intake and output, estimated blood loss and replacement therapy.
Level of consciousness and neuromuscular status	Level of consciousness, orientation to person, place, and time, pupil size and reaction. Ability to respond to commands.
	Assess muscle strength (strong hand grips and leg strength, movement of extremities, sustained eye opening, and ability to lift head off pillow and hold for 5 sec) to determine recovery from neuromuscular blockers.
	If regional anesthetic techniques were used, sensory and motor functions of affected areas are assessed.
Patency of all lines	Assess patency of intravenous lines, type of therapy, and condition of IV site(s).
	Assess patency of urinary catheter, if present, along with amount and type of drainage.
Operative site	Assess dressings, drains, tubes, casts, and other orthopaedic devices. Assess neurovascular status of operative extremity (color, capillary refill, temperature, sensation, movement).
Positioning	Properly position client as indicated by condition, surgery, and anesthetic technique.
Color	Assess color of skin and mucous membranes.
Comfort	Assess both physical and emotional comfort, evaluating need for pain medication. Offer explanations, reassurance, and education.

directed toward the rapid detection of adverse events, thus "rescuing" the client from the consequences.

The tongue is the most common cause of airway obstruction in clients with a decreased level of consciousness. Muscle relaxation causes the tongue to fall back against the posterior pharyngeal wall, particularly in the supine position, impeding airflow. Signs and symptoms include sounds of snoring (there is no sound if obstruction is complete), the presence of respiratory efforts without evidence of exchange, the use of accessory muscles, and other signs of hypoxia. Measures to relieve this obstruction include the use of the head-tilt/chin-lift or jaw-thrust maneuver and use of nasopharyngeal or oral airways. Support of the airway continues until the client recovers enough to breathe spontaneously with a clear, unobstructed airway.

Temporary respiratory depression may result from many anesthetic agents or excessive doses of opioids. Instructions that encourage the client to take full deep breaths can support adequate gas exchange until the agents are sufficiently eliminated, either by being blown off (as with inhalation agents) or with further metabolism. If respiratory depression is caused by excessive doses of opioids, naloxone hydrochloride (Narcan) may be given but must be carefully titrated so that the desired postanesthesia analgesic effects are not overshot or abolished. After naloxone hydrochloride is administered, clients must be observed closely for renarcotization after 20 to 30 minutes because the duration of action of opioids outlasts that of naloxone hydrochloride. Obviously, frank respiratory arrest needs immediate treatment with manual ventilation with a bag-valve-mask. After the client is transferred to the general client care unit, or phase 2 recovery, basic measures to ensure optimal pulmonary function should continue, including frequent repositioning, encouragement of coughing and deep breathing, incentive spirometry, chest physiotherapy (if needed), and adequate control of pain to prevent splinting and anxiety with resultant shallow respirations.

Bronchospasm is a spasmodic contraction of the lower airways and is manifested by wheezing. Severe bronchospasm results in absent breath sounds. Treatment includes the administration of bronchodilators and oxygen therapy as indicated.

Pulmonary edema can develop after laryngospasm and can affect any client who has been intubated. Pulmonary edema after laryngospasm can be self-limiting and usually does not have long-term sequelae; however, it can be potentially life-threatening if unrecognized or misdiagnosed. Postlaryngospasm pulmonary edema (PLPE) is potentially life-threatening and can result in reintubation, mechanical ventilation, admission to an ICU, and a prolonged hospitalization. The exact cause of PLPE is unknown. Alterations in intrathoracic pressure and hemodynamics, thoracic muscle strength, and physiologic pulmonary changes related to the aging process have been associated with the development of PLPE. A

prerequisite for PLPE is a client who is breathing spontaneously against a partially or totally obstructed airway. As the name suggests, laryngospasm is an involuntary contraction of the intrinsic muscles that control the vocal cords or the extrinsic muscles of the larynx. Involuntary contractions result in either a partial or complete closure of the upper airway, obstructing airflow into and out of the lungs. Baltimore (1999) describes treatment as initially directed at relieving the laryngospasm using positive-pressure ventilation with a bag-valve-mask and paralytics. If manual ventilation of the client is ineffective, succinylcholine, a muscle paralytic with a short duration of action, is commonly used to stop laryngospasm. When the client's airway is patent, the focus becomes maintaining the airway patency and delivering oxygen to ensure adequate oxygen saturation of 90% or greater. Reintubation and mechanical ventilation with positive end-expiratory pressure (PEEP) may be necessary for a short time to ensure continued airway patency and oxygenation. Same-day surgery clients with PLPE may need to be admitted overnight, and those who require mechanical ventilation are admitted to the critical care unit.

Aspiration Precautions. Prevention or minimization of risk factors in the client at risk for aspiration is an important function of the anesthesia care provider and the PACU nurse. Acid vomitus can be aspirated or inhaled at any time during the perioperative period. Acid gastric contents can cause physical damage to the lung tissue, which may cause a form of pulmonary edema and subsequent adult respiratory distress syndrome (ARDS). Treatment of ARDS requires mechanical ventilatory support with PEEP.

Risk for Altered Body Temperature

Temperature Regulation. As discussed in the intraoperative section, hypothermia and shivering remain a major problem for postanesthesia clients. On arrival in the PACU, many clients shiver uncontrollably, with such violent contractions that it is sometimes difficult for them to extend an arm to have their BP measured accurately. Shivering may also interfere with an accurate pulse oximetry reading. Shivering represents the body's attempt to generate heat. Exposures to the cold OR environment, vasodilation, neuromuscular paralysis, and suppression of normal temperature-regulating mechanisms by anesthetic agents have all been implicated in postanesthesia hypothermia. Meperidine hydrochloride (Demerol) may be given to control postoperative rigors.

Efforts to attenuate the shivering are required because it increases myocardial oxygen demands fourfold; causes oxygen to bind more tightly to hemoglobin, inhibiting its release to the tissues; and makes the client uncomfortable. Monitoring of temperature and applying warm blankets or a hot air warmer are indicated.

Alteration in Fluid and Electrolyte Balance

Fluid and Electrolyte Management. Fluid and electrolyte balance is critical to proper body function. Alterations may be attributable to preexisting disease, nutritional compromise, drug therapy, overhydration, or underhydration. Treatment should be directed at the cause.

Urinary Retention

Urinary Retention Care. There is ample evidence that certain types of anticholinergics, anesthesia, analgesics, large volumes of IV fluids, pain, and anxiety may predispose clients to urinary retention. Older adults have a higher incidence of urinary retention because of decreased bladder capacity and diminished sensory function. Orthopaedic surgeries involving pelvic structures and total joint arthroplasty of the hip and knee place clients at high risk for urinary retention (Pavlin, Pavlin, Fitzgibbon, Koerschgen, & Plitt, 1999). An enlarged prostate and the inability of male clients to stand to void can also contribute to urinary retention.

Comprehensive urinary assessment includes determining the degree of bladder distention in relationship to IV fluids administered, urinary output, cognitive function, and preexisting urinary problems. Interventions include measures to help the client void spontaneously. If these are unsuccessful, the surgeon should be consulted for an order to catheterize the client.

Nausea

Nausea Management. Postoperative nausea and vomiting (PONV) are among the most common postoperative complaints and can occur after all types of procedures requiring anesthesia or sedation. The development of PONV can lead to serious complications, including aspiration, dehydration, electrolyte disturbances, and disruption of the surgical site. PONV leads to increased cost of treatment and may be associated with increased anxiety, dissatisfaction with the surgical experience, and anticipatory nausea in the future. Preoperative factors associated with an increased risk of PONV include age (young people more often than old people), gender (menses), obesity, previous history of motion sickness or postoperative vomiting, anxiety, gastroparesis, and type and duration of the surgical procedure. Postoperative factors influencing the development of PONV include pain, hypotension, use of opioid analgesia, movement, and oral intake. Despite the advent of new technology and pharmacologic agents, PONV continues to have an incidence of 20% to 30% today (Thompson, 1999). Incidences of PONV greater than or equal to 80% have been reported for clients after undergoing total joint replacement procedures with surgical anesthesia and no antiemetic prophylaxis (Chen, Frame, & White, 1998). Common pharmacologic measures include the administration of droperidol (Inapsine), ondansetron hydrochloride (Zofran), metoclopramide (Reglan), prochlorperazine maleate (Compazine), promethazine hydrochloride (Phenergan), and trimethobenzamide hydrochloride (Tigan).

Although much attention has been paid to the prevention of PONV during the past three decades, little information exists on the efficacy of antiemetic interventions in clients with established PONV. No consensus has emerged in the prophylactic use of antiemetic drugs.

The use of nonpharmacologic techniques to prevent PONV is becoming more prevalent. (Refer to the evidence-based practice table in this chapter.) Lee and Done (1999) performed a meta-analysis of the literature reviewing techniques such as acupuncture, electroacupuncture, transcutaneous electrical nerve stimulation, and acupressure. The main findings of this meta-analysis were that there was a significant reduction in early PONV in adults using nonpharmacologic techniques compared with placebo and that antiemetics versus nonpharmacologic techniques were comparable in preventing early or late PONV in adults. The authors concluded that nonpharmacologic techniques could be recommended in adults as an alternative to no treatment or to first-line antiemetic drugs to prevent early PONV, for example, in clients with known adverse reactions to antiemetic drugs and in those who wish to minimize drug intake in the clinical setting.

The National Institutes of Health (NIH) consensus statement on acupuncture (1998) reported that there is clear evidence that needle acupuncture is efficacious for adult postoperative and chemotherapy nausea. The P6 acupuncture point lies about 4 cm up the arm from the wrist creases and stimulation of this point reduces nausea and vomiting. Lee and Done (1999), in their systematic review, came to the conclusion that stimulation of the P6 point is effective in preventing PONV in adults, but not in children. Recently, a disposable transcutaneous device known as the ReliefBand (Woodside Biomedical, Inc., Carlsbad, California) was approved by the FDA for the treatment and/or prevention of PONV. The device uses low-level electrical current to stimulate peripheral nerves at the palmar aspect of the wrist.

Pain

Pain Management. For clients undergoing surgery, postoperative pain is an anticipated and often feared consequence. Both epidural and patient-controlled analgesia (PCA) are known to reduce stress responses by blocking afferent nociceptive (pain) stimuli, thus reducing neuroendocrine and metabolic responses induced by surgery. Clients should be empowered with the correct knowledge and allowed as much involvement in their pain management as they wish. Pain management is discussed in Chapter 5.

EXAMINING THE EVIDENCE: Moving Toward Evidence-Based Practice
Can Postoperative Nausea and Vomiting Be Reduced by Nonpharmacologic Methods?

AUTHOR(S), YEAR	SAMPLE SIZE	ACTIVITY	DESIGN	OUTCOME VARIABLE	MAJOR FINDINGS
Dundee et al., 1989	$N = 500$ women between the ages of 16–50 yr (45–80 kg) scheduled for minor gynecologic operations scheduled under general anesthesia Premedication was with nalbuphine 10 mg IM 60–90 min before surgery Acupuncture (ACP), in one form or other, was applied at the same time as the premedication	In random order, clients had either P6 acupuncture, "dummy ACP," or no treatment Noninvasive methods of applying the use of a conductive "stud" to the forearm and the final group was the use of "Sea bands"—acupressure Clients were followed at 1 and 6 hr post-treatment Anesthesia was standardized	Randomized, double-blind, controlled study	PONV at 1 and 6 hr	At all times of observation, invasive ACP was followed by a significantly lower incidence of sickness than that in the control group All four ACP treatments, both invasive and noninvasive, were of similar efficacy in reducing sickness during the first hour after operation Invasive acupuncture was followed by less sickness in the 1- to 6-hr period than with the noninvasive approaches
Gunta, Lewis, & Nuccio, 2000	$N = 300$ clients, 18 yr or older, who had surgery with general anesthesia (excluding persons having ear or gastrointestinal surgery)	Closed chart review and data collection by staff nurses assigned to clients in the postoperative period using a standardized data collection tool	Descriptive	Overall nausea and vomiting Surgery greater than 2 hr	39% incidence of nausea and vomiting Women were two times more likely than men to experience nausea and twice as likely to experience severe nausea ($p = .0001$) Persons with surgery lasting 2 hr or greater were twice as likely to experience nausea ($p = .002$)
Ferrara-Love, Sekeres, & Bircher, 1996	$N = 90$ outpatient surgery clients, older than age of 18 yr, excluding thoracic, oral-maxillofacial, ENT, and septoplasty/rhinoplasty	Treatment group received bilateral acupressure elastic bands on wrists Placebo group had elastic bands incapable of acupressure on wrists Control group received routine nursing and medical interventions for nausea and vomiting Antiemetics were prescribed by the anesthesiologist and administered to clients in all three groups if nausea persisted and/or emesis occurred	Single-center, randomized, placebo- and sham-controlled study	Postoperative nausea or vomiting in the operating room, PACU phase I, and PACU phase II	The incidence of nausea and vomiting did not differ overall in the OR or PACU phase I PACU phase II, the incidence was 10% for the treatment group, 20% for the placebo group, and 50% in the control group (overall, $p = .0001$)
Zarate et al., 2001	$N = 221$ outpatients undergoing laparoscopic cholecystectomy with a standardized general anesthetic	A transcutaneous Acupoint electrical stimulation (TAES) device was placed at the P6 Acupoint, whereas in the sham and placebo groups, an inactive device was applied at the P6 Acupoint and at the dorsal aspect of the wrist	Multicenter, randomized, double-blind, placebo- and sham-controlled study	PONV in clients undergoing cholecystectomy	TAES at the P6 Acupoint significantly reduced the incidence and severity of nausea, but not vomiting or retching, after laparoscopic cholecystectomy
Visalyaputra et al., 1998	$N = 125$ clients scheduled to have gynecologic diagnostic laparoscopy, ASA grade 1 or 2, aged 20–40 yr	Randomized into placebo, droperidol, ginger, and ginger plus droperidol Group 1 received two placebo capsules orally with 30 mL of water 1 hr before induction of anesthesia and an injection of normal saline Group 2 received two placebo capsules orally with 30 mL of water and droperidol 1.25 mg IV Group 3 received two capsules of ginger root orally with 30 mL water and normal saline IV Group 4 received two ginger root capsules orally with 30 mL water and droperidol 1.25 mg IV General anesthesia was standardized	Randomized, double-blind study	Post-test in PACU and by phone call at 24 hr postoperative Data collected from both time frames were pooled	There were no significant differences in the incidence of nausea with 32%, 20%, 22%, and 33% for the placebo (group 1), droperidol (group 2), ginger root (group 3), and ginger root and droperidol (group 4), respectively

EXAMINING THE EVIDENCE: Moving Toward Evidence-Based Practice
Can Postoperative Nausea and Vomiting Be Reduced by Nonpharmacologic Methods? **Continued**

AUTHOR(S), YEAR	SAMPLE SIZE	ACTIVITY	DESIGN	OUTCOME VARIABLE	MAJOR FINDINGS
Hinojosa, 1992	N = 40	Charts selected from 1986–1988	Qualitative study using systematic chart review	To identify documented interdependent and independent nursing interventions to prevent or relieve nausea and vomiting during the first 24 hr postoperatively	Nausea and vomiting was documented in only two PACU records and nine postoperative records. There was no way to determine whether this meant no occurrence of nausea and vomiting or just that interventions were not documented. Documented interventions included repositioning clients and administering medications. This study illustrates the need for education about nurses' responsibility to prevent or relieve postoperative nausea and vomiting and the importance in documenting these interventions
Barsoum, Perry, & Fraser, 1990	N = 152 general surgical clients aged 18–84 yr	Group 1 used acupressure elastic bands containing a plastic button to apply sustained pressure at the P6 point. Group 2 used control dummy bands without the pressure button. Group 3 used antiemetic injections of prochlorperazine with each opiate given as required. Bands were applied in the PACU	Randomized, controlled study	PONV measured with linear analogue scale	The severity of nausea was significantly (p = .002) reduced on both days 1 and 2 in comparison to both controls and drug treated clients
Agarwal, Pathak, & Gaur, 2000	N = 200 clients, ASA grade 1 or 2, between ages of 18 and 60 yr, undergoing elective endoscopic urologic procedures	Spherical beads of acupressure wristbands were placed at the P6 points on the anterior surface of both forearms. In group 2, they were placed inappropriately on the posterior surface. General anesthesia was standardized; no antiemetic medication was given before or during operation. The wristband was removed 6 hr postoperatively	Randomized, prospective, double-blind, placebo-controlled study	PONV	In the acupressure group, 25 clients had PONV compared with 29 in the control group, showing the application of acupressure wristbands at the P6 of both forearms 30 min before induction of anesthesia did not decrease the incidence of PONV in clients undergoing endoscopic urologic procedures
Lee & Done, 1999	N = 19 research articles studying the use of nonpharmacologic techniques to prevent PONV	These studies included ACP, electroacupuncture, transcutaneous electrical nerve stimulation, Acupoint stimulation, and acupressure	Meta-analysis	The incidence of nausea, vomiting, or both 0-6 hr (early efficacy) or 0-48 hr (late efficacy) after surgery	Using nonpharmacologic techniques, 20%-25% of adults will not have early PONV as compared with those receiving placebo. This systematic review showed that nonpharmacologic techniques were equivalent to commonly used antiemetic drugs in preventing vomiting after surgery. Nonpharmacologic techniques were more effective than placebo in preventing nausea and vomiting within 6 hr of surgery in adults, but there was no benefit in children

Box continued on following page

EXAMINING THE EVIDENCE: Moving Toward Evidence-Based Practice
Can Postoperative Nausea and Vomiting Be Reduced by Nonpharmacologic Methods? **Continued**

AUTHOR(S), YEAR	SAMPLE SIZE	ACTIVITY	DESIGN	OUTCOME VARIABLE	MAJOR FINDINGS
al-Sadi, Newman, & Julious, 1997	N = 81 clients scheduled for gynecologic laparoscopic surgery	In the study group, after induction of anesthesia but before the start of surgery and before administration of morphine, a sterile acupuncture needle was inserted bilaterally at the P6 point	Double-blind, randomized, controlled study	PONV in the hospital and after discharge	The use of acupuncture at the P6 point reduced the incidence of PONV in the hospital from 65% to 35% compared with placebo and after discharge from 69% to 31% compared with placebo
Fan et al., 1997	N = 200 clients, 108 were in the acupressure group (group 1) and 92 clients were in the control group (group 2), aged 19–59 undergoing outpatient surgery with general anesthesia	In the study group (group 1), spherical beads of the acupressure band were placed at the P6 point on both wrists. In the control group, the acupressure bands were tied loosely and the spherical beads were placed on the dorsum of both wrists. Both groups wore them for 6 hr postoperatively. Anesthesia was standardized and no antiemetic medication was given preoperatively or intraoperatively	Randomized, double-blind study	Observed presence of PONV by blinded researcher and checking of the order sheet for any antiemetics prescribed	In group 1, only 23% had nausea and vomiting as compared with group 2, in which 41% had nausea and vomiting ($p = .0058$)

ASA, American Society of Anesthesiologists; ENT, ear, nose, throat; OR, operating room; PACU, post anesthesia care unit; PONV, postoperative nausea and vomiting.

Phase 1: PACU Discharge Criteria

Once clients recover from the immediate effects of anesthesia and when they are hemodynamically stable, they may be discharged from the PACU back to their rooms or to phase 2. A common scoring system used to determine readiness for discharge from phase 1 is the Aldrete Post Anesthesia Recovery Scoring System (Aldrete & Kroulick, 1970). Scores of 0, 1, or 2 are assigned to the assessment findings of activity, respiration, circulation (BP), consciousness, and color. A score of 10 plus stable vital signs indicate readiness to transfer to phase 2.

Generally accepted criteria for determining readiness for discharge from the PACU are presented in Table 11–6, along with notable exceptions. An anesthesia care provider usually sees and evaluates the discharge criteria and then signs the discharge section of the PACU record.

The nurse who receives the client in phase 2 or on the general surgery care unit should have a full report from the PACU nurse, including information about the surgical procedure; type of anesthesia used; the course of events in the PACU; a description of the client's condition, including vital signs, mental status, and information about the operative site; report on the intake and output; and estimated blood loss. Additional information should include specific nursing care related to the orthopaedic client, including positioning, neurovascular assessment, care of immobilization devices, range-of-motion exercises, and surgeon-specific orders. Administration of medication with special attention to time of administration should be communicated because time of administration

in OR and PACU influence the subsequent medication schedule once the client is transferred.

Inpatient Postoperative Care

Postoperative care of the orthopaedic surgical client begins with transport via cart or hospital bed to the inpatient room. On admission to the surgical unit, the client receives a head-to-toe assessment. Specific nursing care related to the orthopaedic client includes comfort level, positioning, neurovascular assessment, care of immobilization devices, wound care, range-of-motion exercise, and observation for complications. Nursing actions are based on the assessment findings.

Prevention of complications and progression of the postoperative course are of paramount importance for the nurse caring for the hospitalized client. At this point, preoperative education is operationalized, and the client is expected to perform such activities as coughing and deep breathing, incentive spirometry, range-of-motion exercises, turning, positioning, and ambulation with assistive devices as appropriate. Providing education and encouragement empower the client to perform activities of daily living and return home. Information specific to postoperative care of clients undergoing particular surgical procedures may be located in various chapters throughout this book.

Phase 2: Outpatient Postoperative Care

The assessment, implementation, and evaluation process is synonymous with that of inpatient care. In the ambulatory setting, a client receiving local anesthetic agents may go directly to phase 2 of recovery. Clients may be assisted to a recliner, where vital signs are monitored every 30 minutes, and assessment of operative site continues. Analgesics are offered as needed. To prevent severe pain, clients who have received regional blocks should be offered oral analgesics before complete block dissipation.

When clients feel ready to tolerate oral intake, they are offered light snacks, such as clear liquids, toast, soda crackers, and cookies, depending on their condition and preference. Clients are helped to ambulate, using assistive devices as required. The ability to void is assessed, and any IV therapy is discontinued once the client is determined

TABLE 11–6. *Discharge Criteria: Phases 1 and 2*

PARAMETER	ACCEPTABLE CRITERIA	EXCEPTIONS
Phase 1		
Airway	Clear, unobstructed. Gag, swallow, and cough reflexes intact. Respirations unlabored. Able to cough and deep breathe.	Client intubated and being transferred to intensive care unit.
Level of consciousness	Awake and oriented to person, place, and time. Able to respond appropriately. Muscle strength indicates full recovery from neuromuscular blocking agents.	Postoperative deviation from preoperative baseline.
Hemodynamic status	Minimum of three stable vital signs taken 15 min apart. Heart rate between 60 and 100 beats per minute. Normal cardiac rhythm. Blood pressure within normal limits compared with baseline.	Alterations that have been evaluated by the anesthesiologist or surgeon, who clears the client for discharge.
Temperature	Afebrile No hypothermia	Fever that has been evaluated and is being treated.
Urinary output	At least 30 mL if urinary catheter is in place.	Decreased urinary output that has been evaluated by the anesthesiologist or surgeon, who clears the client for discharge.
Surgical site assessments	Dressings dry Drains and tubes patent without excessive drainage. Absence of signs and symptoms of postoperative complications.	Excessive drainage that has been evaluated by the surgeon.
Analgesics and sedatives	At least 30 min following an intravenous dose of medication or 1 hr following intramuscular injection.	Client with patient-controlled analgesia pump or epidural catheter.
Extremities affected by regional anesthetic techniques	Recovery of block with motor control of affected extremities.	None
Phase 2*†	Ability to ambulate. Episodes of nausea, vomiting, and dizziness are minimal. Tolerating clear liquids and light snack. Ability to void without difficulty. Pain controlled with oral medication. No intravenous sedation/analgesia received within 1 hr before discharge. Written discharge instructions and prescriptions given and understood. Escort present.	

*The parameters and criteria of phase 1 must be met along with the phase 2 criteria before discharge.
†Adapted with permission from Wetchler, B. V. (1981, August). Anesthesia for outpatient surgery. *AORN Journal,* p. 295. Copyright © AORN, Inc., 2170 S. Parker Road, Suite 300, Denver, CO 80231.

to be stable. Written discharge instructions are reviewed with clients and care providers. When discharge criteria are met, clients are allowed to go home.

Phase 2: Discharge Criteria

The Joint Commission on Accreditation of Healthcare Organizations and the Accreditation Association for Ambulatory Health Care have set criteria for discharging ambulatory surgical clients (phase 2; see Table 11–6). For orthopaedic clients, special emphasis is given to the assessment of the operative site, neurovascular integrity, and mobility status.

Occasionally, clients who are unable to meet the discharge criteria are admitted to the hospital overnight. Common reasons for unanticipated hospital admissions include bleeding, chest pain, arrhythmia, performance of more extensive surgery than originally planed, aspiration, persistent PONV, severe and uncontrollable pain, prolonged recovery, excessive sleepiness, or lack of an escort.

Discharge Planning. One of the most significant sources of potential liability is the discharge of clients from the ambulatory care setting. The purpose of discharge planning is to prepare the client for transfer outside the health care setting. Discharge teaching enables clients or their responsible escorts to provide postoperative care. Discharge teaching must be provided at a level appropriate for each client. The nursing process of assessment, planning, intervention, and evaluation provides an appropriate framework from which to teach. Remember, however, that teaching does not equate to learning. The nurse teaches, but it is the client who must learn. Many variables can affect learning within the ambulatory surgical setting, including anxiety and environmental distractions. If the client does not speak English, an interpreter is needed and the nurse should document that one was present. In addition, written instructions must be provided so that they can be referenced later. Clear, legible, and concise instructions are mandatory. General areas that typically are addressed in the ambulatory surgery setting of phase 2 are activity, diet, mediations, bathing, wound care, and special instructions and follow-up care. Clients are instructed to call for an appointment if one has not already been scheduled. Any difficulties with voiding, persistent PONV, excessive bleeding, severe pain, or signs and symptoms of neurovascular compromise or infection should be referred to the surgeon after discharge. If clients are unable to contact their doctor, they may contact the ambulatory surgery unit, the facility's emergency department, or the emergency department nearest their home.

Teaching: Prescribed Activity/Exercise. Resuming such activities as work, exercising, weight bearing, and therapeutic exercises or physical therapy is determined by the surgeon. It is important to ascertain that the client understands the treatment plan. Many anesthetic agents have long elimination half-lives, and the client is not considered to be in full control of his or her faculties during this period. Thus, the client should not drink alcohol, drive, operate machinery, perform activities that require high levels of alertness, or make any important personal or business decisions for 24 hours.

Teaching: Prescribed Diet. Many orthopaedic clients are able to progress to a full diet as tolerated. Nutritional status influences both wound healing and immune function, with implications for wound infection. Current suggestions for supporting wound healing include provision of protein 1.5 to 3 g/kg, depending on severity of the wound; 100 to 600 g of carbohydrate/day; and 1% to 5% of daily calories, or one third of nonprotein calories to be supplied as fat. In addition, 1 to 2 g of ascorbic acid and 200% of the RDA for B-complex vitamins are recommended to support healing (Whitney & Heitkemper, 1999).

Incision Site Care. To assist in the avoidance of wound infection, teaching the client about appropriate cleansing, monitoring, and promotion of healing of his or her surgical wound assists in the avoidance of wound infection. The CDC guidelines for infection control (Mangram et al., 1999) suggest that incisions be protected with a sterile dressing for 24 to 48 hours postoperatively. Hands should be washed before and after dressing changes or any contact with the surgical site. Also, client and family education regarding proper incision care, symptoms of SSI, and the need to report such symptoms should be completed. This issues of whether to cover an incision that was closed primarily after 48 hours or on when it is appropriate to shower or bathe with an uncovered incision remain unresolved. Restrictions on bathing are as specified by the surgeon. Most clients are instructed not to get their dressing or wound wet. The surgeon prescribes specific instructions about removing or changing the dressing.

Clients are told that a small amount of bloody drainage is to be expected. If appropriate, the client is taught to elevate the affected extremity, making sure that distal joints are higher than proximal joints and that the extremity is above heart level to promote venous return and decrease swelling. They should receive information related to checking the neurovascular status of the limb. Clients should receive cast care instructions if this type of immobilization device has been applied.

Teaching: Prescribed Medication. Preparing a client to safely take prescribed medications and to monitor for their effects is the nurse's responsibility. New prescriptions for medications such as oral opioid analgesics, antibiotics, or NSAIDs should be given with appropriate instructions. If a dose has already been provided in the ambulatory surgery unit, the client must be told exactly when the next dose is due. In addition, one must consider the client's ability to obtain the necessary medications after discharge. Advanced planning may require sending the escort to have prescriptions filled while the client is recovering.

Clients are told that mild aches and pains are not unusual and can be relieved with acetaminophen or similar nonaspirin analgesics. Aspirin is to be avoided for 7 to 10 days postoperatively because of its anticoagulant effect, unless medical circumstances dictate otherwise and the physician specifically gives this direction.

Clients are usually told to resume their usual medications. Diabetic individuals who take insulin usually require consultation with their medical doctor for necessary adjustments for the rest of the day.

Telephone Follow-up. The postoperative telephone call is an important tool for nurses to use in evaluating a client's ambulatory surgical experience. Monitoring client outcomes is essential in assessing the presence of postoperative complications and in ensuring client comfort, pain relief, and satisfaction (Kleinpell, 1997). A primary responsibility of the nurse during this telephone call is to notify the surgeon of any complications and to instruct the client on appropriate actions to alleviate problems. If the nurse attempts a call but there is no answer or if the nurse leaves a message, this should be documented. If a significant time passes and the nurse is unable to contact the client, the nurse should notify the surgeon and the appropriate supervisor to determine the need for further investigation.

INNOVATIONS AND FUTURE TRENDS

Genetics and robotics are the new areas that will affect orthopaedic surgical clients of the future. Escalating advances are occurring in genetic knowledge. In the near future, it should be possible to describe the complete sequences of genetic events that are involved in the normal development of the skeleton. An example is the use of genes that encode growth factors that promote tissue regeneration after injury or other diseases (Cole, 1999). Recombinant proteins produced after the introduction of the relevant human DNA sequences into cells or whole organisms, such as bacteria or animals, are likely to become commonplace. Orthopaedic surgeons can look forward to administering recombinant proteins to promote regeneration of tissues selectively or to modify other disease processes. Treatment may also be targeted to specific parts of the body by the direct injection of genetically modified somatic cells from the client, for example, synovial cells or chondrocytes into a joint or fibroblasts into tendon (Cole, 1999).

A new robotic method for screw implantation relies on a computed tomography (CT) scans of both vertebrae

and a mold that is reconstructed using a computer-aided engineering (CAE) system. From the reconstructions, the surgeon is able to do preoperative planning, including selection of pedicle screw diameter, direction of screw through pedicle, point of entry, and length of engagement. The three-dimensional models are then meshed to determine positions of the surgeon's preoperative plan relative to the mold (Abdel-Malek, McGowan, Goel, Kowalski, & Smith, 1997). This technology would not be limited to the spine; it should work for fixation anywhere within the body.

In a similar area of research, a technique presented at the XXXII Brazilian Congress in Orthopaedics and Traumatology by Dr. Hammuth Kiefer of Bunde, Germany, uses input from sensors placed above and below the joint (Reuters Health, 2000). A computer shows surgeons the exact position of the mechanical axis of the limb and ensures that the two components of the prosthesis are in perfect alignment. It is theorized that this computerized system can help orthopaedic surgeons position a knee prosthesis with 100% accuracy, thereby reducing the chance of loosening, wear and tear, and the need for revision surgery.

SUMMARY

Knowledge of preoperative, intraoperative, and postoperative nursing care, as well as anesthesia concepts, can enhance the quality of care provided by the perioperative orthopaedic nurse. The information in this chapter is intended as a general guideline for standards of care. Because perioperative practices may vary in different settings, refer to the specific policies at your institution and consult the References for additional information.

INTERNET RESOURCES

A.L.E.R.T., Inc. (a national nonprofit, tax-exempt organization website that provides educational materials, support groups, publications, and product information about natural rubber latex allergy): www.latexallergyresources.org
American Academy of Orthopaedic Surgeons: www.aaos.org/wordhtml/papers/advistmt/wrong.htm
American Society of PeriAnesthesia Nurses: www.aspan.org/PosStmts2.htm
Association of Operating Room Nurses, Inc.: www.aorn.org/patient/rnfafact.htm

REFERENCES

Abdel-Malek, K., McGowan D. P., Goel, V. K., Kowalski, D., & Smith, S. B. (1997). Bone registration method for robot assisted surgery: Pedicle screw insertion. Proceedings of the Institution of Mechanical Engineers. Part H. *Journal of Engineering in Medicine, 211*(3), 221-233.

Agarwal, A., Pathak, A., & Gaur, A. (2000). Acupressure wristbands do not prevent postoperative nausea and vomiting after urological endoscopic surgery. *Canadian Journal of Anaesthesia, 47*, 319–324.

Agu, O., Hamilton, G., & Baker, D. (1999). Graduated compression stockings in the prevention of venous thromboembolism. *The British Journal of Surgery, 86*, 992–1004.

Aldrete, J. A., & Kroulick, D. (1970). A postanesthesia recovery score. *Anesthesia and Analgesia, 49*, 924–933.

al-Sadi, M., Newman, B., & Julious, S. A. (1997). Acupuncture in the prevention of postoperative nausea and vomiting. *Anaesthesia, 52*, 658–661.

American Academy of Orthopaedic Surgeons. (2000). *Advisory statement on wrong site surgery*. Retrieved November 10, 2000. Available at www.aaos.org/wordhtml/papers/advistmt/wrong.htm

American Society of Anesthesiologists (ASA). (1999). *Practice guidelines for preoperative fasting and the use of pharmacologic agents to reduce the risk of pulmonary aspiration: Application to healthy patients undergoing elective procedures*. Retrieved November 4, 2000. Available at www.asahq.org/practice/npo/npoguide.html

American Society of PeriAnesthesia Nurses (ASPAN). (2000). *Standards of perianesthesia nursing practice*. Cherry Hill, NJ: ASPAN.

American Society of PeriAnesthesia Nurses (ASPAN). (no date). *A position statement on fast tracking*. Retrieved November 11, 2000. Available at www.aspan.org/PosStmts2.htm

Aronovitch, S. A. (1998). A 7-day, pilot, comparative, parallel, single center study to determine the safety and efficacy of the MicroPulse system for the prevention of pressure ulcers. *Advances in Wound Care, 11*(3 Suppl), 15–16.

Association of Operating Room Nurses, Inc. (no date). *Registered nurse first assistant consumer fact sheet*. Retrieved November 11, 2000. Available at www.aorn.org/patient/rnfafact.htm

Association of periOperative Registered Nurses (AORN). (1996). Recommended practices for skin preparation of patients. *AORN Journal, 64*, 813–816.

Association of periOperative Registered Nurses (AORN). (1998a). Recommended practices for electrosurgery. *AORN Journal, 67*, 246–255.

Association of periOperative Registered Nurses (AORN). (1998b). Recommended practices for use of the pneumatic tourniquet. *AORN Journal, 68*, 1053–1057.

Association of periOperative Registered Nurses (AORN). (1999). Recommended practices for sponge, sharp, and instrument counts. *AORN Journal, 70*, 1083–1089.

Association of periOperative Registered Nurses (AORN). (2000). Recommended practices for traffic patterns in the perioperative practice setting. *AORN Journal, 71*, 394–396.

Baltimore, J. (1999). Postlaryngospasm pulmonary edema in adults. *AORN Journal, 70*, 467–468, 470–474, 476, 479–484.

Barsoum, G., Perry, E. P., & Fraser, I. A. (1990). Postoperative nausea is relieved by acupressure. *Journal of the Royal Society of Medicine, 83*, 86–89.

Bell, R. D., & Merli, G. J. (1998). Perioperative assessment and management of the surgical patient with neurologic problems. In G. J. Merli & H. H. Weitz (Eds.), *Medical management of the surgical patient* (2nd ed.). Philadelphia: WB Saunders.

Blackburn, E. (1994). Prevention of hypothermia during anaesthesia. *British Journal of Theatre Nursing, 4*, 9–14.

Brazell, N. E. (1997). The significance and application of informed consent. *AORN Journal, 65*, 377–386.

Brumley, C. (2000). Herbs and the perioperative patient. *AORN Journal, 72*, 785–794.

Chen, J. J., Frame, D. G., & White, T. J. (1998). Efficacy of ondansetron and prochlorperazine for the prevention of postoperative nausea and vomiting after total hip replacement or total knee replacement procedures: A randomized, double-blind, comparative trial. *Archives of Internal Medicine, 158*, 2124–2128.

Cole, W. G. (1999). Genes and orthopaedics. *British Editorial Society of Bone and Joint Surgery, 81B*, 190–192.

Donnelly, A. J. (1994). Malignant hyperthermia. *AORN Journal, 59*, 393–405.

Dundee, J. W., Ghaly, R. G., Bill, K. M., Chestnutt, W. N., Fitzpatrick, K. T., & Lynas, A. G. (1989). Effect of stimulation of the P6 antiemetic point on postoperative nausea and vomiting. *British Journal of Anaesthesia, 63*, 612–618.

Dunn D. (1997). Home study program: Malignant hyperthermia. *AORN Journal, 65*, 755–758, 760–762.

El-Gamal, H. M., Dufresne, R. G., & Saddler, K. (2001). Electrosurgery, pacemakers and ICDs: A survey of precautions and complications experienced by cutaneous surgeons. *Dermatological Surgery, 27*, 385–390.

Fan, C. F., Tanhui, E., Joshi, S., Trivedi, S., Hong, Y., & Shevde, K. (1997). Acupressure treatment for prevention of postoperative nausea and vomiting. *Anesthesia and Analgesia, 84*, 821–825.

Ferrara-Love, R., Sekeres, L., & Bircher, N. G. (1996). Nonpharmacologic treatment of postoperative nausea. *Journal of Perianesthesia Nursing, 11*, 378–383.

Friberg, B. (1998). Ultraclean laminar airflow ORs. *AORN Journal, 67*, 841–851.

Garner, J. S. (1982). *Guideline for prevention of surgical wound infections, 1985*. Hospital Infections Program Centers for Infectious Diseases, Center for Disease Control. Available at http://wonder.cdc.gov/wonder/prevguid/p0000420/p0000420.asp.

Gunta, K., Lewis, C., & Nuccio, S. (2000). Prevention and management of postoperative nausea and vomiting. *Orthopedic Nursing, 19*, 39–48.

Hazen, S. E., Larsen, P. D., & Hoot Martin, J. L. (1997). General anesthesia and elderly surgical patients. *AORN Journal, 65*, 815–822.

Hinojosa, R. J. (1992). Nursing interventions to prevent or relieve postoperative nausea and vomiting. *Journal of Post Anesthesia Nursing, 7*, 3–14.

Hoshowsky, V. M. (Ed.). (1995). *Orientation to the orthopaedic operating room*. Pitman, NJ: National Association of Orthopaedic Nurses.

Kent, H. (1999). Built-in antibiotics to help prosthesis patients. *Canadian Medical Association, 161*, 1382.

Kleinpell, R. M. (1997). Improving telephone follow-up after ambulatory surgery. *Journal of Perianesthesia Nursing, 12*, 336–340.

Kurup, V. P., Kelly, T., Elms, N., Kelly, K., & Fink, J. (1994). Cross-reactivity of food allergens in latex allergy. *Allergy Proceedings, 15*, 211–216.

Kurz, A., Sessler, D. I., & Lenhardt, R. (1998). Perioperative normothermia to reduce the incidence of surgical wound infection and shorten hospitalization. *New England Journal of Medicine, 334*, 1209–1215.

Lee, A., & Done, M. L. (1999). The use of nonpharmacologic techniques to prevent postoperative nausea and vomiting: A meta-analysis. *Anesthesia and Analgesia, 88*, 1362–1369.

Lensing, A. W. A., Prandoni, P., Prins, M. H., & Buller, H. R. (1999). Deep-vein thrombosis. *Lancet, 353*, 479–485.

Mangram, A. J., Horan, T. C., Pearson, M. L., Silver, L. C., & Jarvis, W. R. (1999). Guideline for prevention of surgical site infection, 1999. Centers for Disease Control and Prevention (CDC) Hospital Infection Control Practices Advisory Committee. *AJIC American Journal of Infection Control, 27*, 97–134.

McEwen, D. R. (1996). Intraoperative positioning of surgical patients. *AORN Journal, 63*, 1059–1079.

Miller, R. D. (2000a). Preoperative evaluation. In *Anesthesia* (5th ed., pp. 824–884). Philadelphia: Churchill Livingstone.

Miller, R. D. (2000b). Cardiovascular monitoring. In *Anesthesia* (5th ed., pp. 1117–1206). Philadelphia: Churchill Livingstone.

National Institute of Health Consensus Conference. (1998). *Acupuncture, 158*, 2124–2128.

Nichols, R. L. (1996). Surgical infections: Prevention and treatment—1965 to 1995. *American Journal of Surgery, 172*, 68–74.

Nixon, J., McElvenny, D., Mason, S., Brown, J., & Bond, S. (1998). A sequential randomised controlled trial comparing a dry visco-elastic polymer pad and standard operating table mattress in the prevention of postoperative pressure sores. *International Journal of Nursing Studies, 35,* 1932–1933.

Osmon, D. R. (2000). Antimicrobial prophylaxis in adults. *Mayo Clinic Proceedings, 75*(1), 98–109.

Pandit, S. K., Loberg, K. W., & Pandit, U. A. (2000). Toast and tea before elective surgery? A national survey on current practice. *Anesthesia and Analgesia, 90,* 1348–1351.

Pape, T. (1997). Legal and ethical consideration of informed consent. *AORN Journal, 65,* 1122–1127.

Pavlin, D. J., Pavlin, E. G., Fitzgibbon, D. R., Koerschgen, M. E., & Plitt, T. M. (1999). Management of bladder function after outpatient surgery. *Anesthesiology, 91,* 42–50.

Pryor, F. (1997). Key concepts in informed consent for perioperative nurses. *AORN Journal, 65,* 1105–1110.

Reuters Health. (1999, October). *Use of herbal supplements may interfere with surgery outcome.* Retrieved November 4, 2000. Available at http://surgery.medscape.com/reuters/prof/1999/10/10.14/c1101 49h.html

Reuters Health. (2000, November 22). *New technique promises greater accuracy in knee replacement surgery.* Retrieved December 3, 2000. Available at www.reutershealth.com/frame2/arch.html

Rothrock, J. C. (2000). Perioperative patient preparation. In *The RN first assistant: An expanded perioperative nursing role* (3rd ed., pp. 127–150). Philadelphia: Lippincott.

Thompson, H. J. (1999). The management of post-operative nausea and vomiting. *Journal of Advanced Nursing, 29,* 1130–1136.

Visalyaputra, S., Petchpaisit, N., Somcharoen, K., & Choavaratana, R. (1998). The efficacy of ginger root in the prevention of postoperative nausea and vomiting after outpatient gynaecological laparoscopy. *Anaesthesia, 53,* 506–510.

Whitney, J. D., & Heitkemper, M. M. (1999). Modifying perfusion, nutrition, and stress to promote wound healing in patients with acute wounds. *Heart & Lung: The Journal of Acute and Critical Care, 28,* 123–133.

Wymenga, A. B., Van Dijke, B. J., Van Horn, J. R., & Slooff, T. J. (1990). Prosthesis-related infection. Etiology, prophylaxis and diagnosis. *Acta Orthopaedic Belgica, 56,* 463–475.

Zarate, E., Mingus, M., White, P. F., Chiu, J. W., Scuderi, P., Loskota, W., & Daneshgari, V. (2001). The use of transcutaneous Acupoint electrical stimulation for preventing nausea and vomiting after laparoscopic surgery. *Anesthesia and Analgesia, 92,* 629–635.

12

Modalities for Immobilization

SARAH REDEMANN

Methods of immobilization have been used for centuries and play an important role in treating persons with musculoskeletal conditions. Despite modern technology and improvements in materials used, the basic concept of immobilization remains constant. The nurse needs in-depth knowledge of the effects of immobility on all body systems (see Chapter 4) as well as knowledge of the purpose for immobilization, devices available, and possible complications associated with these devices.

The purpose of immobilization is to secure the injured part of the musculoskeletal system to prevent further injury, promote healing, promote a functional result, and reduce pain. The term *immobilizer* has a twofold meaning. It is a generic term to include modalities for securing an injured part (i.e., casts and splints), and it is a specific term referring to a type of immobilizing device such as a knee immobilizer. The various modalities used to obtain adequate immobilization discussed in this chapter include immobilizers, splints, casts, traction, and external fixators. Immobilizers, casts, and splints temporarily immobilize the body part to prevent or correct deformity, maintain support, or protect a fracture or soft tissue injury. Traction uses a pulling force to promote or maintain alignment; realign bone fragments; decrease muscle spasm and pain; and correct, lessen, or prevent deformity. External fixation uses percutaneous pins and a rigid external frame to immobilize fractures, maintaining length and alignment while healing takes place.

Many of these procedures are performed in the outpatient, emergency, or bedside/treatment room setting. Simple orthopaedic procedures such as wound care, fracture or dislocation reduction (manual traction), and placement of traction pins can be accomplished with the client under local anesthesia alone. When more extensive analgesia or muscle relaxation is required, conscious sedation with an intravenous narcotic and tranquilizer is added to the anesthesia protocol. The addition of these medications is beneficial in the reduction of major joint dislocations and long-bone fractures, particularly in counteracting the large deforming forces necessary to facilitate the injury reduction.

IMMOBILIZERS, SPLINTS, AND CASTS

Immobilizers

Immobilizers are a temporary means of securing a part of the body. Immobilizers are removable and are used to maintain support and immobilize injuries, especially injuries to joints. Commonly used commercially available immobilizers include ankle (referred to as 3-D or CAM walker), knee, wrist, elbow, shoulder, and cervical immobilizers. Immobilizers can be removed for range of motion (ROM) of the injured joint, depending on the injury, to allow quicker return of function. Client compliance must be taken into consideration when using removable immobilizers for fracture treatment.

Splints

Splints may be used in all stages of musculoskeletal injuries. Initially, splints may be used for fractures because they are not circumferential, thereby accommodating swelling without risks of constriction. They are easy to apply and remove, allowing for monitoring of soft tissue swelling and skin integrity. A splint may be the definitive treatment for sprains and some fractures. Splints may also be used after initial treatment with casting to provide continued support. There are various forms of splints, ranging from improvised splints made of wood slats to prefabricated splints commercially available. Examples of prefabricated splints and immobilizers are shown in Figures 12-1, 12-2, and 12-3. Some

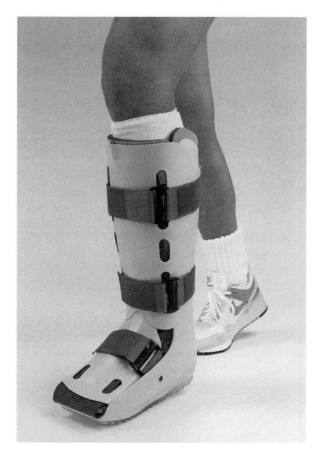

FIGURE 12–1. Pneumatic walker. (Courtesy of AirCast.)

specialized immobilizers provide a means of applying cold or intermittent pressure.

Casts

Casts provide more effective immobilization than splints or immobilizers. Cast types and common uses are described in Table 12–1.

Casting Materials. Casting materials include plaster of Paris and synthetic materials, such as polyester-cotton knit, which is impregnated with polyurethane, fiberglass, or thermoplast. The type of material used is generally based on physician preference. There are significant differences between plaster of Paris and fiberglass cast materials. Plaster of Paris has good molding ability after fracture reduction, is quite messy to apply, takes considerably longer to dry (24 to 48 hours), and is not water resistant; however, it is very cost-effective. Fiberglass materials have molding ability, set up much faster than plaster (5 to 30 minutes), are water resistant, are less messy to apply, and are lightweight; however, these are more expensive.

Cast Application. Cast integrity should be maintained throughout the course of cast therapy. Following application, a plaster of Paris cast is left uncovered to

allow air-drying. The larger and thicker the cast, the longer the required drying time. To prevent indentations in the soft plaster, the cast must be supported and moved with the palms of the hands instead of the fingers. The casted extremity should be placed on a soft, nonplastic surface to prevent flattening of the damp plaster or entrapment of heat. During drying, frequent position change promotes drying of the cast. The client must be turned as a unit, taking care not to use the cast or parts of it (e.g., abductor bars) as movement aids. The cast must be inspected for cracks, softening, or excessive flaking. Weight bearing, if permitted, should not occur until the

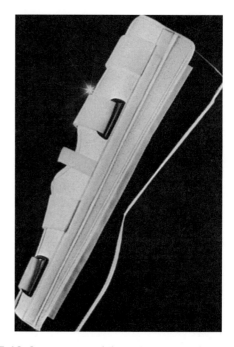

FIGURE 12–2. Knee immobilizer. (Courtesy of Zimmer, Inc., Dover, Ohio.)

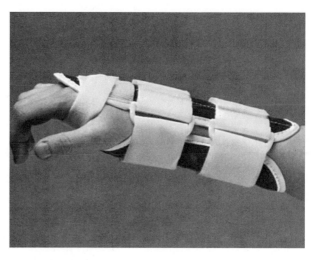

FIGURE 12–3. Wrist immobilizer. (Courtesy of Zimmer, Inc., Dover, Ohio.)

TABLE 12–1. *Cast Types and Common Uses*

TYPE	ILLUSTRATION	BODY PART COVERED	COMMON USES
Short-leg cast		Foot to below knee	Fracture of the foot, ankle, or distal tibia or fibula Severe sprain or strain Postoperative immobilization following open reduction and internal fixation Correction of deformity, such as talipes equinovarus
Long-leg cast		Foot to upper thigh	Fracture of the distal femur, knee, or lower leg Soft tissue injury to the knee or knee dislocation Postoperative immobilization following arthrodesis of the knee
Abduction boots		Feet to below knee or upper thigh	Postoperative immobilization following hip abductor release Maintain abduction
Unilateral hip spica cast		Entire leg and trunk to waist or nipple line	Fracture of the femur Postoperative immobilization following open reduction and internal fixation Correction of deformity, such as congenital soft tissue injury following dislocation of the hip

TABLE 12–1. *Cast Types and Common Uses* Continued

TYPE	ILLUSTRATION	BODY PART COVERED	COMMON USES
Bilateral long-leg hip spica cast		Entire leg bilaterally to waist or nipple line	Fractures of femur, acetabulum, or pelvis Postoperative immobilization following open reduction and internal fixation
Short-leg hip spica cast		Knees or thighs bilaterally to waist or nipple line	Developmental dysplastic hip
Short-arm cast		Hand to below elbow	Fracture of the hand or wrist Postoperative immobilization following open reduction and internal fixation
Long-arm cast		Hand to upper arm	Fracture of the forearm, elbow, or humerus Postoperative immobilization following open reduction and internal fixation
Shoulder spica cast		Trunk and shoulder, arm and hand	Shoulder dislocation Soft tissue injury to the shoulder, such as rotator cuff tear Postoperative immobilization following open reduction and internal fixation

cast is completely dry. A lower extremity plaster cast may not be completely dry for up to 48 hours. Plastic or commercially available cast protectors can protect the cast from wetness during bathing. Other sources of moisture, such as humidifiers, should be avoided.

Synthetic casting materials harden rapidly, thereby facilitating early weight bearing, often within 30 minutes of application. Because the cast dries quickly and can dry during application, synthetic casting materials must be applied rapidly.

Before cast application, the client should be informed that because of the chemical reaction that causes the cast to become hard quickly, heat is produced and it will feel warm. Excessive complaints of burning sensation should not be ignored. Thermal injuries can occur under the cast or splint and result from the water being too warm or the cast being placed on plastic-covered pillows following application. These injuries occur more often when the cast or splint is thick, warm water has been used for dipping the materials, and fast-setting plaster is used. When a cast or splint is applied, the water used for wetting plaster material should be at ambient (room) temperature. The directions for synthetic materials should be consulted before application. The extremity should be placed on a nonplastic surface as the cast or splint dries because plastic can cause heat to be trapped.

Cast Maintenance. Some casting fabrics are loosely woven and tend to be rough, whereas others are tightly woven and feel smooth. If the surface of the cast is rough, a sock or stockinette may be used to protect the opposite limb, prevent snags in clothing, and prevent scratching of furniture. A nail file or emory board can also be used to reduce rough edges.

Skin integrity can be compromised from pressure or rubbing of the cast or immobilizer. Adjacent skin must be cleansed of cast material residue. The client should be instructed to inspect the skin at regular intervals and advised not to place any foreign objects, such as coat hangers or back scratchers, beneath or into the cast.

Synthetic casts may be immersed in water only with specific orders from the physician. Special water-resistant padding can be used for faster drying if the nurse knows that the client will be getting the cast wet. If immersing is permitted, the skin under the cast must be adequately flushed if exposed to chlorine. Drying, a process that can require several hours, can be accomplished with the use of a hair dryer on a low setting. The skin can be burned if the hair dryer is used at a high setting. The physician should be notified immediately if a client complains of a burning sensation under the cast.

An immobilizer in close proximity to the perineal area must be protected from soiling with urine and stool. Plastic should be used to protect cast edges during toileting or bedpan use. A disposable diaper may also be used. The diaper is tucked inside the cast a short distance and then pulled back over the edge of the cast and taped down so that the absorbent side is showing. A disposable diaper can be tucked inside a spica cast for infants and non–toilet-trained toddlers. Only when necessary, a soiled plaster cast can be cleansed with a mild, white, powdered cleanser and a slightly dampened cloth. Commercially available urine-collecting and stool-collecting devices may be necessary for the child or incontinent adult.

Cast Splitting. As a circumferential immobilizer, casts can cause the same effect as a constrictive bandage, that is, pressure or edema or both in the underlying skin and tissues. Casts may need to be opened or replaced to observe the underlying skin or wound or to alleviate pressure in a specific area because of severe swelling. The nurse must be aware of indications for cast splitting (increasing pain, pressure, swelling, and signs of decreased circulation or compartment syndrome). In these cases, casts can be univalved, bivalved, or windowed.

A univalved cast is split anteriorly to facilitate spreading of the casting material and padding beneath it. A bivalved cast is split medially and laterally to create an anterior and a posterior portion. Removal of the anterior portion allows inspection while immobilization is maintained by the posterior portion. Removal of the anterior portion should be done by direction of the physician so reduction is not lost.

In a windowed cast, a specific area is cut out to permit inspection of skin or incision, to remove sutures or staples following surgery, or to relieve pressure without having to replace the entire cast. The window piece of the cast should be saved because it is often reinserted if there is no underlying tissue damage or edema. To restore the integrity of the immobilizer, tape, elastic bandages, or additional cast material is used. Because additional pressure from excessive swelling can cause tissue to protrude into the space where the cast was univalved, bivalved, or windowed, additional padding may be placed into the space before applying tape, elastic bandage, or additional cast material.

Assessment of the Client with an Immobilizer

Nursing assessment begins with the first client contact and follows through until the client achieves maximal return of structure and function. The type and extent of trauma and the underlying structures involved give the nurse clues as to what should be included in the physical assessment.

Because the client and family will be providing care at home, the nurse teaches the family how to assess any and all changes in circulation, motion, and sensation, as well as changes in pain or pressure. The clients should be told about the importance of reporting symptoms. No complaint of pain, pressure, or burning should ever be ignored.

Neurologic Assessment and Intervention. Neurologic evaluation centers on areas where nerve function may be compromised because of the immobilizer or positioning. In lower extremity injuries, the deep and superficial peroneal and the tibia nerves are most at risk. In the upper extremity, the radial nerve and the ulnar nerve should be assessed. Figure 8-6 describes neurovascular assessment of these nerves. There are many individual variations, and tingling or numbness or both may not be present, even with nerve compression. The client should be assessed every 30 minutes for 4 hours after immobilizer application and then every 3 to 4 hours.

Neurovascular status is monitored throughout the course of immobilization. Areas in the extremities that are at particular risk are noted in Figure 12-4. Changes in the client's activity level and increased time in the dependent position can alter neurovascular status. Ice can be applied to minimize edema, thereby decreasing pressure. The extremity should be elevated higher than heart level to prevent and control edema. This is especially important during the first 48 to 72 hours after cast application. Elevation should be continued as long as the client complains of increased pain and swelling when the limb hangs down, which may take a couple of weeks depending on the severity of the injury. (Swelling can occur 6 months to a year after fracturing or severely spraining a joint.) Once the swelling is down and seems to be under control, frequent assessment must be continued to ensure that the cast is not too loose, which could cause skin irritation because of rubbing or possible loss of fracture reduction because of inadequate immobilization. On some occasions, clients have pulled the cast off and put it back on because the cast became loose after the swelling went down after initial application.

The potential for nerve damage is greater when elastic bandages are used to hold splints in place and when immobilizers are applied too tightly. A poorly fitting splint or immobilizer can also impair neurovascular integrity. Special attention should be made when applying a knee immobilizer to ensure that the strap directly below the knee, which usually goes over the fibular head, is not pulled excessively tight thereby putting pressure on the peroneal nerve. The same holds true for a walker used in ankle injuries; the strap at the top and across the ankle at the bottom of the splint must not be applied to tightly. Prefabricated wrist splints need to be observed for constant pressure placed at the base of the thumb, which, long term, can cause nerve damage as well. A well-fitting splint or immobilizer should cause no change in sensation (e.g., numbness) or feeling of pressure.

Circulatory Assessment. Circulatory assessment evaluates the presence or absence of pulse(s), pain, pallor, or coldness. The immobilizer may interfere with evaluation of the pulse, and a Doppler scan may be helpful. The pulse, color, and warmth of the extremity are compared with the noninjured extremity.

Drainage Assessment. If a surgical approach was used or when there is a wound beneath the immobilizer, there may be drainage. Initially, bright red drainage is expected (25 to 48 hours), which gradually turns brownish. During these first 48 hours, assessments should be made every 3 to 4 hours. After 48 hours, drainage may indicate tissue infection or sloughing. The drainage may run or seep through to the dependent part of the immobilizer. No direct relationship exists between the amount of cast drainage observable and the amount of drainage from a wound. Plaster casts are absorbent and act as a sponge, and synthetic casts may act as a wick; therefore, drainage may not be directly apparent near the drainage site. Padding beneath the cast can absorb wound drainage so that it does not appear on the cast itself. Nonetheless, the drainage area on any cast should be measured and documented. Outlining the drainage area on the cast and placing the date and time is a good way to monitor amount and change in drainage. The client should be informed that this is not necessarily something

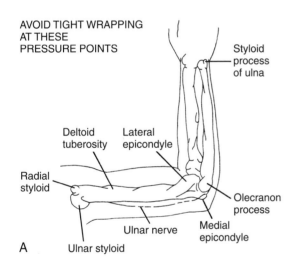

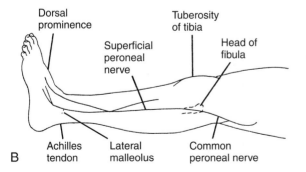

FIGURE 12–4. *A,* Danger points in the upper extremity. *B,* Danger points in the lower extremity. (Courtesy of Zimmer, Inc., Dover, Ohio.)

to be upset about but something that does need to be watched. Any large increase or change in consistency, color, or odor should be reported to the physician immediately.

When there is an immobilizing device encircling the body or an extremity, there is the possibility of skin damage and neurovascular injury. Compartment syndrome, cast syndrome (superior mesenteric artery syndrome), and pressure ulcers are potential complications. Assessment for these complications is described in Chapters 4 and 10 and later in this chapter.

Nursing Management of Client with Immobilizers

Nursing care for the client being treated with immobilizing devices requires attending to comfort, providing education, monitoring for and managing complications, and assisting the client to adapt to functional and body image changes.

Anxiety

Anxiety Reduction. Immobilizing devices affect a client's ability to work, to maintain a home, and to continue normal activities. For the older client, it may contribute to increased disability and risk for additional injuries.

Whether the client is being treated in the ambulatory or acute care setting, anxiety about what will happen at home can be reduced through discussion with the client and family about the anticipated phases of immobilizer use and the perceived problems. Adaptive aids, minor changes in the home environment, and social agencies can be useful in promoting self-care and home care. Major adjustments may need to be made in some cases, for example, the child going home with a body cast. Working with the client and family before the client goes home or eliciting help from home health can decrease anxiety for these clients. Siblings may need to be involved in discussions. Box 12–1 provides educational guidelines for clients in immobilizers.

High Risk for Injury

Cast or Immobilizer Complications. The nurse must be aware of indications for cast splitting (increasing pain, pressure, swelling, and signs of decreased circulation or compartment syndrome). A cast cutter, spreader, large scissors, additional padding, and additional cast supplies or ace bandages should be available for this purpose. The client should be instructed about these symptoms, which indicate complications, and should be advised to seek immediate attention if they occur.

A poorly fitting splint or immobilizer can also impair neurovascular integrity. Special attention should be made when applying a knee immobilizer to ensure that the strap directly below the knee, which usually goes over the

fibular head, is not pulled excessively tight putting pressure on the peroneal nerve. The same holds true for a walking immobilizer used in ankle injuries. The strap at the top and across the ankle at the bottom of the splint should not be applied too tightly. Prefabricated wrist splints need to be observed for constant pressure placed at the base of the thumb, which, long term, can cause nerve damage. A well-fitting splint or immobilizer should cause no change in sensation (e.g., numbness) or feeling of pressure.

When there is an immobilizing device encircling the body or an extremity, there is the possibility of skin damage and neurovascular injury. Compartment syndrome, cast syndrome (superior mesenteric artery syndrome), and pressure ulcers are potential complications. Assessment for these complications is described in Chapters 4 and 10 and later in this chapter.

Pain

Pain Management. Comfort should be promoted with the use of analgesics, particularly after cast application if manipulation or reduction was required. The use of analgesic agents before activity can prevent pain. Elevation and cold therapy can also promote comfort, especially after activity. Progressive pain, pain out of proportion to the injury or treatment, and pain not relieved by comfort measures may be indicative of compartment syndrome (see Chapter 10). Chapter 5 discusses other comfort measures.

Pain that persists several days after reduction or immobilization should be investigated thoroughly. Hot spots or dull pain under an immobilizer may indicate tissue damage. Severe pain expression may suggest inadequate coping, extreme anxiety, further musculoskeletal damage, or injury to underlying parts that was not previously recognized.

Disuse Syndrome

Exercise Therapy: Joint Mobility and Ambulation. Mobility should be promoted within prescribed activity restrictions. Joints above and below the immobilizer should be actively exercised. If the client must be on bed rest, an exercise program for unaffected extremities should be instituted. Isometric exercises of the affected limb are encouraged, as is frequent movement of fingers and toes to reduce swelling and promote circulation. Bath time is a good opportunity to go through passive ROM exercises and evaluate limitation of motion. Because many orthopaedic clients are older adults, concomitant disorders, such as osteoarthritis and osteomalacia, may be present and need to be considered in instituting exercises, turning, and ambulating. Physical therapy is often prescribed following any immobilization treatment to regain function.

BOX 12–1.
Care of the Client Requiring Immobilization

Goal
To maintain immobilizer integrity; to ensure proper circulation, sensation, and motion of the affected body part and to immobilize the affected body part

Patient Education
I. Reinforce physician's explanation of the reason for the cast or immobilizing device and answer any questions for the client
II. Instruct the client and/or family member regarding the following items:
   A. Care of the cast
      1. Keep the cast dry (unless specifically instructed otherwise)
      2. Provide suggestions concerning bathing and showering (e.g., putting plastic bag over cast and applying tape to prevent water from seeping inside, propping affected extremity on something outside the tub or shower)
         a. Plaster casts that do get wet should be left open to the air and physician should be contacted
         b. Fiberglass casts should be dried with a hair dryer on low heat until padding feels comfortable
      3. Prevent soiling of cast: use plastic to protect the edges, especially around the perineum; if cast becomes soiled, wipe off with damp soapy cloth
      4. Check cast for cracks, softening, or flaking
      5. Observe skin around edges of cast to avoid blisters or skin breakdown
      6. Avoid putting anything down in the cast (e.g., using coat hanger or other sharp objects to scratch the skin)
   B. Immobilizer care
      1. The skin covered by removable immobilizers must be assessed for signs of irritation and pressure every 4 hours
      2. The immobilizer must be kept clean and dry; if perspiration accumulates, the device must be permitted to dry thoroughly when not in use
      3. Protect immobilizer from damage when not in use
   C. Elevation/exercise
      1. Elevate the immobilized limb "higher than your heart" to reduce swelling and pain; gravity alone can increase swelling and pain in an immobilized limb that is not elevated
      2. Unless otherwise instructed, you should be exercising your fingers or toes (whichever is affected) to increase circulation and reduce swelling; this should be done initially several times an hour; as time goes by and the swelling is under control, you can reduce this to several times a day
      3. Use your uninvolved arm(s) and leg(s) often; actively exercise joints above and below cast or immobilizer
      4. Once out of the immobilizer you will perform rehabilitation exercises to prevent reinjury
   D. Reportable symptoms
      1. Extreme pain not relieved by elevation or pain medication
      2. Swelling not relieved by elevation
      3. Numbness or tingling
      4. Skin irritation caused by cast/splint
      5. Extreme tightness of cast/splint
      6. Swollen, blue, or cold fingers or toes
   E. Return visits will be necessary for various reasons:
      1. Repeat x-ray films to check alignment of fracture if indicated
      2. Check and cast to make sure it is providing adequate immobilization
      3. Respond to concerns or questions you might have
      4. Change cast if and when necessary throughout the course of treatment
No question or concern should go unattended. Please call if there is anything we can do to alleviate your anxiety.

Impaired Skin Integrity

Skin Surveillance and Cast Care. Skin integrity can be compromised from pressure or rubbing of the immobilizer. Before application of the immobilizer, the skin must be examined and cleansed thoroughly. After application, the edges must be well padded and the skin inspected at regular intervals. Adjacent skin should be cleansed of cast material residue. The client should be instructed not to place any foreign objects, such as coat hangers or back scratchers, beneath or into the immobilizer. After removal of the immobilizer, the skin should be thoroughly cleansed with soap and water and a non-alcohol-based lotion applied.

The skin covered by immobilizers must be assessed for signs of irritation and pressure every 4 hours during the acute phase, which is usually 48 to 72 hours. The immobilizer must be kept clean and dry; if perspiration accumulates, the device must be permitted to dry thoroughly when not in use. Because many of the prefabricated immobilizers have plastic or metal stays to add support, excessive bending or damage to the immobilizer when not in use must be prevented because this could alter alignment when reapplied.

When a cast has been windowed, it is important to retain the piece of the cast removed to create the window so that it can be reapplied following inspection. The window should be replaced promptly after inspection to prevent swelling in the window region, which could cause skin breakdown along the edges of the window. The window piece can be held in place with an elastic bandage or with additional casting material or tape.

Fluid Volume Deficit (Cast Syndrome)

Fluid Management and Electrolyte Management. Fluid loss from cast syndrome can occur in clients with body casts. Cast syndrome (or superior mesenteric artery syndrome) is a serious complication that sometimes follows prolonged supine positioning or spinal instrumentation or the use of a spinal orthosis or body cast. Characterized by nausea, abdominal pressure, and vague abdominal pain, cast syndrome probably results from hyperextension of the spine. Hyperextension of the spine accentuates lumbar lordosis, causing compression of the third portion of the duodenum between the superior mesenteric artery anteriorly and the aorta posteriorly (Fig. 12–5).

Partial duodenal obstruction occurs initially from anatomic compression and progresses to complete obstruction from duodenal edema caused by vomiting and distention. The abdominal window of a body cast must be adequate to facilitate comfort after meals and with position changes. The client should be observed for nausea and vomiting, and the physician should be notified immediately if it occurs. Bowel sounds should be auscultated, and the abdomen should be palpated through the abdominal window when possible. If nausea and vomiting occur, the client should be given nothing by mouth and antiemetics should be avoided. The quality and quantity of emesis, as well as gastric contents if a nasogastric tube is used, should be monitored and recorded.

Intravenous access should be maintained, and the quantity and type of intravenous fluids should be monitored and recorded. The client should be repositioned on the abdomen, if tolerated, to relieve abdominal pressure. Cast removal or bivalving may be necessary. Surgery may be required to release the ligament of Treitz, which immobilizes the fourth portion of the duodenum at its attachment and aggravates distention. Untreated cast syndrome can be fatal because it causes obstruction of the superior mesenteric vein, leading to gastrointestinal hemorrhage and necrosis. It is important to teach clients who

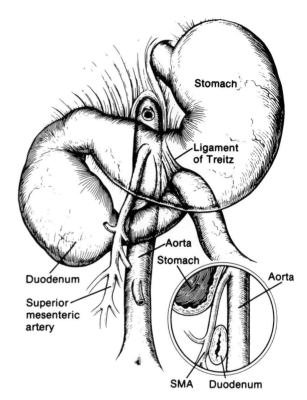

FIGURE 12–5. Cast syndrome. The diagram shows the anatomic relationship of the duodenum, aorta, and superior mesenteric artery (SMA; superior mesenteric artery syndrome). The lateral view suggests a nutcracker effect, with compression of the duodenum between the vascular structures. (From Cohen, L. B., Field, S. P., & Sachar, D. B. [1985]. The superior mesenteric artery syndrome: The disease that isn't, or is it? *Journal of Clinical Gastroenterology, 7,* 113.)

are to be discharged in body jackets or high hip spicas how to recognize cast syndrome, which can develop as late as several weeks or months after application.

Body Image Disturbance

Body Image Enhancement. A positive self-concept can be promoted by preparing the client for what life will be like with an immobilizer. Possible functional deficits imposed by the immobilizer must be anticipated and must be problem solved in advance. Specifically, possible alterations in mobility and social interaction that commonly occur with immobilization must be discussed. The client should be prepared for the appearance of the involved body part after immobilizer discontinuation. The nurse should explain that atrophy of muscles and changes in the appearance of the skin and hair can occur. Because of increased blood supply, hair over the fracture site is often much darker than usual and this color change is surprising to the client when the cast is removed. Hair and skin appearance returns to normal within several weeks of return to normal activity. The client should also be aware that joint stiffness is likely after immobilizer removal but diminishes with exercise.

Knowledge Deficit

Teaching: Procedure/Treatment. The client should be instructed about the potential complications of immobilizer therapy and how these complications should be reported to the physician. Elevation of the extremity during immobilization and following removal of the immobilizer should be encouraged to prevent and eliminate edema. The client should be instructed about the immobilizer and skin care. For infants and children, the parents must be advised on needed car seat adaptation. The client should be prepared for cast removal by explaining that although the cast saw is noisy, the vibrating blade is unlikely to damage the skin. Activity restrictions, exercises for muscle strengthening, and methods to avoid reinjury following immobilizer removal should be discussed. General immobilization instructions are included in Box 12–1.

Noncompliance

Teaching: Prescribed Activity/Exercise. Because the client is often able to remove and reapply splints and immobilizers at will, it may be necessary to evaluate compliance with the prescribed wearing schedule. Compliance is evident from the client's progress or lack of progress. Noncompliance may be attributable to an ill-fitting device or to misunderstandings by the client about the value of the device. Very young children may need some type of restraint to keep them from removing or repositioning the device. The activity needs of children need to be carefully addressed to increase compliance.

TRACTION

Traction, the application of a pulling force to a part of the body, can be used for a variety of reasons. When a bone is fractured or dislocated, traction is used to reduce the fracture, to maintain alignment, or to realign bone fragments until callus forms and calcification begins. Muscle spasm and pain can be alleviated with traction, which also corrects, lessens, and prevents deformities, including contractures. Traction is also used to promote rest and exercise and to maintain the position of a diseased or injured part.

One or a combination of the following mechanisms of force can be provided by traction. A static force promotes immobilization. A dynamic force promotes movement. Running traction exerts a pull in one plane. Balanced suspension uses traction to suspend a part of the body without pulling on the part and can be used in combination with skeletal traction.

Several basic principles are applied to maintain effective traction. Countertraction must always be provided by the client's body weight, the pull of weights in the opposite direction, or elevation of the bed itself. The line of pull must be maintained, and weights must always hang freely. Whether the traction is to be maintained continuously or intermittently should be included in the physician's order for the traction. Nurses must ensure accuracy in the amount of weight used, integrity of the ropes, alignment of traction, position of the client, and the maintenance of countertraction. Some positions are prohibited in different types of traction, and the physician should be consulted before client teaching. For example, the client in halo skeletal traction should not bend forward or twist the body at the waist because this changes the forces in the cervical spine (Botte, Byrne, Abrams, & Garfin, 1995).

Classification of Traction

Skin Traction. Skin traction is maintained by direct application of a pulling force on the client's skin. It is generally used as a temporary measure to reduce muscle spasms or to maintain immobilization before surgery. It should be removed and reapplied at least once a day.

Skin traction can be used for an extended period and is removed and reapplied intermittently as specified by the physician.

Skin adherents may be applied to maintain a steady pull, but they make assessment and reapplication more difficult. Ace wraps, belts, halter, boots, and slings are commonly used as skin traction devices. Between 5 and 8 pounds of weight are generally used in the adult client. Cervical traction, Buck's traction (Fig. 12–6), and Russell's traction are all forms of skin traction.

Complications of skin traction include skin blisters and necrosis, as well as compartment syndrome. Rotation of the extremity and inadequate immobilization, causing damage to the periosteum, can occur (Pierce & Witaker, 1994).

Skeletal Traction. Skeletal traction attaches directly to bone, providing a strong, steady, continuous pull, and can be used for prolonged periods. Weight can be applied with Steinmann pins or Kirschner wires to the extremities or with tongs or halo to the head. Sometimes, pins or wires are incorporated into a cast. The amount of weight used depends on the injury, pathologic condition, body size, and degree of muscle spasm.

Skeletal traction may be the sole treatment or may precede open reduction and internal fixation. Skeletal traction is never removed without a physician's order. Although methods of internal fixation are continuously improving, skeletal traction continues to have a place in the management of fractures with soft tissue injury, deformity, correction, and suspension of burned extremities. Use in older clients is avoided, if possible, because of

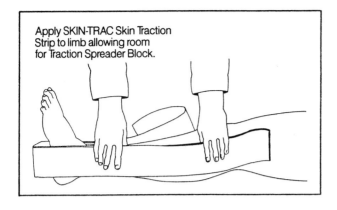

Apply SKIN-TRAC Skin Traction Strip to limb allowing room for Traction Spreader Block.

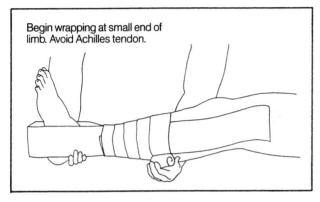

Begin wrapping at small end of limb. Avoid Achilles tendon.

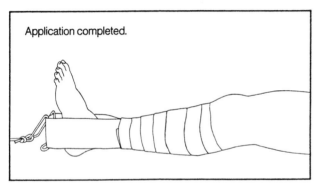

Application completed.

FIGURE 12–6. Buck's traction wrapping. (Courtesy of Zimmer, Inc., Dover, Ohio.)

osteoporosis. Complications specific to skeletal traction are related to hardware use and include pin site infections, neurovascular damage, and osteomyelitis.

Manual Traction. Manual traction is applied with the hands to temporarily immobilize an injured part. A firm, smooth, steady pull is maintained. Manual traction is used during casting, reduction of a fracture or dislocated joint, and halo or tong application. Types of traction, uses, and nursing management are listed in Table 12–2.

Complications

Potential complications from the use of traction include neurovascular compromise, inadequate fracture align-

ment, skin breakdown, and soft tissue injury. Pin tract infection and osteomyelitis can occur with skeletal traction. In addition, complications from immobility (described in Chapter 4) can be encountered, especially with long-term traction and in older adults.

Diagnostics and Assessment

When caring for the client in any type of traction, the nurse must be aware of the client's history, with special emphasis on the reason for traction. Knowledge of the purpose and type of traction and whether the traction is continuous or intermittent is essential. Assessment immediately after the initiation of traction may be more frequent than when the soft tissue injury has subsided.

Physical examination emphasizes the area of the body requiring traction as well as the traction itself. Comparison should be made with the most recent assessment and with the unaffected extremity when possible. Assessment of circulatory status includes obtaining a history of circulatory difficulties that might increase the potential for complications from traction. Assessment of neurovascular status includes evaluating pain, sensation, active and passive ROM, color, temperature, and capillary refill. Although neurovascular assessment includes evaluation of pulses, the nurse must remember that the client with compartment syndrome or nerve palsy can nevertheless have intact distal pulses.

As long as the client is in traction, skin integrity must be assessed and documented, examining especially for redness, bruises, and lacerations. The client's positioning in bed, as well as traction positioning and alignment, requires constant vigilance. The traction ropes and knots must be intact and secure (Fig. 12–7). A photo or sketch of the correct traction setup is most helpful. When the client is immobilized in skin or skeletal traction, gastrointestinal, urologic, and respiratory status must be assessed regularly.

Radiologic evaluation while the client is in traction determines the extent of injury, maintenance of bony alignment, and the progress of healing.

Traction Application

The severity of fracture damage and the extent of soft tissue injury are likely to determine who applies the traction. It may be the physician, technician, or nurse. Physician orders must always include the type of traction, amount of weight to be applied, and whether the traction may be removed for nursing care or mobility activities.

Nursing Management

Anxiety

Anxiety Reduction. Clients are often anxious about the impending application of traction. The nurse must explain the purpose of traction, application procedures, and activity limitations necessitated by the traction.

TABLE 12–2. *Types of Traction*

TYPE	ILLUSTRATION	USES	NURSING MANAGEMENT

Cervical
Skeletal tongs:
  Gardner-Wells
  Crutchfield
  Vinke
	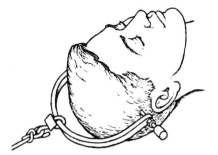
	Gardner-Wells. (Courtesy of Zimmer, Inc., Dover, Ohio.)
		Fractures or dislocation of cervical or high thoracic vertebrae (reduction and immobilization)	1. Maintain constant traction. If pin loosens, apply manual traction. Notify physician immediately. Sandbags or Philadelphia collar may be ordered.
			2. May use turning frames or special beds for positioning.
			3. Assess for correct placement at least every shift. Follow physician directions if tightening required.
			4. Assess pin sites at least every shift. Provide pin care according to physician's order and hospital protocol. Teach client to assess sites and do pin care using mirror.

Halo vest	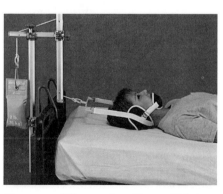	Fractures or dislocation of cervical or high thoracic vertebrae	1. Be prepared for emergency CPR. Tape wrench to front of vest. Familiarize all staff with quick removal instructions. Color code screws to be loosened—nail polish may be used. 2. Check fit of vest. 3. Move client and halo vest as a unit to avoid pressure that may dislodge pins. Never use bars attaching halo to vest for moving client. 4. Provide pin care according to physician order and hospital protocol. 5. Observe skin at edges of vest and where vest overlaps at least each shift. Replace vest liner if it becomes wet or dirty. 6. Help client anticipate situations and problems that may occur at home (e.g., baths, clothes, socialization, fatigue, and sleeping positions)
Skin Chin halter straps	(Courtesy of Zimmer, Inc., Dover, Ohio.)	Severe strains or sprains Torticollis Cervical trauma Nerve root compression	1. Observe for pain and pressure near ears, mandibular joints, chin, and occiput. Mouth guard may prevent jaw discomfort. 2. May protect skin with adherent, thin foam padding. 3. Encourage male clients to shave. 4. Follow physician orders regarding degree of head elevation of bed. 5. Follow physician orders for time client must remain in traction. Clients are usually permitted to remove traction for meals and hygiene. 6. Ensure that client using home cervical traction can correctly demonstrate setup, application, and removal. 7. Establish eye contact by standing where the client can see you.

Table continued on following page

TABLE 12–2. *Types of Traction* Continued

TYPE	ILLUSTRATION	USES	NURSING MANAGEMENT
Lower Extremity Bryant's traction	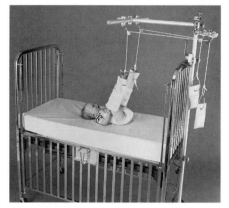 (Courtesy of Zimmer, Inc., Dover, Ohio.)	Femur fracture Congenital hip dislocation	1. Used in children younger than 3 years, weighing less than 30 pounds. 2. Apply bilaterally with hips flexed 45 degrees and legs in extension. 3. Ensure skin integrity and nonadhesive straps and wraps that do not impair neurovascular status. 4. Ensure buttocks are elevated 1–2 inches from mattress. 5. Ensure parents' understanding of the purpose, use, and safeguards of traction. 6. Remove traction, at least daily, to observe skin and provide skin care. 7. Use jacket or vest to prevent child from rotating in bed. 8. Encourage parents to participate in care during hospitalization and point out parallels to home care.
Buck's traction	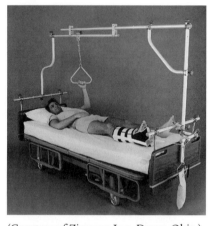 (Courtesy of Zimmer, Inc., Dover, Ohio.)	Hip and knee contracture Preoperative and postoperative positioning and immobilization of hip fractures Muscle spasm, joint rest	1. Ensure skin integrity by avoiding pressure on heel, dorsum of foot, fibular head, or malleolus. 2. Maintain countertraction by elevating foot of bed or keeping head of bed flat. 3. Encourage independence with use of trapeze. 4. Do not put a pillow under the affected limb. 5. Observe skin by removing traction, with someone holding the leg in alignment with manual traction, at least once every shift. 6. A maximum of 10 pounds of traction should be used.
Balanced traction with Thomas ring and Pearson or Brady attachment	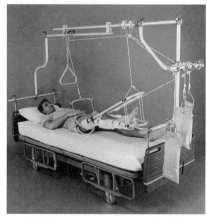 (Courtesy of Zimmer, Inc., Dover, Ohio.)	Older than 3 years of age Used mainly with skeletal pins Supracondylar femur fracture Hip and knee contracture Postoperative positioning and immobilization	1. If skeletal pins are used, give pin care according to physician's order and institutional policy. Be sure pin ends do not come in contact with frame. 2. Provide skin care every 4 hr with assessment. Prevent skin from coming in contact with frame. 3. Ensure that there is no external rotation of the leg because it may put pressure on the peroneal nerve. 4. Do CMS checks every 4 hr. 5. Position slings so that heel and Achilles tendon do not carry the weight of the lower leg. Do quad sets and heel cord exercises 10 times per hr while awake. 6. Observe for pressure at the groin area. Change padding as needed. 7. Pearson attachment should be in line with knee joint.

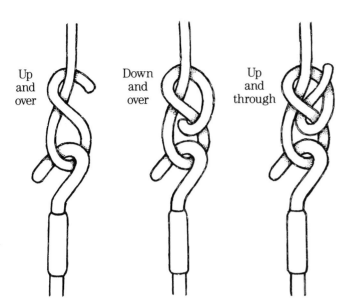

Up and over   Down and over   Up and through

FIGURE 12–7. A traction knot. (Courtesy of Zimmer, Inc., Dover, Ohio.)

When the client's head is immobilized, it is important for the nurse to establish eye contact by standing where the client can comfortably see her or him. The traction apparatus and how it functions must be explained. If traction will be used postoperatively, the client should be allowed to experience the traction and how it feels preoperatively unless this is contraindicated by the client's preoperative condition. Open-ended questions are asked during therapy to determine how the client is reacting to the limitations of traction.

Impaired Skin Integrity

Skin Surveillance and Traction/Immobilization Care. Before traction application, it is important to examine the skin carefully (especially over bony prominences) and to cleanse it thoroughly. Areas where the traction contacts the skin must be well padded to protect the skin, especially in the older client, in whom there is a loss of subcutaneous fat. Following traction application, the client is repositioned at least every 2 hours within the limitations of the traction. Clients are taught how to use the trapeze to exercise and independently change position. Redness after removal of any pressure usually means there is a developing pressure area.

Skin care for the client in skin traction requires special attention to skin and bony prominences. Frequent inspection for sliding, wrinkles, and tenderness under the straps of slings is needed. Skin traction should be reapplied if it becomes nonfunctional and removed for skin care as per protocol. Any redness, irritation, burning sensation, drainage, or foul odor should be reported to the physician. The bed linens should be carefully cleaned of any crumbs after meals or snacks. Straps and padding

should be replaced as they become soiled or wet. Clients should be taught to use the trapeze to facilitate position changes, as their injury allows.

Alteration in Peripheral Tissue Perfusion

Circulatory Care. Tissue perfusion is enhanced by client exercises within the limitations of the traction. Ankle pumps and toe wiggles should be performed 10 times every 1 to 2 hours while awake if allowed. Exercises, regular deep breathing and coughing, adequate fluids, and elastic stockings work together to prevent deep venous thrombosis (DVT). A sequential compression device can be used on the unaffected extremity. Anticoagulants may be used and should be monitored regularly for effectiveness. Client teaching about anticoagulants is essential. Assessment for excessive bleeding includes looking for areas of increased ecchymosis, a pink toothbrush, and blood in the stools. See Chapter 10 for more information on DVT.

High Risk for Peripheral Neurovascular Dysfunction

Peripheral Sensation Management. Application of traction, especially through skeletal pull, increases the risk of neurovascular compromise and compartment syndrome. The pull stretches nerves and blood vessels as well as compartments that may already be tight with blood or fluid. Neurovascular integrity must be monitored and fostered. Accurate assessment of neurovascular status includes evaluating the client's pain, sensation, active and passive ROM, color, temperature, capillary refill time, and pulses. Neurologic impairment specific to the location of the traction should be assessed. The client must be instructed to report changes in sensation promptly because paresthesias are often the first sign of impending impairment. The client must be taught appropriate exercises and must be encouraged to perform them regularly.

High Risk for Injury

Traction/Immobilization Care
Traction Malfunction. Maintaining the mechanics of traction is integral to successful nursing care of the client. The traction must be inspected at the beginning of each shift and after each application or position change. Inspection includes ensuring that all clamps on the traction frame are tight and observing for frayed ropes and insecure knots. Ropes must move freely over pulleys; and weights must hang freely at the ends or side of the bed, not directly over the client. However, when the amount of weight limits the ability of the nursing staff to properly position the client, one individual should support weights and the client should be moved simultaneously by another. The weights should not be removed to facilitate moving the client.

The desired position and alignment of traction must be constantly maintained to promote healing. The nurse must know the proper positioning and alignment needed for various types of traction. It may be necessary for bedside rounds to occur between the off-going and oncoming nurse at shift change to ensure correct positioning in the confused, noncompliant, or active client. Use of restraints ordered by the physician is recommended for uncooperative clients only as a last resort.

Impaired Physical Mobility

Exercise Promotion. Mobility can be encouraged within activity restrictions by fostering independence and instructing the client in repositioning techniques. The client should be allowed as much control as possible in organizing nursing care activities by being given reasonable choices. Exercises and activities that make use of unaffected joints and extremities to maintain ROM and strength should be encouraged. Dumbbells, Silly Putty, foam balls, and elastic pull bands are helpful in the intervals between physical therapy sessions. For some people, a list of the exercises and times to be performed is helpful. A record book may encourage clients to cross off their exercise sessions when finished.

Pain: Acute

Pain Management. Frequent assessment of pain and active listening when the client talks about pain are essential to promote comfort. Asking the client to rate his or her discomfort on a scale of 1 to 10, with 1 being the least and 10 the worst, provides a means of determining whether the pain is getting worse or lessening. The client should be encouraged to talk about his or her pain. The pain experience is extremely individual and does not always appear where and when it is expected. For example, because of the biomechanics of jaw loading in cervical halter traction, the client may develop pain in the ears or mandibular joint. A mouth guard, such as those worn by athletes, can relieve the problem.

Being an active participant in planning and implementing his or her own pain control measures contributes to the client's comfort. Analgesics should be provided promptly, and their effectiveness should be evaluated. An honest discussion about barriers to taking analgesics, such as the fear of addiction, should be initiated if the client seems hesitant about taking or asking for medication. Clients need to know whether analgesics are ordered on a regular schedule or whether they need to ask for them. Clients should be encouraged to take analgesics before the pain becomes severe. It is important to have this discussion with clients who are on patient-controlled analgesia also. A quiet room, a change of position, music, and a foot massage may help the client relax. Prism glasses for those in a halo vest or on flat bed rest may make reading and TV more enjoyable.

Pain unrelieved by analgesics and comfort measures, pain out of proportion to the injury or treatment, and progressive pain necessitate further investigation. See Chapter 5 for further information about pain assessment and management.

Altered Nutrition: Potential for Less Than Body Requirements

Nutrition Management. Adequate nutrition and fluids must be provided to the client in traction. Fluid intake (2000 to 3000 mL), with the higher intake needed in seriously ill clients with drainage, should be provided unless otherwise contraindicated. Output measurement usually suffices to monitor the fluid intake, but the client or family may want to keep a written record.

A dietary consultation is useful because the dietitian calculates the number of calories needed and the proper distribution of the food groups for each client based on weight and height and the client's condition. The importance of maintaining adequate nutritional intake should be stressed. Currently, the normal recommended daily allowance (RDA) of calcium, vitamin D, and phosphorus is thought to be sufficient for bone healing. Megadoses of calcium may be responsible for such complications as hypercalcemia, ectopic calcification and ossification, and nephrolithiasis.

Interval nourishments calculated into the diet provide diversion throughout the day and prevent the feeling of bloating that may occur with inactivity. Eating may be one of the few pleasures the client can enjoy while in traction, but it may be difficult to manage. Finger foods, foods in cups, bent straws, and adapted utensils can help. Food preferences should be adhered to, and regular intake evaluations should be made. Weekly weight measurements are possible with beds that have scales in the frames.

Risk for Infection

Infection Protection and Control. Accurate frequent observations for the signs of infection are imperative. Skin abrasion from skin traction and redness, drainage, or odor from open wounds or pin sites should be looked for and reported promptly. Purulent drainage should be cultured so that antibiotic treatment can be instituted in a timely manner. A mirror can be used to observe skin surfaces not available for direct observation. Routine assessment of vital signs and white blood cell counts also are needed. Some hospital protocols call for the use of foam balls or corks on the ends of traction pins, whereas others do not because foam balls and corks are thought to encourage collection of tissue and promote infection. Strict aseptic technique should be used when changing dressings.

Although pin loosening and pin infections are acknowledged as possible complications of skeletal traction, there is no consensus about prevention or treatment. Edema of the skin at the pin site causes increased pressure. When this pressure exceeds the capillary pressure, the blood supply is reduced, causing the skin to slough. Sterile gauze wrapped securely between the pin insertion site and the skin may decrease pin site motion. Pin care should be performed according to institutional policy and physician preference. When pin care is performed, one must always move in a direction away from the insertion site on the skin and on the pin to avoid a pistoning action, which can carry organisms beneath the pin-skin interface. It is often helpful to teach the client to participate in pin and skin care activities to provide a sense of control. The controversy regarding pin care is discussed in detail in the external fixation section of this chapter.

Constipation

Constipation/Impaction Management. Promoting normal bowel elimination in the client who is immobilized in traction can be challenging. Each bowel movement should be recorded and a schedule maintained that facilitates prompt response to the client's urge to defecate. Using a fracture pan and encouraging privacy and a diet high in fluids and roughage contribute to preventing the complication of constipation. Stool softeners should be ordered routinely, as well as laxatives and enemas for use when necessary.

Altered Urinary Elimination

Urinary Elimination Management. Maintaining normal urinary elimination requires accurate documentation of intake and output as well as assessment of frequency and any complaints the client may have regarding urination. Such complaints might include feelings of urgency, burning, or incomplete emptying of the bladder. Complete emptying of the bladder can be facilitated by elevating the head of the bed, if possible, and using a fracture pan. Fluids must always be encouraged, and excessive intake of calcium products should be eliminated to prevent the formation of renal calculi.

Impaired Gas Exchange

Respiratory Monitoring. A recumbent or semirecumbent position does not favor full diaphragmatic movement. Small tidal and larger residual volumes put the client in traction at risk for respiratory problems. Accurate assessment of breath sounds and documentation and rapid intervention for alterations in respiratory function are critical. Older clients are at special risk for respiratory problems, especially nosocomial pneumonia. These clients also come to their current situation with more chronic respiratory problems.

Frequent repositioning, bed exercises, coughing and deep breathing, the use of an incentive spirometer, elevation of the head of the bed when possible, and adequate fluid intake assist in maintaining adequate gas exchange. Results of arterial blood gas analyses, white blood counts, and radiographic examinations should be followed closely.

Clients with fractures of the long bones and the pelvis are at particular risk for fat embolus syndrome. Any deterioration in mental status, dyspnea, change in vital signs, chest pain, or evidence of neck or chest petechiae requires thorough investigation and rapid intervention. See Chapter 10 for a discussion of fat embolus.

Ineffective Individual Coping and Altered Role Performance

Coping Enhancement and Role Enhancement. Confinement brings with it feelings of loss of control. Being unable to perform many of the activities of daily living independently can precipitate old or new feelings of inadequacy. The loss of privacy can be exceedingly trying. Fears concerning money, loss of a job, and ability to fully recover can be overwhelming, especially for the older client.

Effective coping can be enhanced by allowing the client opportunities to discuss his or her concerns. Open-ended questions should be used to assess emotional status and sexual needs. Uninterrupted private time should be provided to couples, and flexibility in visiting hours should be allowed. Any activity that promotes the client's level of independence and gives him or her a feeling of control over the environment contributes to effective coping. Chapter 2 provides a detailed discussion of coping mechanisms. Continued anxiety may require intervention by social workers or psychologists. Children and their families need special consideration. Behavioral deficits have developed even with the use of simple braces (Dunst, 1990).

Planning ahead for work and home activities, anticipating difficulties, and thinking about ways to handle difficulties should be done in the hospital if possible. Many clients with frames or other external devices find that personal care, fatigue, and finding appropriate clothes are major problems after discharge.

Knowledge Deficit

Teaching: Procedure/Treatment. Client and family teaching and discharge planning begin on the day of admission when the initial client assessment is completed. This assessment includes identifying learning needs of both the client and significant others. Teaching is always individualized, and learning must be evaluated in the continuing process of client education. The special needs of children must be recognized. Each level of development presents special challenges, and the nurse must be cognizant of the behaviors and capabilities associated with various ages.

EXTERNAL FIXATION

External fixation is a method of fracture immobilization in which a system of percutaneous pins or wires is connected to a rigid external frame. It can be constructed in many different configurations and permits three-plane correction of deformities. It is used in massive open comminuted fractures with extensive soft tissue or neurovascular injury in which the risk of infection is high. External fixation is often the treatment of choice in closed fractures that will not maintain position or length, in

arthrodesis, in multiple trauma with a number of fractures, and when comminution requires bone grafting. When urgent transportation of an unstable client is required, external fixation often is the treatment of choice. Such immobilization is most often followed by casting or bracing as soon as sufficient callus has formed to allow for partial weight bearing (called *physiologic loading*), which enhances bone remodeling (Lewallen & Edwards, 1994). External fixation enhances earlier mobilization, but in extremely unstable fractures, weight bearing may be delayed (Pettine, Chai, & Kelly, 1993).

A wide variety of devices are available for use on various body parts, including, but not limited to, fingers, limbs, and the pelvis (Fig. 12–8). The devices

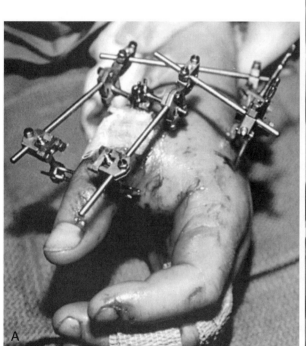

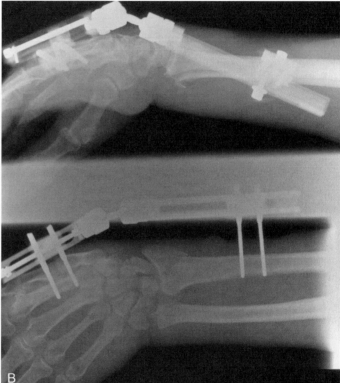

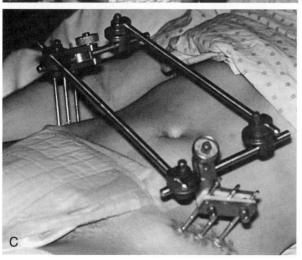

FIGURE 12–8. *A,* Mini-Hoffman external fixator: hand. *B,* X-ray film of forearm with external fixator in place. *C,* External fixator: pelvis. (*A* and *C,* Courtesy of Howmedica, Inc., Pfizer Hospital Products Group. *B,* Courtesy of James Buchanan, MD, Santa Fe, New Mexico.)

TABLE 12–3. *Advantages and Disadvantages of External Fixation*

ADVANTAGES	DISADVANTAGES OR POTENTIAL COMPLICATIONS
Immediate fracture stabilization	Pin loosening and drainage
Rigid fixation with compression to ensure primary bone healing	Pin tract infection
Increased client comfort	Loss of bone stabilization
Facilitation of nursing care	Superficial and deep wound infection in clients with soft tissue injury
Ability to observe soft tissue injury	Skin excoriation and necrosis from the frame
Access to open wounds	Cutaneous nerve injury
Ability to maintain motion of adjacent joints	Muscle impingement
Decreased blood loss when used for pelvic fractures with compression of bleeding sites	Appearance of device may frighten client and family
Decreased risk of sepsis	
Facilitation of vascular and soft tissue reconstruction	
Improved pulmonary function with improved mobility	
Fewer complications of immobility with early mobilization	

are made from materials such as aluminum, titanium, graphite, and lightweight nylon. Pins are of two basic types: transfixing pins (either smooth or with a central threaded section) and half-pins, which are continuously threaded for cancellous bone or interrupted for cortical bone. All pins are self-drilling and self-tapping and are manufactured in various lengths and thread sizes. The advantages and disadvantages of external fixation are listed in Table 12-3.

The Ilizarov external fixation device uses a circular metal frame to increase fixation stability while allowing early ambulation. Through the application of wires, pins, rings, and rods, the device incorporates corticotomy with fixation to encourage new bone growth. It is particularly helpful in treating clients with severe fractures. With its wires, hinges, and distraction and compression rods, the circular external fixator allows correction of three-dimensional deformities, including rotation, angulation, translation, lengthening, and shortening. Fixators are modeled individually for each client depending on correction goals.

Circular fixators also are used to treat unequal or abnormal limb lengths (see Chapter 18) and in the treatment of clients who have had bone segments in the long bones removed because of osteomyelitis or tumors. The Ilizarov method of bone regeneration teases the bone into fetal-like growth of new and viable tissue during the distraction phase. Bone, as well as muscle, blood vessels, nerves, tendons, and skin, has the capacity to grow in response to this same distraction stimulus.

The usual procedure for limb lengthening combines three stages. In the first stage, the external fixator is attached by thin wires through the skin and bone to the circular external frame. Rods that are parallel to the bone are attached to the metal rings. This frame acts as an external scaffolding to provide stability and stimulate the growth process. The second stage involves corticotomy, in which the outer layer of the bone is cut. It is similar to cutting a strip of bark from around the tree but not cutting deeper than the bark. About a week after this surgery, the third stage begins, with the client and family being taught to advance the external fixator to provide the bone distraction, stretching the outer layer of the partially cut bone. Advancement can be done manually or by computer control. The body gradually fills in the gap with healthy new tissue. The process is continued until the desired objective is reached (Lidke, 1989) (Fig. 12–9). A vital characteristic of the Ilizarov procedure is that bone must be distracted at a consistent and steady rate. If more than one or two distraction steps are not performed, the bone may unite prematurely. Clients in whom mental competence or cooperation is lacking are not candidates for this procedure. Compliance, consistency, cooperation, and commitment to the distraction schedule, pin site care, intensive physical therapy, and office visits are prerequisites for a successful outcome.

When the circular external fixator is in place for lengthening, full weight bearing as tolerated not only is permitted but is considered essential to development and consolidation of newly formed bone in the distraction gap (Paley, 1988). Weight bearing is also necessary for utilization of the body's calcium stores (Fig. 12–10). When sufficient new bone has formed at the desired length and it is considered clinically and radiologically strong enough to support unprotected weight bearing, the fixator is removed. Factors influencing growth and consolidation of new bone include age of the client, quality of bone, and rate of distraction. Intensive physiotherapy for all joints and muscles involved is carried out during and after treatment.

Diagnostics and Assessment

Client selection plays an important role in the successful use of external fixation. Potential problems with compliance should be discussed with the client and family. The consequences of noncompliance with the medical regimen can lead to loss of fracture stabilization, pin loosening, and infection.

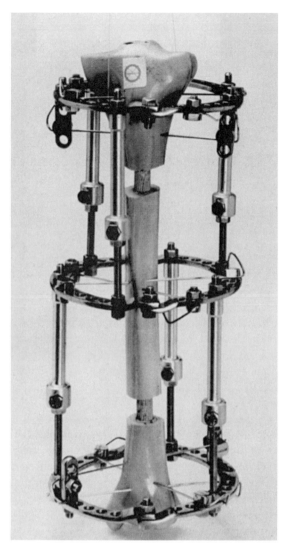

FIGURE 12–9. Bifocal corticotomy. (From Newschwander, G. E., & Dunst, R. M. [1989]. Limb lengthening with the Ilizarov external fixator. *Orthopaedic Nursing, 8,* 17.)

The history should include special emphasis on the condition requiring the use of external fixation and the effects of external fixation on the client's lifestyle. When evaluating effects on lifestyle, one should include the home environment, support systems, previous ambulatory status (when the lower extremity is involved), and ability to carry out activities of daily living and employment.

Physical examination comprises a thorough neurovascular assessment of the affected extremity, evaluation of the appearance of wounds and pin sites, and attention to the signs and symptoms of infection. The results of the examination must be documented thoroughly and in terms other professionals can use after the external fixator is applied.

Radiographs are used to determine fracture alignment and healing. Wound and pin site cultures can be done to establish the presence of infecting organisms. The complete blood count may indicate the need for blood replacement or the presence of infection (elevated white blood cell count).

Following application of the external fixator, specific activity orders are written, with special attention being paid to weight-bearing status when the pelvis and lower extremity are involved. The nurse must be constantly vigilant in assessing correct use of ambulatory aids and adherence to weight-bearing restrictions.

Nursing Management

Nursing care associated with the use of external fixation is similar in many regards to care for clients in traction.

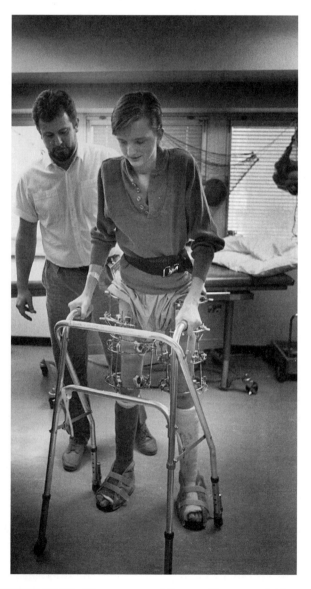

FIGURE 12–10. Ilizarov external fixator. (Courtesy of *Advance Magazine,* University of Michigan Medical Center, Ann Arbor, Michigan.)

High Risk for Peripheral Neurovascular Dysfunction

Circulatory Care. The potential for neurovascular deficit or compartment syndrome is high when external fixation is used because of the extent and type of injury usually managed with this modality. Commonly, clients have extensive soft tissue injury and concomitant intra-compartmental blood loss, blood vessel damage, and nerve damage. Even though the client may have an open fracture, compartment syndrome can occur in another compartment in the same extremity. Maintaining and accurately assessing neurovascular status is of prime importance in caring for the client with an external fixator. Current findings should be compared with baseline data, the involved extremity should be compared with the uninvolved extremity, and clients' reports of changes should be addressed promptly. Edema should be prevented by elevating the affected extremity above heart level. The location, duration, and severity of pain must be assessed, as should the presence of pain accompanying active and passive ROM. Temperature, color, capillary refill time, and pulses are included in the neurovascular assessment. Sensory nerve function should be assessed, and the client should be taught to report promptly any sensation of tingling or decreased feeling.

High Risk for Infection

Infection Control and Prevention. Pin sites and wounds must be observed constantly for signs of infection. Pins should be assessed for loosening. A small amount of bleeding immediately after pin insertion is to be expected and can be controlled with a small pressure dressing. Bleeding that continues for more than 24 hours should be brought to the attention of the surgeon. The nurse should be aware that the metal-adipose tissue interface may produce fatty drainage that mimics pus and occurs from movement of the adipose tissue around the pin. Observations for infection should include determining pin stability; assessing skin tension or puckering at the insertion site; noting odor, color, and characteristics of drainage; and determining whether the skin appears to be growing out on the pins, giving a tentlike appearance. If tenting occurs, the surgeon should be notified so that the wound can be extended.

Factors that are thought to contribute to pin site complications include the type of pin used (smooth vs. threaded) at the pin skin interface, motion at the pin skin interface and pin bone interface, type of fracture (open vs. closed), duration of treatment, and other local factors such as vascularity and skin integrity.

Pin care protocols should identify the method of cleansing (none, soap and water, saline, hydrogen peroxide), dressings (none, dry, or antibiotic), clean versus sterile technique, and frequency of protocol care. Most surgeons recommend pin care that is not abusive to the skin and does not carry organisms beneath the pin-skin interface.

The evidence-based practice table outlines scholarship addressing approaches to pin care. There is very limited evidence to support decisions regarding pin care protocols. No one standard emerges from the literature; rather, there are many different protocols for pin care ranging from no care to basic cleansing through showering and soap and water protocols to use of hydrogen peroxide or alcohol cleansing and application of antibacterial ointments (McKenzie, 1999). Comparative studies have been limited and show no statistical differences in infection rate using the different protocols. Furthermore, the studies have not consistently defined pin tract infections, so it is difficult to determine whether reports include minor pin tract infections versus major ones that require antibiotics, pin removal, or removal of the entire fixators. Multicenter prospective studies to compare different pin care approaches are needed to evaluate the efficacy of pin care protocols.

It is generally agreed that pin tract problems tend to slowly increase the longer the fixator remains in place. Pin loosening should be assessed daily and reported to the physician. Loose pins must be removed to avoid osteomyelitis. The progress of wound healing should be monitored closely, with the appropriate documentation of changes. Antibiotics may be ordered for prophylaxis for 48 to 72 hours after external fixator application.

Impaired Physical Mobility

Exercise Therapy: Joint Mobility and Ambulation. Active and passive ROM exercises often require the assistance of the nurse. They should be integrated into basic care activities when possible, and appropriate reminders should be given to clients about when to exercise. Early consultation to physical therapy for ROM and strengthening of the unaffected extremity can facilitate the clients overall rehabilitation. Attention must be paid to weight-bearing status when transferring clients in and out of bed. Assistance with ambulation following appropriate instruction in the use of assistive devices can help eliminate the complications of immobility. Special attention to ambulatory techniques is especially necessary for clients with lower extremity fixators because the client's balance can be altered by the weight of the frame. Specific direction is necessary from the surgeon to determine if the frame itself can be used to move the affected extremity (DeGeorge & Dunwoody, 1995). The extremity and the external fixator must be moved as a unit. The amount of support that the nurse must provide is determined by the client's ability to control the extremity during movement. If an ankle-foot orthosis is used to prevent foot-drop, a schedule should be established for its application and for appropriate assessment of skin integrity.

EXAMINING THE EVIDENCE: Moving Toward Evidence-Based Practice
Pin Care Protocols

AUTHOR(S), YEAR	STUDY DESIGN	POPULATION	METHODS	RESULTS/FINDINGS
Studies Describing Pin Care Practices				
Sims, 1996	Descriptive survey Examining protocols	68 hospitals	Questionnaire sent to hospitals with orthopaedic surgery services regarding pin care practices	All hospitals clean pins daily Hydrogen peroxide is used most often Majority of hospitals dress pins when they drain Majority remove crusts
Jones-Walton, 1991	Descriptive survey Examining protocols	804 orthopaedic nurses	Survey sent to members of National Association Orthopaedic Nurses	Majority (45%) cleaned pins three times daily Majority (91%) used hydrogen peroxide Most (58%) used clean technique versus sterile 59% reported no standard protocol; more than 1 protocol used on unit Betadine, Polysporin ointment, or alcohol generally used after cleansing three times daily (45%) or twice daily (33%)
Studies Describing Pin Care Complication Rates				
Hutson & Zych, 1998	Descriptive Retrospective 1 group	145 fractures treated with hybrid fixators	Soap and water to remove crusts daily and application of Bactroban	19 (13%) with pin infections needing intravenous antibiotics and/or debridement
Dormans et al., 1995	Descriptive 1 group	37 children, age 3–16 treated in halo vest	Observation of pins and phone questionnaire about complications Varying pin site regimen	59% developed pin site infections Most often at anterior pin sites
Velasquez et al., 1993	Descriptive 1 group	40 clients managed with Ilizarov (skinny wire) fixators	Chart review for complications, as well as direct observation of pin sites for signs of infection No stated protocol for pin care	10 of 40 (25%) developed pin track infections Skin tensions or pins through areas with a large amount of soft tissue such as the thigh had higher infection rates
Gregory et al., 1992	Descriptive	34 pediatric clients with fractures of femur or tibia treated with external fixators	Daily pin care with cooled boiled water Crusted material removed No dressings if no drainage present	Femoral pin sites had an infection rate of 10.3% Tibial pin sites had an infection rate of 2.3% *Staphylococcus aureus* was the most common organism isolated
Studies Comparing Pin Care Protocols and Outcomes				
Gordon et al., 2000	Prospective 1 group compared with other literature findings	27 children with circular external fixators	Observation of pin sites cleaned with daily showering only No physical pin cleaning	4% pin site infection No pins removed because of infection Conclusion: no difference in infection rates compared with complex cleaning regimes
Patterson, 1999	Pilot study of 5 methods of pin care in 1 institution	60 clients with 380 pins	Cleansing with saline, Xeroform wraps Stable dressing, no pin care Saline cleansing, Betadine wraps Half-strength hydrogen peroxide cleaning, Xeroform wraps Half-strength hydrogen peroxide cleansing, Betadine wraps	13% overall infection rate No statistical difference across groups Likely type 2 error because of small sample size Betadine wraps discontinued after 2 clients had a severe skin irritation from this treatment
Sproles, 1985	Prospective Experimental 2 groups	70 clients with either skeletal traction or external fixator	Observation of pin sites of control and experimental groups Experimental group underwent twice-daily pin care, including washing with soap and water and then alcohol Control group had no specific pin care; pins were cleaned per nurse preference	Noted that all clients in study had at least one pin site reaction (not necessarily infection) Experimental group had 13% infection rate Control group had 26.7% infection rate No statistical difference in infection rates between the 2 groups

Self-care Deficit, Body Image Disturbance

Self-care Assistance. Body Image Enhancement. Assistance with activities of daily living is required for the client with an external fixator, especially when the upper extremity is involved. Lack of independence may contribute to frustration and problems with self-image. Body image disturbances may occur because of the visibility of the hardware. Clothes may need to be adapted using hook and loop or Velcro fasteners. Clients with pelvic fixators often prefer large tops to cover the device and bottoms with wide elastic waistlines that will not bind below the fixator.

The nurse must provide support to the client and significant others during the period of adjustment to the external fixation device and the limitations it imposes. Encourage open expression of feelings being careful not to minimize the client's feelings. Focus on the client as a whole person, emphasizing remaining skills and strengths. The client care plan should include ways for the client to regain as much control as possible for the care of the external fixation device.

Pain: Acute

Pain Management. Analgesics are required in the immediate postoperative period. The external fixator generally enhances client comfort, and as the client's activity increases, analgesic use declines. Elevating the limb immediately after application prevents edema and promotes comfort. Slings or balanced suspension can be used to maintain elevation, as well as raising the foot gatch on the bed. Pillows may suffice when extensive soft tissue injury is not present. Padding should be used to protect the uninvolved lower extremity. Pain unrelieved by analgesics, ineffective comfort measures, progressive pain, and pain out of proportion to the injury should prompt further investigation for compartment syndrome (see Chapter 10).

Knowledge Deficit and Potential for Noncompliance

Teaching: Procedure/Treatment. Client and family teaching is of paramount importance in achieving compliance and a successful outcome. By the time of discharge from the hospital or office, the client should begin to accept psychologically the change in body image, have assumed responsibility for pin and wound care, be knowledgeable about the signs and symptoms of infec-

tion, and be safe and comfortable in ambulation. The client must be aware of potential changes in neurovascular and integumentary status and know how to manage the changes with decreased activity and elevation of the extremity. Resumption of sexual activity should be discussed before discharge.

REFERENCES

Botte, M. J., Byrne, T. P., Abrams, R. A., & Garfin, S. R. (1995). The halo skeletal fixator: Current concepts of application and maintenance. *Orthopedics, 18,* 463–471.

DeGeorge, P., & Dunwoody, C. (1995). Transfer techniques of the lower extremity with an external fixator. *Orthopaedic Nursing, 14*(6), 17–21.

Dormans, J., Criscitiello, A. A., Drummond, D. S., & Davidson, R. S. (1995). Complications in children managed with immobilization in a halo vest. *Journal of Bone and Joint Surgery, 77,* 1370–1373.

Dunst, R. M. (1990). Legg-Calve-Perthes disease. *Orthopaedic Nursing, 9*(2), 18–27.

Gordon, J. E., Kelly-Hahn, J., Carpenter, C., & Schoenecker, P. (2000). Pin site care during external fixation in children: Results of a nihilistic approach. *Journal of Pediatric Orthopaedics, 20,* 163–165.

Gregory, R., Cubison, T. C., Pinder, I. M., & Smith, S. R. (1992). External fixation of lower limb fractures in children. *Journal of Trauma, 33,* 691–693.

Hutson, J. J., Jr., & Zych, G. A. (1998). Infections in periarticular fractures of the lower extremity treated with tension wire hybrid fixators. *Journal of Orthopedic Trauma, 12,* 214–218.

Jones-Walton, P. (1991). Clinical standards in skeletal traction pin site care. *Orthopaedic Nursing, 10*(2), 12–16.

Lewalline, D. G., & Edwards, C. C. (1994). Complications of external fixation. In C. Epps (Ed.), *Complications of orthopaedic surgery* (3rd ed.). Philadelphia: Lippincott.

Lidke, K. (1989, Summer). From Siberia with love: The Ilizarov external fixator. *Advance,* 8–12.

McKenzie, L. (1999). In search of a standard for pin site care. *Orthopaedic Nursing Journal, 18*(2), 73–78.

Newschwander, G. E., & Dunst, R. M. (1989). Limb lengthening with the Ilizarov external fixator. *Orthopaedic Nursing, 8*(3), 15–21.

Paley, D. (1988). Current trends of limb lengthening. *Journal of Pediatric Orthopaedics, 8*(1), 73–92.

Patterson, M. (1999*). Comparison of complication outcomes of 5 pin care protocols: A pilot study.* Presented at the National Association of Orthopaedic Nurses Annual Meeting.

Pettine, K. A., Chai, E. Y. S., & Kelly, P. J. (1993). Analysis of the external pin-bone interface. *Clinical Orthopaedics and Related Research, 293,* 18–27.

Pierce, R. A., Jr., & Witaker, J. (1994). Complications of traction, plaster casts and appliances. In C. H. Epps (Ed.), *Complications in orthopaedic surgery* (3rd ed., pp. 69–77). Philadelphia: Lippincott.

Sims, M. (1996). Protocols for the care external fixator pin sites. *Professional Nurse, 11,* 261–264.

Sproles, K. (1985). Nursing care of skeletal pins: A closer look. *Orthopaedic Nursing, 4,* 11–19.

Velasquez, R. J., Bell, D. F., Armstrong, P. F., Babyn, P., & Tibshirani, R. (1993). Complications of use of the Ilizarov technique in the correction of limb deformities in children. *Journal of Bone and Joint Surgery, 75A,* 1148–1156.

13

Modalities for Mobilization

SUSAN M. ADDAMO

Rehabilitation is the restoration of a client's functional status to a preinjury or preoperative level. This rehabilitation process is multifactorial, including exercise programming, the application of physical modalities, functional retraining, client and family education, environmental adaptations, and orthotic prescription for select cases. The structure and strategies of this process are formulated based on the client's age, motivation, cognitive status, and the multiplicity and chronicity of the medical concerns. This comprehensive approach ensures both the safety and efficacy of the individualized rehabilitative treatment program.

Following an orthopaedic procedure, clients may require instruction in appropriate exercises to maintain or increase their flexibility, strength, and dynamic stability. These exercises may be augmented by physical modalities, such as thermotherapy, cryotherapy, electrotherapy, and ultrasound. For example, hydrocollator packs applied to a tight quadriceps muscle before exercise increase circulation and local tissue temperature. The net effect of this heating process is a decrease in pain and a reduction in muscular tension. As a consequence, the client is able to exercise more effectively to restore mobility.

For clients with lower extremity involvement with restricted weight bearing, proper ambulation training with the appropriate assistive device is critical. To ensure client safety during gait retraining and exercise, the client's cardiovascular responses are assessed. Training in functional activities, such as transferring and stair climbing, is also a part of the rehabilitation process and may require a hemodynamic assessment. It is imperative that the client be medically stable before initiation of rehabilitation. This is particularly true in clients with multiple and chronic medical issues, such as concomitant chronic obstructive pulmonary disease (COPD) and coronary artery disease.

Client education is also the key to ensuring successful client outcomes. Rehabilitation staff actively engage the client and family in the teaching process, reinforcing compliance to exercise and ambulation guidelines. In addition, this educational process must address the client's functional needs after discharge, the home environment, and the adequacy of social supports. Issues concerning environmental barriers, home modifications, issuance of durable medical equipment, or provision of home care services must be addressed and resolved before discharge.

Last, many clients with decreased function or stability of a limb may require the aid of an orthotic device to support the body part or to increase its functional capabilities. This specialized service is provided by certified orthotists or other trained health care providers and requires a prescription from a physician.

Although the orthopaedic nurse may not be directly involved in administering many of the exercises and physical therapy modalities described, an understanding of these interventions is important. The orthopaedic nurse is responsible for reinforcement of the rehabilitation process and at some facilities may be responsible for the implementation of selected techniques.

EXERCISE

The goals of therapeutic exercise are to increase joint range of motion (ROM), muscle strength, dynamic joint stability, and cardiovascular endurance. Exercise is also a means of enhancing balance and coordination during mobility and functional activities.

Physiologic Factors Affected by Regular Exercise

Body Density.   Over time, a regular exercise program produces density changes within the musculoskeletal system. The muscles become larger in girth and denser because of an increase in sarcoplasm (the cytoplasm in muscle cells). The amount of adipose tissue is diminished, and the development of connective tissue is augmented within the muscle bundles. The stronger the muscle, the greater the stressors it can withstand.

Exercise also has a positive effect on bone density. Muscular activity or exercise, or both, place additional stress on bones. This stress rearranges the cancellous plates of the bones in a manner directly proportional to the stresses applied, thereby strengthening the bone.

Ligaments also become denser through appropriate therapeutic exercises. To increase the tensile strength of a ligament, a process of minimal stretch followed by release is used. In contrast, a constant prolonged stretch of the fibers weakens them. It is critical, given this stretch response, that the correct exercise and technique be used. If not, one could inadvertently induce ligamentous laxity or joint instability.

Weight changes are also seen with exercise training. An immediate but temporary weight loss occurs as a result of water loss. This weight loss is quickly reversed after eating and drinking. Appropriate nutritional intake is critical when participating in an exercise program. Gradual weight loss occurs as the result of a reduction in fat content. This weight loss occurs as energy utilization exceeds energy consumption. The overall weight loss may decrease as muscle bulk increases in size and density (muscle weighs more than fat).

Muscle Fiber.   Muscle fibers are classified according to two basic types: fast-twitch and slow-twitch. *Fast-twitch* fibers are anaerobic; that is, they do not need oxygen for metabolism. These fibers are responsible for speed or speed-power activities, such as sprinting and weight lifting. Conversely, *slow-twitch* fibers are aerobic. This fiber type requires oxygen for prolonged muscular contractions, as seen in such endurance events as long-distance running and cross-country skiing.

Exercise programs are formulated based on the client's activity demands and the corresponding fiber type. Low-intensity, long-duration exercises develop slow-twitch fibers but fail to adequately strengthen or develop fast-twitch fibers. Specifically, sprinters are trained through short-duration, high-velocity sprints to develop fast-twitch fibers. Marathon runners focus on long distances at a lesser intensity to enhance slow-twitch fiber development.

Muscle Strength.   *Strength* is the capacity to exert force or the ability to do work against resistance. The most noticeable change in muscle from regular exercise is an increase in girth or hypertrophy. *Muscle hypertrophy* occurs as a result of an increase in the size of the muscle fibers, not an increase in fiber number. Capillary or vascular response to exercise is different. Capillary numbers actually increase.

Hypertrophy of the muscle is not always proportional to work. This fact is evident when comparing male and female weight lifters. Male weight lifters develop marked muscular hypertrophy with training, whereas female lifters actualize strength gains with lifting but do not develop hypertrophy. This training effect difference has been postulated to be related to higher levels of testosterone in the male.

Three principles contribute to enhanced muscular strength: the overload, gradual progression, and specificity principles. The *overload principle* states that muscle increases in size and strength only if the workload exceeds previous demands. As the muscle becomes stronger, the amount of stress required to produce gains must rise.

The second principle, *gradual progression,* defines the rate at which resistance is increased. This progression is determined by the client's response, thereby ensuring comfort and safety.

The third and final principle is *specificity.* Training must be structured to mirror the client's activity. Specifically, the velocity and intensity of the movement and its position in space must be replicated to ensure an adequate training effect.

The size of a muscle is not the sole determinant of its strength. Strength differences can also be related to the amount of adipose tissue within the muscle belly. Because adipose tissue is not contractile tissue, it limits the speed and amount of muscular contractility. Thus, a muscle with a limited amount of adipose tissue is stronger and more efficient than a muscle of comparable size with a greater percentage of adipose tissue.

Factors Limiting Exercise

Before an exercise program can be initiated, factors that limit exercise, such as pain and the client's inability to relax, must be addressed. Muscle soreness can be expected with the initiation of an exercise program. An increase in pain that is persistent may be a signal to decrease the difficulty or duration of the exercises. It is important to communicate persistent pain to the physician to ensure adequate medical management and to rule out concerns, such as deep venous thrombosis (DVT) or infection.

Cailliet (1964) graphically described the mechanisms that cause irritation, which result in muscular and joint pain and disability. The progression is shown in Figure 13–1.

Determination of the cause of pain and a means for alleviating it must be the first requirement of an exercise program. The ability to relax can be difficult and may interfere with the correct execution of the exercises. To assist the client to relax, an exercise-relaxation strategy

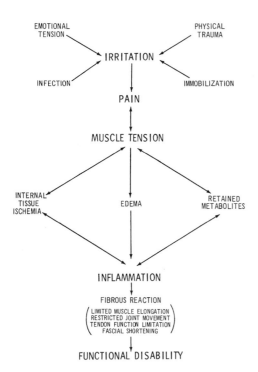

EMOTIONAL TENSION   PHYSICAL TRAUMA

INFECTION   IMMOBILIZATION

IRRITATION

PAIN

MUSCLE TENSION

INTERNAL TISSUE ISCHEMIA   EDEMA   RETAINED METABOLITES

INFLAMMATION

FIBROUS REACTION

LIMITED MUSCLE ELONGATION
RESTRICTED JOINT MOVEMENT
TENDON FUNCTION LIMITATION
FASCIAL SHORTENING

FUNCTIONAL DISABILITY

FIGURE 13–1. Mechanisms leading to pain and disability. (From Cailliet, R. [1964]. *Neck and arm pain.* Philadelphia, FA Davis.)

can be adopted. Specifically, the client should be instructed to rest after each repetition and between each exercise bout. This strategy helps eliminate the tendency to hold the muscle in a partially contracted state, a cause of lactic acid buildup and, ultimately, soreness.

If the client appears tense and has difficulty relaxing, he or she may benefit from frequent short rest periods. If the client's muscle tension is marked, instruction in various conscious relaxation techniques may be indicated. Relaxation techniques are designed to reduce physiologic arousal and increase task-relevant focus (Baechle & Earle, 2000). Diaphragmatic breathing, or belly breathing, is a basic stress management technique. It focuses thought on breathing to clear the mind and therefore increase attention capacity. Jacobson's method is another relaxation technique that uses visualization techniques, or what is also known as *imagery.* An example of Jacobson's method is to tell the client to imagine he or she is melting like butter to facilitate the relaxation response.

The therapist or nurse should be aware of any evidence of marked psychosocial issues or concerns that may be contributing to the client's tension level. These issues may distract the client from the rehabilitation process and adversely affect outcomes. A referral to other health care professionals, such as a social worker or psychiatrist/psychologist, may be appropriate to assist the client.

The exercise activity should be isolated to one area, using only those muscles necessary for the performance of the exercise. Muscle isolation requires special attention

to support and protect both the body segments required for the movement and the inactive muscles and joints.

Rate of Exercise Progression

The appropriate progression of an exercise program is essential. Initial exercises taught to the client should be easy to perform and require a submaximal amount of strength and coordination. Strenuous or complex exercises can be introduced as the client progresses. The progression of exercises must be suited to the individual and instituted based on the client's ability to correctly execute the technique without undue pain or discomfort. If the exercise cannot be performed appropriately, an easier exercise should be substituted. The therapist must constantly assess the client's ability to carry out an exercise and continually adapt the exercise to fit the client's progress.

Client motivation is a key factor in the successful outcome of treatment and may be stimulated in the following ways:

1. Assisting the client to understand both the medical condition and the objective of each exercise
2. Documenting and discussing objective improvement to stimulate further effort; continuously focusing on shortcomings may adversely affect client motivation and outcomes

The client's response to exercise can also be influenced by the attitude and technique of the therapist. Clear, simple instructions often work best. The instructor should give the person his or her full attention and demonstrate a willingness to actively listen. The therapist's own body positioning during the educational process is important. Demonstrating the appropriate positioning techniques facilitates skill acquisition for the client and ensures protection for both the client and the therapist from musculoskeletal strain or injury during physical maneuvers.

No matter what type of exercise is being instituted, the client must be informed of the proper technique and rationale for performing the activity. The physical therapist should demonstrate the exercise to the client using the uninvolved extremity first. Once the client can correctly demonstrate this exercise, the physical therapist should then assist the client to perform the exercise with the involved extremity. The goal of this process is to ensure that the client correctly, safely, and independently executes all exercises.

The client should receive a set of written instructions at discharge, preferably with diagrams, of all prescribed exercises. It is imperative that this information be very specific and contain the proper position, the number of repetitions, the frequency, and the duration for each exercise. These instructions help minimize confusion and reinforce concepts to ensure that established goals are met.

Muscle Contraction

Muscle tissue has the unique ability to produce tension. Muscle contraction involves a shortening of the contractile elements of the muscle. Muscle tissue can produce tension or contract by three different mechanisms. First, *isometric contraction* is when a muscle produces tension equal to the external resistance and no movement occurs. There is no change in the length of the muscle or in the angle of the joint at which the contraction takes place. Second, when a muscle produces tension greater than the external resistance, the shortening movement is termed a *concentric contraction.* Finally, when a muscle produces tension less than the external resistance, the lengthening movement is termed an *eccentric contraction.*

RANGE OF MOTION

The term *ROM* refers to the motion of a particular joint or the ability to move a limb through its arc of motion. ROM exercises can be performed passively or actively to facilitate an increase in flexibility or strength or both. The type of exercise prescribed is based on the severity of the injury, the acuity of the condition, the diagnosis, and the type of surgical procedure. The type, timing, and

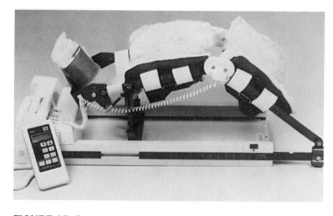

FIGURE 13–2. Continuous passive motion machine. (Courtesy of Sutter Corporation, San Diego, CA.)

exercise progression are often dictated by the physician and by the client's response to treatment.

Passive Range of Motion/Continuous Passive Motion

Passive range of motion (PROM) exercise is the application of an external force without active muscle contraction. This external force can be applied by a therapist, a mechanical appliance, or the client's uninvolved extremity. This form of exercise prevents joint contractures, promotes maintenance of normal joint ROM, and is safely used with weak or paralyzed muscles. After a surgical procedure, PROM reduces adhesions and stimulates healing, resulting in a stronger fixation of the healed structures.

Salter first coined the term *continuous passive motion* (CPM) in 1970, although it was mentioned as early as 1967 by Nickel at Rancho Los Amigos Hospital. The CPM device is an electrically driven apparatus consisting of an adjustable frame, supportive padding, and a control box. This device is used to continuously move an extremity through its ROM. CPM devices are available for both upper and lower extremities (Fig. 13–2).

The CPM device can be applied to the involved extremity immediately after an operative procedure while the client is still under anesthesia. The health care provider is able to lock the CPM device into set limits of motion and control the velocity of the movement. The client has a remote control on/off switch that provides added safety. This ensures that the client can exercise safely, appropriately, and within tolerable limits.

It is unclear how frequently or continuously the CPM device must be applied to obtain its full therapeutic effect and recommendations vary widely. The potential advantages and disadvantages of CPM are listed in Table 13–1. If collagen fibers are left undisturbed, as with immobilization, the cross-linking between fibers can significantly increase. When the close contact between the collagen fibers is disturbed, as with PROM, the cross-linking decreases. This cross-linking has been suggested as the mechanism by which contractures occur, and CPM

TABLE 13–1. *Potential Advantages and Disadvantages of Continuous Passive Motion (CPM)*

ADVANTAGES	DISADVANTAGES
Decrease in disuse atrophy	Cost: health care provider and purchase or rental of the device
Decrease in capsular contractures	Possible increase in postoperative drainage of total knee arthroplasty suture line
Maintenance of articular cartilage	Client's activity is restricted during CPM use
Aids in nutrition of involved tissues	Increased incidence of knee flexion contractures following total knee arthroplasty
Early, continuous mobilization to enhance healing and tissue remodeling	Possible increase in pain and associated analgesic requirements
Decrease in joint effusions and associated pain	
Decrease in joint hemarthrosis	
Reduces the amount of time required to attain knee flexion goal	
Reduction in the incidence of postoperative knee manipulation	

prevents this development. There is evidence that a joint effusion or hemarthrosis can promote muscle atrophy because of the inhibitory effects on muscle contractions. One theory states that early motion serves as a pumping mechanism, decreasing postoperative joint effusions and associated pain.

Because the client must remain supine while the CPM device is functioning, the effects of immobility are one disadvantage of its application. Exercises for the uninvolved extremities must be employed during use of the CPM device to minimize the risk of disuse atrophy of the remaining, inactive muscles. The indications and contraindications for postoperative CPM are listed in Table 13-2.

There is varying evidence about the effectiveness of CPM following total knee arthroplasty (TKA). Studies are described in the evidence-based practice table in this chapter. Short-term increases in joint ROM have been reported for clients who use CPM after TKA (McInnes, Larson, Daltroy, Brown, Fossel, Eaton, Shulman-Kirwan, Steindorf, Poss, & Liang, 1992; Montgomery & Eliasson, 1996; Pope, Corcoran, McCaul, & Howie, 1997; Ververeli, Sutton, Hearn, Booth, Hozack, & Rothman, 1995; Wasilewski, Woods, Torgerson, & Healy, 1990; Yashar, Venn-Watson, Welsh, Colwell, & Lotke, 1997); however, others have not found this short-term benefit (Kumar, McPherson, Dorr, Wan, & Baldwin, 1996). All reports verify that long-term benefits in joint flexion are not achieved with the use of CPM (McInnes et al., 1992; Pope et al., 1997; Ververeli et al., 1995; Wasilewski et al., 1990; Yashar et al., 1997). Reports of other complications, either postoperative or CPM related, have also been

varied. Most researchers have found no additional benefits or complications; however, some researchers report more benefits with CPM while others report more complications with its use. Fewer major wound complications, decreased use of analgesics, shorter hospital stay (Wasilewski et al., 1990), less knee swelling (McInnes et al., 1992; Montgomery & Eliasson, 1996), and fewer knee manipulations (and resulting cost savings) (McInnes et al., 1992; Ververeli et al., 1995) are the purported benefits of CPM. An increase in blood loss (Kumar et al., 1996; Pope et al., 1997) and analgesic requirements (Pope et al., 1997) have been identified as potential disadvantages of CPM. Worland, Arredondo, Angles, Lopez-Jimenez, and Jessup (1998) compared the effectiveness of the CPM machine as a home therapy program versus professional physical therapy following hospital discharge for clients who had TKA. They concluded that the use of the CPM machine after hospital discharge for properly selected clients is an adequate rehabilitation alternative. The cost of CPM was lower than the cost of home professional physical therapy, and there was no difference in results with respect to knee flexion contracture or knee scores.

CPM can be used following ligament surgery, but long-term benefits are questionable. CPM following anterior cruciate ligament (ACL) reconstruction can be used in the hospital or at home after discharge. Initial ROM may be enhanced (Gaspar, Farkas, Szepesi, & Csernatony, 1997), but long-term gains in joint ROM have not been realized (Engstrom, Sperber, & Wredmark, 1995; Gaspar et al., 1997; Richmond, Gladstone, & MacGillivray, 1991; Witherow, Bollen, & Pinczewski, 1993). Reports of additional benefits or disadvantages are varied. Witherow, Bollen, and Pinczewski (1993) report increased analgesic use, more blood loss, and longer length of hospital stay with the use of CPM following ACL repair. In contrast, McCarthy, Yates, Anderson, and Yates-McCarthy (1993) report fewer analgesics being used with CPM during the postoperative period. Use of CPM following rotator cuff repair can result in better short-term ROM (Raab, Rzeszutko, O'Connor, & Greatting, 1996) and less pain (Lastyo, Wright, Jaffe, & Hartzel, 1998; Raab et al., 1996). Lastayo et al. (1998), however, have reported increased cost and no change in function with use of CPM at home after rotator cuff repair.

CPM can benefit the septic joint through intra-articular fluid exchange. Septic joints improve more rapidly with CPM use than with immobilization or prolonged rest.

The current health care trend is toward shorter inpatient lengths of stay and ambulatory care surgeries. Therefore, the way in which CPM is used has changed as well. CPM units may be prescribed for home use or in a subacute rehabilitation setting. Durable medical equipment companies provide units for short-term use, and insurance companies may cover the cost of these units for

TABLE 13-2. *Indications and Contraindications for Continuous Passive Motion (CPM)*

INDICATIONS	CONTRAINDICATIONS
Arthrotomy, capsulotomy, and joint debridements	Unstable fractures
Open reduction and internal fixation of intra-articular fractures	Wound dehiscence
Patellectomy	
Ligamentous repair	
Synovectomy for rheumatoid arthritis and hemophilic arthropathy	
Arthropathy secondary to acute septic arthritis	
Total joint arthroplasty	
Restricted motion secondary to adhesions	
Finger flexor tendon repair	
Knee manipulation	
Septic joints	
Adhesive capsulitis	
Biologic resurfacing for a major defect in a joint surface	

EXAMINING THE EVIDENCE: Moving Toward Evidence-Based Practice
Is Continuous Passive Motion (CPM) Beneficial for Clients Who Have Had Total Knee Arthroplasty (TKA)?

AUTHOR(S), YEAR	SAMPLE	DESIGN/METHOD	OUTCOME VARIABLE	MAJOR FINDINGS
Chen et al., 2000	51 clients receiving inpatient rehabilitation following TKA	2 groups; randomized, prospective Group 1 received CPM 5 hr/day and PT Group 2 received PT alone	Increase in passive ROM from admission, to rehabilitation facility to days 3, 7, and discharge	No differences between groups in ROM increases
Chiarello et al., 1997	45 clients who underwent unilateral TKA	5 groups; randomized, prospective Control (no CPM), short CPM duration (3–5 hr/day) or long duration (10–12 hr/day) with ROM increase 5 degrees bid, short CPM or long duration with ROM increased daily to patient tolerance	Active and passive flexion and extension on each postoperative day by PT Patient preferences for duration and incremental increases	No statistically significant group differences for baseline and final postoperative ROM Most patients preferred CPM duration of between 4 and 8 hr/day Patient-preferred CPM incremental increase in ROM was 6–7 degrees per day
Kumar et al., 1996	83 clients who underwent TKA for treatment of osteoarthritis	2 groups; randomized, prospective Group 1 had CPM Group 2 had early passive flexion (drop and dangle)	Hospital length of stay, wound drainage, ROM at discharge	CPM group had longer hospital stay (1 day), more wound drainage ROM was similar in both groups
Montgomery & Eliasson, 1996	68 clients with primary knee arthroplasties	2 groups; randomized, prospective One group received CPM The other group had active physical therapy	Knee swelling, knee ROM, pain, length of stay	CPM group had less postoperative knee swelling with more rapid initial improvement in knee flexion No differences between groups in knee flexion at discharge, pain ratings, and length of stay
Pope et al., 1997	53 patients (57 knees) who underwent TKA	3 groups; randomized, prospective Group 1 had no CPM Group 2 had CPM 0–40 degrees Group 3 had CPM 0–70 degrees	Knee ROM at 1 week and 1 year, flexion deformity, function, analgesic requirements, blood drainage	Increased ROM in CPM 0- to 70-degree group compared with no CPM group at 1 week No difference in 1-year ROM, flexion deformities, or function Increased analgesic requirement in clients with CPM Increased blood drainage in 0- to 70-degree CPM group compared with other 2 groups
Ververeli et al., 1995	103 clients who underwent primary TKA	2 groups; prospective First 51 patients received CPM Next 53 patients did not receive CPM	Knee ROM at discharge and 2 years postoperatively, pain, knee swelling, wound drainage, pulmonary embolism, length of stay, manipulations	CPM group had greater active flexion at discharge No CPM group had 5 manipulations; CPM group had none No difference in other outcomes
Worland et al., 1998	80 clients (103 knees; 23 clients had bilateral TKA)	2 groups; randomized prospective One group received CPM at home The other group received PT home visits	Knee ROM at 2 weeks and 6 months, cost	Knee flexion was similar in both groups at 2 weeks; there was one flexion contracture in the CPM group No ROM differences at 6 months Cost of CPM was less than that of professional therapy
Yashar et al., 1997	210 clients who underwent TKA	2 groups; randomized, prospective Group I started CPM at 70–100 degrees flexion in PAR Group II started CPM at 0–30 and progressed to 100 degrees	Knee flexion at discharge, 4, 6, 12 weeks, and 1 year. Complications, pain, blood loss	Group I (accelerated flexion) had significantly better flexion at discharge No differences between groups in flexion at other time periods No group differences in complication, pain, or blood loss

postoperative care. Chen, Zimmerman, Soulen, and DeLisa (2000) studied the use of CPM in clients with TKA who were transferred to a rehabilitation hospital. The results indicated no significant difference in PROM between clients who received CPM and physical therapy and clients who received only physical therapy. They concluded that the use of CPM in the rehabilitation hospital is likely of no added benefit to clients admitted after single TKA.

Nursing Care Related to Continuous Passive Motion. Nursing care for the client receiving CPM focuses on proper application, equipment maintenance, client education, and prevention of complications from either the device or immobility. Nursing diagnoses for the use of CPM include high risk for impaired skin integrity, knowledge deficit, and impaired physical mobility.

High Risk for Impaired Skin Integrity

Pressure Management. The client using a CPM device is at risk for altered skin integrity from pressure points and mobility limitations. While using CPM, the client is positioned in the supine position. This prolonged positioning places additional pressure on the sacrum, the unaffected extremity's heel, and the elbows. Careful assessment of these pressure points should be made on every shift. Although the client cannot turn completely, he or she should be encouraged to shift weight and change positioning frequently to decrease pressure.

Areas supported by the CPM device should be assessed frequently for pressure areas as well. The heel and pelvic areas are especially prone to pressure from the device. Adjustments to the CPM or removing the device temporarily may be necessary.

Knowledge Deficit

Teaching: Procedure/Treatment. Instructions about the purpose and use of CPM should be provided. Clients should be reminded to shift their weight frequently and to exercise unaffected extremities. The number of hours per day CPM is to be used and ways to prevent hazards of immobility, such as constipation and skin breakdown, should be discussed.

Impaired Physical Mobility

Exercise Promotion. In addition to being immobile from a surgical procedure, the client using CPM has additional limitations relative to positioning and mobility. The client may be hesitant to ambulate or transfer out of bed because of difficulty getting in or out of the device or the desire to maximize the benefit from the unit. The nurse may also share this hesitation. However, the client should be encouraged to participate in appropriately timed activities, such as physical therapy, walking, and sitting, to prevent the adverse effects of immobility.

Active Assistive Range of Motion

Active assistive range of motion (AAROM) is the active contraction of a muscle with assistance by an external force, such as a therapist, a mechanical appliance, or an uninvolved extremity. This assistance helps support the weight of the limb so that the resistance of gravity is overcome. AAROM can help increase flexibility, strengthen muscles, and improve muscle coordination. When performing AAROM, the client should be encouraged to assist throughout the range. Because excess muscle tension can lead to pain, assistance by an external source prevents a full contraction of the muscle fibers, thereby diminishing the potential for pain.

Active assistive exercise is often the second step in a muscle reeducation and strengthening program. Passive exercise is often indicated initially to ensure pain-free ROM following surgery. Soft tissue structures must be considered sufficiently healed to allow muscle contraction without injury before assistive exercise is allowed. Because strength can be obtained only by active contraction of the muscle, AAROM is the first step toward increasing muscle strength to optimal levels.

Active assistive exercise can be performed with the aid of the therapist or independently by the client. The client has several means of assisting himself or herself. If no equipment is available, the client can use an uninvolved extremity to assist the involved limb through its arc of motion. Once the involved limb has moved to its limit, the uninvolved extremity provides further assistance to end-range. For example, a client with a shoulder problem may clasp hands and assist the involved upper extremity up overhead. In this way, the involved extremity is exercising safely through the support and assistance of the uninvolved extremity. By stretching beyond the client's end-range, joint ROM can be improved.

Examples of active assistive exercise performed with the aid of equipment are wand or cane exercises for the upper extremities (Fig. 13–3) and powder boards (Fig. 13–4) for AAROM for the upper or lower extremities. Following TKA, a client can benefit from the aid of a powder board when initiating active knee flexion and extension while supine. The board reduces friction, thereby assisting the extremity through its arc of motion.

Active Range of Motion

Active range of motion (AROM) exercise is active contraction of the muscle against the force of gravity. Active exercise increases muscle strength and overall function of the extremity. Often, clients are advanced to active exercises once passive and active-assisted exercises are performed easily and painlessly. These exercises can be performed independently and without any costly equipment.

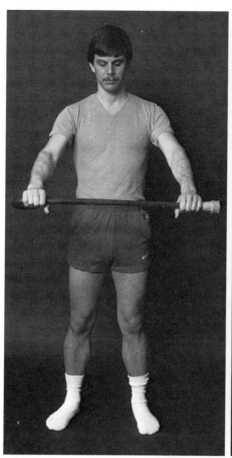
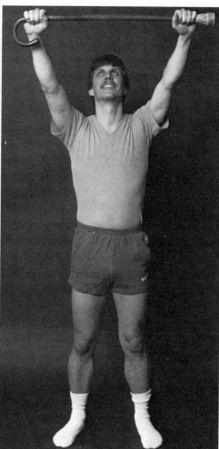

FIGURE 13–3. Cane exercise.

Examples of AROM are straight leg raises (Fig. 13–5A), knee flexion and extension while sitting (Fig. 13–5B), and shoulder exercises while standing. Active exercises are part of the gradual progression of exercises toward an increase in muscular strength and endurance.

Active Resistive Range of Motion

Active resistive exercise (ARROM) is the active contraction of the muscle against some form of resistance. Resistance to the muscle can be increased by weights, equipment, manual resistance, or weight bearing. Active

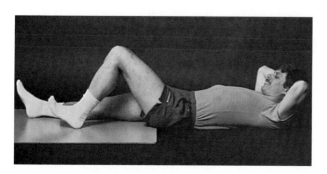

FIGURE 13–4. Powder board.

resistive exercise is used primarily to increase muscle strength and stability.

Therapeutic active resistive exercises can be performed either in an open- or closed-chain position. Open-chain exercises are performed in the non–weight-bearing position. Conversely, closed-chain exercises are performed in a weight-bearing position. An example of an open-chain exercise is a straight leg raise in the supine position. An example of a closed-chain exercise is a partial squat in the standing position. Open-chain exercises are indicated in early phases of rehabilitation because of decreased demands on the muscles and articular surfaces. Closed-chain exercises are added to the program as the client progresses through rehabilitation and is able to tolerate weight bearing. Closed-chain exercises enhance balance, stability, and control and are more functionally based. Closed-chain exercises simulate activities of daily living and the challenges clients may face during recreational or occupational activities. The three basic types of resistive exercise are isometric, isotonic, and isokinetic.

Isometric Exercise. Isometric ("same length") exercise is the active contraction of the muscle with no joint motion or functional movement. The muscle belly increases in size, eliciting a force equal to the resistance produced. An isometric contraction is the result of tension development; it is not an eccentric or concentric contraction. Isometric exercises are useful when the ROM of a joint is limited by injury or immobilization, such as from a cast or brace. These exercises are prescribed when certain points within the ROM of a joint are painful. Tension development through isometric exercise can be performed within the pain-free ranges, avoiding those positions of discomfort.

Isometrics are also indicated for the client with an acutely inflamed joint. An example of isometric exercise is performing sets of quadriceps contractions at various points in the ROM. Quadriceps sets are performed by telling the client to tighten the kneecap and to contract the quadriceps muscle without knee joint motion.

The advantages and disadvantages of isometric exercises are listed in Table 13–3 (Bernhardt, 1986).

Brief repetitive isometric maximal exercise has been shown to be an effective protocol for increasing muscle strength. In this method, the isometric exercise is performed for a 6-second maximal isometric contraction, followed by a 20-second rest. This exercise format should

TABLE 13–3. *Advantages and Disadvantages of Isometric Exercises*

ADVANTAGES	DISADVANTAGES
No equipment necessary	Increases in muscle strength are limited to the angle at which they are performed
Minimal risk of provoking joint irritation	
Appropriate for any muscle	No impact on muscle endurance
Minimizes potential for muscle atrophy	Potential for adverse blood pressure changes
Stimulates mechano-receptors of the joint	

Adapted from Bernhardt, D. B. (1986). *Sports physical therapy* (p. 165). New York: Churchill Livingstone. Reprinted with permission.

be repeated 20 times per day. Other sources state that for maximal safety, the isometric exercise should be performed initially at 75% of maximum and increased to 90% possible tension. Each contraction is held for 6 seconds and repeated at each arc of the motion three to five times. Isometric exercises have a limited strengthening effect. Gains are actualized only in the positions performed. The strength effect does not generalize throughout the entire AROM of the joint.

Isotonic Exercise. An isotonic ("same tension") contraction occurs when the muscle either shortens (concentric) or lengthens (eccentric) against a fixed amount of resistance, and joint motion results. In an isotonic exercise, such as flexing and extending the elbow with a weight, the biceps flexes the elbow through a concentric contraction. The return movement or eccentric contraction occurs as the biceps muscle lengthens from a flexed to an extended elbow position. Eccentric muscle contractions are an excellent way to increase muscle tension but are the main cause of muscle soreness. In turn, this muscle soreness can lead to decreased performance because of pain and biochemical changes. Eccentric contractions often can be performed by the client before concentric contractions and thus can be initiated when concentric movement is too difficult to perform. Because many daily functional activities require eccentric contractions, they should be part of the rehabilitation process.

Isotonic exercise can be broken down further into the categories of constant resistance and variable resistance. *Constant resistance isotonic exercise* is the classic type of isotonic exercise, as in raising and lowering a dumbbell or bench pressing a free weight. The amount of resistance does not change during this type of exercise. The amount of weight prescribed is determined by the maximum amount the client can lift throughout the entire ROM.

Variable resistance isotonic exercise is performed by manual resistance by the therapist or with equipment, such as Nautilus or Universal. A therapist's resistance is

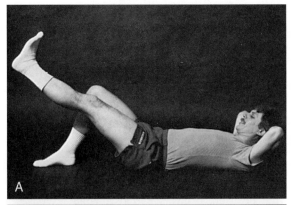
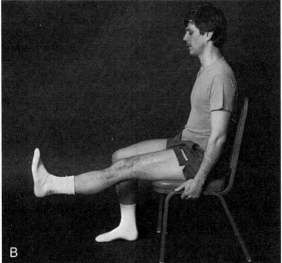

FIGURE 13–5. *A,* Straight leg raise. *B,* Knee flexion and extension.

an excellent way to develop strength in the early stages of rehabilitation, a time when weights may be too risky or difficult to maneuver. This technique is valuable for concurrently assessing and then varying resistance at these specific points in the ROM. Isotonic exercise equipment permits the resistance to vary throughout the ROM by the use of an elliptical cam. The cam provides the least resistance where the ability to produce force is correspondingly lower (early and late in ROM) and the greatest resistance where the muscle is at its optimal length-tension and mechanical advantage (usually mid-range). The acuity of the client's condition, diagnosis, and functional status determine which of these two types of isotonic exercise is most appropriate.

Isotonic exercise protocols differ and date back as early as the 1940s. DeLorme devised a method of progressive resistive exercise, which is the earliest known structured isotonic exercise program. The DeLorme method is based on the 10 resistance maximum (10 RM). The 10 RM is the maximum amount of resistance a person can lift 10 times. The client lifts three sets of 10 repetitions, first at 50% of his or her 10 RM weight, then at 75% of the 10 RM weight, and finally at 100% of his or her 10 RM weight. Many variables, including the number of repetitions per set, the amount and progression of resistance, and the frequency of exercise daily and weekly, determine the outcome of an isotonic exercise program. In general, the more repetitions performed, the greater the endurance. Increasing the amount of weight increases muscle strength. To achieve these gains, isotonic exercise should be performed three to five times per week. The advantages and disadvantages of isotonic exercise are shown in Table 13-4.

TABLE 13–4. *Advantages and Disadvantages of Isotonic Exercises*

ADVANTAGES	DISADVANTAGES
Muscle strength improves throughout the entire range of motion	Equipment can be costly or require excessive space
Enhanced muscle endurance	The resistance/load is limited by the weakest point in the range
Muscle size increases	Typically, muscles are exercised at one velocity, speeds that may not be functionally relevant
Ease of use, low cost	
Exercise is both concentric and eccentric	
Performance can be objectively measured	Increased risk of injury to the extremity (if pain occurs, client is unable to unload weight quickly and safely)
	The eccentric component of isotonic exercise may cause muscle soreness

Adapted from Bernhardt, D. B. (1986). *Sports physical therapy* (pp. 166-167). New York: Churchill Livingstone. Reprinted with permission.

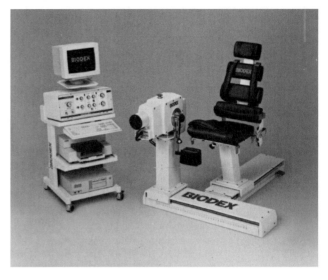

FIGURE 13–6. Biodex. (Courtesy of Biodex, Shirley, NY.)

Isokinetic Exercise. Isokinetic exercise was developed by Perrine in the late 1960s and is exercise at a preset dynamic speed that accommodates resistance to the muscle tension developed at each point of the ROM. Isokinetic exercise uses concentric and eccentric contractions.

Some of the current isokinetic devices on the market are the Biodex (Fig. 13-6), the Cybex II, and the Kin-Com machines. These devices provide computerized, comparative data that either support or refute certain medical diagnoses. Essentially, the isokinetic device has a lever arm that can be moved at a preset speed. The speed remains constant, but the resistance varies and is directly proportional to the force applied on the lever. In this way, the muscles can be maximally overloaded at every point in the ROM. The ability to overload is important when pain or weakness is present. If the client stops or reduces his or her output against the lever, the system adjusts accordingly. This allows the client to continue exercising without trauma or increased pain. In addition, the various speed settings available allow the exercises performed to approximate limb speeds found in functional activities. For example, isokinetic exercise can be used to train athletes at sport-specific speeds that may hasten their return to competition. The advantages and disadvantages of isokinetic exercise are given in Table 13-5.

PROPRIOCEPTION

Proprioception is the ability of muscle to respond to abnormal positions and situations (Baechle & Earle, 2000). It is similar to balance in that it provides a sense of joint position and movement. After an injury or orthopaedic surgery, proprioception, like strength and mobility, is usually impaired. Specific types of exercises improve this sense of position. Lower extremity proprioceptive

TABLE 13–5. *Advantages and Disadvantages of Isokinetic Exercises*

ADVANTAGES	DISADVANTAGES
The muscles are maximally loaded through the entire range of motion	Excessive purchase and maintenance costs of computerized devices
Safety; resistance stops when the client stops contracting because of pain or weakness	Accessories and attachments can be inconvenient and cumbersome to use
Accommodation of resistance, unloads or decreases at the weakest points in the range of motion	Cost of staff education and time
Reduction in joint compression at higher speeds	Single-joint exercise only therefore not the most functional method of strengthening
Exercise can be performed at variable speeds, speeds that mirror functional or recreational activities	
Immediate visual and/or auditory feedback that enhances performance and motivation	
Objective measurement of performance and progress	

Adapted from Bernhardt, D. B. (1986). *Sports physical therapy* (pp. 167–168). New York: Churchill Livingstone. Reprinted with permission.

exercises might include jumping on a minitrampoline or maneuvering on a balance board. An example of proprioceptive training for the upper extremities is push-ups performed on an uneven surface, such as a basketball.

Proprioceptive training is an important part of the rehabilitative process to ensure optimal recovery and minimize the risk of further injury. For example, the client who suffers from chronic ankle sprains must be instructed in proprioceptive exercises in addition to flexibility and strengthening exercises. This proprioceptive retraining helps the client avoid further injury to the ankle.

WEIGHT-BEARING EXERCISE

Ambulation

Ambulation is a complex three-dimensional activity involving the lower extremities, pelvis, trunk, and upper extremities. The following describes the two major phases of the human gait:

1. The *stance phase* of gait encompasses the entire time that the foot is on the ground. It begins with heel strike and ends with toe push off.
2. The *swing phase* is the period of acceleration of the gait cycle. It begins when the foot leaves the ground and lasts through the next heel strike.

During normal walking speed, the stance phase occupies approximately 60% of the gait cycle and the swing phase occupies 40%. Variation from these percentages may be considered pathologic.

Many factors contribute to alterations in the normal gait sequence or pattern. Because gait is an intricate and complex movement involving the musculoskeletal, neurologic, and cardiovascular systems, clinicians need to understand normal physiology, the interplay between systems, and pathomechanics. Cognitive factors, such as mentation and orientation, are critical prerequisites for safe ambulation.

Ambulation should be initiated as early as possible after an orthopaedic injury or surgery to prevent the adverse effects of immobility. Clients who have been on prolonged bed rest have generalized muscle weakness, decreased muscle endurance, decreased cardiopulmonary endurance, and decreased joint flexibility and coordination. Additional complications include, but are not limited to, hypovolemia, orthostatic hypotension, tachycardia, decreased maximal oxygen uptake, pressure sores, and depression. See Chapter 4 for a detailed discussion of the effects of immobility.

To safely mobilize these clients, a progressive program of exercise must be initiated. Because physical challenges can cause adverse cardiopulmonary responses in the deconditioned client, physiologic parameters such as respiration rate or oxygen saturation, heart rate, blood pressure, and electrocardiogram (ECG) should be monitored as appropriate. Client feedback also provides valuable insights into physiologic tolerance. Complaints of nausea, light-headedness, or dizziness can indicate hypotension, hypoxemia, or hypoglycemia, especially in clients with autonomic dysfunction, such as in diabetes.

A graduated, therapeutic exercise program can be initiated at bedside until transfer or gait training is permitted or feasible. PROM and AAROM exercises of all four extremities can be initiated to increase flexibility and strength and progress to resistive exercises as appropriate.

Tilt Table

Weight-bearing activities should be considered a form of exercise for the mobility-impaired client. It is an excellent means of challenging and conditioning the cardiovascular, musculoskeletal, and autonomic systems of the body. To achieve this end, clinicians can use a tilt table. The tilt table is indicated predominantly for the subset of clients who require a slower, more gradual progression to the upright position. Because clients may not initially tolerate the upright position, vital signs and physical signs and symptoms, such as pallor, perspiration, and dizziness, must be monitored. The client should be progressed to the vertical position as signs and symptoms dictate. If the orthopaedic client requires protective weight bearing during the activity because of a fracture or joint replacement, a lift can be placed under the unaffected extremity to prevent or minimize weight bearing on the affected side.

Transfer

When transfer training, the client should transfer toward the unaffected side. The client should sit at the edge of the chair and lean forward. This allows the client to get his or her weight over the lower extremities and reduces the amount of muscular effort required. The client should push up from the arm rests of the chair. The health care provider should not passively pull the client to standing because this may foster dependency and is unsafe for the client as well as the provider (Fig. 13–7).

When providing physical assistance, it is critical that the therapist or nurse follow appropriate safety measures and proper body mechanics. The muscles of the lower extremities should be used whenever possible for lifting, carrying, or pulling activities. The spine should be positioned in extension (erect) for these activities. Serious spinal injuries may be avoided when the appropriate muscles and mechanics are used. Specifically, the health care provider should use a broad base of support by placing feet apart to enhance stability. To reduce the muscular effort and injury potential from lifting, the clinician should instead slide, roll, push, or pull. Based on the level of assistance needed, appropriate devices should be used to transfer clients. Clients should not be lifted or slid up in bed by grasping under the axilla. For non–weight-bearing clients, a mechanical lift with a broad base and the capability of being operated by one person should be employed (Fig. 13–8A). If the client can bear some weight or is unstable, a walking belt with handles and an easy-snap closure (e.g., a Posey ergonomic belt,

Fig. 13–8B) allows the care provider an effective means to transfer the client. A mechanical lift that allows some weight bearing (Fig. 13–8C) is another option for partial weight-bearing or unstable clients.

For horizontal transfers (e.g., the bed to a cart or cardiac chair), the use of specialized sheets (e.g., a Slipp sheet) provides more comfort for the client than transfer boards. There are other devices, such as a Magic Sheet and the Kimbo pelvic lift, that promote ease in lifting clients in bed and in the use of the bedpan. Owen and colleagues (Owen & Fragala, 1999; Owen & Garg, 1993; Owen, Keene, Olson, & Garg, 1995) found that these devices decreased caregiver ratings of perceived exertion in transferring situations, increased client comfort, and lessened the caregiver back injury rate and lost workdays when compared with transferring techniques that did not employ assistive devices. See Chapter 3 for more information on client transfer devices. In addition to assistive devices, appropriate footwear (clinician and client) should be used when transferring or ambulating clients.

Different levels of assist and transfer techniques (described in Box 13–1) are based on the client's condition and the amount of assistance needed.

Weight-Bearing Status

Protective weight bearing is often needed to execute early mobilization safely. The degree of protective weight bearing necessary is determined by the orthopaedic physician, the client's orthopaedic condition, and the surgical procedure. Box 13–2 lists the types of weight-bearing status frequently prescribed by the physician.

Ambulatory Assistive Devices

Assistive devices can provide temporary or permanent assistance by decreasing compressive forces on the lower extremity joints, aiding in balance, and reducing the energy requirements of gait. The type of device selected and the duration of its use depend on the client's

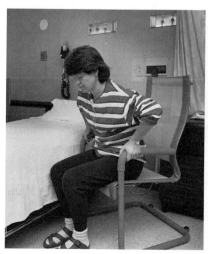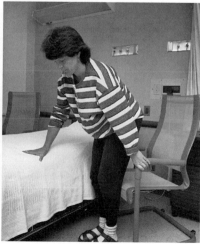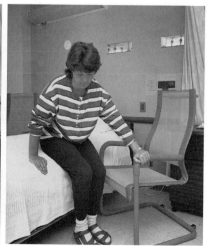

FIGURE 13–7. Chair-to-bed transfer.

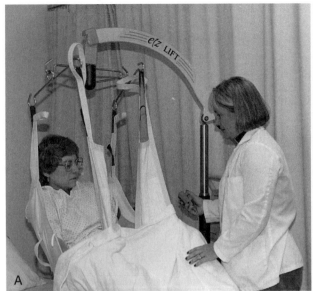

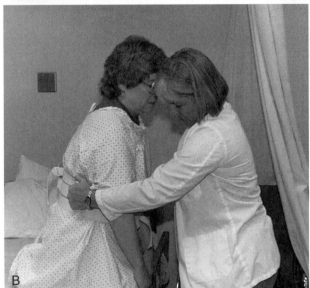

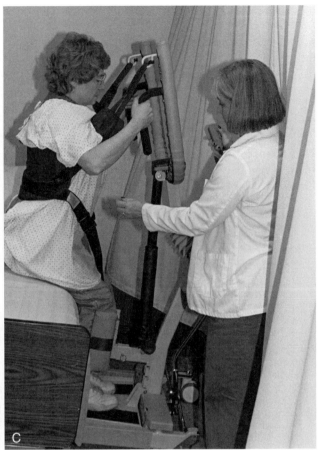

FIGURE 13–8. *A,* Use of a mechanical lift for non–weight-bearing clients. *B,* A walking belt with handles and easy-snap closure (e.g., a Posey ergonomic belt) can be used to assist in transfers when the client is limited to partial weight bearing or is unsteady. *C,* This mechanical lift allows some weight bearing for transfers.

BOX 13–1.

Levels of Assist / Transfer Techniques

Independent

The client requires no assistance, performance is safe.

Standby Assist of 1

The client requires only verbal cuing or direct visual observation. The clinician is ready to assist if the need arises.

Contact Guard of 1

Clinician places hands on client and is ready to provide support if needed. A gait belt should be used.

Physical Assist

The client may require minimal to maximal physical assist of one or more health care providers. Support devices (e.g., a gait belt) or mechanical devices must be considered. The degree of assist or support is determined by the severity of the functional impairment.

Total Assist

Mechanical devices (i.e., electrical or hydraulic lifts) are required to execute transfers.

BOX 13–2.
Weight-Bearing Status

Non–Weight-Bearing Status
No weight is borne by the affected limb.

Touch-Down Weight Bearing
The foot makes contact with the floor, but no weight is borne.

Partial Weight Bearing
The client bears a percentage of weight less than 100% on the affected extremity. The specific percentage is dictated by the orthopaedic surgeon.

Weight Bearing as Tolerated
The amount of weight borne on the extremity is dictated by the client's pain tolerance.

Full Weight Bearing
The client bears weight fully on the affected extremity.

---

diagnosis and overall functional condition. For a subset of clients who cannot ambulate or bear weight bilaterally, a wheelchair may be the mobility aid of choice.

Parallel Bars. If the client's balance, coordination, or muscle strength is questionable, initial trials with ambulation should be done with the parallel bars (Fig. 13-9). Parallel bars provide the client with bilateral upper extremity support during gait training. This added support allows the client to focus on skill acquisition of gait substrates, that is, weight shifting, timing, and motor control. Once the client has demonstrated competency in the parallel bars, gait training is progressed to one of the following assistive devices.

Walkers. Standard walkers are lightweight aids that facilitate partial weight bearing or non–weight bearing of an affected extremity. These devices are also beneficial in enhancing stability for clients with poor balance or risk for falls. Walkers are constructed of aluminum or metal alloys that are able to withstand prolonged use and substantial compressive forces.

Strategies to enhance independence with gait activities begin when the client is hospitalized. For example, upper extremity strength is needed to successfully use a gait aid. The following is a partial listing of specific exercises that can be implemented on admission to strengthen the upper extremities for gait activities.

Biceps: The biceps muscles can be strengthened by the use of the overhead trapeze supplied in many hospital beds.

Triceps: While sitting, the client takes a weight in each hand, with elbows flexed. The client extends his or her elbows so the hands are raised above the head (Fig. 13-10).

Triceps: A book is placed on the bed on each side of the client. The client pushes down on them and lifts his or her buttocks off the bed. It is essential that the client maintain good posture and balance during the exercise.

The non–weight-bearing client ambulating with a walker must follow several steps. First, the client should be supported when attempting to stand from sitting. The client must be stable when standing with a walker before taking a step. Second, the client advances the walker a short distance with the clinician's support as needed. Third, the client transfers all his or her body weight to the arms, keeping his or her elbows fairly straight to absorb body weight. At this time, the client takes a step with the unaffected leg. The client should be reminded to keep the affected leg off the floor with non–weight-bearing restrictions.

Wheeled or rolling walkers may be appropriate for the orthopaedic client who is allowed to bear weight. This type of walker assists the client who has painful lower extremity joints with weight bearing, decreased balance/coordination, or decreased cardiopulmonary function. These walkers are available as two-wheeled, three-wheeled (delta), and four-wheeled walkers (Fig. 13-11). Many accessories for these walkers are available, including hand brakes, built-in seats, and baskets.

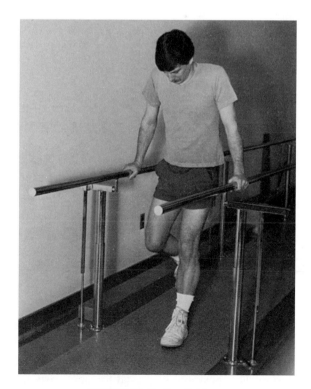

FIGURE 13–9. Parallel bars.

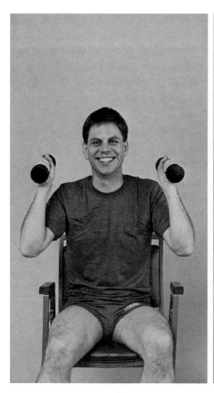
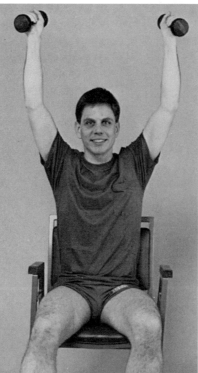

FIGURE 13–10. Triceps strengthening.

Crutches. Crutches can be used temporarily by clients with sprains or casts or after selected surgical procedures. These devices may also be indicated on a permanent basis for clients with congenital or acquired musculoskeletal anomalies, neuromuscular weakness or paralysis, or amputations. When prescribing and adjusting crutches, one must consider the client's overall condition, motivation, age, interests, and goals. The types of metal or wooden crutches commercially available are axillary, forearm, and Lofstrand.

Crutch Length Measurement. Proper fitting of an axillary crutch is essential for avoiding abnormal stresses on the body. An improper fit or usage can result in crutch palsy or back strain. Crutch palsy is caused by constant or prolonged axillary pressure from weight bearing on the crutch pad. Temporary or even permanent numbness in the hands secondary to an irritation of the brachial plexus can occur. The client should be taught to put all of his or her weight on the crutch handgrips. Back strain may occur if the crutch height is set too low, forcing the lumbar spine into forward flexion.

To ensure proper crutch length, the client should assume the tripod position (Fig. 13–12). For safety, the client should wear low-heeled shoes. The handgrip should be adjusted so that the client's wrist is adjacent to the grip with the elbow extended. With the hand on the handgrip, the elbow will be in approximately 30 degrees of flexion. This position is optimal for upper extremity leverage.

Crutch Gaits. Different gait patterns can be used with crutches. The client's diagnosis, weight-bearing status, overall condition, age, and balance dictate which pattern is most appropriate. The following is a list of common gait patterns prescribed:

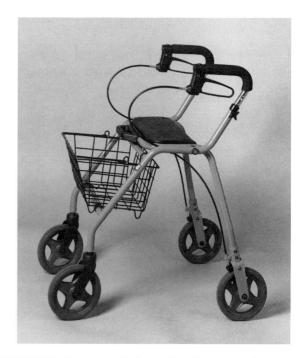

FIGURE 13–11. Four-wheeled walker. (Courtesy of Guardian, Simi Valley, CA.)

affected leg forward, and finally lowers to the seat (Fig. 13–13). To perform the reverse, the client should push off from the armrest or seat with the hand on the affected side and use the contralateral hand to push off from the crutch handgrips.

Surfaces and Stairs. Once the client is able to ambulate effectively on a level surface, negotiating stairs should be taught. When ascending stairs, the unaffected leg advances first up the step while the body weight is supported by the crutches. Full body weight is transferred to this leg once it is safely positioned. The crutches and the affected leg then follow to this same step. When descending, the opposite occurs, the affected leg and crutches lead. The crutches and the affected leg move down one step, the unaffected leg follows. If a single handrail is available, one hand holds the rail and the opposite hand holds the crutches. A similar pattern for ascent/descent is then executed. To ensure client safety while ascending and descending stairs, steps must be uncluttered and well lit.

The health care provider must review with the client the necessary precautionary measures to follow when ambulating on uneven surfaces, sidewalks, and wet or icy pavement. These terrains increase the likelihood of a fall or injury. To enhance safety, the client should be advised to have assistance when attempting these surfaces for the first time. Emphasis should also be placed on durable equipment management, for example, maintaining the crutch components or using ice-grippers during icy weather.

Canes. The client may use one or two wooden or metal alloy canes to enhance stability or to relieve pressure on weight-bearing joints. A cane can reduce only the weight-bearing load on a given lower extremity by up to 30%. The conventional cane style is either a C-curve or T-top. Metal alloy canes are available in single-point (standard) contact, three-point (triangular) contact, or four-point (quadrangular) contact. Before teaching cane-assisted ambulation, the health care provider must assess the client's balance, strength, and confidence to ensure that the appropriate device has been selected. Once the selection has been confirmed, the cane must be correctly adjusted. To measure or adjust a cane, the same technique used for fitting crutches is followed. The handgrip of the cane should be adjacent to the client's wrist with the elbow extended and the client standing erect.

Once the device is correctly adjusted, the client is instructed in the appropriate gait technique. The client should be instructed to completely lift the cane off the floor rather than slide it. This procedure lessens the possibility of a fall as a result of catching the cane tip on the floor. The client using one cane is taught to place the cane close to the body on the unaffected side and is instructed to always advance the cane with the affected

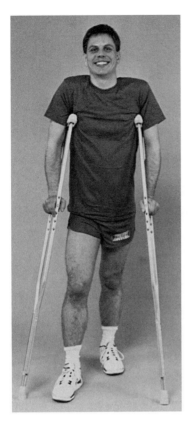

FIGURE 13–12. Tripod position.

1. *Two-point gait:* The opposite arm and leg move simultaneously. The sequence is right crutch and left foot, left crutch and right foot. This pattern is used by clients with bilateral partial weight-bearing limitations, for example, clients with bilateral lower extremity prostheses.
2. *Three-point gait:* Both crutches and the affected lower extremity move simultaneously. This is frequently used when partial or non–weight bearing is desired on the affected leg.
3. *Four-point alternate-crutch gait:* This sequence requires the client to move one crutch or extremity at a time. Specifically, right crutch, left foot, left crutch, and right foot. This technique can be used if weight bearing is allowed. This is a safe gait pattern because three points of support are always on the floor.

Sitting. Clients using crutches must develop independence in rising from the seated position to standing and the reverse, activities commonly known as transitional movements. To safely sit, the client should walk up to the chair and carefully turn around using the crutches. The client should carefully back up to the chair until the unaffected leg touches the seat. The client should grip both crutches in one hand by the handgrips and place them on the unaffected side. After the crutches are securely positioned, the client slowly bends at the waist, places the affected side's hand on the seat, moves the

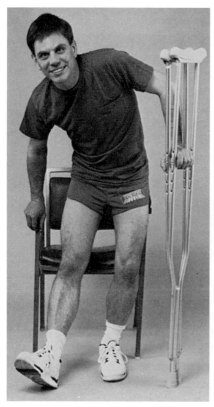
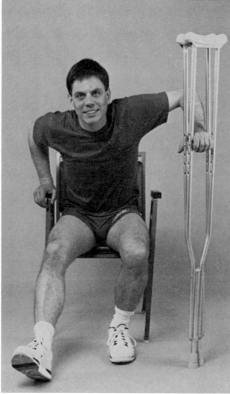

FIGURE 13–13. Stand to sitting with crutches.

leg. If using two canes, the client is instructed in the four-point or two-point gaits as previously described. For ascending steps, the client should step up with the unaffected leg first, then advance the cane with the affected leg. For descending stairs, the client should reverse this process, stepping down first with the cane and affected leg, followed by the unaffected leg.

PHYSICAL MODALITIES

Physical modalities or agents are used in conjunction with therapeutic exercises and functional activities to achieve specific therapeutic goals. The type of agent selected to augment treatment is based on the pathology, the desired tissue effect, the chronicity of the condition, and the client's physiologic status. The specific agents available for the treatment of pain and disability include electricity, sound, cold (cryotherapy), heat (thermotherapy), and light. The focus of this section is limited to those physical agents most commonly used in the orthopaedic setting.

Electric Stimulation

Electric stimulation is the application of low-intensity, pulsed, alternating, or direct currents (Fig. 13–14). This modality can be used to treat neuromuscular, musculoskeletal, soft tissue, and vascular conditions. The indications and contraindications for electrical stimulation are listed in Table 13–6.

There are two types of electric current: galvanic (direct) current and faradic (alternating) current. In direct current (DC) circuits, the electrodes maintain their positive or negative polarity; therefore, when these electrodes are used to stimulate tissues, positive and negative fields are established and maintained under the positive and

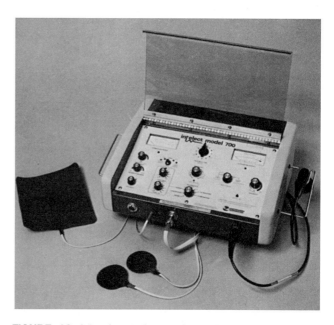

FIGURE 13–14. Electrical stimulator. (Courtesy of Chattanooga Corp., Chattanooga, TN.)

TABLE 13–6. *Indications and Contraindications for Electric Stimulation*

INDICATIONS	CONTRAINDICATIONS
Exercise muscle tissue	Acute inflammation
Decrease or prevent muscle atrophy	Skin abnormalities
Increase circulation	Unstable cardiac pathologic conditions or pacemakers (may stimulate onset of arrhythmias)
Increase tissue temperature	
Reduce adhesions	
Reeducate muscle	Thrombophlebitis or a thrombosis (may cause embolus formation)
Promote healing of peripheral nerve lesions that involve musculotendinous units	
Decrease inflammation	
Decrease edema	
Decrease muscle spasm	
Decrease contracture formation	
Decrease pain	
Treat ulcers	
Increase joint mobility	

negative electrodes, respectively. Alternating current (AC) is a current that changes its direction of flow periodically; therefore, its electrodes change polarity alternately.

High-voltage galvanic stimulation (HVGS) is a form of galvanic stimulation that is more comfortable and therefore is used more frequently than low-voltage galvanic stimulation (LVGS). HVGS has been found to be more comfortable, elicits a stronger muscle contraction, and is preferred by clients over LVGS. High-voltage stimulation has a low-amperage and low-current density, and consists of a twin-pulsed waveform with a pulse duration of up to 200 ms. The voltage of this technique varies between 100 and 500 V.

Physiologic Effects. A number of physiologic effects are induced by electric stimulation to tissues. Specifically, this modality affects the neuromuscular, sensory, and vascular systems and therefore has been used clinically for years in muscle reeducation, wound healing, and pain reduction.

Neuromuscular System. Electric stimulation affects both the sensory and motor systems. Sensory stimulation is the result of excitation of large myelinated sensory A fibers, particularly group II fibers (as seen with transcutaneous electrical nerve stimulation application). These fibers conduct pressure and tactile (touch) input, which are perceived as a tingling sensation by the client. Motor stimulation results when motor nerves are excited through electric stimulation, causing either a twitch or a tetanic muscular contraction. If a client experiences pain with this modality, it may be a result of stimulation of small myelinated A fibers (group III) and nonmyelinated

C fibers (group IV), which conduct predominantly pain and temperature information.

Electric stimulation is an effective adjunct during early and later phases of rehabilitation. The use of HVGS on the quadriceps and hamstrings during immobilization of a client's leg with a cast can help increase thigh girth and maintain limb motor function. Electric stimulation of both agonist and antagonist muscle groups may lessen timing difficulties with sporting events. This technique appears more beneficial than electric stimulation of only the agonist muscle group. These muscle reeducation techniques are better tolerated by the client when the correct electrode size is selected. Specifically, when non-painful stimulation is desired during muscle reeducation, the clinician should select larger electrodes.

Vascular System. HVGS increases blood flow, decreases edema, and facilitates wound healing. An increase in blood flow contributes to pain reduction, decreased muscle spasms, enhanced joint mobility, reduction of edema, and augmented wound healing. Although blood flow is promoted under both poles, the negative pole stimulus provides a better blood flow response than the positive. The blood flow increase seen with HVGS appears to be related to the strength of muscle contraction produced. Types III and IV afferents are thought to be responsible for the reflex cardiovascular changes seen during muscle contraction. These nerves are activated through stimuli, such as muscle pressure, stretch, contraction, and pain.

Edema is an abnormal accumulation of extravascular interstitial fluid. Edema results from an increase in capillary permeability and a rise in the concentration of interstitial protein. An increase in capillary permeability results in leakage of protein and occasionally a gain in leukocytes (part of the inflammatory response). The rise in the concentration of interstitial protein causes an increase in tissue pressure, resulting in expansion in the movement of fluid into the interstitium.

Edema is reduced by restoring normal capillary permeability. This prevents proteins from returning into the capillaries. The proteins in the interstitial space are removed by the lymphatic and proteolytic systems, and interstitial fluid is removed by the lymphatic and vascular systems. Electric stimulation is theorized to facilitate a decrease in edema by promoting blood and lymphatic flow. In addition, this modality reduces the initial loss of fluid to the interstitium by decreasing inflammation. By stimulating these processes, the removal of excess interstitial fluid and protein should be enhanced.

Wound Healing. Low-intensity DC and HVGS enhance wound healing. Physical factors that affect wound healing are the circulatory status, presence of infection, pH of the wound site, client's age, nutritional status, pressure control and dressing interventions, and the client's overall medical condition. These physical factors influence the surrounding tissue fluid medium and cells and the proportional amounts of proteins present. To facilitate timely and appropriate wound healing, all factors must be addressed.

Electric current has been found to affect collagen-producing cells, collagen fibers, charged protein particles, and surrounding tissue fluid. The collagen biosynthesis and increased number of fibroblasts found in previous studies probably shortened wound healing time. We know that the tissues beneath the positive electrode experience vasoconstriction, tissue hardening, sedation, and local analgesia. The negative electrode induces vasodilation, tissue softening, tissue irritation, and decreased swelling. The type of polarity selected for wound healing is dependent on many factors, such as the desired physiologic effect, the presence of eschar or infection, and the type and depth of the wound. Clinicians generally agree that the positive electrical field is more effective for tissue healing and the negative electrical field has a greater bactericidal effect. The average rate of wound healing is 1 mm per day.

Pain Reduction. Electric stimulation provides pain reduction through multiple mechanisms, as previously mentioned. Specifically, reduction in edema, increase in blood flow, control of infection, and facilitation of soft tissue healing ultimately contribute to pain reduction. Again, these outcomes are actualized by the appropriate

TABLE 13–7. *Indications and Contraindications for Iontophoresis*

INDICATIONS	CONTRAINDICATIONS
Arthritic conditions	See contraindications for electric stimulation (see Table 13–6)
Local anesthesia	
Application of steroids to inflamed tissue	History of intolerance to electric stimulation
Antibiotic administration	Pacemakers
Hyperhidrosis (excessive sweating)	Treatment over select thoracic regions (risk of induction of fibrillation)
Calcium deposits	
Tendon adhesions	Drug sensitivity or allergies
Dentistry	Damaged or denuded skin
Ophthalmology	Treatment over temporal or orbital regions

type and parameters of electric stimulation selected by the clinician.

Iontophoresis

Iontophoresis is the use of electric current to transport medications in solution across the skin barrier to affected tissue. Iontophoresis has been in use since 1908, when LeDuc first described this effect. Electric potential causes ions in solution to migrate according to their electric charges.

The Phoresor device (IOMED, Inc.) (Fig. 13–15) is a commercially available iontophoresis system. This device is made up of a 9-V battery, a DC power supply, a controller unit, a disposable electrode assembly, and a high-impedance and low-impedance monitor check (the monitor is a safety mechanism to minimize the potential for electric burns). The intensity of DC is very low and comfortable for the client, specifically 4 mA for a 10- to 20-minute treatment. A number of ions are used clinically for iontophoresis. Two commonly used medications with iontophoresis are lidocaine hydrochloride for local analgesia and dexamethasone sodium phosphate (0.4%) as an anti-inflammatory agent.

Iontophoresis is used primarily to introduce anti-inflammatory agents, analgesics, and antibiotics into the tissue through the skin. It has documented use in a wide variety of medical conditions and tissue types. Indications and contraindications for the use of iontophoresis are listed in Table 13–7.

Physiologic Effects. The positive ions in solution migrate toward the negative pole, causing an alkaline reaction. This reaction creates physiologic effects similar to those found with electric stimulation, for example, increased skin irritation, nerve excitability, and softening of tissues. The opposite effects occur when the negative ions migrate toward the positive pole, for example, a reduction in skin irritation, hardening of tissues, and

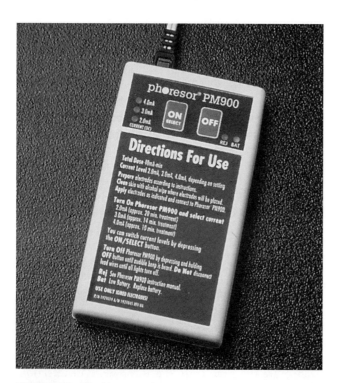

FIGURE 13–15. Phoresor. (Courtesy of IOMED Inc., Salt Lake City, UT.)

diminished nerve excitability. Both poles realize a mild heating effect with transient erythema secondary to vasomotor stimulation. The erythema disappears within 3 to 8 hours under the dispersive electrode, and mottling under the active electrode disappears within several days.

Iontophoresis has several advantages compared with local needle injection. It is sterile (decreased risk for infection), relatively pain free, and noninvasive. Because iontophoresis is applied locally, potential drug toxicity or a systemic reaction is avoided.

The disadvantages and side effects of iontophoresis are few but can include purpura under the treatment electrode and skin irritation or burns if it is used incorrectly. In addition, the effectiveness of this modality is related to tissue depth. It is most effective for the treatment of superficial structures, such as the patellar tendon (tendinitis) and wrist extensors (epicondylitis), and less effective for the treatment of deep soft tissue structures.

Ultrasound

Ultrasound is a form of deep heat, produced by the conversion of electric energy to high-frequency sound energy (Fig. 13–16). Basic research and subsequent clinical application were started in Europe early in the 20th century. The use of ultrasound in the United States followed the European experience in the early 1950s. This modality was used initially for the purpose of pain relief and soft tissue relaxation. Indications and contraindications for ultrasound treatment are shown in Table 13–8.

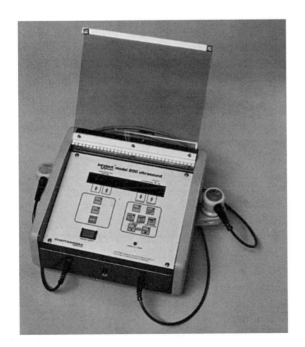

FIGURE 13–16. Intelect model 200 ultrasound machine. (Courtesy of Chattanooga Corp., Chattanooga, TN.)

TABLE 13–8. *Indications and Contraindications for Ultrasound*

INDICATIONS	CONTRAINDICATIONS
Postacute soft tissue trauma	Acute conditions
Tendinitis, bursitis, and fasciitis	Treatment of eyes, ears, or paced heart
Inflammation	Over reproductive organs
Ligamentous or joint contractures	Pregnant uterus
Soften scar tissue	Endocrine glands
Treatment of pressure sores	Central nervous system structures
Facilitate resorption of hematomas	Bony epiphyses or fracture sites
Neuromas	Malignancies
Chronic arthritis	Thrombophlebitis
Sympathetic nervous system disorders (i.e., reflex dystrophies)	Infected tissues
	Areas with a tendency to hemorrhage

Physiologic Effects. The sound waves produced during an ultrasound treatment penetrate tissues approximately 2 inches below the skin, causing a mechanical vibration. This vibration increases local tissue temperature by 7° to 8°F within 20 to 30 seconds, an effect that can last up to 1 hour. In normal application, 50% of the ultrasound energy is transmitted to 5 cm below the skin surface. The sound waves also cause a micromassaging action on cells and enhance cortisol levels when applied to peripheral nerves.

Tissue composition has a direct effect on the therapeutic effect of ultrasound. The more homogeneous the tissue, the less ultrasound energy absorbed. Therefore, subcutaneous fat, which is homogeneous, does not absorb as much ultrasound energy as muscle, a heterogeneous tissue. Because synthetic and metallic implants are also homogeneous, their temperatures rise by only very small increments. Thus, ultrasound treatments can be used safely with obese clients and clients with joint implants.

Ultrasound waves tend to concentrate in junctions between dissimilar tissues, such as the skin-fat and tendon-bone interfaces. This concentration effect leads to an increase in tissue temperature, which can be a concern for specific tissue types, such as tendon and bone, which have a poor blood supply and low water content. Because of this, they are not efficient in disseminating thermal energy. Excessive treatment time or intensity over superficial interfaces can lead to overheating and, ultimately, tissue necrosis. The periosteum is richly supplied with thermoreceptors, sensors that provide feedback regarding excessive tissue temperature. If overheating occurs, the client will feel a deep discomfort. This pain response provides the clinician with immediate and valuable information about the correct intensity and duration.

Treatment Mode. Because air is not an efficient medium for transmitting sound waves, a coupling agent is required between the transducer and treatment site. Coupling agents, such as lotion, gel, mineral oil, or water, can be used. Ultrasound treatment can be given underwater, with the sound head held 0.5 to 1 inch from the skin surface. Underwater treatments are an excellent way of treating bony areas, such as the hands and feet, or irregularly shaped areas where surface contact is difficult to maintain. The sound head should be applied perpendicular to the skin surface using a circular or longitudinal stroking technique. The sound head should be in constant motion; it should never be stationary during treatment.

Ultrasound can be administered using a continuous or pulsed waveform with either a 1- or 3.3-MHz frequency. The clinician selects the appropriate frequency and waveform type based on the desired effect and the location, size, and depth of the tissues treated. Continuous ultrasound produces heat and mechanical vibration, whereas pulsed ultrasound produces mechanical vibration without significant heating. Because of this, pulsed ultrasound is typically used over bony areas to avoid excessive heating in the periosteum-bone interfaces. Frequency selection is based in part on tissue depth. Superficial tissues typically are treated with 3.3 MHz, and deep tissue structures are treated with 1 MHz.

Cryotherapy

Cryotherapy, or cold therapy, used during the first 24 to 72 hours is the most effective method of reducing inflammation from trauma or surgery. Cold constricts blood vessels, and this constriction decreases local tissue blood flow, metabolic activity, and tissue temperature. These physiologic effects reduce edema and anesthetize the affected part by diminishing nerve impulses and conduction velocities. Muscle spasms and tension can be diminished through the lowering of tissue temperature that occurs by the reduction in muscle spindle firing. When pain and muscle spasms are decreased, the pain-spasm-pain cycle can be broken. If edema can be prevented or minimized, the client responds more favorably to exercises needed to restore preinjury function. The combined treatment of rest, ice, compression, and elevation is often referred to as *RICE*.

When using cold applications, the therapist must consider the age of the client, the purpose, and the underlying vascular condition of the tissues treated. Cryotherapy is indicated for soft tissue injuries, such as sprains, strains, contusions, muscle spasms, and chronic inflammatory conditions (e.g., tendinitis, tenosynovitis, fasciitis). Cold is contraindicated for clients with circulatory disturbances, hypersensitivity to cold, intolerance to cold, or Raynaud's phenomenon or over a regenerating peripheral nerve. Prolonged application of cold can cause skin trauma, such as blisters or frostbite.

With the following cryotherapy techniques, the client experiences sensations of intense cold, burning, aching, and eventual numbness. Before initiating any cryotherapy technique, a sensory evaluation must be completed to ensure that the client has adequate sensation to light touch and heat/cold. The treatment should be terminated once the client reports the onset of numbness, typically after 10 to 15 minutes. This is critical to eliminate the potential for thermal injury to soft tissue structures. The cryotherapy technique can be repeated several times daily during the acute phase of injury.

1. *Ice massage:* Paper cups are filled with frozen water, forming an ice cylinder that can be rubbed or massaged directly onto the client's skin surface. Ice massage application is for 5 to 10 minutes or until the client experiences analgesia at the site of application.

2. *Cold immersion:* A whirlpool tank, bucket, or similar container is filled with a mixture of ice and water. Treatment duration depends on the temperature of the water and the client's subjective response. This method is extremely effective for larger areas, such as the ankle, shin, or lower leg. An elastic wrap applied before immersion adds compression to this method.

3. *Ice packs:* Plastic bags filled with crushed ice are placed over a damp towel and then placed over the site of injury. Finer ice chips melt faster but tend to be well tolerated over painful sites.

4. *Chemical cold packs:* Reusable, commercially manufactured packs are placed over a damp towel and then positioned over the affected area. This method is convenient but expensive, and the temperature is not always consistent.

5. *Flexible cold packs:* Refreezable, flexible silicone gel cold packs encased in vinyl are placed over a damp towel and applied to the affected area.

6. *Portable cooling systems:* These systems can be operated either electrically or manually. The electric systems are similar to electric heating pads, providing cooling rather than heat. Manual systems use circulating water to reduce tissue temperature. An example of a manual system is the controlled cold compression unit, which alternately pumps cold water and air into a sleeve that is wrapped around the client's limb.

7. *Evaporative cooling:* Cold sprays (ethyl chloride, dichlorodifluoromethane 15% and trichloromonofluoromethane 85% [Fluori-methane]) evaporate rapidly when sprayed on trigger points and muscle spasms. Unlike the aforementioned techniques, this cooling technique is best suited for the treatment of painful spasms and not for postoperative management or acute injuries. This technique is generally combined with stretching exercises to help reduce the pain-spasm cycle of such soft tissue injuries as low-back strains.

Thermotherapy

Thermotherapy, or heating, improves local circulation by increasing blood flow and dilating closed capillary beds. This process enhances cell metabolism, producing an influx of oxygen and nutrients into the site and encouraging the removal of waste products. Muscle spasms are reduced by inhibiting nerve activity, thereby producing a mild sedative effect with subsequent pain relief. Thermotherapy is very effective in breaking the pain-spasm cycle, particularly in postacute soft tissue injuries, and is often advocated 24 to 72 hours after injuries. Heat application can increase the extensibility of collagenous soft tissue, such as tendon, ligament, scar tissue, or joint capsule, thereby increasing joint ROM and/or decreasing joint stiffness. Heat is contraindicated in acute inflammatory conditions during the first 24 to 72 hours after the injury.

The four major methods of heat application are as follows:

1. *Radiation:* Heat or energy is transferred through space by electromagnetic waves (e.g., infrared lamp).
2. *Conduction:* Heat is directly applied to the body, using hydrocollator packs, hot water bottles, towels, paraffin baths, or electrically heated pads.
3. *Convection:* Heat is transferred via a medium, such as the movement of air or water (e.g., whirlpool bath).
4. *Conversion:* Heat is developed by the passage of sound or electric current through tissue (e.g., electric stimulation, ultrasound, diathermy).

Superficial heat (radiation, conduction, and convection) takes 20 to 30 minutes to produce the desired effect. Temperature elevations are greatest in the skin, with no significant rise 1 to 2 cm beneath the skin surface.

Contraindications to heat use are acute injury or inflammation, recent or potential hemorrhage, thrombophlebitis, impaired sensation, impaired mentation, or malignancy.

The heat applications most commonly used for the orthopaedic patient are described in this section.

Whirlpool bath (a stainless steel tank filled with warm to hot water) is one of the most common forms of heat treatment. A turbine agitates the water, providing tissue massage in addition to the heating effects. Whirlpool is indicated for subacute soft tissue trauma, open wounds or abrasions needing cleansing, and prolonged immobilization of extremities in need of regaining ROM (e.g., after surgery or trauma). Contraindications to hydrotherapy treatments include significant cardiopulmonary disease; active hemorrhaging or swelling; heat stress; and acute contusions, sprains, or strains. Whirlpool treatment duration is typically 20 minutes at a moderate temperature (99° to 104°F) to prevent tissue injury. Clients should never be unattended during treatment because of the risk of heat stress or drowning. The clinician must use approved disinfectants and universal precautions to avoid nosocomial infections or cross-contamination.

A wound care alternative to whirlpool for clients with severe cardiac involvement, moderate to severe peripheral edema, severe peripheral vascular disease (inability to shunt heat from the site), or incontinence is either the Pulsavac System (Zimmer, Inc.) or the use of a hosing technique. Care must be taken to minimize the water pressure with these alternatives because excessive water pressures can interfere with the tissue granulation process and, ultimately, healing.

Hydrocollator packs are moist heat packs used to treat postacute soft tissue injuries, such as contusions, strains, and muscle spasms. These packs contain silicone gel, which absorbs and retains heat. Hydrocollator packs are stored in a heating unit that maintains the temperature at a constant 65.6° to 76.7°C (150° to 170°F). Hot packs are removed from the heating unit, wrapped in several layers of toweling, and applied to the affected part for 20 to 30 minutes. Caution must be observed to prevent thermal burns. To that end, a sensory evaluation must precede its use, and frequent skin inspections must be performed during the treatment. The use of hydrocollator packs is contraindicated for acute injuries, areas with impaired sensation, or tissues compromised by arterial insufficiency or over eyes and genitals.

Paraffin baths provide superficial heat to angular, bony areas of the body, such as the hands, feet, or wrists. A mixture of paraffin and mineral oil (6:1 or 7:1) is used and maintained at 45° to 50°C (113° to 122°F) in a heating unit. Paraffin can sustain heat, promote circulation, and decrease pain and therefore is effective in treating subacute injuries and arthritic conditions. Paraffin baths should not be used when heat is contraindicated, for example, with active hemorrhaging or impaired circulation. In addition, this modality is contraindicated when open wounds are present (the paraffin and mineral oil mixture would be in direct contact with the lesion).

Contrast Baths

Contrast baths alternate cryotherapy and thermotherapy in the postacute phase of injury. This technique is used to relieve local pain and to reduce tissue edema by alternately contracting and relaxing blood vessels. The most common technique uses two whirlpools filled with water, one with cold water at 10° to 18.3°C (50° to 65°F) and the second with hot water at 37.8° to 43.3°C (100° to 110°F). The affected extremity is placed in the cold water for 1 minute, followed by 3 to 5 minutes in the hot water. Cold and hot are alternated for four to five cycles. This technique can be used up to several times a day. Generally, all treatments should end with cold to diminish any swelling the heat produced. Cryotherapy is used exclusively if swelling develops after contrast therapy. AROM exercises can be performed while the affected extremity is in the water to facilitate resorption of edema.

Contraindications for the use of this modality include acute injuries, lesions with active hemorrhaging, and peripheral vascular disease.

Nursing Care for Clients Receiving Cryotherapy or Thermotherapy

Heat/Cold Application. Clients receiving cryotherapy or thermotherapy are at risk for injury to the skin and underlying structures. Considerations for care of these clients are described in Box 13–3.

ORTHOTICS

An orthosis, prescribed by a physician, is an external appliance that applies forces to or removes forces from an area of the body in a controlled manner. Orthotic devices enhance function and mobility, control motion, and provide pressure relief. Optimal client outcomes are best achieved by a multifactorial approach, including rehabilitation techniques, medical management, surgery, and orthotics.

The client's diagnosis, functional status, physical condition, sensorimotor status, and lifestyle must be considered when choosing an orthotic device. The physician must work collaboratively with the therapist, orthotist, and client to create an acceptable device that maximizes function. To ensure client compliance and satisfaction with orthotic interventions, the device must be medically indicated, comfortable, cosmetically acceptable, cost-effective, easily applied and removed, and low maintenance.

Orthotics can be used for one or more of the following reasons:

1. Relief of pain by limiting motion or weight bearing
2. Immobilization and protection of weak, painful, or healing musculoskeletal segments
3. Reduction of axial load, friction, and shear
4. Prevention and correction of deformity
5. Improvement of function or mobility

BOX 13–3.

Nursing Care for Clients Receiving Cryotherapy or Thermotherapy (Cold or Heat Application)

Provide client teaching about the use of the treatment.
Assess for contraindications.
Assess treated skin to minimize potential for thermal injury.
Choose appropriate method of applying heat or cold.
Limit the duration of cold applications and stop when sensation begins to decline.
Do not apply ice packs directly to the skin. Use an insulating material, such as a towel.
Assess and document the client's response to the therapy.

Most health care providers are familiar with common orthotics, such as ankle foot orthoses (AFO), knee ankle foot orthoses (KAFO), custom and noncustom arch supports, forearm supports, and spinal orthotics. For examples of types and specific uses of upper and lower extremity orthotics, see Table 13–9.

Clinicians are becoming familiar with the benefits of pedorthics, an orthotic intervention that addresses complex foot and ankle pathologic conditions. This specialty is invaluable for the management of clients with types I and II diabetes. Foot orthoses relieve pressure, shear, and friction, thereby reducing the potential for diabetic lower extremity amputations.

Many clients with diabetes develop structural foot deformities (e.g., Charcot joints) or lose protective plantar sensation, placing them at high risk for foot ulcerations. Foot orthotics are prescribed as a preventive or corrective measure to eliminate pressure. These devices can be prescribed for open lesions or structures at risk for breakdown. Orthotics, such as custom-molded shoes and inserts, patellar tendon bearing (PTB) orthotics, and noncustom diabetic footwear and inserts, are available to prevent and heal lesions. The type of orthotic prescribed is based on multiple factors, such as the status of protective sensation, type of skeletal deformity, callus location, vascular status, and ulcer grade.

Nursing Care for Clients Using an Orthosis

Circulatory Care, Teaching: Treatment, Skin Surveillance. Nurses need to ensure that orthotics are appropriately applied and fitted. To avoid adverse response, scheduled skin, circulation, and sensory assessments should be performed. The office or clinic nurse may be responsible for checking the fit of the orthosis at intervals, particularly if there has been a change in the client's weight or condition.

The ability of the client to independently don and doff the orthosis should be determined. The orthosis may need to be adjusted for ease of application or pressure relief. Clients should be aware of the number of hours per day the orthosis is to be worn, when it can be taken off, appropriate skin assessment and care, recommended exercises and activities, and how to care for the orthosis. The appropriate prescription, fit, comfort, and training will enhance the client's compliance with orthotic use.

ADAPTIVE EQUIPMENT

Adaptive equipment enables an individual with a physical impairment to function more independently, permitting the performance of an activity of daily living (ADL) that otherwise would be difficult or impossible. Adaptive equipment can reduce the energy and time consumption of a self-care or mobility activity. This benefit is critical for clients with limited cardiopulmonary reserve or musculoskeletal weakness. Issues that influence the prescription

TABLE 13–9. *Types and Uses of Orthotics for Upper and Lower Extremities*

TYPE	USE
Upper Extremity	
Static (resting pan, cock-up, thumb spica)	Optimal positioning, immobilization, and pain control
Dynamic (tenodesis, outrigger, hinged elbow)	Enhance upper extremity function
Lower Extremity	
Hip abduction orthosis	Control selected motions of hip to prevent recurrent dislocations
Hip-knee-ankle-foot orthosis	Stabilize pelvis and lower extremity joints
Knee derotation or hinged orthosis	Provide support and control of the knee with cruciate or collateral ligament injuries
Knee-ankle-foot orthosis	Stabilize hip, knee, or ankle
Ankle-foot orthosis	Stabilize knee, foot, and ankle
Foot orthosis (e.g., custom shoes, shoe modifications, and inserts)	Accommodate foot deformities, relieve pressure, and enhance comfort

and client's acceptance of adaptive equipment include the degree and type of physical impairment, cognitive status, cultural background, and socioeconomic factors.

A client's ADL performance is maximized by the prescription of appropriate, well-fitting devices and comprehensive client education. A complete client evaluation, including assessment of flexibility, strength, functional status, caregiver status, and client's goals, should be performed before issuance of any device. This evaluative process ensures that all issues and functional needs are addressed. In addition, the Joint Commission on Accreditation of Healthcare Organizations (JCAHO) has established criteria that clinicians must address relative to the issuance of durable medical equipment. These standards are directed at ensuring client safety, correct use, and optimal functional outcomes.

A case example that reflects these processes is a total hip replacement procedure. Hip joint replacement surgery restricts hip ROM postoperatively and, subsequently, mobility, toileting, hygiene, dressing, and home management. (See Chapter 16 to review these hip positional precautions.) To minimize the potential of postoperative joint dislocation, hip flexion greater than 90 degrees, hip adduction, and hip internal rotation must be restricted. Several types of adaptive equipment are needed to ensure this end. These include long-handled shoe horns, reachers, and sponges; sock aids; elastic shoelaces; dressing sticks; raised toilet seats; and bath benches.

Toileting

The ability to independently manage toilet activities is critical for successful discharge planning and joint protection. A raised toilet seat reduces the stress on the hips and knees by enhancing mechanical advantage. A commode or toilet allows for optimal positioning for elimination and therefore should be used when possible. To enhance client safety with the use of raised toilet seats or commodes, appropriate handrails can be prescribed. An alternative to these devices is the use of portable urinals

or bedpans. These devices may be easier and safer at night, especially for clients with significant functional impairment, absent caregiver, or sensory loss.

Personal Hygiene

Personal hygiene activities may require adaptive equipment to enable the client to hold, control, or reach. If the client's grasp is absent or weak and the proximal muscles are intact, devices such as toothbrushes, combs, or razors can be adapted with universal cuffs (Fig. 13–17).

Clients may benefit from the use of a bath bench or seat for safe transfers. Nonskid mats or adhesive strips placed on the floor of either a tub or shower can reduce risk for falls. Grab bars provide additional support while performing transfers. A handheld shower allows clients the opportunity to sit and shower. A long-handled sponge enhances independence with bathing if flexibility or strength is limited.

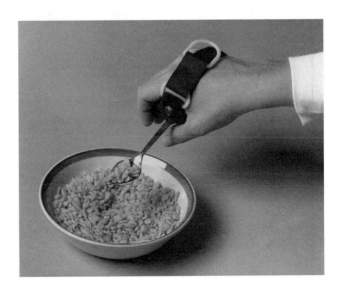

FIGURE 13–17. Universal cuff to assist with activities of daily living.

Dressing

Clients with ROM or strength limitations may have deficits in dressing skills. A variety of dressing aids are commercially available to compensate for these limitations, such as long-handled reachers, dressing sticks, long-handled shoe horns, sock aids, and elastic shoelaces. In addition to these aids, the client should be encouraged to choose clothing with openings and sleeves that are simple to manage and easy to fasten. Specific clothing styles that will facilitate independent dressing include clothes with front openings and wraparound styles. Clothing and shoe wear can be adapted with Velcro closures. Velcro is easier to manage than buttons, hooks, or laces. A number of manufacturers fabricate adaptive clothing for individuals with deficits in strength, coordination, and flexibility. Catalogs for these items can be found in rehabilitation clinics or in some major department stores.

Feeding

Many clients are unable to feed themselves independently because of a loss of grasp, limited ROM, or diminished coordination. Adaptive equipment is com-

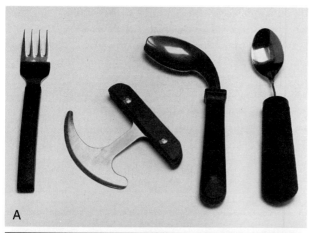

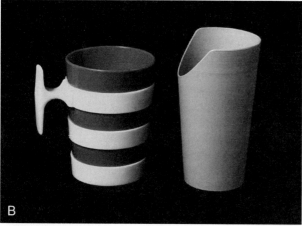

FIGURE 13–18. *A,* Adapted eating utensils for clients with impairment of grasp or reach. *B,* Adapted cups for clients with decreased grasp or loss of cervical extension.

mercially available to compensate for these deficits. Forks, spoons, and knives can be adapted with enlarged handgrips or modified shapes/designs to allow independent use (Fig. 13–18A). Adaptive cups and glasses are available to compensate not only for weak grasp but also for loss of cervical extension, which can interfere with swallowing (Fig. 13–18B).

ENVIRONMENTAL ACCESSIBILITY

Inactivity is one of the most preventable causes of decreased mobility. The ability to remain physically active is determined in part by opportunity. Opportunities must be created for the physically disabled person by compensating for decreased physical capacity and by maximizing existing abilities. Health care providers should create and promote opportunities through client education, the prescription of durable medical equipment, and appropriate referrals to community agencies. A barrier-free surrounding is essential for these individuals.

Adapted housing for the disabled and older person can ensure independent community living. The Americans with Disabilities Act has no legal bearing on single-family residences; however, there are several laws governing accessible housing. The Fair Housing Amendments Act of 1988 affects new construction of buildings with four or more units ready for occupancy after March 3, 1991. All elevator-accessed units and ground floor units in nonelevator buildings must have accessible light switches and electrical outlets, reinforced bathroom walls to allow installation of grab bars, and kitchens and bathrooms usable by people in wheelchairs. Clients with ambulatory limitations or who are wheelchair dependent can benefit from housing adaptations. Specifically, the floor for the ambulatory disabled person should be a nonslip, resilient surface. For the wheelchair user, the surface ideally should be flat and smooth. The wheelchair user also needs larger doorways and lower window sills, countertops, controls, switches, and outlets.

Specific guidelines are available for constructing adaptive housing. For example, an ambulatory person occupies a standing space measuring 18 by 12 inches. In contrast, the ambulatory client with a gait aid requires 26 × 15 inches. This space requirement must be 50% greater for turnabout. A wheelchair user occupies approximately 26 × 48 inches, and turnabout requires approximately 5 × 5 feet. The doorway for the ambulatory person should be 21 inches wide, and for the wheelchair user, it should be 32 inches wide.

The area leading into a building can be the first barrier to the disabled person. To increase accessibility, the ground should be as level as possible and should not exceed a 5% grade. If the slope exceeds 5%, it should be classified as a ramp. To ensure ease and safety of access, the ramp's slope should not exceed 1:12, a grade of 8.33%. It should have a handrail and should be constructed of nonslip materials.

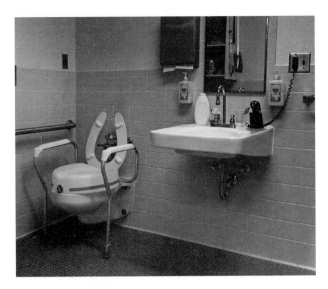

FIGURE 13–19. Adapted bathroom.

Future Trends

Universal design is a term first coined by the architect Ronald Mace (Null & Cherry, 1996). Also known as *life span design,* universal design seeks to create environments and products that are usable by children, young adults, and older adults. These environments and products can be used by people with "normal" abilities and those with disabilities, including temporary ones. A universal design must incorporate four principles: It must be supportive, adaptable, accessible, and safety-oriented. An example of an accessible design is the side-by-side refrigerator freezer. This appliance provides easy access for people of all statures and abilities. Universal design is economical because it uses existing products in different ways but also seeks to standardize those things that can be beneficial to everyone. For example, universal design advocates for a standard door width (3 feet). This would not only provide access for people using wheelchairs and walkers but also save time and money for builders, designers, and manufacturers. Universal design is also aesthetically pleasing and is marketable. As the baby boomers grow older, more money will be spent on products and environments that allow them to maintain their independence.

Special driving and parking privileges have improved access for the disabled, especially in business and school areas. Further progress is needed in residential areas to ensure independent access. Parking spaces for the disabled should be located as close to the entrance as possible to minimize travel distance. Building doors should open easily with one hand and have an entrance opening of 32 inches.

Accessibility in the interior of a home means that the individual is able to travel freely without obstruction. Doors should open away rather than toward an individual. Floors should have a hard, nonslip surface, or if carpeting is present, the pile should be short to reduce wheelchair friction. All throw rugs and clutter pose

hazards and should be eliminated. Handrails should be installed on both sides of the stairs for the client who can negotiate steps. Stairs should be well lit but without dangerous glare.

The bathroom often presents major access barriers for the disabled. The greatest consideration must be given to the placement of the fixtures. Their placement determines the type of wheelchair transfer needed to the toilet, tub, or shower. For greatest convenience, the toilet seat should approximate the height of the seat of the wheelchair. Sinks should be wall-mounted on a bracket or in a countertop not more than 32 to 34 inches high (Fig. 13–19). The shower should accommodate a person in either the standing or sitting position and have a slip-resistant floor. Grab bars help compensate for poor strength, balance, and coordination.

Beds and chairs should be at a specific height and firmness such that a 90-degree angle at the hips and knees is maintained. Chair wedges, chair risers, and thicker cushions can be used to adjust the height, firmness, and slope of chair seats. Armrests facilitate ease of transfers.

The placement of utilities and cabinets affects wheelchair maneuverability and access. In the kitchen, front-opening appliances and equipment are better than top-opening. The optimal height for pullout work tables is 24 inches to accommodate a wheelchair 30 inches. For standing while working, 32 to 37 inches is needed. The refrigerator, stove, and kitchen sink should be arranged to form a convenient work triangle because most trips are made between the sink, refrigerator, and stove. The primary therapeutic goal is simplifying work—a process of improving the job method and adapting mechanical facilities to fit the client's capacity.

Another important issue for the disabled person is transportation. To operate a vehicle, the disabled person must satisfy current and local driving regulations. Automotive driving aids are available to match the disability. The van adapted with a lift is popular because of the ease of entry and exit and reduced physical effort (Fig. 13–20).

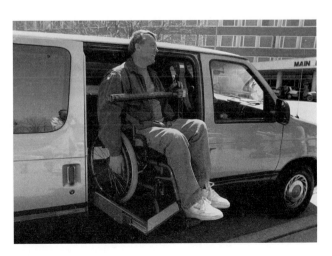

FIGURE 13–20. Van lift for the wheelchair-dependent client.

Public transportation is available for the disabled in many communities. Part I, Title II of the Americans with Disabilities Act (ADA) of 1990 (PL101-336) prohibits discrimination against disabled persons within public transportation programs. Paratransit services have been mandated since January 26, 1995; however, extensions may be granted in cases that present extraordinary difficulties.

SUMMARY

Rehabilitation management of the orthopaedic client requires a comprehensive, interdisciplinary approach for optimal outcome. Health care providers must address the client's physical, functional, and psychological issues to formulate an appropriate therapeutic plan. These issues must be addressed, if feasible, before admission and be continually evaluated during and after hospitalization until the client returns to optimal status. The current health care system of managed care calls for shortened hospital stays for the stable orthopaedic client. Thus, much of the rehabilitative process occurs through outpatient or home physical therapy or at a rehabilitation facility. Clinical decision making for selecting therapeutic interventions must be based on sound clinical and scientific research to ensure both efficacious and safe client care.

INTERNET RESOURCES

American Physical Therapy Association: www.apta.org

Life@Home: www.lifehome.com; home modification products and services for senior citizens and the disabled

McBurney Disability Resource Center: www.dcs.wisc.edu/mcb

National Institute on Disability and Rehabilitation Research: www.ed.gov/offices/OSERS/NIDRR

REFERENCES

Baechle, T. R., & Earle, R. W. (2000). *Essential of strength training and conditioning* (pp. 64–71, 203–204). Champaign, IL.: Human Kinetics.

Bernhardt, D. B. (1986). *Sports physical therapy* (pp. 55–77, 164–170). New York: Churchill Livingstone.

Cailliet, R. (1964). *Neck and arm pain.* Philadelphia: FA Davis.

Chen, B., Zimmerman, J. R., Soulen, L., & DeLisa, J. A. (2000). Continuous passive motion after total knee arthroplasty. *American Journal of Physical Medicine and Rehabilitation, 79,* 421–426.

Chiarello, C. M., Gundersen, L., & O'Halloran, T. (1997). The effect of continuous passive motion duration and increment on range of motion in total knee arthroplasty patients. *Journal of Orthopaedic & Sports Physical Therapy, 25,* 119–127.

Engstrom, B., Sperber, A., & Wredmark, T. (1995). Continuous passive motion in rehabilitation after anterior cruciate ligament reconstruction. *Knee Surgery, Sports Traumatology, Arthroscopy, 3,* 18–20.

Gaspar, L., Farkas, C., Szepesi, K, & Csernatony, Z. (1997). Therapeutic value of continuous passive motion after anterior cruciate replacement. *Acta Chirurgica Hungarica, 36,* 104–105.

Kumar, P. J., McPherson, Dorr, L. D., Wan, Z., & Baldwin, K. (1996). Rehabilitation after total knee arthroplasty: A comparison of 2 rehabilitation techniques. (1996). *Clinical Orthopaedics & Related Research, 331,* 93–101.

Lastayo, P., Wright, T., Jaffe, R., & Hartzel, J. (1998). Continuous passive motion after repair of the rotator cuff: A prospective outcome study. *Journal of Bone and Joint Surgery, 80-A,* 1002–1011.

McCarthy, M. R., Yates, C. K., Anderson, M. A., & Yates-McCarthy, J. L. (1993). The effects of immediate continuous passive motion on pain during the inflammatory phase of soft tissue healing following anterior cruciate ligament reconstruction. *Journal of Orthopaedic & Sports Physical Therapy, 17,* 96–101.

McInnes, J., Larson, M. G., Daltroy, L. H., Brown, T., Fossel, A. H., Eaton, H. M., Shulman-Kirwan, B., Steindorf, S., Poss, R., & Liang, M. H. (1992). A controlled evaluation of continuous passive motion in patients undergoing total knee arthroplasty. *Journal of the American Medical Association, 268,* 1423–1428.

Montgomery, F., & Eliasson, M. (1996). Continuous passive motion compared to active physical therapy after knee arthroplasty: similar hospitalization times in a randomized study of 68 patients. *Acta Orthopaedica Scandinavica, 67,* 7–9.

Null, R. L., & Cherry, K. F. (1996). *Universal design: Creative solutions for ADA compliance* (pp. 1–34). Belmont, CA: Professional Publications.

Owen, B. D., & Fragala, G. (1999). Reducing perceived physical stress while transferring residents. *AAOHN Journal, 47,* 316–323.

Owen, B. D., & Garg, A. (1993). Back stress isn't part of the job. *American Journal of Nursing, 93*(2), 48–51.

Owen, B. D., Keene, K., Olson, S., & Garg, A. (1995). An ergonomic approach to reducing back stress while carrying out patient handling tasks with a hospitalized patient. In M. Hagberg, F. Hoffmann, U. Stöbel, & G. Westlander (Eds.), *Occupational health for health care workers* (pp. 1–4). International Commission on Occupational Health, 2nd International Congress, March 1994, Stockholm.

Pope, R. O., Corcoran, S., McCaul K., & Howie, D. W. (1997). Continuous passive motion after primary total knee arthroplasty. Does it offer any benefits? *The Journal of Bone and Joint Surgery, 79-B,* 914–917.

Raab, M. G., Rzeszutko, D., O'Connor, W., & Greatting. (1996). Early results of continuous passive motion after rotator cuff repair: A prospective, randomized, blinded, controlled study. *American Journal of Orthopedics, 25,* 214–220.

Richmond, J. C., Gladstone, J., & MacGillivray, J. (1991). Continuous passive motion after arthroscopically assisted anterior cruciate ligament reconstruction: Comparison of short- versus long-term use. *Arthroscopy: The Journal of Arthroscopic and Related Surgery, 7*(1), 39–44.

Ververeli, P., Sutton, D., Hearn, S. L., Booth, R. E., Jr., Hozack, W. J., & Rothman, R. R. (1995). Continuous passive motion after total knee arthroplasty. *Clinical Orthopaedics and Related Research, 321,* 208–215.

Wasilewski, S. A., Woods, L. C., Torgerson, W. R., Jr., & Healy, W. L. (1990). Value of continuous passive motion in total knee arthroplasty. *Orthopedics, 13,* 291–295.

Witherow, G. E., Bollen, S. R., & Pinczewski, L. A. (1993). The use of continuous passive motion after arthroscopically assisted anterior cruciate ligament reconstruction: Help or hindrance? *Knee Surgery, Sports Traumatology, Arthroscopy, 1,* 68–70.

Worland, R., Arredondo, J., Angles, F., Lopez-Jimenez, F., & Jessup, D. E. (1998). Home continuous passive motion machine versus professional physical therapy following total knee replacement. *The Journal of Arthroplasty, 13,* 784–787.

Yashar, A. A., Venn-Watson, E., Welsh, T., Colwell, C. W., Jr., & Lotke, P. (1997). Continuous passive motion with accelerated flexion after total knee arthroplasty. *Clinical Orthopaedics & Related Research, 345,* 38–43.

14

Autoimmune and Inflammatory Disorders

PATRICIA A. MacDONALD

The year 2000 not only heralded the new millennium but also marked the "decade of bone and joint disease." The World Health Organization granted this distinction and has turned the world's attention to these "crippling diseases." Autoimmune and inflammatory disorders have been called "the primary crippling diseases" of the developed world, with good reason. The term *arthritis* literally means "inflammation of a joint" but arthritis is actually a collection of more than 100 related, but distinct, conditions. Approximately 49% of all Americans older than the age of 65 believe that they have arthritis. The disease touches 1 in every 7 Americans—1 in every 3 families, or 37 million Americans. Because more than 20% of the U.S. population will be 65 years of age or older by 2035, arthritis will affect even more Americans in the future. Arthritis is the primary reason for work-related disability and is the leading cause of disability among people aged 65 or older.

As the incidence of autoimmune and inflammatory disorders continues to rise, researchers work to uncover the role of overuse, injury, obesity, gene defects, infection, immunosuppression, amino acids, interleukin, and environmental agents in both the development and treatment of these life-altering diseases. In addition, autoimmunity was named a major priority women's health issue by the Office of Research on Women's Health, a unit of the National Institutes of Health, because autoimmune disorders target women 75% of the time.

Rheumatic diseases are characterized by chronic pain and progressive physical impairment of joints and soft tissues. The ultimate goals of the health care team—physicians, nurses, and other health care professionals—are to relieve pain and physical symptoms, assuage psychological distress, improve physical function, and generally aid in the well-being of the client. Equally important, however, are interventions to prevent and ameliorate socioeconomic problems. Indeed, a majority

of the costs, both economic and social, are attributable to lost function rather than to direct medical costs. Until a cure for the many types of arthritis is found or far more effective therapies to prevent joint damage and physical disability are developed, clients will continue to suffer severe, premature economic and social dislocations that will seriously affect their lives. As the population ages, society can expect that these effects will mushroom.

This chapter describes the epidemiology, pathology, clinical presentation, management, and nursing care for the following selected autoimmune or inflammatory arthritic disorders: rheumatoid arthritis (RA); juvenile rheumatoid arthritis (JRA); systemic lupus erythematosus (SLE); psoriatic arthritis (PsA); systemic sclerosis (SS); ankylosing spondylitis (AS); reactive arthritis (Reiter's syndrome); idiopathic inflammatory myopathies, polymyositis (PM), and dermatomyositis (DM); and bursitis. Because RA is both an autoimmune and an inflammatory disease, it is helpful to refer to the discussion of RA while reading about the other disorders.

The American College of Rheumatology (ACR) 20 and the Sharp Score, outcome variables, are the most consistent measures used in the studies. The ACR has accepted the ACR 20 as the basis for improvement. The ACR 20 is defined as a 20% improvement in tender and swollen joint counts and 20% improvement in three of the five remaining core data (Box 14-1). The Sharp Score, named after its originator John Sharp, is a standardized means of scoring the damage done to the joints, joint-space narrowing, and erosions. The lower the Sharp Score, the less damage, erosions, and joint-space narrowing. In early studies, there were no radiographic results listed. Not until the early 1990s were x-ray films taken in clinical trials, and the data were inconsistent and the results difficult to interpret. These same problems are still being addressed. Joint-space narrowing is seen in 83% (Fuchs, Kaye, Callahan, Nance, & Pincus, 1989), and

---

BOX 14–1.

American College of Rheumatology (ACR) Core Data Set and Response Definitions

ACR Core Data Set Component	Validated Measurement Tool
1. Tender joint count	Standardized 68 joint count
2. Swollen joint count	Standardized 68 joint count
3. Subject global assessment of pain	A 0–100 mm visual analog scale
4. Subject global assessment of disease activity	A 0–100 mm visual analog scale
5. Physician global assessment of disease activity	A 0–100 mm visual analog scale
6. Subject assessment of physical function	Modified Health Assessment Questionnaire (MHAQ)
7. Acute-phase reactant value	ESR (Westergren) and C-reactive protein

The ACR 20 definition of improvement is a 20% improvement over baseline in tender and swollen joint counts (1 and 2) and a 20% improvement in three of the five remaining core data set measurements, components 3 to 7.

From Felson, D. T., Anderson, J. J., Boers, M., et al. (1995). American College of Rheumatology preliminary definition of improvement in rheumatoid arthritis. *Arthritis and Rheumatism, 36*(6), 729–740.

---

joint-space narrowing and erosions are seen in 67% (Pincus, Callahan, Fuchs, Larsen, & Kaye, 1995) of clients within the first 2 years of disease. Radiographic progression occurs early and continues over the client's lifetime (Wolfe & Sharp, 1998).

The difficulty in evaluating the results of these clinical trials stems from the differences in designs (single agent vs. combination, active comparator vs. placebo, no prior methotrexate vs. methotrexate failures) and differences in client populations (early vs. late disease, rheumatoid factor positive vs. negative). The radiographic results show that there is slowing of radiographic progression and that all of the drugs cited in the clinical trials function as disease-modifying antirheumatic drugs (DMARDs). None of the studies were read for "healing." Clients treated with methotrexate alone had less damage than those treated with placebo. The addition of the newer medications should limit further damage—as much as 70% less. Methotrexate, etanercept, infliximab, and leflunomide are effective DMARDs, and combination with methotrexate appears to lead to greater efficacy. In the ERA trial, etanercept stopped progression in 63% of clients and 72% of clients achieved an ACR 20 (results at 2 years) (Genovese, Martin, Fleischmann, et al., 2000).

The current trend of standardizing clinical trial designs suggests that in the next 5 years, the efficacy and safety of the treatments for autoimmune and inflammatory disorders will be clearly demonstrated, subjectively as well as objectively. Then evidence-based medicine will truly be practiced.

PATHOPHYSIOLOGY

Relationships between altered immune function and rheumatologic disease are becoming better understood as a result of continued research efforts. *Autoimmune* diseases are conditions in which immunologic self-tolerance has been disrupted, with resultant damage to body tissues or cells normally recognized as self. Autoimmune disorders with muscle and joint involvement include SLE, RA,

DM, scleroderma, Sjögren's syndrome, and mixed connective tissue disease.

To understand systemic, arthritic autoimmune diseases, it is important to briefly review key components of the immune system. The immune system consists of immune cells (primarily B lymphocytes, T lymphocytes, and macrophages) and central and peripheral lymphoid structures. Immune cells are primarily produced in the central immune organs of the bone marrow and thymus. These cells interact with antigens (i.e., substances perceived as foreign to the body) in the peripheral lymphoid structures of the lymph nodes, spleen, tonsils, and other areas where lymphoid tissue is located. As the B and T lymphocytes travel throughout the body, they selectively seek out and destroy foreign antigens, while sparing cells identified as self.

The ability of the immune system to distinguish self from nonself depends in large part on cell-surface antigens. These antigens (which are unique to every person) are encoded by a large cluster of genes called the *major histocompatibility complex* (MHC), which is located on the short end of chromosome 6. Histocompatibility antigens are also more typically referred to as *human leukocyte antigens* (HLA) because they were first discovered on leukocytes. Seven closely related gene loci have been identified: HLA-A, HLA-B, HLA-C, HLA-D, HLA-DR, HLA-DQ, and HLA-DP. Each of these gene loci is occupied by multiple alleles (alternate genes) that code the development of each surface antigen. At least 23 gene products are associated with the HLA-A group, and 47 are associated with the HLA-B group.

Human leukocyte antigens have been categorized into two groups. Found on the surface of nucleated cells, class I antigens include HLA-A, HLA-B, and HLA-C antigens. Class II (D, DR, DQ, and DP) are found on macrophage and B cells, among others (Smith & Arnett, 1991).

As a result of aberrations in HLA activity genetic coding, the body may lose some of its ability to recognize and differentiate self from nonself, resulting in autoimmune disorders. In other words, the body has decreased self-tolerance. However, abnormalities of the HLA system are but one key to the development of autoimmunity. Others involve abnormal T- or B-cell reactivity, resulting in altered recognition of foreign antigens and self by the immune system. For example, altered T-cell function has been implicated in the pathogenesis of arthritic diseases, such as RA (Peacock, Ku, Banquerigo, & Brahn, 1992). Research has begun to identify the specific roles of various T cells in these disease processes. For example, CD4+ T cells have been shown to have a crucial role in the pathogenesis of arthritis, and CD8+ T cells may play an immunoregulatory role (Banerjee, Webber, & Poole, 1992). In addition, research suggests that B cells in the synovial membrane of joints expand as a result of local antigen stimulation (Dybwad, Forre, Natvig, & Sioud, 1995). It is also likely that the immune system can be altered by interactions with chemical, environmental, viral, and bacterial agents.

Another important aspect of autoimmune disease is familial aggregation (or clustering), which suggests that there is a genetic predisposition to the development of specific disorders. This possibility is not surprising because an individual's HLA type is inherited. Indeed, some HLA types appear more commonly in certain disease conditions. For example, in Caucasians, HLA-B27 appears in 80% to 90% of persons with AS but in only 7% to 10% of persons in the general population. For more information on the role of genetics in musculoskeletal disease, see Chapter 7.

RHEUMATOID ARTHRITIS

RA is a chronic, systemic autoimmune disorder whose major distinctive feature is chronic, symmetrical, and erosive inflammation of the synovial tissue of joints. The severity of the joint disease may fluctuate over time, but progressive development of various degrees of joint destruction, deformity, and disability are the most common outcomes of established disease. Associated nonarticular manifestations may include subcutaneous nodules, vasculitis, pulmonary nodules or interstitial fibrosis, and pericarditis. RA is characterized by the presence of rheumatoid factor (RF), an autoantibody directed against the immunoglobulin G (IgG), in more than 80% of those with the disease (Persselin, 1991). In addition to RF, antibodies against collagen, Epstein-Barr virus, encoded nuclear antigen, and certain other antigens have been identified. The role of autoantibodies in RA is still unclear, but research has focused attention on preillness immunologic status in the pathogenesis of RA. Antikeratin antibody (AKA) and antiperinuclear factor (APF) appear to be markers that predict the development of RA in RF-positive clients. However, RA develops in only a proportion of cases (Aho, von Essen, Kurki, Palosuo, & Heliovaara, 1993). Other immunogenetic markers may aid in the identification of clients with early RA with more severe disease (Eberhardt, Grubb, Johnson, & Petersson, 1993). RA may be mild and

relapsing, involving a few joints for a brief period, or it may be markedly progressive, with the development of deformities and severe systemic disease. Overall, the disease is characterized by cycles of exacerbation and remission, the duration of which adds to the feelings of powerlessness and uncertainty that clients with RA often experience. A small percentage of clients have a severely progressive disease that does not respond to aggressive therapy (Paulus, 1991).

Table 14-1 illustrates the 1987 revised criteria for the classification of RA (Arnett et al., 1988). The seven criteria highlight the symmetrical involvement of inflamed joints of the wrist, the metacarpophalangeal (MCP) joints, and the proximal interphalangeal (PIP) joints. Figure 14-1A illustrates the hand joints typically involved in RA, and Figure 14-1B illustrates typical swelling of the hand joint. The distal interphalangeal (DIP) joints are rarely involved in RA and are more commonly affected in osteoarthritis. Four or more of the seven criteria must be met before the disease is classified as RA. In addition, the first four criteria relating to stiffness and swelling must be present for at least 6 weeks, and criteria two through five (swelling and subcutaneous nodules) must be observed by a physician. These criteria remain the hallmark for classification of RA.

Disease Manifestations

Clinical features of RA vary not only from one client to another but also in an individual client over the course of the disease. The most common mode of onset is the insidious development of symptoms over several weeks. Explosive acute polyarticular onset evolving over several days also can occur. RA usually begins gradually, accom-

TABLE 14–1. *1987 Revised Criteria of the American Rheumatism Association for the Classification of Rheumatoid Arthritis**

CRITERION	DESCRIPTION
1	Morning stiffness in and around joints lasting at least 1 hr before maximal improvement
2	Soft tissue swelling (arthritis) of three or more joint areas (including the right and left proximal PIP, MCP, wrist, elbow, knee, ankle, and MTP joints)
3	Swelling of at least one wrist, MCP, or PIP joint
4	Simultaneous symmetric swelling in joints listed in criterion 2
5	Subcutaneous rheumatoid nodules
6	Presence of rheumatoid factor
7	Radiographic erosions and/or periarticular osteopenia in hand and/or wrist joints

*Note: Rheumatoid arthritis is defined by the presence of four or more criteria. Criteria 1 through 4 must have been present for at least 6 weeks.
From Arnett, F. C., Edworthy, S. M., Block D. A., et al. (1988). The American Rheumatism Association 1987 revised criteria for the classification of rheumatoid arthritis. *Arthritis and Rheumatism, 31*(3), 315-324.

panied by systemic manifestations such as anorexia, weight loss, fatigue, muscle aching, and stiffness. Joint pain and swelling are associated with morning stiffness that can last several hours. Joint involvement is usually polyarticular and symmetrical, with the most commonly affected joints being those in the fingers, hands, wrists, knees, and feet.

The bilateral symmetrical involvement of the hands (wrists, MCP joints, and PIP joints) is characteristic of RA.

Inflammation of the PIP joints contributes to the spindle-shaped appearance of the fingers. Tenosynovitis of the flexor tendons of the fingers is common, along with swelling and tenderness of the ulnar styloid process. Decreased dorsiflexion of the wrist occurs early in the disease and can be more painful than changes in the finger joints. With time, progressive synovial damage leads to characteristic deformities of the hands: ulnar deviation of the MCP joints of the fingers and medial

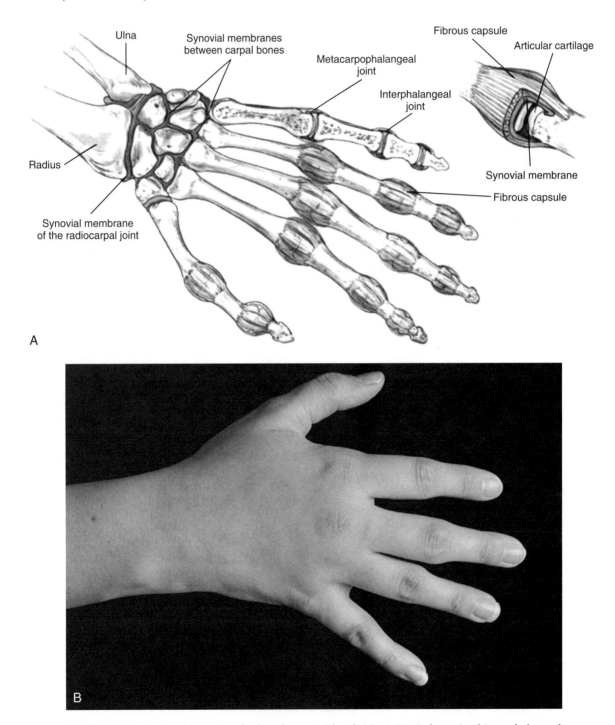

FIGURE 14–1. *A,* Hand joints involved in rheumatoid arthritis. *B,* Typical proximal interphalangeal joint swelling of third finger in early rheumatoid arthritis. (*A,* From Jarvis, C. [1996]. *Physical examination and health assessment* [p. 651]. Philadelphia: WB Saunders.)

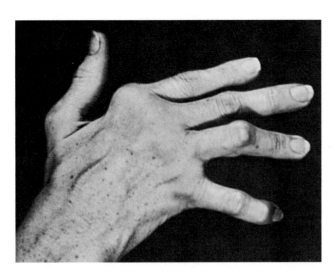

FIGURE 14–2. Radial shift and ulnar deviation of the hand found in rheumatoid arthritis. (From Gartland, J. [1986]. *Fundamentals of orthopaedics* [4th ed., p. 143]. Philadelphia: WB Saunders.)

deviation of the wrist (Fig. 14–2). A swan-neck deformity (hyperextension of the PIP joint with flexion of the MCP and DIP joints) results from contractures of the intrinsic muscles and tendons (Fig. 14–3A). The boutonniere deformity (flexion of the PIP joint and hyperextension of the DIP joint) (Fig. 14–3B) is due to rupture of the extensor tendons over the fingers. Carpal tunnel syndrome, the compression of the median nerve as a result of

tenosynovitis on the volar aspect of the wrist, is fairly common in RA. All of these changes lead to decreased hand strength and decreased ability to maintain a tight pinch.

The shoulders, elbows, and spine are also affected. Shoulder arthritis is seen with late disease, whereas the elbows can become flexed and contracted with early disease. Spinal involvement is usually limited to the cervical area. Atlantoaxial subluxation can lead to tenderness, muscle spasm, persistent head tilt, and occipital headache.

In the lower extremities, RA commonly affects the feet and knees. Cock-up toes result from plantar subluxation of the metatarsal heads. Walking can be difficult because of limited flexion and extension of the ankle. Active synovitis is often seen in swelling over the medial and lateral aspects of the patella. Popliteal cysts (Baker's cysts) can develop behind the knee joint (Fig. 14–4).

As a systemic disease, RA can affect almost every body system. Extra-articular manifestations of RA are summarized in Table 14–2. Three of them, however, are more commonly seen in RA. These include rheumatoid nodules, Sjögren's syndrome, and Felty's syndrome. Rheumatoid nodules, granuloma-type lesions that develop around small blood vessels, can develop in up to 50% of clients with RA. Usually, those affected have high titers of RF (Persselin, 1991). Generally, firm, mobile, and painless, rheumatoid nodules appear over the extensor surfaces of joints, such as elbows and fingers, but may be found

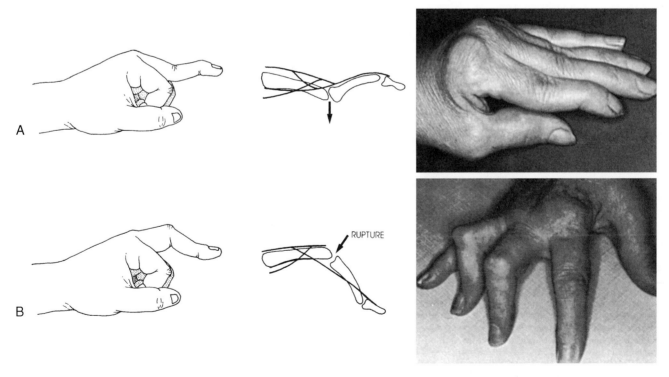

FIGURE 14–3. *A,* Typical swan-neck deformity. *B,* Boutonniere deformity found in rheumatoid arthritis. (*A,* From Magee, D. [1987]. *Orthopaedic physical assessment* [p. 112]. Philadelphia: WB Saunders; *B,* from Kelley, W., Harris, E., Ruddy, S., & Sledge, C. [Eds.]. [1993]. *Textbook of rheumatology* [3rd ed., pp. 961–962]. Philadelphia: WB Saunders.)

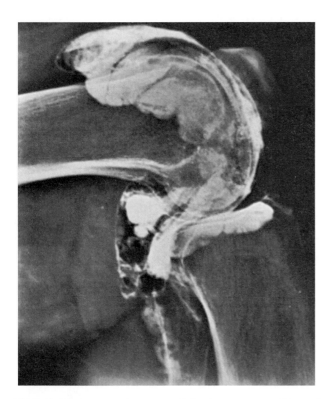

FIGURE 14–4. An arthrogram of the knee in a middle-aged woman with rheumatoid arthritis, demonstrating the formation of a large popliteal cyst. (From Bullough, P., & Bansal, M. [1988]. The differential diagnosis of geodes. *Radiologic Clinics of North America, 26*[6], 1175.)

anywhere in the body, even in the lungs. These can easily break down or become infected. What part these nodules play in RA remains unknown (Halverson, 1995).

Secondary Sjögren's syndrome, keratoconjunctivitis sicca, is seen in about 10% to 15% of clients with RA (Talal, 1988). It may also occur as a disorder by itself or with other connective tissue disease, such as SLE or PM. Clients with Sjögren's syndrome have diminished lacrimal and salivary gland secretion. They may complain of gritty, burning, or sandy eyes, with decreased tearing, itching, and photosensitivity (Halverson, 1995).

Felty's syndrome was originally described as the combination of RA, splenomegaly, leukopenia, and leg ulcers. Subsequent observations have shown an association with lymphadenopathy, thrombocytopenia, and the HLA-DR4 haplotype (Dinant, Mueller, van den Berg-Loonen, Nijenhuis, & Engelfriet, 1980). It occurs most commonly in clients with severe, nodule-forming RA. Other extra-articular problems seen in RA include inflammatory eye disorders, infection, pulmonary disease, vasculitis, and cardiac abnormalities.

Epidemiology

RA occurs worldwide and affects all racial and ethnic groups (Zvaifler, 1988). It can occur at any time of life, but its incidence tends to increase with age, peaking between the fourth and sixth decades. Data from population-

based prevalence and incidence studies have to be interpreted cautiously because there is no unique feature to establish the diagnosis of RA. Women are affected two to three times more often than men. Clients with RA have a substantially reduced life expectancy, and mortality is predicted in most instances by more severe clinical status (Callahan & Pincus, 1995; Myllykangas-Luosujarvi, Aho, & Isomalei, 1995).

The prevalence of RA is estimated to range from 0.5% to 1.5% of the population (Smith & Arnett, 1991). Compared with the incidence found in a study of the years 1950–1974 (Chan, Felson, Yood, & Walker, 1993), the prevalence rate has not decreased. After age 55, the prevalence rates for men and women are estimated to be 2% and 5%, respectively (Neuberger & Neuberger, 1984). Prevalence rates for African Americans are similar to those for Caucasian Americans (Hochberg, Linet, & Silis, 1983). MacGregor, Riste, Hayes, and Silman (1994) found a similar prevalence rate between both African and Caucasian Caribbeans. Studies from Taiwan (Chou, Pei, Chang, Lee, Schumacher, & Liang, 1994) and rural India (Malairya, Kapoor, Singh, Kumar, & Pande, 1993) also found similar prevalence rates for RA among all their populations compared with that among Caucasian persons. RA appears to be a relatively recent disease. It was first described in the mid-18th century and has not been found in skeletal remains from ancient European or Asian civilizations. However, erosive polyarthritis was documented in the skeletons of prehistoric (3000 to 5000 years ago) Native Americans, which might indicate an infectious agent confined to a small geographic area before the 18th century (Schumacher, 1982).

Genetic factors are important in the epidemiology of the disease. A genetic predisposition for RA is seen with a higher concordance rate of 32% in identical twins rather than the 9% rate observed in fraternal twins (Smith & Arnett, 1991). Other research (Nelson, Hughes, Smith, Nisperos, Branchaud, & Hansen, 1993) suggests the reason for consistent reports by female RA clients that joint pain and swelling disappear during pregnancy. It appears that because of genetic differences between a mother and fetus, RA disease activity stops. This remains speculation only but is an exciting area for further research.

The strongest genetic evidence, however, is seen in the association of RA with HLA-DR4, a genetically determined allele of the MHC on the short arm of chromosome 6. Interestingly, although there is an increased prevalence of HLA-DR4 in Caucasian clients with RA, it is not seen in specific populations, such as Ashkenazi Jews, Israeli Jews, and Asian Indians. Other alleles, such as DR1 or A31, may be seen in these ethnic groups (Smith & Arnett, 1991). In a study from South Africa, an association with HLA-DR1O was found among Hindus and Tamils (Moody & Hammond, 1994). Peacock and Cooper (1995) reported an association with HLA-DR1 among Indians living in Britain.

Pathophysiology

The histologic changes in RA are not disease specific but largely depend on the organ involved. The primary joint lesion involves the synovium. RF antibodies develop there against IgG, the largest of the five classes of immunoglobulins, to form immune complexes. Ironically, immunoglobulins are natural human antibodies. It is not clear, however, why the body produces an antibody (RF) against its own antibody (IgG) and, in effect, transforms IgG to an antigen or foreign protein that must be destroyed. The products of macrophages and lymphocytes are thought to have critical roles in the pathogenesis of RA as part of the immune response to an unidentified antigen (Lindley, Ceska, & Peichl, 1991). Moreover, it is the formation of these antibody-antigen immune complexes that leads

TABLE 14–2. *Extra-articular Manifestations of Rheumatoid Arthritis*

FEATURE	ASSESSMENT PARAMETER
General	
Fatigue, fever, myalgias	
Integumentary	
Rheumatoid nodules	Firm, mobile, nontender subcutaneous nodes on the extensor surface of the forearms, legs, occiput, sacrum; may occur wherever there is pressure
Vasculitic skin lesions	Splinter hemorrhages on nails
Purpura	Ecchymosis, bruises, or ischemic involvement, especially on lower extremities
Ocular	
Episcleritis	Pain and visual discomfort
Scleritis	Pain and visual impairment; raised nodules on superior sclerae
Secondary Sjögren's syndrome	Dry eyes, burning, itching, photophobia, decreased tearing
Otolaryngologic	
Rheumatoid nodules on vocal cords	Hoarseness
Secondary Sjögren's syndrome	Dry mouth, decreased saliva
Pulmonary	
Pleuritis, pulmonary fibrosis, pleural effusions	Cough, dyspnea, crackles (fine rales), decreased thoracic expansion
Pulmonary nodules, with or without cavitation	As described above
Cardiac	
Pericarditis, myocarditis	High-pitched, scratchy pericardial friction rubs; may increase in intensity when client leans forward and exhales
Mitral valve disease	Loud, high-pitched blowing murmur characteristic of mitral regurgitation; may have third heart sound (S_3)
Conduction system disease: complete heart block	Apical pulse usually 25–45 beats/min
Gastrointestinal	
Felty's syndrome	Enlarged spleen
Bowel and mesenteric vasculitis	Pain after meals; epigastric bruit
Malabsorption due to amyloid deposits	Frequent loose, watery stools; abdominal distention
Renal	
Proteinuria	Urinalysis
Neurologic	
Myelopathy (C1–C2 vertebral subluxation)	History of transient ischemic attacks (dizziness, numbness, paresthesias, temporary loss of vision)
Carpal tunnel syndrome	Decreased grip strength, thenar atrophy, positive Phalen's test, Tinel's sign
Posterior tibial nerve entrapment	Decreased sensation in first dorsal web space; eliciting numbness and paresthesias after tapping the tarsal tunnel at the ankle joint medial to the dorsalis pedis
Hematologic	
Anemia	
Leukopenia (Felty's syndrome)	

Data from Bennett (1988), Gates & Mooar (1989), Mackenzie (1988), Persselin (1991), and Halverson (1995).

to the activation of the complement system and the release of lysosomal enzymes from leukocytes. Both of these reactions cause inflammation. Initial research has demonstrated that interleukin-8, known as neutrophil-activating peptide-1 (NAP-1), has a definite role in the inflammatory process of RA and that circulating autoantibodies may provide a clinically useful marker for RA severity (Lindley, Ceska, & Peichl, 1991). With the initial formation of immune complexes, synovitis develops as the synovial membrane becomes swollen, irritated, and inflamed.

As the immune complexes are deposited onto the synovial membrane or the superficial layers of the articular cartilage, they are phagocytized by polymorphonuclear (PMN) leukocytes, monocytes, and lymphocytes. Unfortunately, phagocytosis deactivates the immune complexes and simultaneously produces additional enzymes (oxygen radicals, arachidonic acid) that lead to hyperemia, edema, swelling, and thickening of the synovial lining. The hypertrophied synovium literally invades the surrounding tissue, including cartilage, ligaments, joint capsule, and tendons. Eventually, granulation tissue forms to cover the entire articular cartilage, leading to the formation of pannus, a highly vascularized fibrous scar tissue composed of lymphocytes, macrophages, histiocytes, fibroblasts, and mast cells (Cush & Lipsky, 1991). Undoubtedly the most destructive element in RA, pannus can erode and destroy articular cartilage, eventually resulting in subchondral bone erosions, bone cysts, fissures, and the development of bone spurs and osteophytes. Research has identified that tumor necrosis factor (TNF), which is produced by cells at the cartilage-pannus junction, may lead to the cartilage destruction (Chu, Field, Feldmann, & Maini, 1991). Pannus can also scar and shorten tendons and ligaments, conditions that in turn lead to ligamentous laxity, subluxation, and contractures.

The course of RA is variable and unpredictable. Some people experience flares and remissions and others a progressive course. Over the years, structural damage may occur, often leading to articular deformities and functional impairment. In 1987, Yellin, Henke, and Epstein stated that most persons who had RA for 10 years would be unable to work. This is no longer true.

Assessment

Nursing History. Clients with arthritis should have the opportunity to describe complaints and problems from their unique perspective. History questions should focus on specific musculoskeletal complaints according to location, onset, duration, and extent to which function has been affected. General symptoms, such as fatigue, fever, weakness, sleep quality, and mood, also must be addressed. An exploration of the past health history could uncover unusual causes of arthritis. For example, a recent immunization for rubella could precipitate severe joint pain similar to that seen in RA.

Two useful frameworks for organizing the nursing history are the Arthritis Impact Measurement Scales (AIMS), illustrated in Box 14–2, and the *Outcome Standards for Rheumatology Nursing Practice* (American Nurses Association, 1983). The AIMS tool addresses physical, functional, social, and psychological parameters of the assessment process. It is also useful for tracking clients' status over time and can serve as the basis for identifying educational needs or the need for physical therapy, occupational therapy, or social services.

Rheumatology outcome standards identified by the American Nurses Association include (1) pain management deficit, (2) alteration in comfort: stiffness, (3) alteration in energy level: fatigue, (4) self-care deficit, (5) knowledge deficit regarding physical mobility, (6) knowledge deficit regarding self-management decisions, (7) ineffective coping, individual or family, and (8) disturbance in self-concept. These standards relate to the problems that clients and families encounter and can help the nurse effectively organize client assessment data.

Pain. Questions about pain should include the location, type, severity, duration, onset of occurrence, and other related factors, such as swelling or changes in motion. Questions regarding the pattern and timing of pain should be asked. "Is the pain constant, with a gradual onset?" "Does it usually occur in the morning with associated stiffness?" The effect that the pain has had on the client's self-care, work, and leisure activities must be determined. The nurse must find out if the pain occurs with motion or with rest and what self-care activities the client has used to reduce pain (e.g., aspirin, ibuprofen, warm baths). Also, the nurse should ask about specific activities that make the pain worse. Generally, clients with pain associated with RA have a gradual but simultaneous onset of discomfort in symmetrical joints (typically the wrists, PIP joints, feet, and knees), associated swelling of the joints, and the presence of pain at rest.

Stiffness. Questions about stiffness should help clients understand the difference between this gelling phenomenon and pain. The nurse should ask clients when the stiffness first occurred, the location, and the times of the day that it is usually present. Assessing duration of stiffness can be frustrating for the client, so the nurse should ask about its association with activities of daily living (ADLs). In severe RA, it is not uncommon for morning stiffness to last 4 hours or longer.

Fatigue. Information about fatigue should include its effect on the client's ability to work, play, and sleep. Clients may describe themselves as "tired," "worn out," "without energy," or having "no pep." The nurse should determine how severe the problem is and ask what the client does to cope with fatigue (e.g., rest, nap, avoid certain tasks). The nurse should also ask when fatigue

BOX 14–2.
Arthritis Impact Measurement Scales (AIMS)

Mobility
4   Are you in bed or in a chair for most or all of the day because of your health?
3   Are you able to use public transportation?
2   When you travel around your community, does someone have to assist you because of your health?
1   Do you have to stay indoors most or all of the day because of your health?

Physical Activity
4   Are you unable to walk unless you are assisted by another person or by a cane, crutches, artificial limbs, or braces?
3   Do you have any trouble either walking several blocks or climbing a few flights of stairs because of your health?
2   Do you have trouble bending, lifting, or stooping because of your health?
1   Does your health limit the kinds of vigorous activities you can do, such as running, lifting heavy objects, or participating in strenuous sports?

Dexterity
5   Can you easily write with a pen or pencil?
4   Can you easily turn a key in a lock?
3   Can you easily button articles of clothing?
2   Can you easily tie a pair of shoes?
1   Can you easily open a jar of food?

Social Role
7   If you had to take medicine, could you take all your own medicine?
6   If you had a telephone, would you be able to use it?
5   Do you handle your own money?
4   If you had a kitchen, could you prepare your own meals?
3   If you had laundry facilities (washer, dryer), could you do your own laundry?
2   If you had the necessary transportation, could you do shopping for groceries or clothes?
1   If you had household tools and appliances (e.g., vacuum, mops), could you do your own housework?

Social Activity
5   About how often have you been on the telephone with close friends or relatives during the past month?
4   Has there been a change in the frequency or quality of your sexual relationships during the past month?
3   During the past month, about how often have you had friends or relatives to your home?
2   During the past month, about how often have you gotten together socially with friends or relatives?
1   During the past month, how often have you visited with friends or relatives at their homes?

Activities of Daily Living
4   How much help do you need to use the toilet?
3   How well are you able to move around?
2   How much help do you need in getting dressed?
1   When you bathe, by sponge bath, tub, or shower, how much help do you need?

Pain
4   During the past month, how often have you had severe pain from your arthritis?
3   During the past month, how would you describe the arthritis pain you usually have?
2   During the past month, how long has your morning stiffness usually lasted from the time you wake up?
1   During the past month, how often have you had pain in two or more joints at the same time?

Depression
6   During the past month, how often have you felt that others would be better off if you were dead?
5   How often during the past month have you felt so down in the dumps that nothing could cheer you up?
4   How much of the time during the past month have you felt downhearted and blue?
3   How often during the past month have you felt that nothing has turned out for you the way you wanted it to?
2   During the past month, how much of the time have you been in low or very low spirits?
1   During the past month, how much of the time have you enjoyed the things you do?

Box continued on following page

BOX 14–2.

Arthritis Impact Measurement Scales (AIMS) Continued

Anxiety

6   During the past month, how much of the time have you felt tense or high-strung?

5   How much have you been bothered by nervousness and your "nerves" during the past month?

4   How often during the past month have you found yourself having difficulty trying to calm down?

3   How much of the time during the past month have you been able to relax without difficulty?

2   How much of the time during the past month have you felt calm and peaceful?

1   How much of the time during the past month have you felt relaxed and free of tension?

From Meenan, R. F., Gertman, P. M., & Mason, J. H. (1980). Measuring health status in arthritis: The arthritis impact measurement scales. *Arthritis and Rheumatism, 23*(2), 146–152.

usually appears. Unlike stiffness, fatigue generally begins several hours after the client rises, so the later in the day fatigue begins, the less severe the disease.

Mobility and Self-care Deficits. The assessment of self-care deficits and mobility includes those activities that are difficult to accomplish because of pain, fatigue, or stiffness. For example, clients should be asked about problems with dressing, tying shoes, fastening openers, or removing jar lids. The nurse should determine whether painful joints in the knees, feet, or ankles have made it difficult to walk, stand, or climb stairs.

Coping and Self-concept. Throughout the interview, the client's ability to learn and his or her decision-making abilities must be assessed. Coping strategies can be assessed by asking about how the client has managed the stress of the illness and the family's response to the changes in the client's activity level. Nursing research has begun to identify that passive coping styles are associated with negative outcomes and that more assertive or confrontative coping styles are associated with positive outcomes (Downe-Wamboldt & Melanson, 1995). Finally, to assess the effect of the illness on the self-concept, the nurse should note the client's overall appearance and any negative comments about joint changes.

Physical Assessment. The physical examination begins with a thorough assessment of the musculoskeletal system, as outlined in Box 14–3. Detailed examination techniques of musculoskeletal assessment are reviewed in Chapter 8. The following techniques and strategies are useful when examining the client with RA.

The assessment begins with the joints of the upper extremity and then proceeds down to the trunk and lower extremities. Some practitioners prefer to establish muscle strength and range of motion (ROM) as they inspect and palpate each part of the body. Others prefer to incorporate these procedures as part of neuromuscular testing once the assessment of the joints has been completed. The client should be warm, relaxed, and as comfortable as possible so that ROM is accurate. Pairs of joints should be inspected and palpated for symmetry, size, shape, color, appearance, temperature, and pain. Although tenderness is probably the most sensitive physical finding, it is relatively nonspecific for RA (Vollertsen, 1989). Pain with movement is often elicited with examination of the deep socket joints, or it may be present in the wrist or knee early in the disease.

Palpating swollen joints for synovitis is more precise if circumferential palpation is used to examine the PIP and DIP joints (Vollertsen, 1989). This technique is done by placing the thumb and forefinger(s) medially and laterally to enclose the joint capsule. Early synovitis can be detected in the MCP joints by having the client make a fist and then comparing the depression between each joint space. If the client is obese or has pudgy hands or feet, however, it may not be easy to detect mild synovitis.

Particular attention should be paid to the shape and size of the joints of the hands. Spindle-shaped fingers are often seen in the early stages of RA because of the swelling of the PIP joints. A series of jeweler's sizing rings is useful for measuring the size of each DIP and PIP joint. Ulnar deviation of the fingers, muscle atrophy, and the presence of flexion or extension contractures should be assessed for. The nurse should note any deformities, such as swan-neck contractures or boutonniere deformities (see Fig. 14–3), which are present with severe or active disease. Joint destruction and deformity is not reversible.

The nurse must inspect and palpate the elbow using the thumb and fingers of the examining hand to enclose the olecranon process. If synovitis is present, swelling may appear medial or lateral to the olecranon process. Often, synovitis is most readily evident as a thickening or fullness in the medial ulnar groove. The nurse should inspect and palpate the contour of the extensor surfaces of the arm because rheumatoid nodules often begin near the elbow.

The knees must be examined to assess for joint effusion. The bulge sign can be easily elicited by placing the four fingers of the examining hand at the lateral aspect of the knee arching over the suprapatellar pouch. The nurse should apply a quick, firm motion and observe for the movement of fluid from the lateral aspect to the medial aspect of the knee. The fluid can be moved back into the joint through gentle pressure on the medial knee.

The feet and ankles should be inspected and palpated for changes in joint symmetry and configuration. With subluxation of the metatarsal heads, toes can become clawlike and have a cocked-up appearance. The presence of unequal widening between toes must be noted. This finding often indicates early metatarsophalangeal (MTP) joint involvement before other joint changes have occurred (Vollertsen, 1989).

BOX 14–3.
Musculoskeletal Assessment of the Client with Rheumatoid Arthritis

All Joints
Assess for swelling, deformity, warmth, redness, symmetric changes
Palpate surrounding skin for subcutaneous nodules, cysts
Inspect and palpate surrounding muscles for atrophy

Head/Neck
Inspect neck for abnormalities
Palpate temporomandibular joint
Assess tenderness around spinous process and paravertebral muscles
Assess full ROM unless cervical involvement

Hands/Wrists
Inspect for swelling, erythema, deformities
Palpate circumferentially each joint
Assess ROM
Measure and record each joint size using standard jeweler's rings

Elbows
Inspect and palpate olecranon and epicondyles
Assess ROM: flexion, extension, pronation, supination

Shoulders
Palpate shoulder structures, including sternoclavicular joint

Hips
Assess ROM

Knees
Inspect for alignment and quadriceps integrity
Palpate suprapatellar pouch
Inspect for presence of Baker's cysts
Assess ROM

Gait
Assess for abnormalities: short length of stride, slow pace, decreased or prolonged pushoff or heel strike, irregular rhythm
Assess posture

In addition to a full assessment of muscles and joints, clients should be examined for evidence of systemic changes that occur with RA. Although these changes are not usually seen early in the disease, baseline assessment of other body systems is important for monitoring future disease activity and functional abilities. Table 14–2 outlines relevant assessment parameters accompanying extra-articular manifestations.

Diagnostic Evaluation

The 1987 revised criteria for the classification of RA (see Table 14–1) serve as a framework for clinical diagnosis. However, the classification system is not intended to define diagnostic criteria explicitly. Other findings, including the results of laboratory tests, radiologic examination, and synovial fluid analysis, help confirm the diagnosis.

Laboratory Tests. The laboratory evaluation of clients with rheumatic disease is often informative but rarely definitive. Laboratory testing is important in the diagnosis of RA, even though no single set of chemical, serologic, or hematologic tests confirms the diagnosis (Persselin, 1991). Serum and urine chemistries are usually normal in RA. Occasionally, proteinuria and microscopic hematuria are seen as a result of amyloid deposits in the kidney. Elevated erythrocyte sedimentation rates (ESRs) and C-reactive protein (CRP) levels are typical of active disease, with the CRP being a more definitive indicator of inflammation. Hematologic studies often indicate a mild normocytic, hypochromic anemia along with thrombocytosis. An underlying iron deficiency anemia is usually present if the hemoglobin is less than 10 g/mL and ferritin levels are low (Baer, Dessypris, & Krantz, 1990). Low eosinophil counts occur with increased disease activity, and granulocytopenia may indicate Felty's syndrome.

Serologic tests used to confirm the diagnosis of RA include antinuclear antibodies (ANA) and RF. ANA titers are seen in 15% to 20% of clients, more than half of whom have Felty's syndrome. RF, an autoantibody directed against IgM, is positive in only 80% of clients. Higher titers are seen in active disease. However, the presence of IgM RF is not specific for RA. Increased levels can be seen in older adults or after infections or immunizations. RF titers are also present in other rheumatic disorders, including SLE, DM, and SS, and in liver and pulmonary disease. The absence of a positive RF test does not exclude the diagnosis of RA in a client with typical clinical characteristics. Clients can convert from negative to positive when there is an exacerbation in their symptoms. However, clients with seronegative RA have better outcomes and rarely have extra-articular involvement. Recent evidence points to recognition that seronegative and seropositive polyarthritis are separate entities. Table 14–3 lists laboratory tests commonly used in the diagnosis of RA and other rheumatic diseases.

TABLE 14–3. *Common Diagnostic Studies Used in Rheumatic Diseases*

TEST AND PURPOSE	NORMAL VALUE	SIGNIFICANCE
Antinuclear Antibody (ANA) ANAs are gamma globulins that react to specific antigens ANA titer indicates the presence of antibodies that are produced in response to the nuclear part of the white blood cell If antibodies are present, further tests determine the type of ANA circulating in the blood	Titer ≤1:32	A small number of healthy adults have a positive ANA test ANA levels may increase with age, even in those without immune disease Positive titers (1:10–1:30) are associated with SLE, SS, dermatomyositis, and Sjögren's syndrome The higher the titer, the greater the degree of inflammation A negative test for ANA is strong evidence against the diagnosis of SLE
C4 Complement Method to determine serum hemolytic complement activity Complement is a protein that binds antigen-antibody complexes for purposes of lysis Activation of the entire complement system leads to an inflammatory response that destroys/damages cells When the number of antigen-antibody complexes increases markedly, complement is used for lysis, thus decreasing its availability	Men: 12–72 mg/dL Women: 13–75 mg/dL	Increased in active inflammatory disease and in autoimmune disorders (rheumatoid spondylitis, JRA) May be decreased in RA and SLE
C-Reactive Protein (CRP) Indicates presence of abnormal plasma protein (glycoprotein) that appears as a nonspecific response to a variety of inflammatory stimuli	Trace to 6 mg/mL	CRP is a nonspecific antigen-antibody reaction test to help determine the extent/severity of a disease process Elevated measurements indicate active inflammation, both infectious and noninfectious Elevated in RA, bacterial and viral infections, disseminated lupus erythematosus In RA, the test becomes negative with successful therapy, indicating that the inflammatory reaction has disappeared, although the ESR may continue to be elevated
Erythrocyte Sedimentation Rate (ESR) Measures the rate at which red blood cells settle out of unclotted blood in 1 hr	*Wintrobe* Men: 0–7 mm/hr Women: 0–25 mm/hr *Westergren* Men: 0–20 mm/hr Women: 0–30 mm/hr Higher elevations are seen in both men and women older than age 50	Increased rate seen in inflammation and necrotic processes Increase often seen in any inflammatory connective tissue disease An increase often indicates increased inflammation, resulting in clustering of red blood cells, which makes them heavier than normal; the higher the sedimentation rate, the greater the inflammatory activity Particularly useful as a guide to the management of the client with RA Decreased in salicylate toxicity Falsely elevated with excessive exercise, anxiety, pain, or dehydration

TABLE 14–3. *Common Diagnostic Studies Used in Rheumatic Diseases* Continued

TEST AND PURPOSE	NORMAL VALUE	SIGNIFICANCE
HLA-B27 Antigen Measures the presence of HLA-B27, which is used for tissue typing/tissue recognition Five series have been designated for HLA: A, B, C, D, DR, each with 10–20 distinct antigens	Titer $\leq 1:32$	Primary use is to predict the compatibility of donor/recipient tissues and platelets HLA-B27 found in 80%–90% of those with AS and Reiter's syndrome Also found in persons with the pauciarticular subgroup of JRA Presence does not mean disease: HLA-B27 is also seen in 8% of general population

Immunoglobulin Electrophoresis
Measures the values of immunoglobulins, serum antibodies produced by the plasma cells of the B lymphocytes
Five classes:
  IgA—protects mucous membranes from viruses and bacteria
  IgM—first responder to appear after antigens enter body; produces antibody against rheumatoid factor
  IgG—produces antibodies against bacteria, viruses, toxins
  IgD—less active
  IgE—less active
	IgA: 85–385 mg/dL
	IgG: 565–1700 mg/dL
	IgM: 55–370 mg/dL
	IgD: trace
	IgE: trace
		Basic function of immunoglobulins is to neutralize toxic substances (antigens) to allow phagocytosis
		Unique because of their genetic coding: each immunoglobulin interacts with other molecules
		The recognition mechanism of the immunoglobulin forms the basis of the immune response
		Increased levels are found in autoimmune diseases, specifically IgM (lupus, RA), IgG (RA)

LE Prep (LE Test) Measures the number of LE cells, essentially a type of ANA Should be repeated on 3 consecutive days to obtain the most accurate results	Negative	Positive in 75%–80% of clients with SLE Positive results may also be associated with RA and SS
Radioallergosorbent Test (RAST) Measures the quantity and increase of the antigen IgE present in the serum after exposure to a specific antigen	0.01–0.04 mg/dL	Elevated with allergic reactions: asthma, hayfever, dermatitis May be used to evaluate suspected allergic responses in clients on gold therapy
Red Blood Cell Count Measures the number of circulating erythrocytes per cubic millimeter of blood	Men: 4.7–6.1 million (mn)/mm^3 Women: 4.2–5.4 mn/mm^3	Normal values vary according to age When the value is >10% below the normal value, the client is considered anemic Decreased in SLE, RA, chronic inflammation
Rheumatoid Factor (RF) Determines the measurement for RF, a macroglobulin (antibody) directed toward a gamma globulin (IgG) Two tests are used: latex fixation and sheep red cell agglutination	$\geq 1:160$ considered significant in latex fixation $\geq 1:16$ considered significant for agglutination titer	Positive RF present in 70%–90% of persons with RA Negative RF found in 10%–30% of clients with clinical diagnosis of RA Positive RF may also suggest SLE or mixed connective tissue disease The higher the titer (the number to the right of the colon), the greater the degree of inflammation Titer is normally increased in older persons and in those who have had multiple vaccinations or blood transfusions

JRA, juvenile rheumatoid arthritis; RA, rheumatoid arthritis; SLE, systemic lupus erythematosus; SS, system sclerosis; AS, ankylosing spondylitis.
Data from Cella, J. H., & Watson, J. (1989). *Nurse's manual of laboratory tests.* Philadelphia: FA Davis; Pigg, J. S., Driscoll, P. W., & Caniff, R. (1985). *Rheumatology nursing.* New York: Wiley; and Schoen, D. C. (1988). Assessment for arthritis. *Orthopaedic Nursing, 7,* 31–39.

Radiologic Studies. Radiologic findings help in the confirmation of disease activity and the monitoring of treatment results. In the early stages, soft tissue swelling is indicated by increased shadowing on the x-ray film around the affected joint (Fig. 14-5). Massive tissue swelling of the entire joint often precedes further destructive changes, such as periarticular osteoporosis. Subchondral cysts may develop from the invasion of granulation tissue. As the disease progresses, subchondral bone erosions develop (Fig. 14-6), ultimately causing a narrowing of the joint space. In mild disease, erosions may not develop for 6 to 12 months. Initially occurring at the joint margins where the capsule is attached, erosions are first seen in the small joints of the hands and feet, where the bone is less dense. Subluxation and malalignment of the joints can be seen on x-ray film, reflecting the destructive changes seen on physical examination. With advanced disease, subchondral bone destruction and diffuse osteoporosis appear.

Other Procedures. Synovial fluid analysis indicates a change from the normal transparent color to a milky, cloudy, or dark yellow fluid. Arthroscopic examinations typically show pale, thick, edematous synovial villi; cartilage destruction; and fibrous scar formation (pannus). Bone and joint scans can be used to detect early joint changes and more readily confirm the diagnosis.

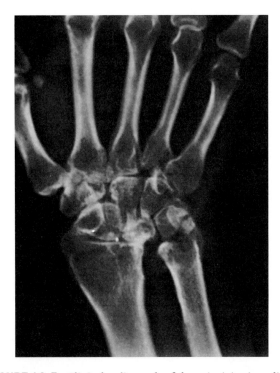

FIGURE 14-5. Clinical radiograph of the wrist joint in a client with early clinical rheumatoid arthritis, showing numerous marginal erosions, particularly in the ulnar styloid process. (From Bullough, P., & Bansal, M. [1988]. The differential diagnosis of geodes. *Radiologic Clinics of North America, 26*[6], 1175.)

Collaborative Treatment

The treatment and management of RA depend on successful collaboration between the client and the entire health care team—physician, nurse, and physical or occupational therapist. Other team members—orthopaedic surgeon, nutritionist, social worker, and orthotist—may be required, as the client's needs change. Figure 14-7 illustrates the approach to RA management. Surgical management is discussed in Chapter 16. The totally dependent RA client is uncommon today, in large part because of advances in joint replacement surgery (Myllykangas-Luosujarvi, Aho, & Isomalei, 1995) and the advent of new therapies. Effective management of RA involves a combination of medications, rest, exercise, and methods of joint protection.

Education is the foundation of the successful treatment of RA. Families must also be educated about the disease process and its effect on the entire family unit. Families must be helped to become partners with the client so that the disease is effectively managed and the client functions at the highest level of his or her abilities.

Collaboration between the nurse and physician, in particular, is necessary for teaching and reinforcing the unpredictable nature of the disease. Clients need to understand that the disease is chronic, characterized by remission and exacerbation in most of those affected, and is therefore somewhat unpredictable. This unpredictability can affect the client's ability to do simple daily tasks. The lack of certainty with which the client and family can plan ahead for outings and special activities can be frustrating for all parties. Individual and family stress can escalate to the point where family counseling is required. Reinforcing positive coping strategies and recommending stress management techniques, however, can help prevent feelings of powerlessness and helplessness.

Key components of client education for those with RA are outlined in Table 14-4. Many of the major content areas, such as fatigue, energy conservation, exercise, and stress management, require considerable follow-up, monitoring, and reinforcement over time.

One important interrelated area of content concerns principles of joint protection and work simplification (Table 14-5). In a multidisciplinary setting, principles of joint protection and work simplification can be taught by the occupational therapist and reinforced by the nurse. Education in these areas can have a positive effect on increased energy levels and decreased fatigue, thereby improving the client's coping abilities and sense of control.

Specific suggestions or anticipatory guidance about self-care can be beneficial. For example, clients should select easy-to-grip combs and brushes with large handles. These devices are readily available at almost all department stores. Using a long-handled bath brush to reach the feet and back during bathing is much less stressful on

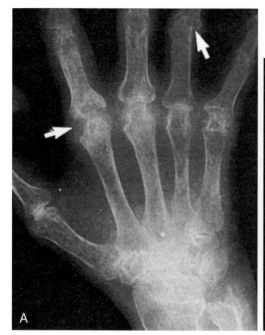
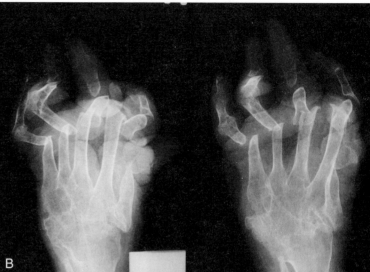

FIGURE 14–6. *A,* Clinical radiograph of the hand in late stages of rheumatoid arthritis. Note the profound osteoporosis. There is proximal interphalangeal (PIP), metacarpophalangeal (MCP), and pancarpal involvement. Note the large subchondral erosion of the second MCP and the fourth PIP joints *(arrows). B,* Additional late stages of rheumatoid arthritis. (*A,* From Brower, A. C. [1984]. The radiologic approach to arthritis. *Medical Clinics of North America, 68,* 1593.)

the joints. Many department stores and mail order catalogs now include a home care section, making it easier to select attractive, adaptable clothing. Jogging suits with pull-on pants and large, easily zippered tops are comfortable and attractive. Adaptive equipment for dressing includes long-handled shoehorns, zipper pulls, and buttoners. Involvement of the feet, including the MTP joints, can seriously affect the ability to ambulate and enjoy life. Referral to an orthotist for proper supportive shoes and or the use of orthotics is essential to reduce pain and prevent further joint damage.

Providing medication instruction is another significant aspect of client education programs. Clients should receive information about the purpose, dose, frequency, and anticipated side effects of each medication they take. Clients need to understand clearly when they are to report adverse symptoms to the health care team and what to do if they miss a dose. Some of the new therapies are self-injectable medications requiring that clients and their families be taught injection and preparation techniques. Preprinted or written instructions are essential to help clients recall the information. Appropriate educational materials on a variety of pharmacologic agents are available from the Arthritis Foundation and the pharmaceutical manufacturers.

Nurses can play an important role in teaching clients to participate in their care by keeping a medication history. Clients can use a notebook or flow sheet to record

essential medication information useful to themselves and other health care providers, such as dentists, other medical specialists, or acute care nurses. It is most helpful for information to be recorded about the medication name, date started, dosage, date discontinued, and reason for discontinuing the drug.

Therapeutic exercise is another important modality in the initial and ongoing treatment of RA. Three types of exercises are typically used: ROM, strengthening, and endurance. The purpose of ROM exercises is to improve joint motion. ROM exercises can be passive, assisted, or active. Carried out by the therapist without any client effort, passive exercises are most often done when the client is totally unable to move the joint because of the

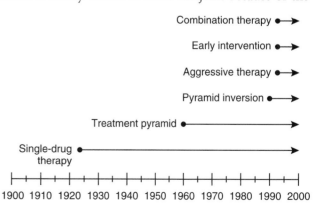

FIGURE 14–7. Changes in treatment approaches.

TABLE 14–4. *Client Education: Rheumatoid Arthritis*

FOCUS	TEACHING POINTS
Pain management	Teach client to distinguish between joint pain and stiffness
	Teach causes of pain: inflammation, mechanical, stress, and decreased stability of tendons, muscles, and ligaments
	Teach purpose of keeping a pain diary or comfort log to monitor progress and effectiveness of medications
	Teach client to define the chronic pain experience so that the warning signal provided by acute pain is heeded
	Reinforce the goal of pain management: to learn how to manage, "live with," or have control over the pain experience
	Teach the use of various relaxation strategies (rhythmic breathing, music, imagery) to decrease pain
	Instruct client to use specific physical modalities (heat, cold, massage, positioning) as adjuncts to pain relief
Fatigue	Teach client about types of fatigue: physical and emotional
	Instruct client that one important source of fatigue—the anemia of a chronic illness—often improves as the disease is better controlled
	Teach client to rest before he or she is fatigued
	Teach and encourage use of assistive devices (e.g., wheeled carts) to conserve energy
Stiffness	Teach client to distinguish between stiffness and joint pain
	Instruct in the use of warm showers or baths to decrease stiffness
	Explain relationship between inflammation and stiffness
Energy conservation	Teach principles and application of energy conservation:
	Keep diary of baseline daily activities for 1 wk. Analyze time needed for energy expenditures and time given to less demanding activities. Make changes in ADLs based on this self-analysis
	Plan ahead by gathering supplies/equipment before starting activity
	Set priorities for work to be done
	Pace activities
	Organize and arrange workspace in the kitchen, laundry area, basement, workshop, and garage
	Use organizers, pegboards, drawer dividers, and small containers to decrease energy required to perform work
	Eliminate any unnecessary steps to perform the activity
	Sit when possible
Sleep/rest	Teach purpose of adequate sleep as a treatment modality to help relieve inflamed joints
	Instruct client in the use of splints as sources of local rest
	Teach client to balance energy-demanding activities with energy-conserving activities
	Teach patient to anticipate need for 10–12 hr of rest with active, systemic disease
	Encourage 8 hr of sleep with at least two 1-hr rest periods during the day
	Teach clients about benefits of emotional rest—diversionary activities that produce emotional well-being
	Instruct client to avoid complete bed rest unless specifically prescribed. Bed rest can quickly lead to weakness, muscle atrophy, and restricted joint movement
Exercise	Teach that primary purpose of an exercise program is to promote, maintain, or restore skeletal and joint function
	Reinforce that exercise programs may not decrease pain
	Instruct client to consult with health care team before proceeding with exercises that cause severe discomfort
	Reinforce three types of exercise:
	Isometric (no joint movement)
	Assisted
	Active
	Teach client that active exercises are not performed when the disease is active because the inflamed joint needs to be rested
	In collaboration with the physical therapist, teach client to take each joint through a full ROM every day, preferably as an active exercise
	Instruct client to use assisted exercises if muscle pain prevents active motion

TABLE 14–4. *Client Education: Rheumatoid Arthritis* Continued

FOCUS	TEACHING POINTS

Exercise *Continued*	Teach guidelines for exercise:
	    Repetitions should vary from 3 to 4 to 10 for each joint
	    Lower number of repetitions but maintain ROM on days when clients have more pain or fatigue
	    Clients should do exercises when least stressed, fatigued, or tired
	    Exercises should be performed in a logical manner, progressing from a supine to a standing position

Knowledge of disease	Reinforce information about the disease: unknown cause, chronic illness, joint and systemic manifestations, course of remissions and exacerbations, control of symptoms
	Instruct client about the purpose, dose, expected benefits, expected onset of action (especially with the slower-acting agents), and the side effects of each medication
	Reinforce the following:
	    Follow-up care (laboratory work)
	    Symptoms to report
	    How to handle missed doses
	Encourage clients to discuss new treatments with health care team

lack of strength or voluntary control. The purpose of passive ROM is to ensure joint movement when there is a risk of developing contractures. Recent research (Rall, Meydani, Kehayias, Dawson-Hughes, & Roubenoff, 1996) has begun to identify a safe role for progressive resistance exercise training in selected clients with well-controlled RA. These exercises lead to significant improvements in strength, pain, and fatigue without exacerbating disease activity or joint pain.

When joint inflammation and flares have diminished, the client performs active ROM exercises as prescribed by the therapist. Although clients may be able to enjoy other

TABLE 14–5. *Principles of Joint Protection and Associated Work Simplification Strategies*

JOINT PROTECTION PRINCIPLES	STRATEGIES TO SIMPLIFY WORK
1. Respect pain (fear of pain can lead to inactivity; ignoring pain can lead to joint damage)	Carry out activities and exercise only to the point of fatigue or discomfort Reduce the time spent in doing painful activities Avoid doing activities (other than gentle ROM) when joints are inflamed
2. Balance work and rest	Rest 5–10 min periodically when doing tasks that take more time Get sufficient sleep Take a 30-min rest during the afternoon
3. Reduce effort to joints	Slide objects rather than lift them Store items at appropriate heights Avoid stooping, bending, or overreaching Sit to work when possible
4. Avoid positions of stress on joints	Avoid tight pinch or grip: use built-up handles and holders for such objects as toothbrushes and pens Avoid turning fingers toward the little finger: turn fingers toward the thumb Avoid wrist flexion and rotation during stirring. *Example:* Use spoon like a dagger Use two hands to lift or carry objects Always consider adaptive devices (jar opener, reachers, built-up keys) to protect joints from deformities
5. Use larger/stronger joints	Lift with palm and forearm instead of fingers Use a backpack, waist pack, or shoulder bag instead of a handbag
6. Use joints in most stable positions	Avoid or minimize excessive stretch of joint ligaments. *Example:* Rise from chair symmetrically and avoid leaning to either side Maintain good posture
7. Avoid remaining in one position	Change position (or stretch) every 20 min Balance sitting tasks with those that require moving around
8. Avoid activities that cannot be stopped	Break activities into defined parts

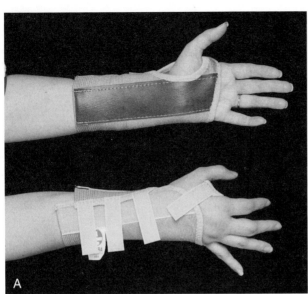 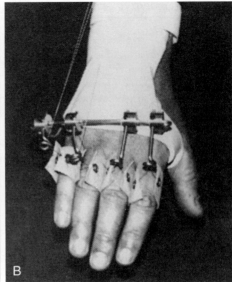

FIGURE 14–8. Static *(A)* and dynamic *(B)* splints used in rheumatoid arthritis or following total wrist replacement.

therapeutic and recreational exercises, they need to understand that engaging in other activities or ADLs is not a substitute for the ROM program. Few daily activities move every joint through a complete ROM.

Strengthening exercises are done to preserve or improve the muscle's ability to perform work. Two types of strengthening exercises are commonly used: isometric and isotonic. With isometric exercises, the muscle is contracted for 5 to 6 seconds, but the joint is not permitted to move. Common isometric techniques include gluteal folds and quadriceps-setting exercises. Isotonic exercises are used carefully in clients with RA because they require repetitive joint motion. However, after joint pain and inflammation have been controlled and the client has achieved increased isometric strength, dynamic, low-resistance exercises are appropriate (Sutej & Hadler, 1991). Appropriate low-resistance exercises for the client with RA include bike riding, swimming, golf, ping-pong, and dance (Banwell, 1984).

Other physical therapy modalities are also useful. For severely inflamed joints, splints appear to help resolve inflammation more quickly than does leaving the joint unsplinted (Fig. 14–8). Heat and cold therapy are important adjuncts to an exercise and rehabilitation program. Superficial heat therapy can be given with hot packs, hydrotherapy, or paraffin baths. Deep heat is achieved through the use of diathermy or ultrasound. Superficial heat appears to cool joints by increasing the local blood flow, but deep heat actually raises the intra-articular joint temperature. As a result, superficial heat is generally preferred to deep heat. Heat seems to be more beneficial in the treatment of chronic conditions characterized by minimal swelling and inflammation. It also permits more effective stretching exercises.

Many persons prefer cold therapy because it appears to provide greater relief of pain and stiffness than heat. However, cold packs should not be used in clients with Raynaud's phenomenon, cold sensitivity, or cryoglobulinemia or in anyone who finds it uncomfortable (Sutej & Hadler, 1991). The Arthritis Foundation has developed a wide selection of literature about RA. Support groups, self-help classes, and water-based or land-based exercises are available. To obtain this information from the Arthritis Foundation, call 800-283-7800 or 404-872-7100. Requests for information can also be mailed to The Arthritis Foundation, 1414 Spring Street, NW, Atlanta, GA 30309 or visit their website at www.arthritis.org.

Pharmacologic Management

The primary goals of RA treatment strategies are to provide pain relief, decrease joint inflammation, maintain or restore joint function, and prevent bone and cartilage destruction. Either a stepwise approach or a modified pyramid has replaced the traditional pyramid of treatment that begins with nonsteroidal anti-inflammatory drugs (NSAIDs) and client education, followed by the addition of methotrexate and then combination therapy. Mild RA is treated with NSAIDs plus hydroxychloroquine. Moderate disease is treated the same, with methotrexate or sulfasalazine added. Low-dose corticosteroids may also be added. Severe disease may require up to three DMARDs in combination with those used to treat moderate disease (Weisman & Weinblatt, 1995). Since 1998 and the advent of the immunomodulator leflunomide (Arava), the biologics etanercept (Enbrel) and infliximab (Remicade), and the medical device the PROSORBA column, the treatment paradigms for severe RA have changed significantly. Figure 14–7 reflects these changes in treatment approaches, from the 1900s to the present. The evidence-based practice table reviews data on new pharmacologic treatments that have made a difference in disease outcome.

NSAIDs are used to treat inflammation and swelling. Following the discovery in 1898 of the first NSAID—aspirin—originally obtained from the bark of the willow tree, NSAIDs have improved the quality of life for millions. NSAIDs suppress inflammation by interfering with the body's production of prostaglandins. Prostaglandins play a major role in the process of inflammation, and NSAIDs act by inhibiting their synthesis. The most common side effects of NSAID therapy occur in the gastrointestinal tract and include nausea and dyspepsia. More importantly, NSAIDs may cause gastric and duode-

nal ulcers. Studies have shown that 10% to 25% of arthritis clients who are on regular treatment with these drugs have NSAID-related ulcers on endoscopy. The primary, serious complications from NSAID-induced ulcers are upper gastrointestinal perforation, obstruction, and hemorrhage. From 2% to 4% of all clients will develop these serious complications (Lichtenstein, Syngal, & Wolfe, 1995).

The key enzyme involved in the production of prostaglandin and that which is inhibited by NSAIDs is cyclooxygenase. There are two forms of this enzyme, cyclooxygenase-1 (COX-1) and cyclooxygenase-2 (COX-2). COX-1 is present in all cells at all times, and its purpose is to produce prostaglandins that regulate normal cellular processes. COX-2 is expressed almost completely in

---

EXAMINING THE EVIDENCE: Moving Toward Evidence-Based Practice
Have New Pharmacologic Treatments for Rheumatoid Arthritis (RA) Made a Difference in Disease Outcome?

AUTHOR(S), YEAR	SAMPLE SIZE	DESIGN	DISEASE DURATION	OUTCOME VARIABLE	MAJOR FINDINGS
Traditional Therapies					
O'Dell et al., 1996	102 clients	MTX 17.5 mg/wk alone vs. sulfasalazine vs. MTX, sulfa, and HCQ Duration of study: 24 mo	Failed 1 DMARD Duration: 9 yr	50% Paulus Sharp Score	MTX, 33%; sulfa + HCQ, 40%; all three, 77% None available
Tugwell, Pincus, & Yocum, 1995	148 clients	CYS + MTX in severe RA—6 mo	Active disease on MTX Duration: 10 yr Function class II or III	ACR 20 Sharp Score	CYS + MTX, 48%; placebo = MTX, 16% None available Toxicity of combination similar to that of single agents
Boers et al., 1997	155 clients	Randomized comparison of combined step-down prednisolone, MTX, and sulfasalazine alone in ERA—56 wk Randomized sulfa 2 g/day, prednisolone 5 mg/day, MTX 7.5 taper to 0 at wk 40	Early disease: <2 yr	ACR 20 Sharp Score	Wk 28 combination, 72%; sulfa, 49%; combination = 2, sulfa = 6, 39% withdrew in sulfasalazine group vs. 8% in combination
Immunomodulators					
Cohen et al., 1999, for the Leflunomide Study Group	199 clients	2-yr treatment of active RA with leflunomide vs. placebo	Active disease on MTX MTX 16.2-16.7 mg/wk	ACR 20 Sharp Score	LEF, 77%; MTX, 60% LEF, 1.6; MTX, 1.2
Kremer et al., 2000	266 clients	Leflunomide + MTX in clients with active RA who are failing on MTX alone—double-blind, placebo-controlled trial, 24 wk		ACR 20, Sharp Score	LEF + MTX, 51.5%; MTX + placebo, 23.3%
Strand et al., 1999		Treatment of active RA with LEF compared with placebo and MTX	Average 7 yr MTX naive		
Aventis Pharmaceuticals, Leflunomide full prescribing information, 2000	MN 301: 350 clients	6 mo—sulfasalazine/LEF/placebo	Average 7 yr MTX naive	ACR 20	Sulfasalazine, 35%; LEF, 41%; placebo, 19%
	US301: 482 clients	12 mo—MTX/LEF/placebo	Average 7 yr MTX naive	Sharp Score	Mean change, $p = .0494$
	MN302: 999 clients	12 mo—LEF/MTX	Average <1 yr	ACR 20 Sharp Score ACR 20 Sharp Score	MTX, 45%; LEF, 49%; placebo, 29% Nonsignificant LEF, 44%; MTX, 57% Nonsignificant

Box continued on following page

EXAMINING THE EVIDENCE: Moving Toward Evidence-Based Practice
Have New Pharmacologic Treatments for Rheumatoid Arthritis (RA) Made a Difference in Disease Outcome?
Continued

AUTHOR(S), YEAR	SAMPLE SIZE	DESIGN	DISEASE DURATION	OUTCOME VARIABLE	MAJOR FINDINGS
Biologic Response Modifiers					
Genovese et al., 2000	632 clients	Etanercept vs. MTX (20 mg/wk) in early RA, 24 mo		ACR 20 Sharp Score	Etanercept, 72%; MTX, 59% MTX, 3.2; etanercept, 1.3
Kremer et al., 2000		Etanercept + MTX			
Moreland et al., 2000	628 clients	Etanercept in DMARD-refractory clients 42 mo of treatment	Mean 12 yr	ACR 20 Sharp Score	Etanercept, 68% No opportunistic or serious infections
Breedveld et al., 1999		Phase III randomized, double-blind, placebo-controlled trial in active RA despite MTX with infliximab	Mean 8–9 yr 99% function class I, II, III		
Lipsky et al., 2000	428 clients	102-wk clinical and x-ray results, 2-yr randomized, phase III trial of infliximab in clients with active RA despite MTX		ACR 20, Sharp Score	MTX + placebo, 20%; MTX + INF, 50% $p < .001$ vs. placebo + MTX
Maini et al., 1999		Infliximab vs. placebo in RA in clients receiving MTX A randomized phase III trial	MTX 15–25 mg/wk		
Weinblatt et al., 1999	89 clients	Etanercept in clients with RA on MTX 6-mo randomized, double-blind, placebo-controlled trial		ACR 20	Etanercept + MTX, 71%; MTX alone, 27%

Note: The ACR 20 and the Sharp Score are outcome variables for improvement of RA symptoms. See discussion on p. 351.
Cys, cyclosporine; LEF, leflunomide; MTX, methotrexate.

response to inflammation. COX-2 produces prostaglandins in the joints and synovium. Evidence suggests that the gastrointestinal side effects of NSAIDs are related to their ability to inhibit COX-1, whereas the beneficial anti-inflammatory effects are primarily the result of inhibition of COX-2 (Patrignani et al., 1994). Two NSAIDs that inhibit COX-2 have been developed. They are celecoxib (Celebrex) and rofecoxib (Vioxx). The COX-2s exhibit anti-inflammatory, analgesic, and antipyretic effects. Efficacy is comparable between the COX-1 and COX-2 medications, with the COX-2s causing less gastrointestinal toxicity.

Second-Level Agents. Because NSAIDs do not alter the course of RA, slow-acting, disease-modifying agents are usually considered when the client does not show an appropriate clinical response (i.e., decreases in pain, swelling, and stiffness) or if x-ray films show evidence of bony erosions within the first 30 to 60 days of onset. Disease-modifying agents act to alter the plasma levels of ESR and CRP, the markers of active inflammation. Second-level disease-modifying drugs commonly include the antimalarial agents (hydroxychloroquine), gold salts, penicillamine, methotrexate, azathioprine, sulfasalazine, and recently cyclosporine (Cash & Klippel, 1994) (Table

14–6). Added to this array there are the immunomodulatory drug leflunomide (Arava) and the biologics etanercept (Enbrel) and infliximab (Remicade).

The antimalarial drug hydroxychloroquine is widely used in treating RA clients. It has a very acceptable toxicity profile and can be safely combined with other DMARDs. Maculopathy occurs almost exclusively at higher-than-recommended dosages (6 mg/kg per day), although eye examinations are recommended every 6 months during therapy. Hydroxychloroquine is particularly effective in the early treatment of clients with mild to moderate and/or seronegative RA. Its true disease-modifying capacity is probably weak, however.

Gold preparations have been used successfully to treat RA since the 1920s, although rarely used today because the onset of action is 3 to 6 months and long-term studies demonstrate clinical efficacy but that erosions continue to develop (Paget, 1997). In the 1960s, a classic double-blind trial confirmed the drug's efficacy (Paulus, 1988). In general, second-level drugs continue to be effective in clients with inactive disease during long-term treatment. Some research (ten Wolde, Breedveld, Hermans, Vandenbroucke, van der Laar, Markusse, Janssen, van den Brink, & Dijkmans, 1996) observed that flare-up of symptoms for rheumatoid clients was more

Text continued on page 375

TABLE 14–6. *Pharmacologic Management of Rheumatoid Arthritis*

DRUG	DOSAGE	SIDE EFFECTS	NURSING CONSIDERATIONS
Analgesics			
Acetaminophen	1000 mg 3–4 times/day not to exceed 3 g/day	Headache, hepatic toxicity and failure, jaundice, chest pain dyspnea, **myocardial damage with dosage >5–8 g/day,** methemoglobinemia, cyanosis, hemolytic anemia, hematuria, anuria, neutropenia, leukopenia, pancytopenia, thrombocytopenia, hypoglycemia, acute kidney failure, renal tubular necrosis, skin rash, and fever	Assess for allergy, impaired hepatic function, chronic alcoholism, pregnancy, lactation Do not exceed recommended dose Avoid using multiple preparations containing acetaminophen—OTC Give with food if gastrointestinal upset noted Not an anti-inflammatory agent Use for acute pain <10 days Report skin rash, unusual bleeding or bruising, yellowing of skin or eyes, changes in voiding patterns
Nonsteroidal Anti-inflammatory drugs (NSAIDs)		Gastrointestinal irritation, fluid retention and edema, diarrhea, interstitial nephritis, CNS changes (dizziness, blurred vision, headaches), hematologic changes, bone marrow depression, prolonged bleeding time, skin reactions and rashes	NSAIDs are generally better tolerated than ASA Therapeutic response may not be seen for up to 2 wk Instruct clients to drive with caution until response to drug is known Give with food or a glass of water Clients should report gastrointestinal distress (heartburn, dyspepsia, nausea, vomiting, abdominal pain) Monitor baseline hematologic, renal, liver, auditory, and ophthalmic functions; repeat periodically Instruct client to report increased bleeding, severe pruritus, weight gain >5 pound/wk, persistent headaches, vision disturbances Client should avoid alcohol because of increased gastrointestinal toxicity
Nabumetone (Relafen)	1000 mg as a single dose or bid may increase to 750 mg bid	See NSAIDs Gastrointestinal: diarrhea, constipation, pain, flatulence Respiratory: dyspnea, hemoptysis, pharyngitis, bronchospasm, rhinitis Aplastic anemia, decreased Hgb or Hct, menorrhagia Dry mucous membranes, stomatitis **Anaphylactoid reactions to fatal anaphylactic shock**	See NSAIDs
Naproxen (Naprosyn) Naproxen sodium (Aleve)	250–1500 mg/day in 2 doses	See NSAIDs	See NSAIDs Aleve—OTC preparation—same side effect profile and nursing considerations

Table continued on following page

TABLE 14–6. *Pharmacologic Management of Rheumatoid Arthritis* Continued

DRUG	DOSAGE	SIDE EFFECTS	NURSING CONSIDERATIONS
NSAID Combinations			
Diclofenac sodium/ misoprostol (Arthrotec)	50–75 mg diclofenac/ misoprostol 200 µg	See NSAIDs May cause diarrhea, abdominal pain, upset stomach and/or nausea Usually develops in the first few weeks of therapy	See NSAIDs **Do not take if pregnant and do not become pregnant; can cause miscarriage, often associated with potentially dangerous bleeding; may result in hospitalization, surgery, infertility, or death** Misoprostol provides protection against the development of stomach and intestinal ulcers resulting from diclofenac use Serious side effects are still possible Avoid the use of antacids containing magnesium to minimize possibility of diarrhea
Ibuprofen (Motrin)	1200–3200 mg/day in 3–6 doses	See NSAIDs Also amblyopia, blurred vision, reduced visual field	Food slows absorption; best given on an empty stomach Clients with visual disturbances should have complete ophthalmoscopic examinations; visual disturbances usually disappear when drug is discontinued
Meloxicam (Mobic)	7.5–15 mg/day	See NSAIDs Gastrointestinal events were the most common reported	See NSAIDs May be taken without regard to timing of meals
NSAID—COX-2 Inhibitors			
Celecoxib (Celebrex)	200–400 mg daily	See NSAIDs Gastrointestinal side effects: ulcers significantly less common than with other NSAIDs Less affect on platelet aggregation; therefore can cautiously be used in clients receiving anticoagulants	See NSAIDs
Rofecoxib (Vioxx)	25–50 mg/day	See NSAIDs Gastrointestinal side effects: ulcers significantly less common than with other NSAIDs Less effect on platelet aggregation; therefore can cautiously be used in clients receiving anticoagulants	See NSAIDs
Antimalarials			
Hydroxy- chloroquine (Plaquenil)	200–400 mg/day	Retinal or visual field changes CNS: vertigo, headaches, confusion Blood dyscrasias, skin rash, pruritus, skeletal muscle weakness, gastrointestinal distress	Gastrointestinal distress: schedule client for baseline and ophthalmoscopic examinations every 6 mo, as well as blood counts Instruct client to report any visual changes, unexplained bruising or bleeding, skin eruptions, or weakness Inform client that full efficacy may not be seen for 6 mo

TABLE 14–6. *Pharmacologic Management of Rheumatoid Arthritis* Continued

DRUG	DOSAGE	SIDE EFFECTS	NURSING CONSIDERATIONS
Disease-Modifying Agents			
Gold compounds Myochrysine, Solganal	Initial dose: 10 mg/wk Second dose: 25 mg/wk Subsequent doses: 25–50 mg/wk	Major: blood dyscrasias, renal impairment, proteinuria, dermatitis Also, CNS effects (sweating, flushing, dizziness), gastrointestinal effects (metallic taste, stomatitis, nausea, vomiting, diarrhea, hepatitis)	Myochrysine is water based; Solganal is oil based Baseline blood counts are essential and periodically should check urine for hematuria and proteinuria before each injection Teach client to report early signs of toxicity: rash, pruritus, stomatitis, metallic taste Discontinue if these appear Monitor for allergic reactions that can occur anytime during therapy Give into gluteus muscle Client to remain flat for 30 min after the injection if dizziness, sweating, or flushing occurs Inform client that benefits may not be seen for 3–4 mo
Auranofin (Ridaura)	6–9 mg/day in 2–3 divided doses	See IM gold Also, diarrhea (dose related), cough, dyspnea	Administer with food and fluids Treat diarrhea if it occurs Inform client that benefits may not be seen for 3–4 mo
Penicillamine (Cuprimine, Depen)	250–750 mg/day	Thrombocytopenia, leukopenia, nephrotic syndrome, skin reactions, gastrointestinal upset, altered taste	Monitor CBC, liver function, urine and platelets weekly for 8–10 wk, then monthly Give on empty stomach (30 min before meals or 2 hr after) Instruct client to report fever, sore throat, chills, bruising, bleeding
Methotrexate	7.5–20 mg/wk (either single dose or 3 doses 8–12 hr apart)	CNS: headache, drowsiness, aphasia, blurred vision, hemiparesis, paresis, seizures, fatigue, malaise, dizziness Gastrointestinal: ulcerative stomatitis, ulceration and bleeding, hepatic toxicity Respiratory: interstitial pneumonitis, chronic interstitial obstructive disease Dermatologic: erythematous rashes, alopecia Other: anaphylaxis, sudden death, chills and fever, metabolic changes, cancer	Monitor renal and hepatic function Give with folic acid 1 mg/day Side effects more evident at higher dosages—may use SC to eliminate or decrease effects Risk of toxicity increased with use of alcohol—clients must refrain Follow CBC, UA, AST, BUN, and Cr every 6–8 wk during therapy Leucovorin may be used 24 hr after MTX dose to ameliorate side effects
Azathioprine (Imuran)	Initial: 1 mg/kg/day as single dose or bid increased at 6–8 wk and every 4 wk if no response Maximum: 2.5 mg/kg/day Clients who do not respond in 12 wk are probably refractory	Gastrointestinal: nausea, vomiting, hepatotoxicity Hematologic: leukopenia, thrombocytopenia, macrocytic anemia Serious infections: fungal, bacterial, protozoal infections secondary to immunosuppression, **may be fatal** Carcinogenesis: increase risk of neoplasia, especially in homograft clients, lymphoma	Take drug in divided doses with food Avoid infections; client must notify doctor if pregnant or wishes to become pregnant Monitor blood counts every 4–6 wk Therapeutic effects are not usually seen for 6–8 wk

Table continued on following page

TABLE 14–6. *Pharmacologic Management of Rheumatoid Arthritis* Continued

DRUG	DOSAGE	SIDE EFFECTS	NURSING CONSIDERATIONS
Alkylating Agents			
Cyclophosphamide (Cytoxan)	50–150 mg/day oral fluid intake (2–3 L/day) and emptying bladder at bedtime are important	Infertility in men and women, loss of appetite, bone marrow suppression, infection, hemorrhagic cystitis, malignancy	Use in severe RA, steroid-resistant SLE: clinical response may not be seen for 3–6 mo Given via IV bolus every 3–4 wk: least toxic route Liver enzymes, CBC, UA and renal evaluations weekly during therapy Counsel men and women about birth control because of associated severe birth defects
Immunomodulators			
Sulfasalazine (Azulfidine)	2–3 g/day in 2–4 doses	Stomach pain, achiness, diarrhea, dizziness, headache, light sensitivity, itching, appetite loss, liver abnormalities, lowered blood count, nausea, vomiting, rash	Slow acting—take with food to decrease gastrointestinal upset; drink 8 glasses of water/day Monitor liver, renal, UA routinely
Cyclosporine (Neoral, Sandimmune)	2.5–5 mg/kg per day in 1–2 doses liquid or capsule	Bleeding, tender or enlarged gums, fluid retention, hypertension, increase hair growth, loss of renal function, loss of appetite, trembling or shaking of hands, tremors	Can be used alone or in combination with methotrexate Monitor liver and renal function routinely Avoid infection Taking dose with food and practicing frequent mouth care may help alleviate tender and bleeding gums Carefully monitor for hypertension and increased creatinine
Leflunomide (Arava)	10–20 mg daily after loading dose of 100 mg/day × 3 days	Diarrhea, elevated liver enzymes (ALT and AST), alopecia, and rash	Monitor liver enzymes monthly initially Cholestyramine 8 g tid for 24 hr in case of toxicity Drug has long half-life: >2 wk
Biologic Response Modifiers			
Etanercept (Enbrel)	25 mg 2 times/wk SC Pediatric dose (4–17 years old): 0.4 mg/kg SC 2 times/wk, with 72–96 hr between doses	Respiratory: URIs, congestion, rhinitis, cough, pharyngitis Gastrointestinal: abdominal pain, dyspepsia Other: irritation at injection site, increased risk of infections, cancers, ANA development, headache, autoimmune diseases	Rotate injection sites Avoid exposure to infections Perform laboratory testing routinely Report fever, chills, lethargy, rash, difficulty breathing, swelling, worsening of arthritis, severe diarrhea Know that this medication is not a cure for RA or JRA
Infliximab (Remicade)	3 mg/kg per infusion given initially, 2 wk, 6 wk, and then every 8 wk	Most common side effects include, dyspnea, urticaria, and headache Lupus-like reactions have been reported Increased risk of infection	Should be given in combination with MTX Observe for reactions during infusion Monitor liver, renal, and CBC every 6–8 wk during therapy
Corticosteroids			
Hydrocortisone (Cortef) Prednisolone (Delta-Cortef) Prednisone (Deltasone)	Highly individualized but the lowest dosage possible is ≤10 mg/day	Osteoporosis, fractures, AVN, gastric ulcers, susceptibility to infection, hyperglycemia, hypertension, cataracts, glaucoma, thinning of skin, acne, hirsutism, moon face, edema, menstrual disorders, emotional lability	Once-daily dosing is preferred (easier to wean) Taper as soon as possible Do not stop drug abruptly Monitor older adults because they are at higher risk of side effects Avoid infections Protect skin from injuries—bruising occurs easily

TABLE 14–6. *Pharmacologic Management of Rheumatoid Arthritis* Continued

DRUG	DOSAGE	SIDE EFFECTS	NURSING CONSIDERATIONS
Combination Therapy	MTX/Hcq/SASA MTX/LEF MTX/ etanercept MTX/ infliximab		

ANA, antinuclear antibody; ASA, aspirin; AST, aspartate aminotransferase; AVN, avascular necrosis; BUN, blood urea nitrogen; CBC, complete blood count; CNS, central nervous system; Cr, creatine; JRA, juvenile rheumatoid arthritis; MTX, methotrexate; OTC, over-the-counter; RA, rheumatoid arthritis; UA, urinalysis; URI, upper respiratory infection.

From Klippel, J. H. (Ed.). (1997). *Primer on the rheumatic diseases* (11th ed.). Atlanta: Arthritis Foundation; and Karch, A. M. (Ed.). (2001). *Lippincott's nursing drug guide*. Philadelphia: Lippincott.

severe after treatment was discontinued than during continuous therapy.

After 20 years of research on the effectiveness of low-dose methotrexate, the drug was approved in 1988 for the treatment of RA unresponsive to second-line agents. Methotrexate was the first agent to demonstrate early onset of action, superior efficacy, and tolerability compared with the classic DMARDs (gold, hydroxychloroquine, and sulfasalazine). Clinical benefit may be seen as early as 3 weeks after initiating treatment, and the maximal improvement is generally achieved by 6 months.

Low-dose methotrexate administered once a week as a single dose (7.5 to 12.5 mg) has been reported to be effective, with little toxicity (Grisanti & Wilke, 1989). Adverse effects have been reported with both low-dose and parenteral administration, but they generally do not require discontinuation of the drug. The most common side effect is gastrointestinal intolerance (e.g., anorexia, nausea, vomiting, diarrhea, weight loss). Other reactions are stomatitis; alopecia; and central nervous system effects, such as headache, dizziness, and depression. As investigated by Moder, Tefferi, Cohen, Menke, and Luthra (1995), hematologic malignancies are uncommon. When bone marrow depression occurs, it is usually associated with renal impairment, folic acid depletion, and the use of trimethoprim-sulfamethoxazole (Wilke, Biro, & Segal, 1987). Opportunistic infections (e.g., *Pneumocystis carinii* infection) also occur in RA clients treated with methotrexate. It is uncertain whether preexisting lung disease predisposes clients with RA to methotrexate pneumonitis (Anaya, Diethelm, Ortiz, Gutierrez, Citera, Welsh, & Espinoza, 1995). It appears that the most vulnerable time for developing infection during methotrexate therapy is in the first year of treatment. Literature also suggests that more methotrexate-associated infections occur in severe RA than in moderate RA (Boerbooms, Kerstens, van Loenhout, Mulder, & van de Putte, 1995).

One advantage of methotrexate is that it can be used for longer-term therapy than many other agents, including gold salts and penicillamine. Drug toxicity, as opposed to lack of response to the medication, is the primary factor limiting clients' continued treatment with

methotrexate (Alarcon, Tracy, & Blackburn, 1989). The probability of developing toxic effects (e.g., hepatotoxicity) when taking methotrexate is significant, especially during the first year of therapy. However, research has shown that folic acid supplementation decreases methotrexate toxicity without compromising efficacy (Morgan, Baggott, Vaughn, Austin, Vertch, Lee, Koopman, Krumdieck, & Alarcon, 1994). However, one study showed a nearly 50% probability of continuing methotrexate up to 6 years after it was initiated (Alarcon, Tracy, & Blackburn, 1989). These results were far superior to the less than 20%, 5-year retention rate of clients taking sulfasalazine, penicillamine, or gold salts (Situnayake, Grindulis, & McConkey, 1987). Methotrexate has become the accepted means of treatment for early RA. In addition, methotrexate in combination with cyclosporine has been shown to be more effective than cyclosporine alone (Tugwell, Pincus, & Yokum, 1995) and will continue to be studied in combination therapy. Folic acid 1 mg/day should be given because methotrexate inhibits folic acid reductase, leading to inhibition of DNA synthesis and inhibition of cellular replications. Concurrent use of folic acid decreases the risk of gastrointestinal and mucocutaneous adverse effects.

Although numerous studies have shown penicillamine to be safe and effective at low dosages (250 mg/day), it is not routinely used to treat RA. Penicillamine has a slow onset of action and a high frequency of side effects, such as leukopenia and autoimmune disorders.

Another slow-acting agent, azathioprine, is metabolized in the body to 6-mercaptopurine, the active form of the drug. Azathioprine inhibits DNA synthesis and both humoral and cell-mediated immune responses. Consequently, B and T lymphocytes are reduced, thereby limiting antibody production. The clinical response to azathioprine is not evident for 3 to 4 months. When azathioprine is used at low dosages of 1 to 2.5 mg/kg per day, most side effects are troublesome but short term; possible side effects include stomatitis, nausea, and vomiting. Bone marrow toxicity can occur, however, so complete blood counts are mandatory to screen for leukopenia. Oncogenesis is a major concern with the long-term use of azathioprine. Transplant clients who receive high dosages of azathioprine have a higher incidence of lymphomas and neoplasms. However, it is not known whether tumor development will occur in RA clients, who typically receive much lower dosages of the drug (Weinblatt & Maier, 1991).

Despite many studies demonstrating the clinical effectiveness of cyclosporine, its cost and potential for irreversible toxicity, even at low dosages (2.5 to 5 mg/kg per day), have limited its use to severe, progressive RA refractory to all other DMARDs (see Table 14–6). A multicenter short-term study comparing RA clients treated with methotrexate alone to those receiving both cyclosporine and methotrexate demonstrated a clinically important (20%) improvement in disease activity, without substantial differences in side effects (Tugwell, Pincus, & Yocum, 1995).

The alkylating agent cyclophosphamide is highly effective for treating RA. However, this drug has been abandoned for routine use because of its high toxicity profile (i.e., oncogenicity, bladder hemorrhage, bone marrow toxicity, and infertility). Cyclophosphamide is the drug of choice in RA vasculitis unresponsive to corticosteroids.

Leflunomide (Arava), a de novo blocker of purine synthesis, has been found to be effective in the treatment of RA. Leflunomide reversibly blocks the enzyme DHODH, which is active in the autoimmune process that leads to RA; blocking this enzyme relieves the signs and symptoms of inflammation and blocks the structural damage caused by the inflammatory response to the autoimmune process.

New biologic response modifiers that target specific cells or cytokines involved in the inflammatory response hold great promise for RA therapy because of their improved efficacy and limited toxicity. The first biologic to be approved by the U.S. Food and Drug Administration (FDA) is etanercept. Etanercept binds specifically to TNF and blocks its interaction with cell-surface TNF receptors. TNF is a naturally occurring cytokine that is involved in normal inflammatory and immune responses. Etanercept consists of genetically engineered (TNF) receptors from Chinese hamster ovary cells that keep the inflammatory response to autoimmune disease in check by reacting with and deactivating free-floating TNF released by active leukocytes. Etanercept is currently indicated for reducing signs and symptoms and delaying structural damage in clients with moderately to severely active RA. Etanercept is a twice-weekly subcutaneous injection of 25 mg. Clients and their families have been very receptive to this form of treatment.

Infliximab, in combination with methotrexate, is currently indicated for the reduction in signs and symptoms of RA in clients who have had an inadequate response to methotrexate. Infliximab (Remicade) is a monoclonal antibody to TNF-alpha. It may be given alone or in combination with methotrexate. This is an intravenous infusion of 3 mg/kg over 2 hours. It is given initially, at 2 weeks, at 6 weeks, and then every 8 weeks.

PROSORBA column, a medical device used in conjunction with apheresis, uses approximately 200 mg of protein A covalently bound to an inert silica matrix that is contained within a 300-mL polycarbonate housing. Each column contains 123 ± 2 g of this matrix. Protein A is a component of certain strains of the *Staphylococcus* bacteria, and it has the propensity to bind IgG and IgG bound to an antigen (i.e., circulating immune complex). The PROSORBA column is indicated for use in the therapeutic reduction of the signs and symptoms of severe RA in adult clients with long-standing disease that has failed treatment or in clients who are intolerant to DMARDs. The procedure requires 12 weekly apheresis procedures. A plasma volume of 1250 ± 250 mL is passed through the column. Clients must have good intravenous access. The therapeutic effect is usually not noticed until completion of the 12-week treatment. There are limited data available regarding repeating the procedure.

Corticosteroids. Corticosteroids produce an immediate and profound anti-inflammatory response in clients with RA. At low dosages, corticosteroids demonstrate characteristics that are primarily anti-inflammatory rather than immunosuppressive. At higher dosages, these agents are immunosuppressive, appearing to exert the greatest suppressive effect on T helper cells. In the 1940s and 1950s, cortisone was almost universally prescribed for the treatment of RA. Its use was quickly modulated by the many adverse effects associated with long-term administration and its lack of effectiveness in preventing disabling deformities. Kirwan and the Arthritis and Rheumatism Council (1995) suggest that adding corticosteroid therapy to slow-acting drugs can improve long-term client outcomes.

More recently, clinicians have been interested in the use of low-dose prednisone as a bridge to carry clients from unsuccessful NSAID therapy until they experience the benefits of the slow-acting, disease-modifying agents (Wilske & Healey, 1989). This time has shortened considerably with the advent of the biologic response modifiers. More recent research (Saag, Koehnke, Caldwell, Brasington, Burmeister, Zimmerman, Kohler, & Furst, 1994) found low-dose long-term prednisone use of less than 5 mg/day to be correlated with the development of adverse effects, specifically serious infections, fractures, and gastrointestinal complications. The initial response to a low dose may be quickly diminished only to be temporarily regained by increased dosages. Daily cortisone therapy can easily become the surviving constant when other agents are discontinued because of toxicity or lack of effectiveness (Paulus, 1991). Clearly, this therapy must be monitored carefully.

Determining which clients are steroid dependent has important implications for those undergoing surgery.

Taking a drug history of the client with RA requires exploration of the use of steroids: when they were initiated, dosage history, and date they were discontinued. Steroid-dependent clients are those currently taking corticosteroids as well as those weaned from chronic corticosteroid therapy within the last year. Other clients at risk of steroid dependency include those who received regular intra-articular injections of steroids, psoriasis clients who routinely used topical steroids on large areas of the skin, and clients with inflammatory bowel disease who routinely used steroid enemas (Paulus, 1991). Steroid-dependent clients who undergo general anesthesia must receive stress doses of corticosteroids to prevent intraoperative shock. Three doses of intravenous hydrocortisone (100 mg each)—one before, one during, and one immediately after the surgical procedure—are usually given (Lockshin, 1985).

Traditional drug combinations for RA include an NSAID, a DMARD, and short intermittent courses of oral corticosteroids. Medications are changed in response to lack of efficacy or if the initial improvement fades.

The use of single-drug therapy has been shown to be of limited efficacy in the treatment of RA. Most clients who are prescribed a single agent are no longer taking the drug 3 years later (Wilke, 1993). However, studies have suggested that combinations of disease-modifying drugs are more efficacious than higher dosages of a single agent. Combination therapy is most effective if introduced within the first 2 years after diagnosis of RA. Methotrexate in combination with the biologics etanercept and infliximab has shown a synergistic effect, as has the immunomodulator leflunomide. In general, however, the superiority of combination therapy over single-drug therapy has been difficult to demonstrate in controlled clinical trials (Paulus, 1993). This remains an area of ongoing clinical research.

Corticosteroids have several unfortunate effects on bone metabolism: decreased calcium absorption, increased urinary calcium excretion, decreased bone formation, and bone resorption that may remain normal or increase. In addition, corticosteroids reduce sex hormone production by reducing adrenocorticotropic hormone (ACTH) levels, which affects adrenal androgen production, and gonad function directly. The use of corticosteroids is associated with rapid bone loss, especially in high-turnover trabecular sites such as the vertebrae and ribs. Bone loss is rapid; prednisone at dosages higher than 7.5 mg/day for 6 months may decrease bone volume by 20%. Treatment guidelines have been published (ACR, 1996). The defect in calcium absorption is treated with daily doses of 1500 mg calcium supplements and 800 IU of vitamin D. Treatment of low gonadotropin levels includes estrogen replacement for women and testosterone replacement for men. The bisphosphonates alendronate sodium and risedronate have taken the lead in treating osteoporosis.

Investigational Agents. Research is currently being conducted using IL-1RA, vaccines, CTLA 4 blockers of CD28, blockers of CD4, and inhibitors of interleukin-1-beta–converting enzyme. Research is focusing on the pathogenesis of disease and in halting the disease progression before damage has occurred.

Outcome Measures

There has been considerable effort devoted to the development of outcome measures in RA. A proposed set of core RA measures includes pain measurement, disability, physician and client global assessment, number of tender and swollen joints, and acute-phase reactants (Bellamy & Bradley, 1996). In addition, the ACR developed a statistically powerful definition of improvement in RA: 20% improvement in tender and swollen joint counts and 20% improvement in three of the five remaining ACR core set measures of client and physician global assessments, pain, disability, and an acute-phase reactant (Felson et al., 1995). These exciting research advances continue to clarify effective and appropriate management strategies for RA clients. At the very least, Pope (1996) suggests that the plan of care for clients with symptoms suggestive of RA should (1) establish a diagnosis of RA as early as possible, (2) determine the stage of disease (joint destruction) and disease activity (inflammation), (3) define relevant factors that will affect prognosis, (4) establish a plan for treatment as early as possible, (5) monitor disease activity and response to treatment, and (6) modify the treatment when client response is absent or inadequate.

Nursing Management

The goal of nursing care for clients with RA should be to promote a healthful, positive life course adaptation. To achieve this goal, the nurse focuses on four domains of human response: comfort, self-care, control, and coping.

Adapting to a chronic illness is a demanding, complex process physically, emotionally, and socially. The energy required to achieve this adaptation can be easily exhausted, especially in the early stages of RA. Achieving normalcy, regulation, or adjustment can become a life-long process, consuming increasing amounts of energy, unless clients learn to participate actively in modulating their responses to the illness. By working together, the nurse helps clients master adaptive strategies in each of the four domains so that physical, psychological, and social energy is renewed.

Alteration in Comfort

Physical Comfort Promotion: Heat Application, Positioning, Pain Management, Sleep Enhancement, Psychological Comfort Promotion: Relaxation, Guided Imagery. Nursing diagnoses of altered comfort include acute or chronic pain, stiffness, fatigue, and sleep pattern disturbance. Achieving a reasonable degree of comfort is a continuous challenge. Pain can be so pervasive and encompassing that it becomes a veil over daily activities, only to lift at unpredictable moments. Clients often use military terms, such as *struggle, battle, siege, in the trenches, attack, fight,* and *surrender,* to describe their experiences with pain and discomfort (Ceccio, 1985). Wiener (1975) emphasized the importance of covering up the pain and keeping up with activities as a means of rejecting or disengaging from the disease. In fact, achieving some degree of comfort is the primary predictor of psychological well-being in women with RA (Lambert, 1985).

Numerous strategies can be used to help clients achieve pain relief. Obviously, teaching clients about their medications and monitoring their response are important nursing responsibilities. Positioning the client, ensuring that the limbs are correctly supported, and reinforcing the use of heat and cold, however, are all important measures for promoting comfort. Some clients find that flannel nightwear, sleeping blankets, and thermal underwear are helpful means of retaining warmth while reducing pain and stiffness.

Modulating the client's response to the experience of joint pain is another key principle of pain management. The uncertainty and unpredictability of the disease, with its concomitant impact on comfort, have been well documented. Mooney (1983) suggests four interventions to help clients with the pain of RA: (1) making them comfortable, according to what has worked for them in the past; (2) listening to and learning from clients; (3) reducing anxiety; and (4) enlisting family and community support. Not all clients with RA have the same pain or the same experience with pain, so it is critical to understand the phenomenon from the individual client's perspective. Attending to anxiety is especially important with hospitalized clients because anxiety levels tend to increase as the number of hospitalizations increases (Muhlenkamp & Joyner, 1986).

Other nonpharmacologic pain management strategies can be useful. They not only can help relieve pain but also can decrease anxiety and thus enhance overall comfort and a sense of control. A variety of relaxation techniques, including imagery, self-hypnosis, and controlled, rhythmic breathing, have been suggested (Johnson & Repp, 1984). An audiotaped relaxation exercise that incorporates the image of a comfortably warm waterfall bathing inflamed joints was useful in relieving pain in 17 older clients with RA (Ceccio, 1985). Progressive muscle relaxation techniques should be used with caution in clients with RA, however, because there is a danger that muscles could be tensed too tightly, thus exacerbating joint and muscle pain (Johnson & Repp, 1984).

Other comfort-promoting activities include the management of stiffness and the promotion of adequate sleep. If these areas are addressed through the nurse/client partnership, fatigue can also be significantly reduced. Clients need to be taught to distinguish between

pain and stiffness and to understand why the nurse is interested in differentiating between the two symptoms. As one of the most important diagnostic criteria of RA (as well as several other arthritic diseases), morning stiffness can vary in duration or quality depending on disease activity. Typically, clients with morning stiffness wake up feeling comfortable until they begin to move (Pigg, Driscoll, & Caniff, 1985). The disabling effects of morning stiffness can be controlled by taking NSAIDs before getting out of bed, sleeping under an electric blanket, or taking a warm bath. If the morning stiffness lasts longer than 1 hour or does not show evidence of decreasing, it is possible that the medication regimen must be altered. When clients have significant morning stiffness (i.e., more than 2 hours per day), they require additional rest and sleep.

Occasionally, if stiffness is severe, family members may need to provide early morning assistance so that the client is prepared for the day ahead. Another option is for clients to begin (or organize) as many tasks as possible the night before so that they have enough time to complete ADLs without rushing or undue anxiety. Clients might also be able to rearrange schedules so that chores normally performed in the morning, when stiffness is most pronounced, are deferred until later in the day. Daytime stiffness can occur, but frequent position changes and pacing or alternating the types of activities usually alleviates it.

One unusual aspect of stiffness is that it is a disabling phenomenon that is not readily understood by other family members. Initially, family and co-workers may wonder if the client is feigning his or her inability to move rapidly or perform optimally in the morning. Helping the client and family understand the need for additional time to complete activities is an important measure in decreasing the family's frustration and the client's anxiety about moving slowly.

Disturbed sleep can significantly affect the client's level of comfort, especially when he or she has a chronic illness. With RA, sleep is often interrupted because of joint pain, excessive fatigue, stiffness, or generalized musculoskeletal aching. Other important causes are anxiety and poor sleep hygiene. Before specific interventions are suggested, the nurse must determine how the sleep has been disturbed—for example, difficulty falling asleep, frequent periods of waking up during the night, or early morning awakening. Often, the nurse's first interventions are to reinforce good sleep habits, such as maintaining a regular sleep schedule, avoiding caffeine or alcohol before bed, or engaging in soothing activities before retiring. Other strategies address specific causes of impaired sleep in persons with RA. For example, warming the bed or taking a bath before bedtime can ease painful joints. Taking the prescribed NSAID (with a light snack of milk and crackers) half an hour before retiring can also promote sleep by relieving joint pain. If clients are awakened during the night because of pain or stiffness, they may need to use a smaller pillow, bed boards, or even lighter-weight blankets. Clients who have difficulty falling asleep because of worries or diffuse anxiety may benefit from using relaxation-imagery exercises.

Self-care Deficit

Self-care Facilitation, Nutrition Support. Self-care includes the nursing diagnoses of self-care deficits, impaired physical mobility, alterations in nutrition, and impaired home maintenance management. Even more important, self-care includes all of those practices that clients undertake to promote their health and well-being despite having a chronic illness. Interestingly, in one study of older clients with arthritic joint pain, the most common self-care practice reported was the administration of prescription or nonprescription medications (Conn, 1990). Other modalities, such as heat, exercise, rest, positioning, or joint protection, were reported occasionally or seldom. Although taking medication is an important aspect of the plan of care for a client with RA, the results of this study emphasize that other beneficial self-care practices must be taught and reinforced to prevent the client from developing self-care deficits.

Nutrition is an important aspect of self-care that is often misunderstood by the client with RA. This misunderstanding can occur because the popular press has promoted nutrition and unique diet therapies as instant cures for arthritis. Clients with RA may become overweight (because of decreased activity or mobility) or underweight (because of the anorexia of a chronic illness, the side effects of medications, or alterations in oral mucous membranes). In addition, diets may not provide sufficient iron to restore the deficit that results from the anemia of a chronic illness.

Clients need to understand that it is just as important to consume nutritionally sound diets as it is to achieve a reasonable body weight. Strategies to promote nutrition in anorexic clients include good oral hygiene before and after meals; small, frequent feedings; and high-calorie snacks. Clients with a dry mouth (xerostomia) benefit from moister foods and extra fluids with meals. Eliminating spicy or acidic foods, sitting upright to eat, and taking all medications with food and a full glass of water can ameliorate gastrointestinal distress. Clients with stiffness or hand deformities need assistive devices to feed themselves or to help with opening cartons or packages.

Control Deficit

Coping Assistance: Hope Instillation, Teaching, Cognitive Restructuring, Decision-Making Support. In general, clients with RA have a difficult time learning to live in partnership with the disease. RA clients may experience the fears of becoming crippled, being perceived as being old and nonproductive, and not being understood by loved ones (Miller, 1983a). As with any chronic illness, clients need to maintain some degree of physical and psychological control over the disabling effects of their symptoms. For some clients, however, the need to exercise control is so great that they can experience extreme powerlessness and helplessness during exacerbations of the illness. Clients who can view their relationship with RA as an evolving partnership have better outcomes, both physically and psychosocially, than clients who perceive the disease to be the "enemy." This sense of partnership helps the client let go (i.e., rest and take care of himself or herself) during exacerbations of the disease yet respond actively by agreeing to engage in health-promoting, self-care practices. It can also help clients not to waste precious energy with anxiety, anger, and unresolved grief or guilt.

Exercising healthful control over the disease may include formulating causes of the illness. In one study, clients who reported causes for their arthritis (e.g., fate, personal habits, heredity, the environment) were less anxious, depressed, and hostile than were those who did not report any cause (Lowery, Jacobsen, & Murphy, 1983). Most likely, clients who continue to ask "Why me?" and who are unable to identify a specific cause of the illness have a more difficult time feeling in control (Salmond, 1989).

Clients with RA who experience loss of control or powerlessness may become "difficult to live with," controlling, demanding, or manipulative (Ignatavicius, 1987). Powerlessness can have physically and mentally detrimental effects on the client and can lead to anxiety, depression, and hopelessness (Stapleton, 1983). The key intervention for powerlessness is to increase the client's active participation in decision making by allowing him or her as many choices as possible, for example, when to take medications or how to perform required ADLs. Helping clients to reframe their relationship with the disease to one of active partnership, as was previously mentioned, can also increase their sense of control.

Two other areas are important to the client's perception of control: client education and hope. Arthritis education provides information that clients can use to make informed decisions about their care. Knowledge about the disease, its course, the appropriate treatment, and what clients can do to promote their well-being increases their mastery of the unknown. Client education in the safe environment of a support group can also decrease the uncertainties of the disease and thus enhance control.

Having a sense of hopefulness about the future is a powerful ally against powerlessness. Everything clients do can be based on some level of hope (Miller, 1983b). Nursing interventions to promote hope include avoiding false reassurance, helping clients to set realistic goals, praising them for all accomplishments (no matter how small), and actively listening. Being sensitive to changes in mood and affect is important, particularly for clients receiving corticosteroid therapy. When clients are receiving steroids, their views about the future often change from hopeful and positive to depressed, despairing expressions about their lives. If medication changes are not possible or if dosage adjustments do not relieve the depression, the nurse should consult the physician about the need for a psychiatric evaluation.

Ineffective Coping

Coping Assistance: Coping Enhancement, Body Image Enhancement, Teaching: Sexuality, Cognitive Restructuring. Coping includes the nursing diagnoses of ineffective individual or family coping, disturbance in self-concept, and altered sexuality patterns. Successful coping strategies help the client with RA integrate the disease into the demands of daily living. Coping strategies can be viewed as either approach (positive or healthful) or avoidance strategies (Salmond, 1989). Healthful approach strategies include seeking out information and assistance, finding strength through spiritual support, verbalizing feelings and concerns, setting goals, expressing positive thoughts, and maintaining realistic independence. The less adaptive, avoidance strategies include denial, excessive sleeping, other passive behaviors, and depression. It has been documented that depression is associated with increased levels of pain and functional impairment and increased use of health care services (Katz & Yelin, 1993). In addition, the relationship between depression and pain may be influenced by the use of adaptive or maladaptive coping strategies and by clients' beliefs about their abilities to control their pain (Keefe, Brown, Wallston, & Caldwell, 1989). Therefore, the nurse's goal is clearly to help the client realize the benefits of the more healthful approach strategies. Healthful coping strategies and the reframing of negative behaviors can be discussed, modeled, and safely tried out in nurse-led client support groups (Cave, 1984).

For some clients, coping may be impaired because of changes in their body image and self-esteem. As the disease progresses, disfiguring joint changes or systemic alterations, such as rheumatoid nodules, may contribute to clients' sensitivity about their appearance and attractiveness. If changes occur in the performance of occupational, family, or social roles, self-esteem can be significantly affected. Fifield, Reisine, Sheehan, and McQuillan (1996) found that men and women with RA were at equal risk of experiencing emotional distress when they maintained employment despite having high levels of functional disability and being exposed to stressful work.

A disturbed self-concept can, in turn, lead to altered patterns of sexuality. The interrelated aspects of these sensitive areas can be hard to assess, and clients may be reticent to share their feelings. Determining clients' perceptions of their body image, however, is essential before the nurse can help them to develop insight, understanding, and a repertoire of self-management skills. Tentative, open-ended questions, such as "Tell me how RA has affected your relationship with your family," may be useful in helping clients explore their feelings and concerns.

One important but often overlooked aspect of coping is sexual expression. Nurses can help clients understand the entire gamut of sexuality, including open communication and touch. Strategies to promote sexual expression include taking a warm bath and pain medication before engaging in sexual activity, using alternative positions to enhance the client's comfort, and timing the activity when the client is well rested.

JUVENILE RHEUMATOID ARTHRITIS

JRA is the most common form of childhood arthritis and one of the more common chronic childhood illnesses. The cause is unknown. Diagnosis requires a combination of data from history, physical examination, and laboratory testing. For most clients, the immunogenetic associations, clinical course, and functional outcome are quite different from those of adult-onset RA. However, approximately 5% to 10% of JRA clients who have RF-positive polyarticular arthritis beginning during adolescence have a disease that resembles adult-onset RA much more than JRA.

JRA is a chronic inflammatory disease of childhood that, in many children, resolves by the time they reach adulthood. Even though the active disease may be ended by adulthood, residual joint damage remains (Fife, 1993). JRA is classified into three major groups according to the mode of onset: systemic, polyarticular (pJRA), and pauciarticular. In addition, pJRA can be divided into seronegative or seropositive subgroups depending on the results of the RF test. Pauciarticular JRA has two subgroups according to the timing of its onset, early (ages 2 to 6) and late (ages 10 to 15). Characteristics common to all groups include (1) symptom fluctuation from severe to mild to absent, (2) morning or inactivity stiffness, and (3) intermittent joint pain and swelling (Page-Goertz, 1989).

The diagnostic criteria for JRA are onset before 16 years of age, persistent arthritis in one or more joints for at least 6 weeks, and exclusion of other types of childhood arthritis. Four key points are often missed, resulting in misdiagnosis. Arthritis must be present and is defined as swelling, effusion, or the presence of two or more of the following signs: limitation of motion, tenderness, pains on motion, or joint warmth. The arthritis, not arthralgias, must persist for at least 6 weeks. All other causes of arthritis in children must be excluded. JRA like RA is a clinical diagnosis. There are no specific laboratory tests that can establish the diagnosis.

The three types of JRA differ as to the number of joints involved, presence of systemic manifestations, complications, disease course, and client outcomes (Table 14–7). The number of joints involved within the first 6 months of diagnosis establishes the specific disease subtype.

Onset Types

Systemic Onset. Approximately 10% of children with JRA have systemic onset. Systemic-onset JRA (sJRA) is characterized by persistent intermittent fever spikes of greater than 101°F and the presence of a characteristic JRA rash. The rash, most commonly found on the trunk, is pale pink, blanching, characterized by small macule or maculopapules, transient (minutes to hours), and non-pruritic in 95% of cases (Lehman, 1997). A hallmark of this fever trajectory is the appearance of subnormal temperature troughs (Page-Goertz, 1989). These daily spiking afternoon fevers, if not adequately controlled by appropriate medication, can be quite disabling. Younger children often become extremely fatigued and irritable as their temperatures rise.

Children with sJRA often have growth delay, osteopenia, diffuse lymphadenopathy, hepatosplenomegaly, pericarditis, pleuritis, anemia, leukocytosis, thrombocytosis, and elevated acute-phase reactants. Positive RF and uveitis are rare. These systemic manifestations are normally present at the onset of the disease and are often

TABLE 14–7. *Classification of Juvenile Rheumatoid Arthritis by Onset Subtypes*

	SYSTEMIC ONSET	POLYARTICULAR ONSET	PAUCIARTICULAR ONSET
Percentage affected	20	40	45
Age at onset	2–15 yr with a bimodal distribution: 1–3 yr 8–10 yr	2–15 yr	2–15 yr Early onset: 2–6 yr Late onset: 10–15 yr
Sexual predominance	Equal predominance	Mostly female (female/male ratio: 2∶1)	Early onset: predominantly female Late onset: predominantly male
Joints involved	Any joint 20% have joint involvement at diagnosis	Five or more joints involved Cervical spine involvement commonly seen Any joints possible: usually symmetrical involvement of small joints	Four or fewer joints during first 6 mo of disease
Fever (°F)	101–105, with subnormal trough	98.6–101	98.6
Rash (% affected)	90	Rarely seen	Absent
Extra-articular manifestations	Myalgia Pleuritis Hepatomegaly Splenomegaly Lymphadenopathy	Growth retardation Malaise, weight loss Adenopathy Rheumatoid nodules and/or vasculitis possible	Early onset: chronic iridocyclitis Late onset: acute iridocyclitis, sacroiliitis; ankylosing spondylitis in many children
Laboratory tests	Elevated ESR Negative RF Rarely positive ANA Anemia Leukocytosis	Elevated ESR Positive or negative RF ANA positive in 25%–40%	Elevated ESR Positive ANA Early onset: positive HLA-DRW5 Late onset: positive HLA-B27
Long-term prognosis	Complete recovery for 50% 1%–2% mortality Severe, chronic arthritis in 25%	Overall, more joint deformities and disabilities RF positive: 50% permanent deformity RF negative: 10%–15% permanent deformity	Expected remission in 60% Early onset: 10% uveitis—blindness Late onset: ankylosing spondylitis

Data from Page-Goertz, S. S. (1989). Even children have arthritis. *Pediatric Nursing, 15,* 11–16, 30; Singsen, B. H. (1988). Pediatric rheumatic diseases. In H. R. Schumacher (Ed.), *Primer on the rheumatic diseases* (9th ed., pp. 160–163). Atlanta: Arthritis Foundation; and Whaley, R. F., & Wong, D. L. (1987). *Nursing care of infants and children.* St. Louis: Mosby.

limited to several months' duration. Although the systemic problems are seldom critical, severe pericarditis or myocarditis requires immediate treatment.

Joint symptoms (e.g., arthralgia, myalgia, transient arthritis) may not be apparent initially but then may occur from weeks to even years after the onset of systemic symptoms. Subjective joint symptoms usually occur first as the joints become painful in association with fever spikes. Swelling, warmth, and tenderness can be observed later. Chronic polyarthritis may continue for years, with or without fever. sJRA may develop at any age, but the peak age of onset is 1 to 6 years old. Boys and girls are equally affected.

Polyarticular Onset. Occurring in about 40% of children with JRA, the polyarticular-onset type involves five or more joints during the first 6 months of illness. Joint involvement is usually symmetrical, but the affected joints may have an asymmetrical or unilateral pattern. Commonly affected joints include the wrists, knees, ankles, and small joints of the hands and feet. Two types of polyarticular onset are differentiated according to the results of the latex fixation test for RF. Girls older than 10 years of age with a consistently positive RF test experience a disease trajectory similar to that of adult RA, including destructive joint changes and the appearance of rheumatoid nodules. Morning stiffness can last from 1 to 3 hours. The onset of joint symptoms can be abrupt and painful. If the disease progresses, hip joint erosion ultimately can require total joint arthroplasty. Thus, this group of children has a 50% risk for developing severe joint deformities (Page-Goertz, 1989).

In clients with pJRA who are negative for RF, the destructive effects of disabling arthritis occur in only 10% to 15% of clients, compared with about half of those with a positive RF (Singsen, 1988). Here, the disease onset can be insidious, with slowly developing joint complaints and early morning stiffness. The child may limp or be reluctant to play or walk.

Pauciarticular Onset. Affecting 30% to 40% of children with JRA, the pauciarticular-onset subtype has arthritis present in one to four joints. There are two major subgroups, which differ in the age of onset and the sexual predominance. The early-onset subgroup occurs most often in females ages 2 to 6. The articular involvement is usually insidious, affecting large joints of the lower extremities. Progression to severe, disabling arthritis is extremely rare. However, flexion contractures are a frequent consequence as the disease progresses. Linear overgrowth of the bones of the involved joints may contribute to these flexion contractures, particularly in the knees. There are no systemic effects.

The major complication occurring in the early-onset subgroup is that of asymptomatic or recurrent chronic inflammatory eye disease (iridocyclitis, iritis, uveitis), which occurs in more than 50% of these clients. Often asymptomatic, iridocyclitis usually follows the appearance of joint symptoms by 1 to 15 years. Photophobia, redness, eye pain, and visual deficits may occur unilaterally or bilaterally. Up to 10% of children with eye involvement develop ocular damage (i.e., cataracts, glaucoma, or band keratopathy) that can lead to blindness (Page-Goertz, 1989). Slit-lamp examination performed by an ophthalmologist every 3 to 4 months is warranted prophylactically to identify early signs of the condition (Cassidy & Petty, 1995).

The second subset of children with pauciarticular JRA includes boys between 10 and 15 years of age who have a positive HLA-B27 histocompatibility antigen associated with an increased risk of developing AS. Initially, these adolescents complain of hip, knee, or ankle pain. After 5 to 10 years, sacroiliac joint changes can be seen on x-ray film. Sacroiliac and back symptoms do not usually occur before the age of 16.

Epidemiology

Incidence. The most commonly cited figure is that there are 70,000 to 100,000 cases (inactive and active) of JRA in the U.S. population under the age of 16 (Lehman, 1997). Using Gere's report on disease persisting into adulthood, an estimated 35,000 to 50,000 Americans older than age 16 have active JRA (Singsen, 1988). JRA affects a smaller portion of the U.S. population than adult-onset RA; however, compared with other pediatric-onset chronic illness, JRA is relatively common. JRA affects approximately the same number of children as juvenile diabetes, at least 4 times more children than sickle cell anemia or cystic fibrosis, and at least 10 times more children than hemophilia, acute lymphocyte leukemia, chronic renal failure, or muscular dystrophy.

Prevalence. The prevalence of JRA in the United States has been estimated to be between 57 and 114 per 100,000 children younger than 16 years of age (Lehman, 1997). All prevalence estimates have wide confidence levels because of the relative rarity of JRA and the small number of actual cases detected in even the largest studies.

Risk Factors. The age of onset has a bimodal distribution, with an early peak (1 to 3 years) affecting primarily girls and a later peak (8 to 11 years) affecting the sexes equally. The overall female/male ratio is 1:1 (Neuberger & Neuberger, 1984). Unconfirmed risk factors include a deficiency of alpha-antitrypsin and a link with the rubella virus. Genetic factors may be important. An increased incidence of late childhood pauciarticular-onset disease, especially in adolescent boys, is associated with the HLA-B27 antigen (Singsen, 1988). Younger children with pauciarticular JRA and uveitis have had an increased incidence of the DR5 and DR8 antigens (Kredich, 1986).

Pathophysiology

The pathophysiology of JRA is similar to that of RA. An inflamed synovial membrane produces increased amounts of synovial fluid, resulting in joint effusion and thickening. The increased blood flow to the joint stimulates the overgrowth of bone, which eventually leads to deformity and ankylosis. These destructive changes occur much later in the course of JRA than they do in RA (Cassidy & Petty, 1995).

Assessment

Nursing History. Taking part in the nursing history of a child with arthritis can be frustrating and problematic for both children and their families. Parents usually have more stress reporting the problems of the younger child because the child is not able to describe symptoms. Older clients can participate in the history-taking process at their appropriate developmental level but may be reticent to describe fully their symptoms or concerns. Parents or caregivers, however, are often the nurse's primary source of information. Questions must be asked with sensitivity because parents can become anxious when they realize they do not remember when symptoms first began. They may not be able to identify specific behaviors but only that the child is "different," "cranky," "listless," or "irritable." Parents whose children have symptoms of sJRA, with daily or twice-daily fevers, may be especially anxious because of the fear that their child has a fatal illness.

Eliciting the history is usually easier when the child or parent is asked about general behavior. The nurse should ask about the child's usual daily routines and how these have changed. For example, the nurse may ask the following: "Has the child been less willing to play specific games or participate in after-school activities?" "Does the child favor or protect an extremity by keeping it flexed (such as an elbow) or by limping?" "Does the child seem to be stiff and move slowly after sitting for an hour?" "Has the child taken more time in the morning to get out of bed, dress, and prepare for the day?" Questions about the difficulty or slowness in tying shoes or fastening buttons in children who have mastered these skills give important clues about the disease activity. When possible, the nurse should try to elicit when specific behavior changes first occurred to help determine more accurately the onset and diagnosis of the disease.

The nurse should ask about the child's general comfort. Young children may express pain through crankiness and irritability, whereas older children may refuse to do painful activities, claiming that the activity is "dumb." The nurse should determine whether the child

has been unusually fatigued or listless or has had difficulty sleeping.

In addition, the nurse should determine whether the child has had any fevers and when they occurred. Their onset, the usual range of temperature, and whether the elevations were accompanied by a rash should be recorded. A pale red macular rash associated with daily temperature spikes is characteristic of sJRA.

Finally, questions about the child's appetite and weight should be asked. Often, children with pauciarticular and pJRA experience decreased appetite. However, children whose activity levels have been significantly affected may begin to gain weight.

Physical Assessment. The physical assessment of the child with JRA focuses on a careful examination of musculoskeletal function. The joints must be inspected and palpated for swelling, tenderness, erythema, and warmth. Inspection must be performed carefully in toddlers and preschool-aged children because their pudgy joints may make it difficult to detect synovitis or swelling. Joint contours must be inspected for the presence of rheumatoid nodules that are occasionally present in polyarticular-onset JRA (pJRA). The nurse should note whether involved joints are symmetrical or asymmetrical in their distribution, as well as the number and exact location. ROM and muscle strength should be screened through age-appropriate activities, if possible, so that early contractures can be identified and treated. A goniometer should be used if there is any question about the extent to which ROM is reduced. It should be noted particularly whether the child prefers to keep joints flexed. Although there may be full ROM, flexed positions can quickly lead to deformities and contractures (Fig. 14–9).

The gait should be assessed to determine the effect of decreased ROM, pain, or weakness on ambulation. If scoliosis or a limp is present, both legs must be measured for a leg length discrepancy of more than 0.25 inches. Although adults can compensate for a 0.5-inch leg length discrepancy, children compensate by developing a flexion contracture of the knee of the shorter leg or by tilting the pelvis into a scoliotic curve (Ansell & Swann, 1983). Children must be assessed and screened for spinal curvatures because scoliosis is a common finding of pauciarticular-onset JRA. The determination of current height and weight is essential, with a review of the child's growth history, because JRA can retard growth.

In addition to a thorough examination of the musculoskeletal system, the child should be assessed for other system changes. The child with sJRA may have an enlarged liver, spleen, or lymph nodes. Cough, rib cage discomfort, and shortness of breath might be seen with pleuritis or myocarditis. When there is a high index of suspicion of pauciarticular-onset JRA, children should be

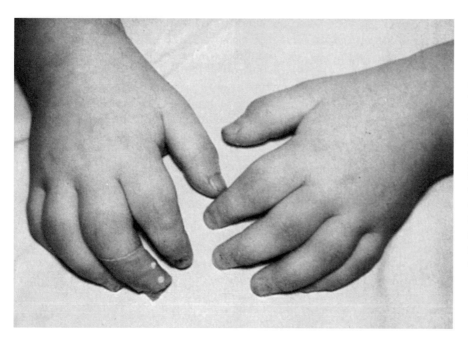

FIGURE 14–9. Hands of a 2-year-old boy with systemic onset of juvenile rheumatoid arthritis (JRA). All the small joints were swollen, warm, and painful. The terminal interphalangeal joints were erythematous. Generalized swelling also involved the digits between the joints. Moderate flexion contractures were already present. (From Kelley W., Harris, E., Ruddy, S., & Sledge, C. [Eds.]. [1989]. *Textbook of rheumatology* [3rd ed., p. 1291]. Philadelphia: WB Saunders.)

screened carefully for iridocyclitis (an inflammatory eye disease that can lead to blindness). Assess the external eyes for redness while questioning the child about photophobia and eye pain.

Diagnostic Evaluation

The diagnosis of JRA is confirmed by the presence of arthritis for at least 6 weeks in one or more joints. Joint pain alone is not sufficient to confirm the diagnosis. There must be objective joint swelling or limited joint motion accompanied by heat, pain, or tenderness. Other causes of joint pain (e.g., SLE, rheumatic fever, AS) must also be excluded before the diagnosis is confirmed. Clinical and laboratory features of the three types of JRA (see Table 14–7) also help establish the diagnosis.

Collaborative Treatment

The standard of care for the treatment of JRA incorporates the comprehensive coordinated efforts of an interdisciplinary team of health care professionals and the family. Comprehensive means addressing all facets of an individual's life that may be affected by a chronic illness such as education, peer relationships, self-esteem, social adjustment, family dynamics, vocational planning, and financial concerns. Treatment begins with diagnosis and can be divided into pharmacologic, physical, and social components.

Pharmacologic Management

The management of JRA begins with pharmacologic agents to reduce inflammation (Table 14–8). Pharmacologic management encompasses treatment of articular, ocular, and other manifestations of JRA. In many clients, the articular manifestations can be treated with NSAIDs. NSAIDs are the first step of treatment. Achieving an

anti-inflammatory effect requires larger doses than are needed for pain control (up to twice the analgesic dose) and consistent ingestion over a longer period. The average time to demonstrate clinical responses to a particular NSAID in JRA clients is 1 month. Many NSAIDs have been prospectively evaluated in clients with JRA, and overall efficacy rates are similar. However, individual responses are idiosyncratic. A favorable response to the first NSAID used occurs in 50% to 60%. About 50% of those demonstrating inadequate clinical response to the first NSAID improve with the next NSAID tried (Ansell, 1984). In general, the selection of NSAID is driven more by logistics than scientific concerns, liquid versus tablets and dosing frequency being the most common. Side effects are similar to those seen in adults and are treated similarly. Celecoxib (Celebrex), naproxen (Naprosyn), tolmetin sodium (Tolectin), and ibuprofen (Pediaprofen) are FDA approved for use in children.

Approximately two thirds of children with JRA are inadequately treated with NSAIDs alone. In a prospective, blinded trial, oral methotrexate given once weekly at 10 mg/m² body surface area (BSA) was well tolerated and significantly more effective than placebo. Methotrexate is used primarily for sJRA or pJRA clients. Overall, 70% to 80% of JRA clients demonstrate clinical improvement on methotrexate therapy, although the rate of response may be lower in sJRA clients who are still demonstrating systemic features (Lang, Laxter, Murphy, Silverman, & Roifman, 1991). In these clients, doses have been increased to 20mg/m² BSA per week and are usually given parenterally. Parenteral administration results in more reliable dosing and generally fewer gastrointestinal side effects. Folic acid is always given with methotrexate to decrease the frequency and severity of side effects. Etanercept (Enbrel) has been approved for the treatment of pJRA. Studies were conducted in children 4 to 17 years of age. Results showed that 74% of clients in initial pivotal trial had a clinical response (Physicians Desk Reference, 2001). In prospective clinical trials, oral gold, D-penicillamine, and hydroxychloroquine showed no greater efficacy than placebo. Injectable gold has never been evaluated in a controlled trial in JRA.

Except for treating the life-threatening complications of myositis or uveitis, corticosteroids are rarely prescribed in JRA because of their adverse effects. The most serious problem is their ability to retard growth, an even more significant problem because marked growth retardation occurs in sJRA and pJRA (Kredich, 1986).

A key component of the collaborative treatment of children with JRA is the design of a therapeutic exercise program, which includes positioning, posture assessment, and the use of heat or cold. Physicians usually prescribe the program; physical or occupational therapists design the individualized schedule; and nurses help follow-up with the implementation, teaching, and evalu-

TABLE 14–8. *Pharmacologic Management of Juvenile Rheumatoid Arthritis*

DRUG	DOSAGE	SIDE EFFECTS	NURSING CONSIDERATIONS
Analgesics			
Acetaminophen	80–325 mg 4–5 times/day depending on body weight	Headache, hepatic toxicity and failure, jaundice, chest pain dyspnea, **myocardial damage with dose >5–8 g/day,** methemoglobinemia, cyanosis, hemolytic anemia, hematuria, anuria, neutropenia, leukopenia, pancytopenia, thrombocytopenia, hypoglycemia, acute kidney failure, renal tubular necrosis, skin rash, and fever	Assess for allergy, impaired hepatic function, chronic alcoholism, pregnancy, lactation Do not exceed recommended dose Avoid using multiple preparations containing acetaminophen—OTC Give with food if gastrointestinal upset noted Not an anti-inflammatory agent Use for acute pain <10 days Report skin rash, unusual bleeding or bruising, yellowing of skin or eyes, changes in voiding patterns
Nonsteroidal Anti-inflammatory Agents (NSAIDs)		Gastrointestinal irritation, fluid retention and edema, diarrhea, interstitial nephritis, CNS changes (dizziness, blurred vision, headaches), hematologic changes, bone marrow depression, prolonged bleeding time, skin reactions and rashes	NSAIDs are generally better tolerated than ASA Therapeutic response may not be seen for up to 2 wk Instruct clients to drive with caution until response to drug is known Give with food or a glass of water Clients should report gastrointestinal distress (heartburn, dyspepsia, nausea, vomiting, abdominal pain) Monitor baseline, hematologic, renal, liver, auditory, and ophthalmic functions; repeat periodically Instruct client to report increased bleeding, severe pruritus, weight gain >5 pounds/wk, persistent headaches, vision disturbances
Naproxen (Naprosyn)	10 mg/kg in 2 doses	See NSAIDs	See NSAIDs
Ibuprofen (Motrin)	30–70 mg/kg/day in 3–4 doses	See NSAIDs Also amblyopia, blurred vision, reduced visual field	Food slows absorption; best given on an empty stomach Clients with visual disturbances should have complete ophthalmoscopic examinations Visual disturbances usually disappear when drug is discontinued

Table continued on following page

TABLE 14–8. *Pharmacologic Management of Juvenile Rheumatoid Arthritis* Continued

DRUG	DOSAGE	SIDE EFFECTS	NURSING CONSIDERATIONS
Disease-Modifying Agents			
Methotrexate	10 mg/m² BSA Maximum 1 mg/kg/wk PO and parenteral	CNS: headache, drowsiness, aphasia blurred vision, hemiparesis, paresis, seizures, fatigue, malaise, dizziness Gastrointestinal: ulcerative stomatitis, ulceration and bleeding, hepatic toxicity Respiratory: interstitial pneumonitis, chronic interstitial obstructive disease Dermatologic: erythematous rashes, alopecia Other: anaphylaxis, sudden death, chills and fever, metabolic changes, cancer	Monitor renal and hepatic function Give with folic acid 1 mg/day Side effects more evident at higher dosages—may use SC to eliminate or decrease effects Risk of toxicity increased with use of alcohol—clients must refrain Follow CBC, UA, AST, BUN, and Cr every 6–8 wk during therapy Leucovorin may be used 24 hr after MTX dose to ameliorate side effects
Biologic Response Modifiers			
Etanercept (Enbrel)	Pediatric dose (4–17 years old): 0.4 mg/kg SC 2 times/wk with, 72–96 hr between doses	Respiratory: URIs, congestion, rhinitis, cough, pharyngitis Gastrointestinal: abdominal pain, dyspepsia Other: irritation at injection site, increased risk of infections, cancers, ANA development, headache, autoimmune diseases	Rotate injection sites Avoid exposure to infections Perform laboratory testing routinely Report fever, chills, lethargy, rash, difficulty breathing, swelling, worsening of arthritis, severe diarrhea Know that this medication is not a cure for RA or JRA
Corticosteroids			
Hydrocortisone (Cortef) Prednisolone (Delta-Cortef) Prednisone (Deltasone)	Highly individualized 0.1–0.15 mg/kg/m²/day	Carefully monitor growth and development Osteoporosis, fractures, AVN, gastric ulcers, susceptibility to infection, hyperglycemia, hypertension, cataracts, glaucoma, thinning of skin, acne, hirsutism, moon face, edema, menstrual disorders, emotional lability	Once-daily dosing is preferred (easier to wean) Taper as soon as possible Do not stop drug abruptly Monitor older adults because they are at higher risk of side effects Avoid infections Protect skin from injuries—bruising occurs easily

ANA, antinuclear antibody; ASA, aspirin; AST, aspartate aminotransferase; AVN, avascular necrosis; BSA, body surface area; BUN, blood urea nitrogen; CBC, complete blood count; CNS, central nervous system; Cr, creatine; JRA, juvenile rheumatoid arthritis; MTX, methotrexate; OTC, over-the-counter; RA, rheumatoid arthritis; UA, urinalysis; URI, upper respiratory infection.

From Klippel, J. H. (Ed.). (1997). *Primer on the rheumatic diseases* (11th ed.). Atlanta: Arthritis Foundation; Karch, A. M. (Ed.). (2001). *Lippincott's nursing drug guide*. Philadelphia: Lippincott.

ation. The keys to any successful program include sound interdisciplinary planning and communication, incorporation of the child and family into the plan, and excellent client and family education (Table 14-9).

Exercises are prescribed and initiated to maintain or increase ROM, to improve muscle strength, and to build endurance. Therapeutic exercises are often incorporated into age-appropriate recreational activities to improve self-esteem and compliance. For example, hand and finger ROM exercises are much more enjoyable when they are part of playing with pull-apart toys, lace-up cards, or clay.

Positioning is also an important aspect of the therapeutic exercise plan. The lower extremities are at high risk for developing flexion contractures, so lying prone for at least 20 minutes daily is highly recommended (Scull, Dow, & Athreya, 1986). Analysis of sitting posture requires assessment by the school nurse to be certain that the child is not using a chair or desk that promotes flexion of the head and trunk. Because more than 30% of the children with JRA have cervical involvement, baseline assessment of sitting posture is essential for the prevention of complications, such as ankylosis.

Splints and braces are important adjuncts to treating the child with JRA. Resting splints are used during the acute stage to immobilize an inflamed joint. The joint is maintained in a functional (or neutral) position rather than one (e.g., flexion) that promotes deformities. Resting splints are worn almost continuously except for bathing and skin care while the joint is inflamed and swollen. Later, once the disease is under control, the splint is worn only at night.

Two commonly used resting splints are the cock-up splint (which supports the wrist in about 20 degrees of extension) and the posterior shell to maintain the knee in extension. Once inflammation has subsided, corrective splints are used to position and hold the joint in its maximum ROM. Sometimes, serial casting is used for corrective splinting, but its main disadvantage is that daily ROM and skin care cannot be done. Functional splints, such as a small wrist support to wear for writing, are used to protect areas from the stresses of performing ADLs.

The use of heat and cold to alleviate pain and stiffness is as important for the child with arthritis as it is for adults with arthritic disorders. Heat therapy includes the use of warm baths, moist warm packs for localized joint pain, and supervised application of paraffin baths to the small joints of the hands. Younger children may be less frightened of paraffin applications if the wax is "painted on" with a small brush. Most children prefer moist heat to cold therapy, and cold packs are used only for acute injuries to decrease swelling (Koch, 1985). If some children prefer cold to heat, however, there is no reason why cold should not be used.

Nursing Management

The child with JRA may experience fatigue, stiffness, impaired physical mobility, and self-care deficits in performing ADLs, just as older persons with arthritis do. However, there are important differences.

One of these differences concerns the impact of the illness on the child's psychosocial well-being. Although the younger client may have difficulties with effective coping and achieving a positive self-concept, the causes of these difficulties are largely related to the achievement of developmental tasks and skills. School attendance, play with other children, and the mastery and enjoyment of individual and group activities are essential for all children. Therefore, it is critical that children with arthritis—no matter what their degree of disability—have opportunities to celebrate success, to develop mastery of low-impact activities, and to be part of normal school and family activities. The nurse can provide anticipatory guidance to the family by suggesting strategies to promote the "work of going to school" (Box 14-4).

Pain is another important area in which there are differences between RA and JRA. Joint pain is highly variable in children with JRA. Children with inflamed joints may report or verbalize less pain than adults. Exactly why this occurs is not easily explained. The child may lack the vocabulary to report the sensation, or he or she may be so easily diverted from the pain by other

TABLE 14–9. *Client Education: Juvenile Rheumatoid Arthritis*

FOCUS	TEACHING POINTS
Disease process	Explain/reinforce type of disease, course, and treatment
	Explain how disease differs from adult rheumatoid arthritis
Pharmacologic management	Instruct in purpose, dosage, and side effects of medications
	Explain how aspirin is superior to acetaminophen because it decreases inflammation
	Instruct child and family not to alter dose without speaking to health care team
	Explain importance of discontinuing aspirin therapy if child is exposed to influenza or varicella
Pain/stiffness	Teach parents to be observant of younger child's behavior as indicator of pain
	Instruct in use of heat or cold therapy
	Teach child to wiggle or stretch while sitting to prevent stiffness
Mobility/exercise	Instruct parents and child in appropriate low-resistance exercises
	Teach child and family importance of resting after school
	Instruct in purpose and use of splints, braces, adaptive equipment, or shoe lifts
	Teach importance of lying prone for at least 20 min/day to prevent contractures
Joint protection	Teach principles of joint protection adapted to child's needs:
	Pick up cups or glasses with both hands
	Use a backpack for school
	Use "fat pens" or felt tip markers
	Wear high-topped canvas athletic shoes
	Squeeze, do not wring, wet objects
	Play scales on the piano to "relax" the fingers
Activity intolerance: school activities	Teach ways to conserve energy to manage schedule of school demands

---

BOX 14–4.

Strategies for School Success in Children with Arthritis

Inform teacher of child's illness; the Arthritis Foundation pamphlet "When Your Student Has Arthritis: A Guide for Teachers" is helpful to school personnel

Have child use a backpack for books and supplies to eliminate strain on small joints

Consider obtaining two sets of books so that child does not have to carry them between school and home

Work with teachers/counselors to schedule rest period after lunch to reduce fatigue

Secure permission for child to use elevators in multistory buildings to decrease stress on joints

Encourage child to wear high-quality canvas running shoes to decrease ankle pain exacerbated by long walks

Prevent pain, stiffness, and fatigue in hand and fingers:
 Use felt-tip pen
 Use built-up pen covered with foam or wedge
 Schedule oral tests (or use tape recorder for responses)
 Use electric typewriter or computer for long reports
 Use chalk in built-up chalkholder for blackboard activities
 Supply flip-chart with felt-tip pen as a substitute for blackboard works

---

activities that the discomfort is ignored (Kredich, 1986). It is also possible that some children have experienced pain for so long that they do not remember what it feels like to be pain free (Page-Goertz, 1989). One major behavioral manifestation of pain is the avoidance of any unusual activity that causes pain. Nurses can work with families to help them understand how to relieve the child's pain. Monitoring the response to anti-inflammatory agents is important, as is working with the child to avoid high-impact activities (e.g., sustained running, football, soccer, jumping rope, weight lifting) that stress joints. Joint splints can help rest inflamed, painful areas by keeping them in a functional, neutral position. Warm baths or hot packs are helpful to children of all ages. Home paraffin baths are not advocated for young children, however, because of the safety hazards (Gorman & Marsh, 1984).

Stiffness presents a special problem because it can prevent the child from fully participating in school and other developmental activities. One way to decrease morning stiffness is to have young preschoolers wear pajama sleepers to maintain body heat overnight. Older children can use a sleeping bag right on top of the bed. It may be advantageous to have the child get up an extra half-hour early in the morning for a 15-minute warm bath to limber up joints before dressing and eating breakfast. At school, stiffness readily develops because of prolonged sitting. Informing teachers about the problem

can help the child or parents negotiate frequent position changes, perhaps by sitting in the back of the room, so that periodic walking or stretching does not disturb other students.

Nutrition should be monitored because children with chronic illnesses need to eat nutritious, well-balanced diets. Nurses need to work with caregivers to ensure that weight is maintained. Children who are stiff and less active have a tendency to gain weight, thus exacerbating the existing stiffness.

Diversional activity deficits can occur in persons with arthritis at any age, but meeting children's needs for diversion and play is essential for their growth and development. The pediatric occupational or physical therapist can suggest excellent age-related activities that are enjoyable and therapeutic.

The effect on the family of any chronic illness in one of the children can be devastating. Parents may feel anxious, guilty, angry, hopeless, and powerless. Nurses must ensure that families fully understand the nature of their child's illness so that lack of knowledge does not contribute to their feelings of powerlessness and diffuse anxiety. Families can be so consumed with the child's illness that they overprotect the child, inhibiting independence in ADLs or the development of self-reliance and autonomy. Parents may restrict play, even when the child is feeling good, thus limiting his or her social contacts. As a result, the child may act out and refuse to cooperate with the treatment regimen. Eventually, the family may pay so much attention to the child with arthritis that the needs of siblings are overlooked. Studies have shown that the negative psychological impact of JRA is greater on the siblings than on the client (Buyon, 1994).

Before family dynamics become seriously impaired, nurses should try to provide anticipatory guidance about the effects of a child's illness on the family. Asking specific questions about other children in the family conveys the nurse's interest in their well-being and acknowledges the importance of the entire family to the child's health. Referring caregivers to professional groups and community agencies for ongoing support and education can help reestablish and maintain the family network.

SYSTEMIC LUPUS ERYTHEMATOSUS

The use of the term *lupus* (Latin for "wolf") to describe various disfiguring cutaneous disorders dates to the medieval period. The first clinical description of rashes that continues to be recognized as lupus was by Biett in 1833 (Klippel, 1990). Credit is usually given to Kaposi for describing the systemic nature of the disease, including fever, weight loss, lymphadenopathy, and mental disturbances. Insights into the pathogenesis of SLE were enhanced by the discovery of the LE cell phenomenon by Hargraves in 1948 and the antinuclear factor by Friou.

SLE is a multisystem, inflammatory connective tissue disorder associated with abnormalities of the immune system. It is a chronic condition characterized by various degrees of increased disease activity that are generally followed by a less active, remitting course. So many classic immunologic abnormalities can be present in SLE that it is considered the prototype of an autoimmune disease. Typically, multiple body organs and systems are affected at different times, thus producing widespread damage to connective tissues, blood vessels, and serous and mucous membranes.

SLE is primarily a disease of young women. Peak incidence occurs between the ages of 15 and 40 during the childbearing years, with a female/male ratio of 5:1 (Pisetsky, 1997). However, the onset can range from infancy to advanced age; in both pediatric and older onset clients, the female/male ratio approximates 2:1. The signs and symptoms vary considerably, from general complaints of fever, fatigue, and malaise to painful, swollen joints to the psychological distress of a variety of skin lesions. The latter can include the classic butterfly rash over the bridge of the nose and cheeks, erythematous discoid lesions (which can result in permanent scars on the scalp, ears, face, or neck), the temporary loss of hair on the scalp, painless mouth ulcers, and cutaneous vascular lesions. Photosensitivity can be especially problematic for some clients with SLE. Sunlight may trigger a local dermatitis or more severe disease activity. Other systemic manifestations (e.g., renal, cardiac, or pulmonary complications) and a variety of serum, immunologic, and antibody abnormalities may be present.

The 1982 revised criteria for the classification of SLE are given in Table 14-10. The diagnosis of SLE is confirmed if a person has any 4 of the 11 criteria present, either serially or simultaneously, during any observation period (Tan, Cohen, Fries, Masi, McShane, Rothfield, Schaller, Talal, & Winchester, 1982).

Epidemiology

In a general outpatient population, SLE affects approximately 1 in 2000 individuals (Ward, Pyun, & Studenski, 1995). Incidence rates have increased over the past 40 years, most likely because of an increased availability of serologic tests and increased awareness of the disease (Klippel, 1990). The disease has a predilection for women in their childbearing years, with young black women being the major group affected. The ratio of females to males affected varies from 3:1 to 8:1 (Hochberg, 1988), with an even higher ratio of 14:1 in Puerto Ricans (Neuberger & Neuberger, 1984).

The prevalence of SLE varies with race, ethnicity, and socioeconomic status. SLE has been estimated to be as high as 50.8 cases per 100,000, with an overall prevalence of 500,000 persons in the United States. Iseki, Miyasato, Oura, Uehara, Nishime, and Fukiyama (1994) reviewed 500 SLE clients over a 20-year period and concluded that

the incidence of SLE was increasing (from 1.6 per 100,000 in 1972 to 4.7 per 100,000 in 1991). The female/male prevalence ratio is 10:1 for women in the childbearing years (Neuberger & Neuberger, 1984). However, men and African American females have been found to have a worse renal outcome (Iseki et al., 1994).

Once considered a fatal disease in young women, SLE now has improved outcomes. More than 85% of persons with the disorder live longer than 15 years after diagnosis (Klippel, 1990). However, increased mortality has been noted in American blacks, Asians, Puerto Ricans, and persons of Hispanic descent living in the southwest United States (Neuberger & Neuberger, 1984). Poor survival has been associated with high serum creatinine, low hematocrit, proteinuria, and the source of medical care funding. The most common causes of death in SLE are active lupus nephritis, vascular events, and infections (Callahan & Pincus, 1995).

An underlying hormonal change may explain why the disease affects so many more women. Genetic factors may also be involved. Familial aggregation occurs in 10% of persons having a first-degree relative with SLE (Hochberg, 1988), including its occurrence in identical twins (Kaplan, 1984). Moreover, in extended families, SLE may coexist with other autoimmune conditions such as hemolytic anemia, thyroiditis, and idiopathic thrombocytopenia purpura. Environmental factors, such as sunlight, burns, and infectious agents, may also contribute to the development of SLE. Acute lupus-like reactions have been reported after taking drugs, such as hydralazine, procainamide, isoniazid, and chlorpromazine. Because at least one food—alfalfa sprouts—can trigger a lupus-like reaction, the question of how many persons develop the disease as a result of chemicals or foods is an important one for future research (Alarcon-Segovia, 1988).

Pathophysiology

The pathologic findings of SLE occur throughout the body and are manifested by inflammation, blood vessel abnormalities that encompass both bland vasculopathy and vasculitis, and immune complex deposition.

SLE results from an abnormal reaction of the body against its own tissues, cells, and serum proteins. In other words, as an autoimmune disease, SLE is characterized by a decreased self-tolerance. In the North American white population, there is a positive association between SLE and two HLA antigens (DR2 and DR3) that are coded by the MHC (Robbins & Kumar, 1987). Persons with SLE have increased numbers of both self and nonself antigens, suggesting hyperactivity of the B cells. Interleukin-6 may have a role in B-cell hyperactivity (Gabay, Roux-Lombard, de Moerloose, Dayer, Vischer, & Guerne, 1993). Abnormal B-cell response, in turn, is due to defective T-cell function. As increased numbers of antigen-antibody complexes form, they deposit on the basement membranes of the capillaries, particularly those of the kidneys, heart, skin,

TABLE 14–10. *1982 Revised Criteria for the Classification of Systemic Lupus Erythematosus*

CRITERION	DEFINITION
Malar rash	Fixed erythema, flat or raised, over the malar eminences, tending to spare the nasolabial folds
Discoid rash	Erythematous raised patches with adherent keratotic scaling and follicular plugging; atrophic scarring may occur in older lesions
Photosensitivity	Skin rash as a result of unusual reaction to sunlight, by client history or physician observation
Oral ulcers	Oral or nasopharyngeal ulceration, usually painless, observed by a physician
Arthritis	Nonerosive arthritis involving 2 or more peripheral joints, characterized by tenderness, swelling, or effusion
Serositis	Pleuritis—convincing history of pleuritic pain or rub heard by a physician or evidence of pleural effusion
	or
	Pericarditis—documented by electrocardiogram or rub or evidence of pericardial effusion
Renal disorder	Persistent proteinuria greater than 0.5 g/day or greater than 3 if quantification not performed
	or
	Cellular casts—may be red cell, hemoglobin, granular, tubular, or mixed
Neurologic disorder	Seizures—in the absence of offending drugs or known metabolic derangements (e.g., uremia, ketoacidosis, or electrolyte imbalance)
	or
	Psychosis—in the absence of offending drugs or known metabolic derangements (e.g., uremia, ketoacidosis, or electrolyte imbalance)
Hematologic disorder	Hemolytic anemia—with reticulocytosis
	or
	Leukopenia—less than 4000/mm^3 total on 2 or more occasions
	or
	Lymphopenia—less than 1500/mm^3 on 2 or more occasions
	or
	Thrombocytopenia—less than 100,000/mm^3 in the absence of the offending drugs
Immunologic disorder	Positive lupus erythematosus cell preparation
	or
	Anti-DNA: antibody to native DNA in abnormal titer
	or
	Anti-Sm: presence of antibody to Sm nuclear antigen
	or
	False-positive serologic test for syphilis known to be positive for at least 6 months and confirmed by *Treponema pallidum* immobilization or fluorescent treponemal antibody absorption test
Antinuclear antibody	An abnormal titer of antinuclear antibody by immunofluorescence or an equivalent assay at any point in time and in the absence of drugs known to be associated with "drug-induced lupus" syndrome

From Tan, E. M., Cohen, A. S., Fries, J. F., Masi, A. T., McShane, D. J., Rothfield, N. F., Schaller, J. G., Talal, N., & Winchester, R. J. (1982). The 1982 revised criteria for the classification of systemic lupus erythematosus (SLE). *Arthritis and Rheumatism, 25,* 1271–1277. Reprinted with permission.

brain, and joints. Immune complexes then trigger the inflammatory response, the primary mechanism by which tissue destruction occurs. The severity of the clinical response and organ destruction is directly related to the intensity of the inflammatory response. Interleukin-1 receptor antagonist (IL-1Ra) concentrations are elevated in most clients with active SLE and may be a good indicator of disease activity (Suzuki, Takemura, & Kashiwagi, 1995). Table 14–11 summarizes the changes in organ systems that occur in SLE.

Along with these changes, LE cells, which are neutrophils resulting from ANAs, develop in the blood. Another antibody, anti-DNA of the IgG type, may be responsible for the development of the engulfed LE bodies in the LE cells. The relationship between the serum LE factor and the pathologic changes that occur with SLE is not clear. However, the absence of the LE factor is a strong indication that the disease is not present. Increased levels of anti-dsDNA antibodies are associated with increased disease activity in clients with SLE (Miltenburg, Roos, Slegtenhorst, Daha, & Breedveld, 1993).

Diagnostic Evaluation

SLE can be differentiated from other connective tissue disorders by the presence or development of glomerulonephritis; photosensitivity; characteristic skin rashes; central nervous system disease; and various cytopenias such as the Coombs'-positive hemolytic anemia, leukopenia, and thrombocytopenia.

The most specific tests for SLE are anti-dsDNA and antibodies to Sm and ribosomal P proteins that are seen exclusively in SLE (Reichlin, 1997). CRP can sometimes be a useful test for distinguishing between a lupus flare and infection. It usually remains normal in a flare but is elevated in infection (Hay & Snaith, 1995).

The most sensitive test for SLE is the relatively nonspecific fluorescent ANA assay. Almost all clients with SLE have a positive ANA test, but it also occurs in many other situations, such as infections, advanced age, and RA, as well as with certain drug therapy regimens. Complement assays for C3, C4, and CH$_{50}$ are useful measures of disease activity.

In clients with suspected systemic rheumatic disease, 15% to 25% of tertiary referrals are clients who do not clearly express the clinical features of any disease or who have partial overlap of features of two or more diseases. These clients usually have symptoms of one or more of the rheumatic diseases and may have autoantibodies that indicate another disease or no disease at all. These clients are usually considered to have undifferentiated connective tissue disease.

TABLE 14–11. *Systems Changes with the Pathogenesis of Systemic Lupus Erythematosus*

SYSTEM	PATHOGENESIS WITH SYSTEMIC LUPUS ERYTHEMATOSUS
Integumentary	Immune complex deposition, inflammation of dermal-epidermal junctions, vasculitis
Gastrointestinal	Collagen degeneration and vasculitis leading to mucous membrane ulcers; vasculitis leading to organ infarction and necrosis
Musculoskeletal	Increased fibrin deposits at synovial surfaces; inflammation of arterioles, venules, and tendon sheaths; eventual necrosis, degeneration, and fibrosis of muscle tissue
Pulmonary	Pleural inflammation; intestinal vasculitis
Cardiovascular	Diffuse vasculitis; inflammation and scarring of atrioventricular and sino-atrial nodes; inflammation of pericardial sac
Renal	Deposition of immune complexes in the glomerular basement membranes
Neurologic	Immune complex deposition; antineuronal antibody activity leading to cerebritis, seizures, organic brain syndrome, and peripheral neuropathies

Assessment

Nursing History. The nursing history of persons with confirmed or suspected SLE must be sufficiently thorough to capture the range of possible symptoms that accompany an autoimmune disease. Clients need to be asked about general problems (e.g., fever, weight loss, fatigue) and about changes in energy levels. A detailed medication history is essential in identifying the need for additional client teaching and in determining that the condition has not been drug induced. Clients should be asked about the names of their current medications, dosage, purpose, side effects, and length of time that they have been taking these drugs. Approximately 25 drugs have been implicated as causing a lupus-like syndrome, but only a few (hydralazine, procainamide, and isoniazid) cause the disorder with any great frequency.

Questions about changes in skin should be asked. The presence, location, and nature of rashes must be explored, as well as association of the rash with exposure to sunlight or even fluorescent lighting. Clients should be asked about changes in their nails (splinter hemorrhages) and nail beds (subungual erythema), loss of hair on the scalp, and development of lesions in the oral and nasal mucosa.

Because SLE is occasionally characterized by generalized cerebritis, careful attention should be paid to the neuropsychiatric system. If seizure activity occurs, it is usually the generalized tonic-clonic type. The client should be asked about visual disturbances, vertigo, facial weakness, and presence of headaches. Changes in emotional status, including anxiety, insomnia, disorientation, and mood swings, are fairly common because of the disease and/or steroid therapy. The client may also complain of impaired cognition, such as mental dullness or a slow reaction time.

Physical Assessment. The nursing assessment should begin with an examination of the integumentary and musculoskeletal systems because clients with SLE have a high percentage of physical changes involving the skin, muscles, and joints. The entire body must be inspected carefully, and the location, nature, and size of cutaneous and vascular lesions should be noted. Transient rashes can appear in any location, particularly after exposure to sunlight. Interestingly, the classic butterfly rash over the bridge of the nose and cheeks affects fewer than half of clients with SLE (Schur, 1983). Discoid lesions, characterized by annular erythematous plaques, can appear as atrophied, scaling areas on the face, neck, and arms. Severe scarring is also possible. Fingers can be affected by erythema under the nail beds or by digital gangrene. Mild to moderate loss of scalp hair can occur when the disease is active. Vascular lesions can include petechiae, purpuric lesions, and Raynaud's phenomenon.

Joint symptoms, with or without active synovitis, occur in more than 90% of those affected (Bunyon & Zuckerman, 1987). Along with Raynaud's phenomenon, these findings are often the earliest features of the disease. Therefore, the musculoskeletal examination should focus on a full assessment of the ROM of all joints, noting the location and presence of synovitis, diffuse swelling, joint and muscle pain, and stiffness. Joint involvement is symmetrical in SLE, but deformities are usually the result of soft tissue stresses rather than erosive changes. One of the more common deformities is Jaccoud's arthropathy, a rheumatoid-like deformity of the hands present in about 10% of clients with SLE (Klippel, 1990). In this condition, the MCP joints are subluxed, ulnar deviation develops, and hyperextension of the PIP joints can be observed.

Because central nervous system involvement is seen in about one third of those with SLE, a complete psychosocial examination should be performed. Questions to identify orientation, mood, affect, changes in cognition, and emotional stability are useful. In persons with frank depression or psychosis, suicidal ideation should be assessed. Other central nervous system assessment parameters include the presence of cranial neuropathies, such as facial weakness, asymmetrical expression, nystagmus, and extraocular muscle weakness.

Assessment of the respiratory system should focus on signs of restrictive lung disease (e.g., tachypnea, cough) and the presence of adventitious lung sounds associated with pneumonia, bronchopneumonia, or pleural effusion. Results of the cardiovascular examination may indicate arrhythmias (associated with fibrosis of the sinoatrial and atrioventricular nodes) and friction rubs accompanying pericarditis. Other physical examination findings may include hepatomegaly, splenomegaly, and lymphadenopathy.

Treatment

The primary management of SLE involves the use of drugs that suppress end-organ inflammation or interfere with immune function. Very few drug therapies have been subjected to randomized clinical trials. Treatment of acute SLE is based on the use of steroids, immunosuppressive agents, and experimental therapies. In the management of these clients, it is critical to be aware of and to aggressively treat the comorbid conditions that commonly occur in SLE: hypertension, infections, seizures, hyperlipidemia, and osteoporosis.

Drug Therapy. NSAIDs are used for musculoskeletal symptoms, mild serositis, and constitutional signs such as fever. Care must be taken when using NSAIDs in clients with SLE. NSAIDs inhibit prostaglandin synthesis within the kidney and impair renal blood flow. Clients with lupus nephritis are particularly susceptible because of a heightened dependency on prostaglandins to maintain renal function that is compromised by glomerular inflammation. Clients should be questioned about their nonprescription use of NSAIDs. Renal abnormalities produced by NSAIDs, particularly impaired renal function, are generally promptly reversible (Klippel, 1997).

Corticosteroids are required to control serious complications, such as thrombocytopenic purpura, hemolytic anemia, myocarditis, pericarditis, seizures, and nephritis. Prednisone is usually given orally at low dosages (up to 15 mg/day), moderate dosages (16 to 40 mg/day), or high dosages (up to 120 mg/day). Divided doses, rather than a single morning dose, are generally administered to ensure more sustained anti-inflammatory action and greater lupus-suppressing activity. Once the disease is under control, however, gradual reduction (tapering) is essential. Clients following a multiple daily-dose regimen must first be converted to a single morning dose before attempting to reduce the actual drug dose. The length of time the client has been taking the drug directly effects the length of drug taper. Many methods have been used with the most common being to decrease the dose by 10 mg in weekly increments.

An alternative to the use of high-dose oral corticosteroids is bolus intravenous steroid pulse therapy. Usually, 1 to 1.5 g of methylprednisolone is given daily for 3 days to persons with severe disease, such as active nephritis, fulminating central nervous system disease, and hematologic crises (Kimberly, 1982). Generally, oral steroids (up to 60 mg/day of prednisone) are also given following this treatment period (Schur, 1983).

According to case reports and uncontrolled studies, pulse therapy can be highly effective in life-threatening SLE. It must be used with great caution, however. Arrhythmias and seizures have been associated with sudden death after administration of pulse therapy. Adverse effects included infections; severe neurologic and cardiovascular complications; gastrointestinal complications, such as perforations or bleeding; and a higher incidence of bone necrosis. Overall, sepsis was the most common serious side effect because infections can go unrecognized in steroid-treated clients.

The antimalarial drug hydroxychloroquine is especially useful in managing cutaneous manifestations of lupus, but this antimalarial compound is also helpful in treating musculoskeletal and constitutional symptoms. An additional benefit is the lowering of serum cholesterol and reducing the risk of venous thrombosis and coronary artery disease. Improvements in cutaneous manifestations, including discoid and subacute cutaneous and erythematous inflammatory lesions, can be remarkably rapid, often evident within days. Discontinuation is associated with an increased risk of lupus flares, including major exacerbations such as vasculitis, transverse myelitis, and nephropathy (The Canadian Hydroxychloroquine Study Group, 1991). As a consequence, there is reluctance to discontinue hydroxychloroquine in stable clients who have clearly benefited from the drug. Low dosages (200 to 400mg/day) are well tolerated and rarely associated with side effects. Ophthalmologic examinations are required before starting drug and every 6 to 12 months thereafter, although the risk of retinal toxicity is extremely small.

The use of immunosuppressive agents has gradually become an accepted therapy for SLE. Methotrexate in low dosages (7.5 to 15 mg/wk) appears to be useful in managing arthritis, skin rashes, serositis, and constitutional signs and symptoms (Wilson & Abeles, 1994). Treatment regimens, including azathioprine (Imuran) or cyclophosphamide (Cytoxan), have been able to halt the progression of glomerulonephritis or result in significantly less renal deterioration (Hay & Snaith, 1995). Azathioprine and intravenous cyclophosphamide can be given. While taking azathioprine, the client should be monitored for skin rash, hepatic toxicity, hyperuricemia, pancytopenia, and gastrointestinal distress. The last three adverse effects, as well as cardiotoxicity, ovarian failure, hemorrhagic cystitis, and a predisposition to cancer occur with cyclophosphamide.

Cyclosporine was used in low dosages (306 mg daily) in both nonrenal manifestations and membranous nephropathy, and the results were encouraging (Radhakrishman, Kunis, D'Agati, & Appel, 1994). Toxicities of the drug were minimal; no nephrotoxicity was observed. However, there is an increased risk of hypertension, and an increase in serum creatinine may be seen.

Danazol, the attenuated androgen, has been shown to be useful in managing lupus thrombocytopenia (West & Johnson, 1988). The mechanism of action has not been defined, but it is thought to involve endocrine influences such as the suppression of pituitary follicle-stimulating hormone and luteinizing hormone actions on immune or reticuloendothelial functions.

Intravenous immunoglobulin has been shown to be useful in managing severe lupus thrombocytopenia. The platelet count rises rapidly within hours of administration; occasionally, extraordinarily high counts are found, making thrombotic events a clinical concern. The rate of relapse after treatment is high. The primary role is to control acute bleeding associated with lupus thrombocytopenia or to rapidly increase the platelet count to allow for splenectomy or other surgery.

Dapsone has been used to manage cutaneous manifestation of lupus, including discoid, subacute cutaneous lupus, bullous, and lupus profundus lesions. Hematologic side effects are common and require close monitoring.

The role of plasma exchange in SLE is limited to rare, acute conditions associated with high mortality, such as thrombotic thrombocytopenia purpura and pulmonary hemorrhage. There is no evidence that plasma exchange is beneficial in the long-term management of lupus, particularly lupus nephritis.

Clients with end-stage lupus nephropathy are managed with dialysis or kidney transplantation. There is a tendency for decreased clinical and serologic lupus activity following the onset of end-stage renal disease. Survival of lupus clients and other end-stage renal clients is comparable. Most studies note an increased incidence of infections among SLE clients receiving dialysis. Kidney transplantation during an acute exacerbation of SLE is controversial and may increase the risk of poor outcome. Recurrence of lupus nephritis in transplanted allografts, often with the same histopathology as in the native kidney, develops in 2% to 4% of transplanted kidneys (Mojcik & Klippel, 1996).

There are several drugs in clinical trials for the treatment of lupus nephritis, including the use of mycophenolate mofetil (CellCept) and tolerogens that arrest the production of dsDNA antibodies. A placebo-controlled trial of DHEA has reported benefits in clients with mild to moderate lupus activity (van Vollenhoven, Engleman, & McGuire, 1995). Experimental research has shown that zileuton (a selective 5-lipoxygenase inhibitor) may be beneficial in treating mild SLE (Hackshaw, Shi, Brandwein, Jones, & Westcott, 1995).

Supportive Therapy. Although drug therapy and the use of experimental treatments play a significant part in the management of SLE, perhaps the more important aspects of treatment are the supportive therapies of physical and emotional rest, diet and nutrition, and skin protection. Nurses have an important role in teaching clients how to manage the daily stress of coping with a chronic illness. Key areas for collaborative education are outlined in Table 14–12.

Nursing Management: Acute Phase

Potential for Infection, Ineffective Airway Clearance, Potential for Injury, Confusion, Fluid Volume Deficit or Excess, Impaired Skin Integrity, Self-care Deficit

Infection Protection, Infection Control, Seizure Management, Acid-Base Management, Delirium Management, Respiratory Management, Skin Care, Skin Surveillance, Self-care Facilitation. The nursing care of clients with SLE can be challenging and demanding. During exacerbations, clients may become acutely and seriously ill. Infectious complications can develop in about half of clients with SLE, especially bacterial infections of the skin, respiratory tract, and urinary tract. Nursing care during this time is directed toward the assessment and management of acute confusional states, the prevention of seizures, the maintenance of skin integrity, the prevention of additional infection, the assessment of renal function, and the management of impaired gas exchange associated with lung disease and infection.

TABLE 14–12. *Client Education: Systemic Lupus Erythematosus*

FOCUS	TEACHING POINTS
Potential for infection	Teach importance of frequent self-monitoring for signs and symptoms of infection, especially if steroid dependent
Skin integrity	Instruct client to avoid drying soaps or powders, irritating perfumes or makeup, and harsh household chemicals
	Suggest use of hypoallergenic makeup
	Suggest cool baths to decrease discomfort and scaling
	Inform client about temporary use of wigs for hair loss
	Teach photosensitive clients to use sunscreens with a sunscreen protective factor (SPF) of at least 15; highly sensitive persons should use a preparation with an SPF of at least 25
	Teach clients to limit sun exposure from 11 AM to 3 PM and wear adequate clothing, hats, and sunglasses
	Teach clients to use corticosteroid creams as directed; emphasize that the cream should be applied sparingly, as a thin layer, so dosage is as uniform as possible; reinforce instruction that cream can be absorbed systemically
Knowledge deficit: current information	Instruct client about the importance of obtaining up-to-date information about the disease from the primary health care providers; excellent information is also available from the Lupus Society and the Arthritis Foundation
Increased disease activity	Teach importance of factors that might lead to flares or increased disease activity:
	Physical or emotional stress
	Medications
	Abrupt discontinuation of medications
	Photosensitivity
	Inform clients to recognize drugs that can contribute to lupus-like syndromes:
	Definite: hydralazine, procainamide, isoniazid
	Possible: dilantin, chlorpromazine, methyldopa, penicillamine, quinidine, propylthiouracil, lithium carbonate
Knowledge deficit of corticosteroids	Teach purpose, dosage, and side effects
	Explain that once remission has been achieved, steroids can be gradually tapered by 5 mg/wk; at 40 mg, the dose can be given as a single daily dose and then tapered to 20 mg/day
	Inform the client that additional tapering can occur from 1 to 2.5 mg/wk until the client is totally weaned
	Explain that if weaning is not possible, the steroid dose is gradually increased to the lowest dosage at which the patient is symptom free
	Instruct client to obtain and wear a MedicAlert bracelet
Knowledge deficit of plasmapheresis	Teach purpose of procedure; reinforce expected benefits
	Teach client and family that repeated treatments are usually given
	Instruct client to keep vascular access site clean and dry and to inspect it regularly for signs of infection

During this acute phase, increased fatigue, joint pain, and stiffness are often present as a result of inflammation and increased disease activity. Nursing activities to manage these acute flares are similar to those used during exacerbations of RA. Self-care deficits are often exacerbated because of the increased disease activity. It is important to help clients maintain as much independence as possible during periods of acute flares so that both self-esteem and physical functions are enhanced. Clients may require considerably more time to complete even one task, so nursing interventions may need to help the client focus on conserving energy and prioritizing self-care actions.

Caring for a client with acutely impaired thought processes can be perplexing. Several factors can contribute to the cause of this nursing diagnosis, including increased inflammation of the central nervous system and psychosis from high doses of steroids. Clients typically have severe throbbing headaches that are sometimes accompanied by generalized tonic-clonic seizures. They may display impaired judgment, inappropriate speech and behavior, difficulty concentrating or comprehending simple instructions, or short-term memory deficits. As the disease progresses, they may have personality changes, with a decreased ability to carry out purposeful activity. Clients with impaired thought processes should be cared for in a quiet environment, particularly when headaches are severe. Clocks and calendars should be provided to help with orientation. Communication must be caring but clear and concise to decrease ambiguity and anxiety.

If clients are prone to seizures, they should be observed carefully for auras or specific activities that might trigger the seizure. During the seizure, the client should be protected from injury by removing dangerous objects, providing padding and blankets, and turning him or her to the side after muscle activity has stopped to prevent aspiration. Restraints should never be applied during the seizure because the intense muscular activity beneath the restraint could lead to fractures.

Another focus of nursing care during exacerbations of the disease is the management of excess fluid volume typically seen in peripheral edema. The goal is to maintain optimal renal function by assessing urinary output and specific gravity every 2 to 4 hours, monitoring fluid intake and electrolyte levels, and assessing changes in the level of consciousness. The skin of a steroid-dependent client with SLE is characteristically tissue thin and fragile, so clients with peripheral edema must be moved and handled gently. The excess osmotic pressure beneath the skin surface can stress it easily, so minimal shearing forces can quickly denude the dermal layers.

Nursing Management: Chronic Phase

Self-esteem Disturbance, Ineffective Coping

Self-esteem Enhancement, Coping Enhancement, Teaching. During the chronic phase of the illness, clients can experience intense frustration because they often do not appear ill. The extreme weakness and fatigue they encounter during exacerbations of the disease, however, can lead to feelings of powerlessness and helplessness, ineffective coping, and a disturbance in self-concept (Halverson & Holmes, 1992). Helping clients with SLE develop a traditional support group is difficult. Lupus clients are often homebound because of extreme fatigue, impaired mobility, and commitment to their roles of spouse and parent. In these situations, the use of telephone support networks or Internet support networks for clients with SLE can be a powerful nursing strategy. At the same time that these networks provide social support and counseling for the homebound, they also encourage personal growth and development among other clients with SLE who have developed positive coping skills. Nurses can play an important role in helping to establish this type of network through the education and support of peer counselors.

During remissions, clients often wonder about whether they can safely have children. This is a natural concern because most clients are women of childbearing age. Because fertility in clients with SLE is comparable to that of the general population (Hay & Snaith, 1995; Wong, Chan, & Lee, 1991), initiating and responding to clients' requests for health information are important functions of the nurse. Relapses of SLE can occur at any time during pregnancy but have not shown an increase in the risk of fetal loss (Lima, Buchanan, Khamashta, Kerslake, & Hughes, 1995). The incidence of relapses during pregnancy has been reported to vary from 22% to

58%. However, most disease exacerbations can be reasonably well controlled with increasing doses of prednisone. Oral contraceptives containing low doses of estrogen are safe with mild lupus but should be used with caution by clients with severe lupus because they can cause a flare-up (Hay & Snaith, 1995). In addition, most studies report good neonatal outcomes in infants born to women with SLE (Wong, Chan, & Lee, 1991), although a high incidence of prematurity has been observed (Lima et al., 1995).

SYSTEMIC SCLEROSIS

Scleroderma—literally meaning hard (*scleros*) skin (*derma*)—encompasses both disease restricted to the skin (localized scleroderma) and disease with internal organ involvement (diffuse scleroderma or SS).

One of the earliest definite descriptions of scleroderma was published by W.D. Chowne (1842, London) pertaining to a child; a description of scleroderma in an adult was published by James Startin (1846, London). Maurice Raynaud (1862, Paris) described the vasospastic phenomenon that bears his name.

SS is one of the least well understood of the rheumatic disorders. It occurs as a multisystem inflammatory connective tissue disease characterized by skin thickening (scleroderma) and deposition of excessive quantities of connective tissue (particularly collagen), which eventually results in severe fibrosis. The skin, blood vessels, synovium, and skeletal muscles are affected along with the microvasculature of internal organs, such as the heart, lung, kidney, and gastrointestinal tract. Widespread vascular involvement, perhaps the earliest and most significant pathologic change, is also a prominent feature of SS (LeRoy, 1985).

SS is considered one of the eight types of scleroderma, the classification of which depends on the degree and extent of skin thickening. The term *scleroderma* was first introduced in the mid-19th century to describe skin induration. Later, others used the term *progressive systemic sclerosis* to reflect its often-generalized multisystem course. Currently, the term *systemic sclerosis* is preferred because many clients have limited skin and organ involvement (Ziegler, 1984). Box 14–5 presents an overview of the classification of scleroderma and SS.

Types

The two major types of SS are classified according to the degree of their skin and systemic involvement. The first type, characterized by diffuse, cutaneous scleroderma, begins with symmetrical widespread thickening of the skin on the extremities, the face, and the trunk. In the early stages of the disease, bilateral symmetrical swelling of the fingers, face, and feet can be seen (Medsger, 1988) and the skin has a tense, wrinkle-free appearance (Fig. 14–10A). As the disease progresses, the skin becomes

BOX 14–5.
Classification of Scleroderma

I. Systemic sclerosis
   A. With diffuse skin thickening: symmetrical, widespread thickening of skin affecting the distal and proximal extremities, face, and trunk; rapid progression of skin changes; early appearance of visceral involvement (gastrointestinal tract, lungs, heart, kidneys)
   B. With limited skin thickening: symmetrical skin involvement restricted to the distal extremities and face; slow progression of skin changes; late appearance of visceral involvement, including distinctive types, such as pulmonary arterial hypertension and biliary cirrhosis; prominence of cutaneous telangiectasias and subcutaneous calcinosis (CREST syndrome)
   C. In overlap: either diffuse or limited skin thickening in association with features of one or more other connective tissue diseases (e.g., systemic lupus erythematosus, polymyositis-dermatomyositis).
II. Chemically induced sclerosis-like conditions
   A. Vinylchloride disease
   B. Bleomycin-induced fibrosis
   C. Trichloroethylene-induced fibrosis
III. Localized form of scleroderma
   A. Morphea
   B. Linear scleroderma (includes *en coup de sabre*)
   C. Diffuse fasciitis with eosinophilia (eosinophilic fasciitis)
IV. Chemically induced forms of scleroderma
   A. Toxic oil syndrome
   B. Eosinophilia-myalgia syndrome
   C. Pentazocine-induced fibrosis
   D. Epoxy resin–induced fibrosis
   E. Scleroderma following autologous bone marrow transplantation (graft-versus-host disease)
V. Diseases with skin changes resembling scleroderma (pseudoscleroderma)
   A. Edematous
       1. Scleredema adultorum of Buschke or associated diabetes mellitus
       2. Scleromyxedema (papular mucinosis)
   B. Indurative and/or atrophic
       1. Lichen sclerosus et atrophicus
       2. Porphyria cutanea tarda
       3. Congenital porphyria
       4. Acromegaly
       5. Amyloidosis (primary and myeloma associated)
       6. Phenylketonuria
       7. Carcinoid syndrome
       8. Localized lipoatrophy, including Gowers' panatrophy of ankles, orbicular lipoatrophy
       9. Congenital poikiloderma, including Rothmund's syndrome, Rothmund-Thompson syndrome
       10. Werner's syndrome
       11. Progeria
       12. Acrodermatitis chronica atrophicans
       13. POEMS (polyneuropathy, organomegaly, endocrinopathy, monoclonal gammopathy, skin changes) syndrome
       14. Digital sclerosis of diabetes mellitus
       15. In carcinomas

From the *Primer on the rheumatic diseases* (10th ed.), Copyright 1993. Used by permission of the Arthritis Foundation. For more information, please call the Arthritis Foundation's information line, 800-283-7800.

more thickened, hidebound, and shiny. Changes in pigmentation (both hypopigmentation and hyperpigmentation) are associated with the loss of normal skin folds. Distal thickening is always more severe than proximal thickening, so the extremities may show more changes than the face. Eventually, the face can become masklike. The mouth is rigid, and the overall expression is blunted or immobile (Fig. 14–10B). Persons with this diffuse type

of SS have a tendency to develop early problems in the gastrointestinal tract, heart, lungs, and kidneys. The esophagus is particularly affected. Because of the early development of visceral changes, the pace, progression, and complications of this type of SS can be rapid.

The second type of SS, limited cutaneous scleroderma, is characterized by skin changes that are usually confined to the fingers and distal portions of the extremities and face. In general, skin changes progress much more slowly than they do in the diffuse type of SS. Truncal scleroderma is absent. Visceral changes (e.g., severe pulmonary arterial hypertension, biliary cirrhosis), if present, are seen late in the course of the disease. Table 14–13 summarizes the visceral and musculoskeletal changes that can occur in limited cutaneous scleroderma.

Persons with the limited type of scleroderma often develop a syndrome that has been abbreviated by the acronym *CREST,* which refers to the following conditions:

*C*alcinosis—calcium deposits in the tissues
*R*aynaud's phenomenon—intermittent vasospasm of the fingertips
*E*sophageal hardening—sclerosis of the esophagus
*S*clerodactyly—scleroderma of the digits
*T*elangiectasias—capillary dilations that form vascular lesions on the face, lips, and fingers

The presence of the CREST symptoms is a poor prognostic indicator. The 10-year survival rate after diagnosis is approximately 65% (Bertsch, 1995).

Raynaud's phenomenon, a generally bilateral vasospastic condition, can be an especially important predictor of scleroderma. Tricolor changes affecting the fingers in Raynaud's disease consist of pallor (white) accompanying vasoconstriction, followed by cyanosis (blue), as capillary blood is desaturated of oxygen and hyperemia (red) secondary to vasodilation. Most clients with Raynaud's phenomenon who develop connective tissue

disease do so within 2 years after the first vasospastic event (Tuffanelli, 1989). However, there is a sizable minority who develop a connective tissue disorder years after the onset of Raynaud's phenomena. Clients with the CREST syndrome often develop painful ulcers on the fingertips or in the areas of calcinosis because of chronic vascular insufficiency. Although not listed in the acronym CREST, there is evidence of pulmonary involvement in most clients but few exhibit clinical symptoms (Bertsch, 1995). An occasional client with limited cutaneous scleroderma develops pulmonary artery hypertension.

Epidemiology

SS is seen worldwide. The incidence for women is more than three times greater than that for men, especially for those between the ages of 14 and 40 years. Black women appear to have a higher risk of developing the disease than do white women. The overall incidence rises with age, with the usual age at onset between 30 and 60 years (Medsger, 1988). SS is rare in children and in men younger than 35 years of age. The prevalence has been calculated to be 10 per 100,000 population (Hochberg, 1988), with a total estimate of 250,000 to 300,000 cases in the United States (Neuberger & Neuberger, 1984). The prevalence in Iceland was found to be 7.1 per 100,000 population, considerably lower than that found in other studies. This suggests that environmental factors, such as pollution, may play a role in the development of SS (Geirsson, Steinsson, Gudmundsson, & Sigurdson, 1994).

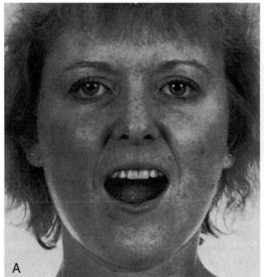 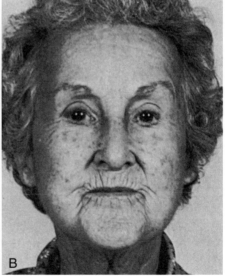

FIGURE 14–10. *A,* The face of a young woman with several months of rapidly progressive scleroderma. The facial skin is taut, with an immobile facies and limitation of the oral aperture. *B,* The face of a woman with long-standing diffuse scleroderma, exhibiting multiple telangiectasias and exaggerated radial furrowing about the lips, resulting in the "bird-face" appearance of the client with progressive systemic sclerosis. (From Kelley, W., Harris, E., Ruddy, S., & Sledge, C. [Eds.]. [1989]. *Textbook of rheumatology* [3rd ed., p. 1218]. Philadelphia: WB Saunders.)

TABLE 14–13. *Visceral, Integumentary, and Musculoskeletal Changes Associated with Systemic Sclerosis*

ORGAN	PATHOLOGIC CHANGES	PHYSICAL CHANGES/DISEASE
Intestinal tract		
Esophagus	Fibrosis and decreased motility	Dysphagia, especially with solids
	Distal esophageal motor dysfunction	Hiatal hernias
	Decreased peristaltic activity	Peptic ulcers
	Gastric reflux	
Small intestine	Loss of smooth muscle due to fibrosis	Intestinal malabsorption, abdominal distention,
	Bacterial overgrowth	diarrhea, weight loss
Large intestine	Patchy atrophy of smooth muscle results in large-mouthed diverticulae	Possible obstipation
Lungs	Interstitial fibrosis	Decreased vital capacity
		Dyspnea
		Pulmonary arterial hypertension
Cardiovascular		
Blood vessels	Epithelium of damaged blood vessels releases vasoactive substances	Raynaud's phenomenon: blanching of fingers associated with complaints of cold, pain, pallor, and possible ulceration of fingertips
	Overproduction of collagen and mucopolysaccharides	
Heart	Patchy replacement of fibrous tissue in the myocardium	Congestive failure
		Atrial arrhythmias
		Ventricular arrhythmias
		Rare: myocarditis and pericarditis
Kidneys	Constriction of renal arteries	Malignant arterial hypertension
	Decrease in cortical blood flow	Rapidly progressing renal insufficiency
	Possible necrosis of blood vessels	
Skin/nails	Edema, fibrosis, collagen thickening	Swelling of hands, feet, digits
		Thickened, hardened, dry skin
		Loss of skin folds
		Changes in pigmentation
		Rigid, masklike expression
		Late: softening and atrophy of skin, especially over joints
		Pitted nails
		Subcutaneous calcium deposits in fingertips
Joints	Synovial effusions	Polyarthritis
	Early: infiltration of lymphocytes and plasma cells with fibrin deposits	Polyarthralgias
	Late: fibrosis of synovial connective tissue	
	Calcific deposits	
Tendons	Fibrin deposits	Carpal tunnel syndrome
	Swollen tendons and tendon sheaths	Leathery friction rubs over extensor and flexor tendons of fingers, forearms, knees, ankles
Bones	Osteolysis: bone resorption of distal phalanges, distal radius/ulna, mandible, ribs	Generalized osteoporosis on x-ray film
Skeletal muscle	Replacement of muscle with fibrous tissue	Disuse atrophy associated with limited joint motion

Data from Medsger, T. A. (1985). Systemic sclerosis (scleroderma), eosinophilic, fascitis, and calcinosis. In D. J. McCarty (Ed.), *Arthritis and allied conditions* (10th ed., pp. 994–1036). Philadelphia: Lea & Febiger; and Medsger, T. A. (1988). Systemic sclerosis and localized scleroderma. In H. R. Schumacher (Ed.), *Primer on the rheumatic diseases* (9th ed., pp. 111–117). Atlanta: Arthritis Foundation.

Several risk factors have been associated with SS. Overproduction of collagen and fibrous skin thickening have been associated with environmental factors (e.g., working with plastics, coal, or silica dust) and a high alcohol intake (Neuberger & Neuberger, 1984). Scleroderma-like conditions can also be present as a result of genetic factors (phenylketonuria), metabolic disorders (Hashimoto's thyroiditis), malignancies, postinfectious disorders, and neurologic conditions (Tuffanelli, 1989).

Pathophysiology

SS is the result of an excessive production of collagen by fibroblasts. It seems likely that lymphocytes accumulate in the lower dermis. These cells, almost entirely T lymphocytes, generate lymphokines, which stimulate fibroblasts to produce excessive amounts of procollagen. After the procollagen is secreted from the cell, it undergoes crosslinking in the extracellular environment to produce mature, relatively insoluble collagen. The skin undergoes fibrotic changes, leading to loss of elasticity and movement.

Vascular changes are also important in the development of SS, particularly in persons with diffuse scleroderma. When the vascular endothelium is injured, damaged blood vessels release vasoactive substances, which are stimulated to overproduce collagen and mucopolysaccharides. Proliferation of the subintimal connective tissue results, along with fibrous thickening and narrowing of the lumina, thus leading to tissue ischemia. A small number of clients with CREST develop pulmonary hypertension and intestinal malabsorption, which are the leading causes of death for these clients (Seibold, 1993).

Assessment

Nursing History. Clients should be interviewed with great sensitivity because of their possible fears about the disease and the changes in body image. The first symptom of SS is often puffiness of the fingers and toes and, in limited scleroderma, Raynaud's phenomenon. Clients should be questioned carefully about their experiences. The nurse should ask them if they have had the sequence of blanching, cyanosis, and erythema associated with periodic vasospasm of the peripheral blood vessels. An inquiry should be made regarding which parts of the body have been affected. Although Raynaud's phenomenon is commonly seen in the hands and toes, it can affect the earlobes, nose, and tongue. It is also important to ask clients under what circumstances (i.e., cold or stress) they have experienced Raynaud's phenomenon.

Clients should be asked about changes in the texture, color, consistency, and moisture of their skin. Because skin changes can be widespread, the nurse should review changes according to body location. Clients should be asked about subcutaneous nodules that they may have noticed under their fingertips.

Other systemic changes to be explored include those associated with the gastrointestinal tract. Clients should be asked about the ease with which they swallow food and the types of food they have had difficulty swallowing. The presence of diarrhea (related to bacterial overgrowth or from malabsorption syndrome), constipation (related to colonic hypomotility), nausea, vomiting, and abdominal distention should be explored within the framework of onset, severity, duration, aggravating factors, and relieving factors. The respiratory system can be affected, secondary to interstitial pulmonary fibrosis. Therefore, clients should be questioned regarding cough, shortness of breath, or dyspnea with activity.

Clients should be asked questions about their musculoskeletal health. The presence of bilateral symmetrical joint pain and swelling should be elicited. Changes in endurance and muscle strength, as indicated by the ability to perform ADLs, should be explored.

Physical Assessment. A careful assessment is required of the entire integumentary system, including the skin on the feet, trunk, and abdomen. The face and lips (as well as fingers, palms, and fingernails) may have telangiectasias (Fig. 14–10B). They are macular dilations of superficial blood vessels that collapse after firm palpation (Tuffanelli, 1989). The hands are inspected and palpated for edema, thickened or hardened skin, loss of skin folds, or wrinkles (Fig. 14–11). Fingers are also inspected and palpated for subcutaneous calcific nodules, dilated capillary loops or venules, or ulcers on the tips of the fingernails. Nail beds are inspected for pitting, changes in contour, and the appearance of suppurative cuticles.

Changes in skin over the forearms, face, legs, and trunk can occur in diffuse cutaneous scleroderma. Therefore, each area should be assessed carefully for edema, thickening, or tightening. The face should be inspected

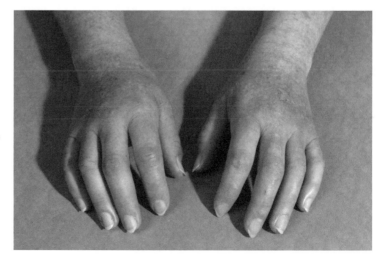

FIGURE 14–11. The hands of a young woman with several months of rapidly progressive scleroderma. The skin is taut and indurated, and there is limitation of both fist closure and finger extension.

for mobility of expression and ability to open the mouth. Persons with SS are often unable to open the mouth fully as the disease progresses. Skin thickening is often accompanied by areas of hypopigmentation and hyperpigmentation, so these changes are most commonly observed on the extremities and chest (Ziegler, 1984).

The musculoskeletal assessment includes a thorough evaluation of ROM because reduced joint mobility and polyarthritis characterize SS. Flexor and extensor tendons should be palpated for the presence of friction rubs. Often, coarse crepitus caused by fibrin deposits can be heard with tendon motion—a sign that is often considered specific for SS. Eliciting Tinel's sign to rule out or confirm carpal tunnel syndrome is useful. Muscle strength should be assessed and graded because SS may have a PM-type myopathy affecting the proximal muscles.

Other body systems should be assessed to provide baseline data or to determine possible organ involvement. The respiratory system should be assessed for the ease and extent of thoracic excursion, presence of dyspnea, and presence of adventitious lung sounds. The heart is examined for changes in rhythm or signs of heart failure. Blood pressure must be monitored closely because sudden malignant hypertension associated with renal disease can occur in SS.

Diagnostic Evaluation

Laboratory findings are relatively normal in persons with scleroderma. Mild hemolytic anemia is often present because of mechanical damage to red cells from diseased small vessels. Mild hypergammaglobulinemia (IgG) and RF are found in 30% of those affected (Medsger, 1988). Slight elevation of the ESR is also common. Proteinuria is common with renal involvement. Most clients have positive titers for ANA. Anticentromere and anticentriole antibodies seem to be relatively specific for scleroderma (Tuffanelli, 1989). Clients with the serum anticentromere antibody have a more favorable prognosis (Bertsch, 1995).

SCL-70, an antibody to topoisomerase, is found in about 35% of persons with diffuse SS but is rarely seen in persons with limited cutaneous involvement and the CREST syndrome. The anticentromere ANA is seen in 80% of those with limited cutaneous involvement and in only 5% of those with diffuse cutaneous involvement (Rocco & Hurt, 1986).

A definite diagnosis of SS requires the presence of one major or two minor criteria. The major criterion is proximal scleroderma with skin thickening and tightening of areas proximal to the MCP joints. These changes can affect the entire extremity, face, neck, thorax, and abdomen. The three minor criteria are (1) sclerodactyly (in which the skin changes are limited to the fingers); (2) digital pitting scars, with depressed areas at the tips of the fingers or loss of fingerpad tissue; and (3) bibasilar pulmonary fibrosis (Masi, Rodnan, Medsger, Altman, d'Angelo, Fries, LeRoy, Kirsner, MacKenzie, McShane, Myers, & Sharp, 1980).

Collaborative Treatment

The treatment of SS involves the shared management of a chronic illness and pharmacologic support. Members of the health care team should educate the client about the nature, course, and treatment of SS; the importance of avoiding cold; stress management techniques as a means to control Raynaud's phenomenon; the prevention of hand contractures and facial rigidity; the nutritional management of constipation and diarrhea and maintenance of ideal body weight; and the prevention of injury (Table 14–14). Protecting digits by wearing gloves or wearing warm socks, avoiding cold temperatures, and not smoking are important self-care measures that may require behavior modification so that the client believes that he or she can have some control over the illness.

Pharmacologic Management

Many drugs are used in SS, but no single agent has been proved convincingly effective. Symptomatic treatment

TABLE 14–14. *Client Education: Systemic Sclerosis*

FOCUS	TEACHING POINTS
Knowledge of disease	Explain chronic systemic nature of disease
Exposure to cold	Discuss how to avoid Raynaud's phenomenon by reducing or eliminating exposure to cold
Mobility	Instruct in individualized exercise program to prevent contractures and decreased muscular flexibility of the face
Pharmacologic therapy	Teach purpose, dosage, and side effects of each medication
Nutrition	Instruct or reinforce the principles of a nutritious, well-balanced diet
	Teach client to increase bulk and fluids to minimize difficulties with constipation
Prevention of injury	Reinforce safety measures to prevent trauma to fingers (e.g., careful handling of sharp, hot, or cold objects) because tightly stretched skin over joint spaces is easily injured
	Teach client to have blood drawn by venipuncture rather than by fingerstick
	Teach client and family to notify health care team if signs of infection are present with ulcerated digits (drainage, odor, elevated temperature)
	Use adult client education principles and behavior modification to help clients stop smoking

and prevention of complications are the current goals of therapy. Three types of therapeutic agents have been used to treat SS: (1) vasoactive agents, (2) anti-inflammatory medications, and (3) immunosuppressive drugs (Tuffanelli, 1989). In Raynaud's disease, calcium channel blockers have become widely prescribed. Nifedipine (10 to 20 mg three times a day) was effective for Raynaud's disease in a controlled, double-blind trial (Rodeheffer, Rommer, & Wigley, 1983). Digital ulcers and digital infarcts have been successfully treated with digital sympathectomies (Zachary, Rice-Puoci, & Ellman, 1997). Corticosteroids are the major anti-inflammatory agent used in SS when clients have significant joint and muscle involvement or extensive skin disease. Low-dose steroid therapy (prednisone, 10 mg per day or every other day) is preferred. Overall, immunosuppressive agents (azathioprine, cyclophosphamide, cyclosporine, and methotrexate) have not consistently been proven effective in the treatment of SS. Cyclophosphamide is often used in clients with progressive lung fibrosis.

Penicillamine, an immunomodulating agent that also interferes with the crosslinking of collagen, is a widely used drug in treating scleroderma. A large, retrospective study showed significant improvement in skin thickening after 2 years of therapy and improved 5-year survival compared with untreated clients (Steen, Medsger, & Rodnan, 1982). Not all clinicians, however, accept penicillamine as established therapy for SS. Initial dosages should be low (125 mg/day), and the dosage should be increased gradually (Tuffanelli, 1989). Reduction of skin thickness requires long-term therapy; therefore, clients need considerable support and monitoring while they are taking penicillamine. In addition, numerous toxic side effects, including lupus-like syndrome, myasthenia gravis, glomerulonephritis, pemphigus, excessive skin wrinkling, and blood and liver dyscrasias, can occur. Clients taking penicillamine must be carefully instructed to report skin rashes, burning, bleeding, sore throats, or fevers that might indicate serious side effects. The nurse and physician must explain the importance of periodic laboratory follow-up of liver, kidney, and renal function to the client.

Various other agents are used to treat specific system problems. Minocycline has been effective in the treatment of diarrhea associated with malabsorption syndrome. This drug may reduce inflammation by blocking metalloproteases. A histamine$_2$-receptor-blocking agent, such as cimetidine, is given for esophageal dysmotility or a proton pump blocker is administered to reduce the acidity of gastric reflux.

Renal crisis and associated hypertension was the most feared complication of SS. The introduction of angiotensin-converting enzyme (ACE) inhibitors, which are capable of reversing underlying hyperreninemia and controlling hypertension, has improved the outcome of renal crisis. Clients now have an 80% 1-year survival and 60% 5-year survival in contrast to 15% 1-year without the use of ACE inhibitors (Steen, Constantino, Shapiro, & Medsgar, 1990).

Unfortunately, no single drug or combination of drugs has proved as successful as the standard treatment in controlled research studies (Medsgar, 1993). Etanercept in a small (10 client), open-label pilot study was encouraging, but further research is necessary (Ellman, MacDonald, & Hayes, 2000). Ongoing clinical trials are rare in this orphan disease.

Nursing Management

Body Image Disturbance, Self-care Deficit, Impaired Skin Integrity, Altered Nutrition, Altered Bowel Elimination

Body Image Enhancement, Self-care Facilitation, Skin Care, Skin Surveillance, Teaching, Nutritional Support. Most clients with SS have significant muscle and joint involvement, including arthralgias, myalgia, and fibrosis of the tendons. When contractures develop, they are often due to the fibrotic changes in the skin. These muscle and joint changes lead to problems often encountered in clients with RA: joint pain, stiffness, fatigue, self-care deficits, and impaired physical mobility.

From the client's perspective, coping with an altered body image that accompanies extensive skin changes can be an overwhelming task. Nurses can help clients understand that successful coping often means assuming responsibility for self-care and the prevention of complications. Therefore, nursing interventions are targeted at maintaining a full ROM of the mouth and hands as well as suggesting creative use of clothing and makeup to enhance the appearance.

Changes in skin integrity require meticulous nursing care. For the acutely ill client, all digits and extremities must be handled carefully and gently. If possible, the client should try to move or reposition himself or herself to minimize discomfort. Debilitated or steroid-dependent clients or those undergoing orthopaedic surgery should be placed on pressure-reducing beds or air mattresses to prevent the development of skin breakdown over bony prominences. Dressings must be removed carefully so that additional trauma does not occur. Although moist dressings are applied to injured areas, they should be dampened with sterile saline if they do not come off easily. Wigley (1992) reported the successful use of a colloid dressing, Mitroflex, to treat digital ulcerations. Tape should be used only when absolutely essential, for example, to stabilize an intravenous catheter needle. Otherwise, all dressings should be secured with stretchable gauze.

When possible, the administration of injections and intravenous therapy should be in sites free of fibrosis and sclerosis. Areas of tough, thickened skin and sclerotic veins cannot be easily punctured. It is also possible to cause additional damage (and create a portal for infection) if needle punctures are not made successfully.

Client education is the cornerstone to effective nursing care of the client with Raynaud's phenomenon. Clients must be assisted to modify their dress and health practices so that all controllable sources of vasospasm are eliminated. Newly diagnosed clients may need anticipatory guidance about how to dress protectively in cold weather and in air conditioning. They may readily recognize the need for gloves but not realize the importance of protecting the head, ears, nose, lips, and feet. Keeping a pair of gloves in a tote bag or pocket is helpful when in air-conditioned stores or when taking frozen items out of the grocery freezer. Clients must maintain their core temperature, always dressing warmly. Clients often must be helped to change their health practices so that they eliminate the use of vasoconstrictive substances, such as alcohol and caffeine. Learning biofeedback or other stress management skills is indicated when clients identify stress as a cause of altered tissue perfusion.

Clients with SS often have difficulty maintaining their weight because of esophageal changes leading to dysphagia, esophagitis, and decreased intestinal motility. Consultation with the dietitian can help the nurse provide appropriate, easy-to-swallow, high-calorie snacks. The dietitian can plan meals to avoid foods contributing to esophagitis and gastric reflux. Remaining upright for 1 to 2 hours after eating also helps prevent esophageal reflux. Avoiding heavy snacks close to retiring, using a large wedge pillow to elevate the head and shoulders, or elevating the head of the bed on shock blocks can prevent bedtime reflux.

The client's ability to chew and swallow dry, compact foods, such as meat and bread, should be evaluated carefully. Often, these foods cause severe choking spells. Clients may moisten them with gravies, sauces, or jellies to improve their tolerability.

The achievement of nutritional goals is often affected by dental hygiene practices. Because of sclerotic skin changes, clients may have a difficult time completely opening the mouth. Mucous membranes may become inflamed or ulcerated because of lack of moisture or inadequate brushing and rinsing. Using a small angled toothbrush or Waterpik can help prevent these problems. Reinforcing the need to perform facial exercises to prevent rigidity of the face and mouth is a priority nursing intervention.

Chronic constipation and diarrhea are two other problems that are usually amenable to nursing intervention. Chronic constipation is associated with the decreased motility of the gastrointestinal tract that accompanies SS. Nursing interventions include eating easy-to-swallow, high-fiber foods and increasing fluids and exercise. The use of bulk stool softeners and suppositories may be needed as part of the bowel program. Diarrhea is associated with malabsorption syndrome. Foods known to precipitate diarrhea should be eliminated from the diet, and natural antidiarrheal agents can be added to meals. When infectious organisms are present, antibiotic agents, often tetracycline, are prescribed.

Nursing care is also directed toward the monitoring and detecting of potential problems. The potential for impaired gas exchange exists when interstitial fibrosis of the lungs occurs. The presence of dyspnea, changes in activity tolerance, and an increased rate and depth of respirations may be noted. Auscultation of lung sounds may indicate fine crackles. Oxygen is usually administered as supportive therapy, and clients are educated about factors (pollen, smoking, humidity) that exacerbate the pulmonary condition.

IDIOPATHIC INFLAMMATORY MYOPATHY (POLYMYOSITIS AND DERMATOMYOSITIS)

Inflammatory diseases of muscle are a heterogeneous group of disorders characterized by proximal muscle weakness and nonsuppurative inflammation of skeletal muscle. Traditionally, the terms *polymyositis* and *dermatomyositis* have been used to represent these diseases. Today it is more appropriate to use the term *idiopathic inflammatory myopathy* to describe the entire group and reserve the terms *polymyositis* (PM) and *dermatomyositis* (DM) for more specific conditions or subsets (Olsen & Wortman, 1997).

The most commonly occurring idiopathic myopathies in adults, PM and DM are diffuse, systemic, inflammatory connective tissue diseases. Although these disorders can have an acute onset and progress rapidly, more typically there is a slower progression. Clients gradually develop significant weight loss, fatigue, and weakness over a period of months, sometimes not even being aware of when the changes began (Cronin, Miller, & Plotz, 1988). Both diseases cause symmetrical progressive weakness of the proximal or limb-girdle muscles and occasionally atrophy of the muscles of the limbs, neck, and pharynx. Decreased muscle strength occurs in the pelvic girdle first, followed by weakness of the legs and shoulders and arms. Weakness of the flexor muscles of the neck occurs in about half of those affected with PM or DM. In acute disease, muscles can be tender or swollen and doughy. When classic skin changes are associated with PM, the disease is classified as DM. A summary of the cutaneous changes seen in DM is outlined in Table 14–15.

The classification of idiopathic inflammatory myopathies, to which PM and DM belong, includes seven groups: (1) PM, (2) DM, (3) amyopathic DM, (4) juvenile DM, (5) myositis associated with neoplasia, (6) myositis associated with collagen vascular disease, and (7) inclusion body myositis.

Epidemiology

The idiopathic myopathies are relatively rare diseases. Accurate estimates of their prevalence are difficult to

TABLE 14–15. *Cutaneous Manifestations of Dermatomyositis*

SKIN FEATURE	DESCRIPTION	LOCATION
Gottron's papules	Violet-colored or erythematous papules or small plaques	PIP joints
Gottron's sign	Reddened, smooth, scaly patches	PIP joints
		Elbows
		Knees
		Ankles
Heliotrope rash	Violet-colored, cyanotic, or erythematous symmetric rash accompanied by edema	Eyelids: more predominant on upper lids
Nail changes	Irregular, thickened, or fissured	Cuticles
	Telangiectasias (dilated vessels)	Nailbeds
	Shiny erythema	Subungual areas
Calcinosis cutis	Calcium nodules of varying size and proximity on the skin surface in long-standing dermatomyositis, especially in children; may be seen in adults	Throughout skin
	In severe cases, the nodules ulcerate, crust over, and even develop eschar	
Poikiloderma	Erythematous, scaling, and atrophic rash	Extensor surface
		Upper back

obtain because the diseases are uncommon and lack universally accepted specific diagnostic criteria. Estimates of incidence range from 0.5 to 8.4 cases per million. The incidence appears to be increasing, although this may simply reflect increased awareness and more accurate diagnosis. Although PM and DM affect all age groups, there is a bimodal distribution of the age of onset, with peaks at ages 10 and 15 years in children and between 45 and 60 years in adults. As with other connective tissue diseases, such as SS and SLE, there is a 2:1 female-to-male predominance in PM-DM with the exception of inclusion body myositis, which affects men twice as often. Racial differences are apparent. In adults, the lowest rates are reported in the Japanese and the highest in African Americans. Although no direct relationships have been established between an inflammatory myopathy and a specific genetic marker, several associations have been recognized. The strongest associations are for HLA-B8, HLA-DR3, and DRW52 phenotypes with PM and DM in all age groups (Olsen & Wortman, 1997).

A subset of clients with inflammatory myopathies develops muscle weakness with an underlying malignancy. The true incidence of this relationship is not clear (Airio, Puklaala, & Isomaki, 1995). Malignancy may precede or follow the onset of muscle weakness. The association is rare in children (Pachman, 1986) but has occurred in clients of all ages in all subsets of disease, although associated malignancy may be more common with DM. Subsequent studies seem to indicate that the types of tumors found roughly paralleled those found in the general population with the exception of ovarian cancer which is over-represented in women with DM (Olsen & Wortman, 1997).

Increased mortality has been associated with DM rather than PM. Mortality in PM is predicted by more extensive clinical involvement and is considerably higher in blacks than in whites (Callahan & Pincus, 1995).

Pathology and Cause

The results of muscle biopsies, usually of the deltoid or quadriceps muscles, have provided useful information about the pathology of the disease. Several changes have been noted, including focal or extensive degeneration of muscle fibers caused by inflammatory infiltrates of lymphocytes and macrophages. In some cases, necrosis of parts or entire groups of muscle fibers can occur. However, fibers can also show evidence of regeneration.

The idiopathic myopathies are believed to be immune-mediated processes that are triggered by environmental factors in genetically susceptible individuals. This is supported by two observations: (1) There is a recognized association with other autoimmune and connective tissue diseases and (2) there is a high prevalence of circulating autoantibodies (Love, Leff, Fraser, Targoff, Dalakas, Plotz, & Miller, 1991; Targoff, 1994). The autoantibodies associated with PM-DM include the myositis-specific autoantibodies (MSAs) found almost exclusively in these diseases. The triggering event of PM-DM is unknown, but viruses have been strongly implicated. The seasonal variation in the onset of disease as well as evidence found in animal models are direct evidence that infectious agents play a role. Genetic factors also play an important role. Individuals with HLA-DR3 are at increased risk for developing inflammatory muscle disease, including PM and juvenile DM. All clients with the anti–Jo-1 antibodies have the HLA antigen DR52, and white clients also have a high prevalence of HLA-B8, HLA-DR3, and DR6. Inclusion body myositis is more likely associated with HLA-DR1, DR6, and DQ1 (Olsen & Wortman, 1997).

Diagnostic Evaluation

Bohan and Peter (1975) describe five criteria that continue to be used for the diagnoses of PM-DM: (1) proximal, symmetrical muscle weakness, with or without dysphagia or respiratory muscle weakness; (2) elevation of serum muscle enzymes; (3) characteristic electromyographic changes; (4) muscle biopsy evidence of myositis; and (5) the typical skin rash of DM. Confidence limits for diagnosing the disease are also defined (Table 14–16). In addition, the diagnosis is confirmed after excluding other neuromuscular diseases, such as myasthenia gravis, amyotrophic lateral sclerosis, polymyalgia rheumatica, and Guillain-Barré syndrome. Research continues to refine the diagnostic criteria for PM-DM, and four additional criteria may become standard in the future (Tanimoto, Nakano, Kano, Mori, Ueki, Nishitani, Sato, Kiuchi, & Ohashi, 1995).

The most important laboratory test is the measurement of the muscle enzyme creatine kinase (CK) (formerly creatine phosphokinase). An elevated CK level indicates muscle injury, but it is not specific to PM-DM. Elevated CK levels can be seen after intramuscular injections, muscle biopsies, or exercise, for example. The level of CK changes according to the activity of the disease (Targoff, 1988). In most cases, other muscle enzymes are also elevated, including aldolase, ALT (alanine aminotransferase, formerly glutamic-pyruvic transaminase [SGPT]), AST (aspartate aminotransferase, formerly glutamic-oxaloacetic transaminase [SGOT]), and lactate dehydrogenase (LDH). The sedimentation rate is normal in 50% of clients.

Electromyographic results often show bizarre, high-frequency discharges with spontaneous fibrillations and positive spikes at rest (Pachman, 1986). Muscle biopsies are done if there is doubt about the diagnosis. The muscle chosen should be affected by the disease but not atrophied. The site should not be one where a previous electromyographic needle has been introduced. When biopsies are performed under general anesthesia, a permanent scar usually forms in a prominent place and the area is sore for several weeks. For these reasons, physicians may prefer not to perform the biopsy unless it is essential

to making the diagnosis (Norins, 1989). Muscle biopsy results, as previously mentioned, show changes associated with necrosis and degeneration as well as evidence of regeneration. Fibrosis may be seen.

Assessment

Nursing History. Eliciting the history of a person with PM-DM begins with the client's perspective. He or she seeks health care because of the nonspecific changes, usually occurring over several months, of increasing fatigue, weight loss, and malaise. When questioned about the nature of the fatigue and how it affects the ability to carry out ADLs, clients usually describe difficulty performing tasks because of muscle weakness. Good screening questions include queries about the changes in ability to perform ADLs that require the use of large muscle groups. Questions about the onset, duration, location, and quality of muscle pain should be asked. Muscle pain or tenderness may or may not be present in the early phases of the disease. The client should be asked about difficulty brushing the hair; reaching over the head for objects on a shelf or when putting on clothes; or performing repetitive chores, such as mowing the lawn, hanging up laundry, or putting away groceries.

For a history of pelvic limb weakness, the nurse should determine whether the client has had difficulty rising from an armless chair, getting out of a car, climbing steps, or riding a bike. The client should be asked about difficulties in raising the neck off the bed or pillow. The client should also be questioned about associated joint pains because arthritis and arthralgia occur in many persons who are in overlap group V (i.e., they have both PM and DM and evidence of another collagen vascular disease, such as RA or SS). Some clients may report a tendency to fall that is unrelated to balance, so changes in gait patterns must be explored with them. Because muscle weakness in the face and larynx is seen in PM-DM, it must be determined whether there has been any difficulty in chewing or swallowing, facial swelling, or hoarseness.

Because PM-DM is a systemic disease, questions must also be included about the integumentary, pulmonary, and cardiovascular systems. The nurse should determine whether the client has experienced any skin or nail changes—rash, reddened areas, scaling—typical of those seen in DM. Common respiratory complications of PM-DM include aspiration pneumonia (because of a weakened cough, slow protective movements with vomiting, and pharyngeal muscle weakness) and interstitial lung disease (Caro, 1989). Questions about previous respiratory diseases, particularly pneumonia and influenza-like illnesses, and about recovery from these illnesses give important information to surgical nurses for preoperative and postoperative pulmonary care. The client's cardiac history should be assessed via questions about arrhythmias and history of a prolapsed mitral valve.

TABLE 14–16. *Confidence Limits for the Diagnosis of Polymyositis and Dermatomyositis*

Definite Diagnosis	
Polymyositis	4 criteria
Dermatomyositis	3 or 4 criteria plus rash
Probable Diagnosis	
Polymyositis	3 criteria
Dermatomyositis	2 or 3 criteria plus rash
Possible Diagnosis	
Polymyositis	2 criteria
Dermatomyositis	1 criteria plus rash

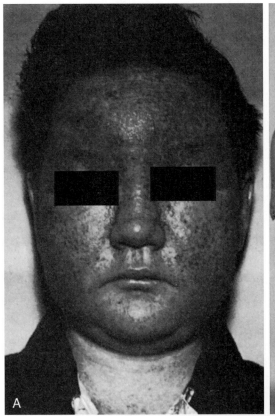
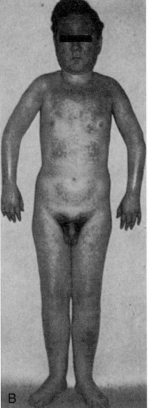
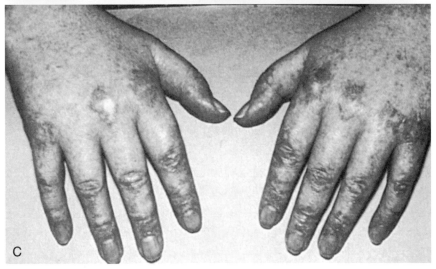

FIGURE 14–12. Views of a 15-year-old boy with severe dermatomyositis showing a very extensive skin rash of the face *(A)*, trunk *(B)*, and knuckles *(C)* in the characteristic distribution despite 3 months of treatment with prednisone. (From Kelley, W., Harris, E., Ruddy, S., & Sledge, C. [Eds.]. [1989] *Textbook of rheumatology* [3rd ed., p. 1276]. Philadelphia: WB Saunders.)

Physical Assessment. The examination of the client with PM-DM requires a meticulous assessment of the skin and nail beds for the presence of erythema, macular-papular rashes, plaques, scaling, and nodules (Fig. 14–12). Skin changes outlined in Table 14–15 can help direct this examination. To confirm the presence of a heliotrope rash on the client's face, the neck and head must be held securely while being lowered off the examination table or the side of the bed. This maneuver elicits increased suffusion to bring out the distinctive bluish red hue of the rash.

Muscle weakness is initially tested by asking the client to walk, to get up from an armless chair, to raise the neck off the bed or table, or to lift a heavy book. Loss of hand strength is less noticeable, but it can be detected by a test of grip strength. Asking the client to shrug the shoulders upward against the nurse's hands can test proximal weakness of the shoulder girdle. Weakness of the masseter muscles (which can be seen in clients who have difficulty chewing) is assessed by palpating their strength when the client clenches the teeth. All muscle groups should be palpated for symmetry, atrophy, pain or tenderness, and the presence of contractures. Atrophy generally appears late in the disease, but contractures develop early if muscle weakness has been severe. As muscles are being assessed, large and small joints should be inspected for erythema, pain, presence of synovitis, and limitations in ROM.

Although the focus of the examination is on the integumentary and musculoskeletal systems, thorough assessment of the cardiopulmonary system is required because of the systemic nature of the disease. The bilateral assessment of chest expansion (diaphragmatic excursion) helps the nurse to know how compliant the muscles of respiration are. The quality of the breathing, the presence of dyspnea with simple activities, and the presence of a cough can indicate an acute or chronic respiratory problem with muscle disease. The quality of the lung sounds should be carefully assessed for fine rales (crackles) because aspiration pneumonia is a common complication of advanced PM-DM.

Pharmacologic Management

The treatment is largely empiric. The treatment of PM-DM usually begins with the daily administration of high doses of oral corticosteroids. Prednisone (1 to 2 mg/kg per day) is given until elevated muscle enzymes begin to decrease toward normal and clients show improvement in their ability to perform ADLs. In severe cases, the daily dose can be divided or intravenous methylprednisolone may be used. Reduction in steroid dosages to alternate-day therapy may not be possible for several months. Some clients require long-term treatment with maintenance doses of steroids because the disease can recur when the steroids are withdrawn. Clients who do not respond to steroids or who cannot tolerate the

high steroid doses usually require the addition of an immunosuppressive agent, such as daily azathioprine (50 to 150 mg/day) or weekly methotrexate therapy (7.5 mg/wk orally or 0.5 to 0.8 mg/kg per week intravenously) (Cronin, Miller, & Plotz, 1988). Other immunosuppressive agents have been used in steroid-resistant clients. Cyclophosphamide, 6-mercaptopurine, chlorambucil, total-body (or total-nodal) irradiation, and intravenous immunoglobulins have also been used. Hydroxychloroquine can be used to treat the cutaneous lesions of DM, although it has no recognized effect on the myositis.

The education of clients receiving high-dose steroid therapy focuses on teaching them about the potential side effects of long-term prednisone use (Table 14–17). Clients should be aware that they have an increased risk of infection and therefore should monitor and report any symptoms such as low-grade fevers, chills, or joint pain to their primary caregivers. Other long-term effects include facial edema, increased appetite, and the development of diabetes mellitus, osteoporosis, and avascular necrosis. Clients should also be instructed to wear a MedicAlert identification tag as long as they are receiving prednisone therapy. Clients must clearly understand that they should never change a dose of prednisone. Steroids must be tapered slowly after high-dose or long-term use because the body cannot respond quickly to changes in cortisol levels. During the period in which high doses of steroids have been administered, the hypothalamus-pituitary-adrenocortical axis has been suppressed, thus leading to negative feedback for the natural production of cortisol. Steroid-dependent clients who abruptly discontinue their therapy can experience an addisonian crisis (characterized by circulatory collapse, vomiting, and severe weakness) with minimal stress.

TABLE 14–17. *Client Education: Polymyositis and Dermatomyositis*

FOCUS	TEACHING POINTS
High-dose prednisone therapy	Instruct client in potential side effects of long-term prednisone therapy: facial edema, diabetes mellitus, osteonecrosis, avascular necrosis, increased appetite, increased risk of infection
	Instruct client never to alter prednisone dose; steroids must be tapered slowly after high-dose or long-term use
	Explain how to maintain medical identification tag (MedicAlert bracelet) and importance of wearing it
	Teach client to be aware of subtle sources of infection: breaks in skin integrity, slow healing of cuts, mouth sores, low-grade fevers, frequent (but painless) urination
	Instruct client to report any nonspecific feeling of being sick
	Teach client that mild weight gain and increased appetite are normal; instruct them to report significant weight gain over 5 pounds/wk
Course of disease	Explain that disease is a chronic one characterized by exacerbations and remissions
	Introduce/reinforce information about the disease:
	Process of muscle fibrosis, necrosis, and regeneration
	Skin involvement
	Other systemic or overlap features
	Control versus cure
	Teach self-management techniques: ROM exercises, resting inflamed muscles, energy conservation, use of assistive devices, and skin care

Nursing Management

Impaired Swallowing, Potential for Injury, Impaired Physical Mobility

Aspiration Precaution, Fall Prevention, Exercise Therapy: Muscle, Exercise Therapy: Ambulation.
Clients with involvement of the pharyngeal and respiratory muscles must be carefully monitored for the prevention of aspiration pneumonia. Helping clients maintain or regain effective swallowing can significantly reduce aspiration. Resting before meals, eating easily swallowed foods (e.g., those of a smooth, slippery consistency), and sitting upright during meals are measures that can enhance the client's ability to swallow.

Clients with PM-DM are also at risk of falling because of muscle weakness, gait changes, and the possibility of osteoporosis from high-dose prednisone therapy. Balancing a muscle-strengthening program with the use of assistive devices and instructions about safe ambulation helps keep the client injury free.

SPONDYLOARTHROPATHIES

The spondyloarthropathies are a group of interrelated disorders that include psoriatic arthritis (PsA), reactive arthritis (Reiter's syndrome), arthritis-associated inflammatory bowel disease, and ankylosing spondylitis (AS). Spondyloarthropathies are distinguished from RA by three characteristics: (1) a negative test for RF, (2) the absence of rheumatoid nodules, and (3) an inflammatory peripheral arthritis that is typically asymmetrical (Vasey, 1984).

Psoriatic Arthritis

Psoriasis is a common skin disorder characterized by stippled nails, pruritus, and silvery scales on bright red plaques, usually on the elbows, knees, and scalp. It is a genetically determined disease associated with several histocompatibility antigens, including HLA-B14, HLA-Bw17, and HLA-Cw6. About 5% to 10% of those with psoriasis develop a distinctive inflammatory arthritis—PsA.

Three to five types of PsA have been proposed (Calin, 1986; Veale, Rogers, & Fitzgerald, 1994). In asymmetrical oligoarthropathy, there is asymmetrical involvement of both large and small joints, and sausage-shaped joints are common (Fig. 14–13). With this type of arthritis, the asymmetrical pattern involves the interphalangeal and MTP joints of the feet and the DIP joints of the fingers. The second type, symmetrical polyarthropathy, closely resembles RA. Arthritis mutilans, a severe form of destructive arthritis, is characterized by telescoping digits also known as the "opera-glass hand." Psoriatic spondylitis is characterized by the sacroiliitis of AS (discussed later in this chapter). Clients with this last type, characterized by DIP joint involvement, often have nail changes such as

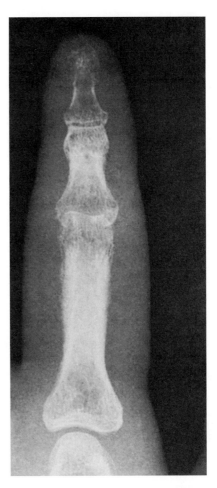

FIGURE 14–13. Psoriatic arthritis in a woman, age 37, manifested by tenosynovitis and production of sausage digit of index finger. The process also features fluffy periosteal new bone of the proximal phalanx. (From Gold, R., Bassett, L., & Seeger, L. [1988]. The other arthritides. *Radiologic Clinics of North America, 26*[6], 1203.)

pitting, transverse depressions, and subungual hyperkeratosis, along with DIP joint disease.

Epidemiology. The overall prevalence of PsA is approximately 0.1% in the United States. Arthritis occurs in approximately 5% to 7% of clients with psoriasis, but it may affect 40% of hospitalized clients with extensive skin involvement (Cuellar, Silverira, & Espinoza, 1994). Two percent of white North Americans and Europeans are believed to be affected with psoriasis, but it is relatively uncommon in Asians. The male/female ratio is equal but varies in subsets of this disease. In contrast to psoriasis, in which the peak age is between 5 and 15 years, the peak age of PsA is between 30 and 55 years, which is similar to the peak age of RA.

Cause. The cause of PsA appears to be a complex combination of immunologic, genetic, and environmental factors (Vasey, 1988). Immunologic changes seen in some clients include elevated titers of IgG and IgA and the presence of immune complexes. There is an increased prevalence of the disease among family members who have PsA. Possible environmental factors include group A streptococci and trauma.

Assessment. The focus of the nursing history for persons with PsA is similar to that for persons with RA. Asymmetrical pauciarticular arthritis, however, often occurs in PsA, so clients should be questioned about the nature, onset, and location of any acutely occurring painful, swollen joints. Questions about back pain and stiffness can help identify psoriatic spondylitis. In addition, clients should be asked about their psoriasis-associated skin changes—location, size, color, and degree of scaling of the plaques—as well as changes in the nail beds of the fingers and the toes. Because the disease seems to be caused by several other factors, clients should be asked about a family history of arthritis, PsA, or psoriasis. The nurse should determine whether they have had a history of severe infection before or after developing symptoms of the disease or any episodes of local trauma to the hands, feet, or spine.

Assessment of the client with PsA begins with a thorough head-to-toe examination of the skin for evidence of psoriatic plaques or nail bed changes. Such completeness is essential because the disease cannot be confirmed, even with characteristic radiologic changes, unless there is evidence of psoriasis. Usually located on extensor surfaces, psoriatic skin lesions are either macular or papular round scales that tend to bleed when they are removed. If clients deny that they have any skin involvement, all areas should be examined carefully, particularly the scalp, axillae, and umbilicus. The nurse should look carefully for pitting nails, which often precede skin rashes and are highly suggestive of psoriasis (Petty & Malleson, 1986).

The assessment of the musculoskeletal system should be deferred until the examination of the integument is complete so that subtle changes in either system are not overlooked. Because the range of joint involvement in PsA is extensive (e.g., asymmetrical or symmetrical, small or large, pauciarticular or monoarticular), each joint must be assessed for swelling, bogginess, and erythema. Particular attention should be paid to the small joints of the hands and feet, watching for swollen, sausage-shaped digits, which result from tenosynovitis of the flexor tendon sheath. The nurse should note whether any of the digits have assumed a spindle or telescopic shape.

Diagnostic Evaluation. The medical diagnosis of PsA is usually confirmed after a positive history of psoriasis and specific x-ray findings. However, it is important to realize that in some clients, particularly children, joint changes precede skin changes (Petty & Malleson, 1986). Nevertheless, most rheumatologists agree that the diagnosis cannot be made without evidence of psoriatic skin or nail changes (Vasey, 1988).

Some changes that appear on x-ray film are suggestive of PsA. In early cases, soft tissue swelling can be seen in clients with psoriasis similar to that observed in RA. Periarticular demineralization of the bone, however, is less common in PsA. Radiologic findings indicative of the disease include erosions of the DIP joints (both hands and feet), which can lead to a whittled, "pencil-in-cup" appearance. Clients with spinal involvement have radiologic evidence of sacroiliitis, but the distribution of the joint changes is less predictable than it is in AS.

Laboratory tests often reveal a slightly elevated ESR and hypochromic anemia. Many clients have mild hyperuricemia; a confusing finding that could initially lead to the diagnosis of gout. Tests for RF are negative in 75% of clients; among the 25% with positive tests, many have coexisting psoriasis and RA.

Collaborative Treatment: Acute and Chronic Phases. Although clients with PsA can have an explosive onset of polyarticular or monoarticular joint pain, erythema, and swelling, treatment goals are directed at the management of a chronic illness. Clients can be confused or discouraged when they first realize their diagnosis. They may perceive themselves as having not just one but two chronic diseases and thus feel increasingly powerless or helpless about their illness. Nurses and physicians must therefore work collaboratively to educate clients about the cause of the disease and the expected course of treatment. As with all other arthritic diseases, engaging the client's interest and partnership in actively managing the disease is essential for the best outcomes.

Nurses work with physicians to educate clients about key treatment strategies (Table 14–18), many of which are similar to those implemented in RA and AS. During exacerbations of the disease, clients must avoid stressing inflamed joints, participate in active assistive ROM exercises to prevent joint contractures, and alternate periods of rest with activity. Those with foot and toenail involvement must be instructed to select appropriate footwear to protect swollen digits and keratotic nail beds.

Pharmacologic Management. The initial treatment for stable plaque psoriasis is topical. However, topical therapy may be impractical for clients with extensive psoriasis (more than 20% involvement), and systemic therapy may be indicated at the outset. Topical treatment includes emollients and keratolytic agents alone or in combination with anthralin, corticosteroids, and vitamin D derivatives. Stress and certain drugs (beta-adrenergic blockers, ACE inhibitors, lithium, and antimalarial drugs) may exacerbate psoriasis and should be used with caution.

In general, PsA is managed following the same principles used to treat RA or spondylitis. Treatment

TABLE 14–18. *Client Education: Psoriatic Arthritis*

FOCUS	TEACHING POINTS
Knowledge deficit of disease process	Teach client about its probable multiple causes and the expected course of treatment
Pain management	Instruct client to avoid stressing inflamed joints during exacerbation of disease
	Explain purpose, action, and side effects of prescribed medications
	Teach client benefit of alternating periods of rest with periods of activity
Altered mobility: prevention of contractures	Teach ROM exercises
Prevention of injury	Teach principles of foot care to persons with foot and nail involvement:
	Inspect feet and nails daily
	Wear cotton socks
	Choose shoes that breathe, with sufficient toe room to accommodate swollen digits
	Check shoes for sharp edges or seams before wearing

depends on the type of joint disease (axial vs. peripheral) and the severity of the joint and skin involvement. Simultaneous joint and skin disease activity has been observed in up to one third of clients, particularly those with nonspondylitis disease. The medical management of PsA begins with the administration of NSAIDs. NSAIDs are effective in most clients.

If the response to NSAIDs is inadequate or if the disease is progressive erosive or polyarticular, DMARDs should be initiated as early as possible. Methotrexate is effective for both the skin disease and peripheral arthritis. Dosage and monitoring is the same as with RA. Sulfasalazine (2 to 3 g/day) is helpful for both axial and peripheral arthritis (Dougados, vam der Linden, Leirisalo-Repo, Huitfeldt, Juhlin, Veys, Zeidler, Kvien, Olivieri, & Dijkmans, 1995). Sulfasalazine has no significant effect on the skin disease. Almost all of the DMARDs have been studied in small open-label, uncontrolled studies and have shown some efficacy.

In a 60-client study, etanercept (Enbrel) has been shown to have significantly improved the arthritis and the skin disease (Mease, Goffe, Metz, VanderStoep, Finck, & Burge, 2000). It is currently being studied in a larger population. See Table 14-6 for more information.

For clients with intractable pain or loss of joint function, surgery may be indicated. Although several reports have raised concerns about a higher risk of infections, recurrent contracture or stiffness, or excessive bone formation after surgery, most of these fears seem ill founded and surgery should not be withheld.

Nursing Management

Impaired Skin Integrity, Body Image Disturbance

Skin Care, Skin Surveillance, and Body Image Enhancement. Nursing interventions are especially important for the client with PsA who is experiencing impaired skin integrity and body image disturbance. Clients with PsA may need basic instruction about how to care for their skin. If skin changes are severe, the client should be referred to a dermatologist or the nurse (and physician) should collaborate with the dermatologist if the client has previously sought care from this specialist. The nurse should review skin care principles, such as the purpose and application techniques of emollients to keep the skin soft; the importance of patting the skin dry after bathing instead of vigorous towel drying; and the correct application of topical ointments with a thin layer, sparingly applied. If the client is hospitalized, it is important that he or she assume responsibility for skin care as soon as it is feasible.

Because of the changes in both the skin and the joints, it is likely that the client has experienced a significant body image disturbance. It is not unusual for persons to be so affected by their appearance that they wear long-sleeved shirts on the hottest days and buy only clothes with pockets to hide their altered fingers. The communication of positive unconditional regard by the nurse—and all members of the health care team—can be a powerful tool to help clients begin to feel comfortable exploring their feelings.

Ankylosing Spondylitis

Formerly called *Marie-Strumpell disease,* AS is a systemic inflammatory disease of the axial skeleton, including the sacroiliac joints, intervertebral disc spaces, and costovertebral articulations. AS is one of the most common seronegative spondyloarthropathies, along with reactive arthritis (Reiter's syndrome) and PsA. The spondyloarthropathies share three characteristics: (1) involvement of the sacroiliac joint, (2) peripheral arthropathy, and (3) absence of RF. Three other features of the spondyloarthropathies have been noted. First, inflammation occurs where the ligament inserts into the bone (enthesis), rather than at the synovium. Extraskeletal changes can occur in the eye, skin, lung parenchyma, or aortic valve. Second, there is considerable overlap between the various spondyloarthropathies. For example, a person with PsA can develop the classic sacroiliitis seen in AS. Finally, there is a tendency toward familial aggregation in the development of the disease (Calin, 1986), with genes other than B27 probably playing a role (Jarvinen, 1995).

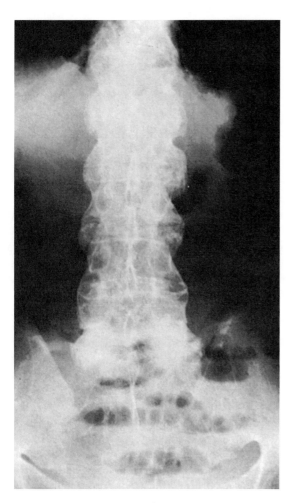

FIGURE 14–14. Late-stage-ankylosing spondylitis. Note the paraspinal ossification and fused sacroiliac joint. (From Kelley, W., Harris, E., Ruddy, S., & Sledge, C. [Eds.]. *Textbook of rheumatology* [3rd ed., p. 1032]. Philadelphia: WB Saunders.)

Literally, AS refers to fusion (ankylosis) of inflamed vertebrae (spondylitis) (Fig. 14–14). The disease typically begins in the spine of young men in their late teens or early 20s. Many clients have bilateral sacroiliitis that causes pain and some degree of restricted motion in the lumbar spine. Peripheral arthritis of the large joints, usually the hips and shoulders and, more rarely, the knees, occurs in 20% to 30% of persons with AS (Arnett, 1987). Small joint involvement is not usually seen. Chest expansion can also be decreased because of an associated costovertebral arthritis. By the time the client is 50 or 60 years old, the fusion of the lumbar spine has proceeded to the cervical region. If AS is not treated, the disease tends to progress with remissions and exacerbations to a final stage of rigid lumbar and thoracic kyphosis that leaves the neck in a flexed position. AS is associated with a shortening of the life span (Callahan & Pincus, 1995).

Several other systemic manifestations of AS can be seen: uveitis, pulmonary fibrosis, inflammatory bowel disease, and aortic insufficiency. Uveitis occurs in up to 25% of all clients with AS, especially in HLA-B27–positive clients with peripheral joint disease, but its incidence seems to be unrelated to the severity of the spondylitis (Calin, 1986). Upper lobe pulmonary fibrosis is rare, but it has been reported. Intestinal inflammation is common in clients with spondyloarthropathy, and one fourth of clients have early features of Crohn's disease (Leirisalo-Repo, Turunen, Stenman, Helenius, & Seppala, 1994). Aortic insufficiency, accompanied by a typical diastolic murmur, occurs in 5% of those with AS, and this problem often leads to the need for an aortic valve replacement. However, cardiac problems do not usually appear for several years.

Epidemiology. It is estimated that the prevalence of AS in white North Americans is 0.1% to 0.2%. In large population surveys in Holland and Australia, 1% to 2% of adults inheriting HLAB27 were found to have AS. Although the usual age of onset has been set between 15 and 35 years, the age group with the highest incidence rate is the 25- to 34-year-old group (Taurog, 1997).

Risk factors associated with AS include gender (with a 3:1 to 4:1 predominance of males to females), the young adult years of adolescence through adulthood (15 to 35 years of age), and a genetic predisposition. A strong tendency toward familial aggregation has been seen (Kelsey, 1982), and a sex-linked hormone may be important (Jiminez-Balderas & Mintz, 1993). The presence of HLA-B27 may also be a risk factor because it commonly appears in the high-risk Indian population but is almost nonexistent in the low-risk U.S. black population. Although the disease is generally seen in men in the third decade of life, the condition may go undetected in women because of its milder course and the usual caution in performing pelvic x-ray examinations in women of childbearing age (Pigg, Driscoll, & Caniff, 1985).

Assessment

Nursing History. Questions should focus on the typical symptoms of pain, stiffness, and fatigue and their effects on performing ADLs, as well as screening for extra-articular involvement. Clients should be questioned about the nature, onset, location, duration, and quality of their pain. The nurse should ask what self-care measures (e.g., use of heat or cold, showers or baths) they have tried to cope with the pain-stiffness-fatigue cycle and which measures have been effective.

The nurse should also determine whether the pain is in the lower back, thorax, or cervical area and whether other large peripheral joints, such as the knees, hips, or shoulders, cause discomfort. During the early phase of AS, clients complain of lumbosacral pain that radiates to the buttocks and thighs. Sleep for clients with AS is different from normal sleep (Jamieson, Alford, Bird, Hindmarch, & Wright, 1995). Therefore, an assessment of sleep patterns should be completed. Clients should be asked if the pain is worse on rising, if it is associated with morning stiffness, and if it decreases with activity. Also, the length of time that the client has been affected with back pain must be determined. These points are important because five features strongly suggest inflammatory spinal disease: (1) insidious onset of discomfort, (2) age younger than 40 years of age, (3) persistence of discomfort for more than 3 months, (4) association with morning stiffness, and (5) improvement with exercise (Calin, 1988).

Clients should also be questioned about fatigue, weight loss, and the presence of a low-grade fever. With advanced disease, cord compression can occur as a result of spinal fractures, so it is important to elicit information about neurologic changes, such as decreased motor activity, paresthesias, numbness, and bowel and bladder incontinence. Because of the possibility of extra-articular disease, it is important to ask clients about their eyes, respiratory status, and heart. Following are suggested screening parameters for each system:

Eyes—presence of blurred vision, decreased vision, pain, excessive tearing, photophobia
Respiratory—presence and quality of cough, sputum production, dyspnea, shortness of breath, smoking history
Cardiovascular—history of murmurs, tachycardia, and extra heart sounds

Physical Assessment. The spinal assessment is often normal early in the disease, or there can be tenderness with deep palpation of the sacroiliac joints. As the disease progresses into the upper spinal segments, loss of the normal lumbar lordosis occurs, followed by decreased flexion, extension, and lateral movement. Asking the client to flex at the waist and observing the flattening of the lumbar spine can assess loss of lumbar lordosis. Tenderness along vertebral structures and marked paravertebral spasm can also be present with decreased lumbar lordosis.

A useful measure of lumbar flexion is the Schober test. With the client standing erect, the nurse makes a mark at the L5-S1 area and another mark 10 cm above it. When the client bends forward in maximal flexion, the distance between the two marks normally should increase to 15 cm (Koerner & Dickinson, 1983). In AS, however, this measurement does not significantly increase. The Schober test is most useful in evaluating young persons because spinal flexion generally decreases with age. An alternative technique to screen for AS is to measure the distance from fingers to floor when the client attempts to touch the toes. Persons with decreased flexion have a greater distance between their fingers and the floor.

The tendency to develop a kyphotic posture in AS is reflected in diminished thoracic expansion. Placing the tapeline at the nipples and then noting the chest measurement with full lung expansion assesses chest expansion. A distance of less than 3 cm, along with other physical signs, is highly suggestive of AS (Arnett, 1984).

As the disease progresses, loss of ROM in the neck leads to a fixed kyphosis that can seriously impair visual function. The serial tracking of measurements of the distance from the client's head to the wall can be used to detect the progression of cervical kyphosis (Arnett, 1984). Positioning the client with the heels against the wall and instructing him or her to extend the neck fully can obtain consistent results.

Clients with AS should also be assessed for two other musculoskeletal changes. The first change is the development of an inflammatory peripheral joint involvement, particularly of the hips, knees, and shoulders. These joints must be assessed bilaterally for changes in ROM, pain, tenderness, and synovitis. Also, the nurse should observe for signs of enthesitis, a problem commonly seen in juvenile AS and occasionally seen in adults. Enthesitis can involve the plantar aspect of the foot (plantar fasciitis), the heel (Achilles tendinitis), and the knee. Other sites include the greater trochanters, superior anterior iliac crests, and ischial tuberosities (Petty & Malleson, 1986). Attachment sites may or may not be swollen, but they are typically extremely painful to palpation.

Because of the potential for developing extraskeletal problems with the eyes, lungs, and heart, these systems should be assessed carefully during the baseline screening. The eyes should be examined for signs of uveitis: edema of the upper lid, excessive lacrimation, small irregular pupil, and swollen iris. The lungs should be assessed for the type and quality of breath sounds. Any cough, sputum production, and dyspnea, which are typically seen in pulmonary fibrosis, should be noted. Also, the nurse should determine whether the client breathes abdominally or diaphragmatically. With pulmonary involvement, diaphragmatic breathing is commonly used to maintain adequate ventilation despite a rigid chest wall.

Heart sounds should be carefully auscultated for the presence of diastolic murmurs associated with aortic insufficiency. The nurse should screen for relatively high-pitched blowing murmurs, which occur as the client leans forward and holds the breath in expiration, by listening at the aortic area and down the left sternal border to the apex.

Diagnostic Evaluation. The diagnosis of AS is based on the results of the history, physical examination, and radiologic findings. Positive physical examination findings include the presence of sacroiliitis, spinal muscle spasms, and decreased hip mobility. Decreased chest expansion is seen later in the disease.

Along with symptomatic sacroiliitis, radiologic confirmation of sacroiliac joint changes is probably the most important finding (Calin, 1986). A scale from 0 to IV is used to rate the degree of joint distortion seen on x-ray film. In many clients, the disease does not progress beyond stage II or III (Calin, 1988). Early in the disease, x-ray films may show no abnormalities, but later, the typical changes of sacroiliitis develop, with patchy sclerosis at the joint margins. Early changes in AS include a squaring off of the anterior lumbar vertebral surfaces. This squaring is caused by erosion of the upper and lower margins of the vertebrae at the site of insertion of the annulus fibrosus. The intervertebral ligaments involved in the inflammatory process heal by ossification, leading to the formation of syndesmophytes in the outer layers of the annulus fibrosus. Eventually, the disc space becomes bridged by these bony syndesmophytes. In end-stage disease, complete spinal fusion (bamboo spine) and fusion of the sacroiliac joints occur along with ossification of all of the ligamentous structures (Shipley, 1985).

Generally, laboratory studies are not helpful in diagnosing AS. Although the HLA-B27 antigen is seen in 90% of clients with AS, it is found in up to 10% of those without the disease, thus limiting its specificity in diagnosis. An elevated ESR is seen in most clients, but it may be normal in those with severe disease. Other findings may include an elevated CK and alkaline phosphatase level, but these are not confirming diagnostic tests (Calin, 1986).

Collaborative Treatment. The treatment goals for AS are to maintain mobility, decrease inflammation, and control pain. As with other chronic conditions, treatment is more successful when clients are engaged in and assume responsibility for health promotion and other self-care activities. Collaborative treatment plans involving the client, physician, and nurse are more successful when the cornerstone is client education. Key concepts in the education of persons with AS are outlined in Table 14–19.

Instructing the client to perform appropriate exercises and to engage in ADLs is critical if he or she is to maintain mobility with minimal spinal curvature. Good posture must be encouraged through exercises that promote stretching and extension of the spine. Swimming is an excellent general conditioner, as is any activity that promotes spinal extension without increased pain. The nurse may need to help the client solve problems about awkward furniture or equipment that reinforces spinal flexion. For example, the client who has a desk job may need to invest in a tilting artist's table so the neck and head are not forced into flexion with constant activity. Selecting ergonomic chairs or ensuring the correct placement of a computer workstation can also be beneficial for the client's comfort. Appropriate sleep posture must be reinforced, particularly in those with mild cervical flexion who are accustomed to sleeping with two pillows. Spinal extension is maximized during sleep if

TABLE 14–19. *Client Education: Ankylosing Spondylitis*

FOCUS	TEACHING POINTS
Impaired mobility	Teach purpose and rationale for ROM and specific therapeutic exercises
Altered comfort	Explain purpose, action, and side effects of prescribed medications
	Instruct client in benefits of alternating periods of rest with periods of activity
	Teach nonpharmacologic pain management strategies: distraction, relaxation, and visualization
Health promotion	Teach benefits of health promotion activities: weight reduction or stabilization, smoking cessation
Avoidance of injury	Teach clients with cervical involvement to keep head erect so if cervical fusion occurs, anterior vision is maintained

clients lie on a firm mattress, preferably with bed boards underneath, in a supine position without a pillow. If the client insists on using a pillow, it should be as flat as possible.

As with many other chronic arthritic conditions, successful pain management depends on reducing inflammation and stiffness. NSAIDs are used to reduce inflammation, and the application of heat (or a warm shower or bath) helps relieve morning pain and stiffness. Dougados and colleagues (1995) found sulfasalazine to be effective in the treatment of active spondyloarthropathy. Methotrexate has also shown beneficial effects in the treatment of severe AS but is not considered standard drug therapy (Creemers, Franssen, van de Putte, Gribnau, & van Riel, 1995).

Nursing Management

Body Image Disturbance, Self-esteem Disturbance, Ineffective Coping, Impaired Gas Exchange

Body Image Enhancement, Self-esteem Enhancement, Coping Support, Airway Management. The nurse plays a key role in educating the client about health-promoting activities, exercise, and the management of pain. One of the most critical areas for skillful nursing intervention involves being attentive to and providing positive, unconditional regard for those persons with changing appearances. If the disease progresses rapidly or if the client has not sought help until skeletal changes are noticeable, he or she may be self-conscious and even depressed about the appearance. Businessmen may have found it increasingly more difficult to find clothing that fits. Some men have been known to avoid buying suits because of their embarrassment about being seen by salespersons or tailors. The client may be so concerned about appearance that he or she avoids social interaction outside of the job. Helping clients who have an altered body image or who are socially isolated is a significant challenge and an opportunity to establish a meaningful, therapeutic relationship. Although specific nursing interventions can be implemented that encourage group participation and interaction, it is often the nurse's positive, unconditional regard that helps the client work toward reintegration of the self. Approximately one third of clients experience depression, and women report more depression than men (Barlow, Macey, & Struthers, 1993).

Another important area for nursing intervention, especially as the disease progresses, is the maintenance of effective breathing patterns and adequate oxygenation. Ongoing assessment of chest wall expansion, instructions in deep-breathing exercises, and the avoidance of smoking and respiratory depressants can help the client maintain optimal breathing. If dyspnea becomes a problem, the nurse should instruct the client in pursed-lip breathing and pacing of activities. For clients with cervical involvement who become acutely ill or require surgery, the anesthesia department must be notified. AS in the cervical area often causes problems with intubation.

Reactive Arthritis (Reiter's Syndrome)

Reactive arthritis and *Reiter's syndrome* are both designations for a form of peripheral arthritis, often accompanied by one or more extra-articular manifestations, which appear shortly after certain infections of the genitourinary or gastrointestinal tracts. Most affected individuals, usually young men, have inherited HLA-B27. Reiter's syndrome originally referred to the clinical triad on nongonococcal urethritis, conjunctivitis, and arthritis that occurred in a young German officer after a bout of bloody dysentery and reported by Hans Reiter in 1916. Because of many overlapping clinical, epidemiologic, and genetic features, reactive arthritis is classified as a seronegative spondyloarthropathy. Box 14-6 lists the current defining characteristics of reactive arthritis. Approxi-

---

BOX 14–6.
Defining Characteristics of Reiter's Syndrome

Seronegative asymmetrical arthropathy (predominantly of the lower extremity)
Plus one or more of the following:
  Urethritis/cervicitis
  Dysentery
  Inflammatory eye disease
  Mucocutaneous disease: balanitis, oral ulceration, or keratoderma

Adapted from Kelley, W., Harris, E., Ruddy, S., & Sledge, C. (1989). *Textbook of rheumatology* (3rd ed., p. 1038). Philadelphia: WB Saunders.

---

mately 80% of clients experience chronic problems marked by periods of remission and exacerbation (Arnett, 1997).

Epidemiology. Reactive arthritis occurs after exposure to a bacterial gastrointestinal or genitourinary infection. Although the exact mechanism remains unclear, certain infective agents and a specific genetic background, HLA-B27, are associated with reactive arthritis. Epidemic reactive arthritis has occurred in association with dysentery. Endemic or postvenereal reactive arthritis is the more common type found in the United States.

Endemic reactive arthritis occurs more commonly in young men (9:1) and is linked to the greater prevalence of HLA-B27 antigen in this population. Cases following food-borne enteric infections affect both genders equally. Whites are affected more commonly than African Americans or other racial groups who have a lower frequency of HLA-B27 (Arnett, 1997). Reactive arthritis is difficult to diagnose and probably occurs more often than reported.

Pathophysiology and Symptoms. Reactive arthritis demonstrates features in almost every system of the body, the most common of which are polyarthritis and urethritis or cervicitis and conjunctivitis.

There is a link between the genitourinary system and reactive arthritis. Urethritis can occur symptomatically (discharge, slight burning on urination) or can be asymptomatic, which is a component in the difficulty in establishing a diagnosis. Reactive arthritis has been reported often in clients with human immunodeficiency virus (HIV) infection. There is a high incidence of prostatitis and acquired immunodeficiency syndrome (AIDS). The role of AIDS in the pathogenesis of reactive arthritis is still being investigated (Altman, Centeno, Mahal, & Bielory, 1994). Urethral infection is commonly accompanied by stomatitis, balanitis, and keratoderma blennorrhagicum. The keratodermal lesions are similar to psoriatic lesions and can appear on the soles of the feet, glans penis, and toes.

Conjunctivitis, considered a classic symptom, is typically a transient, mild phenomenon. If a sterile discharge is present, it subsides within a few days. Uveitis can become a more significant clinical problem in this disorder.

Reactive arthritis is characteristically additive, asymmetrical, and oligoarticular, affecting an average of four joints. The arthritic process generally affects weight-bearing joints, especially of the knees and ankles. Large effusions can accompany it. A sausage toe represents a typical lesion (Fig. 14–15).

Assessment. The history should examine the pattern of orthopaedic pain. Joint pain, back pain, heel pain, and a tendinitis-type pain can manifest in reactive arthritis. Clients with a nonspecific arthritis should be

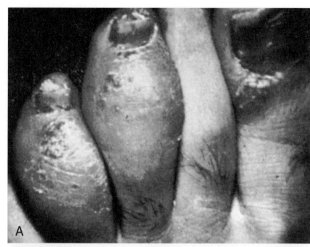

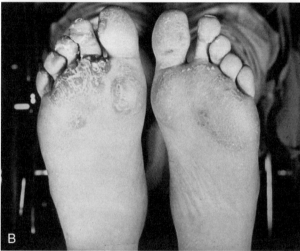

FIGURE 14–15. *A,* Reiter's syndrome. Note the two sausage digits (dactylitis) and the typical nail changes. *B,* Skin on feet also can change. (*A,* From Kelley, W., Harris, E., Ruddy, S., & Sledge, C. [Eds.]. [1989]. *Textbook of rheumatology* [3rd ed., p. 1043]. Philadelphia: WB Saunders.)

questioned about the presence of genitourinary and ocular symptoms. The client should be questioned about any atypical urethral discharge or slight pain or burning on urination for even a few days. An examination of past history of sexually transmitted diseases is important, as is the sexual history in relation to number and frequency of sexual partners. The client should be interviewed for the presence of eye disease. History of recent eye irritation, perhaps attributed to smog or other chemical irritants, should be elicited. The client may have noted dermatologic lesions. The nurse should ask the client about any lesions for which he or she may have used a corticosteroid cream and ask the client about any other vesicle-type lesions.

Physical examination targets the involved joints (see discussions on RA [pp. 353–380] and AS [pp. 409–413]) and inspects for dermatologic lesions and the presence of localized infections.

Diagnostic workup includes x-ray films and laboratory examinations. Early in the disease, there are no radiographic changes. With disease progression, joint-space narrowing and erosive changes can be seen. In advanced disease, the individual may develop sacroiliitis, as found in AS.

Laboratory findings may show an elevated ESR, but the ESR may be normal despite active joint involvement. Mild hypochromic or normochromic anemia may be present. Routine typing for HLA-B27 is unnecessary.

Treatment. Reactive arthritis usually runs a self-limited course of 3 to 12 months in most clients; however, some studies suggest that many clients continue to be plagued by minor musculoskeletal symptoms (Thompson, DeRubeis, Hodge, Rajanayagam, & Inman, 1995). Management of the client targets client education and symptomatic management of symptoms.

Pharmacologic Management. Pharmacologic management is similar to that used for AS. The attacks tend to be self-limiting, lasting 2 to 4 months, with a recurrence rate of 15% per year (Kottke, Stillwell, & Lehmann, 1990).

The use of antibiotic therapy in the prevention or management of reactive arthritis remains controversial. Bardin, Enel, Cornelius, Salski, Jorgensen, Ward, and Lathrop (1992), in a retrospective analysis of 109 clients to determine the efficacy of tetracycline or erythromycin therapy on urethritis, found that only 10% of the sample treated with tetracycline or erythromycin developed a recurrence of articular symptoms, whereas 37% of those who were not treated or were treated with penicillin experienced a recurrence. Other studies have shown that antibiotic therapy did not influence the development of recurrences.

For clients with ocular symptoms, steroid eyedrops or subconjunctival preparations may be needed. Severe uveitis is relatively common and is a difficult clinical management problem.

Small numbers of clients (less than 12) have limited clinical trials in the management of reactive arthritis. Larger randomized, controlled trials are needed.

Physical Therapy. Joint pain and dysfunction are managed with a regimen of physical therapy. Splinting for joint protection along with a managed exercise and activity program are indicated. (See discussion of RA [pp. 353–380] and Chapter 13.)

Client Education. As with any chronic disease, client education plays a crucial role in helping the individual understand and manage the disease. Similar to RA (see prior discussion), clients and their families need information about the disease process and management.

Because of the link to genitourinary pathology, education must target "safe" sexual practices. There is some evidence that use of a condom protects the client from postvenereal exacerbation of reactive arthritis. Clients are advised to avoid multiple sexual partners (Kelley, Harris, Ruddy, & Sledge, 1993).

There is a general recognition that reactive arthritis has a greater propensity for chronicity than previously appreciated, which should temper an overly optimistic prognosis. One study reported that at 1 year, 40% of clients with post–genitourinary-acquired reactive arthritis and 20% of post–gastrointestinal-acquired reactive arthritis still had active disease, but almost all had recovered at 2-year follow-up (Glennas, Kvien, Melby, Overboo, Andrup, Karstensen, & Thoen, 1994).

BURSITIS

Bursitis is a painful inflammation of the bursae, those closed, minimally fluid-filled sacs that are lined with a synovium similar to the lining of joint spaces (Mooar, 1989). The purpose of bursae is to reduce friction between adjacent tissues—tendon and bones or tendons and ligaments—by lubricating these enclosed structures with synovial fluid from the bursal sac. Reilly and Nicholas (1987) identified approximately 150 bursae in the body that typically cover bony prominences, such as the olecranon, trochanter, or patella, or that provide protection between the skin and other structures, such as the calcaneal bursa. They are usually quite thin, but with repeated stress, they can become thickened and filled with fluid secondary to inflammation. Bursitis can be either an acute or a chronic condition.

Epidemiology

It is estimated that approximately 3% of the adult population has painful, symptomatic bursitis (Hollander, 1984). The problem peaks between the ages of 40 and 50, presumably as active adults first experience the beginning of degenerative changes in the joints. However, bursitis is often present in younger adults who are active in sports. The shoulder joint is the most commonly affected, followed by the elbow, knee, and hips. When bursitis involves the upper extremities, the dominant arm is usually affected.

Risk factors associated with the development of bursitis include acute or chronic trauma, typically through participation in mechanical, highly repetitive activities. Other causes include such arthritic conditions as RA, gout, tumors, and degenerative changes associated with increasing age.

Pathophysiology

The inflammation of bursitis usually results from constant friction between the skin and the musculoskeletal tissues around the joint. Generally, it involves sterile or aseptic joint fluid without the introduction of pathogenic organisms. The area around the bursa becomes exqui-

sitely tender, and motion is partially or greatly limited by the swollen, enlarged sac. Tendinitis can be associated with the bursitis, particularly in the shoulder joint.

Bursitis is considered a true inflammatory condition with the classic signs of inflammation, local redness, warmth, and swelling. Microscopic examination may show evidence of edema formation, blood vessel dilation, and inflammatory blood cell infiltration. Obvious cases of inflammation may indicate invasion by bacterial, viral, or fungal agents and thus require appropriate antimicrobial therapy.

Assessment

Typically, the client with acute bursitis complains of exquisite localized pain in the target area. Clients may experience point tenderness; that is, they can point specifically to the spot of greatest discomfort. They may also have diffuse soreness radiating to the tendons at the site. Depending on the location of the bursitis, clients may complain of interrupted sleep (e.g., with subacromial bursitis, calcaneal bursitis), difficulty walking (trochanteric bursitis, calcaneal bursitis), or difficulty performing ADLs (subacromial or olecranon bursitis).

Occupational or avocational activities can also provide insight into the nature of the pain, for example, a woodcarver who has developed acute subacromial bursitis or a businesswoman who walks long distances in medium to high heels. With acute bursitis, clients may be able to identify a specific precipitating event. Clients with chronic bursitis should be asked about the characteristics of previous episodes as well as associated activities or trauma and changes in ROM or muscle strength.

On physical examination, the involved joint in acute bursitis is swollen, warm, tender, and often boggy in consistency (Fig. 14–16). In contrast to the more general tenderness of the rheumatoid joint, the hallmark of bursitis is a localized "trigger-point" tenderness over the involved bursae. At rest, the joint is relatively free of pain, whereas with active motion, the client experiences increased pain, which can radiate to the entire extremity.

With chronic bursitis, joints continue to show signs of swelling, tenderness, and limited ROM because of thickening of the bursal wall, the possible development of adhesions, and increased calcium deposits. Muscle atrophy and weakness, along with an easily palpable, thickened synovial wall, are more apparent in chronic bursitis than they are in the acute type.

Diagnosis and Treatment

The diagnosis of bursitis is generally based on the results of the history and physical examination. Radiographs of the affected joint are usually normal in acute bursitis, whereas in chronic conditions, calcium deposits may be present. Results of laboratory tests and synovial fluid analysis are normal unless the bursa has become infected.

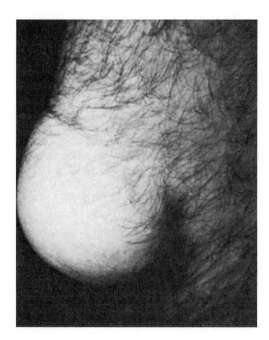

FIGURE 14–16. Distended olecranon bursa. (From Gartland, J. [1986]. *Fundamentals of orthopaedics* [4th ed., p. 146]. Philadelphia: WB Saunders.)

Acute bursitis is treated with rest and immobilization of the affected joint, non-narcotic analgesics, and ROM exercises. In general, the pain of acute bursitis is controlled with NSAIDs. If the condition is treated immediately, intermittent ice applications for up to 48 hours are helpful, just as they are in acute sports injuries. Otherwise, clients are instructed to apply moist heat to the affected joint every 4 hours for 48 hours and to rest or immobilize the joint (with a sling or an elastic bandage, as needed) until pain and muscle spasms subside. Usually, the client is able to begin ROM exercises to maintain or regain motion within 48 hours of the onset of the problem. Client education focuses on the causes of bursitis, the prevention of additional attacks (by avoiding activities that cause constant friction or pressure), the correct application of moist heat, and medication and exercise instruction.

Several types of acute bursitis (subacromial, prepatellar, and trochanteric) also respond well to intra-articular injections of corticosteroids. Bursae are usually injected with 0.5 to 1 mL of hydrocortisone acetate (12.5 to 25 mg) or an equivalent dose of other injectable steroids. Occasionally, clients can develop postinjection flare following intra-articular injections, a condition characterized by erythema, swelling, and tenderness. Postinjection flare can appear a few hours after the injection is given and last up to 2 days. The condition readily responds to the administration of ice packs.

Although the most effective treatment of chronic bursitis is its prevention by avoiding repetitive activities, the chronic type is associated with factors that may be difficult to control. Sudden trauma, infection, and calcium deposits, along with increased age and other chronic conditions, may contribute to the chronicity of bursitis. Treatment includes intra-articular injections of corticosteroids along with rest, immobilization, and therapeutic exercises. Surgery is indicated when calcified deposits or adhesions have significantly impaired the client's function.

Nursing Care

Alteration in Comfort, Impaired Physical Mobility, Temporary Self-care Deficits

Pain Management, Splinting, Medication Administration, and Exercise Therapy: Joint, Work Simplification. Appropriate nursing diagnoses for clients with bursitis include alteration in comfort (acute or chronic pain), impaired physical mobility, and temporary self-care deficits.

Helping clients obtain pain relief is the primary focus of nursing interventions. Without pain relief, joint mobility is impaired through frozen, protective measures. Nurses must instruct clients about the purpose of anti-inflammatory medications as well as the appropriate dose and untoward side effects.

Pain relief is also achieved by resting or immobilizing the joint or by elevating or compressing the involved area to control edema. Teaching clients about the correct application of ice and heat is important so that they receive maximum pain relief. If clients receive intra-articular injections of cortisone, they should be informed about the possibility of a postinjection flare. They should also be reassured that the pain responds quickly to the application of ice packs.

Clients with acute bursitis can easily develop a chronic condition if they do not use the joint after the pain subsides or if they overstress the joint. Exploring their typical daily chores, work, and leisure activities can help identify potentially harmful movements. Suggestions about work simplification techniques, along with appropriate ROM exercises, can help clients regain normal motion in the affected joint.

For athletes or clients who exercise regularly, preliminary stretching, gentle warm-up exercises, and alternate exercises during recovery are strongly encouraged (Cunningham, 1994).

Self-care deficits are usually temporary in acute bursitis. If the condition becomes chronic, clients may experience more difficulties, particularly if the shoulder or elbow is involved. Dressing is easier if oversized garments are worn, especially those with long sleeves or wide pant legs. Shirts and tops that button in the front are also helpful. Clients can be taught to minimize shoulder or elbow pain by putting clothing on the affected arm first and by taking it off the affected arm last.

SUMMARY

Nursing clients with autoimmune or inflammatory disorders that affect the muscles and joints can prove to be a complex and challenging process. Clients can experience acute exacerbations or crises with almost all of these diseases. Systemic manifestations can be as devastating as the musculoskeletal symptoms. The unpredictable nature of these disorders results in considerable uncertainty, which leads to a cycle of ineffective coping, disturbed self-esteem, helplessness, and powerlessness. In many respects, the psychological and social problems associated with these chronic illnesses are more disabling than the physical complaints.

Physiologically, clients with autoimmune or inflammatory joint disorders experience many common problems. The triad of pain, fatigue, and stiffness must be controlled so that function is enhanced or maintained. If this triad, which represents a runaway inflammatory response, is not held in check, essential self-care deficits develop. Difficulty with self-care is usually accompanied by sleep disturbances, altered nutrition, and impaired mobility. All of these problems can adversely affect the individual's self-concept and self-esteem and therefore may lead to social isolation.

Because of the chronicity of these disorders, clients need skilled, knowledgeable nursing care that draws on the disciplines of rehabilitation, counseling, and self-care. The unique role of the nurse for clients with autoimmune or inflammatory diseases is one that assumes accountability and responsibility for guiding and directing the client through the health care maze. Clients with chronic, usually systemic, illnesses require multiple therapies and follow-up appointments for pharmacologic management, nutritional counseling, lifestyle assessment, physical and occupational therapy, and psychological support, to name just a few. The personal and financial cost demanded by the arthritic disorder can exhaust the client's enthusiasm, job security, support systems, and sense of purpose in life. The nurse can provide a sense of consistency, hope, and reassurance that the client can learn to cope with, and positively adapt to, the demands of a chronic illness. Clients with arthritis need the nurse's expertise to teach them how to explore new self-care strategies so that successful adaptation to the disease is a reality. Nurses help clients learn to become partners with the entire health care team as well as with themselves. When clients assume the role of partner, they exhibit greater control, greater accountability, and increased self-esteem as they learn self-management skills. This is nowhere more self-evident than the clients giving themselves their biweekly or daily injections.

Outcomes in autoimmune and inflammatory disease are difficult to predict. The risk factors for poor outcomes in RA are known: high titer RF, nodules, early erosions, shared epitopes HLA-DRB1, educational level, and functional status. It is important to remember that clinical disease does not always correlate with radiographic progression.

Treatment protocols for these disorders, especially those in which clients have early, active disease, are more aggressive than they have ever been. Joint function is more effectively preserved when the disorders are treated early and inflammation is modulated. Treatment in the 21st century is aimed at early, aggressive, and targeted intervention. These new treatments are expensive, but the long-term cost to the client is even higher.

The studies referred to in this chapter point to the necessity for early diagnosis and treatment. It is becoming possible to achieve effective outcomes, slowing the progression of the disease. The costs of these new treatments outweigh the costs of the diseases.

INTERNET RESOURCES

Arthritis Foundation: www.arthritis.org/
Lupus Foundation of America: www.lupus.org/
National Databank for Rheumatic Diseases: www.fibromyalgia.org
Rheumatology Resources: www.rheumatology.org
Scleroderma Foundation: www.scleroderma.org/
Sjögren's Syndrome Foundation: www.sjogrens.org/

REFERENCES

Aho, K., von Essen, R., Kurki, P., Palosuo, T., & Heliovaara, M. (1993). Antikeratin antibody and antiperinuclear factor as markers for subclinical rheumatoid disease process. *Journal of Rheumatology, 20,* 1278–1281.

Airio, A., Puklaala, E., & Isomaki, A. (1995). Elevated cancer incidence in clients with dermatomyositis: a population based study. *Journal of Rheumatology, 22,* 1400–1403.

Alarcon, G. S., Tracy, I. C., & Blackburn, W. D. (1989). Methotrexate in rheumatoid arthritis: Toxic effects as the major factor in limiting long-term treatment. *Arthritis and Rheumatism, 32,* 671–676.

Alarcon-Segovia, D. (1988). Systemic lupus erythematosus: Pathology and pathogenesis. In H. R. Schumacher (Ed.), *Primer on the rheumatic diseases* (9th ed., pp. 96–100). Atlanta: Arthritis Foundation.

Altman, E. M., Centeno, L. V., Mahal, M., & Bielory, L. (1994). AIDS-associated Reiter's syndrome. *Annals of Allergy, 72,* 307–316.

American College of Rheumatology Task Force on Osteoporosis Guidelines. (1996). Recommendations for the prevention and treatment of glucocorticoids-induced osteoporosis. *Arthritis and Rheumatism, 39,* 1791–1801.

American Nurses Association and Arthritis Health Professions Association. (1983). *Outcome standards for rheumatology nursing practice.* Kansas City, MO: American Nurses Association.

Anaya, J. M., Diethelm, L., Ortiz, L. A., Gutierrez, M., Citera, G., Welsh, R. A., & Espinoza, L. R. (1995). Pulmonary involvement in rheumatoid arthritis. *Seminars in Arthritis and Rheumatism, 24,* 242–254.

Ansell, B. M. (1984). Management of polymyositis and dermatomyositis. *Clinical Rheumatology Disease, 10,* 205–214.

Ansell, B. M., & Swann, M. (1983). The management of chronic arthritis of children. *Journal of Bone and Joint Surgery, 65B,* 536–543.

Arnett, F. C. (1997). Reactive arthritis (Reiter's syndrome). In H. R. Schumacher (Ed.), *Primer on the rheumatic diseases* (9th ed., pp. 184–188). Atlanta: Arthritis Foundation.

Arnett, F. C. (1987). Seronegative spondyloarthropathies. *Bulletin on the Rheumatic Diseases, 37,* 1–6.

Arnett, F. C. (1984). Spondyloarthropathies. In G. K. Riggs & E. P. Gall (Eds.), *Rheumatic diseases: Rehabilitation and management* (pp. 429–437). Boston: Butterworth.

Arnett, F. C., Edworthy, S. M., Bloch, D. A., McShane, D. J., Fries, J. F., Cooper, N. S., Healey, L. A., Kaplan, S. R., Liang, M. H., Luthra, H. S., Medsger, T. A., Mitchell, D. M., Nenstadt, D. H., Pinals, R. S., Schaller, J. G., Sharp, J. T., Wilder, R. L., & Hunder, G. C. (1988). The American Rheumatism Association 1987 revised criteria for the classification of rheumatoid arthritis. *Arthritis and Rheumatism, 31,* 315–324.

Aventis Pharmaceuticals. (2000). *Leflunomide full prescribing information.*

Baer, A. N., Dessypris, E. N., & Krantz, S. B. (1990). The pathogenesis of anemia in rheumatoid arthritis: A clinical and laboratory analysis. *Seminars in Arthritis and Rheumatism, 19,* 209–214.

Banerjee, S., Webber, C., & Poole, A. R. (1992). The induction of arthritis in mice by the cartilage proteoglycan aggregen: Roles of CD4+ and CD8+ T cells. *Cellular Immunology, 144,* 347–357.

Banwell, B. F. (1984). Exercise and mobility in arthritis. *Nursing Clinics of North America, 19,* 605–616.

Bardin, T., Enel, C., Cornelius, F., Salski, C., Jorgensen, C., Ward, R., & Lathrop, G. M. (1992). Antibiotic treatment of venereal disease and Reiter's syndrome. *Arthritis and Rheumatism, 35,* 190–194.

Barlow, J. H., Macey, S. J., & Struthers, G. R. (1993). Gender, depression, and ankylosing spondylitis. *Arthritis Care and Research, 6,* 45–51.

Bellamy, N., & Bradley, L. A. (1996). Workshop on chronic pain, pain control, and client outcomes in rheumatoid arthritis and osteoarthritis. *Arthritis and Rheumatism, 39,* 357–362.

Bennett, J. C. (1988). Rheumatoid arthritis: Clinical features. In H. R. Schumacher (Ed.), *Primer on the rheumatic diseases* (9th ed., pp. 97–92). Atlanta: Arthritis Foundation.

Bertsch, C. (1995). CREST syndrome: A variant of systemic sclerosis. *Orthopaedic Nursing, 14*(2), 53–60.

Boerbooms, A. M., Kerstens, P. J., van Loenhout, J. W., Mulder, J., & van de Putte, L. B. (1995). Infections during low-dose methotrexate treatment in rheumatoid arthritis. *Seminars in Arthritis and Rheumatism, 24,* 411–421.

Boers, M., Verhoeven, A. C., Markusse, H. M., et al. (1997). Randomized comparison of combined step-down prednisolone, methotrexate and sulphasalazine alone in early rheumatoid arthritis. *Lancet, 350,* 309–318.

Bohan, B., & Peter, J. B. (1975). Polymyositis and dermatomyositis. *New England Journal of Medicine, 292,* 344–347, 403–407.

Bunyon, J. P., & Zuckerman, J. D. (1987). Articular manifestations of systemic lupus erythematosus. In R. G. Lahita (Ed.), *Systemic lupus erythematosus.* New York: Wiley.

Buyon, J. P. (1994). Neonatal lupus syndromes. *Current Opinions in Rheumatology, 6,* 523–529.

Calin, A. (1986). Seronegative spondyloarthritides. *Medical Clinics of North America, 70,* 323–336.

Calin, A. (1988). Ankylosing spondylitis and the spondyloarthropathies. In H. R. Schumacher (Ed.), *Primer on the rheumatic diseases* (9th ed., pp. 142–147). Atlanta: Arthritis Foundation.

Callahan, L. F., & Pincus, T. (1995). Mortality in the rheumatic diseases. *Arthritis Care and Research, 8,* 229–241.

Caro, I. (1989). Dermatomyositis as a systemic disease. *Medical Clinics of North America, 73,* 1181–1192.

Cash, J. M., & Klippel, J. H. (1994). Second-line antirheumatic drugs for rheumatoid arthritis. *New England Journal of Medicine, 330,* 1468–1477.

Cassidy, J., & Petty, R. (1995). *Textbook of pediatric rheumatology* (3rd ed.). Philadelphia: WB Saunders.

Cave, L. (1984). Lowering the uncertainties of arthritis with a nurse-led support group. *Orthopaedic Nursing, 3,* 39–42.

Ceccio, C. M. (1985). *A taped relaxation/imagery exercise in elderly clients with rheumatoid arthritis.* Unpublished study.

Cella, J. H., & Watson, J. (1989). *Nurse's manual of laboratory tests.* Philadelphia: FA Davis.

Chan, K. W., Felson, D. T., Yood, R. A., & Walker, A. M. (1993). Incidence of rheumatoid arthritis in central Massachusetts. *Arthritis and Rheumatology, 36,* 1691–1696.

Chou, C. T., Pei, L., Chang, D. M., Lee, C. F., Schumacher, H. R., & Liang, M. H. (1994). Prevalence of rheumatic disease in Taiwan: A population study of urban, suburban, rural differences. *Journal of Rheumatology, 21,* 302–306.

Chu, C. Q., Field, M., Feldmann, M., & Maini, R. N. (1991). Localization of tumor necrosis factor in synovial tissues and at the cartilage-pannus junction in patients with rheumatoid arthritis. *Arthritis and Rheumatism, 34,* 1125–1132.

Cohen, S., Weaver, A., Schiff, M., & Strand, V. (1999). For the leflunomide study group. Two-year treatment of active rheumatoid arthritis with leflunomide compared with placebo. *Arthritis and Rheumatism. 42,* S271.

Conn, V. S. (1990). Joint self-care by older adults. *Rehabilitation Nursing, 15,* 182–186.

Creemers, M. C., Franssen, M. J., van de Putte, L. B., Gribnau, F. W., & van Riel, P. L. (1995). Methotrexate in severe ankylosing spondylitis: An open study. *Journal of Rheumatology, 22,* 1104–1107.

Cronin, M. E., Miller, F. W., & Plotz, P. H. (1988). Polymyositis and dermatomyositis. In H. R. Schumacher (Ed.), *Primer on the rheumatic diseases* (9th ed., pp. 120–123). Atlanta: Arthritis Foundation.

Cuellar, M. L., Silverira, L. H., & Espinoza, L. R. (1994). Recent developments in psoriatic arthritis. *Current Opinions in Rheumatology, 6,* 378–384.

Cunningham, M. E. (1994). Bursitis and tendonitis. *Orthopaedic Nursing, 14*(5), 14–16, 70.

Cush, J. J., & Lipsky, P. E. (1991). Cellular basis for rheumatoid inflammation. *Clinical Orthopedics and Related Research, 265,* 9–19.

Dinant, H. J., Mueller, W. H., van den BergLoonen, E. M., Nijenhuis, L. E., & Engelfriet, C. P. (1980). HLA-DRW in Felty's syndrome. *Arthritis and Rheumatism, 23,* 1436.

Dougados, M., vam der Linden, S., Leirisalo-Repo, M., Huitfeldt, B., Juhlin, R., Veys, E., Zeidler, H., Kvien, T. K., Olivieri, I., & Dijkmans, B. (1995). Sulfasalazine in the treatment of spondyloarthropathy. A randomized, multicenter, double-blind, placebo-controlled study. *Arthritis and Rheumatism, 38,* 618–627.

Downe-Wamboldt, B. L., & Melanson, P. M. (1995). Emotions, coping, and psychological well-being in elderly people with arthritis. *Western Journal of Nursing Research, 17,* 250–265.

Dybwad, A., Forre, O., Natvig, J. B., & Sioud, M. (1995). Structural characterization of peptides that bind synovial fluid antibodies from RA clients: A novel strategy for identification of disease-related epitopes using a random peptide library. *Clinical Immunology and Immunopathology, 75,* 45–50.

Eberhardt, K., Grubb, R., Johnson, V., & Petersson, H. (1993). HLA-DR antigens, GM allotypes, and antiallotypes in early rheumatoid arthritis—Their relation to disease progression. *Journal of Rheumatology, 20,* 1825–1829.

Ellman, M. H., MacDonald, P. A., & Hayes, F. A. (2000). Etanercept as treatment for diffuse scleroderma: A pilot study. *Arthritis and Rheumatism, 43,* S392.

Felson, D. T., Anderson, J. J., Boers, M., Bombardier, C., Chernoff, M., Fried, B., Furst, D., Goldsmith, G., Kieszak, S., Lightfoot, R., Paulus, H., Tugwell, P., Weinblatt, M., Widmark, R., Williams, H. J., & Wolfe, F. (1993). American College of Rheumatology preliminary core set of disease' activity measures for rheumatoid arthritis clinical trials. The Committee on Outcome Measures in Rheumatoid Arthritis clinical trials. *Arthritis and Rheumatism, 36,* 729–740.

Felson, D. T., Anderson, J. J., Boers, M., Bombardier, C., Furst, D., Goldsmith, C. H., Katz, L. M., Lightfoot, R., Jr., Paulus, H., Strand, V., Tugwell, P. S. L., Weinblatt, M., Williams, H. J., Wolfe, F., & Kieszak, S. (1995). American College of Rheumatology preliminary definition of improvement in rheumatoid arthritis. *Arthritis and Rheumatism, 38,* 727–735.

Fife, R. Z. (1993). Methotrexate use in juvenile rheumatoid arthritis. *Orthopaedic Nursing, 12*(1), 32–36.

Fifield, J., Reisine, S., Sheehan, T. J., & McQuillan, J. (1996). Gender, paid work, and symptoms of emotional distress in rheumatoid arthritis clients. *Arthritis and Rheumatism, 39,* 427–435.

Fuchs, H. A., Kaye, J. J., Callahan, L. F., Nance, E. P., & Pincus, T. (1989). Evidence of significant radiographic damage in rheumatoid arthritis with the first 2 years of disease. *Journal of Rheumatology, 16,* 585–591.

Gabay, C., Roux-Lombard, P., de Moerloose, P., Dayer, J. M., Vischer, T., & Guerne, P. A. (1993). Absence of correlation between interleukin 6 and C-reactive protein blood levels in SLE compared with RA. *Journal of Rheumatology, 20,* 815–821.

Gates, S. J., & Mooar, P. A. (Eds.). (1989). *Orthopaedics and sports medicine for nurses: Common problems in management.* Baltimore: Williams & Wilkins.

Geirsson, H. A., Steinsson, K., Gudmundsson, F., & Sigurdson, V. (1994). Systemic sclerosis in Iceland: A nationwide epidemiological study. *Annals of Rheumatic Disease, 53,* 502–505.

Genovese, M., Martin., R., Fleischmann, R., et al. (2000). Enbrel (etanercept) vs. methotrexate (MTX) in early rheumatoid arthritis (ERA trial): Two-year follow-up. *Arthritis and Rheumatism, 43,* S269.

Glennas, A., Kvien, T., Melby, K., Overboo, A., Andrup, O., Karstensen, B., & Thoen, J. E. (1994). Reactive arthritis: A favorable 2-year course of outcome, independent of triggering agent and HLA B27. *Journal of Rheumatology, 21,* 2274–2280.

Gorman, T. K., & Marsh, M. E. (1984). Arthritis at an early age. *American Journal of Nursing, 84,* 1472–1477.

Grisanti, J. M., & Wilke, W. S. (1989). New drugs, new therapies for rheumatoid arthritis. *Consultant, 29,* 47–59.

Hackshaw, K. V., Shi, Y., Brandwein, S. R., Jones, K., & Westcott, J. Y. (1995). A pilot study of zileuton, a novel selective 5-lipoxygenase inhibitor, in patients with systemic lupus erythematosus. *Journal of Rheumatology, 22,* 462–468.

Halverson, P. (1995). Extraarticular manifestations of rheumatoid arthritis. *Orthopaedic Nursing, 14*(4), 47–50.

Halverson, P. B., & Holmes, S. B. (1992). Systemic lupus erythematosus: Medical and nursing treatments. *Orthopaedic Nursing, 11*(6), 17–24.

Hay, E. M., & Snaith, M. L. (1995, May). Systemic lupus erythematosus and lupus-like syndromes. *British Medical Journal, 310,* 1257–1261.

Hochberg, M. C. (1988). Epidemiology of the rheumatic diseases. In H. R. Schumacher (Ed.), *Primer on the rheumatic diseases* (9th ed., pp. 48–50). Atlanta: Arthritis Foundation.

Hochberg, M. C., Linet, M. S., & Sills, E. M. (1983). The prevalence and incidence of juvenile rheumatoid arthritis in an urban black population. *American Journal of Public Health, 73,* 1202–1203.

Hollander, J. L. (1984). Injection therapy. In G. K. Riggs & E. Gall (Eds.), *Rheumatic diseases: Rehabilitation and management* (pp. 199–203). Boston: Butterworth.

Ignatavicius, D. D. (1987). Meeting the psychosocial needs of clients with rheumatoid arthritis. *Orthopaedic Nursing, 6,* 16–20.

Iseki, K., Miyasato, F., Oura, T., Uehara, H., Nishime, K., & Fukiyama, K. (1994). An epidemiologic analysis of end-stage lupus nephritis. *American Journal of Kidney Disease, 23,* 547–554.

Jamieson, A. H., Alford, C. A., Bird, H. A., Hindmarch, I., & Wright, V. (1995). The effect of sleep and nocturnal movement on stiffness, pain, and psychomotor performance in ankylosing spondylitis. *Clinical and Experimental Rheumatology, 14*(1), 73–78.

Jarvinen, P. (1995). Occurrence of ankylosing spondylitis in a nationwide series of twins. *Arthritis and Rheumatism, 38,* 381–383.

Jiminez-Balderas, F. J., & Mintz, G. (1993). Ankylosing spondylitis: Clinical course in women and men. *Journal of Rheumatology, 20,* 2069–2072.

Johnson, J. A., & Repp, E. C. (1984). Nonpharmacologic pain management in arthritis. *Nursing Clinics of North America, 19,* 583–591.

Kaplan, D. (1984). The onset of disease in twins and siblings with systemic lupus erythematosus. *Journal of Rheumatology, 11,* 648–652.

Katz, P. P., & Yelin, E. N. (1993). Prevalence and correlates of depressive symptoms among persons with rheumatoid arthritis. *Journal of Rheumatology, 20,* 790–796.

Keefe, F. J., Brown, G. K., Wallston, K. A., & Caldwell, D. S. (1989). Coping with rheumatoid arthritis pain: Catastrophizing as a maladaptive strategy. *Pain, 37,* 51–56.

Kelley, W., Harris, E., Ruddy, S., & Sledge, C. (Eds.). (1993). *Textbook of rheumatology* (4th ed.). Philadelphia: WB Saunders.

Kelsey, J. L. (1982). Epidemiology of musculoskeletal disorders. In *Monographs in epidemiology and biostatistics* (Vol. 3). New York: Oxford University Press.

Kimberly, R. P. (1982). Pulse methylprednisolone in SLE. *Clinics in Rheumatic Diseases, 8,* 261–278.

Kirwan, J. R., & Arthritis and Rheumatism Council Low-Dose Glucocorticol Study Group. (1995). The effect of glucocorticoids on joint destruction in rheumatoid arthritis. *New England Journal of Medicine, 333,* 142–146.

Klippel, J. H. (1990). Systemic lupus erythematosus: Treatment-related complications superimposed on chronic disease. *Journal of the American Medical Association, 263,* 1812–1815.

Klippel, J. H. (1997). Systemic lupus erythematosus: Treatment. In J. H. Klippel (Ed.), *Primer on the rheumatic diseases* (11th ed., pp. 258–261). Atlanta: Arthritis Foundation.

Koch, B. (1985). Rehabilitation of the child with joint disease. In G. E. Molnar (Ed.), *Pediatric rehabilitation.* Baltimore: Williams & Wilkins.

Koerner, M. E., & Dickinson, G. R. (1983). Adult arthritis: A look at some of its forms. *American Journal of Nursing, 83,* 255–262.

Kottke, F. J., Stillwell, G. K., & Lehmann, J. F. (1990). *Krusen's handbook of physical medicine and rehabilitation* (4th ed.). Philadelphia: WB Saunders.

Kredich, D. W. (1986). Chronic arthritis in childhood. *Medical Clinics of North America, 70,* 305–321.

Kremer, J. M., Caldwell, J. R., Cannon, G. W., et al. (2000). The combination of leflunomide and methotrexate in clients with active rheumatoid arthritis who are failing on MTX alone: A double-blind placebo controlled study. *Arthritis and Rheumatism, 43,* Abstract 948.

Kremer, J. M., Weinblatt, M. E., Fleischmann, R. M., Bankhurst, A. D., & Burge, D. (2000). Etanercept (Enbrel) in addition to methotrexate in rheumatoid arthritis: long-term observations. *Arthritis and Rheumatism, 43,* S270.

Lang, B. A., Laxter, R. M., Murphy, G., Silverman, E. D., & Roifman, C. M. (1991). Treatment of dermatomyositis with intravenous gamma globulin. *American Journal of Medicine, 91,* 169–172.

Lambert, V. A. (1985). Study of factors associated with psychological well-being in rheumatoid arthritic women. *Image, 17,* 50–53.

Lehman, J. A. (1997). Connective tissue diseases and non-articular rheumatism. In J. H. Klippel (Ed.), *Primer on the rheumatic diseases* (11th ed., pp. 398–403). Atlanta: Arthritis Foundation.

Leirisalo-Repo, M., Turunen, V., Stenman, S., Helenius, P., & Seppala, K. (1994). High frequency of silent inflammatory bowel disease in spondyloarthropathy. *Arthritis and Rheumatism, 37,* 23–31.

LeRoy, E. C. (1985). Scleroderma (systemic sclerosis). In W. N. Kelly, E. D. Harris, S. Ruddy, & C. Sledge (Eds.), *Textbook of rheumatology* (2nd ed., pp. 1183–1205). Philadelphia: WB Saunders.

Lichtenstein, D. R., Syngal, S., & Wolfe, M. M. (1995). Nonsteroidal anti-inflammatory drugs and the gastrointestinal tract: The double-edged sword. *Arthritis and Rheumatism, 38,* 5–18.

Lima, F., Buchanan, N. M., Khamashta, M. A., Kerslake, S., & Hughes, G. R. (1995). Obstetric outcome in systemic lupus erythematosus. *Seminars in Arthritis and Rheumatism, 25,* 184–192.

Lindley, I. J. D., Ceska, M., & Peichl, P. (1991). Nap-1/IL-8 in rheumatoid arthritis. *Advances in Experimental Medicine and Biology, 305,* 147–156.

Lipsky, P., van der Hiejde, D., St. Clair, W., et al. (2000). 102-week clinical and radiologic results from the ATTRACT trial: a 2 year, randomized, controlled, phase 3 trial of infliximab (Remicade) in clients with active RA despite MTX. *Arthritis and Rheumatism, 43,* S269.

Lockshin, M. (1985). Corticosteroids. In P. D. Utsinger (Ed.), *Rheumatoid arthritis* (pp. 581–600). Philadelphia: Lippincott.

Love, L. A., Leff, R. L., Fraser, D. D., Targoff, I. N., Dalakas, M., Plotz, P. H., & Miller, F. W. (1991). A new approach to the classification of idiopathic inflammatory myopathy: Myositis-specific autoantibodies define useful homogeneous client groups. *Medicine, 70,* 360–374.

Lowery, B. J., Jacobsen, B. S., & Murphy, B. B. (1983). An exploratory investigation of causal thinking of arthritics. *Nursing Research, 32,* 157–162.

MacGregor, A. J., Riste, L. K., Hayes, J. M. W., & Silman, A. J. (1994). Low prevalence of rheumatoid arthritis in black Caribbeans compared with whites in inner city Manchester. *Annals of Rheumatologic Disease, 53,* 293–297.

Mackenzie, A. H. (1988). Differential diagnosis of rheumatoid arthritis. *American Journal of Medicine, 85,* 2–13.

Maini, R., St. Clair, E. W., Breedveld, F., Furst, D., Kalden, J., Weisman, M., Smolen, J., Emery, P., Harriman, G., Feldmann, M., & Lipsky, P. (1999). Infliximab (chimeric anti-tumor necrosis factor alpha monoclonal antibody) versus placebo in rheumatoid arthritis patients receiving concomitant methotrexate: A randomised phase III trial. *Lancet, 354,* 1932–1939.

Malairya, A. N., Kapoor, S. K., Singh, R. R., Kumar, A., & Pande, I. (1993). Prevalence of rheumatoid arthritis in the adult Indian population. *Rheumatology International, 13,* 131–134.

Masi, A. T., Rodnan, G. F., Medsger, T. A., Altman, R. D., d'Angelo, W. A., Fries, J. F., LeRoy, C., Kirsner, A., MacKenzie, A., McShane, D., Myers, A., & Sharp G. (1980). Preliminary criteria for the classification of systemic sclerosis (scleroderma). *Arthritis and Rheumatism, 23,* 581–590.

Mease, P. J., Goffe, B. S., Metz, J., VanderStoep, A., Finck, B., & Burge, D. (2000). Etanercept in the treatment of psoriatic arthritis and psoriasis: a randomized trial. *Lancet, 356,* 385–389.

Medsger, T. A. (1988). Systemic sclerosis and localized scleroderma. In H. R. Schumacher (Ed.), *Primer on the rheumatic diseases* (9th ed., pp. 111–117). Atlanta: Arthritis Foundation.

Medsger, T. A. (1993). Systemic sclerosis (scleroderma), localized forms of scleroderma and calcinosis. In D. J. McCarty & W. J. Koopman (Eds.), *Arthritis and allied conditions* (12th ed., Vol. 2, pp. 1253–1292). Philadelphia: Lea & Febiger.

Meenan, R. F., Gertman, P. M., & Mason, J. H. (1980). Measuring health status in arthritis: The arthritis impact measurement scales. *Arthritis and Rheumatism, 23,* 146–152.

Miller, J. F. (1983a). Energy deficits in the chronically ill: The client with arthritis. In J. F. Miller (Ed.), *Coping with chronic illness: Overcoming powerlessness* (pp. 257–274). Philadelphia: FA Davis.

Miller, J. F. (1983b). Inspiring hope. In J. F. Miller (Ed.), *Coping with chronic illness: Overcoming powerlessness* (pp. 287–289). Philadelphia: FA Davis.

Miltenburg, A. M., Roos, A., Slegtenhorst, L., Daha, M. R., & Breedveld, F. C. (1993). IgA anti-dsDNA antibodies in systemic lupus erythematosus: Occurrence, incidence, and association with clinical and laboratory variables of disease activity. *Journal of Rheumatology, 20,* 53–58.

Moder, K. G., Tefferi, A., Cohen, M. D., Menke, D. M., & Luthra, H. S. (1995). Hematologic malignancies and the use of methotrexate in rheumatoid arthritis: A retrospective study. *American Journal of Medicine, 99,* 276–281.

Mojcik, C. F., & Klippel, J. H. (1996). End-stage renal disease and systemic lupus erythematosus. *American Journal of Medicine, 101,* 100–107.

Moaar, P. A. (1989). The hip and pelvis. In S. J. Gates & P. A. Mooar (Eds.), *Orthopaedics and sports medicine for nurses* (pp. 166–180). Baltimore: Williams & Wilkins.

Moody, G. M., & Hammond, M. G. (1994). Differences in HA-DR association with rheumatoid arthritis among migrant Indian communities in South Africa. *British Journal of Rheumatology, 33,* 425–427.

Mooney, N. E. (1983). Coping with chronic pain in rheumatoid arthritis: Client behaviors and nursing interventions. *Rehabilitation Nursing, 8,* 20–25.

Moreland, L. M., Cohen, S. B., Baumgartner, S. W., et al. (2000). Long-term use of Enbrel in patients with DMARD-refractory rheumatoid arthritis. *Arthritis and Rheumatism, 43,* S270.

Morgan, S. L., Baggott, J. E., Vaughn, W. H., Austin, J. S., Veitch, T. A., Lee, J. Y., Koopman, W. J., Krumdieck, C. L., & Alarcon, G. S. (1994). Supplementation with folic acid during methotrexate therapy for rheumatoid arthritis: A double-blind, placebo-controlled trial. *Annals of Internal Medicine, 121,* 833–841.

Muhlenkamp, A. F., & Joyner, J. A. (1986). Arthritis clients' self-reported affective states and their caregivers' perceptions. *Nursing Research, 35,* 24–27.

Myllykangas-Luosujarvi, R. A., Aho, K., & Isomalei, H. A. (1995). Mortality in rheumatoid arthritis. *Seminars in Arthritis and Rheumatism, 25,* 193–202.

Nelson, J. L., Hughes, K. A., Smith, A. G., Nisperos, B. B., Branchaud, A. M., & Hansen, J. A. (1993). Maternal-fetal disparity in HLA class II alloantigens and the pregnancy-induced amelioration of rheumatoid arthritis. *New England Journal of Medicine, 329,* 466–471.

Neuberger, J. S., & Neuberger, G. B. (1984). Epidemiology of the rheumatic diseases. *Nursing Clinics of North America, 19,* 714–725.

Norins, A. L. (1989). Juvenile dermatomyositis. *Medical Clinics of North America, 73,* 1193–1209.

O'Dell, J. R., Haire, C. E., Erikson, N., Drymalski, W., Palmer, W., Eckhoff, P. J., Garwood, V., Maloley, P., Klassen, L. W., Wees, S., Klein, H., & Moore, G. F. (1996). Treatment of rheumatoid arthritis with methotrexate alone, sulfasalazine and hydroxychloroquine, or a combination of all three medications. *New England Journal of Medicine, 334,* 1287–1291.

Olsen, N. J., & Wortman, R. L. (1997). Inflammatory and metabolic diseases of muscle. In J. H. Klippel (Ed.), *Primer on the rheumatic diseases* (11th ed., pp. 276–282). Atlanta: Arthritis Foundation.

Pachman, L. M. (1986). Juvenile dermatomyositis. *Pediatric Clinics of North America, 33,* 1097–1117.

Page-Goertz, S. S. (1989). Even children have arthritis. *Pediatric Nursing, 15,* 11–16, 30.

Paget, S. A. (1997). Rheumatoid arthritis: Treatment. In J. H. Klippel (Ed.), *Primer on the rheumatic diseases* (11th ed., pp. 168–173). Atlanta: Arthritis Foundation.

Patrignani, P., Panara, M. R., Greco, A., Fusco, O., Natoli, C., Iacobelli, S., Cipollone, F., Ganci, A., Creminon, C., Maclouf, J., et al. (1994). Biochemical and pharmacological characterization of the cyclo-oxygenase activity of human blood prostaglandin endoperoxide synthase. *Journal of Pharmacology, Experimental Therapies, 271,* 1705–1712.

Paulus, H. E. (1988). Clinical pharmacology of the antirheumatic drugs. In H. R. Schumacher (Ed.), *Primer on the rheumatic diseases* (9th ed., pp. 282–288). Atlanta: Arthritis Foundation.

Paulus, H. E. (1991). Current medical approaches to the treatment of rheumatoid arthritis. *Clinical Orthopaedics and Related Research, 265,* 96–102.

Paulus, H. E. (1993). Protocol development for combination therapy with disease-modifying antirheumatic drugs. *Seminars in Arthritis and Rheumatism, 23*(Suppl 1), 19–25.

Peacock, D. J., & Cooper, C. (1995). Epidemiology of the rheumatic diseases. *Current Opinion in Rheumatology, 7,* 82–86.

Peacock, D. J., Ku, G., Banquerigo, M. L., & Brahn, E. (1992). Suppression of collagen arthritis with antibodies to an arthritogenic, oligoclonal T cell line. *Cellular Immunology, 140,* 444–452.

Persselin, J. E. (1991). Diagnosis of rheumatoid arthritis: Medical and laboratory aspects. *Clinical Orthopaedics and Related Research, 265,* 73–81.

Petty, R. E., & Malleson, P. (1986). Spondyloarthropathies of childhood. *Pediatric Clinics of North America, 33,* 1079–1095.

Physician's Desk Reference. (2001). Montvale, NJ: Medical Economics.

Pigg, J. S., Driscoll, P. W., & Caniff, R. (1985). *Rheumatology nursing.* New York: Wiley.

Pincus, T., Callahan, L. F., Fuchs, H. A., Larsen, A., & Kaye, J. (1995). Quantitative analysis of hand radiographs in rheumatoid arthritis: time course of radiographic changes, relation to joint examination measures, and comparison of different scoring methods. *Journal of Rheumatology, 22*(10), 1983–1989.

Pisetsky, D. S. (1997). Systemic lupus erythematosus: Epidemiology, pathology and pathogenesis. In J. H. Klippel (Ed.), *Primer on the rheumatic diseases* (11th ed., pp. 246–250). Atlanta: Arthritis Foundation.

Pope, R. M. (1996). Rheumatoid arthritis: Pathogenesis and early recognition. *American Journal of Medicine, 100*(Suppl 2A), 3s–9s.

Radhakrishman, J., Kunis, C. L., D'Agati, V., & Appel, G. B. (1994). Cyclosporine treatment of lupus membranous nephropathy. *Clinical Nephrology, 42,* 147–154.

Rall, L. C., Meydani, S. N., Kehayias, J. J., Dawson-Hughes, B., & Roubenoff, R. (1996). The effect of progressive resistance training in rheumatoid arthritis. *Arthritis and Rheumatism, 39,* 415–426.

Reichlin, M. (1997). Undifferentiated connective tissue disorders. In J. H. Klippel (Ed.), *Primer on the rheumatic diseases* (11th ed., pp. 244–245). Atlanta: Arthritis Foundation.

Reilly, J. P., & Nicholas, J. A. (1987). The chronically inflamed bursa. *Clinics in Sports Medicine, 6,* 345–370.

Robbins, S. L., & Kumar, V. (1987). *Basic pathology* (4th ed.). Philadelphia: WB Saunders.

Rocco, V. K., & Hurt, E. R. (1986). Scleroderma and scleroderma-like disorders. *Seminars in Arthritis and Rheumatism, 16,* 22–29.

Rodeheffer, R. J., Rommer, J. A., & Wigley, F. (1983). Controlled double blind trial of nifedipine in the treatment of Raynaud's phenomenon. *New England Journal of Medicine, 308,* 880–883.

Saag, K. G., Koehnke, R., Caldwell, J. R., Brasington, R., Burmeister, L. F., Zimmerman, B., Kohler, J. A., & Furst, D. E. (1994). Low dose long-term corticosteroid therapy in rheumatoid arthritis: An analysis of serious adverse events. *American Journal of Medicine, 96,* 115–123.

Salmond, S. W. (1989). Stress and stressors in rheumatoid arthritis. *Journal of Advanced Medical-Surgical Nursing, 1,* 35–43.

Schoen, D. C. (1988). Assessment for arthritis. *Orthopaedic Nursing, 7,* 31–39.

Schur, P. (1983). *The clinical management of systemic lupus erythematosus.* New York: Grune & Stratton.

Scull, S. A., Dow, M. B., & Athreya, B. H. (1986). Physical and occupational therapy for children with rheumatic diseases. *Pediatric Clinics of North America, 33,* 1053–1077.

Schumacher, H. R. (1982). Palindromic onset of rheumatoid arthritis. *Arthritis and Rheumatism, 25,* 361–365.

Seibold, J. R. (1993). Connective tissue diseases characterized by fibrosis. In W. N. Kelley, E. D. Harris, S. Ruddy, & C. Sledge (Eds.), *Textbook of rheumatology* (4th ed., Vol. 2, pp. 1114–1143). Philadelphia: WB Saunders.

Shipley, M. (1985). *Rheumatic diseases.* Baltimore: Williams & Wilkins.

Singsen, B. H. (1988). Pediatric rheumatic diseases. In H. R. Schumacher (Ed.), *Primer on the rheumatic diseases* (9th ed., pp. 160–163). Atlanta: Arthritis Foundation.

Situnayake, R. D., Grindulis, K. A., & McConkey, B. (1987). Long-term treatment of rheumatoid arthritis with sulphasalazine, gold, or penicillamine: A comparison using life-table methods. *Annals of Rheumatic Diseases, 46,* 177–183.

Smith, C. A., & Arnett, F. C. (1991). Epidemiologic aspects of rheumatoid arthritis: Current immunogenetic approach. *Clinical Orthopaedics and Related Research, 265,* 23–34.

Stapleton, S. (1983). Decreasing powerlessness in the chronically ill: A prototype. In J. F. Miller (Ed.), *Coping with chronic illness: Overcoming powerlessness* (pp. 257–274). Philadelphia: Davis.

Steen, V. D., Constantino, J. P., Shapiro, A. P., Medsger, T. A. R. (1990). Outcome of renal crisis in systemic sclerosis: Relationship to availability of converting enzyme (ACE) inhibitors. *Annals of Internal Medicine, 114,* 352–357.

Steen, V. D., Medsger, T. A., & Rodnan, G. P. (1982). d-Penicillamine therapy in progressive systemic sclerosis (scleroderma): A retrospective analysis. *Annals of Internal Medicine, 97,* 652–659.

Sutej, P. G., & Hadler, N. M. (1991). Current principles of rehabilitation for clients with rheumatoid arthritis. *Clinical Orthopaedics and Related Research, 265,* 116–124.

Suzuki, H., Takemura, H., & Kashiwagi, H. (1995). Interleukin-1 receptor antagonist in clients with active SLE. *Arthritis and Rheumatism, 38,* 1055–1059.

Talal, N. (1988). Sjögren's syndrome. In H. R. Schumacher (Ed.), *Primer on the rheumatic diseases* (9th ed., pp. 146–148). Atlanta: Arthritis Foundation.

Tan, E. M., Cohen, A. S., Fries, J. F., Masi, A. T., McShane, D. J., Rothfield, N. F., Schaller, J. G., Talal, N., & Winchester, R. J. (1982). The 1982 revised criteria for the classification of systemic lupus erythematosus (SLE). *Arthritis and Rheumatism, 25,* 1271–1277.

Tanimoto, K., Nakano, K., Kano, S., Mori, S., Ueki, H., Nishitani, H., Sato, T., Kiuchi, T., & Ohashi, Y. (1995). Classification criteria for polymyositis and dermatomyositis. *Journal of Rheumatology, 22,* 668–674.

Targoff, I. N. (1988). Laboratory manifestations of polymyositis and dermatomyositis. *Clinical Dermatology, 6,* 76–92.

Targoff, I. N. (1994). Immune manifestations of inflammatory muscle disease. *Rheumatology Clinics of North America, 20,* 857–880.

Taurog, J. D. (1997). Seronegative spondyloarthropathies. In J. H. Klippel (Ed.), *Primer on the rheumatic diseases* (11th ed., pp. 258–261). Atlanta: Arthritis Foundation.

ten Wolde, S., Breedveld, F., Hermans, J., Vandenbroucke, J. P., van der Laar, M. A., Markusse, H. M., Janssen, M., van den Brink, H. R., & Dijkmans, B. A. (1996). Randomized placebo-controlled study of stopping second-line drugs in rheumatoid arthritis. *Lancet, 347,* 347–352.

The Canadian Hydroxychloroquine Study Group. (1991). A randomized study of the effect of withdrawing hydroxychloroquine sulfate in systemic lupus erythematosus. *New England Journal of Medicine, 324,* 150–154.

Thompson, G. T. D., DeRubeis, D. A., Hodge, M. A., Rajanayagam, C., & Inman, R. D. (1995). Post-salmonella reactive arthritis: Late clinical sequel in a point source cohort. *American Journal of Medicine, 98,* 14–21.

Tuffanelli, D. L. (1989). Systemic scleroderma. *Medical Clinics of North America, 73,* 1167–1180.

Tugwell, P., Pincus, T., & Yocum, D. (1995). Combination therapy with cyclosporine and methotrexate in severe rheumatoid arthritis. *New England Journal of Medicine, 333,* 147–141.

van Vollenhoven, R. F., Engleman, E. G., & McGuire, J. L. (1995). Dehydroepiandrosterone in systemic lupus erythematosus. Results of a double-blind, placebo-controlled, randomized clinical trial. *Arthritis and Rheumatism, 38,* 1826–1831.

Vasey, F. B. (1984). Spondyloarthropathies. *Orthopaedic Review, 14,* 93–97.

Vasey, F. B. (1988). Psoriatic arthritis. In H. R. Schumacher (Ed.), *Primer on the rheumatic diseases* (9th ed., pp. 151–152). Atlanta: Arthritis Foundation.

Veale, D., Rogers, S., & Fitzgerald, O. (1994). Classification of clinical subsets and psoriatic arthritis. *British Journal of Rheumatology, 33,* 143–148.

Vollertsen, R. S. (1989). How to better evaluate the client who complains of joint pain. *Consultant, 29,* 31–46.

Ward, M. M., Pyun, E., & Studenski, S. (1995). Long-term survival in systemic lupus erythematosus. Patient characteristics associated with poorer outcomes. *Arthritis and Rheumatism, 38,* 274–283.

Weinblatt, M. E., & Maier, A. L. (1991). Disease-modifying agents and experimental treatments of rheumatoid arthritis. *Clinical Orthopaedics and Related Research, 265,* 103–115.

Weinblatt, M. E., Kremer, J. M., Bankhurst, A. D., Bulpitt, K. J., Fleischmann, R. M., Fox, R. I., Jackson, C. G., Lange, M., & Burge, D. J. (1999). A trial of etanercept, a recombinant tumor necrosis factor receptor: Fc fusion protein, in clients with rheumatoid arthritis receiving methotrexate. *New England Journal of Medicine, 340,* 253–259.

West, S. G., & Johnson, S. C. (1988). Danazol for the treatment of refractory autoimmune thrombocytopenia in systemic lupus erythematosus. *Annals of Internal Medicine, 108,* 703–706.

Weisman, M. H., & Weinblatt, M. E. (1995). *Treatment of the rheumatic diseases: Companion to the textbook of rheumatology.* Philadelphia: WB Saunders.

Whaley, R. F., & Wong, D. L. (1987). *Nursing care of infants and children.* St. Louis: Mosby.

Wiener, C. L. (1975). The burden of rheumatoid arthritis: Tolerating the uncertainty. *Science and Medicine, 9,* 97–104.

Wigley, F. M. (1992). Treatment of systemic sclerosis. *Current Opinion in Rheumatology, 4,* 878–886.

Wilke, W. S. (1993). Combination therapy for rheumatoid arthritis: New paradigms of treatment. *Cleveland Clinic Journal of Medicine, 60,* 101–102.

Wilke, W. S., Biro, J. A., & Segal, A. M. (1987). Methotrexate in the treatment of arthritis and connective tissue diseases. *Cleveland Clinic Journal of Medicine, 54,* 327–338.

Wilske, K. R., & Healey, L. A. (1989). Remodeling the pyramid: A concept whose time has come. *Journal of Rheumatology, 16,* 565–570.

Wilson, K., & Abeles, M. (1994). A 2-year open-ended trial of methotrexate in systemic lupus erythematosus. *Journal of Rheumatology, 21,* 1674–1677.

Wolfe, F., & Sharp, J. T. (1998). Radiographic outcome of recent-onset rheumatoid arthritis. *Arthritis and Rheumatism, 41,* 1571–1582.

Wong, K., Chan, F., & Lee, C. (1991). Outcome of pregnancy in clients with systemic lupus erythematosus: A prospective study. *Archives of Internal Medicine, 151,* 269–273.

Yellin, E., Henke, C., & Epstein, W. (1987). The work dynamics of the person with rheumatoid arthritis. *Arthritis and Rheumatism, 30,* 507–512.

Zachary, L., Rice-Puoci, F., & Ellman, M. H. (1997). Digital sympathectomy for fingertip ulcerations/infarctions in scleroderma clients. *Arthritis and Rheumatism, 40*(Suppl), S1439, 254.

Ziegler, G. C. (1984). Systemic lupus erythematosus and systemic sclerosis. *Nursing Clinics of North America, 19,* 673–695.

Zvaifler, N. J. (1988). Rheumatoid arthritis: Epidemiology, etiology, rheumatoid factor, pathology, and pathogenesis. In H. R. Schumacher (Ed.), *Primer on the rheumatic diseases* (9th ed., pp. 83–87). Atlanta: Arthritis Foundation.

Metabolic Conditions

CAROL A. SEDLAK and MARGARET O. DOHENY

Metabolic bone disease may result from an inappropriate function of one or several metabolic processes and may be manifested by physical and chemical changes within the bone. Conditions that alter the normal equilibrium existing in bone remodeling, causing metabolic bone disease, include parathyroid malfunction, vitamin or dietary deficiency, estrogen deficiency, and malabsorption syndrome. Often, it is a combination of these conditions that predisposes a person to metabolic bone disease.

This chapter presents the metabolism of bone, followed by a discussion of specific metabolic disorders, including osteoporosis, Paget's disease, osteomalacia, gout, avascular necrosis, hypoparathyroidism, and hyperparathyroidism.

BONE PHYSIOLOGY AND METABOLISM

Bone is not a static mass of hard material. The rigid and seemingly permanent structure of bone is a dynamic system in a state of constant flux. Bone is continually being remodeled. Normally, the deposition (by osteoblasts) and resorption (by osteoclasts) of bone takes place at the same rate, enabling the total mass and composition of bones to remain constant. An alteration in this normal equilibrium constitutes a metabolic bone disease.

Magnesium

Magnesium, an abundant intracellular cation, has an essential enzyme function and plays a key role in the maintenance of healthy bones. About half of the magnesium found in the body is found in bones. The intake of magnesium is directly related to healthful caloric intake. Dietary sources of magnesium include cereal grains, nuts, fruits, legumes, meat, and fish. Magnesium is required for neuromuscular activity, membrane stability, calcium metabolism, calcium channel activity, and ion transport.

Magnesium comprises about 0.5% to 1% of bone ash and influences matrix and mineral metabolism in bone. Oral magnesium supplementation may have beneficial effects in reducing bone loss in osteoporosis, and there is growing evidence that magnesium may be an important factor in the quality of bone and calcium metabolism, especially in growing children and young adults. Researchers cite the need to evaluate magnesium as a potential treatment for postmenopausal osteoporosis (Dimai, Porta, Wirnsberger, Lindschinger, Pampert, Dobnig, Wilders-Truschnig, & Lau, 1998; Sojka & Weaver, 1995).

Calcium

Calcium and vitamin D play vital roles in the formation of bone matrix. Deposits of calcium in the organic matrix of bone add strength and hardness to bone composition. Calcium and vitamin D metabolism involves several metabolic pathways, which are summarized in Figure 15–1.

Calcium is an essential mineral and is present in all body tissue. It is involved in several physiologic processes, including (1) coagulation of blood, (2) maintenance of cardiac rhythmicity, (3) membrane permeability and neuromuscular excitability, (4) formation of bones and teeth, and (5) lactation. Ninety-eight percent of total calcium is stored in bone, and this great reserve of calcium can be released to meet physiologic needs. Calcium can be mobilized from bones to maintain functional levels in other systems at the expense of the bony structures. The body's homeostatic processes help keep the serum calcium at its normal level of 9 to 10.5 mg/dL.

Rich dietary sources of calcium are found in many foods (Table 15–1). Seventy-five percent of daily calcium intake ordinarily comes from dairy products, but many people are unable to ingest dairy products. Dark green vegetables, formerly thought to provide up to 10% of daily

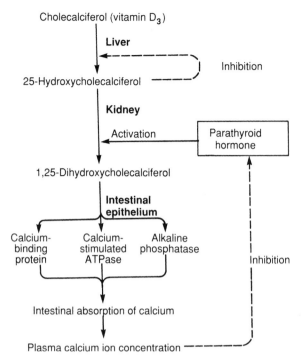

FIGURE 15–1. Vitamin D metabolism. This summarizes the steps that the inactive form of vitamin D, cholecalciferol, must undergo as it is activated to become the final form of vitamin D, 1,25-dihydroxycholecalciferol. (From Guyton, A. C., & Hall, J. E. [1996]. *Medical physiology* [9th ed.]. Philadelphia: WB Saunders.)

calcium intake, are now known to be a relatively poor source of calcium owing in part to the lack of bioavailability of the calcium they contain. Supplements are effective in helping people meet the minimum daily requirements of calcium. Research studies have clarified appropriate forms and daily requirements of calcium (Avioli, 1993; Heaney, 2000; National Institutes of Health [NIH], 1994). Table 15-2 provides the daily adequate calcium intake (AI) levels needed for optimizing health.

Phosphate

Phosphate is an important element in bone metabolism and must be continually replenished to maintain body requirements. Milk, dairy products, and meats are major sources of dietary phosphate.

The crystalline salts deposited in the organic matrix of bone consist mostly of calcium and phosphate. Phosphate and calcium operate in opposition to each other within the kidneys. When phosphate is depleted for any reason, such as in the presence of elevated levels of parathyroid hormone (PTH), the kidneys reabsorb calcium. This feedback system is addressed more thoroughly later in this chapter.

Whereas calcium is poorly absorbed by the intestine, phosphate is readily absorbed, except in the presence of excessive calcium. In the presence of high calcium and phosphate levels, calcium phosphate is formed. Calcium phosphate is poorly absorbed, passes through the intes-

tine, and is excreted in the feces. The major concern in the absorption of calcium and phosphate is a problem of calcium absorption, because if calcium is absorbed, both calcium and phosphate are absorbed. Any condition that alters normal equilibrium in bone turnover can upset the foregoing sequences and lead to metabolic imbalance. Physical findings, assessment, nursing management, intervention, and rehabilitation strategies associated with specific metabolic conditions are discussed later in this chapter.

Vitamin D

Vitamin D is essential in the metabolism of calcium and phosphorus. Calcium is poorly absorbed from the intestinal tract and requires adequate vitamin D to be adequately absorbed and metabolized. Vitamin D itself is not the active substance that actually causes these actions. Vitamin D is converted through a series of reactions in the liver and kidney into the compound, 1,25-dihydroxycholecalciferol, which is the active form of vitamin D that operates in the intestinal epithelium to promote calcium absorption (see Fig. 15-1).

The precursor to vitamin D is present on the skin in the form of a sterol, or lipoid, and the ultraviolet rays of the sun convert this sterol to another product. Further conversion of vitamin D occurs in the liver and kidneys until it reaches its final active form. Therefore, appropriate exposure to sunlight helps prevent vitamin D deficiency and can promote healthy bone metabolism. Individuals who have limited exposure to sunlight (e.g., residents of long-term care facilities, sailors in subma-

TABLE 15–1. *Calcium and Caloric Content of Certain Foods*

FOOD	AMOUNT	Ca (mg)	CALORIES
Dairy Products			
Milk			
Whole, 3.3%	1 cup	291	150
Nonfat (skim)	1 cup	302	86
Buttermilk	1 cup	285	99
Milk chocolate (plain)	1 oz	65	145
Cheese			
Blue or Roquefort	1 oz	150	100
Cheddar	1 cup	815	455
Cottage (4%)	1 cup	135	232
Parmesan, grated	1 oz	390	129
Swiss (natural)	1 oz	219	95
American	1 oz	174	106
Nondairy Products			
Beet greens (boiled)	1 cup	165	40
Sardines (canned)	3 oz	325	177
Broccoli (fresh)	1 cup	42	24

Adapted from Davis, J., & Sherer, K. (1994). *Applied nutrition and diet therapy for nurses* (2nd ed.). Philadelphia: WB Saunders.

TABLE 15–2. *Recommended Daily Adequate Intake (AI) for Calcium*

AGE GROUP	OPTIMAL DAILY INTAKE (mg)
Infants	
0–6 months	210
6–12 months	270
Children	
1–3 years	500
4–8 years	800
9–18 years	1300
Adults	
19–50 years	1000
51 and older	1200
Pregnant and lactating women	
14–18 years	1300
19–50 years	1000

Adapted from the 1997 Institute of Medicine, National Academy of Sciences, report.

rines, residents of northern countries), may experience vitamin D deficiency if oral intake is inadequate.

Certain foods and food products are fortified with vitamin D, but other foods high in natural vitamin D are also high in fat. These foods include fatty fish, cheese, butter, eggs, and liver. Some calcium supplements contain vitamin D and, when used appropriately, can provide the necessary vitamin D to ensure adequate calcium absorption. Placebo-controlled trials have indicated that combination therapy with calcium and vitamin D reduces bone loss and prevents fractures in older adults; however, they also found that discontinuing calcium and vitamin D has little cumulative effect and that bone mineral density (BMD) gains can be lost without the supplementation (Dawson-Hughes, Harris, Krall, & Dallai, 2000). Excessive doses of vitamin D, however, can result in hypercalcemia, hypercalciuria, and demineralization of bone (Lehne, 2000).

Parathyroid Hormone

PTH exerts a potent influence on determining the functional effects of vitamin D in the body, specifically vitamin D's effect on calcium absorption in the intestine and bone. There is an efficient feedback system in operation in the normal adult that accurately maintains proper concentrations of serum calcium. The rate of secretion of PTH is controlled almost entirely by plasma calcium concentration. Hypercalcemia leads to decreased PTH secretion and therefore decreased formation in the kidney of the active form of vitamin D. In other words, hypercalcemia leads to decreased vitamin D formation and decreased intestinal absorption of calcium and the eventual return of the serum calcium level to normal. PTH provides one of the most important mechanisms by which the hormonal system of the body maintains a constant calcium ion concentration (Fig. 15–2).

Calcitonin

Calcitonin, normally secreted by the thyroid gland, provides a second hormonal system control over serum calcium concentration and ultimately over bone metabolism. The effects of calcitonin are opposite to those of PTH. Calcitonin acts to lower plasma calcium concentration by (1) inhibiting osteoclastic bone resorption, (2) increasing osteoblastic activity, and (3) inhibiting the formation of new osteoclasts. Calcitonin is available for therapeutic administration in both parenteral and nasal spray formulations. Both formulations are described in detail later in this chapter.

Estrogen

The ovary is the principal organ of estrogen production. Estrogen plays a vital role in minimizing the loss of bone in women. When estrogen is present, it works to protect the bones in three important ways: (1) by suppressing osteoclastic activity and increasing the number of vitamin D receptor sites on osteoblasts, (2) by promoting renal reabsorption of calcium, and (3) by helping to promote the intestinal absorption of calcium. Research indicates that estrogen also promotes osteoblastic activity, thereby increasing the growth of new

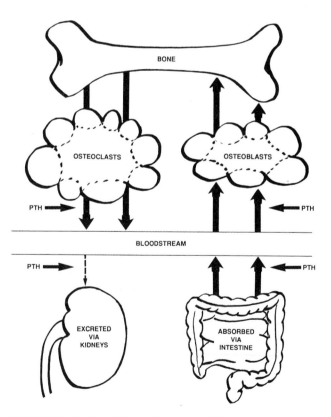

FIGURE 15–2. The effects of parathyroid hormone (PTH) on calcium metabolism. The *solid arrows* illustrate the calcium-saving actions of PTH. Elevated PTH promotes resorption of bone by osteoclasis, inhibits calcium excretion by the kidneys, and promotes calcium absorption from the intestine.

bone and stimulating the thyroid gland to secrete calcitonin, which then provides even more protective action at the cellular level. The absence of estrogen caused by the cessation of ovarian function alters skeletal homeostasis and results in a net loss of bone tissue in the postmenopausal woman. Estrogen is commonly administered to deter the rapid loss of bone mass that occurs at menopause. More about estrogen and bone metabolism is presented in the discussion of osteoporosis.

OSTEOPOROSIS

Osteoporosis has been defined as "a disease characterized by low bone mass and microarchitectural deterioration of bone tissue, leading to enhanced bone fragility and a consequent increase in fracture risk" (Consensus Development, 1993). Osteoporosis and osteopenia (low bone mass) occur when the rate of bone resorption is more rapid than the rate of bone formation. More specifically, osteoporosis is a disturbance of normal osteoblastic and osteoclastic balance in which the mineral and protein matrix components are diminished. In osteoporosis, the trabeculae (thin plates or lattice-like structures in spongy bone) are decreased in numbers and width, and bone mass is decreased (Fig. 15–3). This loss of microarchitectural structure results in fragile bones and fractures. A more recent definition for osteoporosis is based on criteria from the World Health Organization (WHO) and is based on BMD and t-score measurements. A *t-score* is the number of standard deviations (SD) above or below the average BMD value of young healthy white women. Osteoporosis occurs when the t-score is at or below –2.5 SD (Osteoporosis Prevention, 2000; WHO, 1994). Osteopenia is categorized as a value for bone density that lies between 1 and 2.5 SD below the young adult mean value. These parameters provide diagnostic criteria or guidelines to clinicians who make decisions about interventions.

Osteoporosis is the most common metabolic bone disease and is estimated that 1 of every 2 women and 1 in 8 men will suffer an osteoporosis-related fracture in their lifetime (National Osteoporosis Foundation, 2000a). Eight million women and two million men have osteoporosis, and eighteen million more have low bone mass. Osteoporosis is responsible for 1.5 million fractures annually in the United States, and the annual estimated health care costs for this disease approach $14 billion (National Osteoporosis Foundation, 2000a).

There is an age-related pattern of bone loss in the normal older adult, particularly the older woman. At the turn of the 20th century, the average life span of a woman in the United States was just over 50 years, and at that time, few women lived past menopause and did not experience the ravaging effects of osteoporosis. It is now apparent that much of the female population of the United States is living far beyond the age of menopause. Because women now live longer, much attention has been directed to osteoporosis. New options for treatment of osteoporosis are available. Ideally, the best strategy for the eradication of osteoporosis is in prevention rather than treatment.

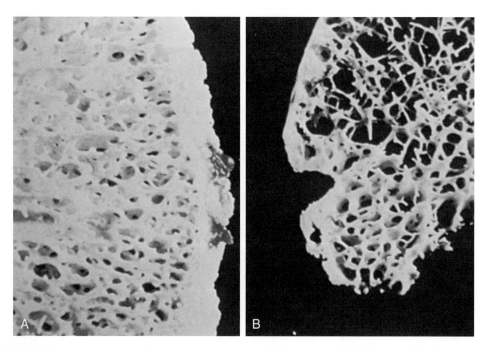

FIGURE 15–3. Normal versus osteoporotic bone. *A,* Microscopic view of normal bone. *B,* Typical osteoporotic bone.

Cause and Incidence

The "silent epidemic" is another label for osteoporosis because the first evidence of osteoporosis is often a painful fracture. The annual incidence of osteoporotic fractures exceeds 1.5 million and includes more than 300,000 femoral fractures and more than 700,000 vertebral fractures, 250,000 wrist fractures, and 300,000 fractures of other bones. Bone mass decreases as one reaches older adulthood and therefore most (but not all) individuals with osteoporosis are old. The risk of a white 50-year-old woman sustaining an osteoporotic hip fracture is equal to her combined risk of breast, uterine, and ovarian cancer (National Osteoporosis Foundation, 2000a).

The exact cause of osteoporosis is unknown. Two major factors contribute to bone mass, or hardness or density of bone: (1) the peak bone mass achieved during young adulthood and (2) the rate of bone loss that occurred after menopause or during late adulthood. Achievement of 100% of optimal peak bone mass occurs by age 35 and is influenced by genetic factors and enhanced by adequate calcium intake, weight-bearing exercise, and the presence of risk factors. The rate of bone loss is strongly influenced by genetics, estrogen, and risk factors.

Risk Factors

The common risk factors for osteoporosis are listed in Box 15-1. The presence of some risk factors can be altered. Women are at a higher risk than men for osteoporosis, and Caucasians and Asians are at higher risk than other ethnic groups. However, approximately 300,000 African American women have osteoporosis (Boyd, 1998; National Research Center Fact Sheet, 1998). Small body structure puts an individual at an even higher risk than an individual with larger bone structure. The presence of a family history of osteoporosis is a major risk factor for the development of osteoporosis.

Estrogen deficiency increases the risks of osteoporosis. Consequently, the postmenopausal woman is at high risk for osteoporosis. Early menopause or surgical oophorectomy without the initiation of hormonal replacement therapy (HRT) has been a well-documented, significant risk factor for osteoporosis. Amenorrhea, in the premenopausal woman, is also considered a risk factor and is usually placed in the changeable category because of the reversibility of the causes and relatively good response to estrogen therapy. Excessive exercise and eating disorders, such as anorexia or bulimia, can also cause amenorrhea and place one at risk. A less common cause of amenorrhea is primary ovarian failure. However, the effects of the diminished estrogen levels associated with this disorder are just as significant as the more common causes of amenorrhea.

Certain medications interfere with bone metabolism and are deemed risk factors. Excessive thyroid administra-

---

BOX 15–1.

Risk Factors for Osteoporosis: Can It Happen to You?

Complete the following questionnaire to determine your risk for developing osteoporosis.

Question	Yes	No
1. Do you have a small frame, or are you Caucasian or Asian?		
2. Do you have a family history of osteoporosis?		
3. Are you a postmenopausal woman?		
4. Have you had an early or surgically induced menopause?		
5. Have you been taking excessive thyroid medication or high doses of cortisone-like drugs for asthma, arthritis, or cancer?		
6. Is your diet low in dairy products and other sources of calcium?		
7. Are you physically inactive?		
8. Do you smoke cigarettes or drink alcohol in excess?		

The more times you answer yes, the greater your risk for developing osteoporosis.

Contact the National Osteoporosis Foundation, 1150 17th Street, Suite 500, Washington, DC 20036. Reproduced courtesy of National Osteoporosis Foundation and U.S. Administration on Aging. (1991). National Osteoporosis Foundation. Reprinted by permission.

---

tion, long-term use of corticosteroids, and use of certain anticonvulsant and certain anticoagulant drugs can increase the risk for osteoporosis (National Osteoporosis Foundation, 2000b). Although glucocorticoids are important in the management of respiratory, joint, and inflammatory bowel disease and other diseases, they inhibit new bone formation at the cellular level. Studies by Lukert (1995) show significant and continuing dose-related bone loss in persons who have taken glucocorticoids for more than 12 months. Other studies show similar results in clients who took corticosteroids for inflammatory bowel disease (Bernstein, Seeger, Sayre, Anton, Artinian, & Shanahan, 1995). Glucocorticoids have an indirect effect on bone by acting on the kidney and the intestine. Urinary calcium loss is increased, and intestinal calcium absorption is decreased in the presence of glucocorticoids.

The other major risk factors for osteoporosis include low dietary intake of calcium, cigarette smoking, excessive consumption of alcohol, and a sedentary lifestyle. Calcium deficiency is a major risk factor for osteoporosis. Calcium is necessary to develop peak bone mass and sustain normal bone remodeling. A low dietary intake of calcium, particularly during the adolescent years, can

EXAMINING THE EVIDENCE: Moving Toward Evidence-Based Practice

For Persons with Risk Factors for Osteoporosis, Will Increasing Dietary Calcium and Weight-Bearing Exercises, as Compared to No Intervention, Increase or Maintain Existing Bone Mass?

AUTHOR(S) YEAR	SAMPLE SIZE	DIAGNOSIS	DESIGN	OUTCOME VARIABLE	MAJOR FINDINGS
Nguyen et al., 2000	1075 women, 690 men >69 yr	Osteoporosis	Cross-sectional epidemiologic	Association between calcium intake and exercise and body mass index	Adequate dietary calcium intake and maintaining physical activity in later life can reduce the risk of osteoporosis
Hunt et al., 1995	62 morning voided urine samples and 50 24-hour urine samples	Spinal cord injury	Determine diagnostic value of urinary pyridinium (Upyr) cross-link by performing urine assays	Levels of Upyr in individuals with impaired physical mobility	Higher-than-normal levels of Upyr found in osteoporotic women. Upyr has the ability to identify states of high bone resorption
Branca, 1999	Review of literature	Osteoporosis	Review of literature	Calcium intake	The increase in bone density in postmenopausal women is positively related to calcium intake when accompanied by exercise
Swezey et al., 2000	Two groups: 20 postmenopausal Caucasian women aged 56-69 in first group, 21 women aged 52-69 in second group	Osteoporosis	Assess effect of resistive isometric exercises over 2 months	Determine whether bone alkaline phosphatase (marker for bone formation and resorption) increases with exercise	10 minutes of daily resistive isometric exercises enhances bone formation
Rutherford, 1999	Literature review of last 20 years	Osteoporosis	Review of literature	Determine whether exercise improves bone mineral density (BMD)	Exercise across the life span can maximize bone mass and maintain muscle strength and balance
Lloyd et al., 1993	94 girls (mean age of 11.9 yr)	Osteoporosis prevention	Randomized, double-blind, placebo-controlled trial	Test effect of 500 mg calcium citrate malate supplementation on bone density of lumbar spine	Supplemental group had greater increases in lumbar spine bone density. Increasing daily calcium intake to 110% of recommended daily allowance can significantly increase bone density in adolescent girls
Dawson-Hughes et al., 2000	295 older men and women (≥68 yr)	Osteoporosis prevention	3-year randomized trial of calcium and vitamin D supplementation followed by 2 years of no supplements	BMD measured by DXA and biochemical markers and bone turnover	Gains in BMD were lost with discontinuation of calcium supplementation. Calcium and vitamin D have limited cumulative effect
Wolf et al., 2000	142 healthy premenopausal and postmenopausal women	Calcium absorption	Determine the efficiency of calcium absorption in women	Calcium absorption values	Calcium absorption values vary widely among women. Women with higher dietary fat had lower calcium absorption ratios. Dietary fat may play a role in determining calcium absorption
Weaver, 2000	Review of literature	Calcium intake	Review of literature	Impact of calcium on BMD	Recommended calcium intakes appear adequate to protect bone health. In postmenopausal women, calcium intake of at least 1 g is needed to impact a positive effect of exercise on BMD
Heaney, 2000	Review of 139 papers	Osteoporosis	Review of 139 papers on calcium intake and bone health	Influence of calcium on bone health	Identified improved bone health, reduced bone loss in older adults, or reduced fracture risk with high intakes of calcium
Osteoporosis Prevention, 2000 (NIH, 1994)	International panel of experts	Osteoporosis prevention and treatment	Panel report from two conferences	Bone development measured by DXA	Developed recommendations for calcium intake and physical exercises to enhance bone development

428

contribute to low BMD. However, adequate intake of calcium does not prevent the accelerated bone loss that occurs with menopause, and a high protein intake causes increased calcium excretion by the kidneys and contributes to the risk of developing osteoporosis.

Smoking has been shown to increase the incidence of osteoporosis by its influence on the onset of menopause and the lowering of BMD. Women who smoke experience an earlier menopause than nonsmoking women and may have lower levels of estrogen (Rapuri, Gallagher, Balhorn, & Ryschon, 2000). Excessive intake of alcohol has been implicated as a risk factor for reduced bone mass. Alcohol has at least two documented deleterious effects on the bone: It interferes directly with bone metabolism at the cellular level by altering the incorporation of calcium into the bone matrix, and it alters the intestinal absorption of calcium. In addition to the effects of alcohol on bone metabolism, high alcohol intake can also alter a person's balance and equilibrium, therefore placing him or her at a higher risk for falls. In the person with existing osteoporosis, this propensity to fall significantly increases the risk of fracturing a bone. It is not known how much alcohol must be consumed before bone mass is reduced (Lappe, 1994).

Immobility has been identified as a risk factor for osteoporosis. Bone requires weight bearing to regenerate, and without the normal stress associated with ambulation, bone demineralizes in a way similar to the atrophy of an unused muscle. Mechanical forces actually promote osteoblast growth and activity. Growth of new bone is further stimulated by changes in the electric charges on bone surfaces created by the stress of exercise. Weightlessness and immobility lead to accelerated bone resorption. This bone resorption rapidly reverses with resumption of normal weight bearing. There has been increased emphasis on the importance of weight bearing after it was determined that astronauts had significant bone demineralization during periods of weightlessness. The weightlessness created in space made weight-bearing exercise impossible, and therefore bone was lost at a rapid rate. Steinberg and Roettger (1993) also cite high rates of bone loss with extended periods of bed rest in hospitalized clients. Whatever the exact mechanism of action, it is well supported that inactivity, as defined by a lack of weight bearing, results in demineralization of bone and loss of bone density (Rutherford, 1999).

Assessment

Nursing History. A comprehensive nursing history is important in the prevention, early detection, and management of osteoporosis. Because the emphasis in care must be prevention and minimizing risks, an accurate and complete history is required. This process is facilitated by use of a risk factor checklist, as presented in Box 15–1. This tool can aid in the evaluation of a client for potential

risks and in the development of a teaching plan specific to the client.

When the nursing history identifies the client as being at high risk for injury secondary to osteoporosis, an expanded assessment emphasizing environmental safety factors should be completed. Box 15–2 presents risk factors that increase the likelihood of falls and injuries. Clients with osteoporosis are at a greater risk for fractures if they fall. If the nursing history indicates a high risk for osteoporosis in a client of any age, further actions, preventive measures, and use of specific diagnostic tools, such as dual-energy x-ray absorptiometry (DEXA), are recommended.

Physical Assessment. Some of the signs and symptoms of osteoporosis can mimic those of other bone diseases (Box 15–3). Specific assessment is necessary for the differential diagnosis. Loss of height may be the first sign of osteoporosis (Hunt, 1996). An annual loss of approximately 0.09% of one's total height is common and expected after age 45. Height loss that exceeds the expected percentage requires further assessment. The loss of height associated with osteoporosis can be quite dramatic. Severe curvature of the spine, particularly of the thoracic area, can be an indication of osteoporosis. Thoracic kyphosis, also called "dowager's hump," may foretell osteoporosis (Fig. 15–4). Low-back pain may be found in osteoporosis, although the differential diagnosis in evaluating the source of the back pain may point to a variety of other disorders. Occasionally, the first sign indicating the presence of osteoporosis may be a fracture. The three most common sites of fracture that occur with osteoporosis are the forearm, femur, and spine. These fractures are common because of the presence of more trabecular or spongy bone, which is more metabolically active than cortical or hard bone, at these sites.

The vertebral body may sustain a crush fracture, or compression fracture, in which the vertebral body collapses on itself (Fig. 15–5). This collapsing of bone accounts for the height loss. Acute onset of severe back pain accompanied by tenderness and voluntary restriction of motion is typical of vertebral compression fractures.

BOX 15–2.
Risk Factors for Falls

Confusion or dementia
Cardiovascular disorders
Decreased mobility
Generalized weakness
Elimination needs
Hypnotics, psychotropics, diuretics, antihypertensives, and other drugs
Environmental hazards
Impaired vision or hearing

BOX 15–3.

Major Assessment Findings with Osteoporosis

Excessive height loss
Thoracic kyphosis
Back pain
Fractures
Dual energy x-ray absorptiometry (DEXA) values >2.5 SD
  below young adult mean value

Minor falls or trauma in the osteoporotic client often cause forearm and hip fractures. The most common forearm fracture is the Colles' fracture, which can be sustained during a simple fall when the client extends an arm for protection. Femoral fractures occur because of the low bone density and the trauma of the fall, or spontaneous fractures may precede the fall if the bone is severely osteoporotic.

Diagnostic Evaluation

New technology has made precise measurement of bone density a reality. With standard x-ray examination, osteoporotic changes cannot be seen until more than 30% of bone mass has been lost. The vertebral compression fracture is demonstrable on x-ray film and appears as a wedge-shaped vertebral radiographic image.

Quantitative computed tomography (QCT) scanning has been widely used to assess BMD of the vertebrae in a three-dimensional manner. The QCT has a precision or accuracy of 3% to 5% but must be calibrated after each use. QCT is accurate but costly and delivers a considerable amount of radiation. For this reason, many clinicians are using other tools.

The newer technique, DEXA, is the most widely used test for osteoporosis. It assesses bone density and is considered the gold standard for BMD. BMD can be measured centrally (hip and spine) or peripherally (pDXA) (forearm, finger, heel). This method is precise and economical and increasingly available. The advantages of DEXA include less radiation exposure, shorter procedure time, superior precision, and higher resolution. The use of DEXA enables clinicians to monitor changes in bone density much more economically than previous technology and provides a logical measure of the outcomes of therapy (Fig. 15–6A). Experts have proposed using the WHO criteria (BMD ≤ 2.5 SD) for diagnosis of osteoporosis. Figure 15–6B shows an example of the output from a DEXA.

Quantitative ultrasound (QUS) offers a low-cost, ultrafast (5 minutes), portable, and radiation-free screening tool for the assessment of density, elasticity, and strength of bone microarchitecture (*Bone mineral density testing,* 1999). Studies indicate that QUS has the ability to predict fractures and that a significant positive correlation exists between DEXA and QUS measurements (Osteoporosis Prevention, 2000).

Diagnostic evaluation of osteoporosis often includes the analysis of serum and urinary markers of bone remodeling. The person with osteoporosis usually has normal serum calcium and phosphorus. These normal levels are maintained because of the body's efficient calcium/phosphorus balance system. Urinary calcium may be elevated. Serum bone G_{la}-protein, also referred to as *BGP* or *osteocalcin,* is synthesized by the osteoblast and is therefore a biochemical marker of bone formation. Osteocalcin is increased in conditions of increased bone turnover, such as Paget's disease or hyperparathyroidism. Osteocalcin is decreased with hypoparathyroidism and in glucocorticoid-treated clients. Other markers of bone formation include serum total and bone-specific alkaline phosphatase and type I collagen propeptide. Biochemical markers of bone resorption include urinary alkaline phosphatase and osteocalcin (indices of bone formation) and urine levels of pyredinolines and deoxypyridinolines (indices of bone resorption). Marker levels do not predict bone mass or fracture risk but may provide perspective on causes of bone loss (Osteoporosis Prevention, 2000).

The use of one or more of these diagnostic tests is common and in many cases may be performed in the office setting. Other tests that are performed in the

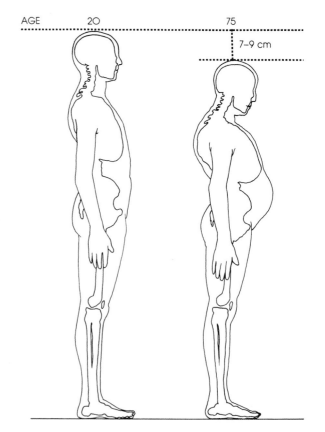

FIGURE 15–4. Loss of height resulting from osteoporosis, leading to dowager's hump. Note the flexed head and protruding abdomen, which occur partially to maintain the center of gravity in its normal position. (From Magee, D. [1992]. *Orthopaedic physical assessment* [3rd ed., p. 585]. Philadelphia: WB Saunders.)

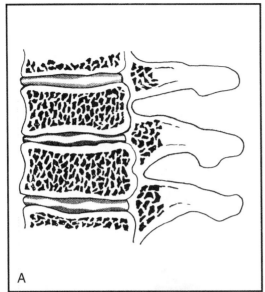
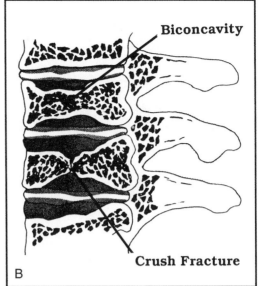
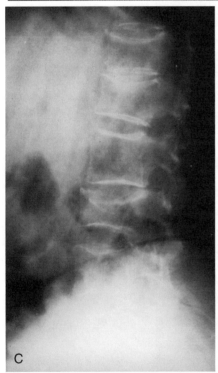

FIGURE 15–5. Effects of osteoporosis on the vertebrae. The normal vertebrae *(A)* differ substantially from the osteoporotic vertebrae *(B)*. Note the compression, or crush, fracture in the middle vertebra pictured. These various abnormalities lead to the shortened stature of the osteoporosis client and can cause both pain and structural changes, such as thoracic kyphosis. *C,* A radiograph of a compression fracture of vertebrae. Note the differences in height and the wedge shape at the site of the compression.

differential diagnosis of metabolic bone disease include spinal radiographs to determine the presence or absence of compression fractures and laboratory tests to determine the levels of serum PTH, serum vitamin D, serum and urinary calcium, and serum creatinine clearance. A complete history and physical examination should precede diagnostic testing.

Pharmacologic Management

Prevention strategies are effective to deter osteoporosis if they are started before bone loss occurs. Ninety percent of peak bone mass is achieved by approximately 20 years of age. The accelerated bone loss that occurs in the first 5 to

6 years after menopause is detrimental to the bony skeleton. Prevention (exercise and adequate calcium intake with vitamin D) and early detection strategies, such as reducing risk factors, must be implemented in youth and before menopause to be effective. If preventive strategies fail, active treatment of osteoporosis is required. Pharmacologic management should be initiated to reduce fracture risk when a woman's BMD t-score is below –2 SD in the absence of risk factors and –1.5 SD with risk factors present (National Osteoporosis Foundation, 2000c).

Three major pharmacologic choices are approved for the management of osteoporosis (Table 15–3).

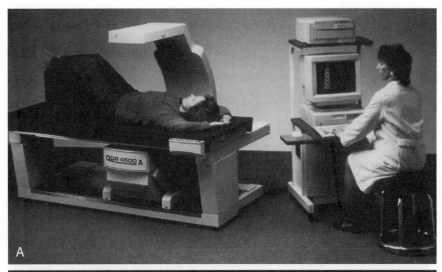

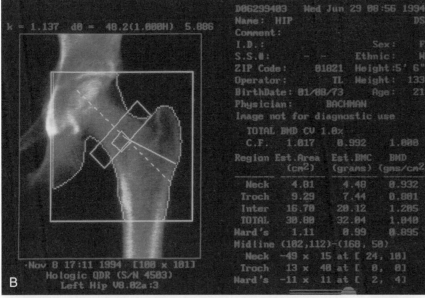

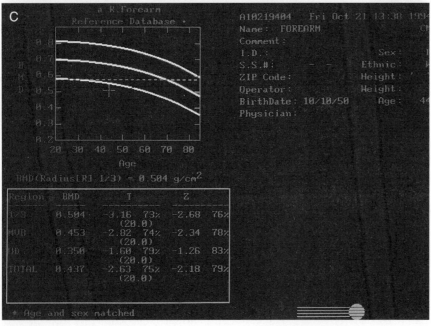

FIGURE 15–6. *A,* Hologic's QDR 4500W. An accepted modality to precisely and rapidly assess bone mineral density. Offers low radiation exposure (10 mrem). The results of the bone mineral density measurement are summarized by a computer and then evaluated by a clinical specialist. *B,* Output from dual-energy x-ray absorptiometry (DEXA) of femur. *C,* Additional output from DEXA. Note the t-score, which is the young adult mean value, and the Z-score, which is the age-matched mean value. (Courtesy of Hologic, Inc., Waltham, MA.)

TABLE 15–3. *Common Medications Used in the Management of Osteoporosis*

AGENT	DOSE/ROUTE	NURSING CONSIDERATIONS AND CLIENT INSTRUCTION
Estrogen	0.3–0.625 mg/day PO *or* 0.05–0.1 mg via transdermal patch, applied twice weekly	Instruct client regarding progesterone (e.g., 10 mg medroxy-progesterone on days 15–25) as prescribed by physician Instruct client regarding monthly breast self-examination, yearly mammography, reporting of any abnormal vaginal bleeding, and gynecologic examinations every 12 months Instruct client to take missed dose as soon as remembered but not to double up to make up for missed doses Review anticipated benefits and possible drug side effects with client Caution clients taking estrogens to stop smoking
Calcitonin	50–100 IU SC or IM daily, or 3 times/wk of salmon calcitonin *or* 0.5 mg SC or IM daily or 2–3 times/wk of human calcitonin	Skin test before initial dose Review anticipated benefits and possible side effects with client and family Side effects include nausea and vomiting, anorexia, mild transient flushing of palms of hands and soles of feet, urinary frequency Recommend that client take at bedtime because this tends to minimize side effects Teach client and family how to administer drug subcutaneously, including injection technique, aseptic technique, accurate dosage preparation, recording of injection sites, rotation of sites Ensure proper nutrition and intake of calcium and vitamin D
Calcitonin nasal spray (Miacalcin)	200–400 IU given in daily doses Alternate nares daily (i.e., use right nare one day and left nare next day)	Skin test before initial dose Side effects include mild nasal discomfort and rhinitis Contraindicated in individuals who were previously allergic to injectable forms of salmon calcitonin Ensure proper nutrition and intake of dietary calcium and vitamin D
Alendronate sodium (Fosamax)	10 mg/day PO (treatment) or 70 mg/wk and 5 mg/day PO (prevention) or 35 mg/wk	To ensure adequate absorption, pill must be taken with 6–8 oz of plain water 30–90 minutes before first food or beverage of the day Take on an empty stomach Client must remain in upright position for 30 minutes after taking medication Side effects include gastric distress, esophagitis, headache Do not take with aminoglycoside antibiotics
Fluoride (slow fluoride)	25 mg bid PO Investigational drug	Review anticipated benefits and potential side effects with client Side effects include gastrointestinal upset (*must* be taken with food), painful joints Monitor serum fluoride levels every 3 months Give with calcium citrate (Pak et al., 1995) Bone mineral density studies at 6-month intervals to document progress of bone density Reinforce importance of adequate calcium intake while taking fluoride
Calcium	1000–1500 mg PO in divided doses	Gastrointestinal distress may occur Free hydrochloric acid is needed for calcium absorption Give calcium with meals Give in divided doses Monitor for history and ongoing presence of hypercalcemia or hypercalciuria
Raloxifene Hcl (Evista)	60 mg/day PO May increase hot flashes Discontinue 72 hours before and during immobilization Do not take with estrogen	Can be taken at any time of day, with or without food Contraindicated in pregnancy and women who are lactating, have history of or active venous thrombosis or pulmonary embolism

Specific doses for the aminobisphosphonate alendronate (Fosamax), selective estrogen receptor modulators (SERMs), and the hormone estrogen have been approved by the U.S. Food and Drug Administration (FDA) for the treatment and prevention of osteoporosis in postmenopausal women. The FDA has approved calcitonin in nasal spray and parenteral forms for the treatment of osteoporosis in both men and women. Newer pharmacologic preparations, including slow-release fluoride, calcitriol, and PTH, are in clinical trials.

Hormonal Replacement Therapy. Estrogen is commonly prescribed for the treatment of postmenopausal osteoporosis. Estrogen deficiency is associated with bone loss, and a woman's bone loss is usually minimized with HRT. The effects of estrogen deficiency on bone are summarized in Figure 15–7, which shows the influence of estrogen in the various metabolic pathways of calcium storage and loss.

Although the exact mechanism by which estrogen suppresses bone mineral loss is unclear, estrogens appear to inhibit bone resorption directly by attaching to specific receptors in bone cells. Estrogens also promote the synthesis of calcitonin. Estrogens have an effect on the intestinal absorption of calcium and enhance the availability of the active metabolite of vitamin D. Activation of this metabolite leads to a decrease in bone resorption.

When a woman enters menopause, the production of estrogen is diminished, leaving her bones unprotected from demineralization. Although not all women experience this demineralization, 25% to 35% are affected. Through bone density measurements and biochemical studies, clinicians can determine whether a woman falls into this high-risk group and whether she is a candidate for HRT. Estrogen replacement commonly minimizes bone loss during the early years after menopause, when an accelerated rate of demineralization occurs. There is also strong evidence that fractures caused by osteoporosis can be prevented in women receiving HRT (Osteoporosis Prevention, 2000).

Estrogen replacement therapy is controversial. Estrogen has been shown to aggravate certain preexisting conditions, including gallbladder and hepatic disease, coagulopathy, and hypertension. Use of the transdermal patch delivery system for estrogen reduces some of these adverse effects because this route bypasses the digestive system and delivers the estrogen directly through the skin and into the vascular system. There is ongoing debate about the use of estrogen in women with a history of breast cancer, and more data are required as to the risk/benefit ratio of prophylactic estrogen and breast cancer. Studies have indicated that HRT can be initiated in vulnerable women many years or even decades after menopause. When estrogen is taken alone, it can increase the risk of endometrial cancer. To eliminate this risk, progestin combined with estrogen is prescribed for women who have not had a hysterectomy.

The orthopaedic nurse's role in caring for the client receiving HRT is primarily educational. Estrogen is not a benign drug, and it can carry with it such adverse side effects as increased vaginal bleeding, headaches, bloating, and weight gain. Breast tenderness and mood swings are common for the woman receiving HRT. A discussion between the woman and her clinician about the advantages, disadvantages, potential side effects, and ongoing surveillance for complications must occur before HRT is initiated. Baseline and annual mammography should be performed on all women who are taking HRT, and these women should perform monthly breast self-examinations. Family history of breast cancer, osteoporosis, and the results of DEXA should also be considered in the decision about HRT. The woman must be well informed about the advantages and disadvantages of HRT and must be assessed at regular intervals for complications.

Antiresorptive Therapy. Alendronate sodium (Fosamax) is approved by the FDA for the treatment of postmenopausal osteoporosis (10 mg daily or 70 mg weekly) and for prevention of osteoporosis (5 mg daily or 35 mg weekly). Alendronate is approved for the treatment

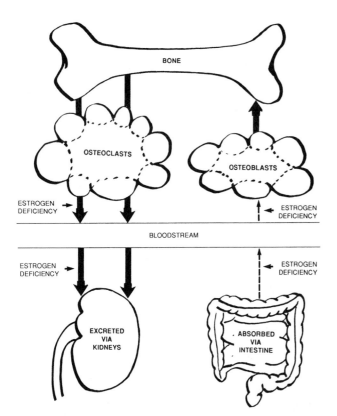

FIGURE 15–7. The effects of estrogen deficiency on calcium storage and loss. Several metabolic pathways of calcium storage and loss are influenced by diminished levels of estrogen. The overall effect is a demineralization of bone.

of steroid-induced osteoporosis in men and women. Alendronate, a bisphosphonate, acts as a specific inhibitor of osteoclast-mediated bone resorption. Studies have shown that subjects who took alendronate for 7 years had increased bone density in the spine and that it is an effective therapy for postmenopausal women with osteoporosis or low BMD (Meunier, Vignot, Garnero, Confavreaux, Paris, Liu-Leage, Sarkar, Liu, Wong, & Draper, 1999; Siris, 2000; Tonino, Meunier, Emkey, Rodriguez-Portales, Menkes, Wasnich, Bone, Santora, Wu, Desai, & Ross, 2000). Alendronate is poorly absorbed from the gastrointestinal tract. Because of this poor absorption, special client teaching must be provided before administration. Client teaching should include the information that alendronate should be taken with 6 to 8 ounces of plain water at least 30 minutes before the first food, medication, or drink of the day. The client should be instructed to remain in an upright position (do not return to bed) for 30 minutes after taking the morning dose.

Currently, concomitant use of alendronate and estrogen is not recommended because of an absence of clinical data to determine the interaction of these drugs. Alendronate is not recommended for clients with renal insufficiency (creatinine clearance less than 35 mL/min) and should be taken with caution by clients with active upper gastric disease. Side effects are relatively uncommon and include abdominal pain and gastric distress. Hypocalcemia should be corrected before initiating therapy, and adequate daily calcium intake must be ensured during therapy. Serum calcium should be monitored during alendronate therapy.

Risedronate (Actonel) is a bisphosphonate that is approved for prevention and treatment of osteoporosis in postmenopausal women and steroid-induced osteoporosis in men and women. It reduced the risk of hip fracture in women with low BMD by 39% (National Osteoporosis Foundation, 2000d).

Calcitonin. Calcitonin, in either the parenteral or nasal spray preparation, is available to treat osteoporosis. Oral administration is inappropriate because calcitonin is a peptide hormone and is destroyed in the gastrointestinal tract. Therein lies the most significant disadvantage of calcitonin therapy other than cost. Until recently, it was necessary to administer calcitonin by the parenteral route. Now, a nasal spray formulation of synthetic salmon calcitonin is approved and is available in the United States. Studies have shown increased vertebral bone mass after long-term therapy with daily nasal spray calcitonin (Avioli, 1995). The nasal spray formulation is contraindicated in anyone with a previous allergy to salmon calcitonin. Use of the nasal spray formulation instead of the parenteral formulation seems to enhance client compliance and minimizes adverse effects.

The nasal spray formulation (synthetic salmon calci-

tonin [Miacalcin]) in daily doses of 200 IU was approved by the FDA in 1995 for the treatment of osteoporosis in women at least 5 years postmenopause who have low bone density and who are not candidates for HRT. Calcitonin is produced in the thyroid and acts to inhibit osteoclast-mediated bone resorption. Calcitonin acts partly by blocking the stimulatory effects of PTH on bone resorption. It is useful in decreasing the rate of bone loss in osteoporosis and may therefore protect the skeleton from fractures. Daily doses of 200 to 400 IU of calcitonin are prescribed to suppress bone resorption.

Some clients develop a resistance to salmon-derived calcitonin after about 2 years, making it ineffective for long-term treatment. This resistance usually subsides if the client is taken off the drug for 6 to 12 months and then resumes therapy. This resistance reportedly does not occur when using human calcitonin, although this form is currently more expensive.

Systemic adverse effects, such as facial flushing, urinary frequency, gastrointestinal distress, nausea, and vomiting, are common with the parenteral formulation. Calcitonin is usually given daily or three times a week by subcutaneous injection. It is reported that fewer side effects occur when the parenteral preparation is administered subcutaneously 2 hours before and after eating and at bedtime (see Table 15–3). The side effects are essentially eliminated with the nasal spray. Nasal discomfort, occasional rhinitis, and itching of the nasal mucosa may occur with intranasal administration.

Education is an essential component when a client begins calcitonin therapy. The orthopaedic nurse can teach the client to self-inject or perhaps teach a family member or friend the technique of subcutaneous injections. It is important to review not only injection technique but also the importance of site rotation and the possible side effects of calcitonin. Teaching for nasal spray administration is less complex. The client should be reminded that the salmon-derived calcitonin must be kept refrigerated if in use for more than 14 days and that the expiration dates should be monitored. Supportive literature and handouts, often available from pharmaceutical companies or created by the orthopaedic nurse, are beneficial in client education.

Sodium Fluoride (Investigational Drug). Sodium fluoride is an investigational drug and shows promise as a potential therapeutic agent for osteoporosis. An FDA advisory committee has recommended the approval of a slow-release formulation of sodium fluoride, taken with calcium. Fluoride can stimulate osteoblastic proliferation and new bone formation. Fluoride therapy requires careful monitoring by a health care provider, however, because it can be toxic. Regular serum fluoride level determinations, BMD studies, fracture history, and biochemical studies need to be routinely performed in persons receiving fluoride therapy.

Selective Estrogen Receptor Modulator. SERMs maximize the effect of estrogen on bone and minimize the negative effects on the breast and endometrium. Raloxifene (Evista) is an example of an SERM and is approved for the treatment and prevention of osteoporosis. In clinical trials, SERM's estrogen-like effect on the skeleton has been shown to reduce the risks of vertebral fractures by 36% and increase the BMD in the spine and femoral neck (Ettinger et al., 1999; Meunier, et al., 1999; Osteoporosis Prevention, 2000). Research continues to determine whether SERMs provide the cardiovascular protective features and cognitive benefits that are associated with HRT.

Calcium and Vitamin D Supplementation. Calcium is not a treatment for osteoporosis, but daily intake of calcium is required to promote optimal bone health and enhance therapeutic outcomes. The need for calcium supplements is nonexistent if the diet contains the normal recommended, age-related, daily allowance of 800 to 1500 mg calcium and 400 to 1000 IU of vitamin D. See Table 15–2 for NIH recommendations for age-related minimum daily requirements (MDR) of calcium. Most individuals do not achieve an adequate daily dietary intake of calcium. A 65-year-old-man requires 1500 mg of daily dietary calcium; he would need to drink five 8-ounce glasses of milk to achieve this daily requirement. Calcium supplements may be used to augment dietary calcium intake. Absorption of the calcium supplements may vary. Calcium carbonate and calcium citrate are two compounds commonly used for supplements. Calcium carbonate may provide more elemental calcium and have more bioavailability. Constipation and bloating may accompany ingestion of calcium carbonate. Adequate intake of water with the supplement may decrease the constipation. Calcium citrate is purported to cause less gastrointestinal distress. A plan for the use of calcium supplements should include the following: awareness of the MDR for specific age groups; selection of a high-quality calcium supplement taken with meals in three divided doses daily; the consumption of 6 to 8 ounces of water with each supplement; and the use of vitamin D–supplemented calcium during intervals of low sunlight exposure (winter months). Research has indicated that individuals from 12 years of age to the very old have benefited from the consumption of adequate intake of calcium.

The use of calcium supplements does have risks. Hypercalcemia, hypercalciuria, and kidney stones are potential side effects of excessive and unsupervised calcium supplementation. Hypercalcemia may cause renal damage. A 24-hour urine collection can be assayed for calcium and creatinine levels before and several weeks after calcium supplementation is begun and repeated about twice yearly to monitor for hypercalciuria. No renal stones were evident in a study of participants who received up to 2.5 g of daily calcium (Avioli, 1993).

Natural estrogens and phytoestrogens from plants (black cohosh, evening primrose oil, soybeans) have weak, estrogen-like effects, but current research does not show any effect on reducing fractures (Osteoporosis Prevention, 2000).

Nursing Diagnoses and Management

Because it is recognized that osteoporosis is both preventable and treatable, the major emphasis of nursing management is on prevention of the disease itself and prevention of injuries in the client with the disorder. Because osteoporosis is seen as a disease of the older adult, it is important that preventive education be instituted before onset or during youth and young adulthood. Education and prevention strategies for learners in all age groups are well within the role of the professional nurse. Client education should target the prevention and the management of osteoporosis for not only women but also for men (Sedlak, Doheny, & Estok, 2000; Sedlak, Doheny, & Jones, 2000) (Table 15-4).

Nursing management of clients with osteoporosis is targeted toward the nursing diagnoses of impaired mobility, nutritional deficit, potential for injury, pain, and alteration in body image. Additional diagnoses may include activity intolerance related to pain and impaired mobility, anxiety related to fear of fractures, ineffective coping related to alteration in body image and chronic disease progression, sexual dysfunction related to back pain, social isolation related to back pain, and fear of falls. Clients with advanced kyphosis may experience problems with constipation and ineffective breathing patterns.

Prevention. Because individuals tend to reach 90% of peak bone mass before the age of 20, education must begin at an early age. School-age children should be taught the importance of calcium intake and exercise in promoting bone health. Individuals should be taught about the complications of osteoporosis and strategies for prevention (Sedlak, Doheny, & Jones, 1998).

Adolescents should be evaluated for their exercise pattern, eating habits, and menstrual status. At particular risk are female athletes (e.g., gymnasts, dancers), who may have limited caloric and calcium intake and an intensive exercise program and may experience amenorrhea. These young women require counseling to assist them in finding a balance between the need to minimize weight gain and to exercise and their physiologic need for calcium balance and bone formation. Young women who have a family history of osteoporosis should be made aware of their risks and informed of long-term strategies for prevention (Hobart & Smucker, 2000).

Teaching individuals to continue regular exercise is a key component in any program for osteoporosis prevention. Weight-bearing exercises (e.g., walking) and weight lifting are important in the prevention of osteoporosis. Swimming and bicycling are good exercises for cardiovascular fitness, but these non–weight-bearing activities are

TABLE 15–4. *Client Education: Osteoporosis*

FOCUS OF TEACHING	TEACHING POINTS
Reducing risk factors	Teach client about the common risk factors for osteoporosis and how to change the modifiable factors
	Modifiable—smoking, high caffeine intake, high protein intake, high alcohol intake, estrogen deficiency, low dietary calcium, inactivity, excessive exercise, anorexia or bulimia
	Nonmodifiable—female, white or Asian, postmenopausal, small bone structure, pale complexion, thin skin, light-colored hair and eyes, genetic predisposition
Exercise	Teach importance of regular, weight-bearing exercise
	Instruct client to engage in appropriate type of exercise for osteoporosis as recommended by physician or physical therapist (avoid high-impact or vertebral spine rotational activities because of fracture risk)
Nutrition	Instruct client about diet, medicinal needs, and calcium supplements
	Provide current information about calcium supplements
	Teach client current recommended dietary allowances for calcium, and review food sources high in calcium
	Recommend lactose-free products to promote intake of milk and dairy products if lactose intolerance is a problem
	Emphasize benefits of exposure to sun for homebound population
Prevention of fractures	Teach client about safety and fall precautions (see Box 15–2), and provide current literature about how to create a safe home environment
	Instruct client about skeletal fragility (low bone mineral density and fracture risks) in relationship to current need to modify activities
	Discuss gradual resumption of selected activities as treatment progresses and skeleton strengthens
	Teach how fractures occur so breaks can be avoided
Pain management	Teach client self-administration of nasal spray calcitonin as ordered by physician, and review its potential analgesic effects
	Review activity tolerance and suggest (with physical therapist consultation) modifications in exercise schedules as indicated

not presumed to promote bone health. Most client education programs for the prevention of osteoporosis now recommend at least 30 to 40 minutes of sustained, weight-bearing activity three to four times per week. The exercise plan for the individual who wants to prevent osteoporosis is very different from the exercise plan prescribed for the individual with osteoporosis. Refer to evidence-based practice question for persons having risk factors for osteoporosis (p. 428).

Consulting a physical therapist on an exercise plan for the person with osteoporosis or low bone density is strongly recommended. Exercises for stretching, strengthening of back extensors, and promoting flexibility are commonly included in the management of these clients. Activities such as lifting, back flexion, or forceful unguarded motions (e.g., opening a window that is stuck or lifting heavy bags of groceries or lifting children) are to be avoided because they may precipitate vertebral and other fractures.

Adults and older adults should be given necessary information on strategies to limit the severity of osteoporosis through diet and activity. The belief that osteoporosis is an inevitable part of aging must be extinguished. The National Osteoporosis Foundation, a not-for-profit organization, provides excellent support, information, and educational materials about osteoporosis (Table 15–5).

High Risk for Impaired Physical Mobility

Exercise Promotion. Although the elite athlete with rigorous exercise regimens may experience the damaging effects of demineralization related to altered estrogen balance, the major activity problem in the development of osteoporosis is the lack of weight-bearing exercise. The beneficial effects of exercise on bone have been well established. Client education must emphasize that bones require a weight-bearing state to develop, grow, and remodel. The mechanical force of weight bearing promotes bone growth, and just as muscles atrophy without use, bones weaken and demineralize without exercise.

Client education programs for the prevention of osteoporosis recommend regular and sustained weight-bearing activity. Walking is one of the easiest and most beneficial forms of exercise for bone health and can be tolerated by most age categories. Jogging tends to be too high impact, and swimming does not provide the weight bearing necessary for bone stimulation. Also, specific strengthening exercises may be indicated to provide increased strength and support.

For the client with advanced osteoporosis, the goal is to maintain independence in activities of daily living (ADLs). Attaining this goal is likely to prevent the complications of immobility (see Chapter 4). The client

TABLE 15–5. Osteoporosis: Nursing Management

NURSING PROBLEM	NURSING INTERVENTIONS
Pain	Promote comfort
	Teach client self-administration of calcitonin as ordered by physician, and review its potential analgesic effects
	Review activity tolerance, and suggest (with physical therapy consultation) modifications in exercise as indicated
	Advise client about outpatient physical therapy schedule for heat, massage, and back-strengthening exercise
	Instruct client to avoid sudden forceful back flexion
	Avoid lifting anything greater than about 10 pounds
Self-image	Promote positive self-image
	Assess anxiety and response to diagnosis, injury, and pain
	Suggest osteoporosis support group, if available, for psychosocial help in dealing with effects of osteoporosis (consider referral for private counseling if indicated)
	Provide realistic, yet optimistic, feedback to client about loss (of height, of bone integrity) and the potential outcomes of treatment
Knowledge deficit	Provide information on the disease and treatment
	Assess current knowledge base, and correct misconceptions about prognosis
	Discuss modes of treatment, and outline personal treatment plan with specific time frame for introduction of each prescribed treatment or intervention
	Provide current client education literature, and refer to osteoporosis lecture series (where available) for further information
	Provide or show appropriate videotapes (where available) on osteoporosis and related issues, and discuss content with client after viewing
	Inform about National Osteoporosis Foundation, 1150 17th Street, NW, Suite 500, Washington, DC 20036; telephone 202-223-2226, fax 202-223-2237; website: www.nof.org
Nutrition	Instruct on dietary, medicinal needs, and calcium supplements
	Provide current information on calcium supplements, and recommend calcium citrate to alleviate gastrointestinal problems (gas)

can be assisted in reaching this goal by using certain assistive or adaptive devices (see Chapter 13). Mechanisms to assist with ADLs, such as adaptive clothing, safety bars, and ambulatory aids, may support the client's independence. Collaboration with the occupational therapist and physical therapist is essential in promoting the goal of maximum mobility and independence.

Nutritional Deficit: Calcium Balance

Nutritional Counseling. Nutritional deficits in the client at risk for osteoporosis center on the amount of calcium and vitamin D in the diet. Many Americans consume far too little calcium (NIH, 1994). The average daily intake of calcium in the American woman is estimated to be about 500 mg, in contrast to the recommended level of 1000 to 1500 mg. Education must be targeted toward helping individuals of all ages realize the important relationship between adequate calcium intake and strong bones. Without adequate amounts of calcium, the body robs the bones to supply calcium for physiologic needs.

In 1994, the NIH Consensus Development Conference on Optimal Calcium Intake was held. Conclusions from this conference of experts included (1) that a large number of Americans fail to achieve optimal calcium intake, (2) that optimal daily intake should range from 400 mg/day for infants to 1500 mg/day for men and women older than 65 years of age, and (3) that total intake of up to 2000 mg/day appears to be safe for most individuals (NIH, 1994). See Table 15–2 for specific recommendations across the life span.

Calcium assimilation within the body can also be jeopardized by certain dietary practices that are common among Americans. Diets high in protein, fiber, sodium, and carbohydrates diminish the ability to maintain total body calcium stores. Individuals having these dietary patterns along with low dietary calcium intake require nutritional counseling. Table 15–1 lists calcium-rich foods. Adequate vitamin D must be consumed for the metabolism of calcium.

High Risk for Injury

Safety and Fracture Prevention. Osteoporosis predisposes the client to fractures, and prevention of falls is critical in caring for vulnerable clients. Helping the client balance optimal activity with fall prevention actions can be beneficial in minimizing injury. A tendency to fall can be a result of the natural processes of aging, but additional factors commonly affect the risks of falling and concomitant fracture among clients of all ages (see Box 15–2). The nurse must remain cognizant of these factors by integrating three themes into client education: (1) optimal management and follow-up care of clients with disorders that disturb balance or cause visual or hearing loss; (2) educational counseling on the need to limit the use of balance-disturbing drugs, including alcohol and psychotropic drugs; and (3) thorough and appropriate client and family education regarding the risks of falling, including reduction of environmental hazards.

Assessment must be made to identify those clients who, out of fear of falling, severely limit their activity. These clients may be at greater risk for fractures secondary to the lack of activity (National Osteoporosis Foundation, 2000e).

Residents of long-term care facilities and retirement communities are at particularly high risk for falls and the resultant fractures that contribute to mortality and morbidity. Research indicates that use of a fall risk assessment tool can accurately predict which clients are at risk to fall and the time intervals when falls are most common—1200 to 0300 and 1500 to 1800 hours (McFarlane & Melora, 1993). Implementation of fall risk strategies can reduce the incidence of falls. These strategies include using a fall risk appraisal instrument, admitting a high-risk client to a room that is in close proximity to the nurses' station, assisting with elimination in a safe and timely manner, and making frequent visits or rounds to client rooms. The use of alarm systems that gave warning when a client left the bed did not reduce the number of falls in one study (McFarlane & Melora, 1993). Other research-based fall prevention strategies include the use of deep seat chairs (38% of falls are caused by sliding from chairs) and distribution of an educational leaflet to teach the client and the caregiver strategies to decrease the incidence of falls (Sweeting, 1994). Exercise regimens that improve balance are also effective in decreasing falls. A collaborative plan of care that includes the client, significant other, nurse, physical therapist, and others may be required in the client who is at high risk for falls.

Some compression fractures occur with lifting of heavy objects, such as bags of groceries or grandchildren. The client with established osteoporosis should avoid lifting more than 5 to 10 pounds. This restriction prevents the lifting of children. The adult can avoid lifting but still snuggle the child by requesting that the child crawl or climb into the adult's lap or be placed there. This approach avoids lifting but still allows one to hold young children.

Pain Related to Back Discomfort, Compression Fracture, and Impaired Mobility

Pain Management. Osteoporotic fractures can be very painful, and clients with advanced disease can become completely immobile. Pain management is addressed in Chapter 5. Typically, clients with osteoporosis experience acute pain when there is a fracture, especially a compression fracture of the vertebrae. Acute pain is treated pharmacologically with both non-narcotic and narcotic analgesics. Nonsteroidal anti-inflammatory drugs (NSAIDs) are useful in the management of acute and chronic pain. Muscle relaxants can be used to decrease the muscle spasm that accompanies the compression fracture. Careful assessment of the client who is

receiving analgesic medication is required to detect side effects that could potentiate falls. Application of heat to the back may reduce pain in the lower back. The short-term use of back braces may also offer some pain relief after compression fractures. Long-term use of braces or corsets promotes muscle wasting and can be harmful. A balance between rest, pain relief, and mobility is required but difficult to attain after compression fracture.

Altered Body Image Related to Kyphotic Changes

Promote Positive Self-image. Clients with advanced osteoporosis can experience body image changes because of dowager's hump and height loss. Obtaining clothing that fits properly may be difficult. For some individuals, the altered body image and increased safety risks because of potential for fracture can precipitate a withdrawal from normal social activities. Alterations in sexuality can occur as a result of mobility deficits, discomfort, and poor self-esteem. See Chapter 2 for a discussion of body image. The management and prevention of pain in the client with osteoporosis is a worthwhile goal and one that is amenable to nursing interventions (Table 15-5).

PAGET'S DISEASE OF BONE

Paget's disease of bone (osteitis deformans) is a skeletal disorder that results from excessive osteoclastic activity. This increased osteoclastic resorption leads to a compensatory increase in bone formation and acceleration of bone remodeling. The resulting bone is highly vascular, structurally weak, and susceptible to deformity and fracture. The long bones, pelvis, lumbar vertebrae, and skull predominantly are affected.

Cause and Incidence

The cause of Paget's disease is unknown, but it is the second most common bone disease after osteoporosis in the geriatric population. There is evidence of a familial tendency; 25% to 40% of clients with Paget's disease have at least one relative with the disorder (Ankrom & Shapiro, 1998). Paget's disease is rare before age 40 and increases from about 3.5% of the population older than 50 years of age to about 12% after age 80. It is more common in men than in women (Tiegs, Lohse, Wollan, & Melton, 2000). Researchers speculate that Paget's disease may be caused by infection from certain blood-borne viruses, and that following the acute viremia, osteoclasts or their precursors become chronically infected, thus stimulating osteoclastic proliferation (Kaplan & Singer, 1995; Siris, 1995a). However, recently, a gene for Paget's disease has been localized, indicating a genetic basis of Paget's disease (Nance, Nuttall, Econs, Lyles, Viles, Vance, Pericak-Vance, & Speer, 2000).

Assessment

Clients with Paget's disease of bone may be asymptomatic. In clients who are symptomatic, the symptoms are often vague and difficult to distinguish from those of other diseases. The most common complaints are pain, bone deformity, and increased tendency to fracture. Deep aching bone pain is present, and it often is aggravated by weight bearing. Pagetic lesions lead to deformities that are demonstrable on x-ray film (Fig. 15–8). Joint destruction and arthritis also occur because the pagetic joint deformity can invade the joints and contribute to osteoarthritis. Pagetic lesions in the spine can lead to degenerative arthritis, spinal stenosis, and nerve root impingement and may cause pain that radiates from the spine to the lower extremities (Kaplan, 1999a; Lewis, Tesh, & Lyles, 1999).

Additional symptoms of Paget's disease include bony deformities of the skeleton, particularly in the skull. Progressive enlargement of the skull takes place over many years, resulting in a soft, thick, and enlarged skull (Fig. 15–8C). Blood flow to pagetic bone is also greatly increased. The affected areas are warm to the touch because the increased vascularity may cause a rise in local temperature of up to 5°F (Mirra, Brien, & Tehranzadeh, 1995). Paget's disease of the spine can lead to the development of kyphosis and height loss from vertebral compression fractures. Bowing in the long bones of the arms and legs, with subsequent varus (turned inward) deformity of the elbows and knees, may occur. In the lower extremities, a bowing deformity of the tibia is common (Fig. 15–9). A pathologic fracture of the tibia may be the first indicator of the presence of Paget's disease of bone. These fractures are typically transverse, have minimal comminution, and resemble a snapped piece of chalk. They are called *chalkstick fractures* (Fig. 15–10).

A less common complication is a decrease in auditory acuity that occurs as the skull enlarges in the region of the temporal bone. These deficits may include impairments

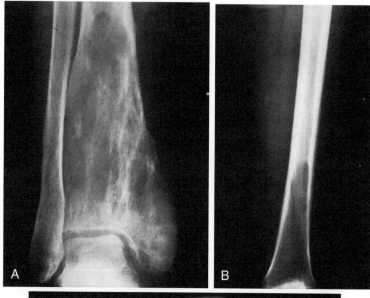

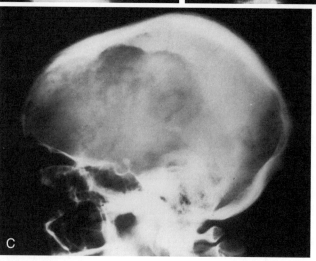

FIGURE 15–8. Radiographs and bone scans of various forms of pagetoid bone. *A,* Radiograph of tibia, demonstrating severe osteolytic activity. *B,* Radiograph of femur demonstrating osteolytic and sclerotic foci in the same bone. *C,* Lateral radiograph of skull demonstrating osteoporotic type lesions called osteoporosis circumscripta, a common manifestation of Paget's disease. (Courtesy of The Paget Foundation.)

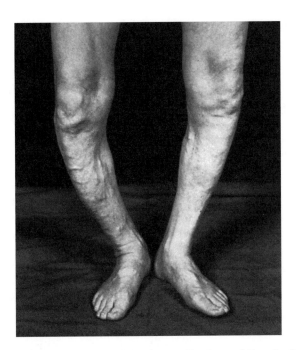

FIGURE 15–9. Musculoskeletal complications of Paget's disease of bone. Severe bowing of the right tibia indicates asymmetry of Paget's disease of bone. Severe bowing causes knee and ankle pain. Minimal bowing of the right tibia did not indicate pagetic lesions. (Courtesy of The Paget Foundation.)

in vision, eye and facial muscles, hearing, swallowing, speech, and balance.

A rare complication in the older pagetic client is congestive heart failure that develops as the overworked heart attempts to pump blood through the increased mass of blood vessels in active pagetic bone. This high-output cardiac failure occurs when more than one third of the skeleton is affected by Paget's disease. Other cardiovascular abnormalities associated with Paget's disease include hypertension, atherosclerosis, systolic murmurs, and aortic valve calcification. A most alarming complication of Paget's disease is the development of a malignant bone tumor. Certain malignancies, primary or secondary, may develop in a preexisting pagetic lesion (Kaplan & Singer, 1995). A marked increase in pain or deformity may herald this latter complication. This acute increase in severity of symptoms indicates the need for radiologic assessment and possible bone biopsy.

Diagnostic Evaluation

Laboratory Findings. Serum alkaline phosphatase (ALP) levels are characteristically elevated in clients with Paget's disease and indicate excessive osteoblastic activity. Normal serum ALP is 30 to 115 IU/L. In Paget's disease, the level can range from high normal to more than 2000 IU/L. Serum ALP is a commonly used blood chemistry indicator, and a good correlation exists between the extent and activity of the disease and the level of serum ALP. However, the value of ALP is diminished in the presence

of liver disease and pregnancy. Certain drugs also alter serum ALP levels. Clients with end-stage Paget's disease have characteristically low ALP levels. The urinary excretion of pyridinoline crosslinks correlates well with clinical symptoms but is somewhat costly to use to monitor the progress of the disorder (Siris, 1995a). Serum calcium, phosphorus, and albumin levels should be assessed but are usually normal (Mirra, Brien, & Tehranzadeh, 1995).

Expert clinicians recommend annual assessment of serum ALP in asymptomatic clients and three or four times per year for clients undergoing pharmacologic treatment (Siris, 1995a). Annual x-ray studies are recommended for clients with active osteolytic disease.

Timely assessment of calcium levels is also essential. The client with Paget's disease who has an acute episode of immobility is particularly prone to hypercalciuria, hypercalcemia, and renal stones (Mirra, Brien, & Tehranzadeh, 1995). Hyperuricemia and gout may be associated with Paget's disease because of increased purine metabolism. Approximately 10% of individuals with Paget's disease have evidence of hearing loss, and about 1% experience severe hearing loss (Monsell, 1995). Therefore, the pagetic client older than age 50 should have regular audiograms to promote early detection of hearing loss.

Radiographic Findings. Radiologic examination of the skeleton is the primary means of confirming the diagnosis of Paget's disease. In the early phases of the

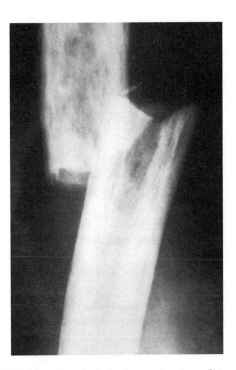

FIGURE 15–10. Musculoskeletal complication of Paget's disease. Chalkstick fracture. Fractures are common with Paget's disease of bone. The pagetic fracture is usually transverse, has minimal comminution, and resembles the snapping of a carrot or piece of chalk. (Courtesy of The Paget Foundation.)

disease, there are characteristic osteolytic lesions, most commonly observed in the long bones and skull (see Fig. 15-8). Later, an adjoining overgrowth of bone appears, providing a coarse irregular appearance and enlargement of bone contours. After symptoms are present, the weakened bone usually shows the characteristic mosaic pattern. Long bones may have tiny cracks, and the surface of the skull may appear irregular because of the varying thickness of the bone (see Fig. 15-8C) and low-density lesions.

A radioactive bone scan may be done to evaluate the metabolic activity of a pagetic lesion. A radioactive isotope with an affinity for bone is injected intravenously, and the radioactive substance collects in the areas of active Paget's disease and can be detected by the scanner. Because of the isotope's inclination to be deposited at the sites of high bone turnover, these isotopes are useful in defining the number, extent, and metabolic activity of the pagetic lesions (Mirra, Brien, & Tehranzadeh, 1995). Technetium-labeled bisphosphonates are commonly used in radioisotope scanning. The bone scan is used to determine whether a particular lesion seen on x-ray film is still active. An inactive lesion does not show an increased uptake of isotope. Magnetic resonance imaging (MRI) of the skull may be used in the assessment of the client with Paget's disease and would probably indicate extreme thickening of the bone.

Bone Biopsy. In most clients suspected of having Paget's disease, the history, physical examination, biochemical studies, and radiologic examination should be adequate to confirm the diagnosis. Occasionally, it is necessary for the clinician to perform a bone biopsy to clarify an unusual clinical or radiologic finding. A high suspicion for malignant changes, as indicated by recent increase in pain or deformity and radiologic indications, in a preexisting pagetic bone lesion may require a bone biopsy. Details about bone biopsy are described in the section on osteoporosis.

Treatment Modalities

Asymptomatic clients with Paget's disease require no treatment, and mildly symptomatic clients usually are treated successfully with analgesics, anti-inflammatory drugs, and aspirin. NSAIDs, such as ibuprofen, and aspirin may be used to minimize the arthritis associated with the joint destruction that may occur with Paget's disease. When the pain is severe or disabling and when neurologic or cardiac complications develop, treatment involves the use of more specific therapeutic agents. Indications for drug therapy in Paget's disease include bone pain, impending surgery, hearing loss, spinal stenosis, high-output congestive heart failure, fracture prevention, and rapidly progressive osteolytic lesions (Kaplan & Singer, 1995).

The vigorous treatment of Paget's disease includes the use of suppressive agents, such as calcitonin. Calcito-

nin is one of the treatments of choice because it inhibits osteoclastic resorption of bone, which therefore leads to a decrease in bone turnover. The parenteral formulation of calcitonin is approved for treatment of Paget's disease. Table 15-6 discusses the use of calcitonin in the section on osteoporosis.

Bisphosphonates constitute a second category of suppressive agents that are effective in the treatment of Paget's disease. Etidronate disodium (Didronel) blocks bone resorption and bone formation by coating the bone surfaces with a slippery, soaplike substance. It has the distinct advantage of being available in tablet form and can be especially useful in treating clients who have developed a resistance to calcitonin. A principal disadvantage is that etidronate usually should not be taken for longer than 6 months at a time because of the high incidence of side effects. Some clinicians use a multiyear regimen in which etidronate is given for 6 months (on) and avoided for 6 months (off). Nausea and cramps can occur early in treatment but can be reduced by taking the drug on an empty stomach and delaying eating for 2 hours after a dose. Calcium and iron supplements may decrease the absorption of etidronate. Large doses or prolonged use of bisphosphonates have been known to increase the risk of osteomalacia and pathologic fractures. Bisphosphonates should not be used in the immobilized client or the client with a fracture because they inhibit new bone formation. Etidronate should not be taken within 2 hours of taking any food or medications.

Alendronate sodium (Fosamax) is an aminobisphosphonate approved for the treatment of Paget's disease of bone. This drug decreases the rate of bone resorption, resulting in decreased bone formation. The recommended dosage of alendronate for Paget's disease is 40 mg once daily for 6 months. This drug must be taken on an empty stomach and before any food. For a more in-depth discussion of alendronate, see the section on osteoporosis and Table 15-6.

Plicamycin is an antineoplastic antibiotic that may inhibit PTH's effect on osteoclasts. This drug has been used to treat the symptoms that may occur with Paget's disease, but it has a high toxicity and is rarely used (Gennari, Nuti, Agnusdei, Camporeale, & Martini, 1994; Siris, 1995a).

Pamidronate disodium (Aredia) is a bisphosphonate compound approved for the treatment of Paget's disease. Pamidronate is given intravenously. It is a potent suppressor of bone resorption because of its inhibitory effect on osteoclasts, its ability to bind calcium phosphate crystals in the bone, and its ability to block calcium reabsorption. Pamidronate remains bound until the bone is remodeled (Lehne, 2000). The use of pamidronate has resulted in more normal serum ALP levels and calcium levels as well as prolonged remissions in many clients (Mazieres, 1995). Adverse effects of pamidronate include fever, chills, nausea, general malaise, and thrombophlebitis at the infusion site. Daily oral calcium supplements

TABLE 15–6. *Medications Used in Paget's Disease*

NAME	DOSAGE	CONTRAINDICATIONS	SIDE EFFECTS	ROUTE	NURSING IMPLICATIONS
Salmon calcitonin	50–100 IU/day	Clinical allergy to salmon calcitonin Skin test before first dose	Nausea, flushing, feeling of warmth, urinary frequency	SC	Skin test before first dose; teach about self-injection, site rotation, and timing
Calcitonin, human	0.25–0.5 mg	None known	Nausea, flushing, feeling of warmth, urinary frequency	SC or IM	
Alendronate (Fosamax)	40 mg/day	Severe renal insufficiency (creatinine clearance < 35 mL/min)	Abdominal pain, esophagitis, gastritis, nausea and vomiting	PO take only with plain water	Take with 6–8 oz of plain water, and on an empty stomach at least 30 min before first food or drink of day; remain in upright position after taking
Etidronate disodium (Didronel)	5 mg/kg for 6-mo periods	Large doses increase chance of pathologic fracture, osteomalacia; should not be used in immobilized client or client with a fracture	Nausea, cramps, diarrhea (give on empty stomach and do not eat for 90 min after dose); may be taken with juice	PO	Take in divided daily doses?
Pamidronate (Aredia)			Hypocalcemia and second-degree hyperparathyroidism; flulike symptoms; thrombophlebitis at IV site	IV	Also take oral calcium supplements 500 mg bid
Tiludronate (Skelid)	400 mg for 3 mo			PO	Take with 6–8 oz of plain water and *not* within 2 hr of meals

(500 mg twice daily) may prevent the hypocalcemia and secondary hyperparathyroidism that are common during pamidronate therapy (Siris, 1995a).

Serum calcium and phosphate levels, complete blood count, temperature, pulse, respiration, and renal function should be monitored during pamidronate therapy. Indications of hypocalcemia, including perioral tingling, numbness, paresthesia, and a positive Chvostek's sign or a positive Trousseau's phenomenon, should be assessed and reported to the primary practitioner immediately.

Surgical procedures may be required to manage the symptoms and arthritic changes related to Paget's disease. Tibial osteotomy may be performed to realign the knee and relieve pain (Kaplan, 1999b). Total joint replacement and spinal decompression are beneficial in alleviating the severe pain associated with Paget's disease (Lewallen, 1999). Excessive blood loss during surgery is a concern because of the highly vascular bone. Thus, before surgery, a vigorous course of calcitonin is administered to de-

crease bone remodeling and minimize blood loss during surgery (Kaplan, 1999b). Rapid mobilization after surgery assists in preventing the bony demineralization associated with disuse and the resultant hypercalcemia and risk for renal stones that may occur in these vulnerable clients.

Nursing Diagnoses and Management

The goals of nursing intervention for the client with Paget's disease focus on pain control; prevention of deformity, injury, and fractures; education about the disease process; and the availability of specific therapies. Table 15-7 summarizes the teaching suggested for the client with Paget's disease.

As in other metabolic disease of bone, the primary nursing diagnoses seen in clients with Paget's disease are alterations in comfort, impaired mobility, potential for injury, alteration in body image, and alteration in coping. Additional diagnoses that may occur, especially in advanced disease, include fear related to potential falls or

TABLE 15–7. Client Education: Paget's Disease

FOCUS OF TEACHING	TEACHING POINTS
Pain management	Teach client to take medications as prescribed and to position self with care in bed or chair
	Instruct client to move slowly and with measured steps; no abrupt movements
Self-care and medications	Educate client about the disease process and the drugs client will be taking:
	Describe pagetic process to client and provide information about The Paget Foundation (120 Wall St., Suite 1602, New York, NY 10005; telephone 1-212-509-5335, fax 212-509-8492; website: www.paget.org; e-mail pagetfdn@aol.com)
	When taking calcitonin:
	Teach self-injection and site rotation
	Warn about side effects and that they are mild and infrequent and usually diminish with continued use of calcitonin
	When taking alendronate or etidronate:
	Teach client to take medication on empty stomach, first thing on arising in the morning
	Instruct client to take bisphosphonate with 6–8 oz of plain water, not to eat for 30 min after morning dose, and to remain in upright position after taking bisphosphonate
	Tell client to report any abdominal cramps, diarrhea, new bone pain, or fractures
	Explain importance of completing regular follow-up laboratory tests

fractures, self-care deficit related to deformity, social isolation related to self-care deficit, sexual dysfunction related to bone pain and deformity, and sensory or perceptual alterations (visual and auditory) related to cranial nerve damage.

Pain Related to Bone Deformities

Pain Management. Although most Paget's disease clients are asymptomatic, the most common symptom is pain. This pain is usually a deep, aching bone pain and can be worsened by weight bearing when either the spine or the lower extremities are involved. Simple analgesics or anti-inflammatory medications usually control the pain in early Paget's disease. However, in more advanced stages of the disease, therapy with bisphosphonates (alendronate and etidronate), pamidronate, or calcitonin is required. Nonpharmacologic strategies for pain relief may also be helpful. Heat therapy and gentle massage can alleviate mild discomfort. Bracing can assist to immobilize and support the extremity or vertebrae, thus reducing the pain. Exercise protocols and activity regimens should be carefully planned to prevent injury and minimize the experienced sense of fatigue. For clients with advanced Paget's disease involving the joint, joint replacement surgery may be indicated. Avoidance of long-term immobility is important.

Impaired Physical Mobility

Exercise Promotion and Assessment. Most clients with Paget's disease are encouraged to remain as active as possible. Simple strengthening and weight-bearing exercises may be taught, and a physical therapy consultation provides advice on walking aids, heel lifts, and possibly corsets to help improve function and mobility. It is important that the nurse assess the client for any new areas of restricted movement as well as for any limitations in ability to carry out normal ADLs. Assessing for evidence of hypercalciuria, hypercalcemia, and hematuria should be implemented with periods of immobility for the client with Paget's disease.

Potential Injury: Fractures Related to Impaired Metabolism

Safety and Fracture Prevention. The client with Paget's disease is at risk for experiencing fractures, especially during the active phase of the disease. Care is similar to the interventions for preventing injury in the client with osteoporosis and osteomalacia. The environment should be assessed for potential hazards. Client teaching should emphasize safety and fall precautions. The goal should be for the client to proceed with an activity program with an awareness of areas of potential hazard.

Altered Body Image

Promotion of Positive Self-image. Once deformities occur in Paget's disease, they are irreversible. Bony deformities (cranial changes resulting in an enlarged, soft cranium and hearing loss; long bone changes resulting in bowing; and vertebral changes resulting in kyphosis) can affect the person's self-concept and may require integration of a revised body image. If the individual's independence and mobility are maintained, the individual is more likely to cope effectively with the body image disturbance.

Altered Individual and Family Coping

Education and Counseling. Education and emotional support provide the foundation for helping the client and family cope with the impact of Paget's disease. A discussion of the pagetic process and its (limited) tendency to progress, along with a description of the (low) probability of encountering life-threatening or life-limiting complications, can be beneficial and encouraging to the client with Paget's disease.

In providing support and education to clients with Paget's disease, it is helpful to give them information about The Paget Foundation (see Table 15-7). This nonprofit organization publishes a valuable newsletter, provides a wealth of current information, and carries out public awareness campaigns.

There is no cure for Paget's disease, but as indicated, treatment is available to relieve the pain and discomfort of the disease and to retard disease progression. Medications used in the treatment of Paget's disease need to be discussed with the client, and a thorough review of proper dosage, administration, and possible side effects must occur. At-risk family members of individuals with Paget's disease should be advised to have serum ALP assessed every 2 to 3 years after age 40 (Siris, 1995b).

OSTEOMALACIA

Osteomalacia literally means "softening of bones," and it occurs when calcified bone mass is decreased and calcium and phosphorus fail to be deposited in the bone matrix. Osteomalacia is characterized by inadequate concentration of calcium or phosphorus and inadequate mineralization of bone matrix (Roberts & Lappe, 2001). There is a greatly increased amount of osteoid, or perosseous matrix, in various parts of the skeleton and a resultant decrease in mineralization. The absence of adequate calcium or phosphorus to promote the mineralization of bone leads to the softened skeletal structure. This softening causes marked deformities of weight-bearing bones, distortion in bone shape, and pathologic fractures. Assessment of the client with osteomalacia usually reveals bone pain, myopathy, and skeletal fractures (Reginato, Falasca, Pappu, McNight, & Agha, 1999). Individuals who are taking medications such as phenytoin and those who have limited exposure to sunlight are at risk for osteomalacia and may require vitamin D supplements.

Osteomalacia is often confused with osteoporosis because these disorders share many clinical manifestations and can occur together. However, osteoporosis is decreased bone mass predominantly related to lack of calcium and bone mass. Osteomalacia is demineralized bone primarily related to a lack of vitamin D. Medications that are known to cause osteomalacia include aluminum, antacids, anticonvulsants, etidronate, and fluoride (Bohannon & Lyles, 1994). Other clinical situations in which osteomalacia occurs are listed in Box 15-4. Whereas osteoporosis is considered to be predominantly irreversible, osteomalacia is considered reversible with treatment. Table 15-8 clarifies the differential features of osteoporosis and osteomalacia and Paget's disease.

Cause

Osteomalacia, often called the adult form of rickets (see discussion on rickets at the end of this section), results

from a vitamin D deficiency. Osteomalacia is a mineralization defect that occurs in bone remodeling after the epiphyseal plates have closed, whereas rickets is a deficit in the growing bone, specifically in endochondral bone formation. Some industrialized nations have regulations that require milk to be fortified with vitamin D. Therefore, the incidence of vitamin D–deficient rickets and osteomalacia is low in these nations. However, both rickets and osteomalacia persist, albeit in lower frequencies. Adulthood osteomalacia causes less severe clinical features than does childhood rickets. In the mature skeleton, 5% to 10% of total calcium is newly laid down each year. Consequently, a mineralization defect in adults must be present for several years to produce clinical manifestations.

In the United States, genetically acquired derangements of vitamin D and phosphate metabolism have been identified as the most common cause of underlying osteomalacia. Vitamin D deficiencies can be found with intestinal or renal disease or after major intestinal surgery. Lack of exposure to sunlight can occur with the homebound or institutionalized older person. Inadequate intake of fortified foods in this same population further aggravates the condition.

Assessment

The clinical manifestations of osteomalacia are subtle. The client may complain of bone pain ranging from mild aching to extreme tenderness when weight or pressure is

---

BOX 15–4.

Clinical Situations in Which Osteomalacia May Occur

Vitamin D disturbances
  Inadequate production of vitamin D
    Inadequate sunlight exposure, dietary deficiency
  Abnormal metabolism of vitamin D
Drug therapy
  Phenytoin
  Fluoride
Hepatic disease
Renal disease
Inadequate absorption of vitamin D
  Gastrectomy
  Gastric or intestinal bypass surgery
  Malabsorption syndrome
  Inflammatory bowel disease
  Renal disease
    Chronic renal failure
    Tubular necrosis
    Hypophosphatemia
  Familial metabolic disorders
    Familiar hypophosphatemia

Adapted from Ignatavicius, D. D., Workman, M. L., & Mishler, M. A. (1995). *Medical-surgical nursing* (2nd ed.). Philadelphia: WB Saunders.

applied to the affected bones. Poorly localized muscle pains and weakness may accompany the bone pain. The pelvic region and the dorsolumbar area are usually affected. Clients may complain of low-back pain and difficulty with position change. In addition, muscle weakness contributes to a waddling, unsteady gait and high risk for falls. Loss of vertebral height causes kyphosis. A history of multiple fractures may be present.

Skeletal discomfort may be vague and generalized. The spine, ribs, pelvis, and lower extremities are most often affected. As the disease progresses and is untreated, minor trauma can cause fractures, and bowing of bones (particularly long bones) and shortening of stature can occur (Fig. 15–11).

Assessment must include a thorough pain history as well as complete dietary, gastrointestinal, and renal history so that any potential causative factors can be highlighted. The nurse may be the one to determine the causative factor, which might be gastric bypass surgery. Duration of exposure to sunlight and intake of vitamin D also should be assessed.

Diagnostic Evaluation

Significant osteomalacia can exist without radiographic manifestations. Radiographic images may show compression fractures of the vertebrae as well as generalized demineralization of bone, along with loss of transverse trabeculae and severe osteopenia (Fig. 15–12). Areas of spongy bone show a decreased trabeculae with a coarsened and unsharp appearance. Osteoid may be deposited

in excessive amounts at various sites, particularly in the vertebral bodies and pelvis. Although this osteoid remains relatively mineral deficient per unit area, the total excess amount can cause areas of increased radiographic density. Bending and bowing deformities of long bones may be evident on x-ray examination in long-standing disease, as can the appearance of biconcave vertebrae and a distorted appearance of the pelvic outlet.

A radiologic diagnostic finding for osteomalacia is the presence of radiolucent bands, called *Looser's zones.* These pseudofractures are considered a type of stress fracture and may precede other radiographic changes in osteomalacia. Pseudofractures occur at sites of increased stress and therefore accelerated bone turnover. There is a defect in the mineralization of the osteoid laid down in the replacement process that accounts for the lucent radiographic appearance. Looser's zones are most often found along the concave side of the femoral neck, the pubic rami, the ribs, the clavicles, and the lateral aspects of the scapulae.

Biochemical findings vary, depending on the stage of the disease and its cause (see Table 15–8). Vitamin D–deficient osteomalacia is characterized by a low or low-normal serum calcium level, low serum phosphorus level, elevated serum (ALP) level, increased PTH level, and decreased urinary calcium level.

Because of the difficulty in diagnosing osteomalacia in adults, a bone biopsy may be indicated. A rib and the iliac crest are sites from which the biopsy sample is generally taken. Depressed appositional rate, increased

TABLE 15–8. *Differential Characteristics of Osteoporosis and Osteomalacia and Paget's Disease of Bone*

CHARACTERISTIC	OSTEOPOROSIS	OSTEOMALACIA	PAGET'S DISEASE
Definition	Bone density value of >2.5 SD below the young adult mean value	Demineralized bone	Disorder of skeletal remodeling in which there is an increase in bone formation resulting in structurally weak, fracture-prone bones
Pathophysiology	Loss of microarchitecture of bone, frequently with fractures	Vitamin D deficiency	Active and inactive phases occur; late in the active period, osteoblastic bone formation predominates
Assessment findings	Very low DEXA values, fractures after minimal or no trauma	Pseudofractures, Looser's zones	Bone pain, pathologic fractures, bone enlargement
Calcium	Serum normal Urinary decreased	Serum normal or decreased	Serum increased or normal
Phosphate	Serum normal	Serum normal or decreased	Serum normal
Parathyroid hormone	Serum normal	Serum normal or increased	—
Alkaline phosphatase	Serum normal	Serum increased	Serum greatly increased
Pyridinoline crosslinks	Serum increased Urinary increased	—	Serum increased Urinary greatly increased
Bone biopsy	Decreased mass of normally mineralized bone	Demineralization of bone; increased quantity of uncalcified matrix	Disordered remodeling; giant osteoclasts, increased osteoblastic and osteoclastic activity

If altered renal function is the primary cause of osteomalacia, a review of how the kidneys increase their urinary excretion and why calcium is lost is required. A loss of calcium or phosphorus during pregnancy or lactation may be an underlying cause, and a description of this specific physiology is required to assist the childbearing woman to participate in her plan of care.

Client teaching and nursing management for the client with osteomalacia are shown in Table 15-9. Simple nutritional vitamin D deficiency responds to oral doses of 2000 to 5000 IU/day of vitamin D, taken for several months, followed by replacement doses of 200 to 400 IU/day. Clients with malabsorption may require large doses of oral vitamin D (25,000 to 100,000 IU/day) or may require parenteral administration of the vitamin.

Because therapeutic doses of vitamin D are high, clients need to be counseled about the potentially toxic effects that may occur with excessive intake of vitamin D. Teaching the client about the clinical indicators of hypercalcemia—dehydration, confusion, muscle weakness—and which indicators require immediate medical interventions is necessary. (See the discussion

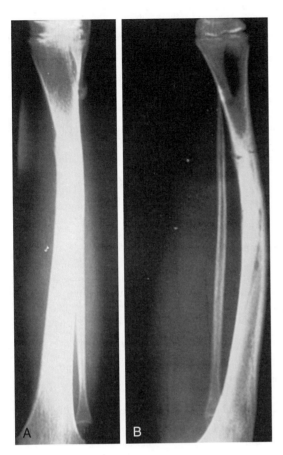

FIGURE 15-11. Osteomalacia. *A,* Normal tibia. *B,* Bowing of the tibia in a client with osteomalacia. (From Steinberg, M. [1991]. *The hip and its disorders* [p. 614]. Philadelphia: WB Saunders.)

mineralization lag time, and reduced calcification may distinguish osteomalacia from other metabolic bone disorders.

Nursing Diagnoses and Management

Much of the orthopaedic nurse's role in assessing and treating osteomalacia is collaborative. The goal in treating osteomalacia is to normalize the clinical, biochemical, and radiologic abnormalities without producing hypercalcemia, hyperphosphatemia, hypercalciuria, nephrolithiasis, or ectopic calcification. The primary nursing responsibility, after assessment of causative factors, is client education.

If the cause of osteomalacia is related to a simple dietary deficiency of calcium or vitamin D, these deficiencies need to be resolved. Client education is useful in resolving such insufficiencies as well as educating the health care community and families at risk (Hartman, 2000). In the more complex gastrointestinal etiology, such as malabsorption syndrome or inflammatory bowel disease, a multispeciality focus is needed in which the nurse collaborates with the client and the gastroenterologist and dietitian.

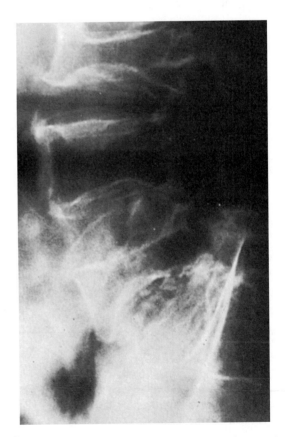

FIGURE 15-12. Adult osteomalacia shows only occasional severe osteopenia on radiographs, a finding difficult to distinguish from osteoporosis or other causes of diminished bone mass. (From Mankin, H. [1990]. Rickets, osteomalacia, and renal osteodystrophy. *Orthopaedic Clinics of North America, 21,* 81-96.)

TABLE 15–9. *Client Education: Osteomalacia*

FOCUS OF TEACHING	TEACHING POINTS
Self-care	Teach client about modes of treatment and prognosis
	Review sources of dietary calcium, phosphorus, and vitamin D
	Teach client about high-vitamin, high-protein, low-fat diet
	Instruct client in importance of maintaining adequate nutritional balance, and provide consultation with appropriate specialists, as indicated (e.g., dietitian, psychiatrist, gastroenterologist)
	Review kidney function and how calcium is lost via kidney, if altered kidney function is primary cause of osteomalacia
	Recommend LactAid to promote intake of milk if lactose intolerant
	Refer for dietary consultation and follow-up to assess and monitor nutritional status and calcium balance
Maintaining mobility	Teach client how to use ambulatory devices, with physical therapist's assistance, as necessary
	Instruct client about spacing of activities for energy conservation
Prevention of injury	Teach client about high fracture risk, even with minor trauma, related to fragile bone status
	Instruct about environmental hazards (e.g., scatter rugs, phone cords, small animals under foot)
	Teach client necessary safety measures and methods to acquire safety aids for home (e.g., shower bars, toilet seat extenders, and stool-side bars/support)
Pain management	Teach client to space activities and move slowly (avoid abrupt motions, especially pivotal or rotational maneuvers)
	Suggest special back and neck support when sitting, lying down, or driving
	Review prescribed medications with client and discuss pain management versus control
Impaired mobility	Promote optimum physical mobility, within limitations
	Review importance of regular, weight-bearing exercise
	Discuss types of exercise recommended by physical therapist, and support prescribed exercise schedule
	Review limitations in ADLs and promote ongoing independence in ADLs within scope of limitations
	Reinforce regular self-administration of nasal spray calcitonin, as prescribed, and present expected outcomes
Safety and fracture prevention	Prevent further injury to skeleton
	Review safety and fall precautions, and provide current literature about occurrence of falls and how to create a safe home environment
	Recommend reduction of daily alcohol intake
	Discuss skeletal fragility and meaning of low bone mineral density (including fracture risks) in relationship to current activities; avoid lifting over 5–10 pounds
	As treatment progresses, as evaluated by serial bone mineral density scans, discuss gradual resumption of selected activities
	Recommend extra precautions in walking dog in neighborhood and possibly walking on flat surfaces
Health-seeking behaviors (multigenerational)	Client and daughter will be aware that maternal history of osteoporosis is a major risk factor for daughter's bone health
	Schedule counseling session with client and daughter
	Inform daughter of her risk for osteoporosis and assess her desire to decrease risks
	Inform client and daughter of resources of National Osteoporosis Foundation

ADLs, activities of daily living.

of hyperparathyroid states for more details on hypercalcemia.) Clients must be advised to follow up with their clinician to obtain radiologic and biochemical evidence of satisfactory clinical outcomes.

Nursing care in osteomalacia is similar to care of the client with osteoporosis, and the reader is referred to that section for a complete discussion of nursing management. Attention to nutritional deficits is required in the therapeutic regimen for osteomalacia.

Nutritional Deficit: Vitamin D, Calcium, and Phosphate Balance

Nutritional Counseling. When the cause of osteomalacia is nutritional, dietary considerations are an integral component of the regimen and may require consultation with a dietitian. As noted in the osteoporosis section, the North American diet is notoriously low in calcium. This is only a minor factor in the osteomalacia pathophysiology, however, because the primary culprit is usually vitamin D deficiency. Adequate vitamin D can be obtained from proper exposure to the ultraviolet rays of the sun. Homebound and institutionalized clients, who typically receive less exposure to the sun, should have a regimen in which direct skin exposure to the sun is implemented.

Clients should be instructed on foods rich in vitamin D, such as eggs, swordfish, herring, sardines, and chicken liver. In addition, milk and dairy products, as well as some cereals, are fortified with vitamin D. Many of these foods are high in cholesterol, and individuals with concerns about hypercholesterolemia may need additional dietary counseling.

RICKETS

Cause

Common rickets (vitamin D–deficiency rickets) is a bone disorder affecting children; it results from a deficiency in vitamin D. Common rickets is characterized by deficient mineralization of the osteoid formed by the growth plate (the epiphysis). The fortification of dairy products with vitamin D has all but eliminated common rickets in the United States, although it is still prevalent in other parts of the world. Children susceptible to common rickets include children of vegetarian parents who avoid milk products and breast-fed children who are not weaned to vitamin D–supplemented milk. Breast milk may not contain enough vitamin D to protect infants, particularly dark-skinned children and those living in cloudy, northern U.S. cities (Feldman, Marcuse, & Springer, 1990). A careful dietary history that assesses for milk intake is essential in the evaluation for rickets.

Nutritional rickets can be manifested between the ages of 6 and 24 months and somewhat earlier in premature infants, who often have small adipose deposits and delayed maturation of the hepatic enzymes that catalyze 25-hydroxylation of calciferols (Aurbach, Marx, & Spiegel, 1992). In the United States, most cases of rickets have been among African Americans living in the north or northeast. African American infants need considerably more sun exposure than Caucasian infants to derive the same benefits in terms of vitamin D.

Assessment

Certain assessment findings are typical with childhood rickets. Decreased linear growth is common, as are radiographic signs of failure of the bone matrix to mineralize. Palpable knobs at the costochrondal margin, called *rachitic rosary*, are seen with rickets. Epiphyseal widening is especially prominent at the wrist and ankles. Bones exhibit excessive plasticity, causing bowing of the legs and the formation of a depression or groove (Harrison's groove) at the lower edge of the thorax. Bossing, or

protrusion or enlargement, of the forehead may also be evident.

Progressive bowing deformity in toddlers is often the presenting feature that may signal the possibility of rickets. Inadequate linear growth, especially during early childhood, indicates a low percentile on the height assessment charts and may trigger alarm in parents or clinicians. This low percentile of expected height may indicate a need for assessment for the presence of rickets.

Pathologic fractures can occur. Decreased mineralization can result in delayed dental eruption and delayed fontanelle closure. Because rickets is a systemic disorder, general manifestations include lethargy, listlessness, weakness, hypotonicity, and irritability.

Diagnostic Evaluation

Although laboratory findings vary depending on the underlying cause, serum calcium and phosphate levels are usually low. The resulting hypocalcemia can cause tetany or seizures. The presence of a positive Chvostek's sign or a positive Trousseau's sign gives evidence of hypocalcemia. Increased levels of PTH are common because this hormone is secreted in response to the low calcium levels. Serum ALP levels are elevated.

Radiographic findings show changes at open growth plates, which are best seen in those areas showing most active growth. Abnormalities reflect the disordered increase in cell growth along with deficient mineralization. Common findings include flaring, cupping, and decreased mineralization of the distal metaphyses. The deformities vary depending on the child's age because stress and strain are applied differently with age-related posture and activity changes. During the first months of life, the cranium is particularly affected because the skull must accommodate the rapidly growing brain. Excess osteoid formation manifests as a squared configuration of the cranium known as *craniotabes*. During infancy and early childhood, the long bones show the greatest deformity, both at the cartilage-shaft junctions and in the diaphyses. The infant with severe rickets often sits all day long for months with legs crossed, tailor-fashion, leaning slightly forward and supporting the body on outstretched hands. Bowing is also a result of displacement of the growth centers. With increasing age, the effects of weight bearing manifest as scoliosis coupled with bowing deformities of the long bones (Pitt, 1991).

Nursing Diagnosis and Management

Altered Growth and Development Related to Altered Nutrition (Vitamin D Deficiency)

Treatment for rickets is to provide adequate levels of vitamin D. Because nutritional beliefs or practices of the individuals or significant others may not support the incorporation of fortified milk, oral replacement of vitamin D may be necessary. A single oral dose (200,000 to 500,000 IU) of vitamin D can be given. This dose is generally not associated with toxicity and should last for about 3 months. Instead of a high, single dose, 5000 IU of vitamin D daily can be given for 1 to 2 months.

Once therapy has been initiated, the child should be re-evaluated at 1 month for evidence of healing and other outcomes. Healing is demonstrated by calcification of the previously uncalcified epiphyseal line. The ALP level drops back to normal as the skeleton heals. Once healing has occurred, the child must continue to receive the recommended daily allowance of 400 IU of vitamin D from either diet or vitamin supplementation. Parental education must focus on the role of vitamin D and how this nutrient relates to the child's musculoskeletal health.

If this treatment is not successful, other causes of rickets must be evaluated. For the child with X-linked hypophosphatemic rickets, vitamin D alone does not resolve the condition. A combination of vitamin D and phosphate is the therapy of choice. The child receiving this regimen must be followed closely because the combination of vitamin D and phosphate can cause the accumulation of calcium in the kidneys (nephrocalcinosis), which can lead to kidney failure.

To prevent vitamin D–deficiency rickets, the American Academy of Pediatrics recommends routine vitamin D supplementation for the breast-fed infant whose mother's nutrition is inadequate. Vitamin D supplementation is recommended for the infant who does not benefit from exposure to ultraviolet radiation because of dark skin color or minimal sunlight exposure (Hartman, 2000). The minimum daily requirement for infants (beginning at birth to 2 months of age) for vitamin D is 200 to 400 IU.

GOUT

Gout is a metabolic condition of altered uric acid metabolism characterized by the deposition of urate salts in articular, periarticular, and subcutaneous tissues. *Gout* is an umbrella term for a group of at least nine metabolic disorders characterized by an elevation in the serum uric acid concentration (hyperuricemia); gout affects about 840 in 100,000 people (American College of Rheumatology, 2000).

Cause

Although its cause is unknown, primary gout is linked to genetic defects in purine metabolism, which cause overproduction or retention of uric acid. This overproduction promotes the deposition of crystalline sodium urate in the soft tissues (particularly the synovial joint) and creates an inflammatory response and severe joint pain. Secondary gout occurs during treatment with such drugs

as cyclosporine, hydrochlorothiazide, or furosemide. These drugs interfere with urate excretion. Secondary gout also occurs as a result of certain acquired disorders, including states of increased cell turnover or breakdown and impaired renal function. Examples include malignant disease, myeloproliferative disorders, and hemolytic anemia (Box 15–5).

Prolonged use of certain diuretics can lead to hyperuricemia and gout, as can the prolonged ingestion of a variety of other common medications (Box 15–5). Because the kidneys are damaged, the ability to excrete uric acid is diminished. As the uric acid accumulates in the bloodstream, it tends to precipitate and form deposits at sites where blood flow is less active, such as in cartilaginous tissue. These accumulations of sodium urate crystals are called *tophi* (Fig. 15–13A), and they tend to form near joints. The duration of gout in the client as well as the degree of hyperuricemia and renal function status seem to determine the course of development of tophi. The affected joints become red, hot, and painful (Fig 15–13B).

Gout frequently occurs in middle-aged men but may develop in postmenopausal women and in organ transplant recipients (Jones & Ball, 1999). Risk factors for gout include male gender, obesity, excessive alcohol intake, hyperlipidemia (type IV), occupational and environmental lead exposure, hypertension, renal insufficiency, use of diuretic drugs, and familial history (Careless & Cohen, 1993; Rasaratnam & Christophidis, 1995). Gout can affect any joint but tends to occur in the feet and legs, predominantly the great toe (see Fig. 15–13). Gout

---

BOX 15–5.

Major Factors Influencing Hyperuricemia and Gout

Increased Production of Uric Acid
Lymphoproliferative disorders
Chronic hemolytic anemia
Excessive alcohol intake
Radiation therapy or chemotherapy

Decreased Renal Excretion of Uric Acid
Acidosis
    Excessive alcohol intake
    Starvation
Renal failure
Medications
    Cyclosporine
    Diuretics
    Low-dose salicylates
    Ethambutol
    Nicotinic acid
    Others

Stages and Presenting Symptoms

There are four stages of clinical progression in gout (Table 15-10). In the first, asymptomatic, stage, serum urate levels increase but no symptoms occur. About 5% of clients with first-stage gout progress to the second stage, acute gouty arthritis. This stage is often precipitated by surgery, trauma, drugs, alcohol, or emotional stress. Acute attacks have a rapid onset, usually involve one joint (especially the great toe and joints in the foot and leg), and are exquisitely painful. During this stage, the urate crystals and infiltrating leukocytes damage the intracellular phagolysosomes. Lysosomal enzymes in the synovial fluid cause tissue damage and inflammation. The affected joint is swollen and painful to touch and motion. The client may have initiated physiologic splinting to decrease joint motion and pain.

The third stage, the intercritical period, is the interval following the acute stage when the client is essentially symptom free. This phase may last for months or even years before the occurrence of another acute attack. In the fourth stage, chronic gout, the person has experienced several episodes of acute gout and now experiences persistent pain. In this stage, sodium urate crystal deposits are observed in the earlobes, fingers, hands, knees, feet, ulnar sides of forearms, Achilles tendons, and internal organs. Major assessment findings for the stages of gout are included in Table 15-10.

Diagnostic Evaluation

A complete nursing history should be completed on the client with gout, with special emphasis on onset, frequency, severity, age of the client, and location of symptoms. A pain history is helpful, as is assessment of calorie and protein intake and alcohol intake patterns. It is useful to determine a family history of gout as well as any pertinent medication history that may have increased the client's risks for secondary gout. Diuretic use, hypertension, and renal impairment may be associated with gout (van Doornum & Ryan, 2000). Few clients with gout require hospitalization. Although the course of gout is variable, with proper treatment the acute attacks of gout can be infrequent and crippling deformities can be decreased.

The physical, laboratory, and radiographic findings in gout are listed in Table 15-10. X-ray analysis may be deceiving in the diagnostic evaluation of gout. A gouty joint may look normal at first and may later progress to a joint that appears "punched out." This appearance is related to the presence of the urate crystals in the bony structure. Eventually, the cartilage is destroyed, the joint narrows, and degenerative changes occur. Arthrocentesis (i.e., aspiration of synovial fluid) is occasionally done to diagnose gout, and analysis of the specimen may reveal needlelike intracellular crystals of sodium urate. Specific

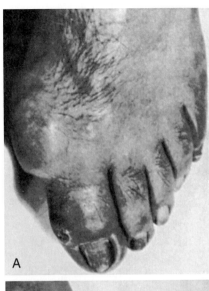
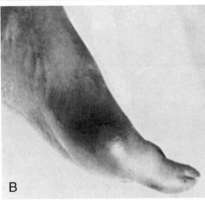

FIGURE 15-13. *A,* Tophi with chronic gout. Hard, painless nodules (tophi) over metatarsophalangeal joint of the first toe. Tophi are collections of sodium urate crystals as a result of chronic gout. They sometimes burst, with a chalky discharge. *B,* Acute gouty arthritis. Episode of gout here involves the first metatarsophalangeal joint. Clinical findings consist of redness, swelling, heat, and extreme tenderness. (From Jarvis, C. [1992]. *Physical examination and health assessment* [p. 724]. Philadelphia: WB Saunders.)

symptoms progress as urate crystal deposits are surrounded by an inflammatory process, which leads to a collection of fibrous tissue, giant cells, and local necrosis in or near the joint.

Individuals who have had organ transplants, particularly renal and cardiac allografts, are a new category of individuals who may develop gouty arthritis. The increased frequency of gout in these individuals is related to the use of cyclosporine and diuretics (Rosenthal & Ryan, 1995). Prophylactic use of probenecid or low-dose oral colchicine may be considered for these vulnerable individuals. In addition, ongoing monitoring of serum uric acid and renal function and assessment of joint appearance is recommended after organ transplant (Rosenthal & Ryan, 1995).

TABLE 15–10. *Major Assessment: Diagnostic and Physical Findings with Gout*

	PHYSICAL FINDINGS	LABORATORY FINDINGS	RADIOGRAPHIC FINDINGS
Stage 1: Latent asymptomatic hyperuricemia	Asymptomatic	Hyperuricemia, 7–10 mg/dL	Joint looks normal
Stage 2: Acute gouty arthritis	Sudden-onset intense pain, generally monoarticular; swelling and tenderness usually of great toe and metatarsophalangeal joint; other possible joint involvement in fingers, knees, ankles, wrists, elbows; fever possible, as are headache, tachycardia, and hypertension	Hyperuricemia, >10 mg/dL Albuminuria, >100 mg/24 hr Increased erythrocyte sedimentation rate Increased urinary uric acid Leukocytes >11,000/mm^3	Joint looks punched out as urate crystals replace bony structure
Stage 3: Intercritical	Asymptomatic	Same as stage 2	Same as stage 2
Stage 4: Chronic gout	Pain, aching, stiffness, and nodular joint swelling; tophi on olecranon bursa, Achilles tendon, extensor surface of forearm, infrapatellar bursa, and helix of ear	Same as stage 2	Narrowed joint with cartilage destroyed; degenerative arthritic appearance

guidelines for the management of gout in primary care are available (Carew & Roberts, 1999; Pal, Foxall, Dysart, Carey, & Whittaker, 2000). Reliance on serum uric acid levels for diagnosis of gout may be misleading (Corkill, 1994) even though the plasma urate concentration is an important determinant of the risk of developing gout (Rasaratnam & Christophidis, 1995). The presence of urate crystals in synovial fluid aspirate can confirm the diagnosis of gout (Corkill, 1994).

Pharmacologic Management

Pharmacologic management is the focus of treatment. Treatment goals include terminating the acute phase and preventing recurring attacks and complications from urate crystal deposits (Pittman & Bross, 1999). Drugs to manage gout may be categorized as those used for the treatment of acute gout and those used in the prevention of recurrent gout and hyperuricemia. Combination drug treatment is common. Colchicine and NSAIDs are the mainstay of treatment in second-stage gout. With recurring acute attacks, allopurinol may be given to suppress uric acid production. Uricosuric agents, such as probenecid or sulfinpyrazone, may be used to increase excretion of uric acid. Corticosteroids may be given to control inflammation, particularly if symptoms are resistant to the milder drugs. Table 15–11 presents the common medications used in the management of gout.

Nursing Diagnoses and Management

The management of gout is aimed at reducing pain and immobilizing the painful joint. Client teaching is summarized in Table 15-12.

Pain Related to Inflammation

Pain Management: Physical Comfort Promotion. Bed rest, including immobilization of the affected joint or extremity, is the usual treatment for gout. Either hot packs or ice packs, depending on client and physician preference, can be applied to the affected joint. Clients with severe pain may be unable to tolerate any pressure over the affected gouty joint. A cradle over the affected extremity promotes comfort by keeping bed linens off the painful and inflamed area, and simple analgesics may be used to relieve the discomfort of a mild attack.

Alteration in Nutrition

Nutritional Counseling. There are differing opinions as to the appropriate dietary therapy to prescribe for the client with gout. A review of many scholarly papers on the management of gout did not reveal any that included dietary restriction in the therapeutic regimen (Gray, 1993). Recently, more clinicians have been moving away from the dietary restrictions of the past (low-purine diet) and recommend either no restrictions or only decreased intake of alcohol and red and organ meats (Pittman & Bross, 1999).

Excessive alcohol intake is to be avoided because it can precipitate an acute attack of gout. Fad starvation diets have also been linked to the precipitation of an acute gout episode. The client should be counseled to avoid sudden and severe dietary modifications.

TABLE 15–11. *Medications Used with Gout*

NAME/ACTION	USUAL DOSAGE/ROUTE	INDICATIONS	CONTRAINDICATIONS	SIDE EFFECTS	CLIENT EDUCATION
Colchicine Action: an anti-inflammatory drug specific for gout (not commonly used)	0.5 or 0.65 mg PO qh until symptoms subside or until nausea, vomiting, abdominal cramping, diarrhea occur; total dose should never exceed 10 mg (Rasaratnam & Christophidis, 1995); maintenance dose, 0.5 mg 1–4 times/wk	Acute gout (stage 2)	Administer with caution in older or debilitated clients, especially with renal, gastrointestinal, or heart disease	At or near full dose, nausea, vomiting, diarrhea (although it is generally necessary to reach full dose for adequate therapeutic effects)	Instruct client to begin medication at first warning of acute gout attack, and follow physician's therapy thereafter Drink at least 2 L fluid daily to prevent crystal precipitation and possible stone formation
Allopurinol (Zyloprim) Action: inhibits production of uric acid	Based on serum uric acid levels, 200–300 mg/day PO for mild gout, 400–600 mg/day for moderately severe tophaceous gout, usually tapered weekly	Chronic gout (stage 4) Primary or secondary gout Primary or secondary uric acid nephropathy, with or without accompanying symptoms of gout Treatment of recurrent uric acid stones	Children and nursing mothers Renal impairment Drug sensitivity Inhibits metabolism of warfarin; dosage of warfarin may need to be decreased	Skin rash (discontinue immediately) Drowsiness Nausea and vomiting, diarrhea, abdominal pain	Instruct client to complete prescribed follow-up blood and urine tests (e.g., liver function studies) Precautions about driving if drowsiness occurs Divide doses throughout day Administer with meals Increase daily fluid intake to 3 L
Probenecid (Benemid) Action: acts on renal tubules to inhibit reabsorption of uric acid	0.25 g (½ tablet) bid for 1 wk, then 0.5 g (1 tablet) bid thereafter; increase by 0.5 g every 4 wk up to 2 g/day	Hyperuricemia associated with gout and gouty arthritis Chronic gout (stage 4)	Do not give with ASA (offsets action of probenecid) Do not give to children younger than 2 Blood dyscrasias or uric acid kidney stones	Occasionally mild gastrointestinal upset (may subside by reduction of dose) Constipation Headache Urinary frequency Flushing	Instruct client to avoid alcohol Have serum uric acid levels determined every 6 mo Take with food and in divided doses May decrease excretion of certain drugs (i.e., indomethacin, antibiotics, rifampin, and NSAIDs); dosages of these other drugs may need to be decreased
Sulfinpyrazone (Anturane) Action: reduces hyperuricemia in chronic gout	200–400 mg/day in 2 divided doses; increase to full maintenance dose within 1 wk (400 mg/day) Supplied in 100- and 200-mg tablets	Chronic tophaceous gout	Active peptic ulcer May potentiate hypoglycemic action of sulfonylurea agents and insulin Do not give with aspirin (antagonizes action of sulfinpyrazone) Can inhibit metabolism of certain drugs (e.g., warfarin); dosage of warfarin may need to be decreased	Upper gastrointestinal disturbance Tinnitus	Instruct client to increase fluid intake Take medication with food or milk
NSAIDs (e.g., indomethacin, ibuprofen, ketoprofen) Action: provide symptom relief	Indomethacin recommended dosage is 50 mg, then 25 mg tid or qid	Severe pain and other symptoms of gout; inhibits production of stable prostaglandins; has anti-inflammatory effects	Poor renal function, gastric ulcer disease, elevated blood pressure, cardiac failure	Gastric disturbances, nausea and vomiting; may cause constipation	Instruct client to take with food Have adequate fluid intake Pain should be relieved within 2–4 hr Joint swelling decreased in 3–5 days
Glucocorticoids Action: powerful anti-inflammatory agent; rarely used except in clients refractory to treatment	Oral prednisone 20–50 mg/day for 3–5 day, then in weaning doses for about 10 days *or* Triamcinolone (50 mg one time IM, *or* intra-articular (0.5–1 mL into the joint)	Used for refractory cases of polyarticular acute gout Intra-articular steroids used with single joint involvement	Infection or diabetes mellitus	Retention of sodium and water	May cause gastric distress when taken orally

NSAIDs, nonsteroidal anti-inflammatory drugs.
Data from Conaghan, R. G., & Day, R. O. (1994). Risks and benefits of drugs used in the management and prevention of gout. *Drug Safety: An International Journal of Medical Toxicology and Drug Experience, 11,* 252–258; Lemone, P., & Burke, K. M. (1996). *Medical-surgical nursing.* New York: Addison-Wesley; Lehne, R. A. (2000). *Pharmacology for nursing care.* (3rd ed.). Philadelphia: WB Saunders; Murtagh, J. (1995). Acute gout in the great toe. *Australian Family Physician, 24,* 437; and Rosenthal, A. K., & Ryan, L. M. (1995). Treatment of refractory crystal-associated arthritis. *Rheumatic Disease Clinics of North America, 21,* 151–161.

TABLE 15–12. *Client Education: Gout*

FOCUS OF TEACHING	NURSING INTERVENTIONS
Pain management	Promote comfort
	Administer pain medications as needed and other medications as ordered; monitor for side effects of drugs
	Apply ice and hot packs as ordered
	Provide comfort and immobilization of extremity as needed
	Encourage bed rest and use cradle to keep sheets off feet
Skin integrity	Assess skin for tophi formation
	Apply lotions for dryness
	Turn and position client when immobile
Prevention of recurrence	Assess knowledge of treatment regimen and teach accordingly
	Instruct client on low-purine diet (as indicated) and the avoidance of alcohol
	Instruct client on proper medication sequence and advise to report side effects immediately
Prevention of renal complications	Encourage client to drink up to 3 L of fluids a day (if adequate kidney function)
	Monitor intake and output
	Monitor serum uric acid level regularly

Alteration in Skin Integrity Related to Tophi Formation

Maintenance of Skin Integrity. Skin integrity is an important concern, especially in the client with chronic tophaceous gout. The client must be instructed in ongoing self-care, particularly in areas of tophi development. Lotions can be applied for dryness. The client should be instructed to avoid irritation and trauma to the area because the tophi may perforate and become infected. Wearing protective or special footwear may be advised to protect from injury and trauma.

High Risk for Alteration in Urinary Elimination Due to Stone Formation or Renal Failure

Urinary Elimination Promotion. Adequate fluid intake is critical in the client with gout, particularly once pharmacologic treatment has begun. As the uric acid levels are diminished in the blood by the antigout medication, high levels of uric acid are eliminated in the urine. Without adequate fluid to promote this elimination, uric acid crystals may accumulate and precipitate in

the urinary tract and lead to stone formation. The client with gout and normal renal function should be advised to consume 2.5 to 3 L/day of fluid. Intake and output should be monitored, and serum uric acid levels should be assessed regularly.

With proper treatment, gout rarely leads to any permanent arthritic changes. Because few clients today are hospitalized with a primary diagnosis of gout, the nursing interventions delineated within this chapter are often carried out by the client, family, or home health nurse. Therefore, client teaching is very important (see Table 15–12).

AVASCULAR NECROSIS

Avascular necrosis (AVN) of bone results from temporary or permanent loss of blood to the bones. AVN typically occurs in people between 30 and 50 years of age, with about 10,000 to 20,000 developing AVN each year (NIH, 2000).

Cause

The pathogenesis of AVN is circulatory compromise to the blood supply of the bone. The pathologic condition that follows the compromise, ischemia, or infarction includes a necrotic collapse of the bony architecture with fragmentation. The fragmentation and collapse are followed by a deformity that leads to pain and subluxation of the bone from the joint. Joint function, joint mobility, and range of motion (ROM) are affected with AVN. Arthritis may follow. Early diagnosis and treatment of AVN may prevent irreversible joint changes and decrease the need for surgical intervention.

The causes of the circulatory compromise (ischemia) that precipitates AVN have been identified. They include prior fracture with blood flow disruption to bone, trauma, exposure to radiation or chemotherapeutic agents, corticosteroid treatment, Gaucher's disease, sickle cell disease, alcohol abuse, pancreatitis, and decompression disease (NIH, 2000). AVN of the femoral head may be an iatrogenic complication when positional abduction restraints are used in the treatment of neonatal hip dysplasia (Bearcroft, Berman, Robinson, & Butler, 1996). AVN may occur at any age and in any bone, but the area of the femoral head is the most common site. AVN is also found in the humeral head, carpal scaphoid (navicular), and astragalus (talus) and after segmental fractures or with gout. Idiopathic AVN has also been observed and is probably nontraumatic in origin.

The orthopaedic nurse is most familiar with AVN as a complication of femoral neck fracture. Nearly 20% of clients with femoral neck fracture develop AVN at some point after their injury, and the chances of AVN are dramatically increased if treatment of a femoral neck fracture is delayed for 24 hours. AVN may also follow bone transplantation, when the newly transplanted bone fails to develop adequate circulatory support.

Recently, steroid-induced AVN has received much attention, and although many theories have been proposed about why corticosteroids predispose bone to AVN, the actual etiology remains unclear. The theories regarding steroid-induced AVN include lipid transport alteration, vasculitis, abnormalities of coagulation, and stress fracture involving osteoporotic bone. Long-term steroid therapy has proved detrimental to bones in several ways, and even short courses of high-dose steroids have been associated with the development of AVN.

Assessment

Nursing History. Many of the signs and symptoms of AVN are similar to those of other disorders, and a complete history is vital in evaluating these clients. The underlying causative factor may be elicited during history taking, and any specific incidents that may be associated with AVN must be explored in depth. A client may report continued pain after a fracture, or there may be a complaint of decreased ROM noticed with use of the affected part. Gait disturbances (limping) may be present if AVN affects bones of the lower extremity. Any of these disturbances should signal the possibility of AVN, and physical assessment should then focus on specific examination of the affected bone or joint.

Physical Assessment. AVN of the femoral head may first be suspected when the client complains of inguinal pain, possibly radiating to the thigh or knee. Pain with any motion is a common complaint, and approximately two thirds of clients with AVN experience pain at rest. One third of the affected clients report pain at night. On physical examination, limitations in internal rotation and abduction of the affected leg are present. However, ROM may be normal if assessment is performed before the onset of degenerative changes. A gait analysis of the client with AVN by the orthopaedic nurse often reveals a gluteus medius limp.

Diagnostic Evaluation

If AVN is suspected after clinical assessment, radiologic assessment is required. Plain radiographs of the affected femoral head reveal an increase in the density of the superior portion of the femur, with a radiolucent zone present between the avascular segment and the adjacent bone (Mercier, 1991). Computed tomography (CT), scintigraphy, and conventional and dynamic MRI are used to detect and stage the degree of severity of AVN. Figure 15-14 illustrates radiographic and MRI changes seen with osteonecrosis. MRI of the affected bone has the ability to precisely delineate the avascular area. MRI is the standard tool used for diagnosis of AVN.

Power Doppler sonography has been used to assess femoral head blood supply in neonates (Bearcroft et al., 1996). More invasive procedures to detect AVN, such as a bone marrow biopsy, are rarely used because they require surgery.

Treatment Modalities

Treatment of AVN depends on the pathogenesis, but the goal is to stop further damage and promote bone and joint survival. Factors that are considered for treatment include client age, stage of the disease (early or late), location and amount of bone affected, and cause of AVN (NIH, 2000). Conservative management of AVN is implemented early in the course of this complication and includes avoidance of weight bearing on the affected joint for periods up to 6 months and the use of anti-inflammatory medications. Most clients eventually need surgery to repair the joint.

Conservative management has not always been beneficial in managing AVN; therefore, various surgical proce-

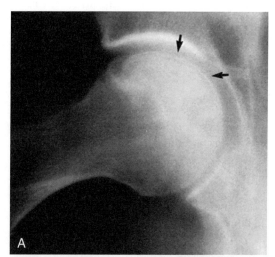
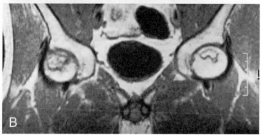

FIGURE 15–14. *A,* This is an early radiographic change characteristic of avascular necrosis (AVN; osteonecrosis). The femoral head of this asymptomatic client shows characteristic changes of advanced AVN *(arrows).* This lesion was discovered accidentally in a radiograph taken after a fall. *B,* Early changes of AVN in both femoral heads using special magnetic resonance imaging. (From Chang, C. C., Greenspan, A., & Gershwin, M. E. [1993]. Osteonecrosis: Current perspectives on pathogenesis and treatment. *Seminars in Arthritis and Rheumatism, 23,* 47-69.)

dures have been proposed to treat this problem. Surgical interventions may include core decompression, osteotomy, bone graft, and arthroplasty (NIH, 2000).

Joint Replacement.   Total hip arthroplasty or hemiarthroplasty is often used by the orthopaedic surgeon for treatment of AVN. In the older client, these procedures often represent the best solution for providing pain relief and restoring ROM. Figure 15–15 illustrates the radiologic appearance of the bipolar device after surgery for AVN. In the younger client, osteotomy can be used, particularly if some normal femoral head cartilage exists (see Chapter 16 for nursing care following total joint replacement).

Joint Fusion.   In young, active clients, arthrodesis (i.e., surgical immobilization of a joint) has been recommended as an alternative to total joint replacement. It is difficult to achieve union in areas of avascular bone, but this treatment modality is still advocated by some as a beneficial option in young clients with unilateral post-traumatic AVN. When bilateral hip involvement is present, as with alcohol-related or steroid-induced osteonecrosis, arthrodesis is uncommon.

Nursing Diagnoses and Management

Nursing management depends on diagnosis as well as medical management. Alteration in ROM and pain are the two most common nursing diagnoses for the management of AVN.

Impaired Mobility Related to Pain and Treatment Regimen

Pain Management.   The client with AVN often experiences gait disturbances and constant aching pain, which is unrelieved by rest or analgesics. Movement of the affected part can be painful, and the client is reluctant to move for fear of increasing discomfort. The management goal is to achieve maximum mobility. Protective weight bearing, using appropriate ambulatory devices, must be taught. Pain management in the client with AVN includes the use of NSAIDs and other analgesics, as well as nonpharmacologic strategies (see Chapter 5 for discussion of pain). Because surgery is common soon after medical diagnosis, nursing management is also related to the particular surgical intervention (see Chapter 16 for surgical procedures of the hip).

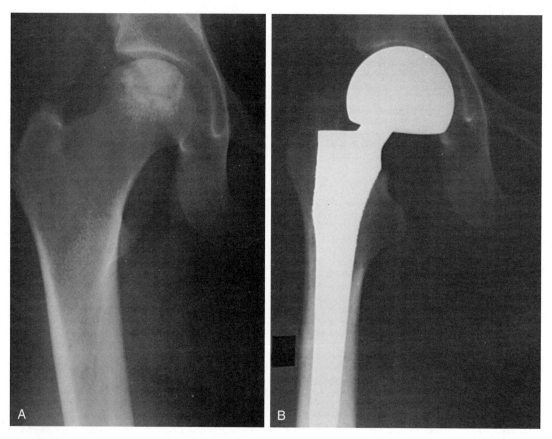

FIGURE 15–15. *A,* Avascular necrosis. *B,* After treatment with a cementless bipolar device. (From Steinberg, M. [1991]. *The hip and its disorders* [p. 841]. Philadelphia: WB Saunders.)

Summary

No completely acceptable treatment exists for AVN. There remains a high failure rate with conservative management, and surgical intervention short of total joint replacement leads to inconsistent results. Assessment, diagnostic evaluation, and treatment are a challenge in AVN. Although this problem has been recognized for many years, the actual pathophysiology remains uncertain.

HYPOPARATHYROIDISM AND HYPERPARATHYROIDISM

Parathormone

Parathormone, or PTH, plays a significant role in metabolic bone physiology and bone disorders. PTH is secreted by the parathyroid glands, the small round bodies—about 6 mm by 3 mm by 2 mm in size—that are attached to the posterior surfaces of the four lateral lobes of the thyroid gland. These glands are the overall regulatory organ for calcium homeostasis (Hellman, Carling, Rask, & Akerstrom, 2000). The primary function of PTH is to control bone calcium and bone phosphate and to maintain homeostasis of blood calcium concentration. A polypeptide, PTH binds to specific cell surface receptors, leading to mobilization of intracellular calcium (Mihai & Farndon, 2000). This polypeptide hormone regulates calcium and phosphate levels by three actions (see Fig. 15–2):

1. PTH stimulates bone breakdown or resorption, thereby releasing calcium and phosphate from the bones into the blood or extracellular fluid.
2. PTH acts on the intestines to increase calcium absorption. This is accomplished by increased renal formation of 1,25-dihydroxycholecalciferol from vitamin D.
3. PTH acts on renal tubules to accelerate excretion of phosphates from the blood into the urine and at the same time to accelerate calcium absorption from the tubules back into the blood.

A negative feedback mechanism operates between the parathyroid glands and serum calcium. When an excess amount of PTH is secreted (hyperparathyroidism), serum calcium levels rise. When hypercalcemia is present, a well-controlled feedback mechanism enables the body to respond by activating several feedback processes designed to lower the serum calcium (see Fig. 15–2). The thyroid secretes calcitonin, which in turn reduces resorption of bone at a cellular level. Estrogen has a positive effect on the secretion of calcitonin from the thyroid gland, thereby enhancing this calcium-regulation feedback system. The healthy body efficiently maintains a normal blood calcium level of 9 to 11 mg/dL, owing to the feedback loop. A failure at any point along this loop alters the metabolic balance of serum calcium, resulting in several potentially life-threatening disorders. There is evidence that serum levels of PTH rise with aging (Horowitz, Wishart, Need, Morris, & Nordin, 1994). The rest of this section addresses alterations that occur in the hyperparathyroid and hypoparathyroid states.

Hyperparathyroidism

Hyperparathyroidism occurs when there is an excessive secretion of PTH, often from the enlargement of one or more of the parathyroid glands. The resulting rise in PTH causes rapid absorption of calcium salts from the bones, producing a higher-than-normal blood concentration of calcium (hypercalcemia). Primary hyperparathyroidism has been frequently associated with bone loss in cortical bone (Khan & Bilezikian, 2000). The skeletal and renal systems are the two major sites of involvement in primary hyperparathyroidism, but bones and other organs also may be involved. One study indicated that postmenopausal women with primary hyperparathyroid disease experienced more fractures and height loss than did controls (Kenny, MacGillivray, Pilbeam, Crombie, & Raisz, 1995). The detection of hypercalcemia by commonly used automated blood chemistry tests has increased the diagnosis of hyperparathyroid disease (Kim, 1994). Hypercalcemia is a common assessment finding in the client with hyperparathyroidism.

Hypercalcemia causes significant alterations in several body systems and is responsible for many of the signs and symptoms present in hyperparathyroidism. The clinical signs and symptoms of increased calcium levels begin to appear when the serum calcium rises above 12 mg/dL, and they can become quite pronounced as the calcium level rises above 15 mg/dL. Box 15–6 lists the signs and symptoms of hypercalcemia.

Cause and Incidence. The most common cause of primary hyperparathyroidism is a single adenoma of the parathyroid, but it may also occur with genetic or multiple endocrine disorders. A familial pattern of occurrence has been noted.

Primary hyperparathyroidism occurs in 1 of every 1000 individuals. It affects women twice as often as men and generally occurs between the ages of 30 and 60 years. Primary hyperparathyroidism can also occur in children and older adults.

Secondary hyperparathyroidism occurs in abnormalities that increase resistance to the metabolic action of PTH, such as in chronic renal failure, vitamin D deficiency, osteomalacia, intestinal malabsorption syndrome, and rickets.

Assessment. The client with hyperparathyroidism is assessed for the two major types of clinical manifestations: those resulting from the hypercalcemia and those

---

BOX 15–6.
Major Assessment Findings with Hypercalcemia

Renal
Polyuria, polydipsia, marked dehydration
Renal insufficiency, renal calculi
Renal failure

Neurologic
Slowing of thought, irritability
Confusion, lethargy
Stupor to coma

Gastrointestinal
Nausea and vomiting, abdominal distention, atonic ileus

Musculoskeletal
Muscle weakness and fatigue, hypotonia
Bone pain, fractures

Cardiovascular and Electrocardiographic Changes
Increased PR interval and decreased QT interval
Increased bradyarrhythmias, heart block, cardiac arrest
Hypertension

Other
Increased serum calcium (>11 mg/dL)
Increased urinary phosphate, increased osteoclastic activity
Decreased serum phosphate

Data from Edelson, G. W., & Kleerekoper, M. (1995). *Medical Clinics of North America, 79,* 79-106; Harvey, H. A. (1995). The management of hypercalcemia of malignancy. *Supportive Care in Cancer, 3,* 123-129; and Kaplan, M. (1994). Hypercalcemia of malignancy: A review of advances in pathophysiology. *Oncology Nursing Forum, 21,* 1039-1046.

---

resulting from the associated bone disease—excessive bone resorption by osteoclasts. This investigation involves an accurate assessment of the skeletal, renal, gastrointestinal, and central nervous systems. The most common physical findings are listed in Box 15-7 and Table 15-13. When hypercalcemia is present, it is important to determine the exact cause. Malignancies, such as multiple myeloma, may also precipitate hypercalcemia and require persistent and deliberate diagnostic investigation.

Nursing History. Nursing history of parathyroid function includes gathering information on previous alterations in function of the parathyroid glands and any familial patterns of occurrence. Because parathyroid gland dysfunction can be an insidious process, the client often is unaware of any problem until he or she is quite symptomatic. A history of kidney stones may be related to mild hyperparathyroidism. Often, the symptoms of bone disease occur after a longer and more severe alteration in parathyroid gland function.

Physical Signs and Symptoms

Bones. Extreme osteoclastic activity occurs in the bones of a client with hyperparathyroidism, resulting in an osteodystrophy, a defect in bone development. PTH increases the number, formation, and activity of osteoclasts and also transiently depresses osteoblastic activity. The late effect of hyperparathyroidism on the bones is both osteoblastic and osteoclastic. Overall, there is more osteoclastic bone absorption than osteoblastic bone formation, particularly in severe cases of hyperparathyroidism. This imbalance between osteoclastic absorption and osteoblastic formation accounts for the eventual decrease in bone density. The client with hyperparathyroidism is at risk for cortical bone loss (Fuliehan, Moore, LeBoff, Hurwitz, Gundberg, Angell, & Scott, 1999). X-ray examination or bone density measurements (DEXA) are recommended. Plain radiographs show extensive decalcification and occasionally large punched-out cystic areas of bone that are filled with giant cell tumors. This cystic bone

---

BOX 15–7.
Major Assessment Findings with Hyperparathyroidism

Renal
Flank pain
Polyuria, polydipsia
Renal calculi
Azotemia

Skeletal
Chronic low-back pain
Fractures
Bone tenderness

Gastrointestinal
Severe epigastric pain
Pancreatitis
Peptic ulcers
Nausea, constipation
Decreased motility

Neuromuscular
Marked muscle atrophy and weakness

Central Nervous System
Stupor, coma
Depression, psychosis
Paresthesias

Other
Cataracts
Acidosis, weight loss
Cardiac arrhythmias
Hypertension
Dental changes

TABLE 15–13. *Major Diagnostic Findings in Primary Hyperparathyroidism and Hypoparathyroidism*

DIAGNOSTIC PROCEDURE	TYPICAL RESULTS FOR HYPERPARATHYROIDISM	TYPICAL RESULTS FOR HYPOPARATHYROIDISM
Serum		
Calcium	Increased: >10 mg/dL in 95% of clients	Decreased: tetany occurs at 6–7 mg/dL
Phosphate	Decreased: usually falls below 1.8 mg/dL because of inverse relationship with calcium	Increased: >5.4 mg/dL
Magnesium	Decreased: directly affects PTH secretion; when <1 mg/dL, PTH secretion is impaired	Increased
Chloride	Increased: >102 mg/dL because of high urinary bicarbonate losses and metabolic acidosis	Decreased
Uric acid	Decreased	Increased
Alkaline phosphatase	Increased: elevated with osteoblastic activity but nonspecific because any disease process that causes hypercalcemia can lead to elevated levels	Decreased
PTH radioimmunoassay	Increased	Decreased: used as a measure of chronic hypoparathyroidism as well
Creatinine	Decreased	Increased
Vitamin D	—	Levels are low
Urinary		
Calcium	Increased: levels usually <25 mg/dL	Decreased: in an attempt to balance the system by preserving calcium
Phosphorus	Decreased: levels usually <1.8 mg/dL	—
Bacteriologic culture	When pyuria, renal lithiasis, or nephrocalcinosis is present	—
Routine urine	Alkalosis	—
Skeleton		
Radiographs	Radiographs of the hands, clavicle ends, and skull may show demineralization, decreased bone density, cyst formation	Increased bone density is a late manifestation of chronic hypoparathyroidism
Bone mineral density	Shows decreased bone density	Increased bone density with chronic hypoparathyroidism; may not provide valuable information in the acute client
Kidneys		
Excretory urogram	May show renal calculi with possible obstruction	—
Parathyroid		
Parathyroid ultrasound	May show enlargement of one or more of the parathyroid glands	—
Heart	—	Prolonged ST and QT intervals

PTH, parathyroid hormone.

disease is called *osteitis fibrosa cystica.* The results of the DEXA are low bone density.

Kidneys. Even in mild hyperparathyroidism, when few physical signs and symptoms are evident, there is a profound tendency to form kidney stones. These stones may be formed as the kidneys attempt to excrete the excess calcium and phosphate released from the bones. In addition to the increased volume of urine (polyuria) and the higher urinary concentration of calcium and phosphate, crystals of calcium phosphate tend to precipitate in the urinary tract and form calcium phosphate stones. These crystals form stones more readily in an alkaline medium. Interventions include drugs and dietary modifications that lower the urinary pH because acidic urine is not conducive to stone formation. After urinary pH is adjusted, other treatment modalities are initiated to prevent and treat the renal calculi.

Kidney stones are among the most common complications of primary hyperparathyroidism. Because of early detection of hypercalcemia, the skeletal complications are less common in the United States. The implementation of appropriate management of hyperparathyroidism has also contributed to the diminished incidence of some of its common complications. Additional signs and symptoms related to hyperparathyroidism include urinary obstruction, urinary tract infection, and possible renal failure.

Heart. Electrocardiograph changes, such as shortened QT interval and prolonged PR interval, arrhythmias, heart block, or cardiac arrest, may occur (Edelson & Kleerekoper, 1995) with hypercalcemia. These arrhythmias may be life-threatening. Management of both the arrhythmias and the hypercalcemia is required. High levels of PTH have been associated with hypertension in women (Jorde, Sundsfjord, Haug, & Bonaa, 2000).

Central Nervous System. The nervous system is depressed in the presence of hypercalcemic states, and reflex activities of the central nervous system become sluggish. Muscles become weak and hypotonic because of the effects of elevated calcium on the muscle cell membranes.

Gastrointestinal System. A major finding in hypercalcemia is the marked dehydration that dominates the clinical assessment (Edelson & Kleerekoper, 1995). Hypercalcemia can also cause anorexia, nausea, vomiting, and constipation, most likely because of the diminished contractility of the muscular walls of the gastrointestinal tract. There is also an increased incidence of pancreatitis in clients with hyperparathyroidism and resultant hypercalcemia, as well as a higher incidence of peptic ulcers, in part because of an increased secretion of gastrin and pepsin. More recent clinical data question the high incidence of peptic ulcers and report that the frequency of gastrointestinal complications in hypoparathyroid clients appears to be approximately the same as in the general population.

Diagnostic Evaluation. Box 15–7 and Table 15–13 summarize suggested assessment for diagnostic evaluation in primary hyperparathyroidism.

Laboratory Findings. An elevated plasma (ionized) calcium level (greater than 10.5 mg/dL) alerts the practitioner to the possibility of primary hyperparathyroidism. See Box 15–6 for assessment findings with hypercalcemia. Urinary calcium is usually low. Serum phosphorus is usually low because of this element's reciprocal relationship to calcium. Serum magnesium may be low. Elevated PTH levels lead to high serum chloride levels because of the effect PTH has on the kidney. Hyperchloremic acidosis can occur in the presence of moderate to marked (greater than 11.5 mg/dL) hypercalcemia. Serum ALP is usually high as a result of the increased osteoblastic activity that occurs as the body attempts to form new bone as rapidly as old bone is absorbed.

Radiographic Findings. In milder cases of hypercalcemia caused by hyperparathyroidism, biochemical studies may not accurately reflect ongoing bone resorption, but by the time this process can be seen on standard radiographs, rather advanced bone demineralization has occurred. Bone density measurements (DEXA) are required and are invaluable in determining the degree of bone loss in hyperparathyroidism because bone loss appears to be accelerated in untreated primary hyperparathyroidism (Orr-Walker, Evans, Clearwater, Horne, Grey, & Reid, 2000).

Treatment Modalities. Medical management of hyperparathyroidism is aimed at controlling the secretion of PTH and managing the symptoms of hypercalcemia. Many technologic advances have influenced the diagnosis and treatment of clients with hyperparathyroidism (Irvin & Carneiro, 2000). Actual hypercalcemic crisis is uncommon in clients with hyperparathyroidism. This crisis is more common with certain malignancies. Several intervention methods are used to return the elevated serum calcium levels to normal. For many postmenopausal women with mild hyperparathyroidism, estrogen replacement promotes the return of serum calcium levels to a more normal value and reduces bone turnover (Marcus, 1995). See Table 15–14 for nursing interventions and client teaching for the client with hyperparathyroidism.

Hydration Therapy. In the hypercalcemic state, the kidneys attempt to achieve homeostasis by excreting large amounts of calcium in the urine. This attempt results in polyuria, hypercalciuria, and severe dehydration. Therefore, hydration therapy is essential, and fluid intake is increased up to 2000 to 4000 mL/day. The goal is to lower the serum calcium by 1.5 to 2 mg/dL in 24 to 48 hours (Edelson & Kleerekoper, 1995). Magnesium and potassium supplementation may be required.

Pharmacologic Management. Severe hypercalcemia can become life-threatening and must be treated as a medical emergency when it occurs. Intravenous normal saline is rapidly infused in an attempt to expand fluid volume and inhibit renal resorption of calcium. Furosemide, a loop diuretic, is given (20 to 80 mg every 1 to 8 hours intravenously or orally) to promote the delivery of filtered urine to the distal tubule, which helps swamp the calcium resorption mechanism and thereby prevent even more calcium from being resorbed.

TABLE 15–14. *Nursing Interventions and Client Teaching: Hyperparathyroidism*

FOCUS OF TEACHING	NURSING INTERVENTIONS

Calcium balance	Reduce serum calcium levels:
	    Monitor strict intake and output
	    Hydrate client per physician orders
	    Monitor for signs of fluid overload:
	        Respiratory assessment, abnormal lung sounds (crackles)
	        Peripheral edema, daily weights, intake and output
	    Replace urinary losses as ordered
	    Administer diuretics and antihypercalcemic agents as prescribed
	Discuss how to obtain Medic-Alert bracelet

Promoting urinary elimination	Prevent or alleviate urinary elimination disorders:
	    Diet as ordered
	    Force fluids: at least 2 L/day unless contraindicated
	    Ambulate client as much as possible
	    Strain all urine
	    Strictly record intake and output
	    Assess for evidence of urinary tract infection and urinary stasis

Mobility	Promote mobility within limitations:
	    Schedule activities of daily living with rest periods and short periods of activity
	        Provide analgesics and comfort measures as needed
	        Assist client with transfers and ambulation as needed

Self-care	Increase client's knowledge of prescribed treatment and follow-up:
	    Emphasize need for regular follow-up blood and urine tests
	    Teach client to avoid calcium-containing antacids, thiazide diuretics, and vitamins A and D
	    Teach client about limitations of dietary calcium intake
	    Teach client to return for bone density testing as prescribed

Other agents used to decrease serum calcium levels include pamidronate and calcitonin. Calcitonin is usually given by intramuscular or subcutaneous injection every 6 to 8 hours. The blood calcium levels begin to fall within 2 hours of calcitonin injection, and a peak effect usually occurs after 6 to 10 hours. The hypocalcemic effect of parenteral calcitonin is transient (Shane, 1996). Few data are available regarding the use of nasal spray calcitonin with hypercalcemia. Inorganic phosphate can also be used because it decreases serum calcium by complexing it

and depositing it in the bone. Intravenous pamidronate, a bisphosphonate, is also effective in the pharmaceutical management of hypercalcemia. Pamidronate is infused over 2 to 4 hours. It is discussed under "Paget's Disease of Bone."

Surgical Treatment. Surgical treatment of hyperparathyroidism usually involves removing part of the parathyroid glands and the tumor or adenoma that caused the problem. There are NIH guidelines for surgery for hyperparathyroidism. Emphasis is on the early treatment and surgical intervention for primary hyperparathyroidism (Walgenbach, Hommel, & Junginger, 2000). Once abnormal parathyroid tissue is surgically removed, rapid improvement usually occurs. An improvement in BMD was documented in one study of hyperparathyroid clients who met guidelines and had surgical parathyroidectomy (Silverberg, Gartenberg, Jacobs, Shane, Siris, Staron, McMahon, & Bilezikian, 1995).

Nursing Diagnoses and Management. Nursing care of the client with hyperparathyroidism focuses on the major clinical manifestations of the disease. Hypercalcemia, dehydration, and the associated bone loss must be treated. Table 15–14 highlights the nursing care of the client with hyperparathyroidism.

Altered Fluid and Calcium Balance Related to Parathyroid Hormone Secretion

Electrolyte Management. Hydration therapy is prescribed for hypercalcemia, and the nurse plays a key role in ensuring strict adherence to the prescribed regimen. In an effort to reduce serum calcium levels created in the hyperparathyroid state, close monitoring of the client's fluid balance must occur. Intake and output and daily weights are monitored carefully, and any assessed signs of fluid overload, such as pulmonary crackles, are documented and reported to the primary caregiver. Urinary losses are replaced as ordered, and specific antihypercalcemic agents and diuretics are administered. The collaborative goal is to achieve and maintain a eucalcemic state.

Altered Urinary Elimination Patterns Related to Fluid and Electrolyte Imbalance

Urinary Elimination Promotion. Unless contraindicated, up to 2.5 to 3 L of fluid per day is encouraged to prevent further urinary elimination disorders. All urine is strained for evidence of stones, and any stones or sediment is saved for laboratory analysis. Because urinary tract infections are common in the presence of hyperparathyroidism, any signs of urinary stasis, hematuria, or dysuria need to be assessed, documented, and reported.

Renal stone formation is increased in the presence of an alkaline urine. Cranberry juice in amounts of 1 L/day is still recommended by some clinicians to help lower the urinary pH, although its effectiveness is not consistent. Consultation with a dietitian about dietary modifications to maintain urine with a low pH (acid) is recommended.

Altered Mobility Related to Bone Demineralization and Pain

Exercise Therapy: Ambulation. If the client is ambulatory, mobility is encouraged to maintain musculoskeletal and renal function. Routine ADLs should be scheduled with frequent rest periods to conserve energy. Mild analgesics should be provided as ordered. Optimum mobility must be maintained to prevent the bone demineralization that occurs with bed rest. Nursing interventions that promote optimal mobility and avoid dehydration are appropriate for the client with hypercalcemia.

Knowledge Deficit Regarding Treatment and Ongoing Monitoring of Condition

Teaching. Regular follow-up visits are scheduled for monitoring serum calcium and creatinine clearance levels, and the client is instructed to return at the appropriate intervals. Urinary calcium, phosphate, and creatinine levels are obtained and analyzed for significant changes; and clients are instructed to avoid certain medications, vitamins, and dietary supplements. Clients should be followed at 6-month to yearly intervals with assessments of physical changes, blood chemistry, urinary calcium and urinalysis, BMD measurements, and PTH immunoassay levels.

Hypoparathyroidism

Cause. Hypoparathyroidism occurs when the parathyroid glands do not secrete adequate PTH. This can occur suddenly, as when the parathyroid glands are removed or injured (e.g., during thyroid surgery). Idiopathic atrophy of the parathyroid gland and congenital hypoparathyroidism may also occur. Acquired reversible hypoparathyroidism can result from any condition that causes hypomagnesemia, such as alcoholism or malabsorption syndrome. Hypoparathyroidism can also result from any disorder that limits vitamin D availability, such as pancreatitis, hepatic or renal disease, gastric or intestinal surgery, or small intestine malabsorption.

Assessment. Nursing history is targeted toward assessment of possible causes, as well as assessment of subjective symptoms. The nurse should assess for any history of intestinal diseases, alcohol abuse, recent neck irradiation or surgery, or a family history of hypoparathyroidism. The physical signs and symptoms of hypoparathyroidism are related to the effects of the diminished PTH levels. The serum level of phosphate rises (hyperphosphatemia), and the serum level of calcium falls

(hypocalcemia). The hypocalcemia is the result of the lack of PTH influence in its primary sites of action. Decreased PTH causes (1) a decrease in intestinal absorption of calcium because of the accelerated synthesis of vitamin D, (2) a decrease in the resorption of calcium from bone, and (3) a decrease in the resorption of calcium through the renal tubules. Hyperphosphatemia is in part caused by the decreased renal excretion of phosphate.

The hypocalcemia of hypoparathyroidism causes irritability of the neuromuscular system (Box 15–8). This hypocalcemia in turn contributes to the clinical signs, which include paresthesias, muscle spasm and tension, increased deep tendon reflexes, and tetany. Hypocalcemia often occurs insidiously, and vague symptoms of anxiety and other mental status changes may appear. Skin changes can also be associated with chronic hypocalcemia. Eyebrow hair may become sparse, and nails and other hair may become dry and brittle. *Candida* infections may affect mucous membranes, probably because of the immunodeficiency associated with idiopathic hypopara-

---

BOX 15–8.
Major Assessment Findings with Hypocalcemia and Hypoparathyroidism

Neuromuscular
Irritable skeletal muscles
  Twitches, cramps, tetany
Paresthesias
  Tingling and numbness sensations
  Positive Chvostek's sign
  Positive Trousseau's phenomenon
Hyperactive deep tendon reflexes
Laryngospasm

Central Nervous System
Mood disorders
Syncopal spells
Seizures

Cardiovascular
Electrocardiogram abnormalities
  Prolonged QT interval
  Prolonged ST interval
  Tachycardia
  Decreased cardiac output

Gastrointestinal
Increased gastric motility
Hyperactive bowel sounds
Abdominal cramping and diarrhea

Skin
Dry, flaking skin
Brittle nails and hair
Thinning eyebrows

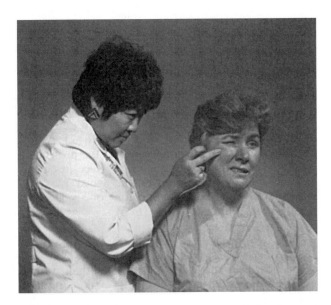

FIGURE 15–16. Chvostek's sign. Spasm of facial muscle elicited by tapping over the facial nerve, indicative of hypocalcemia. (From Ignatavicius, D. D., Workman, M. L., & Mishler, M. A. [1995]. *Medical-surgical nursing* [2nd ed.]. Philadelphia: WB Saunders.)

thyroidism. Mild metabolic alkalosis usually occurs as well and may be evidenced by the tingling and clawing of hands and hyperventilation.

In the early stages of hypocalcemia, the client may complain of numbness, tingling, and cramps in the arms and legs as well as stiffness in the hands and feet. Two classic assessment signs of hypocalcemia are Chvostek's sign and Trousseau's phenomenon. Chvostek's sign is positive when a sharp tapping on the side of the face in front of the ear and over the facial nerve elicits muscle twitching around the mouth, nose, and eye (Fig. 15–16).

To assess for Trousseau's phenomenon, a blood pressure cuff is inflated around the arm to slightly above the systolic pressure. After 1 to 3 minutes, the reduced blood flow precipitates localized neural irritation. In the presence of hypocalcemia, this neural irritation causes the wrist and metacarpophalangeal joints to flex while the fingers abduct (Fig. 15–17). This response constitutes a positive Trousseau's phenomenon and suggests latent tetany and hypocalcemia.

Assessment of hypoparathyroidism often can be difficult because of the vague symptoms of aches and pains as well as the ill-defined symptoms of anxiety and emotional manifestations that occur. A nursing history may elicit important clues, and hypoparathyroidism should be suspected in clients with a history of intestinal disease, alcohol abuse, or recent neck irradiation or surgery. In addition to the aforementioned signs and symptoms of hypocalcemia, the client may also have abdominal pain and cardiac arrhythmias, along with decreased muscle strength that can lead to congestive heart failure and respiratory insufficiency caused by laryngospasm. These last few symptoms are rare but can occur at very low serum calcium levels. Because hypocalcemia can be life-threatening at such low levels, rapid assessment and interventions are critical.

Diagnostic Evaluation. The same laboratory tests used to investigate hyperparathyroidism are used in the assessment of hypoparathyroidism (see Table 15–13). The findings are reversed. Serum calcium is decreased, and tetany begins to develop when the calcium level reaches about 6 to 7 mg/dL. Serum phosphorus increases in hypoparathyroidism, and PTH levels are low. In kidney failure, however, clearance of PTH is slowed, and the serum PTH may be higher than expected.

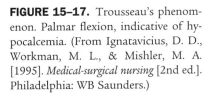

FIGURE 15–17. Trousseau's phenomenon. Palmar flexion, indicative of hypocalcemia. (From Ignatavicius, D. D., Workman, M. L., & Mishler, M. A. [1995]. *Medical-surgical nursing* [2nd ed.]. Philadelphia: WB Saunders.)

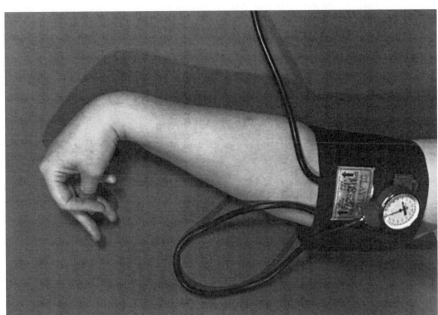

In hypoparathyroid states, the levels of vitamin D are low. In addition to its ability to promote calcium absorption from the gastrointestinal tract, vitamin D also has an effect similar to that of PTH on the bones. That is, PTH promotes calcium and phosphorus absorption. When PTH is not used to treat hypoparathyroidism, high dosages of vitamin D may be used and can effectively control the calcium levels in the extracellular fluid of the hypoparathyroid client. Urinary calcium levels are low in the hypoparathyroid client because the kidneys attempt to balance the system by conserving calcium.

Medical Management. Acute hypoparathyroidism is a medical emergency. Treatment must be initiated to control the tetany and prevent the laryngeal spasms, which could obstruct the airway and cause respiratory arrest and death. Immediate therapy includes intravenous calcium, usually in the form of calcium gluconate. Diazepam, anticonvulsants, and certain sedatives may be given to control the seizures or muscle spasms that occur during a severe hypocalcemic state. Respiratory support may be required.

Nursing Diagnoses and Management. Because hypoparathyroidism can lead to life-threatening complications in a short time, an important focus of nursing management is assessment and treatment of the resultant hypocalcemia and seizures that may occur (Table 15–15). The high risk for physical injury related to seizures necessitates special safety precautions, and an optimal activity level can be achieved only with progressive, supervised, and guided increases in activity.

Alteration in Neuromuscular Status Related to Hypocalcemia

Safety Precautions, Airway Management. Serum calcium levels are treated in the acute hypocalcemic client by the intravenous administration of calcium, usually in the form of calcium gluconate. Cardiac and respiratory function must be monitored carefully throughout this acute phase, and the goals of management are to control tetany and prevent laryngeal spasms and seizures as the client's serum calcium level is restored to a normal level.

Because hypoparathyroidism is often a chronic condition, the client must be instructed about the symptoms of hypocalcemia and hypercalcemia. This symptom recognition is critical to the early recognition and prevention of any acute crisis resulting from calcium imbalance. Clients and their families should be taught to assess for Chvostek's sign and Trousseau's phenomenon and what symptoms require urgent communication with the primary health provider. Follow-up appointments to monitor the various laboratory and diagnostic imaging parameters of hypoparathyroidism also need to be made, and the client must be reminded of the potential life-threatening nature

TABLE 15–15. *Nursing Interventions and Client Teaching: Hypoparathyroidism*

GOALS	NURSING INTERVENTIONS

Maintaining optimal calcium levels and intake	Increase serum calcium levels and prevent cardiopulmonary arrest
	   Administer intravenous calcium as prescribed
	   Monitor cardiac function and respiratory function
	   Administer calcium supplements and vitamin D as ordered

Prevention of seizures and injury	Prevent injury during seizures
	   Maintain seizure precautions
	   Pad client's side rails
	   Keep suction equipment at bedside
	   Administer anticonvulsant drugs as prescribed

Management of pain and spasms	Increase activity tolerance
	   Prevent muscle spasm with heat and gentle positioning
	   Teach client to avoid positions that aggravate muscle spasms (e.g., leg crossing)
	   Assist the client to establish alternate periods of mild exercise and rest

Nutrition	Educate client
	   Foods high in calcium: milk, yogurt, dark green leafy vegetables
	   Foods with added calcium: some orange juice, cereals
	   Calcium supplements to be taken with meals

of this illness as well as the importance of follow-up care. Clients are encouraged to wear some form of identification, such as a Medic-Alert emblem, or some identification in the wallet to ensure prompt treatment in an emergency. Appropriate methods of communication between the client and the clinician must be made available in cases of labile serum calcium.

High Risk for Physical Injury Related to Seizure Activity

Seizure Precautions, Seizure Management. Provision of a safe environment for potential seizures is paramount in the nursing management of the hypocalcemic client. Minimizing noises, bright lights, sudden movements, and temperature changes is advised because of the client's neuromuscular irritability. The possibility of injury during a seizure is decreased by the institution of seizure precautions and the availability of suction equipment. Anticonvulsant drugs are administered as prescribed. Both sedatives and anticonvulsants are often used to help control spasm until serum calcium levels return to normal.

Individuals living with chronic hypoparathyroidism must be assisted to provide adequate information to employers about the condition. Because of the possibility of seizures with severely low calcium levels, there is concern when the affected individual works with heavy machinery or drives a motor vehicle. Many of these affected individuals choose to focus on educating employers that hypoparathyroidism is a controllable chronic problem that may not affect job performance. These vulnerable clients require frequent monitoring and tight control of their calcium levels. Discussion of potential neurologic or cardiac side effects is often framed in terms of late complications that can be prevented by early symptom recognition and ongoing monitoring. Clients can become proficient at detecting changes in their own assessment status if they are provided with good teaching.

METABOLIC CONDITIONS: INNOVATIONS AND FUTURE TRENDS

Direction for future trends in metabolic conditions that affect bone can be directly addressed through nursing and medical research. For example, the NIH Consensus Statement on Osteoporosis (Osteoporosis Prevention, 2000) identified the following areas for further research:

1. What strategies optimize peak bone mass in young girls and boys?
2. What is the impact of calcium deficiency and vitamin D deficiency in childhood?
3. What are the best ways to identify and intervene in disorders that impede the achievement of peak bone mass in ethnically diverse populations?
4. What pharmacogenetic approaches are available for identifying and targeting specific genetic factors predisposing to osteoporosis?
5. What are the psychosocial and financial effects of osteoporosis on caregivers and family members?
6. What is known about the causes of osteoporosis in perimenopausal women?
7. Determine successful methods of educating the public about prevention, diagnosis, and treatment of osteoporosis.

It is hoped that in time these questions will be answered and that the incidence of osteoporosis will decrease.

INTERNET RESOURCES

American College of Rheumatology: www.rheumatology. org/patients/factsheet/gout.html; provides information about gout

National Institutes of Health: www.nih.gov/niams/ healthinfo/avnecqa.htm; questions and answers about avascular necrosis

National Osteoporosis Foundation: www.nof.org

Osteoporosis Prevention, Diagnosis, and Therapy: NIH Consensus Statement: http://odp.od.nih.gov/ consensus/cons/111/111_statement.htm

REFERENCES

American College of Rheumatology. (2000). *Gout.* Available at www. rheumatology.org/patients/factsheet/gout.html

Ankrom, M. A., & Shapiro, J. R. (1998). Paget's disease of bone (osteitis deformans). *Journal of the American Geriatrics Society, 46,* 1025–1033.

Aurbach, G. D., Marx, S. J., & Spiegel, A. M. (1992). Metabolic bone disease. In J. D. Wilson & D. W. Foster (Eds.), *William's textbook of endocrinology* (8th ed., pp. 1477–1518). Philadelphia: WB Saunders.

Avioli, L. V. (1993). Calcium and bone: Myths, facts and controversies. In L. V. Avioli (Ed.), *The osteoporotic syndrome* (3rd ed., pp. 109–122). New York: Wiley-Liss.

Avioli, L. V. (1995). New nasal spray calcitonin for treatment of postmenopausal osteoporosis. *Osteoporosis Report, 11*(3), 4.

Bearcroft, P. W., Berman, L. H., Robinson, A. H., & Butler, G. J. (1996). Vascularity of the neonatal femoral head. *Radiology, 200,* 209–211.

Bernstein, C. N., Seeger, L. L., Sayre, J. W., Anton, P. A., Artinian, L., & Shanahan, F. (1995). Decreased bone density in inflammatory bowel disease is related to corticosteroid use and not disease diagnosis. *Journal of Bone and Mineral Research, 10,* 250–256.

Bohannon, A. D., & Lyles, K. W. (1994). Drug-induced bone disease. *Clinics in Geriatric Medicine, 10,* 611–623.

Bone mineral density testing. (1999). Whitehouse Station, NJ: Merck & Co.

Boyd, J. L. (1998). Osteoporosis in African American women: Dilemma or challenge? *The Journal of Multicultural Nursing and Health, 4,* 20–24.

Branca, F. (1999). Physical activity, diet, and skeletal health. *Public Health Nutrition, 2,* 391–396.

Careless, D. J., & Cohen, M. G. (1993). Rheumatic manifestations of hyperlipidemia and antihyperlipidemia drug therapy. *Seminars in Arthritis and Rheumatism, 23*(2), 90–98.

Carew, M., & Roberts, K. (1999). Care of the patient with gout. *Geriatric Nursing, 20*(3), 156–157.

Conaghan, R. G., & Day, R. O. (1994). Risks and benefits of drugs used in the management and prevention of gout. *Drug Safety: An International Journal of Medical Toxicology and Drug Experience, 11,* 252–258.

Consensus Development Conference: Diagnosis, prophylaxis, and treatment of osteoporosis. (1993). *American Journal of Medicine, 94,* 646–650.

Corkill, M. M. (1994). Gout. *New Zealand Medical Journal, 107,* 337–339.

Davis, J., & Sherer, K. (1994). *Applied nutrition and diet therapy for nurses* (2nd ed.). Philadelphia: WB Saunders.

Dawson-Hughes, B., Harris, S. S., Krall, E. A., & Dallai, G. E. (2000). Effects of withdrawal of calcium and vitamin D supplements on bone mass in elderly men and women. *American Journal of Clinical Nutrition, 72,* 745–750.

Dimai, H. P., Porta, S., Wirnsberger, G., Lindschinger, M., Pampert, L., Dobnig, H., Wilders-Truschnig, M., & Lau, K. H. (1998). Daily oral magnesium supplementation suppresses bone turnover in young adult males. *Journal of Clinical Endocrinology and Metabolism, 83,* 2742–2748.

Edelson, G. W., & Kleerekoper, M. (1995). *Medical Clinics of North America, 79,* 79–106.

Ettinger, B., Black, D. M., Mitlak, B. H., Knickerbocker, R. K., Nickelsen, T., Genant, H. K., Christiansen, C., Delmas, P. D., Zanchetta, J. R., Stakkestad, J., Gluer, C. C., Krueger, K., Cohen, F. J., Eckert, S., Ensrud, K. E., Avioli, L. V., Lips, P., & Cummings, S. R. (1999). Reduction of vertebral fracture risk in postmenopausal women with osteoporosis treated with raloxifene: Results from a 3-year randomized clinical trial. Multiples outcomes of raloxifene evaluation

(MORE) investigators. *Journal of the American Medical Association, 282,* 637–645.

Feldman, K. W., Marcuse, E. K., & Springer, D. A. (1990). Nutritional rickets. *American Family Physician, 42,* 1311–1318.

Fuliehan, G. E., Moore, F., LeBoff, M. S., Hurwitz, S., Gundberg, C. M., Angell, J., & Scott, J. (1999). Longitudinal changes in bone density in hyperparathyroidism. *Journal Clinical Densitometry, 2,* 153–162.

Gennari, C., Nuti, R., Agnusdei, D., Camporeale, A., & Martini, G. (1994). Management of osteoporosis and Paget's disease. *Drug Safety, 11*(3), 179–195.

Gray, M. A. (1993). Antigout medications. *Orthopaedic Nursing, 12*(4), 53–55.

Guyton, A. C., & Hall, J. E. (1996). *Medical physiology* (9th ed.). Philadelphia: WB Saunders.

Hartman, J. (2000). Vitamin D deficiency, rickets in children: Prevalence and need for community education. *Orthopaedic Nursing, 19*(1), 63–69.

Harvey, H. A. (1995). The management of hypercalcemia of malignancy. *Supportive Care in Cancer, 3*(2), 123–129.

Heaney, R. P. (2000). Calcium, dairy products, and osteoporosis. *Journal of the American College of Nutrition, 19*(2 Suppl), 83S–99S.

Hellman, P., Carling, T., Rask, L., & Akerstrom, G. (2000). Pathophysiology of primary hyperparathyroidism. *Histology and Histopathology, 15,* 619–627.

Hobart, J. A., & Smucker, D. R. (2000). The female athlete triad. *American Family Physician, 61,* 3357–3364, 3367.

Horowitz, M., Wishart, J. M., Need, A. G., Morris, H. A., & Nordin, R. E. (1994). Primary hyperparathyroidism. *Clinics in Geriatric Medicine, 10,* 757–775.

Hunt, A. H. (1996). Height change and bone density: A nursing study. *Orthopaedic Nursing, 15*(3), 57–66.

Hunt, A. H., Civitelli, R., & Halstead, L. (1995). Evaluation of bone resorption: A common problem during impaired mobility. *SCI Nursing, 12*(3), 90–94.

Ignatavicius, D. D., Workman, M. L., & Mishler, M. A. (1995). *Medical-surgical nursing* (2nd ed.). Philadelphia: WB Saunders.

Irvin, G. L., & Carneiro, D. M. (2000). Management changes in primary hyperparathyroidism. *Journal of the American Medical Association, 248,* 934–936.

Jarvis, C. (1992). *Physical examination and health assessment* (p. 74). Philadelphia: WB Saunders.

Jones, R. E., & Ball, E. V. (1999). Gout: Beyond the stereotype. *Hospital Practice, 34,* 95–102.

Jorde, R., Sundsfjord, J., Haug, E., & Bonaa, K. H. (2000). Relation between low calcium intake, parathyroid hormone, and blood pressure. *Hypertension, 35,* 1154–1159.

Kaplan, F. S. (1999a). Severe orthopaedic complications of Paget's disease. *Bone, 24*(5 Suppl), 43S–46S.

Kaplan, F. S. (1999b). Surgical management of Paget's Disease. *Journal of Bone and Mineral Research, 14*(Suppl 2), 34–38.

Kaplan, F. S., & Singer, F. R. (1995). Paget's disease of bone: Pathophysiology, diagnosis, and management. *Journal of the American Academy of Orthopaedic Surgeons, 3,* 336–344.

Kaplan, M. (1994). Hypercalcemia of malignancy: A review of advances in pathophysiology. *Oncology Nursing Forum, 21,* 1039–1046.

Kenny, A. M., MacGillivray, D. C., Pilbeam, C. C., Crombie, H. D., & Raisz, L. G. (1995). Fracture incidence in postmenopausal women with primary hyperparathyroidism. *Surgery, 118,* 109–114.

Kim, T. S. (1994). Primary hyperparathyroidism. *Orthopaedic Nursing, 12*(3), 17–28.

Khan, A., & Bilezikian, J. (2000). Primary hyperthyroidism: Pathophysiology and impact on bone. *Canadian Medical Association Journal, 163*(2), 184–187.

Lappe, J. M. (1994). Bone fragility: Assessment of risks and strategies for prevention. *Journal of Obstetrical and Gynecological Nursing, 23,* 260–268.

Lehne, R. A. (2000). *Pharmacology for nursing care* (4th ed.). Philadelphia: WB Saunders.

Lemone, P., & Burke, K. M. (1996). *Medical-surgical nursing.* Menlo Park, CA: Addison-Wesley.

Lewallen, D. G. (1999, December). Hip arthroplasty in patients with Paget's disease. *Clinical Orthopaedics and Related Research,* 243–250.

Lewis, T., Tesh, A. S., & Lyles, K. W. (1999). Caring for the patient with Paget's disease of the bone. *Nurse Practitioner, 24,* pp. 50, 53, 57–58.

Lloyd, T., Andon, N. B., Rollings, N., Martell, J. K., Landis, J. R., Demers, L. M., Eggli, D. F., Kieselhorst, K., & Kulin, H. E. (1993). Calcium supplementation and bone mineral density in adolescent girls. *Journal of the American Association, 270,* 841–844.

Lukert, B. P. (1995, November). *Glucocorticoid-induced osteoporosis.* Paper presented at the meeting of the National Osteoporosis Foundation conference on bone mass measurement, Los Angeles, CA.

Magee, D. (1997). *Orthopaedic physical assessment* (3rd ed.). Philadelphia: WB Saunders.

Mankin, H. (1990). Rickets, osteomalacia, and renal osteodystrophy. *Orthopedic Clinics of North America, 21,* 81–96.

Marcus, R. (1995). Bones of contention: The problem of mild hyperparathyroidism [Editorial]. *Journal of Clinical Endocrinology and Metabolism, 80,* 720–722.

Mazieres, B. (1995). Treatment of Paget's disease of bone with bisphosphonates. *Expansion Scientifique Francaise, 62*(2), 72–77.

McFarlane, M. A., & Melora, P. S. (1993). Decreasing falls by the application of standards of care, practice and governance. *Journal of Quality Nursing Care, 8*(1), 43–50.

Mercier, L. A. (1991). *Practical orthopaedics* (3rd ed.). St. Louis: Mosby.

Meunier, P. J., Vignot, E., Garnero, P., Confavreux, E., Paris, E., Liu-Leage, S., Sarkar, S., Liu, T., Wong, M., & Draper, M. W. (1999). Treatment of postmenopausal women with osteoporosis of low bone density with raloxifene. *Osteoporosis International, 10,* 330–336.

Mihai, R., & Farndon, J. (2000). Parathyroid disease and calcium metabolism. *British Journal of Anesthesia, 85,* 29–43.

Mirra, J. M., Brien, E. W., & Tehranzadeh, J. (1995). Paget's disease of bone: Review with emphasis on radiologic features, Part I. *Skeletal Radiology, 24,* 163–172.

Monsell, E. M. (1995). Hearing loss in Paget's disease. In *A client's guide to Paget's disease of bone* (pp. 29–30). New York: Paget Foundation.

Murtagh, J. (1995). Acute gout in the great toe. *Australian Family Physician, 24,* 437.

Nance, M. A., Nuttall, F. Q., Econs, M. J., Lyles, K. W., Viles, K. D., Vance, J. M., Pericak-Vance, M. A., & Speer, M. C. (2000). Heterogeneity in Paget disease of the bone. *American Journal of Medical Genetics, 92,* 303–307.

National Institutes of Health (NIH). (1994). *Optimal Calcium Intake Consensus Statement, 12*(4), 1–31.

National Institutes of Health (NIH). (2000). *Questions and answers about avascular necrosis.* Available at www.nih.gov/niams/healthinfo/avnecqa.htm

National Osteoporosis Foundation. (2000a). *Fast facts.* Available at www.nof.org

National Osteoporosis Foundation. (2000b). *Medications and bone loss.* Washington, DC: Author.

National Osteoporosis Foundation. (2000c). *Physician's guide to prevention and treatment of osteoporosis.* Washington, DC: Author.

National Osteoporosis Foundation. (2000d). *News release.* Available at www.nof.org

National Osteoporosis Foundation. (2000e). *Client information.* Available at www.nof.org

National Research Center Fact Sheet (1998). Osteoporosis and African American women. *National Research Center Fact Sheet,* pp. 1–12.

Nguyen, T. V., Center, J. R., & Eisman, J. A. (2000). Osteoporosis in elderly men and women: Effects of dietary calcium, physical activity, and body mass index. *Journal of Bone and Mineral Research, 15,* 322–331.

Orr-Walker, B. J., Evans, M. C., Clearwater, J. M., Horne, A., Grey, A. B., & Reid, I. R. (2000). Effects of hormone replacement on bone mineral density in postmenopausal women with primary hyperparathyroidism: Four-year follow-up and comparison with healthy postmeno-pausal women. *Archives of Internal Medicine, 160,* 2161–2166.

Osteoporosis Prevention, Diagnosis, and Therapy. (2000, March 27–29). *NIH Consensus Statement, 17*(1), 1–36.

Pak, C. Y. C., Sakhaee, K., Adams-Huet, B., Piziak, V., Peterson, R. D., & Poindexter, J. R. (1995). Treatment of postmenopausal osteoporosis with slow-release sodium fluoride. Final report of a randomized controlled study. *Annals of Internal Medicine, 123,* 401–408.

Pal, B., Foxall, M., Dysart, T., Carey, F., & Whittaker, M. (2000). How is gout managed in primary care? A review of current practice and proposed guidelines. *Clinical Rheumatology, 19,* 21–25.

Pitt, M. (1991). Rickets and osteomalacia are still around. *Radiologic Clinics of North America, 29*(1), 97–118.

Pittman, R. R., & Bross, M. H. (1999). Diagnosis and management of gout. *American Family Physician, 59,* 1799–1806, 1810.

Rapuri, P. B., Gallagher, J. C., Balhorn, K. E., & Ryschon, K. L. (2000). Smoking and bone metabolism in elderly women. *Bone, 27,* 429–436.

Rasaratnam, I., & Christophidis, N. (1995). Gout: A disease of plenty. *Australian Family Physician, 24,* 849–860.

Reginato, A. J., Falasca, G. F., Pappu, R., McNight, B., & Agha, A. (1999). Musculoskeletal manifestations of osteomalacia: report of 26 cases and literature review. *Seminars in Arthritis and Rheumatism, 28,* 287–304.

Roberts, D., & Lappe, J. (2001). Management of clients with musculo-skeletal disorders. In J. Black, J. Hawks, & A. Keene (Eds.), *Medical-surgical nursing clinical management for positive outcomes* (6th ed., pp. 551–585). Philadelphia: WB Saunders.

Rosenthal, A. K., & Ryan, L. M. (1995). Treatment of refractory crystal-associated arthritis. *Rheumatic Disease Clinics of North America, 21,* 151–161.

Rutherford, O. M. (1999). Is there a role for exercise in the prevention of osteoporotic fractures? *British Journal of Sports Medicine, 33,* 378–386.

Sedlak, C., Doheny, M., & Estok, P. (2000). Osteoporosis in older men: Knowledge and health beliefs. *Orthopaedic Nursing, 19*(3), 38–46.

Sedlak, C., Doheny, M., & Jones, S. (1998). Osteoporosis prevention in young women. *Orthopaedic Nursing, 17*(3), 53–60.

Sedlak, C., Doheny, M., & Jones, S. (2000). Osteoporosis education programs: Changing knowledge and behaviors. *Public Health Nursing, 17,* 398–402.

Shane, E. (1996). Hypercalcemia. In M. J. Fauvus (Ed.), *Primer on the metabolic bone diseases and disorders of mineral metabolism* (3rd ed., pp. 177–181). New York: Raven.

Silverberg, S. J., Gartenberg, F., Jacobs, T. P., Shane, E., Siris, E., Staron, R. B., McMahon, D. J., & Bilezikian, J. P. (1995). Increased bone mineral density after parathyroidectomy in primary hyperparathy-roidism. *Journal of Clinical Endocrinology and Metabolism, 80,* 729–734.

Siris, E. (2000). Alendronate in the treatment of osteoporosis: A review of the clinical trials. *Journal of Women's Health Gender Based Medicine, 9,* 599–606.

Siris, E. S. (1995a). Paget's disease of bone. *Journal of Clinical Endocrinology and Metabolism, 80,* 335–338.

Siris, E. S. (1995b). Paget's disease in families. In *A client's guide to Paget's disease of bone* (pp. 5–6). New York: Paget Foundation.

Sojka, J. E., & Weaver, C. M. (1995). Magnesium supplementation and osteoporosis. *Nutrition Reviews, 53*(3), 71–74.

Steinberg, F. U., & Roettger, R. F. (1993). Exercise in prevention and therapy of osteoporosis. In L. V. Avioli (Ed.), *The osteoporotic syndrome* (3rd ed., pp. 171–184). New York: Wiley-Liss.

Steinberg, M. (1991). *The hip and its disorders.* Philadelphia: WB Saunders.

Sweeting, H. L. (1994). Client fall prevention—A structured approach. *Journal of Nursing Management, 2,* 187–192.

Swezey, R. L., Swezey, A., & Adams, J. (2000). Isometric progressive resistive exercises for osteoporosis. *Journal of Rheumatology, 27,* 1260–1264.

Tiegs, R. D., Lohse, C. M., Wollan, P. C., & Melton, L. J. (2000). Long-term trends in the incidence of Paget's disease of bone. *Bone, 27,* 423–427.

Tonino, R. P., Meunier, P. J., Emkey, R., Rodriguez-Portales, J. A., Menkes, C. J., Wasnich, R. D., Bone, H. G., Santora, A. C., Wu, M., Desai, R., & Ross, P. D. (2000). Skeletal benefits of alendronate: 7-year treatment of postmenopausal osteoporotic women. Phase III osteo-porosis treatment study group. *Journal of Clinical Endocrinology and Metabolism, 84,* 3109–3015.

van Doornum, S., & Ryan, P. F. (2000). Clinical manifestations of gout and their management. *Medical Journal of Australia, 172,* 493–497.

Walgenbach, S., Hommel, G., & Junginger, T. (2000). Outcome after surgery for primary hyperparathyroidism: ten-year prospective follow-up study. *World Journal of Surgery, 24,* 564–569, 569–570.

Weaver, C. M. (2000). Calcium requirements of physically active people. *American Journal of Clinical Nutrition, 72*(2 Suppl), 579S–584S.

Wolf, R. L., Cauley, J. A., Baker, C. E., Ferrell, R. E., Charron, M., Caggiula, A. W., Salamone, L. M., Heaney, R. P., & Kuller, L. H. (2000). Factors associated with calcium absorption efficiency in pre- and perimenopausal women. *American Journal of Clinical Nutrition, 72,* 466–471.

World Health Organization (WHO). (1994). Assessment of fracture risk and application to screening for postmenopausal osteoporosis. *WHO Technical Report Series, 843.* Geneva, Switzerland: Author.

Degenerative Disorders

DOTTIE ROBERTS

Arthritic disorders affect nearly 43 million Americans and represent the leading cause of disability in the United States. Arthritis includes a variety of diseases and conditions, but the most common cause of joint pain is osteoarthritis (OA). Previously known as *degenerative joint disease,* OA is a slowly progressive disorder characterized by deterioration of articular cartilage. The estimated cost of OA is $15.5 billion annually, more than half of which is attributed to sick days from work (Kee, 2000). These figures are especially significant to nurses when combined with the fact that the number of older adults, who are most affected by arthritis, is increasing at a rapid rate both numerically and as a proportion of the total population. Preserving function, preventing disability, and managing arthritis pain represent an imposing challenge to those who care for aging people.

In addition to OA, the degenerative disorders of chondromalacia patellae (patellofemoral pain syndrome), Charcot joints (neuropathic arthropathy), and bunions may have marked social and economic impact. These varied conditions, which share many similarities in nursing diagnoses and interventions with OA (Table 16–1), are also discussed in this chapter.

OSTEOARTHRITIS

Over the past 20 years, understanding of OA has increased substantially. It is no longer considered a wear-and-tear condition that occurs as a normal part of aging. In fact, changes found in cartilage of asymptomatic older individuals are quite different from those seen in osteoarthritic cartilage. OA is now viewed as a process in which new tissue is produced as a result of joint insults and cartilage destruction. Systemic involvement is not a feature of the disease.

Among the controversies that still surround OA is one question about the character of the disease: Is it an inflammatory disease or a pain syndrome? In affected clients, evidence suggests that synovial cells and chondrocytes contain increased levels of inflammatory agents as well as the products of inflammation. Because nonsteroidal anti-inflammatory drugs (NSAIDs) may work more effectively than pure analgesics in OA symptom management, an inflammatory etiology is suspected. A counter argument holds that OA is actually a repair process in damaged joints. Although low-grade inflammation is anticipated during the various phases of repair, the role of synovitis in OA is minimal. Other factors, such as decreased muscle strength and obesity, are strongly associated with disease development. Although NSAIDs may help reduce the pain of OA, simple analgesics have also been effective. In addition, the disease responds to nonpharmacologic interventions such as physical therapy and weight reduction, which have no anti-inflammatory effects. Although both arguments concerning the pathogenesis of OA have merit, additional work is clearly needed to allow complete understanding of disease development.

Classification

Formerly known as primary OA, *idiopathic osteoarthritis* occurs in individuals who have no history of joint injury or disease or of systemic illness that may contribute to the development of arthritis. Aging certainly influences the decreasing quality and quantity of proteoglycans in the cartilage of arthritic joints. Additional evidence points to the existence of an autosomal-recessive trait with gene defects that cause premature cartilage destruction.

Secondary osteoarthritis, on the other hand, has an identifiable cause. Any condition that directly damages articular cartilage, subjects joint surfaces to excessive or abnormal forces, or causes joint instability can lead to arthritic changes. Research on the occurrence of knee OA

TABLE 16–1. *Common Nursing Diagnoses, Outcomes, and Interventions for the Degenerative Disorders*

NURSING DIAGNOSES	OUTCOMES	INTERVENTIONS
Pain: acute or chronic	Pain is managed or minimized	*Provide comfort measures to alleviate pain* Assess level of pain related to joint disease, surgery Assess for limited joint motion and proper functional alignment Instruct client in proper body mechanics, maintenance of good posture Instruct client in use of assistive devices as indicated Discuss less stressful or fatiguing ways of performing tasks Encourage client to avoid forceful or repetitive movements Encourage use of physical modalities for pain relief and joint protection (i.e., heat, splinting) before and after activity Instruct client in use of analgesics and NSAIDs before activity and at bedtime
Impaired physical mobility	Client achieves optimal mobility and muscle strength, with joint deformity prevented or minimized	*Promote mobility and muscle strength within restrictions* Assess degree of functional limitations related to pain, stiffness, deformities, limited ROM, operative procedures Instruct client in use of orthotics and assistive devices Discourage periods of prolonged inactivity Discuss use of environmental modifications to overcome barriers to mobility (i.e., ramps, handrails) Encourage exercise and activity program to strength muscles and maintain function, using physical therapy consultation as indicated Encourage achievement of ideal body weight to facilitate mobility
Activity intolerance	Client tolerates activity with minimal fatigue or pain	*Develop a plan to balance rest and activity* Encourage verbalization of emotions related to pain, fatigue, activity restrictions Assist client in identifying specific physical and psychosocial activities that are fatiguing Assist client in reorganizing daily activities to optimize rest periods, avoid acute pain episodes Instruct client in principles of energy conservation, work simplification, joint protection, alternative methods of performance Reinforce the client's abilities rather than disabilities Promote participation in a fitness or conditioning program to maximize endurance Discuss need to avoid social withdrawal and isolation Encourage resumption of normal social activities within the rest/activity cycle
Sleep-pattern disturbance	Client experiences adequate sleep and rest	*Promote sleep and rest* Teach relaxation methods to promote sleep Instruct client in use of analgesics or NSAIDs at bedtime Discuss use of bedtime routine (e.g., warm bath) to promote sleep
Self-care deficit: bathing/hygiene, dressing/grooming	Client demonstrates optimal independence in activities of daily living (ADLs)	*Promote independence in ADLs* Assess home environment for barriers to independent performance of ADLs Provide and instruct in use of assistive devices as needed to perform self-care activities (e.g., raised toilet seats, handrails and shower bench, long-handled shoehorn, sock donner) Arrange in-home assistance as needed
Alteration in self-concept	Client verbalizes positive self-concept	*Promote positive image of client appearance and abilities* Emphasize that client is more than a diagnosis of chronic illness Discuss effects of disease on client's body image and self-esteem Encourage positive coping mechanisms (e.g., participation in support group)

Table continued on following page

TABLE 16–1. *Common Nursing Diagnoses, Outcomes, and Interventions for the Degenerative Disorders* Continued

NURSING DIAGNOSES	OUTCOMES	INTERVENTIONS
Altered sexuality	Client expresses comfort with sexual function	*Promote optimal sexual role functioning* Discuss attention to details that reinforce overall sense of sexuality (i.e., grooming, hygiene, communication/relationships) Encourage use of analgesics or NSAIDs and relaxation strategies (e.g., warm bath) before sexual activity Provide information on alternative sexual positions that may be less stressful on affected joints Encourage discussions with partner on adaptive positions, alternate timing, increasing awareness of client's needs
Altered nutrition: more than/less than body requirements	Client attains or maintains optimal nutrition	*Promote optimal nutritional status* Develop a weight reduction plan and activity prescription for overweight client Assess for lack of appetite, anorexia, anemia in client with systemic disorder Assess for underlying depression or grief, which may contribute to dietary imbalances Integrate client's personal, cultural, age-related food preferences, eating patterns into dietary planning
Altered role performance	Client manages home and work roles	*Promote optimal role functioning* Assess functional deficits that may require vocational or lifestyle adjustments Assess economic impact of treatments, functional impairments (i.e., insurance coverage, loss of income) Discuss appropriate adaptations when symptoms interfere with role performance Encourage verbalization about role changes, impact on self-concept
Ineffective coping: individual and family	Client and family cope positively with changes imposed by illness and treatment regimen	*Promote positive coping and family functioning* Instruct client and family about disease process, therapeutic regimen, possible disease complications Review factors that increase personal and family stress and explore effective coping strategies for each one Assist with problem-solving in face of perceived difficulties Assist client and family with identifying available support systems, community resources (e.g., support groups, self-help groups, educational resources) Discuss nonprescription remedies marketed in popular media and personal options concerning alternative treatments Encourage verbalization of emotions related to client's attempts to live successfully with chronic disease

in women, which occurs twice as often as in men, has suggested an interesting correlate for occurrence of the disease: walking in high-heeled shoes. Kerrigan, Todd, and O'Riley (1998) demonstrated 23% greater torsional forces applied across the knee during walking in high-heeled shoes compared with walking barefoot. They concluded that use of high-heeled shoes might predispose a woman to degenerative changes in the knee. Other typical causes of secondary disease are listed in Box 16–1.

OA is also classified on the basis of joint involvement. Localized disease affects only one or two joints. With generalized OA, three or more joints are involved. *Nodal*

(hand involvement) and *non-nodal* (without hand involvement) generalized arthritis are additional terms used to classify the extent of disease. Nodal generalized arthritis has been labeled *menopausal osteoarthritis* because of its frequent onset in women at the time of menopause. Nodal disease may affect the knees, hips, and cervical and lumbar spine as well as the hands.

Epidemiology

OA is the most common articular disease among adults. Its prevalence varies among different populations, but it is a universal problem among humans. The process of OA may actually begin by ages 20 to 30. More than 90% of individuals are affected by age 40, but few experience symptoms until after age 50 or 60. Before the age of 50, men are affected more often than women. Incidence of disease in persons older than the age of 50, however, is twice as great in women (Kee, 2000; Roberts, 2001). In younger individuals, OA is most commonly due to trauma, repetitive occupational stress, joint hemorrhage, or infection.

The search for a single cause of OA has been unsuccessful, but multiple risk factors and influences have been linked to the development and progression of the disease. Sex hormones and other hormonal factors may play a role in the onset of arthritis. The increased incidence of the disease in aging women is believed to result from estrogen reduction at menopause. Women are more likely to develop OA of the hands, with inflammation in the distal interphalangeal (DIP) and proximal interphalangeal (PIP) joints, which produces Heberden's and Bouchard's nodes, respectively. Excessive production of growth hormone may also lead to arthritis development by contributing to increased bone overgrowth. In addition, increased secretion of parathyroid hormone leads to hypercalcemia and subsequent skeletal changes that can affect disease onset.

Genetic factors appear to contribute strongly to the risk for OA. For example, the incidence of Heberden's nodes (nodal OA in the DIP joints) is three times higher among sisters than in the general population. Inherited metabolic conditions such as hemochromatosis or ochronosis have also been linked to severe OA. In addition, mutations in the type II collagen gene have been identified within families whose affected members generally exhibit chondrodysplasia and severe polyarticular OA at an early age. Although families with these gene mutations account for a relatively small proportion of the total OA population, their experience offers profound insight into disease development.

Because of the chronicity of OA, a great deal of effort has been expended on identification of modifiable risk factors. Excessive weight has long been accepted as a contributor to OA. Research has consistently demonstrated an increased incidence of knee OA in overweight individuals. Obesity also contributes to development of hip OA, but the association is weaker and less consistent than with knee OA. This variation is related to the different amount of force exerted across the two joints when an individual stands or walks; the knee bears up to six times the body's weight, but only three times that weight is born by the hip (Roberts & Lappe, 2001). Hand OA is also weakly associated with obesity, suggesting that metabolic factors may contribute to disease development in overweight individuals.

Level of activity is another modifiable risk factor. Moderate recreational exercise has been shown to decrease both the likelihood of developing OA and the progression of arthritic symptoms. It first strengthens the muscles, tendons, and ligaments that support the joint. By driving synovial fluid through the cartilaginous matrix, exercise also stimulates growth of avascular articular cartilage. The mechanical process of joint movement is therefore critical to cartilage regeneration and joint mobility. Finally, because regular exercise helps with weight control, it also indirectly promotes joint health.

On the other hand, greater incidence of OA has been associated with strenuous, high-intensity, repetitive exercise. For example, research has demonstrated an increased risk for development of OA following involvement in competitive athletics that expose joints to high levels of impact and torsional stress, such as running, soccer, and football (Kee, 2000). Many individuals who develop OA after sports participation do not have a clear history of joint injury. Because cartilage lacks innervation, however, its damage does not cause pain directly and injuries may go undetected. In addition, individuals probably vary in their susceptibility to joint degeneration because of multiple personal differences, including genetically determined cartilage composition and tissue response to

---

BOX 16–1.
Causes of Secondary Osteoarthritis

Secondary osteoarthritis is caused by any condition that damages cartilage directly; applies chronic, excessive, or abnormal forces to joints; or causes joint instability
Trauma: sprains, strains, dislocations, fractures (with potential for avascular necrosis, osteonecrosis)
Mechanical stress: long-term participation in repetitive physical activities (e.g., athletics, repetitive task performance as part of occupation)
Inflammation in joint structures: inflammatory cells releasing enzymes that digest cartilage
Joint instability: damage to supporting structures (e.g., ligaments, tendons)
Neurologic disorders: pain, deficient proprioceptive reflexes leading to increased tendency for abnormal movement, positioning, weight bearing (e.g., Charcot neuropathy)
Congenital/acquired skeletal deformities: varus leg deformity, dislocated hip, joint laxity, Legg-Calvé-Perthes disease
Hematologic/endocrine disorders: hemophilia with chronic bleeding into joints; hyperparathyroidism with calcium loss from bone
Use of selected medications: activity of collagen-digesting enzymes stimulated in synovial membrane (e.g., colchicine, indomethacin, steroids)

Adapted from Roberts, D. (2001). Arthritic and connective tissue disorders. In D. Schoen (Ed.), *NAON core curriculum for orthopaedic nursing* (4th ed.). Pitman, NJ: National Association of Orthopaedic Nurses.

exercise. Joint instability or mechanical problems resulting from loss of normal ligament or meniscal function may also accelerate the development of degenerative changes with sports participation.

Quadriceps weakness may be another factor in the development of OA of the knee. Commonly associated with knee OA, quadriceps weakness has been widely believed to result from disuse atrophy secondary to pain in an affected joint. However, Slemenda, Brandt, Heilman, Mazzuca, Braunstein, Katz, and Wolinsky (1997) found that quadriceps weakness might be present in individuals who have OA but have neither knee pain nor muscle atrophy. Data collected on 462 community-based arthritic volunteers were consistent with the possibility that quadriceps weakness is indeed a primary risk factor for knee pain, disability, and progression of joint damage.

OA demonstrates site specificity, with certain synovial joints showing high prevalence of disease: weight-bearing joints (hips, knees); cervical and lumbar spine; DIP, PIP, and metacarpophalangeal (MCP) joints in the hands; and metatarsophalangeal (MTP) joints in the feet (bunion deformity, or hallux valgus). The hips are more often affected in men and the hands in women, especially after menopause. Some clients have a variant form of the disease called *generalized osteoarthritis*, in which Heberden's nodes on the DIP joints are accompanied by polyarticular disease in three or more sites. Although OA is typically asymmetrical, the generalized form is often symmetrical in distribution. Another disease variant is erosive OA, seen in clients who have bony erosions at the interphalangeal joints.

The disability associated with OA is easily understood when these commonly affected joints are considered. Arthritic changes in the feet and knees, for example, can lead to an unstable gait and an increased risk for falls. In the hands, arthritis can limit fine motor movements and create difficulty with dressing or other self-care tasks. Arthritis in the shoulders and elbows may have similar effects on hygiene and grooming. The emotional impact of arthritis can be further disabling if depression results from dealing with the pain, chronicity, and physical limitations of OA.

Pathophysiology

Healthy articular cartilage is smooth, white, glistening connective tissue that covers synovial joint surfaces. It demonstrates extremely low friction with movement. Articular cartilage also possesses a unique shock-absorbing capacity related to its characteristic compressibility and viscoelasticity. Chondrocytes, the cellular component of cartilage, produce type II collagen and proteoglycans to create a matrix that protects the bone ends in a joint; lesser amounts of types I, IX, and XI collagen are also present. The proteoglycans possess unique hydrophilic properties that further increase the ability of the cartilage to resist wear with heavy joint use.

OA results from a joint insult that leads to deterioration of the cartilage matrix followed by the body's subsequent ineffectual attempts at repair. Damage to the cartilage triggers a massive metabolic response at the level of the chondrocytes. Initial enzymatic tissue breakdown results in a decrease in proteoglycan content in the matrix, in turn causing cartilage softening and loss of elasticity. As the body tries to compensate for these changes, proliferating chondrocytes increase their synthesis of collagen and proteoglycans. However, this increase cannot keep pace with the progressive destruction by lysosomal enzymes, and the cartilage becomes increasingly susceptible to joint friction.

The decrease in proteoglycan content results in loss of support for collagen fibrils, allowing even more damage to the articular cartilage from forces of joint friction. Changes in collagen synthesis also occur, with a fibrous tissue replacing the typical type I collagen. Decreased cushioning results from this change in collagen, and the cartilage loses its ability to resist wear with heavy use. Concurrently, proteoglycans lose some of their hydrophilic properties and the matrix becomes less permeable. Nutrients from synovial fluid have increased difficulty reaching deep layers of cartilage, making repair of joint damage even more unlikely.

Alterations in the collagen structure lead to loss of support, and cartilaginous fibers begin to rupture. Fissuring, fibrillation, and erosion cause the articular cartilage to become yellowish, dull, and granular in appearance. This softened, fibrillated cartilage eventually becomes abraded to subchondral bone in the center of the joint surface. In the peripheral joint area, the body responds with a proliferation of fibroblasts and new bone formation that results in bony outgrowth and spur development at the joint margins. The loss of central cartilage and increase in peripheral cartilage create an incongruity in joint surfaces, changing the normal stress distribution across the joint and leading to motion restriction. Small pieces of cartilage (osteophytes) may shear off the joint surface, creating pain and further limitation in movement. Osteophytes also attract phagocytic cells that attempt to cleanse the joint of loose debris. A secondary synovitis can result, creating an enlarged joint capsule. The localized inflammatory response also leads to increased production of synovial fluid and further joint swelling.

The early pain and stiffness of OA stem not from the primary disease itself but from the secondary effects of synovitis, joint capsule distention, bony proliferation, and damage to adjacent articular structures. Cartilage lacks a nerve supply and the joint surfaces themselves do not become painful until subchondral bone is exposed in later stages of the disease.

Once the process of OA is initiated, it continues unchecked. Cartilage architecture changes, and the mechanics of joint use are further altered. The result is more

TABLE 16–2. *Differential Diagnosis of Osteoarthritis and Rheumatoid Arthritis*

	OSTEOARTHRITIS	RHEUMATOID ARTHRITIS
Pathology	Central cartilage destruction with bone growth at joint periphery; localized inflammation possible	Synovial membrane inflammation with cartilage/bone erosion leading to joint capsule destruction; damage to ligaments, tendons; characterized by remissions and exacerbations
Joints affected	Weight-bearing joints (hips, knees, spine), DIP and PIP joints; asymmetrical joint involvement	Wrists, knees, PIP and MCP joints; symmetrical joint involvement
Effusions	Localized inflammatory response may lead to increased synovial fluid production and mild joint swelling	Characteristic of disease
Symptoms	Localized pain and stiffness; Heberden's and Bouchard's nodes; mild swelling possible; pain with activity that improves with rest	Swelling, redness, warmth, pain, tenderness; nodules over extensor surfaces; fatigue, muscle aches; pain at rest, especially at night; elevated ESR, may have positive RF
Other systems affected	None	Lungs, heart, skin
Body size	May be overweight	Usually average to underaverage weight for size
Age at onset	4th to 5th decades	Young to middle age
Gender	2:1 female	3:1 female
Heredity	Genetic factors appear to contribute strongly	Familial tendency
Tests	X-ray films; laboratory studies, synovial fluid analysis to rule out other causes of joint pain	X-ray films; positive RF (80%); positive ESR; synovial fluid analysis to rule out other causes of joint pain
X-ray findings	Subchondral cysts, sclerosis, osteophytes, joint space narrowing	Erosions, osteoporosis
Treatment	Weight control, exercise, joint protection; adjunctive therapies such as heat, cold; medication; surgery	Inflammation reduction; balance of activity and rest; joint protection; splint to minimize joint deformity; balanced diet; adjunctive therapies such as heat, cold; medication; surgery

stress, additional joint damage, and the release of degradative enzymes. OA becomes a self-perpetuating disease process.

Assessment

Clinical features of OA are highlighted in a definition of the disease that was first published in the proceedings of a 1994 conference jointly sponsored by the American Academy of Orthopaedic Surgeons and the National Institutes of Health (Keuttner & Goldberg, 1995): When clinically evident, OA is characterized by joint pain, tenderness, limitation of movement, crepitus, occasional effusion, and variable degrees of local inflammation. The nurse must carefully assess the client with musculoskeletal symptoms to differentiate OA from rheumatoid arthritis or other arthritides (Table 16–2). Box 16–2 describes multiple signs and symptoms of OA that can guide a complete history, physical examination, and functional assessment for each client.

Nursing History. Joint pain is often the dominant symptom and the usual reason for seeking medical evaluation. The pain is typically mechanical in nature, often described as "aching," and is one way by which OA is differentiated from inflammatory arthropathies. The

BOX 16–2.

Characteristic Signs and Symptoms of Osteoarthritis

Objective

Joint crepitation with motion; client may complain of audible "popping, cracking, grinding"

Limited ROM, which continues to decrease with disease progression; may be due to incongruous joint surfaces, osteophytes, joint contracture

Affected joints become unstable and "give way" with weight bearing, making client fearful of falling

Enlarged joints because of formation of spurs and enlarged, boggy synovium with disease progression

Joint deformity because of loss of articular cartilage, collapse of subchondral bone, bone overgrowth, atrophy of adjacent muscles

Subjective

Deep, aching, localized joint pain; morning pain and pain with use typical of early disease; late disease causes pain at rest, which may affect sleep pattern

Pain with joint palpation

Involved joints become stiff with inactivity or changes in weather affected client typically describes localized, asymmetrical pain that increases with joint use and is relieved by rest, particularly in early stages of the disease. Night pain or pain at rest may occur with disease progression. Pain may also increase with the fall in barometric pressure that precedes inclement weather. Because the onset of pain is typically insidious, the client may not be able to recall exactly when it began. In addition, the client with probable hip OA may develop a limp as a result of referred pain around the groin and inner thigh radiating to the buttocks, knee, and outer thigh. The pattern of pain and stiffness is likely to be different for each involved joint, so specific questions are needed to elicit the information that will help in diagnosis. The experience of pain is not necessarily related to other evidence of disease severity but reflects the individual client's pain threshold and his or her use of the affected joint. A visual analogue scale should be used with the initial assessment to gauge the client's current pain and to serve as a benchmark for future changes.

Complaints of joint stiffness range from slowness of movement to pain on initial activity. Early morning stiffness is common in OA clients, but the duration is often less than 30 minutes, again differentiating OA from active rheumatoid arthritis. Stiffness after periods of rest or inactivity (articular gelling or gel phenomenon) is also characteristic of OA but typically resolves within several minutes. The client may describe a squeaking, creaking, or grating with movement (crepitus), which indicates the presence of loose cartilage particles in the joint capsule. He or she may note a worsening of symptoms in cool, damp, and rainy weather; this complaint is due to changes in intra-articular pressure associated with changes in the atmospheric pressure. Finally, overactivity can cause a moderate effusion that exacerbates joint stiffness. Complaints of weakness or numbness in the arms or legs should be noted as suggestive of possible nerve root impingement by osteophytes in OA of the spine.

The nurse should also question the client about general symptoms such as malaise and fatigue that provide evidence of living with chronic illness. The client's emotional response to illness should be assessed as well, to include his or her coping pattern, knowledge and acceptance of illness and treatment regimen, and changes in mood associated with disease progression. In addition, the nurse must determine the impact of arthritis symptoms on the client's ability to perform activities of daily living (ADLs) and to serve in roles such as parent or provider. An arthritis impact scale can be used to assess functional ability by targeting the impact of the disease on role functioning and on some self-care skills.

Because of the evidence for a genetic predisposition to disease development, the nurse should ask the client about a family history of OA. Questions about occupational and recreational activities can help determine whether any joint has been subjected to repetitive stress or injury, and questions about past weight changes can ascertain the possible role of obesity in joint changes.

Physical Examination. Physical findings are usually localized to symptomatic joints and vary with disease severity. Examination should proceed in a logical way, from the joints of the upper extremities down to the trunk and lower extremities. The client should be warm, relaxed, and as comfortable as possible to ensure accuracy of the range-of-motion (ROM) assessment. Pairs of joints should be compared for symmetry, size, shape, color, appearance, temperature, and pain.

Affected joints are likely to be tender to palpation. Capsular or joint line tenderness suggests a capsular or intracapsular origin for pain consistent with OA. Point tenderness away from the joint line is typical of periarticular lesions (e.g., bursitis) rather than arthritis and is an important finding in differentiating possible musculoskeletal diagnoses. The nurse may feel crepitation in the arthritic joint during passive movement, indicating loss of cartilage integrity; this sign is present in more than 90% of clients with OA of the knee (*Osteoarthritis,* 1997). Reduced ROM, extremely common in osteoarthritic joints, is a principal feature or contributor to the client's overall disability. Any resulting loss of function is more important than a measurement of the precise loss of motion. Limited movement or locking during movement occurs mainly because of osteophyte encroachment, joint remodeling, and capsular thickening. However, it may be accentuated by mild effusion and soft tissue swelling.

Examination may detect deformity or instability peculiar to the affected joint. Heberden's nodes on the DIP joints of the hands indicate osteophyte formation and loss of joint space. They can occur as early as age 40 and tend to be seen in affected members of the same family. Bouchard's nodes on the PIP joints indicate similar involvement to Heberden's nodes (Fig. 16–1). Almost 50% of clients with OA of the knee have a joint malalignment that most commonly occurs as a varus deformity because of cartilage loss in the medial compartment. Leg length discrepancy may be noted because of loss of joint space in advanced hip OA. In addition, muscular atrophy may be seen in advanced disease secondary to joint splinting for pain relief.

Joint warmth and soft tissue swelling can indicate local inflammation that may accompany or precede signs of joint damage. Inflammation is most evident at the knee or during early stages of OA development in the fingers. In the knee, mild synovitis with slight to moderate effusion can create a positive bulge sign. Large effusions are uncommon with OA, however, and their presence should suggest another pathologic condition. Differential diagnosis is critical because hot, markedly swollen joints may be caused by septic arthritis, gout, pseudogout, or basic calcium phosphate arthritis.

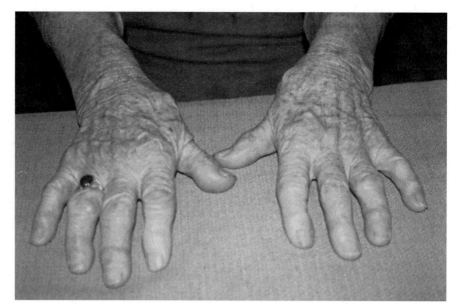

FIGURE 16–1. Both hands show evidence of osteoarthritic changes characterized by multiple nodules on the DIP joints (Heberden's nodes) and PIP joints (Bouchard's nodes).

Diagnostic Evaluation

Both clinical and financial pressures influence the need for prompt recognition and management of mild OA. Timely, cost-effective use of diagnostic tools aids in confirming the diagnosis and in initiating appropriate treatments that will allow the client to maintain an optimal level of function.

Laboratory Tests. Because the diagnosis of OA can almost always be made by history and physical examination, routine laboratory tests are typically useful only in screening for associated conditions and in establishing baselines before initiation of therapy. For example, a baseline complete blood count (CBC) is suggested for the client who will be taking NSAIDs for arthritis symptom management. After the client begins NSAID therapy, additional CBCs should be routinely ordered to screen for anemia related to occult gastrointestinal bleeding. Renal and liver function tests are also suggested before initiation of aspirin or NSAID therapy in the older client. Additional tests should be ordered every 6 months during treatment to monitor for occasional side effects such as renal insufficiency, hepatitis, and electrolyte imbalance.

Tests for rheumatoid factor (RF) and erythrocyte sedimentation rate (ESR) are often routinely ordered for clients with joint complaints. However, about 20% of healthy older individuals are RF positive (*Osteoarthritis,* 1997). In addition, ESR tends to rise with age. Neither value would therefore exclude a diagnosis of OA in the older client. However, the client with a markedly elevated ESR needs evaluation to rule out polymyalgia rheumatica, chronic infection, or an underlying malignancy such as multiple myeloma.

Radiographic Studies. Although radiography of affected joints is important in confirming the diagnosis

of OA, findings do not always correlate with the severity of clinical symptoms. The American College of Rheumatology (ACR) developed the following criteria that continue to guide disease diagnosis (Hochberg, Altman, Brandt, Clark, Dieppe, Griffin, Moskowitz, & Schnitzer, 1995a, 1995b):

- For knee OA, the presence of knee pain and radiographic osteophytes and at least one of the following: age greater than 50 years, morning stiffness lasting less than 30 minutes, and crepitus on motion
- For hip OA, the presence of hip pain and at least two of the following: ESR of less than 20 mm/hr, radiographic femoral or acetabular osteophytes, and radiographic joint space narrowing

As OA progresses, asymmetrical joint space narrowing increases as a result of loss of articular cartilage or progression of bone remodeling (Fig. 16-2A and B). Later radiographic changes include the formation of subchondral cysts and an alteration in the shape of bone ends that provides additional evidence of bone remodeling. Central erosions and cortical collapse in the DIP and PIP joints may be seen on radiographs in some clients with erosive OA. However, marginal erosions and bone demineralization are not features of OA and should suggest a diagnosis of rheumatoid arthritis or other inflammatory disease.

Among other possible radiographic studies, a bone scan can be used to determine the skeletal distribution of OA. It is especially sensitive to the changes of early disease. Magnetic resonance imaging (MRI) is much more sensitive than plain x-ray films in identifying the progression of joint destruction by providing a detailed view of thinning cartilage, capsular edema, and subchondral cysts. Optical coherence tomography (OCT) is another radiographic technique that has shown great sensitivity

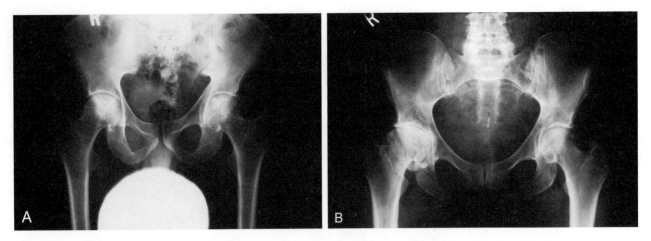

FIGURE 16–2. *A,* An anteroposterior (AP) view of a normal hip joint, with no evidence of arthritic changes. *B,* An AP view demonstrates radiographic changes consistent with advanced osteoarthritis, including a narrowed joint space and cystic formations within the bone.

and reproducibility in measuring articular cartilage changes. OCT allows a noninvasive study similar to ultrasound; instead of sound waves, however, it measures the back-reflection of infrared light.

Because radiographic changes indicative of OA are common in the general population, the nurse must be aware that the client's pain may not in fact be caused by OA. Even if radiographic evidence of OA is present, the client's pain may realistically arise from a periarticular source, such as anserine bursitis of the knee or trochanteric bursitis of the hip. In addition, pain may be the result of problems with tendons, ligaments, or menisci.

Synovial Fluid Analysis. Analysis of synovial fluid is a reliable method for differentiating OA from other forms of arthritis. In the osteoarthritic joint, the synovial fluid is clear yellow. It demonstrates high viscosity resulting from the presence of a normal amount of hyaluronic acid. The white blood cell (WBC) count is low, and the glucose level equals that of the client's serum.

Collaborative Treatment: Nonpharmacologic Office and Community Interventions

Management of OA requires commitment from the client and collaboration with members of the health care team. As the client's needs change, various providers may become involved in his or her care: physician, nurse, physical and occupational therapists, dietitian, social worker, orthotist, and orthopaedic surgeon. Treatment goals include the following:

- Management of pain and inflammation
- Maintenance or improvement of joint function
- Limitation of disability through prevention or correction of deformity
- Achievement of optimal role function and independence in self-care
- Avoidance of adverse drug events

- Acceptance of chronic illness and its associated therapeutic regimen
- Use of positive coping strategies

Most OA clients experience success with conservative disease management that includes physical therapy, pharmacologic interventions, and self-care modifications. Care is focused on helping the client and family understand the disease process, the suggested treatments, and any necessary alteration in performance of ADLs. Surgical intervention would be considered if the client has unrelieved pain, especially pain that interferes with rest; diminished ability to perform ADLs independently; and progressive loss of joint function despite maximal medical therapy. Possible surgical procedures include osteotomy, debridement, cartilage implantation, arthroplasty, and arthrodesis; the choice would be based on factors such as disease progression, client age, and desired activity level.

Client Education. Education and cognitive-behavioral interventions to support education are the foundation of successful OA management. An informed client is more likely to collaborate with the health care team in creating a treatment regimen that minimizes or eliminates risk factors. Current, well-written pamphlets or brochures should be shared with the client and family members, and time should be allowed during regular visits to discuss questions they may have. Client-nurse discussions should focus on explanations of the development and progression of OA, pain management and medication use, the importance of exercise, sound nutritional choices for weight management, joint protection and the use of appropriate body mechanics, stress management and coping with chronic illness, and complementary and traditional treatment options.

In addition, the client can gain understanding of the disease and support in coping efforts through community resources such as the Arthritis Foundation. Self-management programs such as the Arthritis Self-Help Course are administered by local chapters of the Arthritis Foundation. Research has demonstrated that the client who participates in this program has better outcomes and lower health care costs than the client who relies on traditional care alone (*Osteoarthritis*, 1997). Chapter 2 provides further information on educational and cognitive-behavioral strategies to assist clients in coping with their illness and treatment regimen.

Nutritional Counseling. For the client who requires weight reduction to alleviate arthritis symptoms and slow disease progression, nutritional counseling is a key strategy. Because obesity is related to an increased incidence of OA, the nurse or dietitian must help the overweight client evaluate his or her current diet and make appropriate low-calorie changes. Assessment of personal resources must be completed to determine whether the client will be able to follow a recommended food plan. Finances may be limited, for example, or the client with poorly fitting dentures may have problems with chewing. Age-related changes in taste and smell may also make some foods less appealing. Individualized counseling is important to the success of a weight reduction program.

Exercise. Exercise has been identified by the ACR (2000) as an integral part of OA management. Joint loading and mobilization are essential to maintenance of articular cartilage integrity. Quadriceps muscle weakness, which can contribute to progressive articular damage, can also be decreased with regular exercise. Research has shown that programs for specific muscle strengthening and aerobic conditioning can result in a modest reduction in the pain and disability of knee OA (Cooper, 1999). The benefit may be relatively short lived, however, because of a steady decline in the number of clients who continue to exercise over time. The nurse should encourage the client to exercise regularly and should then contact him or her frequently to increase the likelihood of adherence to the activity plan. The client must also be counseled to follow a careful progression in activity level. Some exercises, for example, are too vigorous and therefore likely to aggravate arthritis symptoms. Other exercises may be too gentle and unlikely to have a positive effect on muscle strength or joint ROM.

An exercise prescription should include components that focus on cardiovascular conditioning, improved strength and flexibility, and increased joint mobility. Aerobic or resistance exercises have led to improvements in physical performance and pain, as well as reports of decreased disability. Strength training and weight-bearing ROM exercises have been shown to improve gait and overall function. Low-impact, gravity-limiting exercises such as bicycle training have increased muscle tone and strength and improved neuromuscular function and cardiovascular endurance without applying excessive force across joints. High-impact activities should be avoided unless appropriate adaptations can be made. These activities include jogging or jumping that jars the joints, activities that require lifting or manipulating equipment (tennis), and highly competitive or contact sports.

Gradual progression is the key to the success of an exercise program, starting at the client's current level of performance and increasing the number of repetitions as the client is able. Small gains should be encouraged and overexertion avoided. Referral to a physical therapist may help facilitate exercise and control joint symptoms. The client should also be encouraged to time analgesics appropriately to participate more comfortably in exercise sessions.

Joint Protection. Joint protection is another non-pharmacologic intervention used to relieve pain and to improve joint biomechanics and function in the client with OA. A good understanding of principles of joint protection is important, including the need for a balance of rest and activity. The client must learn to rest the affected joint during episodes of acute inflammation, maintaining it in a functional position through the use of splints or braces if necessary. Weight bearing is also typically restricted for the inflamed joint. Because stiffness results from rest, however, joint immobility should not exceed 1 week. Modification of occupational and recreational activity also protects the joint from stress. The client with knee OA, for example, should avoid prolonged standing, squatting, kneeling, or sitting in low chairs. The use of assistive devices, such as canes, crutches, or walkers, reduces the biomechanical forces across the joint. Use of orthotics or shock-absorbing shoes may also be beneficial.

Thermal Applications. Applications of heat and cold may help alleviate pain and stiffness. Ice is not used as often as heat in the treatment of OA, but it can be helpful during periods of acute inflammation. Heat therapy may be particularly beneficial for stiffness by increasing collagen elasticity and flexibility. It is available in various modalities, including hot packs, ultrasound, whirlpool, paraffin wax, and massage.

Complementary and Alternative Therapies. Complementary and alternative approaches to symptom management have become increasingly popular with clients seeking relief of arthritis symptoms (Kuhn, 1999). Total visits to practitioners of alternative medicine in the United States increased by almost 50% between 1990 and 1997, exceeding visits to all primary care physicians and representing an estimated $21.2 billion for services ("Alternative Medicine on Rise," 2000). Some modalities, such as copper or magnetic bracelets, are harmless and possibly worthless, supported solely by anecdotal evidence. Other treatments, such as bee stings, may lead to severe toxicities. A few therapies have been proven to have modest beneficial effects. Acupuncture, for example, has been determined in randomized clinical trials to be a legitimate, useful, and safe method for pain management (Horstman, 1999).

Tai chi is a conservative, economical movement therapy that has become popular as a low-impact form of exercise for arthritis. This ancient Chinese martial art and meditation combines a choreographed series of slow movements with mental concentration and coordinated breathing. Tai chi can be performed by anyone, regardless of age, and can even be done in a wheelchair. Jacobson, Cheng, Cashel, and Guerrero (1997) studied films of individuals practicing the original 108 forms of tai chi and concluded that it presents a low-stress method to enhance stability, improve kinesthetic sense, and strengthen knee extension. Lumsden, Baccala, and Martire (1998) found that tai chi enhanced mobility for clients with OA without activating joint pain. Because of its slow and gentle movements, performance of tai chi carries no specific dangers. However, the nurse should reinforce the importance of warming up before practice to prevent stretching injuries. To decrease the risk of falls, use of nonskid footwear is also important during performance of tai chi.

Among the most popular alternative modalities is the use of herbal supplements. Since 1991, when Kwai garlic was first sold in a drugstore, herbal products have moved beyond health food stores to become readily available in discount stores, groceries, and pharmacies (O'Koon, 1999). Supplements such as Echinacea, ginkgo, and St. John's wort have become household names to the millions of people who seek improved health. The nurse and the arthritis client need reliable information about herbal products to make appropriate treatment choices. Among the products identified by the Arthritis Foundation (Horstman, 1999) as potentially useful for the pain or inflammation of arthritis are ginger, turmeric, and cayenne red pepper.

Ginger, a common ingredient in Asian cooking, has long been used to calm an upset stomach. Ginger is believed to have anti-inflammatory properties, and because it inhibits production of prostaglandins and leukotrienes that contribute to pain and swelling, it is also a potential analgesic. Ginger can be administered in several forms. A pain-relieving tea can be made by steeping 1 teaspoon of fresh grated ginger in a cup of water, and powdered ginger can be given in capsules or tablets. A hot compress that includes ginger root can be applied to painful joints. The arthritis client should avoid tinctures, which can contain 50% grain alcohol and have interaction potential with other prescriptive medications. Although ginger is fairly benign, the arthritis client should be aware that very large doses can have gastrointestinal effects similar to NSAIDs. Ginger can also increase bleeding risks for the client who is taking an anticoagulant.

Turmeric, a root similar to ginger, has been used in Ayurvedic medicine to treat inflammation and in Chinese medicine to treat arthritis pain. The active ingredient is curcumin, which is believed to inhibit production of prostaglandins and stimulate production of cortisol. The usual dosage of turmeric is 400 mg in capsules or tablets given three times a day. It can also be added to food during cooking to provide flavor and color. Scientific evidence is not complete, but turmeric has no known side effects and may provide some relief for the arthritis client. Turmeric should not be taken by a client who has gallstones or is pregnant because of the unknown effects in these populations.

Cayenne red pepper (*Capsicum* species) contains capsaicin that prompts the release of pain-relieving endorphins. Evidence gathered over two decades also points to the ability of capsaicin to block pain by interfering with substance P, which is responsible for transmission of pain impulses. The ACR recommends capsaicin as a topical cream in the treatment for knee OA. Although a concentrated product is available by prescription, creams of 0.025% to 0.075% capsaicin are sold over-the-counter (OTC). After the cream is applied to affected areas, the arthritis client experiences a transient burning sensation before capsaicin starts to decrease joint discomfort. Because of the risk of skin injury, the cream should not be used with an external heat source such as a pad or hot water bottle. The client should apply capsaicin to a small area first as a test and discontinue the product if the skin is sensitive to its effects; the cream should also not be applied to irritated or broken skin. The nurse should instruct the client to practice good handwashing after application before touching the eyes or other parts of the body (Rains, 1995).

Counseling on the use of these or other herbal products is a responsibility of the interdisciplinary team. Chapter 2 addresses issues related to counseling regarding herbal therapy. The client with arthritis should be cautioned against believing any label or brochure that promises a cure for arthritis. Although complementary therapies may have a place in arthritis management, the nurse should also educate the client about the implications of delaying medical care or using unproven remedies to the exclusion of proven arthritis treatments.

Collaborative Treatment: Pharmacologic Management

Pharmacologic therapy should serve as an adjunct to nonpharmacologic approaches to arthritis management. Because no drug can reverse the structural and biochemical abnormalities of OA, therapy is aimed at pain management. Older adults, who represent the largest population affected by OA, may also have other chronic diseases and take multiple medications. The nurse and other health care providers in all settings must be aware of factors that affect the success of arthritis drug therapy in older adults. For example, the client may self-medicate with OTC drugs that can adversely interact with the recommended arthritis regimen. Because the client often receives health care from multiple providers, he or she is also more likely to experience the phenomenon of polypharmacy or to take duplicate medications. The older client also experiences changes in body composition and a functional decline that affect the way the body absorbs and metabolizes medications. Safe, effective pharmacologic treatment must be based on the maxim, "Start low and go slow."

Analgesics and Nonsteroidal Anti-inflammatory Drugs. Acetaminophen is now recommended by the ACR (2000) as the initial drug of choice for symptomatic OA. A dosage of up to 1000 mg four times daily is suggested. Adverse effects from acetaminophen are generally mild, with a very low incidence of toxic effects on the liver and kidneys, occurring primarily in clients who drink large amounts of alcohol. For acute exacerbations of pain, acetaminophen can be supplemented in the short-term with opioid analgesics such as propoxyphene, codeine, or oxycodone.

If acetaminophen proves inadequate for control of arthritis pain, low-dose OTC ibuprofen (up to 400 mg four times daily) or nonacetylated salicylates are part of the ACR recommendations for clients with normal renal function and no history of gastrointestinal problems. If pain persists, prescriptive doses of NSAIDs may be indicated. The analgesic effect of NSAIDs is exerted by inhibition of prostaglandin synthesis through inactivation of cyclooxygenase (COX) enzymes. Traditional NSAIDs such as ibuprofen or naproxen sodium reduce prostaglandin levels in the stomach and kidneys through COX-1 inhibition, creating a risk for gastric ulceration or renal impairment. The older client is particularly prone to these side effects because of diminished physiologic reserve and the likelihood of multiple chronic conditions. Careful monitoring of hemoglobin and hematocrit is critical during NSAID treatment to detect potential gastrointestinal bleeding, which can be life-threatening. The use of traditional NSAIDs results in approximately 107,000 hospitalizations and 16,500 deaths annually in the United States, costing more than $1 billion ("Hospital Extra," 1999).

Newer NSAIDs with COX-2 selectivity (e.g., celecoxib, rofecoxib) have demonstrated their anti-inflammatory effects with less gastrointestinal toxicity. These drugs are currently more expensive than first-generation NSAIDs, but the cost savings from reduced gastrointestinal effects should offset the initial higher cost. Once-daily dosing with a COX-2 inhibitor may also be a potential advantage in prescribing for the arthritis client who has difficulty managing a more complicated drug regimen. However, the differences between the two types of medications must be carefully examined in terms of interaction

potential with other drugs the client may receive, including methotrexate, warfarin, lithium, and angiotensin-converting enzyme (ACE) inhibitors (Simon, 1999).

Prophylactic use of gastrointestinal-protective medications is suggested with moderate- to high-dose traditional NSAID therapy in clients older than 60 years of age who have a history of peptic ulcer disease and when therapy is anticipated to last more than 3 months. Proton pump inhibitors and histamine-2 blockers have both been effective in reducing the risk of ulceration, perforation, or bleeding from NSAID use.

For unremitting pain, an opioid analgesic can be safely added to an NSAID or simple analgesic for up to 2 weeks. In one study, oxycodone added to NSAID therapy was shown to reduce OA pain and improve quality of sleep. The controlled-release form of the drug caused fewer side effects than the immediate-release medication (Caldwell, Hale, Boyd, Hague, Iwan, Shi, & Lacouture, 1999).

Biologic Agents. The idea of cartilage regeneration has received considerable attention in the consumer literature, and two nutritional supplements have rapidly gained popularity as treatments for OA. Glucosamine sulfate has been perceived as a "building block" for regeneration of glycosaminoglycans in articular cartilage. Chondroitin sulfate acts as a connecting matrix between protein filaments in cartilage, and its availability is believed to stimulate matrix synthesis and accelerate the healing process. Because neither agent is directly incorporated into the extracellular matrix, their rapid onset of action suggests an anti-inflammatory effect. Research on chondroitin sulfate is ongoing, with some controversial outcomes regarding its role in arthritis treatment. On the other hand, glucosamine has been found in several short-term European trials to be better than placebos and some NSAIDs in relieving both pain and inflammation associated with OA (Rehman & Lane, 1999). Intramuscular and intra-articular glucosamine injections also appear to be well tolerated, but further studies are needed to determine various dosing regimens and potential long-term effects. Routine use of glucosamine sulfate or other nutritional supplements as a primary therapy for OA is not recommended until well-designed trials can determine their efficacy.

Another dietary supplement, S-adenosylmethionine (SAM-e), has also attracted consumer attention. Unlike many supplements, SAM-e is neither an herb nor a hormone. It is a naturally occurring substance that is believed to play a role in biochemical reactions such as methylation, which helps the body grow and repair cells. Although SAM-e has been prescribed in Europe for three decades, it did not became available as a supplement in the United States until the spring of 1999. The Arthritis Foundation ("SAM-e," 2000) reported that "there is sufficient information to support the claim that SAM-e provides pain relief for osteoarthritis." However, the foundation cited no scientific evidence to support claims of at least one manufacturer that SAM-e contributes to "joint health." Although experts say the evidence supporting the benefits of SAM-e is extensive compared with other supplements, the known risks, benefits, and costs must be examined before recommending or proceeding with treatment (Ramos, 2000).

In clinical studies, these supplements had to be taken for 3 to 4 weeks before providing any pain relief. Because of this delayed effect, the client with OA should continue conventional medications at least a month before attempting to reduce his or her usage. Any changes in the therapeutic regimen should be attempted only with a medical recommendation.

Other supplements, such as vitamins C and D, received public notice for treatment of knee arthritis following publication of findings from the classic Framingham Osteoarthritis Study (McAlindon, Felson, Zhang, Hannan, Aliabadi, Weissman, Rush, Wilson, & Jacques, 1996). Results suggest that vitamin D might reduce radiographic progression of arthritis. Participants with low levels of serum 1,25-hydroxyvitamin D showed three times the risk of radiographic disease progression. In addition, the study showed that antioxidants may play a role in delaying OA. Through its effect on the vitamin C–dependent enzyme lysyl hydroxylase, vitamin C is needed for the stabilization of mature collagen. In the Framingham Study, clients with low oral vitamin C intake had a threefold increase in radiographic progression of knee OA. Referral to a dietitian may help the arthritis client maintain appropriate vitamin intake.

Viscosupplementation. Hyaluronic acid has been used in treatment of knee OA because of its characteristic viscoelasticity and its potential to supplement joint lubrication by synovial fluid. It may also have an anti-inflammatory effect, although clinical studies have produced mixed results with this costly intervention. Although some studies have shown reduced pain after injection of hyaluronic acid, a significant placebo effect has been documented. The drug has not been shown to alter the progression and extent of OA or to stimulate cartilage regrowth.

Two formulations, sodium hyaluronate and hylan G-F-20, have been approved by the U.S. Food and Drug Administration (FDA). Both are contraindicated for clients who have allergies to avian proteins, feathers, and egg products. A weekly dose of 2 mL is administered via intra-articular injection into the affected knee; notable side effects include pain and swelling at the injection site. Most clients do not notice therapeutic effects until several weeks after the last dose has been administered. Some clients have reported a sustained response of 3 to 5 months, but additional well-controlled, long-term studies are needed to confirm the efficacy of the two drugs.

Corticosteroid Therapy. Systemic corticosteroid therapy is not indicated in OA because of its side effects. However, intra-articular injections of glucocorticoids are often used to treat OA, particularly in joints that show signs of inflammation. Multiple studies have demonstrated that the effect of injection is short lived (3 to 4 weeks) but positive, with a powerful placebo response. Injections in single weight-bearing joints should be separated by 3 to 4 months because of the possibility of damage to intra-articular structures by residual corticosteroid crystals. Injection may be a useful adjunct for the client with limited therapeutic options.

Topical Analgesics. Studies have shown that topical analgesics can provide some pain relief for the OA client. Capsaicin cream in particular has demonstrated significant reduction of knee pain when used along with regular arthritis medications. However, the necessity for several applications a day often leads to poor compliance. The nurse should ensure that the client understands the need for multiple applications to get best results with any topical analgesic.

Nursing Management

Nursing care for the client with OA promotes a healthy, positive adaptation by focusing on three domains of human response: comfort, self-care, and coping. The nurse and client work collaboratively to promote use of adaptive strategies in each domain (see Table 16–1).

Comfort. The domain of comfort includes the nursing diagnoses of pain (acute or chronic) and sleep-pattern disturbance.

Pain

Promotion of Physical Comfort, Pain Management. Pain and stiffness are the predominant clinical features of OA. Pain is often described as deep and aching. Early in the disease, it occurs with overuse of affected joints. Later, pain may occur even at rest. Stiffness is limited to the involved joints and is usually of short duration (30 minutes after arising), typically following periods of immobility or occurring in response to changing barometric pressure.

Complaint of pain is often the initial reason that an OA client seeks medical evaluation. Although the client's primary goal is pain relief, members of the health care team know that prevention of disability and deformity, preservation or restoration of function, and prevention of psychosocial complications are related to pain control and integral to effective management of OA.

Untreated pain may lead to the client's decreased use of an affected joint, fear of the possible crippling effects of OA, loss of independence, and depression. The nurse helps the client adapt to chronic illness by teaching methods to (1) minimize pain and stiffness, (2) maintain optimal mobility, (3) prevent or minimize deformity, and (4) preserve normal family and social role function. Ongoing teaching focuses on the disease process, development of skills to cope with chronic illness, self-care measures to preserve role function and self-esteem, and traditional and nontraditional methods of pain relief.

A thorough nursing history determines the effects of pain and stiffness. Questions focus on the location of complaints, duration, and aggravating and alleviating factors. Pain intensity is most effectively measured with a visual analogue scale or with a functional assessment tool, such as the Stanford Arthritis Disability and Discomfort Scale. The Stanford Scale, which includes a pain analogue scale, may be preferable because it gives a more inclusive picture of the impact of arthritis pain. After completion, the tool can be attached to the client record in the hospital or office to serve as a baseline in evaluating treatment outcomes. As the client completes additional tools at scheduled times during treatment, qualitative and quantitative changes in functional status can be noted. Documented improvements can serve as a powerful incentive for the client's continued adherence to the prescribed regimen. Lack of improvement helps in determining the need for a change in treatment.

After assessing the client's pain experience and joint mobility, the nurse can provide instruction on individualized pain management strategies that include prescribed analgesics, joint rest, weight loss, use of heat and cold, and alternative modalities. Discussion of joint protection strategies, gait training, and energy conservation is critical to the client's ability to minimize pain and maintain a functional joint. For example, a client with OA of the hip may benefit from partial weight bearing or a toe-touch gait achieved with use of a cane or walker. The assistive device shifts some of the body weight to the upper extremities and decreases loading across the hip. Other joints may be splinted or braced in a neutral position for brief periods to relieve stress. Prolonged immobility or bed rest is not typically recommended, however, because of the risk for increased disability, loss of strength, and development of muscle atrophy or contractures. The client who complains of morning stiffness should be encouraged to avoid activities early in the day and to mix activity and rest during the remainder of the day. Isometric exercises may also help increased joint mobility and muscle strength.

In addition to teaching about prescribed medications, the nurse should suggest strategies that allow the client to be an active partner in pain management. Use of a pain journal helps the client monitor the effects of activity as well as personal response to medications or other treatments. It also teaches the client to recognize and interpret body cues. The pain journal assists the health care team in determining treatment changes based on an accurate record of the client's day-to-day arthritis

experience, a system proven to be more effective than simple recall of events.

Other modalities such as phonophoresis or transcutaneous electric nerve stimulation (TENS) may prove helpful in pain management (see Chapter 5 for complete discussion of pain and pain management). The client can also learn to use nontraditional pain management strategies effectively; these strategies include relaxation techniques, guided imagery, therapeutic touch, self-hypnosis, and controlled rhythmic breathing.

Sleep-Pattern Disturbance

Sleep-Enhancing Interventions. Managing pain and stiffness helps greatly in promoting adequate sleep. The nurse can reinforce good sleep habits by teaching the client to avoid caffeine or alcohol before bedtime. Soothing activities, such as reading or taking a warm bath, may also be effective in promoting sleep. Simple analgesics or NSAIDs can minimize pain and stiffness when taken at night, further enhancing the sleep cycle.

Self-care. The domain of self-care includes the nursing diagnoses of alterations in nutrition, impaired physical mobility, self-care deficits, and impaired home maintenance.

Alterations in Nutrition

Nutrition Management, Counseling for Weight Reduction. The focus of nutritional counseling should be the promotion of a sound diet with achievement and maintenance of a reasonable body weight. Weight control is critical to decreasing pain, joint stress, and destruction. To promote success in weight reduction, both the client and the family must receive instruction on any suggested diet alterations. To keep the client from feeling victimized, flexibility in menu planning combines use of favorite foods with the ability to dine in restaurants. Short-term, easily obtainable goals should be set for weight loss. Recommended diet changes should also be simple enough to encourage compliance.

The client may have questions about the possible relationship of foods and arthritis. Practitioners of conventional medicine have been hesitant to admit that arthritis symptoms may be triggered by food allergies. Alternative medicine practitioners, however, have long held the belief that symptoms worsen in response to specific foods. The nightshade vegetables are considered a common source of allergens. These include white potatoes, tomatoes, eggplant, and green and red peppers. Other possible triggers are dairy products, wheat, eggs, oranges, nuts (especially peanuts), green beans, beef, yeast, chocolate, sugar, corn, and yellow wax beans (Zampieron & Kamhi, 1999). An elimination diet can be suggested to help the client determine whether any foods do in fact trigger increased arthritis symptoms; referral to a dietitian would ensure that elimination of foods is done in a way that does not compromise general health.

Impaired Physical Mobility

Activity and Energy Management. Impaired mobility may result from the pain and stiffness typical of OA. As described previously, an important part of the therapeutic regimen is the development of an activity plan that balances appropriate exercise with needed periods of joint rest. Exercises should be planned for the time of day when the client is least tired and is experiencing the least amount of pain and stiffness. Pain management interventions performed before activity may make it easier for the client to complete the prescribed exercises.

Self-care Deficits and Impaired Home Maintenance

Assistive Devices. Impaired mobility related to advanced OA may lead to self-care deficits and interfere with normal role performance. Referral to an occupational therapist will help the client through prescription of assistive devices that facilitate self-care activities. The nurse should remember that self-care deficits and impaired home maintenance may also affect the client's self-image. Visible hand deformity and the loss of hand strength, which limit activities such as opening jars or writing a check, can lead to decreased self-esteem and must be considered in any care plan.

Most clients with mild arthritis are able to continue to work at their jobs with minor adaptations, such as scheduled rest periods and frequent position changes. However, younger clients who engage in heavy labor may need referral to a vocational counselor for job retraining. Although older clients may not work outside the home, they may require assistance with everyday tasks. Family members often become caregivers for a client with worsening OA, and their needs must also be considered. Respite from another family member, friend, or nursing assistant will make the return to caregiving responsibilities easier. In addition, the respite provider offers a unique socialization opportunity for the client.

Coping. The domain of coping includes the diagnoses of ineffective coping, impaired adjustment, and altered sexuality.

Ineffective Coping

Promotion of Positive Coping and Family Functioning. Coping with a chronic illness such as arthritis may require the client to work through stages of grieving similar to those experienced by a dying individual. Visiting different physicians in hopes of another diagnosis or following popular treatments that promise a quick

cure may all indicate the client's difficulty in accepting the presence of OA. The client who is in denial should receive accurate information in response to questions. As the nurse focuses on arthritis symptoms and their effect on the client's daily activities, the client learns ways in which he or she can be successful in disease management.

Family members may experience the same stages of grieving as they begin to recognize the lifestyle changes that accompany a diagnosis of OA. Through active listening and empathy, the nurse responds therapeutically to family expressions of frustration. With an understanding that acceptance cannot be hurried, the nurse provides information at appropriate times to allow both client and family members to progress through the grief process and ultimately cope successfully with the presence of chronic disease.

Impaired Adjustment

Education and Counseling. Impaired adjustment is a state in which the client is unable to modify his or her lifestyle and behavior in a manner consistent with a change in health status (North American Nursing Diagnosis Association [NANDA], 1999). The client characteristically refuses to participate in care or to implement the suggested therapies. Historically, a large percentage of clients have been identified as having adjustment issues.

The nurse must first recognize the difficulty that the arthritis client and involved family members may have in accepting a diagnosis and following a treatment regimen. Advice regarding career or activity changes may seem unreasonable to the client. The client may become disappointed with a health care system that, in general, poorly manages chronic disease. Finally, family members may resent a disease process that makes the client less available for shared pastimes. The nurse must carefully structure educational encounters to ensure that the client and family receive appropriate information at the time when it will be most useful to them.

Altered Sexuality

Promotion of Optimal Sexual Role Functioning. OA causes pain and stiffness that may interfere with sexual performance, particularly if affected joints include the spine, hips, and knees. If the client also develops a negative self-image as the result of joint deformities, depression and decreased libido may result from a feeling of reduced physical desirability. Fatigue related to living with chronic illness interferes with normal sexual function. In addition, if family discord has resulted from the diagnosis of OA, the relationship between the two partners may be altered and the desire for intercourse decreased.

After receiving information about the disease process, the client should be counseled on alternative positions that promote comfort during intimacy. For example, a spoon position allows a posterior approach for intercourse that reduces pressure on affected joints. This side-lying position may be the most comfortable for clients with spinal involvement and related back pain. Analgesics, a warm bath, or a glass of wine before intercourse may also help alleviate pain and stiffness that inhibit performance. If intercourse becomes too difficult, the client and partner should be urged to continue holding and caressing to promote positive self-image and a satisfying relationship.

Surgical Management

Surgical treatment for OA is indicated when conservative management fails to control pain and when the effects of arthritis on normal living become intolerable. Although total joint arthroplasty (TJA) is a popular intervention, the surgeon may first consider other procedures that preserve natural tissues and have less associated morbidity, such as debridement, cartilage transplant, osteotomy, or arthrodesis (fusion). Joint arthroplasty has been traditionally reserved for older clients, who typically place fewer demands on the prosthesis, decreasing the risk of loosening and breakage. Younger clients with knee OA are often candidates for a wedge osteotomy, a procedure that typically alleviates arthritis symptoms in the short term. If client condition dictates, however, a joint arthroplasty may be performed on a younger individual with the full expectation that revision will be necessary at some future time.

General Surgical Concepts. Because TJA eliminates the pain of arthritis, the client's functional status and quality of life are enhanced. A successful outcome is based on many factors, including the commitment of client and family to a postoperative rehabilitation program. Pain relief is a major goal of surgery, but correction of deformity and the return of self-care capability are also very important. The surgeon discusses the risks and benefits of joint arthroplasty with the client, giving consideration to the client's age, occupation, disease severity, and individual motivation. Contraindications to TJA include active infection within the affected joint, abnormal joint sensation as with neuropathic arthropathy, and arterial impairment to the extremity. Other factors that may also influence the likelihood of surgical success include history of infection in the affected joint, severe compromise of muscular control around the joint, and inability of the client to perform or cooperate with the necessary postoperative rehabilitation regimen.

Preoperative education may occur in a variety of settings. The office nurse may review information about the surgery, including joint anatomy and surgical instrumentation. Many hospitals or large surgical practices offer a joint replacement class that further discusses the client's preadmission testing and preoperative course. Postoperative expectations regarding mobility and pain management are discussed, often including a demonstration of muscle strengthening exercises and of assistive devices, such as the walker or crutches. The possibility of transfusion, use of drains, use of devices such as a continuous passive motion machine or abductor wedge, and the client's elimination needs should also be discussed. Direction should be provided regarding cessation of NSAIDs, aspirin, or anticoagulants at a prescribed preoperative date. Discussion of expected hospital length of stay and discharge needs helps the client make arrangements for transportation and family support. The working client must be asked to arrange sick leave and possibly delay vacation plans for several months. The client who lives alone may need a short stay in a rehabilitation facility or may require the assistance of home health services.

The client's nutritional status should be assessed for factors that may affect wound healing, including diabetes, obesity, anemia, malnutrition, and smoking. Dietary counseling includes the need to maintain good diabetes control, avoid smoking, lose weight, treat anemia, and optimize malnourished states. Supplemental nutrition may be indicated, for example, to prepare the malnourished client for the challenge of surgery. The nurse must remember that the obese client is not necessarily well nourished; depletion of visceral protein (serum transferrin, serum albumin, serum prealbumin) is typical in this client and can result in delayed healing or infection.

After surgery, referral to a physical therapist provides the client with instruction in exercise and mobility. Exercise increases muscle strength, prevents contractures, and improves joint ROM. The plan of care is based on the client's general health, including the presence of other chronic diseases, and the expected postoperative activity level.

Preoperative Evaluation of the Total Joint Arthroplasty Candidate. To minimize the morbidity of TJA, the surgeon must correlate possible risks with the client's medical history in performance of a thorough medical evaluation (Table 16–3). The nurse must recognize that the average client undergoing TJA is an older individual at higher risk for medical complications because of preexisting chronic conditions such as hypertension, coronary artery disease, and chronic obstructive pulmonary disease.

Postoperative Considerations. Postoperative complications occur in approximately 25% of TJA clients older than 65 years of age. The in-hospital mortality rate is less than 1% and usually related either to myocardial infarction with cardiac arrest or pulmonary embolism (Roberts & Lappe, 2001). Most complications are transient and reversible. These include heart failure, atelectasis, and

TABLE 16–3. *Preadmission Evaluation for Total Joint Arthroplasty*

POTENTIAL PROBLEM AREAS	INTERVENTIONS	OUTCOMES
Cardiovascular	Evaluate angina, coronary artery disease, chronic obstructive pulmonary disease, hypertension	Stabilize existing conditions
Wound healing	Evaluate diabetes mellitus	Control diabetes mellitus
	Evaluate nutritional status	Weight reduction for obese client; improved nutrition for malnourished client
Musculoskeletal	Evaluate muscle strength and ROM, refer to physical therapy for conditioning	Improved upper extremity strength to use assistive devices; able to participate in postoperative therapies
Thromboembolic events	Discuss prior history of deep venous thrombosis, pulmonary embolism; evaluate coagulability; determine appropriate postoperative prophylaxis	No thromboembolic complications

pneumonia. Infection and thromboembolic complications remain the greatest threat to the arthroplasty client.

Deep Venous Thrombosis and Pulmonary Embolism. Thromboembolic events are the most common medical problems encountered after TJA. The incidence of deep venous thrombosis (DVT), for example, may be as high as 57% in total hip arthroplasty (THA) and 84% in total knee arthroplasty (TKA) among clients who had not received prophylactic treatment (Brander, Kaelin, Oh, & Lim, 2000).

To prevent the development of potentially fatal blood clots, the client is mobilized early in the postoper-ative course and treated prophylactically with any combination of a number of agents: anticoagulants (low-dose heparin, warfarin, aspirin, or low-molecular-weight hepa-rin [LMWH]), foot pumps (Fig. 16–3A) or pneumatic compression stockings (Fig. 16–3B), and antiembolic stockings (TEDS). To reduce thromboembolic risk, the Fourth AACP Consensus Conference on Antithrombotic Therapy specifically recommended early mobilization, intermittent pneumatic compression, and epidural anes-thesia when appropriate in all clients undergoing major lower limb orthopaedic surgery. The nurse should also encourage the client to perform flexion and extension exercises of the feet and ankles (ankle pumps) at least 10

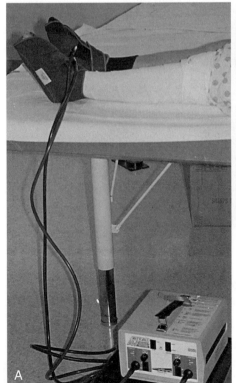

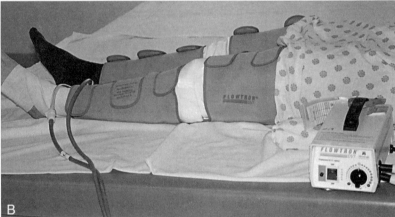

FIGURE 16–3. *A,* Foot pumps may be used postoperative to promote venous return from the lower extremities. *B,* Pneumatic compression stockings are often used to decrease the risk of deep venous thrombosis following total joint arthroplasty.

times every 1 to 2 hours while awake to prevent venous stasis. Chapter 10 discusses assessment and intervention for the client experiencing DVT.

Infection. Infection is classified as early, delayed, or late depending on the timing of its development after surgery. Early infection occurs in the first 3 months, delayed infection occurs between 3 months and 1 year, and late infection occurs more than 1 year postoperatively.

Early infection can be either superficial or deep. Delayed wound healing is often a sign of superficial infection. Early deep infection is typically the result of contamination at the time of surgery, as is delayed infection. The client complains of mild to moderate pain in the involved joint and the ESR may be elevated, but other signs of infection are often not present. Diagnosis is made through joint aspiration followed by culture and sensitivity testing. Late infection appears to occur from hematogenous seeding. Treatment in all cases depends on the causative organism. Parenteral antibiotics and surgical debridement are usually necessary. In addition, the prosthetic implant must often be removed.

Joint Instability and Loosening. Joint instability and prosthesis failure are other postoperative concerns. Unstable joints have a tendency to dislocate, most commonly at the hip and elbow. Joint reduction (manipulation to relocate the joint) is necessary, sometimes followed by bracing.

Loosening of components may become a problem 5 to 15 years after implantation. Loosening occurs at the bone-cement interface of cemented prostheses, possibly related to mechanical stresses placed on the joint. Progressive implant instability leads to client complaints of increasing pain.

Impact of Health Care Reform. Although shorter hospital stays for joint arthroplasty clients have been the norm for several years, the Balanced Budget Act of 1997 directed additional attention to acute care and posthospital costs for 10 diagnostic-related groups (DRGs) that included DRG 209 (total hip and knee). When posthospital services such as rehabilitation or home health care were ordered, the act limited hospital payment to a blend of the usual DRG payment and a lower transfer payment amount. The change was intended to correct perceived lower hospital costs connected with higher use of post-acute care providers. It provided an acute care length-of-stay goal of 4 days for the TKA or THA client and sparked increased scrutiny of resource utilization. Discharge planning is vital in light of this short length of stay.

Discharge Planning. Discharge planning should realistically begin at the time of preadmission evaluation with an anticipation of rehabilitation needs. Preparing the client for discharge requires a multidisciplinary approach to ensure a smooth transition from hospital to home, inpatient rehabilitation, skilled nursing facility, or extended care setting. The nurse provides information that will help the client prepare the home environment by anticipating postoperative needs and limitations. Education also focuses on prevention of infection, necessary precautions based on surgical approach, and the need for follow-up care. Specific discharge needs are discussed under the types of joint arthroplasty.

Education. Members of the health care team begin anticipating discharge even before surgery. However, the client may experience pain and anxiety during the first 1 or 2 days after surgery that interfere with the ability to learn more than the skills needed for immediate health maintenance. By the third or fourth postoperative day, the client can be more attentive to discussions about the home exercise regimen and guidelines for a return to normal activity. A clinical pathway often identifies common topics for discussion and guides the nurse in reviewing pertinent information with the client and family. Educational points for TJA clients are included in Figure 16-4A and B, Table 16-1, and the Total Hip Arthroplasty Clinical Pathway.

Environmental Management. Some hospitals or physicians arrange a preadmission visit by a nurse or physical therapist to assess the home environment for client safety and mobility. For example, scatter rugs should be removed, and bars may need to be installed adjacent to the toilet or shower. The need for other assistive devices or medical equipment, including a raised toilet seat for the hip arthroplasty or bilateral knee arthroplasty client, can also be reviewed. Recommendations can be made regarding the need for home assistance after discharge, or discussion can begin about client placement in another setting for additional therapy after acute hospitalization. If a home visit cannot be scheduled, the client should receive information about environmental management from the office nurse or in a preoperative class.

Postoperative Expectations. The client needs reassurance that the surgeon and office staff will be available to answer any questions that arise after discharge. The schedule for postoperative office visits, which varies with individual surgeons, should be explained. A typical schedule includes an initial visit at 3 to 6 weeks after discharge followed by visits at 3, 6, 12, and 24 months. Radiographs are also taken at regular intervals to evaluate for bone resorption and implant loosening, which may necessitate revision surgery. Between office visits, the nurse should encourage the client to call if uncertain about any proposed activity or physical discomfort. In addition, the client needs a written statement or identification card

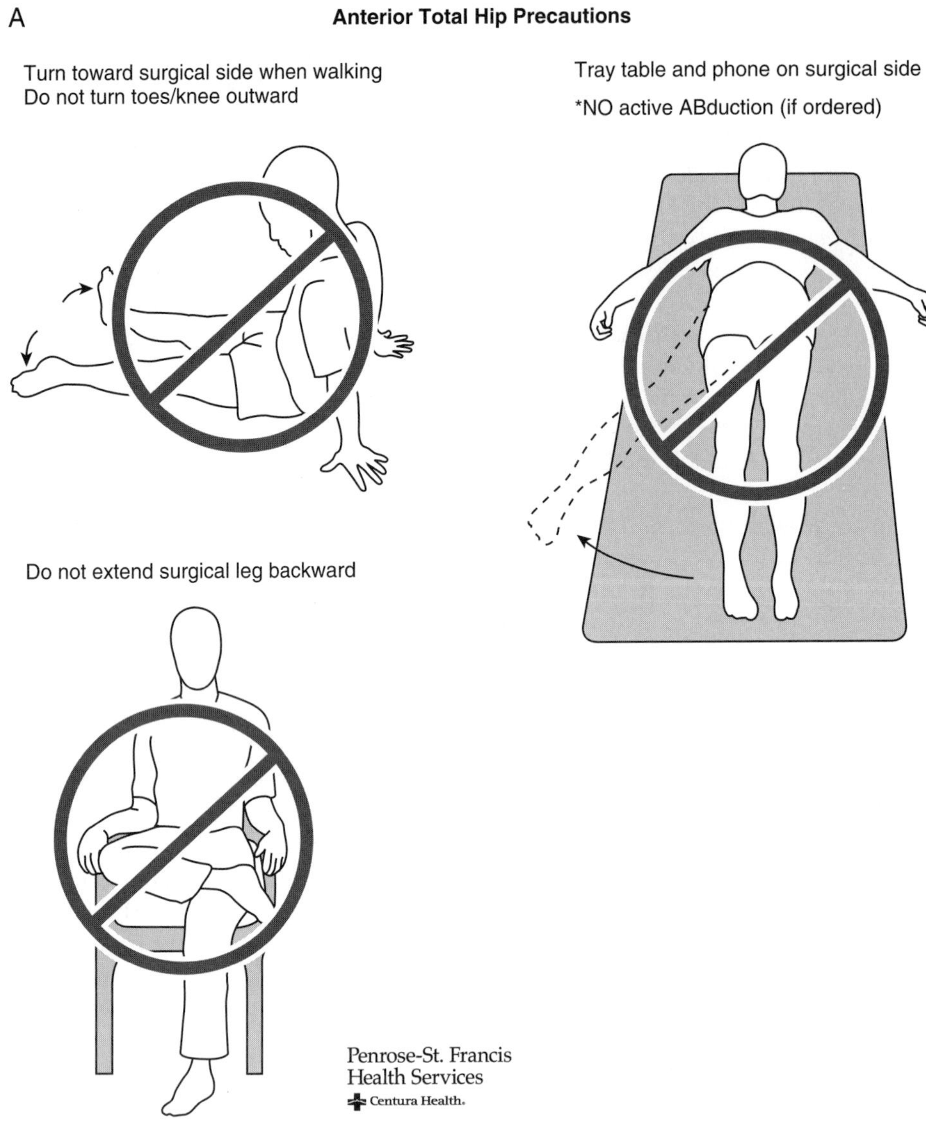

A

Anterior Total Hip Precautions

Turn toward surgical side when walking
Do not turn toes/knee outward

Tray table and phone on surgical side

*NO active ABduction (if ordered)

Do not extend surgical leg backward

Penrose-St. Francis
Health Services
✚ Centura Health.

FIGURE 16–4. *A,* Instructional sheet to guide client in precautions following THA performed using anterior approach.

that will allow later passage through airport security checkpoints.

Management of Infection Risk. The client should remain alert to signs of infection anywhere in the body, seeking immediate medical evaluation and treatment to decrease the risk of seeding the arthroplasty site. The client must be aware of the need for adequate antibiotic prophylaxis before procedures such as instrumentation of the genitourinary tract, administration of a barium enema, or removal of an ingrown toenail. Following TJA, the client has also traditionally been told to take prophylactic antibiotics before dental cleaning because of the risk of component infection from bacteria entering the bloodstream. Orthopaedic guidelines for routine dental work have now changed to recommend antibiotics only in the client who received a total joint implant within the

previous 2 years, had a prior joint infection, or has weakened immunity.

Osteoarthritis of the Hip

History. In addition to assessing general pain characteristics as previously discussed, the nurse must determine pain symptoms that specifically indicate hip involvement. Pain may be present at the groin (femoral nerve), the buttock or lateral thigh (sciatic nerve), or the anterior thigh or ipsilateral knee (obturator nerve). It may interfere with the client's mobility and affect conduct of normal business or personal activities. The history should reveal any predisposing factors for hip disease: alcohol abuse or steroid use that may be associated with avascular necrosis of the femoral head, history of hip dislocation, or history of childhood or adolescent hip difficulties that suggest a congenital or developmental cause.

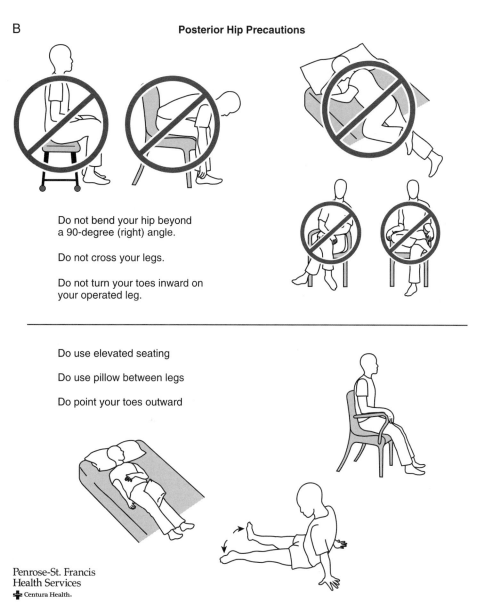

B

Posterior Hip Precautions

Do not bend your hip beyond
a 90-degree (right) angle.

Do not cross your legs.

Do not turn your toes inward on
your operated leg.

Do use elevated seating

Do use pillow between legs

Do point your toes outward

Penrose-St. Francis
Health Services
✚ Centura Health.

FIGURE 16–4 *Continued.* B, Postoperative precautions for client after THA performed using posterior approach.

Physical Examination. The examination should be started with the client standing. A positive Trendelenburg test demonstrates sagging of the pelvis during ipsilateral single stance and indicates pelvic muscle weakness on the side of the affected hip. The nurse should evaluate the client's gait with and without assistive devices. During the early stages of hip disease, an antalgic gait may be evident; the client demonstrates a shortened stance phase and shortened length of stride on the affected extremity. The typical gait with hip disease is a lurching gait, commonly described as a Trendelenburg gait. With disease progression, the abductor muscles function less efficiently, and a tilting of the pelvis away from the affected hip results during the stance phase of the gait. These signs suggest an underlying mechanical problem in the hip.

A gradual loss of motion at the hip results from additional cartilage deterioration. The position of most comfort for the client with hip OA is often one of slight hip flexion, which relieves pressure on the irritated joint capsule. As this position is assumed more and more often, the hip flexors overpower the extensors and a flexion contracture of the joint results. Internal rotation is commonly lost during late stages of hip OA, and external rotation and abduction are often compromised. Because passive ROM often exacerbates disease symptoms, the client may describe pain that radiates into the groin or thigh with extremes of joint motion. Shortening of the affected extremity may also occur because of progressive erosion of the joint's bony anatomy.

Total Joint Class date: _____	SPAT Visit 4-7 Days Pre-Op: ☐ Type & cross if needed Date: _____ ☐ UA ☐ CBC Init.: _____ ☐ Renalytes ☐ EKG per anesthesia guidelines	AM Admit Unit: Baseline P.Ox _____ ☐ T&C 2 units blood ☐ H&H Date/Initial:
OR: Approach: ☐ Anterior ☐ Posterior ☐ Foley inserted (optional) Date/Initial:	PACU: ☐ Portable hip x-ray Date/Initial:	

DATE/SHIFT (each 8h)				DATE/SHIFT (each 8h)				DATE/SHIFT (each 8h)			
PHASE 3 - Operative and 1st 24 hrs; stabilization **Advance to next phase when all outcomes are met. Shaded column indicates length of stay exceeding expectations for this phase. Call Case Mgr. if in this phase > 24hrs.**				**PHASE 4** - Post-op; initial mobilization **Advance to next phase when all outcomes are met. Shaded column indicates length of stay exceeding expectations for this phase. Call Case Mgr. if in this phase > 48 hrs.**				**PHASE 5** - Post-op; initial mobilization **Advance to next phase when all outcomes are met. Shaded column indicates length of stay exceeding expectations for this phase. Call Case Mgr. if in this phase > 48 hrs.**			
Titrate O_2 via P.Ox to 90% or pre-op baseline P.Ox, then d/c; TCDB for first 24h				Titrate O_2 via P.Ox to 90% or pre-op baseline P.Ox, then d/c							
Assessment: Post-op protocol for VS and CMS checks				VS and CMS q4h				VS bid; CMS q shift			
Neurological				Neurological				Neurological			
Sleep/Rest				Sleep/Rest				Sleep/Rest			
Cardiovascular				Cardiovascular				Cardiovascular			
Respiratory				Respiratory				Respiratory			
Gastrointestinal				Gastrointestinal				Gastrointestinal			
Integumentary/Skin Assessment				Integumentary				Integumentary			
Musculoskeletal				Musculoskeletal				Musculoskeletal			
Neurovascular				Neurovascular				Neurovascular			
Psychosocial				Psychosocial				Psychosocial			
Spiritual				Spiritual				Spiritual			
Learning Readiness				Learning Readiness				Learning Readiness			
Pt. perceives pain relief w/meds				Pt. perceives pain relief w/meds				Pt. perceives pain relief w/meds			
Assess pain q2h				? Pain assessment							
Surgical dressing/incision				Surgical dressing/incision				Surgical dressing/incision			
Discontinued IV site				Discontinued IV site				Discontinued IV site			
Current IV site/saline lock				Current IV site/saline lock				Current IV site/saline lock			
IV: D5LR @75cc/h Other IV: _____				IV d/c'd when taking p.o. fluid, p.o. pain meds, antibiotics complete, & no potential for transfusion							
				IV to saline lock if antibiotics not complete, getting IV meds, potential for transfusions exists							
PCA: MS 1mg/h with 1mg q6min demand (or alternative if MS contraindicated)				PCA if still needed; d/c if tolerating p.o. pain meds							
MS 6-10mg IM q3-4h if PCA interrupted and when PCA d/c'd				MS if still needed							
Other analgesic:											
Inapsine .25-.5cc IV q4-6h prn N/V											
Vicodin 1-2 tabs q3-4h prn pain				Vicodin 1-2 tabs q3-4h prn pain				Vicodin 1-2 tabs q3-4h prn pain			
Autologous blood as ordered											
Cefazolin 1gm q8h X 3 doses											
Coumadin or Lovenox per guideline for prevention of DVT (no Toradol, no NSAIDS); daily PT if on Coumadin				Coumadin or Lovenox per guideline for prevention of DVT (no Toradol, no NSAIDS); daily PT if on Coumadin				Coumadin or Lovenox per guideline for prevention of DVT (no Toradol, no NSAIDS); daily PT if on Coumadin			
Advance diet as tolerated to patient's usual diet				Advance diet as tolerated to patient's usual diet				Patient's usual diet			

√- standards met * = significant finding, see Focus Note

ADDRESSOGRAPH

Total Hip Arthroplasty
Clinical Pathway

DATE/SHIFT (each 8h)				DATE/SHIFT (each 8h)				DATE/SHIFT (each 8h)			
PHASE 3				**PHASE 4**				**PHASE 5**			
If Foley inserted in OR, d/c in Phase 3 or 4 per patient need				If Foley inserted in OR, d/c in Phase 3 or 4 per patient need							
If unable to void, straight cath q8hX3											
Prevention of constipation: Pericolace 1 p.o. bid				Prevention of constipation: Pericolace 1 p.o. bid							
Bowel Program - see Phase 4 ?				Laxative at HS prn if no BM during Phase 4							
				AM suppository prn if no BM during Phase 4							
Elevated toilet seat placed in BR											
I&O				d/c I&O when continuous IV d/c'd				d/c I&O when continuous IV d/c'd			
Bed with trapeze				Bed with trapeze				Bed with trapeze			
Pillow between knees				Pillow between knees				Pillow between knees			
Hemovac (optional)				DC when < 30cc/shift							
Dressing intact				Dressing change qd and prn							
				OOB ? chair 3 times daily				OOB ? chair 3 times daily			
Teaching: Pain reporting using a 0-10 scale				Teaching: Pain control				Teaching: Reinforce hip precautions			
Bedpan use				Hip precautions				Reinforce other teaching as needed			
Trapeze use				Use of BSC				Discharge:			
				Use of elevated toilet seat				Print Discharge Order Set for			
Ankle pumps				Bowel program				physician review			
Respiratory hygiene				Print Discharge Order Set for				Written discharge instructions sent			
Post in pt. room "My Daily Goals"				physician review				with patient			
Describe Lovenox injection technique				↵⟋Coumadin ↵⟋ Lovenox Observe self-injection				Reinforce Lovenox injection or Coumadin teaching			
RN Initials:											
Anticipate discharge setting.				Discharge assessment by Case				Transfer to: ↵⟋Home w / OP therapy			
Evaluate insurance for Lovenox. Discuss with physician.				Mgr.; arrange transfer to next level of care				↵⟋Home ↵⟋SNF ↵⟋Nursing Home			
				Order equipment				↵⟋Home with Homecare			
								↵⟋Acute rehabilitation			
Care Management Initials								↵⟋Order services			
P.T. evaluation				Advance Exercises				Progress exercise to pt. tolerance			
Dangle on bedside				Gait training with walker				Instruct on home exercise program			
Begin gentle exercises/ankle pumps				Weight-bearing status				Family training			
				Progress ambulation				Car transfer training			
Chair and ambulate in AM post-surgery	SEE P.T. FLOW RECORD				SEE P.T. FLOW RECORD			Ambulation on uneven levels	SEE P.T. FLOW RECORD		
Instruct on weight-bearing status											
P.T.											
				O.T. Evaluation	SEE O.T. FLOW RECORD			Practice precautions during dressing, toileting, tub/shower transfers with appropriate ADL and DME; recommendations for other equipment	SEE O.T. FLOW RECORD		
				Review THR precautions							
				Review ADL equipment and home DME (bathing, showering)							
O.T.											
				Pastoral Care visit							
Chaplain Initials											

RNs: Advance patient to next phase when the following outcomes are met. DC previous orders in PCSS and enter new phase orders when advancing patient to the next level.

Outcomes: Pain controlled ≤ level 3 within 24 hrs of surgery				Outcomes: Verbalizes goals to be met each day				Discharge/Transfer Outcomes:			
								ADLs: I S M			
Tolerates oral fluid without N/V				Has had a BM				Transfer in/out of bed: I S M			
Hemodynamically stable: VS stable, H&H stable				Tolerates usual diet				Transfer toilet: I S M			
				Stable H&H				Transfer car: I S M			
Participates in gentle exercise; OOB to chair				Reaches baseline P.Ox and O$_2$ d/c'd				Stairs #_____: I S M			
								Gait #_____: I S M			
				Relief with p.o. pain med				*Legend:*			
				Temperature <101? for 8 hrs				*I = independent*			
				Void s difficulty; Foley out				*S = supervised*			
				Able to self-inject Lovenox or verbalize appropriate				*M = minimal assist*			
RN Initials				Coumadin use				**Case Manager Initials:**			

Reprinted with permission from Penrose—St. Francis Health Services, Colorado Springs, Colorado.

Radiographic studies should be regularly scheduled to track progression of joint degeneration. Joint space narrowing, loss of articular cartilage, osteophyte and cyst formation, and evidence of subchondral collapse should be evaluated. Radiographic findings were discussed earlier in this chapter.

Conservative Management. General conservative management of OA was discussed earlier in this chapter. A balance of rest and exercise provides relief of discomfort for most clients. To minimize stress across the hip joint, the client may use a cane held in the contralateral hand.

Surgical Management. If conservative measures fail to relieve symptoms or if symptoms interfere significantly with the client's day-to-day life, surgical intervention may be considered. Possible procedures include osteotomy of the femoral neck, hip fusion, and THA. The excision arthroplasty (Girdlestone), which was used for OA treatment before the advent of hip implants, is now mainly used as a salvage procedure for failed THA and not as a primary procedure.

Proximal Femoral Osteotomy. In early hip OA, when joint congruency still exists and motion is relatively normal, a proximal femoral osteotomy realigns the femoral neck and redistributes mechanical stress across less worn areas of the femoral head. The younger client, the heavier client, or the client who is inappropriate for arthroplasty because of activities or lifestyle may be a perfect candidate for osteotomy. A wedge of bone is removed from the proximal femur, typically in the area of the lesser trochanter, to realign the angle of the femoral neck relative to the femoral shaft. Fixation is accomplished with a plate and screws to allow healing at the osteotomy site. To facilitate healing at this high-stress region of the femur, the client generally remains on crutches with only partial weight bearing for at least 3 months.

Proximal femoral osteotomy is successful in the vast majority of cases. A successful procedure allows more vigorous activities with fewer restrictions than TJA and thus remains an attractive alternative for the younger, more active client. Because OA symptoms continue to progress gradually, up to 75% of clients need additional surgery, such as joint arthroplasty within 10 years of the osteotomy.

Hip Fusion. Fusion of the femoral head to the acetabulum eliminates motion across the hip joint and thus relieves the pain of hip OA. The extremity is fused in a position of approximately 30 degrees of flexion, neutral abduction, or adduction and 5 degrees of external rotation. Increased motion at the knee and in the lumbar spine compensates for loss of flexion through the hip

joint following fusion. Once successful fusion is achieved, the client has no extraneous activity limitations.

Hip fusion is performed by dislocating the hip, stripping all remaining cartilage from the femoral head and acetabulum, reducing the hip joint, and then maintaining its position with a variety of internal fixation devices to allow bone fusion to occur. Further immobilization in a body cast (spica) is required in most cases during the healing process (see Chapter 12 for a complete discussion of nursing management for the casted client). Despite aggressive internal fixation methods and postoperative use of a spica cast, fusion failure may occur in up to 50% of clients and necessitate repeat surgery.

Because hip fusion results in shortening of the affected extremity by 1 to 1.5 inches (2.5 to 4 cm), the client must be informed preoperatively of the need for a shoe lift to minimize disruption in the gait pattern after surgery. Following hip fusion, increased stress on the ipsilateral knee may contribute to development of knee OA over the next 10 to 20 years. Hip fusion also causes additional stress on the lumbar spine, which may result in increasing low-back pain as the client ages. Considerations such as these may require the client and surgeon to consider a reconversion of the hip fusion to a THA. Arthroplasty restores hip motion and can also significantly decrease back and knee pain.

Although there are obvious disadvantages to hip fusion, the procedure remains a viable surgical option for the young client with advanced unilateral hip OA. The young client often leads a vigorous, active life through work and recreational activities, and hip fusion allows a return to a more normal lifestyle than does THA.

Total Hip Arthroplasty. Charnley pioneered artificial replacement of the hip joint in the late 1960s, using a stainless steel femoral component and a polyethylene socket fixed to the surrounding bone with a plastic cement (polymethyl methacrylate [PMMA]). In the United States today, more than 200,000 THAs are performed annually. More than 1 million arthroplasties are believed to exist throughout the world, making the procedure one of the most common implant operations performed. THA is performed by resecting the femoral head and neck and then preparing the acetabulum with reamers to create a hemispheric surface onto which the acetabular prosthesis is fixed.

Cemented and noncemented arthroplasties. The use of PMMA bone cement allows immediate fixation of the femoral and acetabular components in THA. Cemented components are typically used for the older client or the client who has compromised bone strength because of osteoporosis or other conditions (Fig. 16–5A). Cemented THAs loosen at a rate of approximately 1% per year, generally resulting from failure of the PMMA bone cement. This failure can be hastened in a heavier client or

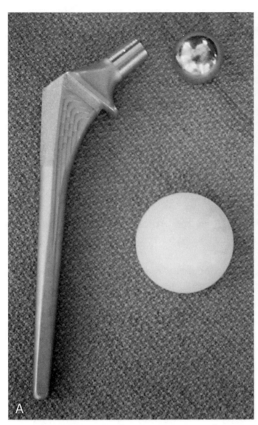

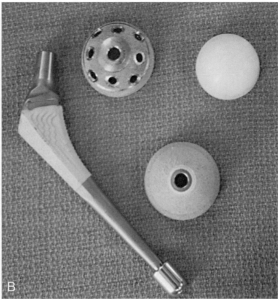

FIGURE 16–5. *A,* Coated femoral head and all-polyethylene acetabular cup for cemented THA. *B,* Porous femoral stem and two types of acetabular components with femoral head for cementless THA.

a younger, more active client. For the younger client, noncemented components may therefore be indicated (Fig. 16–5*B*). Use of a prosthesis with porous surfaces allows bony ingrowth into the implant itself and may provide better long-term outcomes.

Surgical technique. Although a number of vendors have developed THA components, a common three-part set includes the femoral neck and stem, a slide-on femoral head, and a metal acetabulum with or without fixation screw holes. Hip prostheses may be constructed of several different metal alloys that determine their relative lightness and durability.

Depending on physician preference and the type of exposure required for the procedure, the surgical approach for THA may be anterolateral, direct lateral, transtrochanteric, or posterolateral. The nurse must know the surgical approach to understand the position used to dislocate the operative hip. If that position is replicated postoperatively, the client's risk for hip dislocation increases. With an anterolateral position, the client lies supine on the table and the operative hip is externally rotated and extended with the knee flexed. With the posterolateral position, the client lies on his or her side with the operative hip flexed, adducted, and internally rotated. Many surgeons use the posterolateral position for either the anterior or posterior approach.

After the hip has been exposed through an incision of approximately 10 inches in length, an osteotomy of the

femoral neck is performed to expose the acetabulum. To prepare the acetabulum for reaming and for fitting with the prosthesis, the surgeon removes osteophytes and cysts. Trial prostheses are placed and their fit evaluated before the surgeon makes a final choice of appropriately sized components. If the prosthesis will be press-fit (noncemented), the bone is prepared for pegs or spikes. The surgeon presses the cup firmly into place, evaluating its apposition to the bone. If a cemented prosthesis is to be used, the surgeon drills anchor holes into the iliac subchondral bone. After cleaning the bone thoroughly with a pressure-pulsed lavage, the surgeon cements the acetabular cup into position.

In preparing the femur, the surgeon reams the bone's intramedullary canal to form a tunnel. A trial prosthesis is placed and the hip is reduced to assess for motion, stability, and length. If results are acceptable, trial components are removed. For the press-fit prosthesis, the surgeon presses the femoral stem into the reamed intramedullary canal. For a cemented prosthesis, the femur is cleansed and the canal plugged to keep the cement from traveling too far distally. The surgeon fills the canal with cement, inserts the femoral stem, and then places the femoral head. After reducing the hip, the surgeon performs a final evaluation for motion, stability, and length.

Before closure, the surgeon may place a closed wound drainage system, such as a Hemovac. Drainage systems have been used historically because of the belief that they prevented development of hematomas, which appeared to negatively affect wound healing and increased the risk for infection. However, use of wound drainage systems has recently decreased because research has demonstrated their ineffectiveness in preventing hematoma formation. Results indicate that drain usage may actually lead to increased blood loss and wound contamination (see the evidence-based practice table that follows).

Revision total hip arthroplasty. Before initial arthroplasty, the surgeon should discuss the possibility of prosthetic loosening with the client. All mechanical components have a limited life span, but awareness of the possibility of implant failure does not prepare the client for the course of revision surgery. Surgical time may be considerably longer and blood loss greater with revision surgery than with the primary arthroplasty. Comfort, gait, and ROM may not be as good as after the initial arthroplasty. However, failure of the first procedure means that revision may be better than the primary result.

Assessment of the candidate for revision surgery includes a thorough evaluation of pain and joint function. For example, constant deep pain that is aggravated by weight bearing suggests infection. Pain secondary to

loosening is quite similar but more likely to be relieved by rest than pain resulting from infection. Pain experienced in the groin is probably due to a loose socket, and pain in the upper thigh or midthigh is attributable to a loose femoral component. Physical examination also helps determine the cause of failure. The push-pull test (alternately pushing and then pulling on the extremity in a longitudinal direction with the hip in full extension) may be helpful in evaluating for loose components. Pain with this maneuver suggests a loose prosthesis. Pain with passive internal rotation also implies loosening of femoral components. Laboratory analysis is typically indicated to distinguish septic from aseptic loosening; tests include ESR, C-reactive protein, WBC count, and differential. If infection is suspected, joint aspirate is analyzed for cell count and a culture performed. Staphylococci are the most common infecting organisms, but infection with anaerobic organisms is also possible. Radiographic studies also help determine the cause of increased pain or decreased function.

Indications for revision THA include fracture of the femoral shaft, repeated dislocation (Fig. 16-6A), hardware failure (Fig. 16-6B), infection, incorrect placement of

EXAMINING THE EVIDENCE: Moving Toward Evidence-Based Practice
Studies of Closed-Suction Drainage after Total Joint Arthroplasty

AUTHOR(S), YEAR	SAMPLE SIZE	DESIGN	OUTCOME VARIABLES	MAJOR FINDINGS
Ritter, Keating, & Faris, 1994	N = 415 TKA and THA	Random assignment Group I: closed wound drainage system Group II: no postoperative drainage	Postoperative drainage that required cessation of ROM exercises, amount of transfused blood, preoperative and postoperative hemoglobin levels, ROM for TKA clients	No significant difference between groups on all variables
Holt et al., 1997	N = 136 TKA	Random assignment Group I: closed-suction, non-reinfusable wound drains Group II: undrained wound	Blood loss, blood transfusion requirements, postoperative pain, postoperative swelling, number of dressing reinforcements required, ecchymosis, ROM, time to active straight leg raises, length of stay, hospital costs, incidence of complications	No significant difference in blood loss, transfusion requirements, pain, swelling, ROM, time to active straight leg raises, length of stay, hospital costs, incidence of complications 40% of dressings in undrained group required reinforcement; no dressings in drained group required reinforcement ($p < .001$) 39% of drained group developed ecchymosis, compared with 69% of undrained group ($p < .001$)
Adalberth et al., 1998	N = 90 TKA	Random assignment Group I: no drain Group II: autotransfusion system Group III: standard disposable closed-suction drainage system	Hemoglobin/hematocrit values, drainage volumes, homologous/autologous transfusions, ROM, knee swelling, length of stay Parameters recorded preoperatively, days 0–8, and 4 months postoperatively	No significant difference among groups on all variables
Crevoisier, Reber, & Noesberger, 1998	N = 98 TKA or THA	Random assignment Group I: suction drainage Group II: no wound drainage	Wound healing, severity of hematoma, postoperative transfusion requirement, ROM, length of stay	No significant difference between groups on all variables

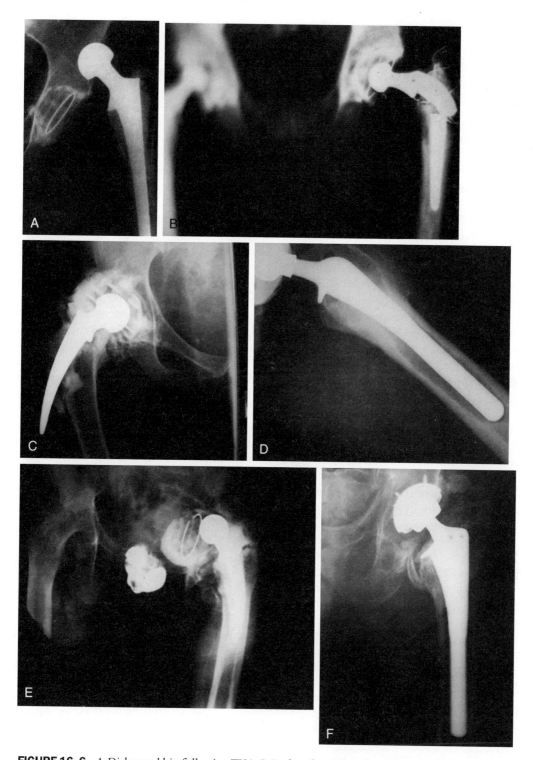

FIGURE 16–6. *A,* Dislocated hip following THA. *B,* Broken femoral component in THA client. *C,* THA demonstrating a femoral stem placed through the lateral cortex of the proximal femur. *D,* Osteolysis around the femoral component of THA. *E,* Protrusion of the acetabular cup through the pelvis of a patient following THA. *F,* Heterotropic bone formation around the hip joint after THA.

prosthesis (Fig. 16–6C), osteolysis (Fig. 16–6D), acetabular protrusion (Fig. 16–6E), heterotrophic bone formation (Fig. 16–6F), and loosening (Fig. 16–7). With the increased use of press-fit components and improved tech-

niques for cement insertion, loosening now occurs less commonly following THA.

When revision surgery is first considered, the surgeon makes plans to revise the acetabular component or the

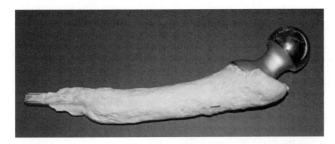

FIGURE 16–7. A femoral component that had loosened and was easily removed during revision arthroplasty. Because cement still adheres to the femoral stem, it appears that loosening occurred at the bone-cement interface.

femoral component or both. Final determination of involved components cannot be made until the hip is opened and each area is assessed. Gross loosening of components typically occurs at the bone-cement interface and is quite obvious at the time of revision. If cemented components are being revised, both cement and hardware must be removed. More recently, revision prostheses have been designed to achieve bony ingrowth fixation rather than cemented fixation.

Nursing Management during Postoperative Period. Acute postoperative care focuses on managing pain, assessing neurovascular status in both lower extremities, monitoring fluid balance and vital signs, assessing dressings and drains for excessive output, directing the client in performance of pulmonary hygiene, encouraging leg exercises while the client is awake, changing position every 1 to 2 hours, following hip precautions to avoid dislocation, and initiating physical therapy. Use of a clinical pathway (see the THA Clinical Pathway) provides coordinated care from a multidisciplinary approach. The pathway should have been initiated when the client decided to have surgery, continued through preoperative education, and used postoperatively to ensure appropriate use of rehabilitation services. Including client goals (Box 16–3) in the pathway encourages a more collaborative approach to postoperative care.

Pain (Acute): Related to Surgery

Pain Management, Analgesia. Although a short period of acute postoperative pain is expected, the client often describes actual relief of pain compared with his or her preoperative experience with arthritis. Opioid analgesics are delivered via various modalities, including patient-controlled analgesia (PCA) and epidural analgesia, for the first 24 to 72 hours after surgery. Oral opioids, sometimes in combination with NSAIDs, are ordered as the client tolerates fluids intake. (See Chapter 5 for discussion of pain management considerations and Chapter 2 for coping.)

Impaired Physical Mobility: Related to Postoperative Pain or Fear of Movement

---

Mobility and Activity Patterns. The client's degree of mobility impairment following THA may be affected by pain and fear of movement, as well as by arthritic limitations in other joints. The nurse must first address pain management needs and then be aware of any weight-bearing limitations ordered for the client. Following use of cemented components, the client is often allowed to bear as much weight as desired on the operative extremity. The surgeon writes the activity order as weight bearing as tolerated (WBAT) or full weight bearing (FWB). Although incisional pain may inhibit movement, the client can safely direct weight through the operative leg without affecting placement of the prosthesis. If the client is not allowed to bear weight (non–weight bearing [NWB]), the nurse must carefully monitor the operative leg during transfers and ambulation to ensure adherence to activity orders. Appropriate staff assistance and instruction in the use of walker or crutches will help the client gain confidence. Scheduled physical therapy for exercise and mobility training also are invaluable as the client seeks independence.

In addition to postoperative limitations, the client may have arthritis pain in other joints, affecting his or her ability to use a walker or crutches to transfer from bed to chair or to ambulate. If the client is unable to lift a conventional walker because of arthritis in the hands, elbows, or shoulders, for example, a platform or wheeled walker may be needed. The nurse must consistently address sources of chronic pain to enable the client to participate fully in postoperative recovery.

Risk for Peripheral Neurovascular Dysfunction: Related to Pressure or Swelling

---

Assessment of Neurovascular Status. Any orthopaedic surgery carries a risk for neurologic or vascular impairment. The nurse should be aware of the potential for compartment syndrome or nerve injury related to edema or extremity positioning. Commonly affected nerves include the sciatic, femoral, obturator, and peroneal nerves. The client experiences persistent pain and, with sciatic nerve injury, motor weakness. Vascular complications are relatively rare with THA and more likely to be found after revision surgery because of difficult dissection procedures.

The nurse should assess neurovascular status of the operative extremity at least every 4 hours or more frequently as directed by the surgeon or indicated by client condition. Findings must be compared with the nonoperative extremity. Assessment includes the presence and quality of bilateral pedal pulses, skin color and temperature, capillary refill of the toes, sensation and movement of the toes, and the client's ability to perform dorsoplantar flexion of the foot. Any pallor or coolness, numbness or tingling, or decreased ability to move the extremity must be reported immediately to the surgeon.

Risk for Injury: Related to Prosthesis Dislocation

Education: Avoiding Extreme Positions. Because the hip remains unstable until the surrounding soft tissue is healed, the client must be taught to avoid positions that would increase the risk for prosthesis dislocation. Following THA, the nurse or physical therapist can remind the client of appropriate precautions by using instructional handouts or fliers that can be posted near the bed (see Fig. 16-4*A* and *B*). Performance of exercises such as gluteal isometrics also strengthens the muscles that surround the joint capsule and decreases the risk of dislocation.

Postoperative positioning depends on the surgical approach. If the surgeon used a posterolateral approach, the client must not flex the hip beyond a 90-degree angle. He or she should not bend at the waist, for example, to lace or slip on shoes. The client should also not reach for linens that are fan-folded at the bottom of the bed or chair. In addition to flexion limits, the client should not cross the operative leg past the body's midline (adduction) and should not inwardly rotate the replaced hip. To maintain these precautions, the client should be coached to point the toes on the operative leg outward slightly when ambulating.

BOX 16–3.

My Daily Goals: Total Hip Replacement

Day of Surgery	Day 1	Day 2	Day 3	Day 4
Begin gentle exercises with physical therapy and/or stand at the bedside	Begin additional exercises Start gait training with a walker Up in a chair	Walk with the walker Up in a chair three times Increase "range of motion"	Able to move in and out of bed Able to transfer on/off toilet Able to use mobility equipment	Able to do car transfers Able to climb stairs Able to dress my lower body
Tolerating oral fluids without nausea	Make progress with food intake	Eating my usual diet Have a bowel movement		
Pain relief/control		If a urinary catheter has been removed, able to urinate without difficulty	Continue to walk and sit in a chair several times a day	Transfer out of acute care to: Home with family help Home with home care physical therapy visits Acute rehabilitation Nursing home/skilled nursing facility Other
Learn about the following: Reporting pain to the nurse How to use the bedpan How to use the trapeze Why the head of my bed is rolled up How to do ankle pumps How to breathe deeply and cough	Learn about the following: Pain control Hip precautions Use of the bedside commode Use of the elevated toilet seat Nurse will describe home Lovenox injection (shot) or warfarin pill for blood anticoagulation	Learn about the following: More about hip precautions Equipment to be used at home for dressing, bathing, toileting, etc. How to give myself a Lovenox injection (shot) or how to take the warfarin pill correctly	Learn about the following: More about hip precautions How to give myself a Lovenox injection (shot) or how to take the warfarin pill correctly	Learn about the following: Discharge instructions Prescription for Lovenox or warfarin

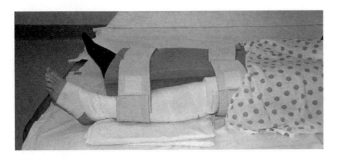

FIGURE 16–8. Abductor wedge assists client in maintaining correct position following THA performed by posterior approach.

After surgery with a posterolateral approach, the client's leg should be maintained in external rotation, abduction, and hip extension. Use of a triangular abductor pillow or wedge between the client's legs helps maintain position (Fig. 16–8). When placing the wedge, the nurse must ensure that the straps do not place pressure on the client's peroneal nerve. Balanced suspension or traction may also be used to keep the leg in abduction. If the client's leg is especially weak, placement of a trochanter roll will help align the extremity. In addition, an occupational therapist may suggest several assistive devices to allow the client more independence in self-care while still maintaining appropriate precautions. A long-handled shoehorn, sock donner, and reachers help the client avoid extremes of hip flexion. To further avoid extremes of flexion, the client needs an elevated toilet seat (at least 21 inches high) and a shower bench or chair.

Precautions following an anterolateral surgical approach are nearly opposite those used after the posterolateral approach. For example, the client is able to sit upright at 90 degrees after THA with an anterolateral approach. The client should avoid active abduction, maintaining the legs side-by-side without a wedge or pillow between them. With walker use, the client should be reminded to avoid turning the toes and knee outward. The operative leg should also not be extended backward. The nurse can help the client maintain anterolateral precautions by placing the tray table and phone on the operative side.

Risk for Altered Tissue Perfusion: Related to Surgical Procedure and Immobility

Assessment of Neurovascular Function, Administration of Blood Transfusion. Venous thromboembolism, the most common complication after THA, can present as either DVT or pulmonary embolism (PE). The incidence of DVT in THA clients not receiving prophylaxis may be as high as 57% (Brander et al., 2000). To decrease the risk of emboli formation, the health care team uses a variety of interventions. Early ambulation is critical to clot prevention. In addition, flexion/extension exercises of the ankles (ankle pumps) cause muscle

contractions in the calves and assist in venous blood return to the heart. Elastic antiembolism stockings (TEDS) may also be used, alone or in combination with pneumatic compression devices. Stockings or pneumatic compression devices must be worn whenever the client is in bed or in a chair until he or she is fully ambulatory and removed only for brief periods to allow for bathing and skin assessment.

A prophylactic anticoagulant such as low-dose heparin, warfarin, aspirin, or LMWH is typically initiated 12 to 24 hours after surgery. The client who receives warfarin typically is given a 7.5- to 10-mg loading dose, followed by daily dosing based on prothrombin times. Efficacy of low-dose heparin is determined through the partial thromboplastin time. Both medications are continued until the surgeon determines that client mobility has improved sufficiently to minimize the risk for venous thromboembolism. LMWH, on the other hand, requires no laboratory monitoring and typically is administered for only 10 to 14 days after surgery. Occasionally, the surgeon may choose to initiate both warfarin and LMWH on the evening following surgery. LMWH works quickly to anticoagulate the client and, in this case, is discontinued when the client leaves the hospital. Warfarin, which is slower to reach therapeutic levels in the blood, is less expensive and easier for the client to use after discharge than LMWH.

Client education about anticoagulants is critical to their successful use. The nurse should inform the client of signs of internal bleeding such as abdominal or flank pain, coughing up or vomiting blood, rust- or tea-colored urine, and tarry stools. The client also must understand that even a minor cut will bleed for a longer time and must be instructed to apply direct pressure following a shaving cut or nick with a kitchen knife. The nurse must stress the need for the client to seek immediate evaluation of any head injury because of the risk of intracranial bleeding. For the client taking warfarin, the nurse should reinforce the need for consistent intake of foods that contain vitamin K (e.g., green leafy vegetables). Many of these foods are an important part of a nutritionally sound diet and should not be eliminated, particularly by the client who also follows a low-fat diet. If the client is being discharged with a prescription for LMWH, instruction on injection technique should be started early enough in the hospitalization to allow sufficient time for practice and reinforcement.

Blood administration during or after THA may be indicated. Because joint arthroplasty is an elective procedure, autologous blood transfusions or blood salvage procedures may easily be accomplished (see Chapter 10). Serial hematocrits may be performed for several days after surgery to monitor the client's response to blood loss and to determine the need for transfusion. Because surgical time and accompanying blood loss have continued to decrease, many surgeons no longer routinely ask the client to provide autologous blood preoperatively.

Instead, they recommend iron supplementation before and after surgery to ensure a normal hemoglobin and hematocrit.

Risk for Infection: Related to Surgical Procedure or Prosthesis

Observation, Prophylactic Antibiotics. Following THA, the possibility of infection is a great concern. Joint infection can lead to osteomyelitis or to possible surgical failure that necessitates the removal of prosthetic components. Incidence is fortunately low, at 1% or less (Roberts & Lappe, 2001); however, careful monitoring is still required to keep the rate of infection to a minimum. The thin client, who has poor soft tissue coverage over the hip components, is more prone to infection than the heavier client. The client who has undergone revision THA is also at increased risk for infection because of the longer surgical exposure and operative time.

Because poor dentition is a potential source of bacteria, the client should be encouraged to achieve and maintain good oral hygiene preoperatively. Prophylactic antibiotics are routinely administered to the THA client, with the first dose given shortly before the incision is made. Dosing continues for 2 to 3 days postoperatively. If a surgical drain has been inserted to remove wound exudate, it should be emptied at least once a shift using aseptic technique. Because wound drainage can harbor pathogens, the nurse should assess its color and odor and promptly report any abnormalities to the surgeon. Routine assessment of the surgical site for redness or purulent drainage is also essential. Use of staples for wound closure has been associated with a lower deep infection rate, but delays in healing can indicate a superficial infection. Dressing changes must be accomplished using strict aseptic technique. The client's temperature must also be taken at regular intervals and a careful assessment done to identify the cause of any elevation.

After superficial wound healing has occurred, the presence of increasing joint pain may indicate a delayed, deep infection. As the client prepares for hospital discharge, the nurse should ensure that he or she understands the significance of increasing pain and of the need to report its occurrence promptly to the surgeon. In addition, the client should be reminded to discuss the possible use of prophylactic antibiotics for future surgical procedures that can cause a transient bacteremia.

Altered Nutrition (Greater Than Body Requirements): Related to Need for Weight Maintenance

Education. One contributor to the success of THA is the client's ability to maintain normal weight. If calorie reduction and weight loss are indicated, the client should be instructed to initiate diet changes 3 to 4 weeks postoperatively on the surgeon's advice. Before that time, the client should not attempt to decrease calories but should instead focus on maintaining a high carbohydrate and high protein intake that is critical to wound healing.

Self-care Deficit: Related to Limitations Following Surgery

Assistance with Care Needs. The THA client is generally hospitalized for 4 to 5 days after surgery. Although additional services may be needed in a rehabilitation hospital, skilled nursing facility, or extended care setting, the client may still be discharged with self-care deficits. If hip precautions preclude the client from performing foot care, referral to a podiatrist may be indicated. An available family member may alternatively be able to perform foot and nail care. Although a family member can also help the client to put on socks and shoes, use of an assistive device, such as a sock donner or long-handled shoehorn, will allow the client to maintain more independence in self-care. The client is typically able to shower but may need a bench or handbars for safety. Tub baths are not recommended because of the difficulty of getting in and out of the tub. In addition, the healing incision should not be wet for an extended period.

Osteoarthritis of the Knee

After the spine and hip, the knee is the third most common site of OA involvement. The knee is an extremely complex joint that actually demonstrates movement in three separate planes: flexion/extension, abduction/adduction, and internal/external rotation. During normal walking, a force of about three times the client's body weight is transmitted through the knee. Force is unevenly distributed, with a large amount transmitted to the medial side of the knee. Going up and down stairs increases the force transmitted through the knee to approximately four to five times body weight (Roberts & Lappe, 2001).

History. The client most often complains of pain with accompanying stiffness. The nurse evaluates the degree of pain and the extent of any related functional disability. History of any injury is important as a possible precipitating factor in the appearance or increase of pain. The nurse should also ask if the client has experienced an increase in activity level that may precipitate symptoms. A history of locking, catching, or joint effusion may indicate internal derangement in addition to OA.

Physical Examination. With the client standing, the nurse should grossly evaluate leg alignment. A valgus deformity (knock-knee) indicates destruction of the lateral knee compartment (Fig. 16–9, *left*), and a varus deformity (bowleg) indicates pathology in the medial knee compartment (Fig. 16–9, *right*). Disease in either compartment may affect a femoral condyle, a tibial plateau, and the articulating segment of the patella. After evaluating

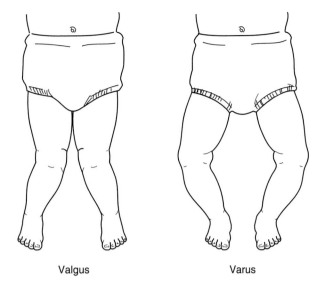

Valgus   Varus

FIGURE 16–9. Valgus and varus deformities that may result from compartmentalized osteoarthritis.

alignment, the nurse can assess gait by asking the client to walk across the room. The presence of limping, lateral joint thrust, shortened stride, or fixed flexion deformity should be noted.

With the client on the examination table, the knee joint can be evaluated for ROM and measurement of the Q angle. Palpation may detect the presence of effusions, tenderness, cysts, and osteophytes. Radiographic evaluation is an essential diagnostic step in determining the appropriate therapeutic regimen for the client.

Conservative Management. Knee OA appears to be better tolerated than hip disease because the knee is not usually painful at rest. Conservative treatment is similar to that for hip OA. Weight loss, activity modification, use of assistive devices, and use of analgesics or anti-inflammatory medications may help decrease disease symptoms. Use of topical capsaicin cream has also provided transient relief from the pain of knee OA. In addition, physical modalities such as heat or ice may be useful for pain treatment. Use of a shoe wedge may be a simple intervention that affects joint pain by changing the load distribution on the knee with weight bearing.

Surgical Management. Surgery may be an appropriate intervention if conservative measures no longer control the client's symptoms. Alternatives include autogenous cartilage implantation, osteotomy, fusion, and TKA.

General preoperative evaluation was reviewed earlier in this chapter. In addition to assessing pain and functional disability, the surgeon determines current knee ROM as a guide for the surgical approach. Use of a clinical pathway guides care of the TKA client beginning with the preoperative evaluation (see the TKA Clinical Pathway).

Autologous Cartilage Implantation. Although not indicated for all clients with knee OA, autologous cartilage implantation has shown encouraging results for treatment in the client with normal knee alignment and no evidence of ligamentous instability or of arthritis on the corresponding tibial surface. An autogenous cartilage biopsy specimen of approximately 200 to 300 mg of articular cartilage is obtained arthroscopically. The specimen is then enzymatically digested, and the chondrocytes are cultured in the laboratory. Autologous cartilage implantation techniques currently require arthrotomy of the knee joint to expose the lesion. At the time of surgery, the focal area of arthritis on the femoral condyle or trochlear groove is debrided to a rim of normal healthy cartilage and a template is made of the defect. The template is then used to obtain a periosteal graft, usually from the proximal tibia. The graft is sutured to the ends of the articular cartilage defect. After verification of a watertight seal, the suture repair is reinforced with autogenous or commercially prepared fibrin glue and the cultured chondrocytes are injected under the periosteal graft.

Postoperatively, the client is required to pursue a specific rehabilitation program and is generally allowed to return to full activities 1 year after surgery. In the United States, 2-year outcome studies have revealed significant improvement in client function and symptoms compared with the preoperative condition. The incidence of failure is 5.8% after 2 years (LaPrade & Swiontkowski, 1999).

Osteotomy. Early to intermediate stages of knee OA typically involve one side of the joint more than the other. Normally, the knee exhibits 7 degrees of valgus alignment. A varus deformity results from a wear process in the medial aspect of the joint, which is the compartment that is affected most often. Progression of disease leads to loss of the normal valgus alignment and causes increased stress on the medial knee compartment. During early disease, medial OA can be managed by performing a proximal tibial osteotomy. Osteotomy is particularly indicated for the young, active, or heavy client who has OA confined to the medial compartment. The procedure has a high degree of success in relieving knee pain. Because about 50% of clients experience recurrence of joint symptoms within 10 years, however, the procedure is generally considered a precursor for knee arthroplasty.

Proximal tibial osteotomy is performed by cutting a laterally based wedge of bone from the proximal tibia and restoring the normal valgus alignment of the knee joint. The first tibial cut is made about 2 cm below the joint line, and a second cut is made at approximately a 10-degree angle to the first for removal of a wedge of

Total Joint Class date: _____	SPAT Visit 4-7 Days Pre-Op: ☐ Type & cross if needed Date: _____ ☐ UA ☐ CBC Init.: _____ ☐ Renalytes ☐ EKG per anesthesia guidelines	AM Admit Unit: Baseline P. Ox_____ ☐ T&C 2 units blood ☐ H&H Date/Initial:
OR: ☐ Foley inserted (optional) Date/Initial:	PACU: Date/Initial:	

PHASE 3 - Operative and 1st 24 hrs; stabilization **Advance to next phase when all outcomes are met. Shaded column indicates length of stay exceeding expectations for this phase. Call Case Mgr. if in this phase > 24hrs.**	DATE/SHIFT (each 8h)			PHASE 4 - Post-op; initial mobilization **Advance to next phase when all outcomes are met. Shaded column indicates length of stay exceeding expectations for this phase. Call Case Mgr. if in this phase > 48 hrs.**	DATE/SHIFT (each 8h)					PHASE 5 - Post-op; initial mobilization **Advance to next phase when all outcomes are met. Shaded column indicates length of stay exceeding expectations for this phase. Call Case Mgr. if in this phase > 48 hrs.**	DATE/SHIFT (each 8h)					
Titrate O_2 via P.Ox to 90% or pre-op baseline P.Ox, then d/c; TCDB for first 24h				Titrate O_2 via P.Ox to 90% or pre-op baseline P.Ox, then d/c												
Assessment: Post-op protocol for VS and CMS checks				VS and CMS q4h						VS bid; CMS q shift						
Neurological				Neurological						Neurological						
Sleep/Rest				Sleep/Rest						Sleep/Rest						
Cardiovascular				Cardiovascular						Cardiovascular						
Respiratory				Respiratory						Respiratory						
Gastrointestinal				Gastrointestinal						Gastrointestinal						
Integumentary/Skin Assessment				Integumentary						Integumentary						
Musculoskeletal				Musculoskeletal						Musculoskeletal						
Neurovascular				Neurovascular						Neurovascular						
Psychosocial				Psychosocial						Psychosocial						
Spiritual				Spiritual						Spiritual						
Learning Readiness				Learning Readiness						Learning Readiness						
Pt. perceives pain relief w/meds				Pt. perceives pain relief w/meds						Pt. perceives pain relief w/meds						
Assess pain q2h				↓ Pain assessment												
Surgical dressing/incision				Surgical dressing/incision						Surgical dressing/incision						
Discontinued IV site				Discontinued IV site						Discontinued IV site						
Current IV site/saline lock				Current IV site/saline lock												
IV: D5LR @75cc/h Other IV: _____				IV d/c'd when taking p.o. fluid, p.o. pain meds, antibiotics complete, no potential for transfusion												
				IV to saline lock if antibiotics not complete, getting IV meds, potential for transfusions exists												
PCA: MS 1mg/h with 1mg q6min demand (or alternative if MS contraindicated)				PCA if still needed; d/c if tolerating p.o. pain meds												
MS 6-10mg IM q3-4h if PCA interrupted and when PCA d/c'd				MS if still needed												
Other analgesic:																
Inapsine .25-.5cc IV q4-6h prn N/V																
Vicodin 1-2 tabs q3-4h prn pain				Vicodin 1-2 tabs q3-4h prn pain						Vicodin 1-2 tabs q3-4h prn pain						
Autologous blood as ordered																
Cefazolin 1gm q8h X 3 doses																
Advance diet as tolerated to patient's usual diet																

√ - standards met   * = significant finding, see Focus Note

ADDRESSOGRAPH

Total Knee Arthroplasty
Clinical Pathway

Box continued on following page

DATE/SHIFT (each 8h)					DATE/SHIFT (each 8h)					DATE/SHIFT (each 8h)				

PHASE 3					PHASE 4					PHASE 5				
If Foley inserted in OR, d/c in Phase 3 or 4					If Foley inserted in OR, d/c in Phase 3 or 4									
If unable to void, straight cath q8hX3														
Prevention of constipation: Pericolace 1 p.o. bid					Prevention of constipation: Pericolace 1 p.o. bid									
Bowel Program - see Phase 4 →					Laxative at HS prn if no BM during Phase 4									
					AM suppository prn if no BM during Phase 4									
Elevated toilet seat place in BR as needed					Elevated toilet seat placed in BR as needed									
I&O					d/c I&O when continuous IV d/c'd					d/c I&O when continuous IV d/c'd				
Bed with trapeze					Bed with trapeze					Bed with trapeze				
CPM as ordered by physician					CPM as ordered by physician					CPM as ordered by physician				
Hemovac (optional)					DC when < 30cc/shift									
Dressing intact					Dressing change qd and prn									
					OOB → chair 3 times daily					OOB → chair 3 times daily				
Teaching: Pain reporting using a 0-10 scale					Teaching: Pain control					Teaching: Reinforce teaching as needed				
Bedpan use					Use of BSC					Discharge:				
Ankle pumps					Use of elevated toilet seat					Print Discharge Order Set for physician review				
Respiratory hygiene					Bowel program					Written discharge instructions sent with patient				
SCD/Flowtron compression to calves					Print Discharge Order Set for physician review									
Post in pt. room "My Daily Goals"														
Describe Lovenox injection technique					⤷Coumadin ⤷ Lovenox Observe self-injection					Reinforce Lovenox injection or Coumadin teaching				
RN Initials:														
Anticipate discharge setting.					Discharge assessment by Case Mgr.; arrange transfer to next level of care					Transfer to: ⤷Home w / OP therapy				
Evaluate insurance for Lovenox. Discuss with physician.										⤷Home ⤷SNF ⤷Nursing Home				
					Order equipment					⤷Home with Homecare				
										⤷Acute rehabilitation				
										⤷Order services				
Care Management Initials														
Inpatient evaluation					Advance Exercises					Progress exercise to pt. tolerance				
Begin gentle exercises/ankle pumps					Gait training with walker					Instruct on home exercise program				
Knee immobilizer		SEE P.T. FLOW RECORD			Weight-bearing status		SEE P.T. FLOW RECORD			Family training		SEE P.T. FLOW RECORD		
CPM as ordered by physician					Progress ambulation					Car transfer training				
Instruct on weight-bearing										Ambulation on uneven levels				
Dangle on bedside														
OOB to chair and ambulate in AM post-surgery														
P.T.														
					O.T. Evaluation		SEE O.T. FLOW RECORD			Practice dressing, toileting, tub/ shower transfers with appropriate ADL and DME; recommendations for other equipment		SEE O.T. FLOW RECORD		
					Review ADL equipment and home DME (bathing, showering)									
O.T.														
Chaplain Initials					Pastoral Care visit									

RNs: Advance patient to next phase when the following outcomes are met. DC previous orders in PCSS and enter new phase orders when advancing patient to the next level.

Outcomes: Pain controlled ≤ level 3 within 24 hrs of surgery				Outcomes: Verbalizes goals to be met each day					Discharge/Transfer Outcomes: ADLs: I S M				
Tolerates oral fluid without N/V				Has had a BM					Transfer in/out of bed: I S M				
Hemodynamically stable: VS stable, H&H stable				Tolerates usual diet					Transfer toilet: I S M				
				Stable H&H					Transfer car: I S M				
Participates in gentle exercise; OOB to chair				Reaches baseline P.Ox and O₂ d/c'd					Stairs #_____: I S M				
				Relief with p.o. pain med					Gait #_____: I S M				
				Temperature <101° for 8 hrs					*Legend:*				
				Void s difficulty; Foley out					*I = independent*				
				Able to self-inject Lovenox or verbalize appropriate					*S = supervised*				
RN Initials				Coumadin use					*M = minimal assist*				
										Case Manager Initials:				

Reprinted with permission from Penrose—St. Francis Health Services, Colorado Springs, Colorado.

bone. During the early stages of healing, the client wears a knee immobilizer or cylinder cast and initially uses crutches or a walker to maintain partial weight bearing. Complications of osteotomy are relatively uncommon but include peroneal palsy, compartment syndrome, and delayed union or nonunion of bone.

A distal femoral osteotomy is performed for treatment of lateral compartment OA in the young, active, or overweight client. A wedge of bone is removed from the distal femur in the supracondylar region, and the bone is fixed in place with screws and a plate. The procedure restores the knee to a more neutral alignment and decreases mechanical stress on the lateral joint. Partial weight bearing is required for several months after surgery to allow healing of the osteotomy site. If internal fixation is successful, use of a knee immobilizer or cast is not necessary. Relief of OA symptoms may last for 5 years after this procedure.

Fusion. Knee fusion results in an immobile joint fixed in extension. The procedure is indicated for the young, active client who is a poor candidate for joint replacement surgery. Fusion also may be performed on the client whose disease is too advanced for osteotomy or on the client who has septic arthritis or severe post-traumatic arthritis.

Knee fusion results in shortening of the extremity by approximately 0.5 inch, which does not usually present a significant dysfunction for the client. A knee fixed in extension may produce minor inconvenience in some situations, but no severe restrictions in activity are required after successful knee fusion. This procedure has an exceedingly high long-term success rate in relieving knee pain. Although it is technically possible to convert a fused knee to a total arthroplasty, this action is generally discouraged because knee function is often less than optimal.

In the performance of knee fusion, the surfaces of the distal femur and proximal tibia are trimmed to provide flat surfaces across which fusion can occur. The affected extremity is generally immobilized, either with external clamps attached to pins inserted through the proximal tibia and distal femur or with a variety of internal fixation devices. Knee fusion typically requires 3 months or more of postoperative immobilization, and the client must maintain partial weight bearing with the use of an assistive device until successful fusion has occurred.

Total Knee Arthroplasty. For clients 65 years and older who no longer receive benefit from conservative arthritis management, the procedure of choice is resurfacing of the affected joint with metal-on-plastic prosthetic components. The goal of TKA is to recreate the motions of flexion, extension, abduction, adduction, and rotation that may have been lost with progressive osteoarthritic joint changes. TKA also relieves pain and corrects joint deformity. The 10-year success rate for the procedure is 98%.

Indications and contraindications. A client younger than 65 years of age who weighs more than 200 pounds or is exceedingly active is probably better served by other alternatives. Recently, however, the success of traditional TKA has steadily extended the indications for this procedure to younger age groups. Presence of diabetes mellitus or peripheral vascular disease increases the client's risk for infection and delayed wound healing. Other contraindications are similar to those for THA.

Surgical procedure. Knee prosthetics most commonly have three components: the femoral component, the tibial plate, and the patellar button (Fig. 16–10*A*

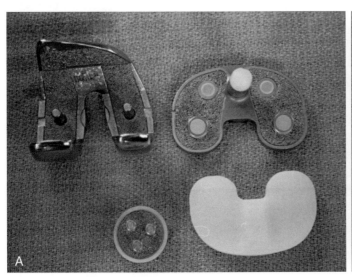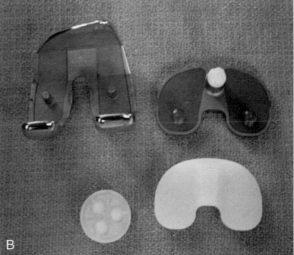

FIGURE 16–10. *A,* Prostheses designed for cementless TKA and bony ingrowth fixation. *B,* Components for cemented TKA.

and *B*). These tricompartmental prostheses come in various sizes to ensure the most accurate fit for each client. Some parts may be specific to the right or the left knee. A unicompartmental prosthesis is rarely used; it replaces the femoral and tibial surfaces on only one side of the knee.

The surgical incision for TKR extends from 4 or 5 inches above the patella to 2 or 3 inches below it. The standard approach is either medial parapatellar or lateral parapatellar. Soft tissue is balanced across the joint to correct any existing flexion contractures. The proximal tibia and distal femur are trimmed to fit the chosen prosthesis. After osteotomy, the bone surfaces are prepared to accept the prosthesis based on the choice of cemented or press-fit (noncemented) components. The patella is resurfaced with a polyethylene button after the surgeon ensures that the patellar prosthesis tracks normally during knee flexion and extension. Wound drains may be placed before closure of the incision. A bulky pressure dressing is applied unless the client is to start continuous passive motion (CPM) immediately, in which case a lighter dressing is used.

Bilateral arthroplasty. The client with severe OA in both knees may be a candidate for bilateral TKA (Fig. 16–11*A* and *B*). Performance of arthroplasty on only one knee would unnecessarily stress the other knee. The bilateral procedure allows even, partial weight bearing on each extremity.

Hemiarthroplasty. If OA is limited to either the medial or lateral knee compartment, hemiarthroplasty may be indicated. Many surgeons consider hemiarthroplasty an alternative to osteotomy for the client with knee OA. Like TKA, the procedure also uses a metal resurfacing of the femur articulating with a polyethylene tibial insert. Results are clearly better in the client who weighs less than 180 pounds and has a relatively sedentary lifestyle. Recovery is generally quicker than from either osteotomy

or TKA, and hemiarthroplasty does allow conversion to TKA if necessary in the future. Because the success rate of hemiarthroplasty is greater than 95% after 5 years, this procedure can be considered as an alternative to TKA when a less radical form of arthroplasty is appropriate for a client.

Revision. As with any joint replacement, the knee may require revision. One indication for total knee revision is prosthesis failure (Fig. 16–12). Other indications include mechanical failure of the interface, failure of the initial fixation, instability, and stiffness with decreased ROM.

Nursing Management during Postoperative Period. With the exception of differences in mobility management and of a lessened chance for dislocation, management of the client following TKA is similar to that following THA. Nursing diagnoses of pain, risk for altered tissue perfusion, risk for infection, and altered nutrition are managed in the same way as for THA.

Impaired Mobility: Related to Surgical Implant

Mobility and Activity Pattern. When there is not excessive postoperative bleeding, the client may begin immediate CPM using a machine that gently flexes and extends the knee through an ordered ROM (Fig. 16–13). CPM has been believed to minimize the risk of postoperative stiffness and enhance remobilization of the joint after TKA, but additional research provides mixed results and has led many surgeons to forego this intervention (see the evidence-based practice table that follows).

When it is used, the CPM apparatus may be applied in the postanesthesia care unit or on the inpatient unit in the first 24 hours after surgery. It moves the knee slowly through an arc of motion. Resistance to motion by muscle guarding interrupts the cycle. ROM, speed, and

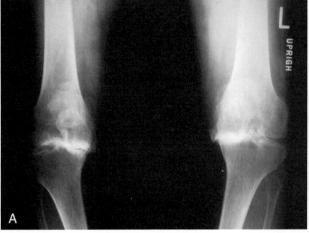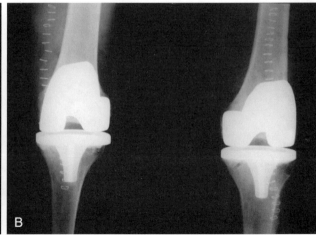

FIGURE 16–11. *A,* Advanced bilateral knee arthritis. *B,* Postoperative x-ray film demonstrates placement of bilateral knee prostheses on same client.

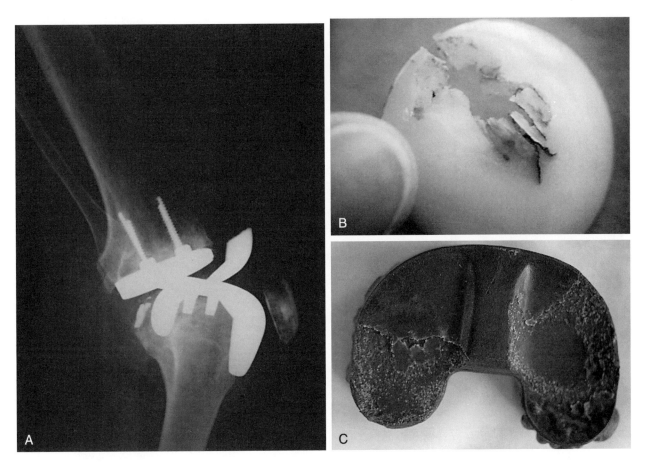

FIGURE 16–12. *A,* X-ray evaluation of TKA shows broken, rotated femoral component anterior to knee. *B,* Deterioration of tibial component was not evident until its removal at the time of revision knee arthroplasty. *C,* Destruction of the patellar component progressed from anterior to the back of the component, wearing completely through the polyethylene.

resistance are adjustable. Settings vary according to physician preference, but a common regimen allows the client to begin at 0 degrees of extension and 35 to 40 degrees of flexion. ROM is gradually increased, with a goal of 90 degrees of flexion. To maximize the benefit of therapy, CPM should be used a minimum of 6 to 8 hours daily. Longer use can be based on client tolerance or desire and surgeon orders.

The CPM apparatus is placed on the bed in a slightly abducted position. The femur bar is adjusted based on the length from the client's greater trochanter to the axis of knee motion. The axis may be marked to facilitate proper positioning in the machine. (For a complete discussion of CPM, see Chapter 13.) When the client is not undergoing CPM, the surgeon may order application of a knee immobilizer to keep the leg in extension. A pillow may be placed under the foot for comfort.

Because some surgeons do not order CPM, a postoperative regimen of regular exercise for muscle strengthening and ROM is essential for a successful outcome for the client. ROM exercises may be followed by prolonged stretching to increase knee flexion or extension. Exercises to strengthen the quadriceps, hamstrings, and gluteal

muscles are also initiated. These consist of isometrics and bilateral straight leg raises. Active knee extension is encouraged to prevent flexion contracture. Home exercises may be ordered, to include active-assisted ROM and mild isometric quadriceps strengthening. To obtain optimal knee function, the client should continue the exercise program for at least 6 weeks postoperatively.

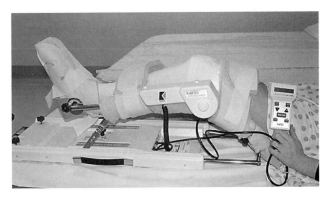

FIGURE 16–13. Continuous passive motion (CPM) machine assists TKA client in achieving increased ROM.

EXAMINING THE EVIDENCE: Moving Toward Evidence-Based Practice
Studies of Continuous Passive Motion (CPM) after Total Knee Arthroplasty

AUTHOR(S), YEAR	SAMPLE SIZE	DESIGN	OUTCOME VARIABLES	MAJOR FINDINGS
McInnes et al., 1992	$N = 102$	Random assignment Group I: CPM within 24 hours of surgery, ROM increased as tolerated Group II: standardized rehabilitation program alone	Pain, active and passive ROM, swelling, quadriceps strength at 7th postoperative day, complications, length of stay, active and passive ROM, and function at 6 weeks	Use of CPM increased active flexion, decreased swelling No significant effects on pain, active and passive extension, quadriceps strength, length of stay At 6 weeks, no differences between groups in either ROM or function
Kim & Moon, 1995	$N = 68$	Random assignment Group I: alternate flexion and extension splinting Group II: CPM	Postoperative ROM	ROM of alternate flexion and extension splinting group significantly greater than that of CPM group ($p < .01$)
Ververeli et al., 1995	$N = 103$	First 51 clients received CPM initiated in recovery room; next 52 clients did not receive CPM Both groups underwent identical physical therapy protocol starting on 1st postoperative day	Active flexion, pain, wound healing, knee swelling, wound drainage, pulmonary embolism, length of stay Parameters measured at discharge, 6 weeks, 6 months, and 2 years postoperatively	At discharge: no significant difference between groups on pain, healing, swelling, drainage, pulmonary embolism, length of stay Significant increase in active flexion in CPM group ($p < .0001$) At 6-week, 6-month, and 2-year intervals: no significant difference between groups
Kumar et al., 1996	$N = 83$	Random assignment Group I: CPM use Group II: early passive flexion of knee (drop and dangle protocol) Postoperative physical therapy regiments otherwise identical	Length of stay, extension range, wound drainage Parameters measured at 5th postoperative day, 6 weeks, 3 months, and 6 months postoperatively	Clients in drop and dangle group discharged 1 day earlier ($p = .01$), had better extension range at 6-month interval ($p = .03$) No significant difference between groups on other variables at other intervals
Montgomery & Eliasson, 1996	$N = 68$	Random assignment Group I: CPM Group II: active physical therapy Rehabilitation initiated 1st postoperative day in both groups	Knee swelling, knee flexion, pain, length of stay	CPM group sustained less postoperative swelling, more rapid initial improvement in knee flexion No differences between groups in knee flexion at discharge No differences between groups in pain, length of stay
Pope et al., 1997	$N = 53$	Random assignment Group I: no CPM Group II: CPM at 0 to 40 degrees Group III: CPM at 0 to 70 degrees CPM clients had machine for 48 hours; all clients had identical physical therapy regimen	Flexion, overall ROM, functional results, analgesic requirement, blood loss Parameters measured preoperatively, at 1 week and 1 year postoperatively	Significant increase in flexion in 0 to 70 CPM group compared with no CPM group at 1 week At 1 year, no significant difference in flexion, overall ROM, functional results among groups Significant increase in analgesia requirement ($p = .04$) in CPM groups Increased blood drainage postoperatively in 0 to 70 CPM group compared with no CPM ($p = .005$) and 0 to 40 CPM groups ($p = .01$)
Chen et al., 2000	$N = 51$	Random assignment Group I: CPM for 5 consecutive hours per day plus physical therapy Group II: physical therapy only	Flexion measured on admission, 3rd and 7th postoperative days, discharge	No significant difference in flexion between groups

The client's activity generally begins with sitting and then standing at the bedside, perhaps on the evening of surgery or on the morning of the first postoperative day. Within 24 to 48 hours after surgery, the client is able to ambulate with assistance. Weight bearing on the operative extremity is determined by surgeon order and based in part on the choice of cemented or noncemented components. Immediate weight bearing to client tolerance is generally allowed, for example, with cemented prostheses. Use of walker or crutches is continued until quadriceps function is sufficient to allow ambulation with a simple cane.

Risk for Injury: Related to Prosthesis Dislocation

Client Education. Dislocation is not a common occurrence following TKA. The client has few positioning limitations but should be encouraged to avoid prolonged knee flexion to decrease the risk for contracture. In addition, the nurse should instruct the client to limit kneeling and deep knee bends indefinitely.

Osteoarthritis of the Shoulder

OA of the shoulder often results from either significant trauma or a chronic rotator cuff tear. Its presence is associated with significant loss of ROM, which complicates disease management and may compromise the result of any chosen therapy. Because of the relatively unconstrained articulation between the spherical humeral head and the minimally concave glenoid, the shoulder is the most mobile joint in the body. Shoulder motion is provided by the rotator cuff and deltoid muscles. The rotator cuff is a confluence of the subscapularis, supraspinatus, infraspinatus, and teres minor tendons. Large acute tears in the supraspinatus tendon often produce immediate pain and loss of the ability to abduct or elevate the shoulder. With pain comes decreased motion, leading to fairly rapid contracture of the shoulder capsule that further affects ROM. Attempts to restore shoulder motion or use the joint normally often exacerbate the pain, resulting in a vicious cycle marked by additional pain and ROM limitations. Management of shoulder OA must therefore have two goals: restoration of motion toward a normal range and treatment of the arthritis itself.

Surgical repair of the rotator cuff is clearly indicated in the client younger than 40 years of age. For the client older than 40 years of age, the likelihood of success with surgery slowly decreases. The unrepaired tendon appears to be associated with arthritic changes in the glenohumeral joint, possibly influenced by altered mechanical stress across the joint because of the absence of rotator cuff function. If the client has poor nutritional status, further degeneration of the articular cartilage in both the glenoid and the humeral head may result.

History. The client with early OA describes the shoulder pain as mild, with intermittent morning stiffness and limited motion. Onset of symptoms is slow, but as the disease progresses, night pain becomes a predominant occurrence that often awakens the client from sleep. As pain increases in frequency, the client describes more and more difficulty in the performance of personal hygiene and grooming, such as combing the hair. The nurse must determine whether the pain is linked to a recent or past trauma and whether it occurs in a single joint or in both shoulders.

Physical Examination. Inspection of the shoulder may reveal erythema, soft tissue and bony swelling, and fluid bulging (usually anteriorly). The nurse should compare the affected shoulder with the unaffected joint. Structures around the shoulder should be palpated for tenderness and swelling. As the client is assisted with ROM, the nurse should note the presence of crepitus and joint noises. Pain is usually elicited with both passive and active motion, which are limited. Weakness in abduction or forward flexion of the joint is also typical.

Laboratory analysis aids in ruling out systemic disease such as infection and hypothyroidism and also assists in differentiating inflammatory arthritis from OA. Radiographic evaluation includes an anterior and posterior view of the glenohumeral joint in internal and external rotation, as well as an axillary lateral view. The axillary view, which aids in detection of anterior or posterior dislocation or subluxation, is important in primary OA because posterior wear on the glenoid allows the humeral head to subluxate posteriorly. MRI has proven useful in determining the integrity of the rotator cuff.

Conservative Management. In addition to interventions discussed previously in this chapter, physical therapy is particularly helpful in evaluating joint damage and treating shoulder OA. Isometric muscle strengthening exercises using a resistive exerciser (Fig. 16–14) often help the client regain some shoulder motion. Instruction on joint protection measures is also an important part of therapy. Local injections of intra-articular corticosteroids may be useful for their anti-inflammatory and analgesic effects. Injections are most effective when combined with a regular physical therapy program.

Surgical Management. If conservative measures fail to relieve the client's symptoms, surgical alternatives may include shoulder fusion and either hemiarthroplasty or total shoulder arthroplasty (TSA). The client's motivation and expectations are critical factors in the choice of surgical procedure.

Shoulder Fusion. Glenohumeral fusion is performed almost exclusively in the young client who has post-traumatic arthritis, is engaged in heavy labor or other activities that require vigorous use of the upper extremities, or has septic arthritis. In addition, the client with severe rotator cuff disease and the individual who lacks the motivation for postoperative rehabilitation following TSA may also be candidates for shoulder fusion. For all others, prosthetic replacement is typically the procedure of choice. If fusion is indicated, however, it provides a predictable and durable result.

Shoulder fusion is performed by denuding the glenoid and humeral head of any remaining cartilage and

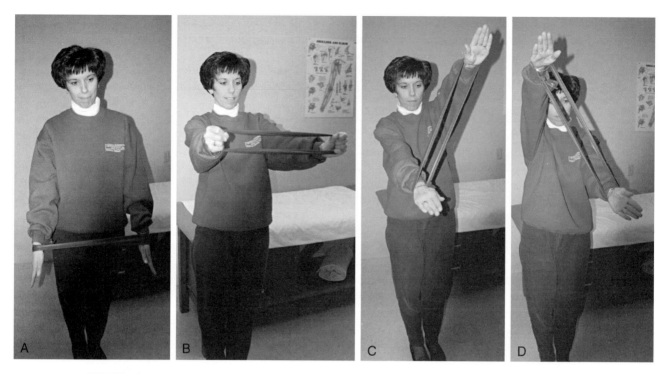

FIGURE 16–14. Use of resistive exercise band to improve muscle strength. *A* and *B,* Resistive shoulder abduction. *C* and *D,* Band is stretched in one direction, held for a count of five, then stretched in the opposite direction and held for a count of five.

internally fixing the humerus to the glenoid, often using autogenous bone graft. The humerus is fused in the position of a "saluting soldier," that is, 30 to 40 degrees of abduction, 30 degrees of forward flexion, and 45 degrees of internal rotation. After successful fusion, motion in the upper extremity is achieved through scapulothoracic motion. Scapular mobility gradually increases during the first 12 to 18 months after fusion, allowing 50% to 60% of normal motion to aid in performance of most ADLs.

For about 3 months postoperatively, the client must wear a brace to maintain the arm in the desired position. The nurse should inform the client that, during the first 6 to 12 months after brace removal, some aching pain is typical as muscles attached to the scapula adapt to the increased activity that occurs through scapulothoracic motion. When successful shoulder fusion has occurred, however, no limitations are placed on the client's upper extremity use. Complications of shoulder fusion are relatively rare. They include possible nerve injury during the operative procedure itself or failure to obtain successful fusion.

Total Shoulder Arthroplasty and Hemiarthroplasty. Experts continue to debate the indications for hemiarthroplasty (humeral component replacement alone) versus TSA (replacement of both humeral and glenoid components). Because the shoulder is not a weight-bearing joint, however, hemiarthroplasty may be an appropriate surgical treatment for OA. If extensive erosion of the glenoid exists, it may also be resurfaced with a polyethylene concave component to accomplish TSA (Fig. 16–15). For the client older than age 40, TSA is often a consideration.

Primary OA and rheumatoid arthritis account for about 85% of all TSAs; the remaining procedures are performed for secondary arthritis (Cuomo & Checroun, 1998). The most common indication for TSA is pain relief. Restoration of motion and strength is a less consistent accomplishment, particularly in the client who has irreparable defects in the rotator cuff. Rotator cuff disruption is not a contraindication for TSA, but the client must understand that return of motion will be less than optimal.

Three basic types of prostheses are used. An unconstrained prosthesis is used when the client has an intact, functioning rotator cuff. A constrained prosthesis may be used in a client with continued severe pain in an unstable shoulder without a rotator cuff. A semiconstrained prosthesis is primarily dependent on the rotator cuff mechanism but has some constraint built into its design. Postoperative dislocation and glenoid component loosening have decreased with the use of semiconstrained or unconstrained prostheses that provide larger surfaces for anchoring in the scapula with methylmethacrylate. Ingrowth of bone and initial screw fixation have also decreased the risk of dislocation.

Preoperative nursing care. Referral to physical therapy for exercise instruction is essential. The client is taught exercises that must continue for 6 to 12 months after surgery to ensure optimal motion at the glenohumeral joint.

Surgical procedure. The operative arm is suspended in a stockinette sling to allow exposure posteriorly, anteriorly, and laterally. The incision corresponds to the deltopectoral interval, which splits the deltoid and pectoralis major muscles from each other without damaging them. Only the subscapularis muscle is actually cut during the procedure, and this division is made near its attachment to the proximal humerus. To ensure optimal deltoid function, that muscle is not detached from its origin on the clavicle or acromion.

The glenoid component is inserted first and cemented into place with methylmethacrylate. The glenoid is checked after insertion; if it is found to be loose, recementing is essential. The humerus is cut at the level of the anatomic neck, and the prosthesis is inserted into the humeral shaft, with or without cement. Component size is based primarily on the rotator cuff, and the largest size that permits closure of the cuff is chosen. Careful closure of the anterior capsular structures and subscapularis muscle is critical to prevention of anterior dislocation.

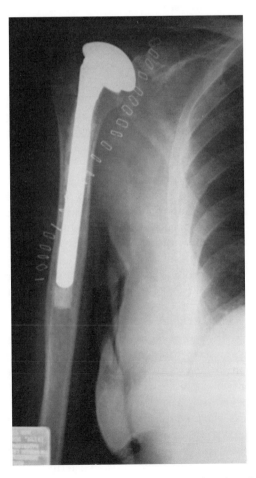

FIGURE 16–15. Cemented TSA in radiographic view 6 weeks postoperatively.

Nursing Management during Postoperative Phase. As with all joint arthroplasty procedures, postoperative nursing care focuses on managing pain, assessing neurovascular integrity, assisting the client to adapt to self-care deficits imposed by the procedure, and identifying early complications.

Risk for Peripheral Neurovascular Dysfunction: Related to Intraoperative Nerve Injury

Neurovascular Assessment. Nerve injury is rarely reported after TSA but, because of the proximity of the brachial plexus to the surgical site, the nurse should regularly assess the client for postoperative palsy. Traction placed on the brachial plexus for surgical positioning appears to be the most common mechanism of injury. The nurse evaluates motor function of the radial nerve by having the client move the thumb toward the palm and back again (thumb abduction). To assess motor function of the ulnar nerve, the nurse asks the client to abduct or spread the fingers wide against pressure. Cutaneous nerve function is assessed by having the client raise the forearm (biceps flexion), and the axillary nerve is assessed by asking the client to push the elbow outward against pressure. Palpation of the deltoid for contraction also evaluates axillary nerve function.

Impaired Physical Mobility: Related to Surgical Implant

Client Education, Rehabilitation. Rehabiliation is essential to the success of TSA. The client must be an informed, motivated participant in the postoperative course of treatment. A stiff, possibly painful joint may result if physical therapy is not performed as recommended for the first 6 to 12 months after surgery. Careful attention to postoperative therapy, however, can potentially lead to near-normal shoulder motion and function. Individualized exercises are ordered by the surgeon and are typically taught and monitored by the physical therapist. Pendulum ROM exercises are generally initiated at 3 to 5 days after surgery (Fig. 16–16*A*). The client bends forward at the waist, allowing the arm to hang passively and vertically to the floor. He or she then swings the arm in increasingly wide circles to gently restore joint motion. Pendulum exercises do not place significant strain on the reconstructed subscapularis tendon or rotator cuff. With the help of an outpatient physical therapist, the client begins passive ROM through rope and pulley exercises approximately 2 weeks after surgery (Fig. 16–16*B* and *C*). At about 6 weeks after surgery, exercises to strengthen the shoulder muscles will be initiated.

Passive ROM may be initiated in the immediate postoperative period through the use of the shoulder CPM machine. This apparatus provides passive motion in

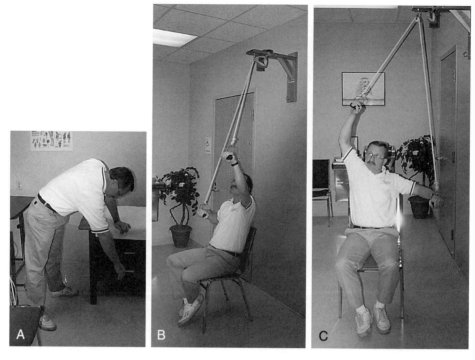

FIGURE 16–16. *A,* For pendulum exercises, the client bends forward at the waist, first circling the operative arm inward with the palm facing backward, then circling the arm in an outward direction with the palm facing forward. *B* and *C,* Rope and pulley exercises are used to passively elevate the operative arm to stretch out adhesions and promote gliding of soft tissue planes past each other. The unaffected arm is used to pull the operative arm upward in the scapular plane.

all three planes of the shoulder, although only forward flexion and external rotation are used initially.

Discharge Precautions. The nurse emphasizes the client's abilities, suggesting safe activities once recovery is complete. With surgeon approval, the client may be able to throw a ball and play tennis or golf. The nurse should caution the client against participation in activities that cause uncontrolled impact loading on the shoulder, such as contact sports or skiing.

Complications. Infection, dislocation, and failure to restore motion may be complications of TSA. Postoperative infection is possible following TSA, but the risk is less than that of knee or hip arthroplasty. Instability represents 38% of all TSA complications (Cuomo & Checroun, 1998), resulting from poor balance of soft tissue surrounding the shoulder. Poor prosthesis alignment, a deficient glenoid or a severely destroyed rotator cuff, and late infection may also increase the risk for dislocation. Other late complications include prosthesis or bone fracture and prosthesis loosening.

Osteoarthritis of the Elbow

OA of the elbow is typically related to injury to the humeral, ulnar, or radioulnar joint. Despite radiographic evidence of disease severity, symptoms are generally mild

because the elbow is a slight weight-bearing joint when compared with the joints in the lower extremities. However, the pain and limited motion caused by OA of the elbow can be disabling in athletes and laborers who extensively use their upper extremities.

History. The client complains of pain and stiffness with loss of motion and strength. As the nurse asks the client about limitations in daily activities, the type and extent of motor deficits become evident. The client may describe difficulty in lifting or receiving an item into the hand (supination); in writing (pronation); or in eating, dressing, and grooming (flexion). Few activities require elbow extension.

Physical Examination. Limitations of pronation and supination may be noted on ROM examination in early elbow OA, followed by deficits in flexion and extension in later disease. The nurse should determine whether pain is greater with supination and pronation or with flexion and extension because the difference determines the client's treatment. Examination generally reveals no palpable or visible swelling at the joint.

Radiographs should include anteroposterior, lateral, and radial head–capitellum views to determine the degree of joint involvement. Joint damage must always be correlated with the client's clinical presentation. In addition, synovial fluid should be analyzed to rule out sepsis and inflammatory disease.

Conservative Management. Measures for management of elbow OA are similar to those for other joints, but they tend to be more successful than conservative interventions for weight-bearing joints such as the knee or hip. If conservative management fails, surgical intervention may become necessary.

Surgical Management. Various operative procedures have been performed for elbow OA. These include arthroplasty with resection of the articular surface, interposition arthroplasty using fascia or an artificial membrane, open debridement arthroplasty, arthroscopic debridement with spur resection and removal of loose bodies, and total elbow arthroplasty (TEA).

Replacement components for TEA (Fig. 16–17) are available in two forms: semiconstrained or nonconstrained. Because the semiconstrained prosthesis is basically a hinge, it is indicated only rarely for the very old client with severe loss of bone density or joint instability following trauma. The semiconstrained prosthesis does not allow for much rotation and has been associated with a high incidence of loosening. The nonconstrained prosthesis resurfaces the ends of the bones to form the joint with a combination of metal and polyethylene similar to that of TKA. Because these components have had a high frequency of loosening, TEA has usually been indicated for the client with rheumatoid arthritis or the individual older than the age of 65 years who expects to place only minimal demands on the joint after surgery. Research continues to evaluate component use with OA.

Surgical Procedure. TEA is most often performed through a lateral or posterior approach that allows

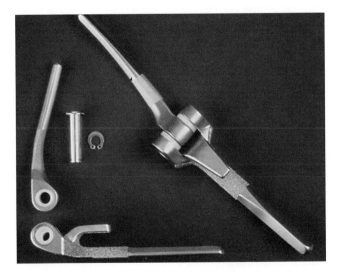

FIGURE 16–17. Prosthetic components for total elbow arthroplasty.

exposure of the radius, ulna, and humerus. The lateral approach minimizes the risk of ulnar nerve damage, hematoma formation, and dislocation. Technique generally includes elbow synovectomy and radial head resection to relieve pain and enhance joint motion.

Preparation for placement of a nonconstrained prosthesis begins with debridement of the capitellum and trochlea of the humerus and the trochlear notch of the ulna to allow healthy bone to come in contact with the components. The humeral and ulnar medullary canals are reamed to accept the component stems, which are secured with cement. After inserting the prosthesis, the surgeon reduces the elbow and evaluates ROM. A wound drain may be inserted at the time of closure. The elbow is maintained in a posterior splint at 90 degrees of flexion unless the triceps has been spared, in which case the extremity may be splinted in extension.

Complications. Following TEA, the client may experience incomplete and unpredictable relief of pain, subluxation or dislocation, infection, and temporary or permanent ulnar nerve palsy.

Nursing Management

Risk for Peripheral Neurovascular Dysfunction: Related to Intraoperative Nerve Injury

Neurovascular Assessment. Because of the risk of ulnar nerve injury, the nurse should routinely evaluate motion and sensation of the fourth and fifth digits in the hand on the client's affected side. Immediately following surgery, pain and edema may minimize the client's ability to abduct and adduct the fingers. Numbness may continue for 6 to 8 weeks after surgery.

Impaired Physical Mobility: Related to Surgical Implant

Client Education, Exercise. Postoperatively, the affected extremity is maintained in abduction and neutral-to-internal rotation. Abduction and external rotation are avoided. The client should be instructed not to use the affected arm for pushing up in bed or in a chair. In addition, the client should be advised to avoid extending the arm (90-degree abduction) from the side of the body to pick up items that are not easily within reach. To avoid this motion in ADLs, the client should be taught to maintain the elbow in adduction and to reach forward, not to the side. Because of the client's restricted movement, the nurse should place personal items within easy reach of the unaffected extremity.

Gentle active-assisted ROM exercises for flexion, extension, and forearm rotation begin within 1 to 3 days after surgery. Active ROM of proximal and distal joints is practiced to prevent loss of motion and to aid in edema control. Compressive gloves, wraps, or sleeves may also be ordered for treatment of edema. As healing progresses, home strengthening exercises for the biceps and triceps muscles are added to the regimen. Heavy lifting and contact sports are prohibited.

CHARCOT JOINTS (NEUROPATHIC ARTHROPATHY)

The name of Jean-Martin Charcot became associated with neuropathic joints following his 1868 report on arthropathies seen in persons with central nervous system lesions. Since the publication of Charcot's original work, neuropathic joints have been identified in multiple conditions that produce reduced pain sensation. These include diabetes mellitus, tertiary syphilis and tabes dorsalis, syringomyelia, multiple sclerosis, peripheral nerve lesions, and congenital insensitivity to pain. Charcot neuropathy occurs most commonly in diabetes, with an incidence of up to 2.5% (Bayne & Lu, 1998).

Neuropathic joints are a rare disorder characterized by distal bone and joint destruction, subluxation and dislocation, and a hypertrophic periosteal reaction. The foot and ankle are most commonly affected, although cases involving the knee and non–weight-bearing joints such as the wrist and shoulder have been identified. Charcot spine has also been noted, not only in association with diabetes and syphilis but as a late complication of traumatic spinal cord injury.

Cause

Charcot's neuropathy results from disruption in a joint's normal sensory innervation. The exact cause is unclear, but it is believed that development of Charcot joint requires three forms of neuropathy: autonomic, motor, and sensory. Loss of vascular tone because of autonomic neuropathy leads to vasodilation and increased perfusion, which allows for bone demineralization. Loss of muscular support and joint instability results from motor neuropathy. Sensory deficits have two roles in the development of neuropathy. First, loss of protopathic sensibility prevents a client from detecting trauma that can precipitate the neuropathy. This deficit may also lead to a delay in treatment because the client is unaware of injury and continues to bear weight on the affected joint. Second, loss of proprioception can worsen the instability of motor neuropathy. It can also lead to increased load on the joints of the foot as the client unconsciously applies more force to the affected extremity in an attempt to gain more proprioceptive information. Prognosis for Charcot neuropathy is poor. With few salvage procedures available, amputation has been a common treatment.

Assessment

A careful history generally reveals a long course of decreased sensitivity to heat and cold. For example, the client may report burns from hot liquids that would cause blisters but no pain. Although the client becomes insensitive to temperature and pain, awareness of light touch is generally preserved. Loss of sensation allows repeated injury to the joint that further contributes to degeneration and laxity. Swelling and deformity of the affected joint typically result from rapid joint destruction. Pain occurs secondary to inflammation but is much less than would be expected given the degree of degeneration apparent on radiographs. Pulses are palpable.

Diagnostic Studies

Radiographs reveal severely destructive arthritis with subchondral sclerosis, massive marginal osteophytosis, and possible subluxation. Osteochondral fragmentation and debris formation are also typical. Electromyograms and nerve conduction studies confirm the presence of severe sensorimotor peripheral neuropathy. MRI studies may be ordered to confirm or rule out syringomyelia or spinal cord lesions.

Conservative Management

Management of Charcot neuropathy focuses primarily on protecting the joint from repeated injury. Immobilization through casting or bracing and use of orthotics will maintain proper alignment and appropriate stress distribution across the joint. Although there is no definitive cure, it is possible in some cases to halt bone and soft tissue destruction. For example, intravenous bisphosphonates (e.g., pamidronate) have been administered to inhibit the bone resorption of Charcot neuropathy. Low-intensity ultrasound therapy, which has been used as an adjunct to fracture healing since 1988, has also been used with startling success in recent clinical trials for treatment of recalcitrant cases of Charcot neuropathy. Continued multicenter studies may prove that this therapy enhances healing and offers economic benefits for both client and payer.

Combined magnetic field (CMF) bone growth stimulation is another promising adjunct in the treatment of neuropathic arthropathy. The effects of this treatment modality on bone healing are well documented. Because there is no difference in the mechanism of healing for fractures associated with Charcot neuropathy and other fractures, use of CMF should also be expected to accelerate the healing rate of Charcot fractures. In a pilot study performed by Hanft, Goggin, Landsman, and Surprenant (1998), 21 clients received daily treatments of 30 minutes in duration with a CMF bone growth stimulator. CMF bone stimulation significantly accelerated the process of consolidation in study participants when compared with 10 control participants.

Surgical Management

Fusion is the treatment of choice for unstable joints, but it is difficult to achieve. Absence of protective sensation often allows the client to overuse the joint in the early postoperative period, compromising the surgical result. Amputation may become necessary if other interventions fail.

Nursing Management

Education to prevent joint destruction is the nurse's primary focus. The nurse explains the use of casts, splints, braces, orthotics, or other assistive devices prescribed for joint protection. He or she should help the client understand that immobilization will decrease joint inflammation, which is critical to a successful outcome. Immobilization also helps minimize joint deformity.

CHONDROMALACIA PATELLAE (PATELLOFEMORAL PAIN SYNDROME)

Chondromalacia patellae is actually a pain syndrome rather than a single diagnosis. Found in all ages beginning with adolescence, it is characterized by patellofemoral joint pain that results from softening with fissure formation on the undersurface (articular cartilage) of the patella. It is also known as *patellofemoral arthralgia* or *patellofemoral pain syndrome*.

Cause

Although some cases of patellofemoral pain syndrome have no identifiable cause, others are clearly linked to trauma. For example, long-distance running can result in repetitive trauma that leads to chronic inflammation. Direct trauma to the patella may cause a chondral fracture and subsequent anterior knee pain. Other causes of patellofemoral pain include lateral subluxation of the patella owing to excessive valgus alignment of the knee, increased femoral neck anteversion, increased tibial torsion, and lateral placement of the tibial tubercle. Underdevelopment of the quadriceps muscles may be a predisposing factor in the development of patellofemoral pain syndrome.

Assessment

The client generally complains of slight swelling and aching knee pain after prolonged standing or walking or after any activity that requires repeated knee flexion and extension. Prolonged sitting with the knee flexed at 90 degrees can also create a dull pain that is often referred posteriorly to the popliteal fossa. Pain usually subsides with movement or straightening the leg. Physical examination may reveal lateral tracking of the patella during active extension of the knee. When the client rises from a chair, the nurse may also note excessive forward bending because of knee pain. Significant disease is associated with quadriceps atrophy. If patellar subluxation is a contributing factor, the nurse will observe a positive apprehension sign when attempting to push the kneecap laterally while the leg is passively extended; the client with

a history of prior subluxation or dislocation of the patella often stops the examiner from continuing because of fear of repeated effects. Crepitus, which is often present during ROM, may be painful.

Diagnostic Studies

Standard anteroposterior and lateral radiographs of the knee are not helpful in diagnosing patellofemoral disease. Axial radiographs (sunrise views) need to be included with the knee in 30, 60, and 90 degrees of flexion. These films may demonstrate changes in the articular surface and abnormal tracking patterns of the patella. MRI and bone scanning may also aid in diagnosis. Because symptoms do not necessarily correlate with the degree of articular softening, diagnostic arthroscopy has mixed benefits.

Conservative Management

The first step is identifying and treating possible causes of the syndrome. A progressive resistance exercise prescription includes isometric quadriceps exercises and isotonic hamstring exercises 2 to 3 days each week. NSAIDs are taken for pain and inflammation, and ice may be used for local effects. With perseverance, most clients respond to conservative treatment.

Surgical Management

If symptoms persist after 6 months of treatment, surgery may be considered. Patellar debridement may bring good or excellent results to as many as 60% of clients, but functional limitations may continue after the procedure (Federico & Reider, 1997). If subluxation occurs during active extension, the lateral retinaculum may be released either arthroscopically or through an incision. More severe cases of lateral dislocation generally require either medical translocation of the tibial tubercle or a combination of lateral retinacular release and medial plication or tightening of the medial retinaculum. For severe patellofemoral arthritis, tibial tubercle elevation may be helpful in decreasing joint reactive forces.

Nursing Management

The client and significant others need thorough instruction in the prescribed regimen of NSAIDs and exercise. The nurse should remind the client to avoid stair climbing, squatting, kneeling, running, and prolonged sitting.

BUNIONS (HALLUX VALGUS)

Bunions are a foot deformity involving the first MTP joint in the great toe. Occurring nine times more often in women than in men, bunions may be the result of a congenital disorder or may be acquired during periods of active growth in adolescence. They can also occur at any time throughout the aging process. Bunions may appear on one foot or on both feet because of either degenerative conditions within the MTP joint or maladaptive remodeling of the metatarsal head caused by locally applied irritation generally associated with footwear. The term *hallux valgus* is used to describe the lateral deviation of the great toe (Fig. 16–18). The resulting malalignment associated with hallux valgus can be associated with OA of the MTP joint, known as *hallux rigidus*.

Assessment

The client with hallux valgus generally complains of pain resulting from irritation of the metatarsal head as it pushes against the inside of the shoe. Physical examination reveals enlargement of the dorsomedial aspect of the first metatarsal head. Painful calluses may be present under the second and third metatarsal heads as a result of a shift in weight bearing. ROM may be decreased, and hammer toes may also be present.

Diagnostic Studies

Standard anteroposterior and lateral radiographs are ordered. Exostosis of the first metatarsal head with subluxation or dislocation is a typical finding.

Conservative Management

Initial treatment may consist entirely of obtaining footwear with a wider toe box to allow sufficient space for the forefoot and to decrease pressure over the bunion. If this is unsuccessful, orthotics and steroid injections of the MTP joint may be considered. Failure of conservative treatment or the desire for a cosmetic correction will lead to surgical intervention.

Surgical Management

When severe, progressive hallux valgus affects the position and function of the lateral four toes, surgical

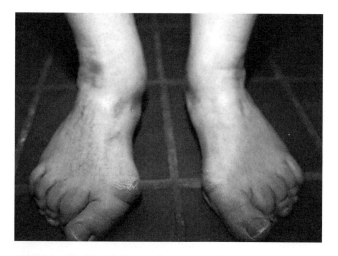

FIGURE 16–18. Hallux valgus, lateral deviation of the great toe.

alignment of the great toe is required. The exostosis is removed, the deformity corrected, and the mechanics of the foot improved by surgery. Osteotomy of the metatarsal or proximal phalanx of the hallux or fusion of the MTP joint may be performed. Choice of procedure is dictated by the degree of deformity, the severity of the valgus angle, and the surgeon's preference. The goal is pain reduction and restoration of the foot's anatomic position. Implant arthroplasty was once a common treatment, but the lack of long-term durability for silicone implants has forced this procedure into relative disfavor.

Complications related to bunion surgery include limited ROM in the MTP joint because of adhesions and scar tissue forming on the extensor or flexor hallucis longus tendon, paresthesias of the great toe because of compromise of the medial dorsal cutaneous nerve, recurrence of deformity, overcorrection of deformity leading to altered foot biomechanics, and dorsal nerve impingement or inadvertent tendon injury. Many of these complications require additional surgery to correct.

Nursing Management

General postoperative care includes emphasis on pain management and neurovascular assessment. The operative foot is initially elevated to decrease edema and pain. When the client is allowed to ambulate, crutch training is ordered and a postoperative wooden shoe is used to minimize pressure over the surgical site.

SUMMARY

Chronic diseases, such as OA and related degenerative disorders, can lead to significant disability that affects both the client and the family. Varied treatments focus on symptom management because, for most degenerative conditions, a cure does not exist. The nurse's role is to help the client accept the disease and live with it proactively by becoming a partner in treatment decisions. This chapter offers an integrated approach to medical and nursing management of OA and associated degenerative disorders. It includes a detailed discussion of TJA, which remains the best surgical alternative when conservative management fails.

After years of being accepted as an inevitable part of aging, OA is now the thrust of research efforts on many fronts. New treatments are being developed and current treatments evaluated more stringently for efficacy. The disease process itself is also being studied extensively in hopes of decreasing the occurrence of OA.

Acknowledgments

The author thanks Steven Myers, MD; Geri Tierney, RN, ONC; and Mrs. Lyn Owen for provision of multiple radiographs used in this chapter.

INTERNET RESOURCES

American College of Rheumatology: www.rheumatology. org

Arthritis Foundation: www.arthritis.org

FocusOnArthritis.com: www.aboutarthritis.com

Mayo Clinic: www.mayoclinic.com

Medical College of Wisconsin Physicians and Clinics: HealthLink: www.healthlink.mcw.edu

National Institutes of Health/National Institute of Arthritis and Musculoskeletal and Skin Diseases: www.nih.gov/niams/healthinfo

National Library of Medicine/MEDLINEplus Health Information: www.nlm.nih.gov/medlineplus

PodiatryNetwork.com: www.podiatrynetwork.com

REFERENCES

Adalberth, G., Bystrom, S., Kolstad, K., Mallmin, H., & Milbrink, J. (1998). Postoperative drainage of knee arthroplasty is not necessary. *Acta Orthopaedica Scandinavica, 69,* 475–478.

Alternative medicine on the rise in the US. (1998). *Science News* [On-line]. Available at www.abc.net.au/science/news/stories/s14424.htm

American College of Rheumatology (ACR) Subcommittee on Osteoarthritis Guidelines. (2000). Recommendations for the medical management of osteoarthritis of the hip and knee: 2000 update. *Arthritis & Rheumatism, 43,* 1905–1915.

Bayne, O., & Lu, E. J. (1998). Diabetic Charcot's arthropathy of the wrist: Case report and literature review. *Clinical Orthopaedics and Related Research, 357,* 122–126.

Brander, V. A., Kaelin, D. L., Oh, T. H., & Lim, P. A. C. (2000). Rehabilitation of orthopedic and rheumatologic disorders: Degenerative joint disease. *Archives of Physical Medicine and Rehabilitation, 81*(Suppl 1), S67–S72, S78–86, S101–102.

Caldwell, J. R., Hale, M. E., Boyd, R. E., Hague, J. M., Iwan, T., Shi, M., & Lacouture, P. G. (1999). Treatment of osteoarthritis pain with controlled release oxycodone or fixed combination oxycodone plus acetaminophen added to nonsteroidal anti-inflammatory drugs: A double blind, randomized, multicenter, placebo controlled trial. *Journal of Rheumatology, 26,* 862–869.

Chen, B., Zimmerman, J. R., Soulen, L., & DeLisa, J. A. (2000). Continuous passive motion after total knee arthroplasty. *American Journal of Physical Medicine and Rehabilitation, 79,* 421–426.

Cooper, S. M. (1999). Improving outcomes in osteoarthritis: How to help patients stay a step ahead of the pain. *Postgraduate Medicine, 105*(6), 29–38.

Crevoisier, X. M., Reber, P., & Noesberger, B. (1998). Is suction drainage necessary after total joint arthroplasty? A prospective study. *Archives of Orthopaedic & Trauma Surgery, 117,* 121–124.

Cuomo, F., & Checroun, A. (1998). Avoiding pitfalls and complications in total shoulder arthroplasty. *Orthopedic Clinics of North America, 29,* 507–518.

DiNubile, N. A. (1997). Osteoarthritis: How to make exercise part of your treatment plan. *The Physician and Sports Medicine, 25*(7), 47–57.

Federico, D. J., & Reider, B. (1997). Results of isolated patellar debridement for patellofemoral pain in patients with normal patellar alignment. *American Journal of Sports Medicine, 25*(5), 663–669.

Hanft, J. R., Goggin, J. P., Landsman, A., & Surprenant, M. (1998). The role of combined magnetic field bone growth stimulation as an adjunct in the treatment of neuropathy/Charcot joint: An expanded pilot study. *The Journal of Foot and Ankle Surgery, 37,* 510–515.

Hochberg, M. C., Altman, R. D., Brandt, K. D., Clark, B. M., Dieppe, P. A., Griffin, M. R., Moskowitz, R. W., & Schnitzer, T. J. (1995a). Guidelines for the medical management of osteoarthritis: Part I. Osteoarthritis of the hip. *Arthritis & Rheumatism, 38,* 1535–1540.

Hochberg, M. C., Altman, R. D., Brandt, K. D., Clark, B. M., Dieppe, P. A., Griffin, M. R., Moskowitz, R. W., & Schnitzer, T. J. (1995b). Guidelines for the medical management of osteoarthritis: Part II. Osteoarthritis of the knee. *Arthritis & Rheumatism, 38,* 1541–1546.

Holt, B. T., Parks, N. L., Engh, G. A., & Lawrence, J. M. (1997). Comparison of closed-suction drainage and no drainage after primary total knee arthroplasty. *Orthopedics, 20,* 1121–1124.

Horstman, J. (1999). *The Arthritis Foundation's guide to alternative therapies.* Atlanta: Arthritis Foundation.

Hospital extra: New drugs. Celecoxib (Celebrex): A new 'super NSAID.' (1999). *American Journal of Nursing, 99*(4), 24b.

Jacobson, B. H., Cheng, H. C., Cashel, C., & Guerrero, L. (1997). The effect of T'ai Chi Chuan training on balance, kinesthetic sense, and strength. *Perceptual & Motor Skills, 84*(1), 27–33.

Kee, C. C. (2000). Osteoarthritis: Manageable scourge of aging. *Nursing Clinics of North America, 35,* 199–207.

Kerrigan, D. C., Todd, M. K., & O'Riley, P. (1998). Knee osteoarthritis and high-heeled shoes. *Lancet, 351,* 1399–1401.

Keuttner, K. E., & Goldberg, V. (Eds.). (1995). *Osteoarthritic disorders.* Rosemont, IL: American Academy of Orthopaedic Surgeons.

Kim, J. M., & Moon, M. S. (1995). Squatting following total knee arthroplasty. *Clinical Orthopaedics and Related Research, 313,* 177–186.

Kuhn, M. (1999). *Complementary therapies for health care providers.* Philadelphia: Lippincott Williams & Wilkins.

Kumar, P. J., McPherson, E. J., Dorr, L. D., Wan, Z., & Baldwin, K. (1996). Rehabilitation after total knee arthroplasty. *Clinical Orthopaedics and Related Research, 331,* 93–101.

LaPrade, R. F., & Swiontkowski, M. F. (1999). New horizons in the treatment of osteoarthritis of the knee. *Journal of the American Medical Association, 281,* 876–878.

Lumsden, D. B., Baccala, A., & Martire, J. (1998). Tai Chi for osteoarthritis: An introduction for primary care physicians. *Geriatrics, 53*(2), 84, 87–88.

McAlindon, T. E., Felson, D. T., Zhang, Y., Hannan, M. T., Aliabadi, P., Weissman, B., Rush, D., Wilson, P. W., & Jacques, P. (1996). Relation of dietary intake and serum levels of vitamin D to progression of osteoarthritis of the knee among participants in the Framingham study. *Annals of Internal Medicine, 125,* 353–359.

McInnes, J., Larson, M. G., Daltroy, L. H., Brown, T., Fossel, A. H., Eaton, H. M., Shulman-Kirwan, B., Steindorf, S., Poss, R., & Liang, M. H. (1992). A controlled evaluation of continuous passive motion in patients undergoing total knee arthroplasty. *Journal of the American Medical Association, 268,* 1423–1428.

Montgomery, F., & Eliasson, M. (1996). Continuous passive motion compared to active physical therapy after knee arthroplasty. *Acta Orthopaedica Scandinavica, 67,* 7–9.

North American Nursing Diagnosis Association (NANDA). (1999). *Nursing Diagnoses: Definitions and Classification, 1999–2000.* Philadelphia: Author.

O'Koon, M. (1999). Shopping for a "cure." *Arthritis Today* [On-line]. Available at www.arthritis.org/ReadArthritisToday/1999_03_04.shopping.asp

Osteoarthritis. (1997). In J. H. Klippel (Ed.), *Primer on the rheumatic diseases* (11th ed.). Atlanta: Arthritis Foundation.

Pope, R. O., Corcoran, S., McCaul, K., & Howie, D. W. (1997). Continuous passive motion after primary total knee arthroplasty. *The Journal of Bone and Joint Surgery, 79B,* 914–917.

Rains, C., & Bryson, H. M. (1995). Topical capsaicin: A review of its pharmacological properties and therapeutic potential in postherpetic neuralgia, diabetic neuropathy and osteoarthritis. *Drugs and Aging, 7,* 317–328.

Ramos, L. (2000). Beyond the headlines. SAMe as a supplement: Can it really help treat depression and arthritis? *Journal of the American Dietetic Association, 100,* 414.

Rehman, Q., & Lane, N. E. (1999). Getting control of osteoarthritis pain: An update on treatment options. *Postgraduate Medicine, 106*(4), 127–134.

Ritter, M. A., Keating, E. M., & Faris, P. M. (1994). Closed wound drainage in total hip or total knee replacement. *The Journal of Bone and Joint Surgery, 76A*(1), 35–38.

Roberts, D. (2001). Arthritic and connective tissue disorders. In D. Schoen (Ed.), *Core curriculum for orthopaedic nursing* (4th ed.). Pitman, NJ: National Association of Orthopaedic Nurses.

Roberts, D., & Lappe, J. (2001). Management of clients with musculoskeletal disorders. In J. Black, J. H. Hawks, & A. Keene (Eds.), *Medical-surgical nursing: A psychophysiologic approach* (6th ed., pp. 551–586). Philadelphia: WB Saunders.

SAM-e (S-adenosylmethionine). (2000). *Arthritis Foundation* [On-line]. Accessed at http://www.arthritis.org/resource/statements/sam%5Fe.asp

Simon, L. S. (1999). Arthritis: New agents herald more effective symptom management. *Geriatrics, 54*(6), 37–42.

Slemenda, C., Brandt, K. D., Heilman, D. K., Mazzuca, S., Braunstein, E. M., Katz, B. P., & Wolinsky, F. D. (1997). Quadriceps weakness and osteoarthritis of the knee. *Annals of Internal Medicine, 127,* 97–104.

Ververeli, P. A., Sutton, D. C., Hearn, S. L., Booth, R. E., Jr., Hozack, W. J., & Rothman, R. R. (1995). Continuous passive motion after total knee arthroplasty. *Clinical Orthopaedics and Related Research, 321,* 208–215.

Zampieron, E., & Kamhi, E. (1999). *Arthritis: An alternative medicine guide.* Tiburon, CA: AlternativeMedicine.com Books.

17

Disorders of the Spine

MARY FAUT RODTS

Spinal problems are the result of many different underlying diagnoses, such as deformity, fracture, osteomyelitis, tumors, and degenerative disease. The spine is intimately involved with the neural structures. Thus, an understanding of the neurologic implications of any spinal problem is considered a priority of the orthopaedic nurse. Every spinal problem should be considered simultaneously from the orthopaedic and neurologic point of view. Some spinal diagnoses, such as fracture, tumor, or infection, should heighten the awareness of the nurse that a problem with instability of the spine is a significant concern. Before a plan of care is embarked upon, a determination about spinal stability must be made.

The difference between a stabilized spinal problem and instability is the ultimate concern of the nurse. Understanding anatomy assists nurses in planning appropriate and safe nursing care for all individuals with spinal problems (see Chapter 6). Underlying spinal stability and stability gained through surgical intervention are key factors in the progression of rehabilitation programs for these clients. Rapid and active nursing care and rehabilitation may be undertaken only if a client's spine is stable. If the spine of a neurologically normal client is not stable, the primary nursing goal is to prevent deterioration of neurologic function and to maintain general physical conditioning within the parameters established for each client.

The nursing plan for all spine conditions should be developed based on evidence that certain interactions optimize client care and recovery. Nurses must look to the literature and research to offer rationale for nursing interventions. At the same time, it is an opportunity to identify research questions for clinical nursing practice.

SPINAL COLUMN DEFORMITIES

Scoliosis

The spine, in the coronal plane, should appear completely straight. The term *scoliosis* is used to describe a lateral curvature of the spine, with vertebral body rotation (Fig. 17–1). Curvature is classified as structural or nonstructural in origin. A *structural curvature* of the spine is a curve that does not correct itself on forced bending against the curvature and has vertebral rotation. A *nonstructural curvature* is one that is easily corrected on forced bending or in the supine position and does not have rotation of the vertebral bodies. See Box 17–1 for the method of measuring spinal x-ray films.

Idiopathic Scoliosis. The most common form of scoliosis is idiopathic scoliosis. This term has been applied because the exact cause is unknown. Idiopathic scoliosis occurs in normal, healthy, growing children who have no other apparent health problems. The incidence of idiopathic scoliosis is less than 1% (Bridwell & DeWald, 1997). It occurs most often in preadolescents and adolescents. Although it was once thought to be primarily a problem in females, school screening studies have demonstrated that equal numbers of boys and girls show small degrees of abnormal spinal curvature. From 3% to 5% of children screened for scoliosis have positive findings. Progressive idiopathic scoliosis occurs more often in girls; therefore, girls more often require treatment. Until it is proved that a curvature is not progressive, both boys and girls should be observed. Progression of idiopathic scoliosis is possible until skeletal maturity is reached. Continued progression is even possible after maturation if the curvature is greater than 40 to 45 degrees. Curves less than 20 degrees in a growing child require

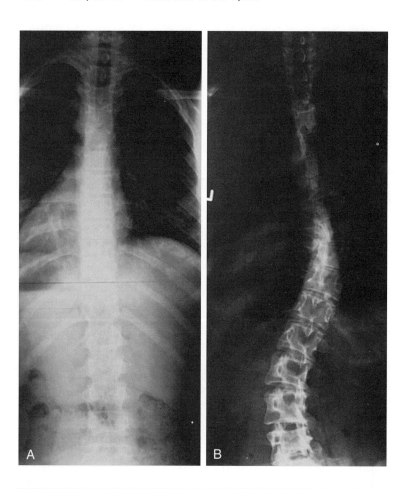

FIGURE 17–1. X-ray film of a normal *(A)* and scoliotic *(B)* spine in the posteroanterior projection.

BOX 17–1.
Measuring Spinal X-ray Films

The scoliotic angle of the spine is determined by the Cobb method of measurement. The larger curve is identified, and a line (A) is drawn at the top of the most proximal vertebra that is tilted maximally into the concavity of the curve. A similar line (B) is drawn at the bottom of the distal vertebra that is tilted maximally into the concavity of the curve. The angle thus created (<C) is measured in degrees and represents the scoliotic measurement.

In practicality, the lines often extend beyond the edges of the x-ray film, requiring that perpendicular lines be erected to lines A and B. <D, created by these perpendicular lines, is equal to <C.

---

observation for progression and no treatment in a skeletally mature individual. Individuals with curves between 20 and 40 degrees and those who are skeletally immature require brace management. Curves greater than 45 degrees require surgical intervention (Table 17–1).

Congenital Scoliosis. Congenital scoliosis is malformation of the bony vertebral segment of the spine. Because embryonic development of the vertebrae takes

place before 8 weeks of gestation, such a defect is often present before a woman becomes aware that she is pregnant. The cause of congenital scoliosis is unknown.

Congenital scoliosis can be divided into failures of formation and failures of segmentation. Failure in either category can cause significant scoliosis. *Failure of formation* refers to the absence of a portion of a vertebra. *Hemivertebra* refers to the absence of an entire side of a vertebra. A *wedge vertebra* is missing only a portion of one side of the vertebra. *Failure of segmentation* refers to the absence of the normal separations between vertebrae (Fig. 17–2). Congenital deformities can also be the result of a combination of defects. The incidence of congenital scoliosis is less than 0.5%.

Decision making for the treatment of congenital scoliosis is difficult. Each anomaly must be identified to fully understand how it interacts or balances others. A

TABLE 17–1. *Idiopathic Scoliosis*

	ANGLE OF CURVATURE (DEGREES)	SUGGESTED THERAPY
Children	0–20	Observation
	20–40	Bracing
	>40	Surgery
Adults	<50	Observation
	>50	Surgery

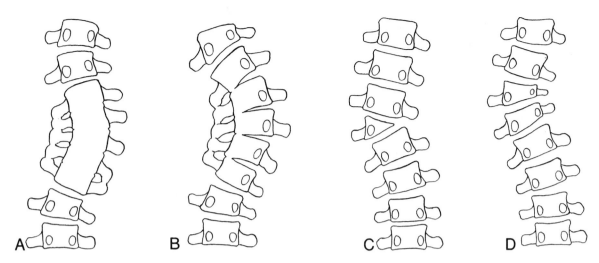

FIGURE 17–2. Drawing demonstrating different congenital anomalies. *A,* Block vertebra. *B,* Bar. *C,* Hemivertebra. *D,* Multiple hemivertebrae.

child with an isolated hemivertebra may have a worse prognosis than one with multiple congenital vertebral anomalies. Congenital scoliosis, when identified, should be followed closely and monitored for progression. Bracing is rarely definitive treatment. Surgical intervention is necessary for progressive congenital scoliosis and should, if possible, be performed before major deformity develops.

Neuromuscular Scoliosis. Many different neuromuscular conditions are associated with spinal deformities: cerebral palsy, syringomyelia, polio, myelomeningocele, spinal muscular atrophy, spinal cord tumors, trauma, and various myopathic conditions (e.g., muscular dystrophy, arthrogryposis, myotonia, hypotonia). Partial or complete paralysis of the trunk musculature can cause a long, sweeping scoliosis. In contrast to those with idiopathic scoliosis, most individuals with neuromuscular scoliosis have compromised health. These clients are often frail and have decreased pulmonary function. The use of a brace is generally contraindicated, and surgery is the treatment of choice. Surgery is undertaken cautiously, however, and meticulous postoperative nursing care is mandatory to anticipate and prevent problems after surgery.

Spina Bifida, Meningocele, and Myelomeningocele. The term *spina bifida* is used to describe a defect in the vertebral arches or the lamina. The incidence of spinal dysraphism is 1 in 1000 live births. Often, this is an incidental finding, one that produces no symptoms and requires no treatment (Table 17-2). A meningeal sac that protrudes through such a laminar defect but contains no nerve tissue is called a *meningocele.* If the sac contains neural elements, the term *myelomeningocele* applies. Such a condition almost invariably leads to neurologic deficit. Spinal deformities secondary to myelomeningocele are

common and are among the most difficult spinal problems to treat. Therefore, differentiation among spina bifida, meningocele, and myelomeningocele is necessary for ascertaining prognosis.

An infant born with meningocele or myelomeningocele should be evaluated and treated immediately by the neurosurgical service in an effort to prevent or limit neurologic deficit and complications such as meningitis and hydrocephalus. Neurologic impairment varies from

TABLE 17–2. *Classification of Spina Bifida*

CLASSIFICATION	CHARACTERISTICS
Spina bifida occulta	Incomplete closure of laminae, one or more vertebrae
	Absence of protrusion of intraspinal contents to surface
	Possible overlying cutaneous defect, neurologic deficit, spinal cord dysplastic changes
Meningocele	Unfused vertebral arches
	Visible meningeal sac filled with cerebrospinal fluid and composed of dura mater or arachnoid, no nerve tissue
	No myelodysplasia of spinal cord
	Sensory, motor, reflex status intact
	No sphincter disturbance
Myelomeningocele	Unfused vertebral arches
	Cystic distention of meninges, nerve tissue within or adherent to sac
	Spinal cord myelodysplasia
	Neurologic deficits (sensory, motor, reflex, sphincter) caudal to level of lesion

Adapted from Tachdjian, M. (1990). *Pediatric orthopedics* (2nd ed., pp. 1773, 1886). Philadelphia: WB Saunders.

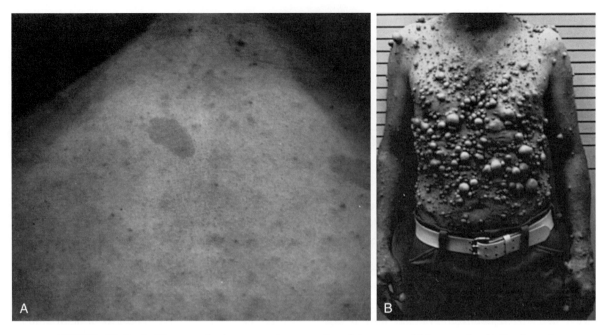

FIGURE 17–3. *A,* Photograph demonstrating a café-au-lait spot, which may be indicative of neurofibromatosis if five or more are present. *B,* Client with multiple neurofibromas.

minimal foot deformity to paraplegia with bowel and bladder incontinence.

The specific cause of these spinal defects is not known. However, they occur early in embryonic development, often within the first weeks of gestation. Amniocentesis, serum alpha-fetoprotein determination, and ultrasonography are tests that can provide further information about the presence of a neural tube defect in utero (see Chapter 18).

Neurofibromatosis. Neurofibromatosis is a disease that is genetically transmitted from one generation to the next. The incidence is 1 in 2500 to 1 in 3300 live births (Bridwell & DeWald, 1997). It is characterized by an abnormal proliferation of normal neural tissue and can affect any area of the body. There is a high degree of association between this condition and scoliosis and kyphoscoliosis.

Diagnosis of neurofibromatosis is based on certain physical findings, the most common of which is the café-au-lait spot. A café-au-lait spot appears on the skin as a light brown patch (Fig. 17-3A). An isolated spot is not indicative of neurofibromatosis, but such a diagnosis should be considered in a client with five or six café-au-lait spots. Multiple neurofibromas are also associated with this disease (Fig. 17-3B).

Clients with neurofibromatosis often have sharp, angulated scoliotic curves, which is a difficult type of spinal defect to treat. This type of curve is called *dystrophic* and requires aggressive surgical management because conservative methods generally fail. On the other hand, some of these clients have an idiopathic type of curvature

that is more amenable to conservative treatment (i.e., bracing).

Marfan's Syndrome. Marfan's syndrome is a mesenchymal disorder that is associated with a defect of the connective tissues. Disruption of mesenchymal tissue is seen in the cardiovascular and ocular systems as well as in the musculoskeletal system. These clients exhibit a high incidence of scoliosis and kyphoscoliosis, and reports of incidence vary from 34% to 73% (Bridwell & DeWald, 1997). Initial diagnosis is often made after routine history and physical examination, which reveal a tall, slender client with long fingers and a positive history of similar family characteristics. Associated characteristics include marked ligamentous laxity, dislocated ocular lens, and dilation of the aorta (which often results in aortic aneurysms).

Tumors. Spinal tumors can be associated with development of spinal deformities. The diagnosis of a spinal tumor is often made when there is a history of back pain and an associated onset of spinal deformity. Scoliosis in young clients is rarely accompanied by pain. If pain is present and consistent, further diagnostic efforts should be undertaken to rule out spinal tumors.

Osteoid osteoma, a benign bone tumor, often occurs first as a painful scoliosis. After further evaluation, a small tumor composed of osteoid and atypical bone is found. Such a tumor is commonly located in the posterior element of a vertebra. Often, accurate diagnosis is delayed because initial x-ray films appear normal. The practitioner should be suspicious, however, if a client complains of localized back pain that is exacerbated at night but can be relieved with salicylates.

Postirradiation Scoliosis. Spinal deformities may develop after radiation therapy for a variety of conditions, especially following radiotherapy for Wilms' tumor or neuroblastoma. Radiation, necessary for obliteration of these tumors, often produces asymmetrical growth in adjacent growth plates and soft tissues, leading to subsequent spinal deformity. Because this has been identified as a problem, radiation oncologists are often able to plan treatment to prevent the development of spinal deformity.

Nonstructural Scoliosis. *Nonstructural scoliosis* is scoliosis that completely resolves when the client bends to the affected side and that exhibits no vertebral rotation. Poor posture, leg length discrepancy, and visual problems may each cause an apparent scoliosis. Various treatment modalities (e.g., physical therapy, shoe lifts, corrective eyeglasses) alleviate these types of nonstructural scoliosis.

Hysterical scoliosis has been documented on rare occasions (Blount, 1974). This form of scoliosis is characterized by a long, sweeping curvature, with significant decompensation and shoulder asymmetry. The client often maintains this posture throughout an entire physi-cal examination. Diagnosis is confirmed by placing the client under general anesthesia, when pathologic curvatures resolve. Hysterical scoliosis requires psychiatric management.

Nonstructural scoliosis may also occur secondary to nerve root irritation. A herniated nucleus pulposus, spinal cord tumor, spondylolysis, or spondylolisthesis may irritate a spinal nerve, causing pain and subsequent scoliosis. Following relief of the nerve irritation, this type of scoliosis usually resolves.

Kyphosis

Kyphosis describes a posterior rounding at the thoracic level of the spine. A certain degree of kyphosis is normal (Fig. 17–4), but curvatures greater than 45 degrees are generally considered excessive. Further investigation as to the cause of this degree of kyphosis should be undertaken. Kyphosis is said to be postural if a client can voluntarily hyperextend the spine to correct the curvature and there is no radiologic evidence of structural change.

Scheuermann's Disease. Scheuermann's disease presents with a structural kyphosis of greater than 45 degrees, irregular vertebral endplates, disc space narrowing, wedging of three or more thoracic vertebrae, and often pain. In mild cases, initial treatment consists of

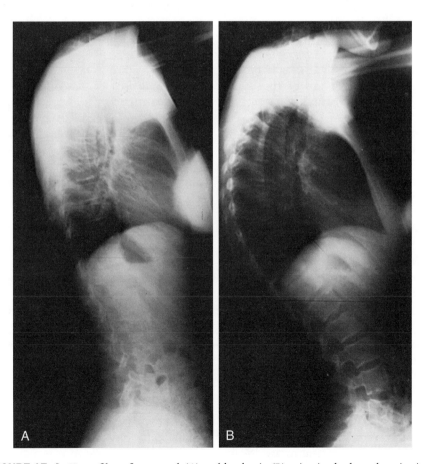

FIGURE 17–4. X-ray film of a normal *(A)* and kyphotic *(B)* spine in the lateral projection.

hyperextension exercises. If the curvature increases, however, correction with a Milwaukee brace (worn 23 hours/day) in conjunction with an exercise program is necessary. More severe kyphosis requires anterior and posterior spinal fusion, with appropriate prosthetic implants to correct the deformity and to maintain spinal alignment.

Congenital Kyphosis. Congenital kyphosis is produced if a malformation of the vertebral structure occurs in utero. As in congenital scoliosis, failure of formation or segmentation may be responsible for the deformity. Because there is a high incidence of neurologic problems associated with this condition, aggressive treatment may be necessary if the curvature is progressive.

Neuromuscular Kyphosis. Kyphosis is sometimes associated with neuromuscular disorders, such as cerebral palsy, spinocerebral degeneration, spinal muscle atrophy, muscular dystrophy, and other myopathic conditions. Under these circumstances, curvature results from poor muscle control, that is, control that is necessary to hold the spine in an erect position. Typically, these clients require the use of both arms to support the torso in an upright position. The use of a brace may be contraindicated because clients often have decreased pulmonary function secondary to underlying disease processes. Modified or part-time braces may be used to allow additional spine growth before spinal fusion. If curvature progression is documented, however, bracing must be discontinued and surgery must be undertaken. Surgery is recommended to provide spinal stability; to improve balance in the sitting position; and to regain use of the upper extremities, which had been used for trunk support.

Postsurgical Kyphosis. Kyphosis may occur secondary to multilevel laminectomy for excision of spinal cord tumors or cysts. Progressive deformity is almost certain in young, growing children and is occasionally seen in adults. Anterior and posterior spinal fusion is necessary to prevent increasing deformity if the prognosis for the original disease process is good.

Postirradiation Kyphosis. Radiation for treatment of tumors can alter vertebral growth plates and soft tissues, causing spinal deformity. As in postirradiation scoliosis, radiation oncologists are cautious in planning radiation treatment to avoid this problem if possible.

Metabolic Disorders. Metabolic disorders, such as osteoporosis and osteomalacia, are often precursors to the development of kyphotic deformities. Compression fractures, attributable to demineralization of the bone, are noted in the spinal column. Such fractures cause pain, deformity, and sometimes neurologic deficits. Osteoporotic fractures account for millions of health care dollars spent each year.

Encouraging research has identified new drugs, such as alendronate (Fosamax) and raloxifene (Evista), that appear to increase the strength of bone and reduce fracture. Health education to reduce the incidence of osteoporosis should be a prime focus of all health care providers. Programs to teach young children about the importance of calcium and vitamin D intake as well as the need for daily exercise will help decrease the number of people affected by osteoporosis in future generations.

Evaluation by an endocrinologist is necessary for determining the appropriate medical management and protocols for increasing bone density. For the client with progressive kyphosis, prophylactic posterior spine stabilization in conjunction with anterior spinal fusion may be recommended. Difficulties arise when bone integrity is insufficient to support prosthetic implants.

Kyphoplasty for the treatment of osteoporotic vertebral fractures appears to be a promising treatment for painful, spinal fractures. A hollow needle is placed into the fractured vertebra with a balloon used to restore near-normal vertebral shape. Bone cement is then placed into the vertebra, giving it instant stability (Fig. 17–5A and B). The procedure is less invasive than major reconstructive procedures and can be accomplished much more easily. Long-term follow-up is necessary to fully evaluate its efficacy.

Clients with isolated spinal fractures secondary to osteoporosis are treated for traumatic fractures, with special consideration given to underlying disease processes.

Ankylosing Spondylitis. Ankylosing spondylitis (Marie-Strumpell disease) is an arthritic disorder that results in autofusion of the joints of the spine, sacroiliac, and hip. Initially, clients have significant back pain and stiffness. In the early stages, radiographic findings are negative. At one time, such clients were rarely diagnosed and were often told to seek psychiatric evaluation and counseling for their back pain. As the disease progresses, x-ray films reveal bony ankyloses leading to the pathognomonic bamboo spine.

Treatment for the early phases of ankylosing spondylitis includes maintenance of normal spinal posture through physical therapy and appropriate medical management (anti-inflammatory and pain medications). Spinal joints still ankylose but in correct orientation, thereby preventing the significant deformities often seen with this disease. For clients first seen at later stages of the disease, spinal osteotomy, instrumentation, and fusion are often needed to realign the spine.

Assessment

Nursing History. The nurse observing the client for a spinal deformity should be concerned with the client's developmental milestones, onset of deformity, leg length discrepancies, and symptoms of pain or weakness. Table

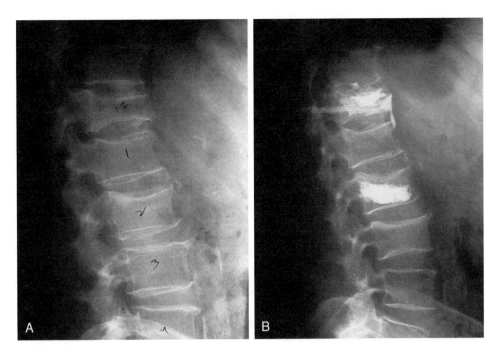

FIGURE 17–5. Preoperative and postoperative lateral x-ray films of the spine demonstrating T12 and L2 osteoporotic spine fractures. (Courtesy of Howard An, M.D.)

17–3 describes key assessment findings for clients with spinal disorders. Establishment of a family history of spinal deformity and past treatment modalities for family members may determine the extent of the problem. The nurse should elicit the client's perception of the problem, concerns about body image, and apprehension over possible treatment (see Chapter 2 for psychosocial concerns).

Physical Assessment. All clients being evaluated for spinal deformity should have a complete orthopaedic and neurologic examination performed. Any evidence of unusual gait, weakness, or abnormal reflexes or sensation should be a cause for concern and should be fully evaluated. Intraspinal problems, such as cysts, tumors, or herniated nucleus pulposus, can be the cause of spinal deformity.

The physical assessment remains the same for both the child and the adult. Because the anterior and posterior torso must be evaluated, care should be taken to protect the client's privacy by providing an examination gown that can be easily moved to view the spine. The client should not be examined while clothed. Various health care providers, including the physician, nurse, and physical therapist, can perform screening for spinal deformity.

Before the client undergoes screening, the examination should be explained so that the client is at ease, thus providing a more accurate examination. When the assessment is being performed in the school setting, appropriate information about clothing should be given to the

children before the screening. Boys should wear gym shorts, and girls should wear a two-piece bathing suit or a plain one-piece suit. Stripes, diagonal prints, and ruffles make it difficult for the observer to assess the contours of the back. Children with shoulder-length or longer hair should be asked to pull the hair up in a barrette or rubber band. The child cannot hold the hair up for the examination.

Even though proper clothing is being worn, girls and boys should be screened separately. It is best to have the child brought to the examiner, who is either in a separate room or in a room that is screened off for privacy. Another person can be the recorder of information or provide the assessment form to the screener to help expedite the process. When the child enters the screening area, the screener should provide a reassuring review of what will be done.

The child is first observed from the back. The child stands with equal weight on both feet, arms hanging freely at the sides and relaxed. The screener evaluates symmetry of the shoulders, scapula, and waist creases, as well as arm lengths (Fig. 17–6A). The child is then directed to place fingertips together as if diving into a pool and bend forward slowly. The examiner observes for thoracic rib prominence or paravertebral muscle prominence in the lumbar spine (Fig. 17–6B). A scoliometer to quantify the rib or paravertebral prominence can be used. The scoliometer is placed at the apex of the curvature, and a measurement is obtained. A scoliometer reading of above 5 degrees warrants referral. This completes the observation from the back.

The child is then asked to turn and face the screener, with equal weight on each foot. The screener looks for symmetry of the shoulders, breasts, anterior rib cage, waist creases, and arm lengths (Fig. 17-6C). The child is then asked to bend forward to identify any asymmetry of the thoracic or lumbar spine (Fig. 17-6D). The final part of the assessment is to view the child from the side, looking for increased thoracic rounding or lumbar sway-back. This should be looked for in both the standing and the forward-flexed position (Fig. 17-6E).

The use of a scoliometer helps the screener quantify the deformity and communicate with other professionals with a consistent measurement tool. The screener has the client perform a forward-bend test and then places the scoliometer at the point of greatest prominence (Fig. 17-7). A reading is then obtained and recorded. A measurement of greater than 5 degrees should be indicative of a possible curvature of the spine, and the client should be referred for further evaluation.

Any child who has positive findings should be referred to the primary care physician, pediatrician, or nurse practitioner for further evaluation. Some schools have a rescreening program that is conducted by the screener and a local physician to facilitate the referral.

TABLE 17-3. *Assessment of Spine Disorders*

DISORDER	HISTORY	PHYSICAL FINDINGS	DIAGNOSTIC EVALUATION
Scoliosis	Idiopathic type is rarely accompanied by pain Nonstructural type may involve a history of nerve root pain	Asymmetry of shoulders, scapular, waist creases Thoracic rib prominence or paravertebral muscle prominence on forward bend	Structural: lateral curvature and vertebral rotation on posteroanterior x-ray film Nonstructural: curve corrected on forced bending or in supine position; no rotation of vertebral bodies Congenital: malformation of bony vertebral segment of spine
Kyphosis	May complain of thoracic back pain	Posterior rounding at the thoracic level	Kyphotic curve of more than 45 degrees on x-ray film
Herniated nucleus pulposus	May recall specific incident that precipitated pain May be gradual but persistent radicular pain Increased pain with sneezing, coughing, or Valsalva's maneuver	Limited straight leg raise May have decreased reflexes May have muscle weakness Signs depend on the level of herniation	Myelogram shows decreased dye flow at affected level(s) MRI or CT shows bulging or extruded disc material and narrowed canal
Spondylolysis	Complaints of low-back pain May isolate specific incident that brought on back pain Often associated with athletic activity (e.g., gymnast, football lineman, wrestler)	Acute muscle spasm present May list to one side	Oblique x-ray film shows defect or break in neural arch between superior and inferior articulating processes "Scotty dog with a collar" appearance of posterior elements
Spondylolisthesis	Low-back pain sometimes radiating to lower extremities May be history of specific incident that precipitated pain	Increased lumbar lordosis Waddling gait Decreased ability to touch the toes Limited straight leg raising Mild scoliosis May have bowel and bladder problems May have decreased motor reflex and sensation	Lateral x-ray film shows forward subluxation of one vertebra on another
Spinal stenosis	Usually older than 60 years of age Leg pain after walking short distance Needs frequent rest to relieve pain	Gait is crouched over, with lumbar spine flexed forward	X-ray film, myelogram, CT, MRI, show bony narrowing of canal

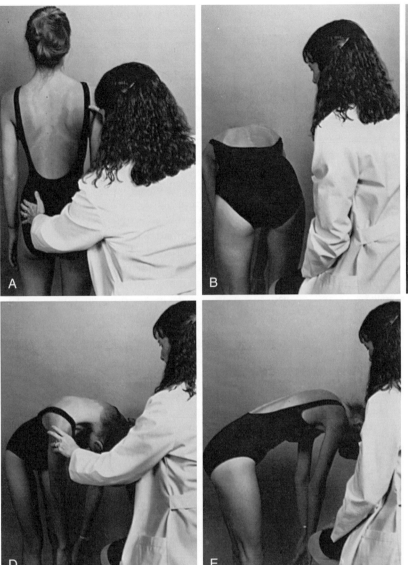

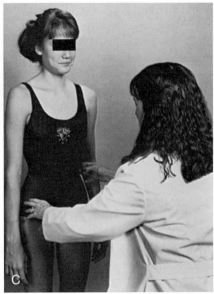

FIGURE 17–6. School screening of a child for spinal deformity from the back *(A);* bending *(B);* from the front looking for anterior chest deformity and asymmetry *(C);* bending toward the examiner, which may help visualize particular curves better *(D);* and from the side in both standing and bending positions to visualize increased kyphosis or lordosis *(E).*

Any child with a positive examination should be referred to an orthopaedic surgeon who has knowledge of spinal deformity treatment. The key to a good screening program is consistency and accurate record keeping.

Diagnostic Evaluation. Upright posteroanterior and lateral radiographs are generally recommended to confirm the diagnosis of scoliosis or kyphosis. However, special concern arises for children requiring long-term monitoring of spinal deformities. Radiologic evaluation is the only exact diagnostic tool available for monitoring changes in deformity, but excessive radiation exposure of children is inappropriate. Because breast tissue is in close proximity to the spine, inadvertent exposure occurs. Shielding helps prevent this problem, but in more severe scoliosis, breast shields do not allow full visualization of

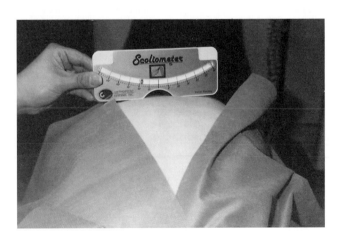

FIGURE 17–7. Proper placement of the Scoliometer on the rib prominence.

the spinal column. Obtaining x-ray films in a posteroanterior orientation has been shown to decrease radiation exposure to the breasts and is generally recommended (DeSmet, Fritz, & Asher, 1981). Recent research studies indicate that there may be a slight increased risk of breast cancer in women who were treated for idiopathic scoliosis and had multiple radiographic examinations (Bone & Hsieh, 2000; Morin, Lonstein, Stovall, Hacker, Luckyanov, & Land, 2000). Radiographs should be obtained only when an increase in curvature is suspected for follow-up in this client population. Clinical evaluation should guide the use of radiographs.

Treatment Modalities and Related Nursing Management

Nonsurgical Treatments for Spinal Deformities.
Nonsurgical treatment programs for clients with spinal deformity consist of observation, braces, and exercise regimens. Generally accepted criteria for specific treatments exist (Table 17–4). However, each client must be individually evaluated, not only for the particular medical problem (e.g., scoliosis vs. kyphosis) but also for individual ability to cope with potential treatments. One client may refuse to wear a brace under any circumstances. Another child may insist on treatment for even a slight curvature. Individual traits and personalities must be taken into consideration if treatment is to be successful.

Braces. Many different types of orthoses have been developed over the years for treatment of spinal deformities. The best known is the Milwaukee brace (Fig. 17–8A). This type of brace was first used as a means of providing postoperative immobilization for spinal fusion clients. Indications for its use increased, however, and for 20 years it was the most commonly used brace for both scoliosis and kyphosis. Today, the primary indication for this type of brace is the treatment of kyphosis. The Milwaukee brace consists of a pelvic girdle, three bars (two posterior and one anterior) attached perpendicular to the girdle, a throat ring, and strategically placed pads at the apex of the curve (these help initiate active correction by the client). Clients wearing this type of brace are directed to pull up and out of the brace and away from the pads to achieve correction of their curvature. In contrast to scoliosis, correction of kyphosis is often maintained after use of the brace is discontinued.

Because of its visibility, the Milwaukee brace was not appealing to most children, so other methods were sought to prevent increased deformity. Although it is commonly agreed that the Milwaukee brace is necessary for control of kyphosis, underarm braces (e.g., the Lyon or Wilmington brace, Fig. 17–8B) have been used to prevent progression of thoracic or thoracolumbar scoliosis. Cosmetically, these braces are more acceptable and allow near-normal adolescent activities. A brace developed at Boston Children's Hospital (Fig. 17–8C) is used for correction of lumbar curves and thoracolumbar curvatures that have their apices below the level of T9. The Boston brace is also accepted more readily by clients.

A new brace, called SpineCor, was developed in Canada and is currently under investigation. This brace is appealing because it is a flexible brace that allows for virtually free, unhampered movement. Consisting of a vest, pelvic band, and a series of straps (Fig. 17–8D), it is more acceptable to the children than the previously used braces. The indications for its use are still being developed, but it appears to be a promising alternative to the traditional care for this adolescent problem.

Bracing is instituted after progression of a deformity has been documented. A part-time bracing program (12 hours per day) may be recommended if the curvature is between 15 and 20 degrees, progression is seen, or there is a positive family history of scoliosis. In most cases, however, full-time bracing is required until signs of skeletal maturity are evident. Maturation signals include development of secondary sexual characteristics and, in females, the onset of menses. Radiologic evidence of maturation can be seen on hand x-ray films when the epiphyses have closed (Fig. 17–9A) or pelvic x-ray films when complete excursion and fusion of the iliac apophyses have occurred (Fig. 17–9B). Spinal muscle strengthening exercise is an important adjunct to all full-time (23 hours per day) brace programs. Without it, trunk musculature loses tone and, after prolonged bracing, requires extensive rehabilitation.

Nursing Management.
Bracing for scoliosis or kyphosis is a complex undertaking for the health care team, client, and family. A full-time bracing program places tremendous emotional stress on the client, and some children simply cannot deal with it in addition to the stresses of adolescence. Table 17–5 provides client guidelines for bracing for spinal deformity. To prevent psychological problems, signs of problems need to be recognized early and bracing programs must be modified or discontinued. Discontinuation of treatment protocols and possible consequences (e.g., a possible need for surgery at

TABLE 17–4. *Treatment Options for Scoliosis and Kyphosis*

	OBSERVATION	EXERCISE	BRACING AND EXERCISE	SURGERY
Scoliosis	5–20 degrees	Not recommended	20–40 degrees	>40 degrees
Kyphosis		40–50 degrees	50–70 degrees	>70 degrees

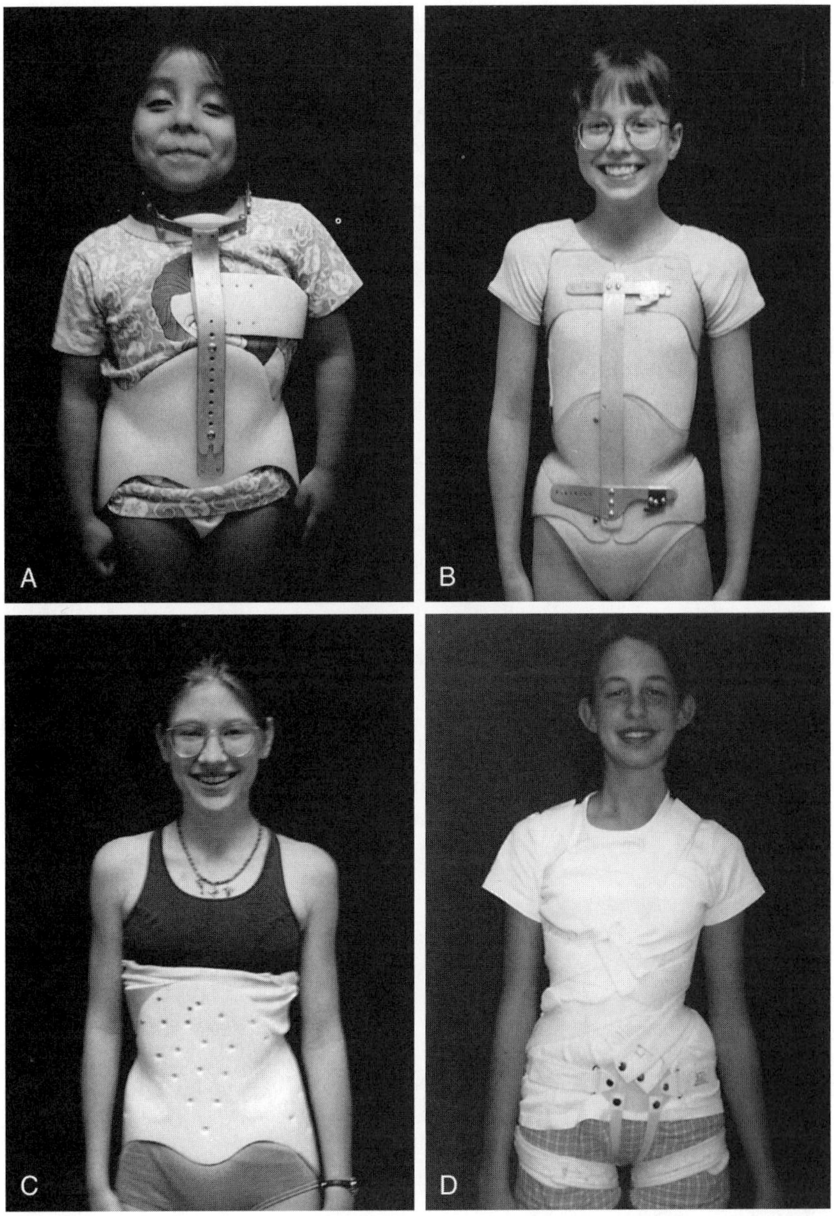

FIGURE 17–8. *A,* The Milwaukee brace is most commonly used today for the treatment of thoracic kyphosis. *B,* The Lyon brace is one of many underarm braces available for the treatment of thoracic, thoracolumbar, and thoracic/lumbar curvatures. This brace avoids the unsightly neck ring that most clients find difficult to cope with. *C,* The Boston brace is used for curves of the thoracolumbar and lumbar spine with an apex below T9. *D,* The newest brace available to control both thoracic and lumbar scoliosis, the SpineCor Flexible brace is under investigation to ensure its efficacy.

some future date) need to be explained to clients and families.

The most common problem associated with corrective braces is skin irritation and breakdown. Both can be avoided by meticulous skin care. Smooth cotton T-shirts or cotton tubes should be worn under braces at all times to avoid direct skin and brace contact. This garment should be changed daily and laundered. If a skin rash develops, laundering with a mild soap (e.g., Ivory, Dreft) often alleviates the problem. In warm climates, the undergarment should be changed more frequently. Body lotions and powders are discouraged. These products can combine with perspiration to form a sticky buildup, which may irritate the skin.

Clients are told to gradually increase the time spent each day wearing the brace, so that by 10 days after receipt of the brace, the prescribed duration per day has been achieved. Redness of the skin under the pads is expected. Rubbing the reddened areas with alcohol after a daily shower or bath helps toughen skin and allows it to withstand the pressure. Rarely, clients may have continued skin problems and may develop an allergy to the pad material, necessitating a change in padding.

Some clients have difficulty eating if an orthosis is tight. In most cases, the brace can be loosened during meals and for the first 30 minutes after each meal to allow adequate nutritional intake. Clients wearing the Milwaukee brace have the additional concern of the neck ring, which limits their range of motion. Difficulties encountered with school activities (e.g., reading, writing) may be alleviated with the use of a slant desk or podium placed on the desk to bring school materials to eye level.

One of the most difficult problems with wearing a brace is finding suitable clothing to go over the brace. Loose-fitting shirts or shirts with buttons down the front work well, as do pants or skirts with elastic waists. To protect clothing from brace hinges and screws, the client should be instructed to cover the hinges and screws with tape or Molefoam (Dr. Scholl product), which is used to protect the feet from shoe pressure points. The client guidelines (see Table 17–5) summarize client education for the client wearing a brace.

Surgical Treatment for Spinal Deformities. Surgical intervention for spinal deformity is recommended only after thorough evaluation of each client's clinical indications (diagnosis, degree of curvature, deformity, decompensation, and neurologic status) and other pertinent data (age, health status, social history, emotional stability, and readiness to undergo a major surgical procedure). There are general guidelines for surgical intervention, but these can be altered depending on individual circumstances. Surgical treatment is recommended when scoliotic curves are greater than 45 degrees and progression is noted. Kyphosis requires surgical intervention when the curvature measures greater than 65 degrees.

The surgical approach to the spine can be posterior or anterior depending on diagnosis and location of deformity. In almost all cases, spinal fusion is the ultimate goal. Spinal fusion is the healing of one vertebra to an adjacent one, so as to prohibit motion between them. A bone graft is taken from another area of the body (e.g., iliac crest, fibula, tibia, rib) and is used to create a bony ankylosis (fusion) from one vertebra to the next.

The spinal surgeon may recommend any combination of surgical procedures. Once the surgical plan has been established, a detailed explanation should be provided to all involved. The spinal surgery client and family often benefit from speaking with clients who have already completed the proposed plan. The client should be referred to another person who has undergone the exact program that is being proposed. Because of the complex nature of these procedures, clients may become confused if counseled by someone who has even a slightly different problem.

Posterior Approach. The posterior approach consists of a long, straight, midline incision extending one to two levels above and below the segments to be fused. The musculature is retracted, and the posterior elements are decorticated to provide a better environment for bone healing. Most commonly, an iliac bone graft is obtained either through the same incision or through a separate incision made over the iliac crest. The graft is placed next

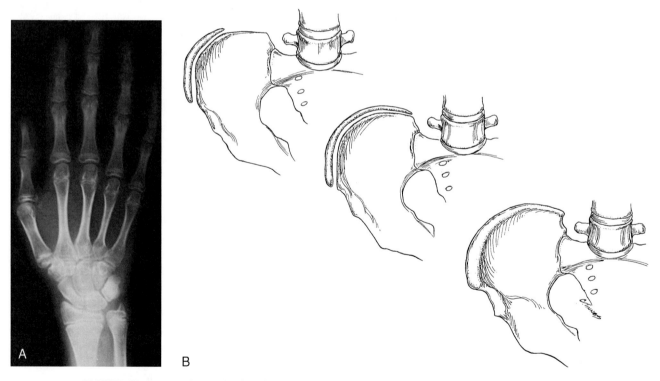

FIGURE 17–9. *A,* Radiograph of the hand taken to evaluate skeletal maturity. *B,* The iliac apophysis is another indicator of growth. The apophysis is first seen at the lateral aspect of the pelvis, with completion of growth expected when the iliac apophysis is completely across and fused to the pelvis. (*A* from Greulich, W. W., & Idell Pyle, S. [1959]. *Radiographic atlas of skeletal development of the hand and wrist* [2nd ed.]. Stanford: Stanford University Press. With the permission of the publishers, Stanford University Press. © 1950 and 1959 by the Board of Trustees of the Leland Stanford Junior University.)

TABLE 17–5. *Client Guidelines: Bracing for Spinal Deformity*

	FITTING FOR BRACE	DURING BRACE TREATMENT	AFTER DISCONTINUATION OF BRACE USE
Setting	Orthotist's office	Physician's office	Yearly follow-up
Activity		Gradual increase in wearing time	Continue full activity with no restriction
		Trunk muscle strengthening exercises	
		Removal of brace and full participation in physical education class	
		Removal for 1 hour per day for hygiene and exercises	
Tests		Radiographs are taken 1 month in brace to ensure maintenance and partial correction of curve in brace	Radiographs taken at yearly follow-up examinations
Diet	Normal diet	Normal diet	
		If difficulty arises when eating, loosen brace during the meal and for the first 30 min after	
Teaching	Discuss the brace molding process	Hygiene—daily shower and change of T-shirt or tube	Immediately following brace removal there may be slight discomfort noted, which will disappear within a few days
	All efforts are made to protect your privacy	Watch for skin irritation	
	Bring a jogging suit with you to the orthotist's office to wear with the new brace	If a sore develops, discontinue brace and call the nurse or physician immediately	
		If the skin is reddened, alcohol may be used	
	Do not buy new clothing until you have the brace to ensure the correct size	Do not use lotion or powder under the brace	
		Allergy to the brace padding is unusual but may require changing of the pad material	
	Do not be discouraged; the first few days of bracing are tough, but it does get better!	Bracing is necessary until growth is complete, which usually occurs 2 years after the onset of menses in females and when the Risser sign is 4	
		Wear loose-fitting shirts or shirts with buttons down the front	
		Wear pants, skirts, or shorts with elastic waists Cover brace hinges and screws with tape or Molefoam to protect clothing	

to the decorticated spine to create the environment for fusion. Spinal fusion begins to occur from the operative day, although radiographic evidence of fusion may take 4 to 6 months to appear.

Various types of instrumentation are used to stabilize and obtain some correction of the deformity. Surgeons choose the type of instrumentation based on the following considerations: (1) diagnosis, (2) magnitude of curvature, (3) flexibility of the curve, (4) age of the client, (5) inherent strength of bone, (6) the client's ability to wear postoperative immobilization devices, and (7) the surgeon's familiarity with the instrumentation system.

Segmental instrumentation provides multiple points of fixation along the spinal column, allowing earlier return to activity, often without bracing. The Cotrel-Dubousset (CD) system was the first such system to be developed. Other segmental fixation instrumentation systems include the Texas Scottish Rite Hospital (TSRH), ISOLA, and Moss-Miami methods.

Each of these systems provides multiple points of

fixation and thus achieves greater postoperative stability than those previously used. Each system consists of a minimum of two rods, multiple hooks, and a transverse coupling device (Fig. 17–10). Although the surgical implantation of segmental instrumentation is technically more difficult, the system's greatest asset is that no postoperative immobilization is required. Clients are ambulatory on the second postoperative day and are discharged within 1 week after surgery. In spine centers where numerous surgical procedures are performed weekly, there does not appear to be any increased risk associated with this procedure. A brace may be prescribed (Fig. 17–11) after surgery.

Used less today are the Harrington rod system and the Luque system. The Harrington system is still used, partly because of its availability and because many practitioners are familiar with it. This system was developed in the early 1960s and has been the cornerstone on which advancements in spinal surgery have been built (Dickson & Harrington, 1973). The simplest of Harrington systems consists of one rod and two hooks. However,

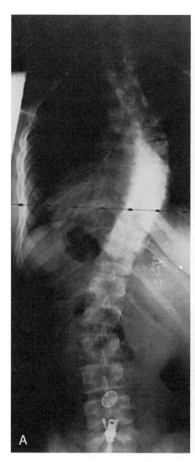
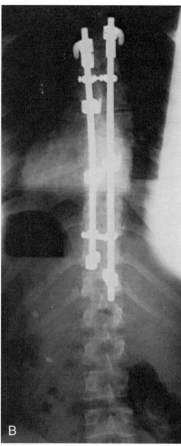

FIGURE 17–10. Preoperative *(A)* and postoperative *(B)* posteroanterior x-ray films with Cotrel-Dubousset instrumentation.

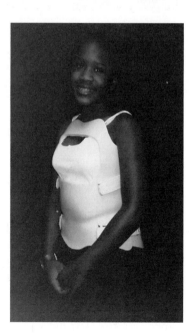

FIGURE 17–11. Thoracolumbar sacral orthosis.

these can be augmented by placement of spinous process wiring. Wires placed through the base of spinous processes and around the Harrington rod provide multiple points of fixation.

The Luque system is an alternative type of posterior instrumentation. This system consists of two rods with sublaminar wires placed at every vertebral level. The Luque system offers significant stability, but there is an increased incidence of neurologic problems attributable to passage of the sublaminar wires. This system is used most often in clients who are already neurologically compromised (e.g., neuromuscular disease, paralysis).

A posterior or anterior osteotomy is performed when the spine has autofused or has previously been surgically fused and mobility of the spine is necessary for further correction of deformity. An *osteotomy* is defined as cutting through a previous fusion mass to provide mobility. Extreme care is needed to avoid contact with neural structures.

Anterior Approach. The anterior approach to the spine is often used, especially under the following conditions: (1) lumbar scoliosis in an adolescent client, (2) lumbar scoliosis in an adult client (in the first of a two-stage procedure), and (3) kyphosis in both adult and adolescent clients (to provide anterior fusion and anterior column stability).

A thoracotomy or thoracoabdominal approach is performed, and a rib is removed. The thoracic or abdominal contents are retracted to allow visualization of the spine. The discs are then removed and replaced with autogenous rib bone grafts, rib strut grafts, or fibular strut grafts, depending on the specifics of the surgical procedure. Often, no instrumentation is placed anteriorly, and correction is achieved through posterior instrumentation. This may be accomplished by turning the client after closing the anterior incision and doing a posterior approach under the same anesthetic. Another option is to wait a few days and perform a posterior approach as a separate procedure.

If instrumentation is used, the most common types of anterior instrumentation are the Zielke, Harms, Moss, and Kaneda systems. After disc excision, screws are placed across vertebral bodies generally at 4 to 6 levels, and a rod is placed through the ends of the screw heads. The rod is then tightened to achieve maximum correction of the deformity. These instrumentation systems provide better control over maintenance of sagittal alignment and are therefore commonly used (Fig. 17–12).

Thoracoscopic approach to the spine is becoming more common (Connelly & Manges, 1998; Kuklo & Lenke, 2000; Nymberg & Crawford, 1996; Picetti, Blackman, O'Neal, & Luque, 1998; Regan, Ben-Yishay, & Mack, 1998). This allows the spinal surgeon to perform an anterior disc excision and fusion using the same principles as arthroscopic surgery. Through strategically placed portals, the anterior spine is approached, allowing disc excision and fusion. Initial work is being done with the placement of spinal instrumentation to correct spinal deformity. Still a new procedure, this may be a trend in the future care of certain spinal deformities.

In selected clients, anterior and posterior spinal fusion may be performed simultaneously. An advantage to this approach is shorter hospitalization and less time spent in bed with possible subsequent problems. The disadvantage is the magnitude of anterior and posterior spinal fusion with instrumentation for deformity. Postoperative pain management, pulmonary hygiene, and mobilization require expertise.

Traction. Although traction is not used often today, severe deformities may require the slow, closely monitored correction that this technique provides. This system consists of a halo (a round metal band that is affixed to the outer table of the skull by four screws) and weights that are suspended from the halo. Body weight thereby provides countertraction. The benefit of halo-gravity traction is that the client can be mobile either when in a wheelchair or when using a walker (Fig. 17–13). A radiograph of the cervical spine should be obtained at intervals to guard against overdistraction. A neurologic assessment should be performed every 4 hours and after

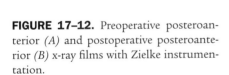

FIGURE 17–12. Preoperative posteroanterior *(A)* and postoperative posteroanterior *(B)* x-ray films with Zielke instrumentation.

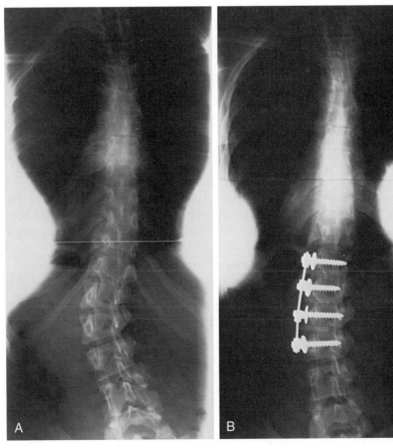

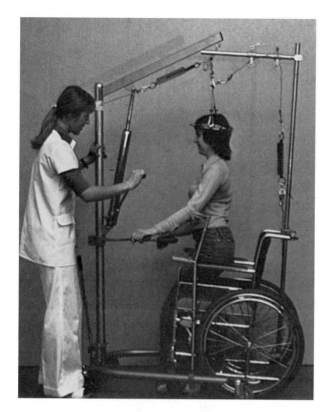

FIGURE 17–13. A client in halo-gravity wheelchair traction being transferred to a halo-gravity walker. (Photograph courtesy of Klause Zielke, M.D.)

any change in traction position. This should include examination of cranial nerves to discern subtle changes in neurologic status while halos are in place. If changes are seen, weights should immediately be decreased and the orthopaedic service notified.

Meticulous care of pin sites should be taken to avoid pin site infection or subsequent loosening, which would necessitate premature removal of halo traction. Controversy exists over the best method of pin care. In our medical center, halo pin sites are cleansed every 8 hours with sterile water. A small amount of antibiotic ointment is placed around each pin site. At the next cleansing, all antibiotic ointment is removed and is not allowed to become encrusted. To facilitate observation of the pin and pin care, the hair should be kept closely trimmed around the pin. If the pin site becomes reddened, swollen, painful, or loosened, the pin must be relocated. For further discussion of pin care, see Chapter 12.

The client in halo-gravity traction requires close nursing supervision and assistance for all activities, including hygiene and nutrition. Because of significant limitations, the client requires maximal assistance. Secondary to limited range of motion of the cervical spine, all intake should be monitored and nausea or vomiting prevented. If nausea or vomiting occurs, the client should not be allowed any nutrition by mouth until the situation has been corrected. The surgeon should be consulted as to whether slight elevation of the head of the bed or the

side-lying position can be instituted to facilitate oral nutrition.

An explanation before surgery of postoperative traction techniques is necessary to alleviate fear. Traction is often applied 2 or 3 days before the initial surgical procedure in an effort to increase client and family understanding of the process. Constant reassurance by the nurse and availability of nursing personnel are mandatory until the client is comfortable and confident in the traction system.

Complications. As with any surgical procedure, there are potential complications. In addition to the complications discussed in Chapter 10, specific concerns as they relate to spinal surgery need to be understood. The most devastating complications in spinal surgery are death and paralysis. The 1999 Scoliosis Research Society Morbidity and Mortality Report revealed that out of the 16,053 spinal surgeries performed by 48% of its members, there were 37 deaths (0.0023% incidence). In that same review, 3550 clients underwent spinal surgery for scoliosis and 9 deaths were reported (0.0025% incidence). All clients undergoing major spinal surgery should be evaluated for potential risk factors, such as decreased pulmonary function and coagulation disorders. The necessary steps should be taken to avoid intraoperative or postoperative complications (Bridwell, Lenke, Baldus, & Blanke, 1998).

Neurologic loss following scoliosis surgery has been reported. In this same review, a 0.67% incidence of neurologic loss was noted in scoliosis surgery (Morbidity and Mortality Committee Report, 1999). An overall complication rate in adolescent idiopathic scoliosis of 7.3% was reported, which included death, neurologic compromise, deep infection, superficial infection, urinary tract infection, respiratory problems, spinal fluid leakage, excessive blood loss, and implant problems.

Techniques available for intraoperatively monitoring spinal cord function include somatosensory-evoked potentials (SSEPs), motor-evoked potentials (MEPs), and the Stagnara wakeup test. SSEPs are the electrophysiologic responses of the nervous system to sensory stimulation. Stimulation of lower extremity peripheral nerves (posterior tibial nerve) is recorded from the cerebral cortex. Intraoperative tracings are compared with baseline recordings made before surgery. Changes in amplitude or latency may be the result of anesthetic agents, technical difficulties, or neurologic compromise. Knowledgeable anesthesiologists or neurologists can detect changes in SSEP or MEP tracings and the potential neurologic problems they may reflect.

The Stagnara wakeup test is an additional method for evaluating spinal cord function. The client, under close observation by the anesthesiologist, is awakened enough to follow verbal commands. For example, to demonstrate neurologic motor integrity, the client is asked to move each foot in a certain direction. This test is performed after placement of corrective spinal instrumentation or manipulation of the spine before closure. Clients must be observed closely throughout these maneuvers, however, because there have been reported cases of self-extubation, with subsequent respiratory arrest.

Respiratory problems (e.g., pneumonia, hemothorax, pneumothorax), wound infection, urinary tract infection secondary to catheterization, phlebitis and its sequelae, and significant blood loss are all potential complications of spinal surgery. In clients requiring spinal fusion and instrumentation, there is the additional concern of instrument failure and pseudarthrosis. This complication is identified several months after surgery and often requires reoperation for replacement of instrumentation and augmentation of the spinal fusion. In rare cases, instrumentation may become dislodged, causing problems such as dural leak or nerve entrapment. All spinal surgical clients should be monitored closely for signs and symptoms of complications after surgery.

LOW-BACK DISORDERS

Various disorders affect the lower back. The most common are low-back strain, herniated nucleus pulposus, spondylolysis, spondylolisthesis, and spinal stenosis. Each causes some degree of back pain, which may or may not be associated with leg pain.

Low-Back Strain

Low-back strain is by far the most common cause of back pain. Typically, it occurs following a change in activity, not necessarily related to significant trauma to the lower back. An activity as common as house cleaning may trigger a bout of low-back pain. In the United States

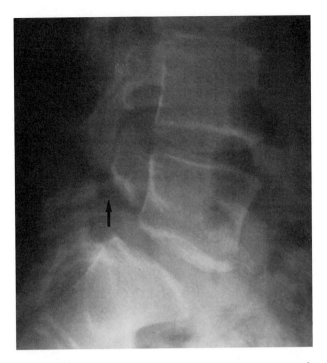

FIGURE 17–15. Lateral x-ray film demonstrating a spondylolysis.

today, low-back strain is the leading cause of days absent from work.

Herniated Nucleus Pulposus

As the annulus fibrosis ages, it loses its ability to contain the nucleus pulposus. The nucleus pulposus can then extrude through the annulus fibrosis. This pathologic condition is known as a herniated disc (Fig. 17–14). Narrowing of the canal and bulging or extrusion of the disc material into the canal are demonstrated most commonly by magnetic resonance imaging (MRI), myelogram (decreased dye at the affected level[s]), or computed tomography (CT) scan. The disc then exerts direct contact on neural structures. Initially, the nucleus pulposus may be termed *bulging*, which may or may not cause significant symptoms. The size of the spinal canal, the location of the defect, and the relative quantity of nucleus pulposus present all play roles in the treatment plan. Conservative management is often attempted in an effort to decrease symptoms, such as back and leg pain, but if neurologic deficit is present (e.g., marked weakness, bowel or bladder difficulties), surgical intervention may be necessary.

Spondylolysis

Spondylolysis is a defect or break in the neural arch between the superior and inferior articulating processes. The union between these two areas is normally bone. However, in spondylolysis, it is composed of fibrocartilaginous tissue. The client with spondylolysis does not have a forward slip visible on x-ray film, but on oblique views, the characteristic "Scottie dog with a collar" appearance of the posterior elements is observed (Fig. 17–15). Because

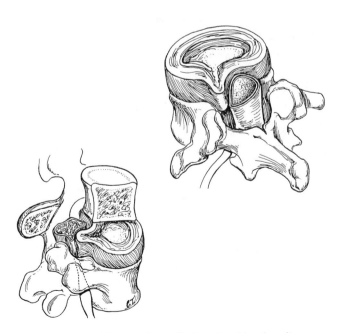

FIGURE 17–14. Drawings of a herniated lumbar disc.

of the inherent weakness in the lower spine, this condition may progress to spondylolisthesis. If an acute spondylolysis is diagnosed, management with an orthosis can sometimes aid in healing of the fracture.

Spondylolisthesis

Spondylolisthesis describes the forward subluxation of one vertebra on another, most often within the lumbosacral region of the spine (Fig. 17–16A and B). This condition may develop at an early age, but it generally does not become symptomatic until later childhood or adolescence. Various authors have discussed five different types of spondylolisthesis: congenital, isthmic, traumatic, degenerative, and pathologic. Congenital spondylolisthesis is characterized by an elongated pars interarticularis, with no other apparent defect. Isthmic spondylolisthesis occurs when there is a defect in the pars interarticularis. Traumatic spondylolisthesis is detectable as a fracture of the pars interarticularis following trauma. Degenerative spondylolisthesis is seen in the presence of degenerative facet joints and discs. The final form of this disorder, pathologic spondylolisthesis, is rare and occurs only secondary to infection or tumor.

To better understand the severity of spondylolisthesis, one must first understand the classification commonly used to describe the subluxation. Myerding (1938) developed a technique of dividing spondylolisthesis into four grades, with grade IV describing nearly complete forward slippage (Fig. 17–17A). Newman (1965) later described a system for classifying the degree of forward as well as downward slippage of affected vertebrae (Fig. 17–17B).

Spinal Stenosis

Spinal stenosis is a narrowing of the spinal canal (Fig. 17–18A and B). CT scan or myelogram can best demonstrate this narrowing. Stenosis can be either congenital or acquired (e.g., degenerative) and can occur in any region of the spine. Congenital spinal stenosis can be problematic if any other pathologic condition becomes apparent (e.g., an acute herniated disc). Significant neurologic compromise may occur if a narrowed canal is invaded by disc material.

Typically, spinal stenosis is a problem of older adults (older than 60 years of age) and is a consequence of the natural degeneration of the discs that occurs with age and any associated arthritic changes. The client's medical status and the presence of other spinal pathologic conditions determines whether conservative or surgical treatment should be undertaken.

Assessment

Nursing History. The nursing history for problems in the lower spine should focus on the chief complaint;

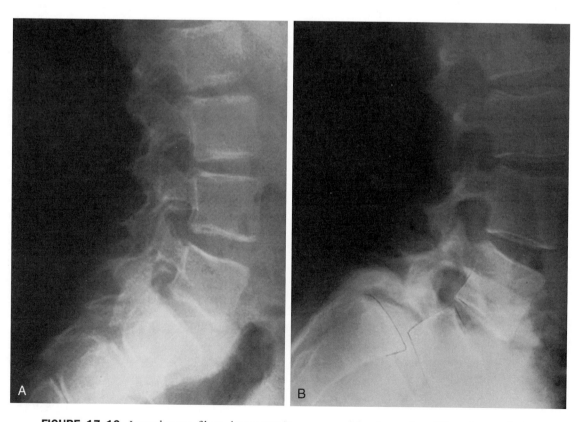

FIGURE 17–16. Lateral x-ray films demonstrating a normal lumbar spine *(A)* and a grade IV spondylolisthesis *(B)* with the forward slip of L5 on the sacrum.

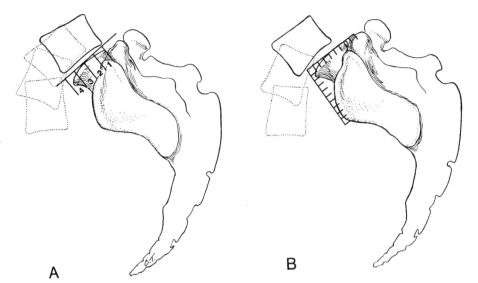

FIGURE 17–17. The Myerding (A) and Newman (B) classifications of spondylolisthesis.

symptoms, including back or leg pain, numbness, weakness, or list; the exact location of the pain or numbness; duration of symptoms; mechanism of injury; previous nonsurgical or surgical treatment; affect on occupation and family; and whether litigation is pending (see Table 17–3).

A history of how well the client is coping with the problem or disability is important. The client with chronic pain often has a difficult time coping with the situation and may warrant referral for psychological assistance and chronic pain management.

Physical Assessment. All clients being evaluated for a problem of the lower spine should have a complete orthopaedic and neurologic examination (see Chapter 8). The client should be observed for the ease with which he or she is able to move about the examination room. The client should be asked to walk normally, giving the

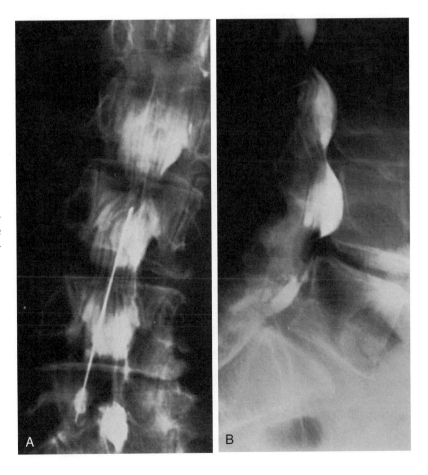

FIGURE 17–18. Anteroposterior (A) and lateral (B) x-ray films demonstrating a severe spinal stenosis. Note the irregular flow of contrast material.

examiner the opportunity to evaluate gait, specifically looking for an antalgic gait, limp, lurch, weakness, or list. Reflex testing should include patellar, Achilles, Babinski's, and clonus. Motor strength testing of all muscle groups in the lower extremities as well as pulses of the lower extremities should be performed. Pain secondary to vascular disease can mimic spinal radiculopathy. Straight leg raising should be tested with the client in the lying position and validated while the client is in the sitting position (see Table 17–3).

The client with a herniated nucleus pulposus may describe a specific incident that caused immediate leg pain and is typical of the acute disc rupture. A small tear in the annulus may allow the nucleus to rupture slowly, giving a picture of gradual but persistent onset of radicular pain. The client may also note increased pain with sneezing, coughing, or Valsalva's maneuver.

Spondylolisthesis clients usually have a history of low-back pain, sometimes radiating into the lower extremities. Increased lumbar lordosis and a waddling gait are common with more severe subluxation. Most clients are unable to touch their toes, and straight leg raising is limited. Mild scoliosis, secondary to the spondylolisthesis, may also be present. Bowel and bladder difficulties, as well as decreased motor reflex and sensation, may be present. A complete neurologic examination should be performed.

The client may first seek medical attention for increased back pain after physical activity or for attention focused on an unusual gait by family or peers. In some cases, specific situations such as a slip during a gymnastic stunt or a fall during a tennis match may be directly related to the onset of symptoms.

A client with spinal stenosis describes leg pain that begins after walking a short distance. The client walks crouched over, with the lumbar spine flexed forward, and requires frequent rest periods to achieve relief. Clients often state that they cannot shop unless they are able to bend over a grocery cart.

Diagnostic Evaluation. Radiographs, CT scan, MRI, and electromyography are helpful in identifying a problem in the lower spine. A myelogram is reserved for preoperative evaluation to further identify the pathologic condition. A discogram is used to determine the health of the disc. The injection of contrast material into the nucleus allows the disc to be visualized. Differential nerve blocks can also prove helpful in identifying difficult nerve root entrapment problems. Under x-ray visualization, a suspected nerve root sleeve is injected with dye and an x-ray film is obtained. An anesthetic agent is then injected, and pain relief is monitored. If complete pain relief is achieved, the offending nerve has been identified. If no pain relief is obtained, an additional nerve root may be tested. This technique is used only for diagnostic evaluation. Permanent relief is not intended.

Treatment Modalities and Related Nursing Management

Nonsurgical Treatments for Low-Back Disorders.
One in seven people will be affected by low-back pain. Between $20 to $50 million are lost in wages each year (Biggos, 1994). Because of the impact that low-back pain has on the general population, much attention has been placed on identifying the best treatment modalities. From assessment to treatment, this client population requires astute assessment and intervention.

Assessment. The initial assessment of the client with low-back pain should be comprehensive to determine whether a serious pathologic condition is present. Because low-back pain represents the largest group of clients requesting treatment of musculoskeletal disorders and the greatest amount of dollars being spent, numerous attempts have been made to set standards or protocols for treatment. See, for example, the Agency for Health Care Policy and Research (AHCPR) algorithms for the management of acute low-back problems in adults on pages 535 to 539. With use of a standardized method for assessment and treatment, a more consistent time frame for wellness can be established and anticipated.

Any algorithm for care must be used under the supervision of the physician or nurse with the knowledge base to determine when a treatment plan must be revised. Inconsistencies in either the history or physical examination should be viewed carefully. The use of even the simplest of modalities in an unwarranted situation may sustain the illness.

Rest. Following a complete orthopaedic and neurologic examination and the elimination of serious pathology, nonsurgical treatment programs for clients with acute low-back disorders are the first course of treatment (AHCPR, 1994). The client is placed on limited activity, with adjunctive medications and physical therapy depending on symptoms. If severe symptoms are present, a short course of bed rest may be prescribed. In most cases, side-lying with hips and knees flexed or semi-Fowler's position provides the most comfort. This regimen may be attempted for 5 to 7 days if gradual improvement is noted. Worsening of back or leg pain and worsening neurologic status are indications for re-evaluation and further diagnostic workup.

Corsets and Orthoses. Corsets may be recommended for short-term use in clients with acute low-back pain. A lumbosacral corset may be as simple as an elastic garment encircling the abdomen and lower back or as complex as a device consisting of elastic with posterior steel stays. Clients may find corsets useful for pain relief but should be cautioned not to depend on the corset because maintaining muscle tone is important for future rehabilitation.

Text continued on page 539

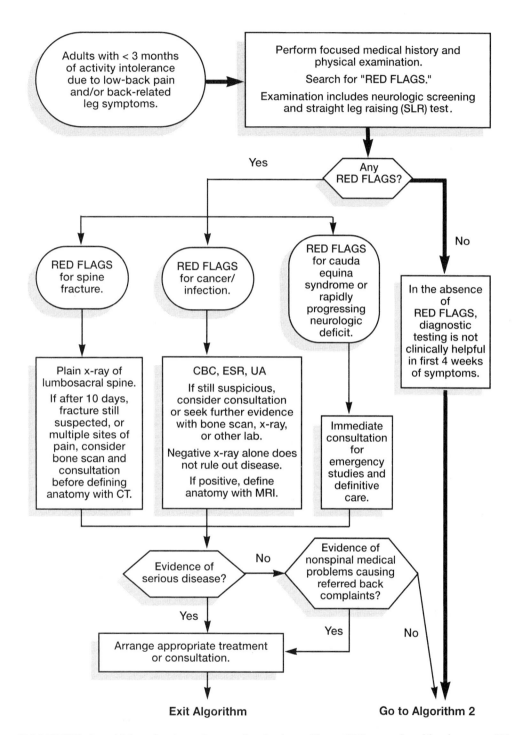

ALGORITHM 1. Initial evaluation of acute low-back problem. CBC, complete blood count; CT, computed tomography; ESR, erythrocyte sedimentation rate; UA, urinalysis. (From Agency for Health Care Policy and Research [AHCPR]. [1994]. *Algorithms for the management of acute low back problems in adults.* Clinical Practice Guideline 14, Attachment A, Publication No. 95-0642. Rockville, MD: Author.)

Initial visit

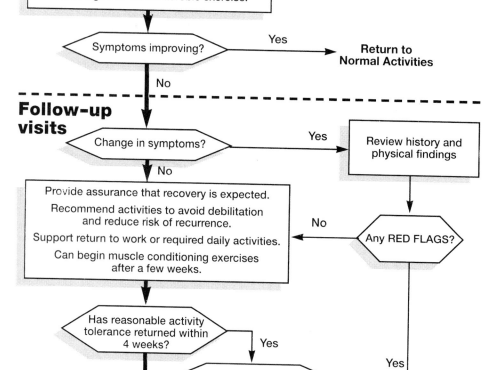

ALGORITHM 2. Treatment of acute low-back problem on initial and follow-up visits. (From Agency for Health Care Policy and Research [AHCPR]. [1994]. *Algorithms for the management of acute low back problems in adults.* Clinical Practice Guideline 14, Attachment A, Publication No. 95-0642. Rockville, MD: Author.)

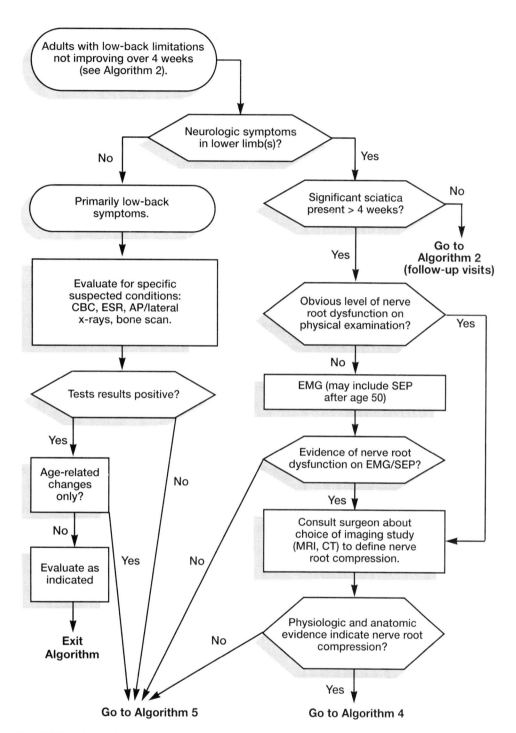

ALGORITHM 3. Evaluation of the slow-to-recover client with low-back problem (symptoms more than 4 weeks). AP, anteroposterior; CBC, complete blood count; ESR, erythrocyte sedimentation rate. (From Agency for Health Care Policy and Research [AHCPR]. [1994]. *Algorithms for the management of acute low back problems in adults.* Clinical Practice Guideline 14, Attachment A, Publication No. 95-0642. Rockville, MD: Author.)

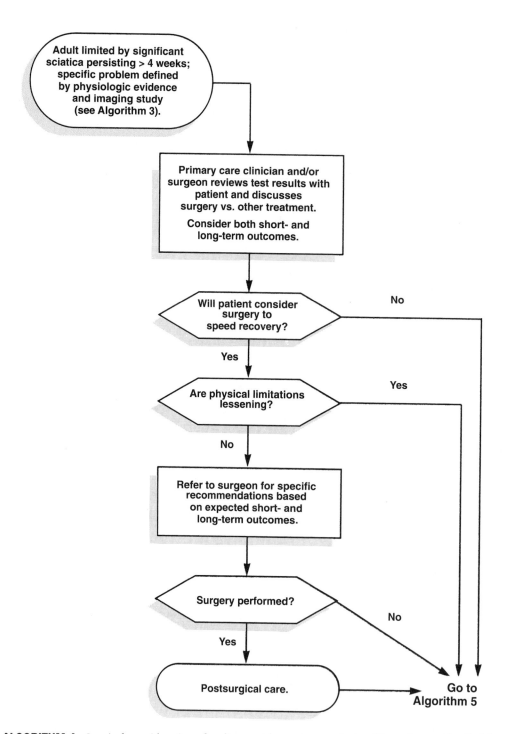

ALGORITHM 4. Surgical considerations for clients with persistent sciatica. (From Agency for Health Care Policy and Research [AHCPR]. [1994]. *Algorithms for the management of acute low back problems in adults.* Clinical Practice Guideline 14, Attachment A, Publication No. 95-0642. Rockville, MD: Author.)

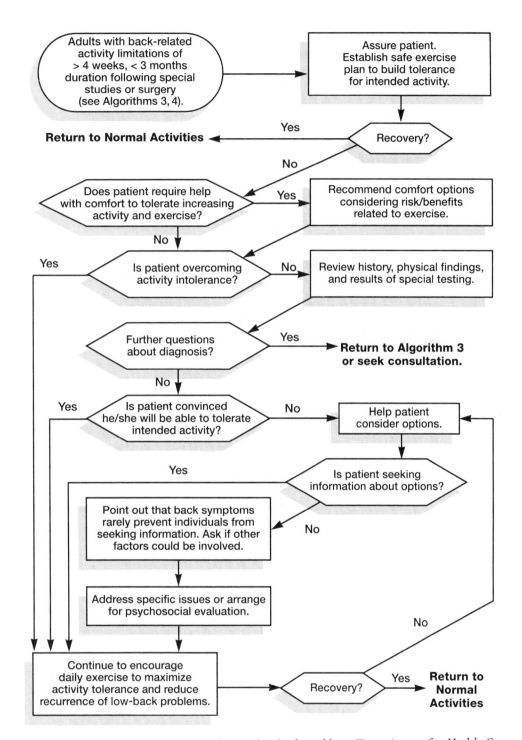

ALGORITHM 5. Further management of acute low-back problem. (From Agency for Health Care Policy and Research [AHCPR]. [1994]. *Algorithms for the management of acute low back problems in adults.* Clinical Practice Guideline 14, Attachment A, Publication No. 95-0642. Rockville, MD: Author.)

A lumbosacral orthosis is often used after surgery for spinal fusion clients. It may consist of a chair back brace or a custom-molded plastic brace (Fig. 17–19). Such an orthosis may be used as a nonsurgical treatment modality if a client's health status does not allow a major surgical procedure.

Epidural Steroid Injections. Epidural steroid injections may also be used to treat low-back and leg pain. In many centers, anesthesiologists evaluate clients and perform these injections. After sterile preparation of the posterior lumbar site, a needle is placed into the epidural space and a solution of corticosteroids is injected. This

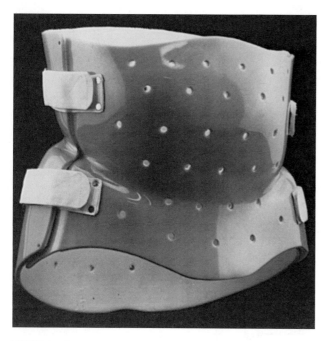

FIGURE 17–19. Custom-molded orthosis for low lumbar spine immobilization.

solution is used to bathe the spinal nerves and roots in an effort to decrease swelling and inflammation. Client responses to epidural injections vary. Some require as many as three injections at 2-week intervals, others receive complete relief with a single injection, and still others receive no relief or the pain increases.

Activity Resumption Program. Many different approaches have been used over time for the treatment of acute low-back pain. Historically, this client population was placed at bed rest for prolonged periods. These clients developed significant weakness and rehabilitation became prolonged. Today the approach ranges from the early institution of physical therapy to having the client rapidly return to routine activities. In a review of recent literature (see the evidence-based practice table in this chapter), bed rest was confirmed to increase rehabilitation time. Early increased activity showed improved outcomes, a faster rate of recovery, and a reduction in chronic pain. Specific exercises for acute pain have been found not to be as effective as early resumption of regular activities. For the client with chronic pain, exercise and alternative therapies may be beneficial.

Alternative Therapies. Different approaches such as massage therapy (Preyde, 2000), use of herbals (Chrubasik, Eisenberg, Balan, Weinberger, Luzzati, & Conradt, 2000), acupuncture, and magnet therapy have all been under evaluation as possible treatment for low-back pain. Varying results are reported, and efficacy is still being determined. It appears that increased back pain

has not occurred after use of these modalities, and some relief has been noted. Therefore, further research is needed in these areas.

Rehabilitation Programs. The management of low-back disorders has become a priority to health care professionals. Because of the large number of people who are affected by low-back pain at one time or another, either by work or recreational injuries, an increasing amount of resources are being used to identify ways to effectively treat this client population (Rodts, 1999). A comprehensive rehabilitation program should consist of a multifaceted approach utilizing the expertise of a wide range of caregivers such as physicians (physiatrists, surgeons, psychiatrists), nurses, pain management specialists, physical therapists, occupational therapists, psychologists, and social workers. A well-organized assessment program should be developed, and state-of-the-art therapy facilities should be used.

If conservative nonsurgical treatment has been successful and pain has been reduced, clients are usually placed on a rehabilitative program, sometimes referred to as "back school." The goals of this program are (1) to provide education on the anatomy of the spine and on appropriate techniques to decrease the probability of recurrence; (2) to strengthen the lower back and abdominal musculature and to regain mobility of the lumbar spine; and (3) to regain muscle tone and stamina gradually, allowing return to normal activities. A well-organized therapy program is needed to achieve maximum results.

Functional capacity evaluations help the rehabilitation nurse formulate a plan to return the client to the previous occupation or prepare the client for a new occupation. Work hardening programs are designed to simulate the job setting and gradually increase work tolerance. Elaborate work training centers exist that help facilitate return to gainful employment. Rehabilitation physicians and physiatrists now offer additional insight into this client population and often provide the necessary supervision for the more complex client.

The client with chronic pain presents a difficult management problem. The client may be postsurgical or suffering from a problem for which surgery is not indicated. These clients often benefit from participation in a pain management program. These programs use a multidisciplinary approach, including a physician, pharmacologist, psychologist, nurse, physical therapist, and social worker. The impact of potential lifelong disability secondary to pain is devastating. Every effort must be made to develop a guided program, which may consist of medications; alternative modalities such as biofeedback, massage, heat/cold therapy; counseling; and most important, an exercise program individually designed to help improve and maintain as much strength and stamina as possible within the limitations of the client's disability.

Pain management in this group of clients is essential and must be coordinated and managed by professionals who understand chronic pain, not by those who believe that all clients with chronic pain have drug-seeking behaviors. Physicians and nurses with expertise in pain management are integral to the development of a plan of care that allows the client comfort and the ability to participate in some activities of daily living.

Surgical Treatment of Low-Back Disorders. The surgical treatment of low-back disorders can be divided into those requiring posterior versus anterior approaches. Posterior surgical procedures include disc excision, percutaneous disc excision, decompression, and decompression and fusion with or without instrumentation. The anterior approach is used for anterior disc excision, placement of prosthetic devices, and anterior spinal fusion. There are

EXAMINING THE EVIDENCE: Moving Toward Evidence-Based Practice
Management of Acute Low-Back Pain

AUTHOR(S), YEAR	SAMPLE SIZE	DIAGNOSIS	DESIGN	OUTCOME VARIABLE	MAJOR FINDINGS
van Tulder et al., 2000	N = 39 randomized controlled trials	Acute and chronic low-back pain	Meta-analysis Assessing exercise for low-back pain		Specific exercises are not effective for the treatment of acute and low-back pain. Exercises may be helpful for chronic back pain and may help clients return to normal activities of daily living (ADLs)
van Tulder et al., 1998	N = 150 randomized controlled trials	Acute and chronic low-back pain	Meta-analysis Acute low-back pain = 150 trials Chronic low-back pain = 81 trials Both = 1 trial	Quality of methodology Data extracted to look at therapy, pain intensity, improvement, functional status, and positive or negative study conclusions	Acute group—nonsteroidal anti-inflammatory drugs (NSAIDs) and muscle relaxants more effective than placebo; bed rest and exercises were not effective. Chronic group—manipulation, back school, and exercise are more effective
Waddell, Feder, & Lewis, 1997	N = 18 randomized controlled trials	Acute low-back pain	Meta-analysis Evaluated the difference between bed rest and immediate activity		8 of 10 bed rest trials showed bed rest to be ineffective. 8 of 8 activity trials showed improved outcomes. 3 of 4 activity trials showed a faster rate of recovery. 4 of 5 activity trials showed less chronic pain or disability with routine activity. None of the activity trials showed activity led to adverse outcomes
Faas et al., 1995	N = 473	Acute low-back pain	Group I = no therapy (155) Group II = placebo ultrasound (162) Group III = exercise (156)	Number and duration of pain episodes; change in functional health status	No difference in all 3 groups in regards to pain recurrence or duration. Group III were less tired than Group I. No difference existed in functional status among all groups. Exercise therapy was no more effective than no therapy
Malmivaara et al., 1995	N = 186	Acute low-back pain	Group I = bed rest (67) Group II = exercise (52) Group III = control (67)	Duration of pain, pain intensity, lumbar flexion, Oswestry back-disability index, days absent from work	Bed rest group recovered more slowly in regard to pain, lumbar flexion, Oswestry back-disability index, and sick days. Exercise group had slower recovery in lumbar flexion, number of sick days. Physician visits less in control group. Maintaining regular activity and avoiding bed rest and exercises led to a more rapid recovery

specific diagnostic indications for each procedure. Important to each is accurate diagnosis regarding the level and location of the problem and verification at the time of surgery that the level can be surgically invaded.

Posterior Approach

Interdiscal electrothermal annuloplasty. Interdiscal electrothermal annuloplasty is the latest in minimally invasive procedures being developed to treat spine pain. A catheter and thermal coil are placed directly into the disc. With the client awake and the area anesthetized, heat is then introduced into the disc to shrink the nucleus pulposus and seal the outer layer of the annulus. The study results vary; more research is necessary to assure its efficacy.

Percutaneous disc excision. A small scope device is placed posteriorly into a disc and is used to vacuum disc material out. This technique is most appropriate for contained lateral discs. It is not indicated for extruded discs.

Laminectomy. The standard surgical therapy for lumbar disc disease is still limited laminectomy and disc excision. A small posterior approach laminectomy or partial laminectomy is performed to allow appropriate visualization and removal of disc material. Removing only the necessary bone during laminectomy is important to help maintain structural stability.

Recovery after either of these procedures is rapid and requires a minimal hospital stay. Clients should be warned, however, against increasing activities too quickly. For approximately 3 weeks after discharge, they should be restricted in the length of time they are allowed to remain in a sitting position (e.g., bathroom activities plus sitting periods of no more than 15 to 20 minutes). This allows the affected nerve root to maximally recover.

Decompression. Posterior decompression is recommended if neural contents are compressed secondary to spinal stenosis. This procedure requires a posterior midline approach, with removal of offending bony structures. Laminectomy alone may be adequate, but further lateral decompression may be necessary depending on the exact location of the defect. If stenosis occurs at more than one level, multilevel decompression may be necessary.

Fusion. Once the posterior elements have been removed and neural structures are freed of compression, the stability of the spine must be determined. When the spine is in jeopardy of increased motion, spinal fusion on affected segments is performed, using either autologous bone graft or allograft.

Instrumentation may be indicated as an adjunct to help immobilize the spine. Pedicle screws are currently being used with many different devices available. After a posterior incision is made, screws are placed through the pedicles and into the vertebral body. Plates or rods are

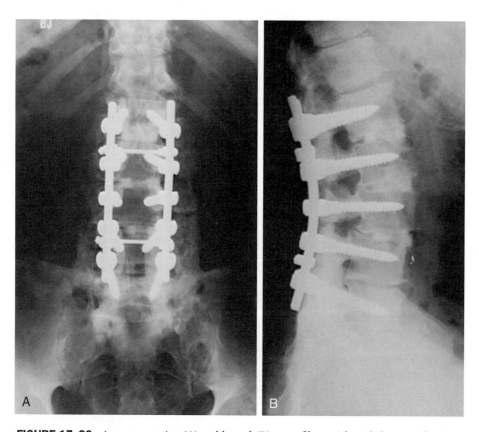

FIGURE 17–20. Anteroposterior *(A)* and lateral *(B)* x-ray films with pedicle screw fixation.

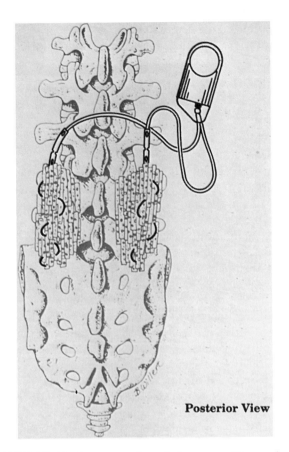

FIGURE 17–21. Demonstration of placement of internal spinal stimulation leads. (Courtesy of EBI Medical Supplies, Parsippany, New Jersey.)

used to connect the screws with cross-linking devices to add further stability (Fig. 17–20). Many surgeons believe that increased stability allows for earlier ambulation and rehabilitation and decreases the incidence of complications. In the hands of competent spinal surgeons, pedicle screws are the best alternative for lumbar fixation. A posterior lumbar interbody fusion (PLIF) may also be performed when the cauda equina is mobile and when fusion of the anterior column of the spine would be beneficial. This allows for placement of bone graft or prosthetic device that provide structural support. Braces are often used after surgery to provide additional support.

Anterior Approach. An anterior approach to the lumbar spine is often used to help achieve fusion healing in clients who have not previously achieved fusion. It may also be used as an initial approach if the potential for posterior fusion healing is decreased, for example, in severe spondylolisthesis. The level or levels that need to be fused determine the surgical approach. An increased risk of retrograde ejaculation in males has been reported after anterior lumbosacral spine fusion (Bradford, Lonstein, Ogilvie, & Winter, 1987). General surgeons are usually present for this type of procedure, and male clients

should be counseled regarding the possibility of postoperative sterility. The anterior approach allows direct placement of bone graft or prosthetic devices into the disc space.

Spinal electric stimulation as an adjunct to spinal fusion to enhance fusion rate has been proven to be successful. Both internal and external devices are available. Internal leads are placed during a surgical procedure or during a second surgical procedure if a spinal fusion is not successful (Fig. 17–21). The external system consists of a corset-like appliance worn by the client for a minimum of 3 hours per day (Fig. 17–22). The client can be ambulatory and participate in regular activities while wearing the stimulator. This is often the preferred method for bone stimulation because it does not require an additional surgical procedure.

CERVICAL SPINE DISORDERS

As in other areas of the spine, strains, herniated nucleus pulposus, degenerative disc disease, and spinal stenosis are also possible in the cervical spine. The anatomy of the cervical spine is much different from that of the thoracic or lumbar spine. The cervical spine is reliant on the tendons, muscles, bony anatomy, and disc bonds for stability. It does not have the additional protection of the visceral organs, ribs, and large groups of muscles, as are found in the thoracic and lumbar spine. The cervical spine canal has the smallest diameter; therefore, a pathologic condition that develops can cause problems easily. In addition, cervical spine disease is associated with potential catastrophic outcomes if undetected and untreated.

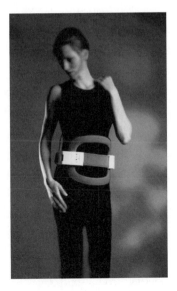

FIGURE 17–22. Client wearing an external bone stimulator. (Photo courtesy of Orthofix Inc.)

Assessment

Nursing History. In addition to the history discussed previously for problems in the lower spine, the client should be questioned about any areas of weakness, sensory changes, or upper extremity pain.

Physical Assessment. As stated earlier, the client should have a complete orthopaedic and neurologic examination. Specific attention should be focused on the upper extremities, looking for reflex, sensory, or motor changes.

Diagnostic Evaluation. Radiographs, CT scan, MRI, and electromyography help identify cervical spine problems. An invasive procedure, such as a myelogram, is used less often since the emergence of MRI.

Treatment Modalities and Related Nursing Management

Nonsurgical Treatments for Cervical Spine Disorders

Rest. Almost everyone will experience an episode of neck pain at some point. The client who awakes with neck pain can often be adequately treated with rest and modalities. The person who has sustained an injury in which instability of the cervical spine has been ruled out benefits by a course of rest, modalities, and sometimes physical therapy.

Orthoses. A soft cervical collar provides support to the neck and should be used for short-term treatment. If cervical spine instability is suspected and surgery to stabilize the spine is not possible, stability must be achieved by an orthosis, such as a Philadelphia collar, SOMI brace, or halo and vest. The client must be educated about the importance of following instructions about brace removal. If instability of the spine is present, the brace should not be removed unless the physician so instructs.

Cervical Traction. Cervical traction can be used for both stable and unstable cervical spine problems. For the client who has a strain, home cervical traction can often provide comfort during the initial postinjury phase. Cervical traction in the hospital setting is often used to immobilize the client while other injuries are being tended to and before application of an orthosis or surgical intervention.

Surgical Treatment. Both the posterior and anterior spine approaches can be used in the cervical spine. Although surgical decompression and fusion can be performed without instrumentation, instrumentation such as wires, plates, screws, and cages often is used to help stabilize the spine and facilitate fusion healing.

Depending on the degree to which the spine is stabilized, an orthosis or halo may be necessary after surgery.

COMMON NURSING CONCERNS FOR THE CLIENT WITH A SPINE DISORDER OR SPINAL SURGERY

Rehabilitation and prevention of complications are the orthopaedic nurse's primary responsibility. In this role, the nurse has the opportunity to direct and coordinate, in conjunction with other members of the health team, some of the most important aspects of spinal nursing care.

Rehabilitation begins immediately after a client makes the decision to participate in a treatment program. If the treatment consists of surgery, a presurgical and postsurgical plan can be developed. Presurgical plans range from simple to complex, depending on the magnitude of surgical intervention. General presurgical considerations include (1) general medical clearance and investigation of potential problems (e.g., pulmonary status, coagulopathy), (2) complete explanation of the treatment plan, (3) physical therapy to increase stamina, (4) autologous blood donations, and (5) discharge requirements (e.g., assistance devices for home use, day care for the children of an adult client, temporary day care for siblings [if the client is a child], home tutors, home health aides for families who cannot take time away from jobs). Clarifying early what will be required and making appropriate arrangements prevent later problems and facilitate early discharge.

Nursing Management

Knowledge Deficit

Teaching: Disease Process and Procedure/Treatment. The client and family must have a thorough understanding of the spinal problem, the proposed plan of care and time frame to complete that plan of care, the importance of compliance with the treatment regimen, and the repercussions of treatment failure. Because many spinal problems are not emergent, a logical and well-planned course can be developed to provide all the necessary information to the client.

Successful treatment is based on client compliance. Compliance is often difficult because of the length of treatment, as in bracing for scoliosis or avoidance of recreational activities after spinal surgery. Identification of methods to help follow the treatment plan and not compromise it should be explained to the client; for example, the client may be allowed to remove a brace used for the nonoperative treatment of scoliosis for a special function. This gives the child the opportunity to participate in peer activities with the understanding that this is a special allowance.

Pain

Pain Management. In the course of treatment, every client with a spine disorder has alteration in comfort ranging from discomfort secondary to the application of a brace to postoperative pain. Management is based on the problem and the severity of the discomfort. Children wearing braces for management of deformity can easily be managed by a gradual, increasing brace-wearing schedule. At most, the child may require acetaminophen.

The surgical client requires the use of intravenous opioids for 24 to 72 hours after surgery, depending on the surgical procedure. Patient-controlled analgesia (PCA) with a continuous infusion of morphine is the preferred method of postoperative pain management. With client education and parental and nurse encouragement, young children have been successful using PCA. Although some physicians were concerned about an increased incidence of ileus using PCA, this has not been validated. Once the client is tolerating a liquid diet, pain management can be achieved by oral analgesics, such as acetaminophen with codeine or hydrocodone bitartrate. Adjunctive therapy with muscle relaxants, such as diazepam, is also indicated. The postoperative client requires pain management for a minimum of 2 to 3 weeks after spinal surgery. A gradual reduction of opioids is indicated after long-term use. On occasion, the postoperative spinal surgery client has persistent pain, and consultation with the pain management center is a benefit to both the client and the staff. Because many spine surgical clients have had long-term pain problems, it is imperative to have knowledgeable health care providers with an expertise in pain management as part of the spine care team. Consistent and continued pain management support are critical for optimal results.

Alteration in Nutrition: Less Than Body Requirements

Nutrition can be affected by a tight orthosis, nothing-by-mouth (NPO) status following surgery, anesthetic agents, loss of appetite or nausea secondary to opioid use, and ileus. Maintenance of nutrition is managed in the new brace wearer by allowing the brace to be loosened for a short time during and after meals.

Diet Staging. The postoperative client requires precise nutritional management to prevent nausea and vomiting. Frequent monitoring of bowel sounds is performed. A slow resumption of diet is encouraged once bowel patency has been ensured. Ileus may develop secondary to opioid use or tightened structures following correction of deformity. If distention, nausea, or vomiting is present, diet should be restricted until the symptom subsides. In the client who has significant vomiting, a superior mesenteric artery syndrome (cast syndrome) should be suspected (see Chapter 12). Treatment consists of NPO status, sedation, and stomach decompression by nasogastric tube to low suction. Generally, within 48 to 72 hours, the ileus or obstruction abates, and the diet may be slowly increased.

Risk for Wound Infection

Infection Protection and Control. As in any surgical procedure, astute intraoperative and postoperative nursing care is necessary to protect the client from wound infection. Maintenance of a sterile environment in the operating room and protection of the surgical site in the early postoperative period are mandatory. The client's vital signs and laboratory values should be examined for signs of infection (e.g., elevated temperature, rising white blood cell count or erythrocyte sedimentation rate). The wound should be observed for any signs of infection (e.g., redness, fluctuation, drainage, an inordinate amount of pain). Wound and blood cultures may be indicated if positive findings are noted.

Fluid Volume Deficit

Blood Products Administration. The client requiring a multilevel spinal surgical procedure often has a shift in fluid balance secondary to blood loss and the use of hypotensive anesthesia. It is common for blood replacement to be necessary. Because of increasing concerns about human immunodeficiency virus (HIV) and non-A, non-B hepatitis, autologous blood donations before elective spinal surgery may be considered. Surgeons should estimate the total number of units of blood that may be needed. Clients are then given the option of donating blood for the surgery. If only 1 to 3 pints of blood is needed, clients are usually able to donate the blood within 35 days of surgery (within that period, the blood can be kept whole and the freezing process can be avoided). Clients undergoing multiple surgeries, however, may require 6 to 8 pints of blood. These clients may be able to donate a pint of blood at 7-day intervals, with the earliest donations frozen for later use. Although each blood bank has its own guidelines, these clients should be given iron supplements.

Children may successfully donate blood for elective spinal surgery (Murray, Forbes, Titone, & Weinstein, 1997) provided that a protocol is established to determine the amount of blood to be drawn at each time in relation to the child's weight. The process of blood donating also helps the child prepare for the surgery and believe that he or she has an active participatory role rather than a passive role.

Autotransfusion. Autotransfusion devices are also an option for blood replacement in the operating room and postoperatively. See Chapter 10 for a further discussion of these devices.

Fluid Management. Fluid imbalance can occur as a result of hypotensive anesthesia, which causes temporary renal slowdown, with decreased urinary output. Increasing fluid intake only results in fluid overload and generalized edema. Diuresis occurs within 48 hours, and urinary output returns to normal.

High Risk for Peripheral Neurovascular Dysfunction

Neurologic Monitoring. As in any major surgical procedure, close postsurgical monitoring is necessary to prevent potential complications. After assessment of vital signs, the neurologic examination is most important (see Chapter 8). An examination of both the upper and lower extremities should be performed after any spinal surgical procedure to determine any changes that may be a result of the surgical procedure or a result of positioning on the operative table. Once the upper and lower extremity neurologic examination is determined to be normal, a more focused examination should be conducted. In any client having cervical spinal surgery, both the upper and lower extremities should be assessed. For lumbar surgery, the examination can be focused on the lower extremities. Any deviation from normal should be reported and documented in the client's record. As simple a comment as "My legs are heavy" should spark another neurologic examination. Sensory and motor function should be assessed every 2 hours in the first 24 hours after surgery. There have been reported cases of neurologic loss 36 hours or more after surgery, so neurologic evaluations should be made every 4 to 8 hours until discharge. The nurse can identify changes in neurologic status while performing such procedures as log-rolling and placement of suppositories.

Ineffective Breathing Pattern

Respiratory Monitoring. Because of general anesthesia, opioids, and postoperative pain, respiratory problems may arise. Pulmonary hygiene should begin immediately to prevent atelectasis and pneumonia. Hemothorax and pneumothorax have occurred after corrective surgery for deformity, even with a posterior approach, and should be suspected as possible causes if respiratory status deteriorates. Close monitoring of breath sounds alerts the nurse to these conditions as well as atelectasis and pneumonia. Deep breathing exercises and application of an incentive spirometer should be done every 1 to 2 hours for the first 24 to 48 hours after surgery and every 2 to 4 hours thereafter until the client is ambulatory.

High Risk for Disuse Syndrome

Exercise Therapy. Clients undergoing a single-level disc excision generally require little preoperative physical therapy but do require therapy in the form of exercise, back school, and possibly, work hardening in the future. Children wearing a brace for nonoperative treatment of deformity or those undergoing a spinal fusion for scoliosis also require minimal physical therapy and rehabilitation. In contrast, clients requiring multiple surgical procedures for severe scoliosis, who have become sedentary because of disability or disfigurement, do much better after surgery if they have strengthened themselves preoperatively. Clients may be asked to perform 6 to 12 months of general physical conditioning and strengthening exercises as well as spine flexibility exercises. This type of program must be individualized within the restrictions imposed by a client's symptoms and disabilities. A valuable asset to the health care team is a physical therapist, who can help identify appropriate goals and the regimen to meet such goals. It is then the nurse's responsibility to encourage and support clients to follow their conditioning programs.

Bed Rest Care. The problems of immobility have been greatly decreased by better spinal instrumentation and early mobilization using proper technique (Figs. 17–23 and 17–24). In selected cases, however, bed rest may be required, increasing the risk of complications

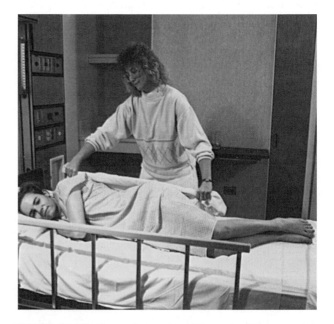

FIGURE 17–23. Draw sheet, placed from shoulders to pelvis, provides uniform support for the back as the client is turned from side to side. (From Rodts, M. F. [1997]. Nursing care of the spinal surgery patient. In K. Bridwell & R. DeWald [Eds.], *The textbook of spinal surgery* [2nd ed., p. 26]. Philadelphia: Lippincott.)

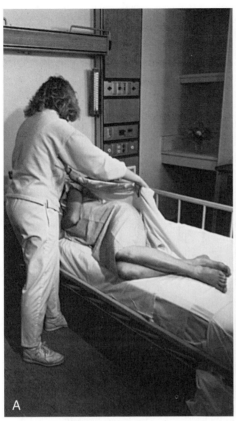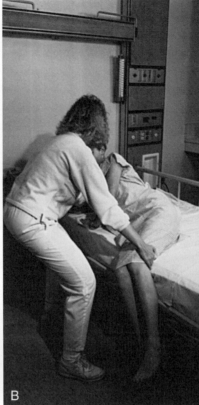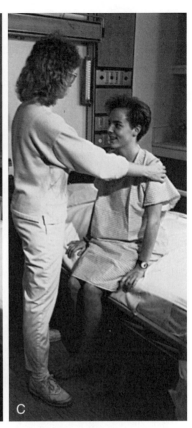

FIGURE 17–24. *A,* With the use of an appropriately placed draw sheet, the client is turned to the side-lying position. *B* and *C,* The client pushes up with the arms as the legs swing over the side of the bed in one motion. (From Rodts, M. F. [1997]. Nursing care of the spinal surgery patient. In K. Bridwell & R. DeWald [Eds.], *The textbook of spinal surgery* [2nd ed., p. 27]. Philadelphia: Lippincott.)

such as phlebitis, blood clots, pulmonary embolism, and decubitus ulcers. Prevention of these is a nursing responsibility. See Chapter 4 for a complete discussion of immobility.

Alteration in Body Image/Self-esteem Deficit

Body Image Enhancement/Self-esteem Enhancement. The client with spinal deformity or back pain with associated limitation of activities may experience an inability to cope and a diminished self-concept. Deformity is often misunderstood and misinterpreted by the health care team as not being important. Although most clients insist that the deformity is not the reason for seeking treatment, in many cases, the concern over body image is real and should be addressed. Assessing whether the client has unrealistic goals about treatment and its outcome is necessary. Early identification of grandiose expectations helps alleviate disappointment following the completion of treatment.

Role Enhancement. The client with either acute or chronic low-back pain has the fear that returning to normal work and recreational activities will not occur. In some cases, this is a valid assessment and alternatives should be discussed early in treatment.

Coping Enhancement. Many clients benefit from a psychological evaluation to help develop reasonable strategies to assist with coping and acceptance of long-term restrictions.

EXPECTED OUTCOMES

Discharge requirements can be anticipated by the orthopaedic nurse familiar with spinal surgery clients. At the time of discharge, most clients are ambulatory and have had physical therapy instructions for getting in and out of bed, gait, stair climbing, and mild upper and lower extremity exercises. Clients should be almost independent in hygiene activities, but standby assistance for showers is always a good idea for the first week after discharge (or longer if needed).

Wounds should be dry and intact at discharge. They do not require nursing evaluation unless they become swollen or reddened, drainage develops, or fever occurs. Any one of these signs may represent potential problems, and clients should be advised to call the surgeon or nurse.

A home care nurse may be appropriate if there is concern about the wound.

Nutrition is an important aspect of the recovery and healing of postsurgical clients. Wound healing requires a well-balanced diet. Clients should be discouraged from dieting during the initial recovery phase and should be encouraged to consume approximately 1200 mg of calcium per day to aid bone healing.

Return to normal activity levels as soon as possible is a major goal. Home tutors for children should be anticipated and used for the first 2 to 3 weeks after discharge. In most cases, children are allowed to return to school 3 or 4 weeks after surgery. Children who undergo more than one surgical procedure may require an additional 3 to 4 weeks at home.

Recovery in adult spinal surgery clients varies depending on the number of surgical procedures performed. A single surgical procedure generally requires 6 weeks of recovery time, and multiple surgical procedures may require 2 to 3 months. Preoperative health status significantly influences postoperative recovery.

During the first month of recovery, clients are asked to increase endurance gradually through a walking program. Starting with a distance of just 100 feet and progressing to several blocks is advised. Sitting for longer than 30 minutes is discouraged after lumbar spine surgery, which causes increased pain secondary to spinal alignment in this position. Driving is discouraged until stamina has returned and clients no longer require pain medications or muscle relaxants.

Special arrangements need to be made for clients who do not have family or other support people to oversee their first 2 to 3 weeks at home. Postsurgical clients do not require skilled nursing care but clearly

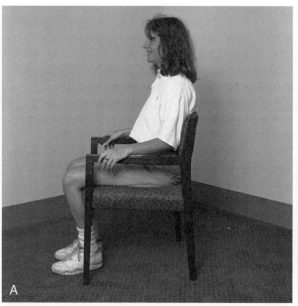

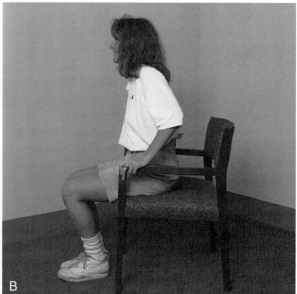

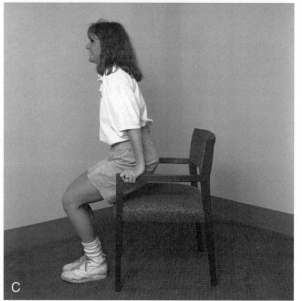

FIGURE 17–25. *A,* Client sitting correctly in a suitable chair with armrests. *B,* Preparing to rise, the client moves the buttocks to the front edge of the chair. *C,* Using the arms and legs, the client rises, keeping the back straight. (From Rodts, M. F. [1997]. Nursing care of the spinal surgery patient. In K. Bridwell & R. DeWald [Eds.], *The textbook of spinal surgery* [2nd ed., p. 28]. Philadelphia: Lippincott.)

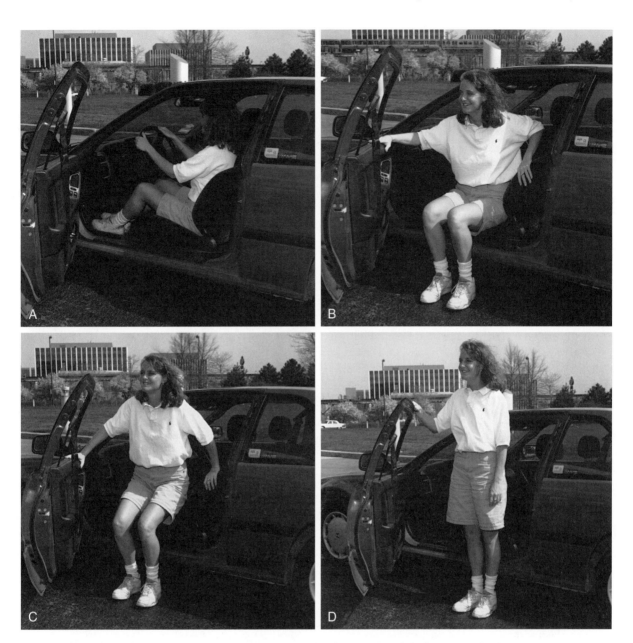

FIGURE 17–26. *A,* The client should have proper lumbar support while driving. *B,* The client prepares to exit the car by turning the entire body to place both feet firmly on the ground. *C,* Identifying stable points on the car, the client uses the upper and lower extremities to stand, limiting the amount of forward flexion. *D,* Standing is accomplished with as little lumbar flexion as possible. (From Rodts, M. F. [1997]. Nursing care of the spinal surgery patient. In K. Bridwell & R. DeWald [Eds.], *The textbook of spinal surgery* [2nd ed., p. 29]. Philadelphia: Lippincott.)

benefit by having someone available to make meals; take care of household duties; and provide child care, if needed.

Clients must be discouraged from lifting more than 5 or 10 pounds and from participating in strenuous activities. Six weeks after surgery, clients are usually allowed to increase lifting but are restricted from work and recreational activities that cause stress to the spine. Excessive bending, twisting, and stooping are discouraged. Although surgeons should provide a list of their favorite restricted activities following spinal surgery, the

most common are gymnastics, tumbling, wrestling, horseback riding, bowling, roller or ice skating, snow or water skiing, tobogganing, amusement park rides, and competitive team sports. Activities such as swimming (without diving), biking in the erect position, and walking are encouraged.

A simple activity, such as getting up from a chair (Fig. 17–25) or getting out of a car (Fig. 17–26), can be difficult for both the nonsurgical and surgical spine client. All spine clients should be instructed on the proper way to perform these activities.

INNOVATIONS AND FUTURE TRENDS

The future in spinal care will be geared toward finding ways to approach the spine through less invasive procedures. Examples of this are kyphoplasty (p. 520) and thoracoscopic spinal surgery (p. 529). Both procedures will be perfected and provide an alternative to the current surgical procedures.

SUMMARY

The spinal client has requirements for many different levels of care. Orthopaedic nurses must have an understanding of many different aspects of nursing care. Adolescents may require emotional support for brace treatment, whereas the adult undergoing multiple reconstructive surgeries for low-back pain will have different needs. As better surgical techniques develop, clients with more difficult problems are being treated surgically in an effort to better their quality of life. Nursing skills need to meet these demands to provide safe, comprehensive, orthopaedic nursing care.

INTERNET RESOURCES

Scoliosis Research Society: www.srs.org
Spine Universe: www.spineuniverse.com
Spine-health.com: www.spine-health.com

REFERENCES

Agency for Health Care Policy and Research. (1994). Acute low back problems in adults: Assessment and treatment. *Clinical Practice Guidelines, Quick Reference Guide for Clinicians, Dec*(14), iii–iv, 1–25.

Biggos, S. (1994). *Acute low back problems in adults* (AHCPR Publication No. 95-0642).

Blount, W. P. (1974, September). *The diagnosis of "hysterical" (conversion) scoliosis.* Proceedings of the ninth annual Scoliosis Research Society Meeting, San Francisco.

Bone, C. M., & Hsieh, G. H. (2000). The risk of carcinogenesis from radiographs to pediatric orthopaedic patients. *Journal of Pediatric Orthopaedics, 20,* 251–254.

Bradford, D., Lonstein, J., Ogilvie, J., & Winter, R. B. (1987). *Moe's textbook of scoliosis and other spinal deformities* (2nd ed.). Philadelphia: WB Saunders.

Bridwell, K., & DeWald, R. (Eds.). (1997). *The textbook of spinal surgery* (2nd ed.). Philadelphia: Lippincott.

Bridwell, K., Lenke, L., Baldus, C., & Blanke, K. (1998). Major intraoperative neurologic deficits in pediatric and adult spinal deformity patients. Incidence and etiology at one institution. *Spine, 23,* 324–331.

Chrubasik, S., Eisenberg, E., Balan, E., Weinberger, T., Luzzati, R., & Conradt, C. (2000). Treatment of low back pain exacerbations with willow bark extract: A randomized double-blind study. *American Journal of Medicine, 109,* 9–14.

Connelly, C. S., & Manges, P. A. (1998). Video-assisted thoracoscopic discectomy and fusion. *AORN Journal, 67,* 940–948.

DeSmet, A., Fritz, S. L., & Asher, M. A. (1981). A method for minimizing the radiation exposure from scoliosis radiographs. *Journal of Bone and Joint Surgery, 63A,* 156–158.

Dickson, J. H., & Harrington, P. R. (1973). The evolution of the Harrington instrumentation technique in scoliosis. *Journal of Bone and Joint Surgery, 55A,* 993–1002.

Faas, A., van Eijk, J. T., Chavannes, A. W., & Gubbels, J. W. (1995). A randomized trial of exercise therapy in patients with acute low back pain. Efficacy on sickness absence. *Spine, 20*(8), 941–947.

Kuklo, T., & Lenke, L. (2000). Thoracoscopic spine surgery: Current indications and techniques. *Orthopaedic Nursing, 19,* 15–22.

Malmivaara, A., Hakkinen, U., Aro, T., Heinrichs, M. L., Koskenniemi, L., Kuosma, E., Lappi, S., Paloheimo, R., Servo, C., & Vaaranen, V. (1995). The treatment of acute low back pain—Bed rest, exercises, or ordinary activity? *New England Journal of Medicine, 332*(6), 351–355.

Morbidity and Mortality Committee Report. (1999). Rosemont, IL: Scoliosis Research Society.

Morin, D. M., Lonstein, J. E., Stovall, M., Hacker, D. G., Luckyanov, N., & Land, C. E. (2000). Breast cancer mortality after diagnostic radiography: findings from the U.S. scoliosis cohort study. *Spine, 25,* 2052–2063.

Murray, D. J., Forbes, R. B., Titone, M. B., & Weinstein, S. L. (1997). Transfusion management in pediatric and adolescent scoliosis surgery: Efficacy of autologous blood. *Spine, 22,* 2735–2740.

Myerding, H. W. (1938). Spondylolisthesis: An etiologic factor in backaches. *Journal of the American Medical Association, 111,* 1971.

Newman, P. H. H. (1965). A clinical syndrome associated with severe lumbosacral subluxation. *Journal of Bone and Joint Surgery, 47B,* 472.

Nymberg, S. M., & Crawford, A. H. (1996). Video-assisted thoracoscopic releases of scoliotic anterior spines. *AORN Journal, 63,* 561–562.

Picetti, G., Blackman, R. G., O'Neal, K., & Luque, E. (1998). Anterior endoscopic correction and fusion of scoliosis. *Orthopedics, 21,* 1285–1287.

Preyde, M. (2000). Effectiveness of massage therapy for subacute low-back pain: A randomized control trial. *Canadian Medical Association Journal, 162,* 1815–1820.

Regan, J. J., Ben-Yishay, A., & Mack, J. J. (1998). Video-assisted thoracoscopic excision of herniated thoracic disc: Description of technique and preliminary experience in the first 29 cases. *Journal of Spinal Disorders, 11,* 183–191.

Rodts, M. F. (1997). Nursing care for the spinal surgery patient. In K. Bridwell & R. DeWald (Eds.), *The textbook of spinal surgery* (2nd ed.). Philadelphia: Lippincott.

Rodts, M. F. (1999). Lumbar spine. In C. Crowther (Ed.), *Primary orthopaedic care.* St. Louis: Mosby.

Tachdjian, M. (1990). *Pediatric orthopedics* (2nd ed., pp. 1773, 1886). Philadelphia: WB Saunders.

van Tulder, M. W., Malmivaara, A., Esmail, R., & Koes, B. W. (1998). Exercise therapy for low back pain. *Cochrane Database System Review,* (2), CD000335.

Waddell, G., Feder, G., & Lewis, M. (1997). Systematic reviews of bed rest and advice to stay active for acute low back pain. *British Journal of General Practice, 47*(423), 647–652.

18

Congenital and Developmental Disorders

Pediatric musculoskeletal disorders cover a wide spectrum of acute and chronic problems that may be present at birth or develop during infancy, childhood, or adolescence. There are three broad categories that these disorders fall into:

1. Conditions that will correct spontaneously with little or no medical intervention
2. Those that necessitate treatment to prevent permanent deformity or sequelae that may affect the child's growth and development
3. Chronic conditions that may require ongoing intervention beginning in infancy and extending throughout childhood and adolescence

Regardless of the nature of the problem, the nurse caring for a child with a musculoskeletal problem must remain cognizant that the entire family is the client. Identifying the family and assessing the impact of the problem on family members is an important step in the care of the pediatric client. Any problem that affects one family member can influence the entire family. Involving and supporting the family from the beginning increases their understanding, helps relieve anxiety, and facilitates optimal outcomes.

INFANTS

In the following section, the musculoskeletal problems and conditions of infants are discussed. To understand these problems it is important to begin with a knowledge base of normal findings in the neonate. Regardless of whether an abnormality is recognized at birth, every newborn should have a thorough musculoskeletal examination.

The newborn has a convex spine, with the scapulae, shoulders, and trunk musculature all appearing symmetrical. The neck rotates in all directions. The baby should be interactive and able to focus on faces or objects. The facial features are symmetrical, and the size of the limbs is equal on both sides of the body. The infant should move all extremities and have a substantial amount of strength in the legs. The lower extremities may have a considerable amount of deformity, which is normal because of the child's intrauterine position. The foot should be flexible, point straight, and move in all directions when stimulated. The heel should be well formed. All five toes should be separated. The infant's foot is flat without an arch (Alexander & Kuo, 1997).

Congenital Muscular Torticollis

Torticollis is a unilateral contracture of the sternocleidomastoid muscle that causes the head to tilt to the contracted side and the chin to turn to the contralateral side. The problem is present at birth, although it is often missed and not diagnosed until the child gains head control. The problem can result in limited range of motion (ROM) of the neck and facial asymmetry.

Etiology. The restricted neck movement and shortening of the sternocleidomastoid muscle is caused by a muscular fibrosis involving one side of the neck. The actual cause of the fibrosis is unknown, although the problem may be the result of intrauterine positioning. Pressure against the sternocleidomastoid may cause a local venous occlusion that leads to compartment syndrome in the neck and the resulting fibrosis.

Assessment

Subjective Assessment: Nursing History. Torticollis is often noted by the clinician while examining the child for some other reason. If a limitation in neck movement is suspected, the parents should be asked whether they have observed the infant turning his or her head from side to side. Often, they mention that the child favors looking in one direction.

As with all problems, the nurse should begin with a birth history and inquire whether the child was lying breech or whether there were problems with the delivery. The developmental history is very important. Visual problems, especially strabismus, can cause a torticollis. The nurse should ask if the child tracks with the eyes or has any other type of medical problems.

Objective Assessment: Physical Examination. The clinician should note the position of the head and neck. The neck ROM should be tested. The infant's neck should rotate 70 degrees bilaterally. Lateral flexion is normally 40 degrees bilaterally. With torticollis, the neck rotation is decreased toward the side of the deformity and lateral flexion is restricted on the opposite side. When the child has torticollis, the area over the sternocleidomastoid should be palpated for the presence of a hard mass (often referred to as a "tumor") felt over the distal portion of the muscle near the clavicle.

The entire spine should be examined for any deformity. The clinician should rule out scoliosis and any type of spine anomaly such as a hemivertebra. The upper extremities should be examined, with the clinician specifically looking for the presence of a hand grasp reflex and symmetrical movements in both extremities. The clinician should note the child's facial features and determine whether both sides of the face are symmetrical. The examiner should also check whether the child tracks with both eyes.

There is a strong association between torticollis and hip dysplasia. Therefore, the child with torticollis should have his or her hips examined throughout the first year of life.

Diagnostic Evaluation. Radiographs of the cervical spine should be taken to rule out any structural deformities such as a hemivertebra, Klippel-Feil syndrome, or some other congenital deformity of the neck. If visual problems are suspected, the child should be referred to an ophthalmologist for further evaluation.

Treatment Modalities and Related Nursing Management. The first intervention to be instituted is physical therapy. This should consist of passive stretching exercises and a home program to be performed by the parents on the days that the baby does not attend therapy. The sooner the therapy is begun, the less chance the child will have any residual asymmetry in the facial features and the greater likelihood the problem will be corrected with conservative measures.

For those with a mild residual deformity and no further improvement after physical therapy, a head-neck-chest orthosis can be used to hold the head straight or in

a slightly overcorrected position. This sometimes places enough stretch on the soft tissues to eliminate what is left of the deformity. Severely affected children older than 1 year of age, those who were diagnosed late, and/or those refractive to conservative treatment require surgery. A surgical release of the sternocleidomastoid is performed. The child is then put in a head-neck-chest orthosis to maintain the position for approximately 2 months; the child then undergoes more physical therapy. This is usually the definitive treatment, although the deformity can recur as the child grows older.

Nursing Management. For the newly diagnosed infant, the nurse should educate the parents about the deformity, the need for treatment, and the consequences of noncompliance. If a brace is necessary, the nurse should check the brace to ensure that it fits properly and does not irritate the skin.

The postoperative management is routine care of the incision and pain management. Again, it is the nurse's role to educate the family about having the child wear the brace consistently and properly.

Summary. Torticollis is a unilateral contracture of the sternocleidomastoid muscle that restricts neck movement and can result in facial asymmetry. Early intervention involves physical therapy. Cases that are detected after the first few months of life may be slow to respond to therapy or may require surgery. There is an increased incidence of hip dysplasia associated with torticollis.

Developmental Dysplasia of the Hip

Definition. *Developmental dysplasia of the hip* (DDH) is a nonspecific term indicating abnormal development of the hip joint. It may refer to an anomalous relationship of the head of the femur to the acetabulum, or it may be used to describe the abnormal development of the acetabulum. *Congenital dislocated hip* is a term no longer used because the disorder is not always present at birth and the hip is not always dislocated. The child may be born with the femoral heads lying in the correct position within both sockets; however, during the first year of life, one or both acetabula may cease to develop and the hip(s) become dysplastic.

Several other terms are used to describe the types of hip dysplasia that may exist. A *dislocated* hip is one in which the femoral head lies completely outside the acetabulum. A *dislocatable* hip is one in which the femoral head lies within the socket but can be manually displaced out of the acetabulum. The *subluxed* or *dysplastic* hip is one in which the femoral head lies within the acetabulum; however, the acetabulum may be shallow and may not completely cover the femoral head. A *teratologic dislocation* is one that has displaced before birth and is often associated with other congenital anomalies.

Incidence and Etiology. The incidence of hip dysplasia is approximately 10 per 1000 live births. The incidence of frank dislocation or a dislocatable hip is 1 per 1000. The left hip is involved in 60% of cases, the right hip in 20%, and both hips in 20%. Hip dislocations are 5.5 to 8 times more prevalent in girls than in boys. Caucasians have a higher incidence of developmental dysplasia than other groups.

Although the exact cause of developmental dysplasia is unknown, a number of risk factors have been identified. First, DDH has a known hereditary component. The incidence is higher in individuals with a family history and in identical twins. Generalized ligamentous laxity, also a hereditary condition, puts individuals at risk for DDH. In addition, the maternal hormones relaxin and estrogen, which are present during labor to relax the maternal pelvis for delivery, increase the laxity of the infant's hip joint. Girls are more susceptible to the effects of these hormones, which may explain why the incidence of DDH is higher in girls than in boys. Approximately 30% to 50% of children with DDH have a history of breech presentation. Restricted fetal movement increases the incidence of this disorder; thus, first-born children are at higher risk probably because tighter uterine muscles restrict fetal movement.

The presence of other congenital anomalies, especially torticollis and clubfoot, is strongly associated with an increased incidence of DDH. For this reason, the hips of these clients should be examined carefully. A screening x-ray film of the pelvis at age 3 to 4 months should be obtained to rule out DDH.

Pathophysiology. In the mildest type of hip dysplasia, the hip is unstable or dislocatable. The increased laxity of the joint capsule allows the hip to be displaced in a posterior and lateral direction to the rim of the acetabulum when adducted. This problem persists only for a short amount of time. The hip then stabilizes as surrounding soft tissue strengthens and tightens or the subluxation progresses. If the hip is not corrected, the joint capsule stretches in a lateral direction, the femoral head moves further toward the rim of the acetabulum, and the fibrocartilage labrum and cartilaginous tissue of the acetabular rim become deformed. The capsule over the medial part of the acetabulum is constricted, and the acetabular floor may fill with fatty tissue, preventing a spontaneous reduction of the femoral head. If the head is allowed to remain in a lateralized position, the development of the superior rim of the acetabulum will be affected. If the head is dislocated for a prolonged period, it becomes embedded in the muscle or begins to form a secondary or false acetabulum.

Hip dysplasia can result in a delay in the ossification of the femoral head. A prolonged dislocation can lead to the head becoming flattened against the iliac wing, a decreased distance between the femoral head and greater trochanter, and a reduction in the height of the capital femoral epiphysis (Tachdjian, 1997).

Assessment

Subjective Assessment: Nursing History. The clinician should start with questions regarding the child's birth, especially whether the child was lying in the breech position. Any family history of DDH should be noted. The child's development and overall health, including any other problems or congenital anomalies, should be included as a part of the history.

Objective Assessment: Physical Examination. In addition to the hips, the neck, spine, and upper and lower extremities should be examined. The practitioner should remain cognizant that one thorough hip examination is not enough. Because hip subluxation or dislocation can present in older infants who had a previously normal hip examination, it is important to assess the hips at every checkup throughout the first year of life.

The hip examination. The infant must be relaxed and quiet for the hip examination to be reliable because the practitioner may fail to note an abnormality if the child is moving and crying. The examination requires gentle maneuvers. The child should be lying supine on a firm surface with the pelvis stabilized.

Hip abduction. The amount of abduction in both hips is observed. Both hips and knees are flexed to 90 degrees and gently abducted. In an infant, both hips should abduct approximately 90 degrees from the midline. Any decrease in the amount of abduction or asymmetry should be noted.

Ortolani's sign. A positive Ortolani's sign is indicative of a dislocated hip. The examining maneuver, illustrated in Figure 18–1, relocates the dislocated femoral head back into the socket. The infant's hips and knees are flexed to 90 degrees. The examiner's thumb is placed over the lesser trochanter and the remaining four fingers placed on the greater trochanter. The examiner then abducts one hip while applying a gentle upward pressure on the greater trochanter. If the sign is positive, the examiner will feel and may hear a significant "clunk" as the femoral head enters the acetabulum.

Barlow's sign. A positive Barlow's sign is indicative of an unstable hip. As illustrated in Figure 18–2, the examiner attempts to sublux or dislocate the femoral head out of the acetabulum during the maneuver. With the child supine, the hips and knees are flexed to 90 degrees. The examiner's fingers are placed in the same position, with the thumb on the lesser trochanter and the remaining four fingers over the greater trochanter. The examiner adducts the hip with a gentle downward pressure on the lesser trochanter. The femoral head slipping out of the acetabulum is palpable when the test result is positive.

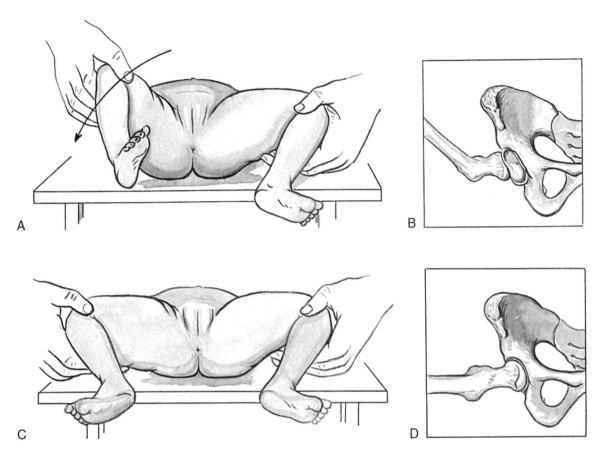

FIGURE 18–1. *A–D,* Ortolani's test. See text for explanation. (From Tachdjian, M. O. [1990]. *Pediatric orthopedics.* Philadelphia: WB Saunders.)

Galeazzi sign. Because a dislocated hip often presents with femoral shortening, the examiner should observe the child for the presence of a positive Galeazzi sign. This is manifested by a shortening of the femur on the side of the dysplastic hip. Both hips and knees should be flexed to 90 degrees. The examiner should then observe the height of both femurs at the knees. Any asymmetry should be noted.

Telescoping sign. The examiner should assess the overall laxity of the hip joint. A loose hip is one at risk for a dislocation. With both hips and knees flexed to 90 degrees, the examiner should place his or her fingers in the same position and gently move the hip up and down to assess whether any laxity exists within the joint. Generally, the femoral head should be well seated and stable within the acetabulum. Newborns may exhibit some increased laxity in the hip joint because of the presence of the maternal hormones and the practitioner should closely monitor this. Resolution should be noted within 1 month after birth.

Asymmetry of gluteal folds. Asymmetry of the gluteal folds can be a sign of DDH. Although this is not as definitive of a sign as those listed previously, it should elicit suspicion when noted in conjunction with other signs. Asymmetry of thigh folds is a common occurrence and not a sign of DDH.

The Ortolani's and Barlow's signs begin to disappear after the age of 3 months and become less reliable indicators. After this age, the examiner should expect to find a hip adduction contracture or a leg length discrepancy (positive Galeazzi sign) if the child has a hip dislocation. When a toddler or older child has a waddling gait, leg length discrepancy, or positive Trendelenburg's sign (the child is unable to hold the pelvis level when standing with weight on the affected leg) (Fig. 18–3), the examiner should be suspicious that the child may have DDH.

Diagnostic Evaluation. In the newborn period, diagnosis is made primarily on the basis of physical examination. Radiographs of the hips during this period are difficult to interpret because the cartilaginous femoral head is not evident until it begins to ossify at age 3 to 4 months (Fig. 18–4). Until that time, ultrasound is the best method for diagnosing DDH. Using ultrasonography, one can determine the relationship of the femoral head to the acetabulum, the development of the acetabulum, and the amount of laxity in the hip joint. Between the ages of 3 and 4 months, when the ossification of the femoral head begins, radiographs become the diagnostic method of choice.

Treatment Modalities and Related Nursing Management. The goals of treatment are to restore the normal relationship between the femoral head and the acetabulum and to promote the development of the acetabulum. The long-term goal is a hip that functions normally for life. Early identification and treatment of the condition is imperative to achieve optimal outcome and prevent complications. The older the infant is at the time of diagnosis, the more complicated the treatment.

Neonatal Period. The first-line of treatment is the use of a Pavlik harness. The harness maintains the hips in a position of flexion and abduction and allows the hip capsule to tighten with the hip in the acetabulum. This not only maintains the femoral head in the correct position but also promotes the development of the acetabulum. The Pavlik harness is an extremely effective method for treating newborns with developmental dysplasia (Fig. 18–5). Treatment should begin as soon as the diagnosis is made. The length of treatment varies depending on how quickly stability is achieved and usually takes 6 to 12 weeks. It is recommended that the parents be

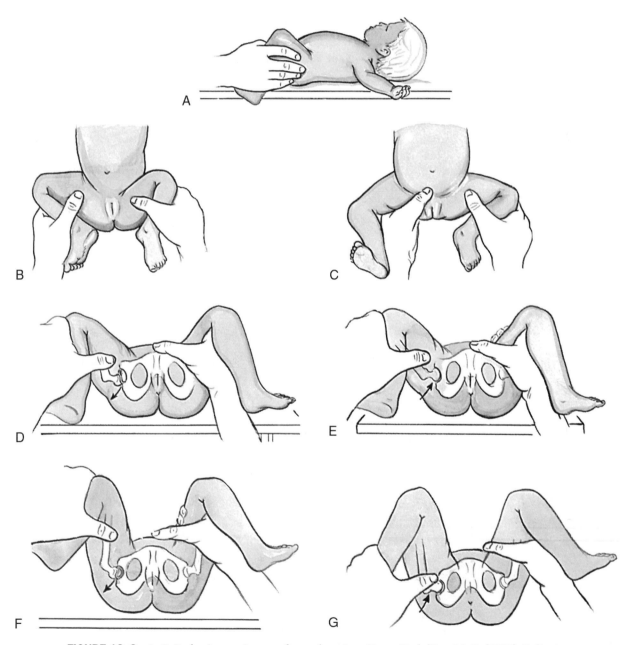

FIGURE 18–2. *A–G,* Barlow's test. See text for explanation. (From Tachdjian, M. O. [1990]. *Pediatric orthopedics.* Philadelphia: WB Saunders.)

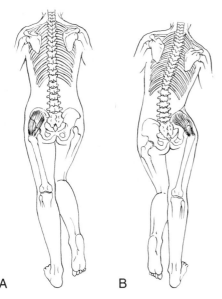

FIGURE 18–3. *A–B,* Trendelenburg lurch. (From Tachdjian, M. O. [1990]. *Pediatric orthopedics.* Philadelphia: WB Saunders.)

allowed to remove the harness for no more than 30 minutes a day to bathe the child and check the skin. Education of the parents is important. If the parents do not leave the harness on as instructed or if they change the adjustments of the straps or handle the baby incorrectly, the effectiveness of the harness is diminished. Boxes 18–1 and 18–2 and Figure 18–6 discuss instructions to parents.

A potential complication of the harness is avascular necrosis of the femoral head. If the hip is maintained in too much flexion or abduction, the blood supply to the femoral head can be compromised. To prevent this, the harness should be applied and adjusted by an experienced nurse or physician who has an understanding of the hip abduction and flexion parameters. Careful fitting with follow-up visits for readjustments to accommodate the

newborn's growth is mandatory. It is important to emphasize to the family the reason for the importance of the entire treatment regimen. After the age of 6 months, the infant is too large for the harness and other types of hip abduction orthoses are used.

After the age of 6 months, treatment becomes more difficult because the ligamentous laxity of the newborn is no longer present and contractures of the soft tissues about the hip have developed. The older the child, the greater the difficulty in relocating the hip and the greater the chance of complications.

If the hip cannot be reduced with the Pavlik harness or if the child is too large for the harness (usually beyond age 6 months) the next procedure is a closed reduction. The hip is manually reduced under general anesthesia, and a hip spica cast is applied. An arthrogram is performed during the procedure to outline the cartilaginous structures of the hip. If the adductors of the hip are tight, an adductor tenotomy is performed to reduce the risk of avascular necrosis and increase hip ROM. The child remains in the cast for 6 weeks, with the hips and knees in flexion and abduction. The cast is then changed under anesthesia and replaced by a hip spica with the hips and knees in extension. Casting is often followed by a hip abduction brace for approximately 6 months.

If the closed reduction is not successful, an open reduction is performed. The hip joint is opened, and the femoral head and acetabulum are visualized. The femoral head is placed in the acetabulum, the incision closed, and a hip spica cast applied. An open reduction may be accompanied by a femoral shortening procedure that facilitates a concentric reduction, decreases the pressure exerted on the femoral head, and reduces the risk of avascular necrosis. Casting is maintained for 12 weeks, followed by bracing with a hip abduction orthosis.

Once the hip is located in the socket, the child enters a waiting period; during this time, periodic x-ray films and examinations are done to determine whether the

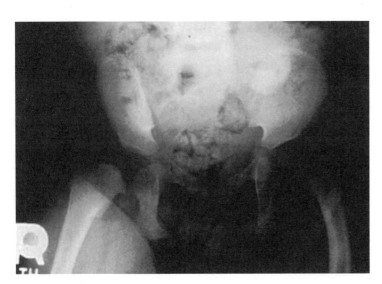

FIGURE 18–4. Radiographic example of developmental dysplasia of the hip. Note the lack of ossific nucleus and acetabular dysplasia. (From Ozonoff, M. B. [1992]. *Pediatric orthopedic radiology* [2nd ed.]. Philadelphia: WB Saunders.)

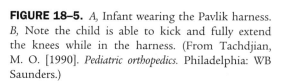

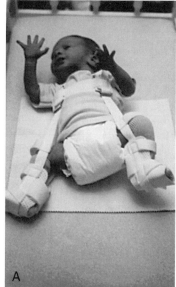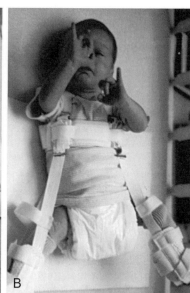

FIGURE 18–5. *A,* Infant wearing the Pavlik harness. *B,* Note the child is able to kick and fully extend the knees while in the harness. (From Tachdjian, M. O. [1990]. *Pediatric orthopedics.* Philadelphia: WB Saunders.)

acetabulum is developing correctly. There are two components to normal hip development: The femoral head must be located within the acetabulum, and the acetabulum must form correctly to contain the femoral head. If the acetabulum fails to properly develop by 4 years of age, the child undergoes a pelvic osteotomy. The Salter osteotomy, the procedure of choice in young children, is usually the definitive procedure for these clients. The distal segment of the iliac bone is divided and rotated laterally and downward. This provides complete coverage of the acetabulum over the femoral head. A bone graft is placed, and pins maintain the new position until healing is complete. The child is placed in a hip spica cast for 6 weeks.

BOX 18–1.

Information for Parents: Care of Their Infant in the Pavlik Harness

General Care

1. Handling your child may seem awkward at first. You will become more comfortable with experience. Treat your child normally. Do not be afraid to handle and cuddle your child.

2. Your child may look uncomfortable in the harness, but he or she is not. This is a natural position for a baby, especially when the baby is on his or her stomach. When awake, your child should spend most of the time on his or her stomach, if possible, because this is the best position for the hips.

3. Do not readjust the harness in any way unless you have been instructed to do so. You can change your child's clothes and diaper without removing the harness. Ask your baby's doctor whether you may take off the harness once a day for bathing or if it must be in place at all times. You will have a chance to practice handling your child, to dress him or her in the harness, and to remove and put on the harness.

4. Clothes worn over the harness will keep the harness clean. Make sure the diaper is tucked underneath all of the straps. Clean all soiled areas with a damp cloth as soon as they are soiled. If the harness can be removed, wash it in cold water only. Do not put it in the dryer.

Skin Care

1. Skin irritation from the harness can be a problem for your baby. A T-shirt and socks (preferably cotton) should be worn under the harness. Change them daily or as needed. T-shirts with snaps or ties at the side are easier to manage than those that go on over the head. Socks should be long enough to reach above the footpiece of the harness and should not have a tight elastic band at the top.

2. Keep the skin clean and dry at all times. It is especially important to check the skin creases at the thighs, behind the knees, and the neck.

3. Avoid the use of powders, creams, and lotions on the skin covered by the harness. These can soften the skin and cause more irritation.

4. Inspect the skin carefully for signs of irritation. Call your doctor or nurse if the skin is irritated.

Handling and Positioning

1. Your child may be positioned on his or her back or stomach, not on the side.

2. Do not hold or position the baby so that his or her legs are pushed together. Be careful when wrapping him or her in quilts or blankets that the legs remain apart.

BOX 18–2.

Fitting the Pavlik Harness

(See Fig. 18–6)

1. Lay the harness on the examining table or bed and then lay the infant on top of the harness.
2. Adjust the chest strap so that it is at the baby's nipple line and fasten across the chest. Be sure that the strap is not too high, or it will rub under the arms. If the chest strap is too low, the flexion and abduction straps will be difficult to adjust correctly (see Fig. 18–6*A* and *B*).
3. Fasten the shoulder straps to the chest strap.
4. Place the feet in the footpieces and adjust the anterior (flexion) strap so that the hip is flexed to 100–110 degrees (see Fig. 18–6*C* and *D*).
5. Turn the baby onto his or her stomach to adjust the posterior (abduction) straps. The abduction straps should be adjusted so that some adduction is allowed but the knees cannot be brought completely together (see Fig. 18–6*E* and *F*). Turn the baby back onto his or her back and check the amount of adduction this adjustment allows. When the hips are in the correct position, the nurse should not be able to elicit a positive Ortolani's sign. Excessive abduction of the hips, however, can cause an avascular necrosis.
6. Mark the straps with indelible ink when they are adjusted.
7. Explain to the parents about diapering, dressing, undressing, and removal and reapplication of the harness.
8. Instruct the parents not to cut off excess length of the straps because this length will be needed to make future adjustments. The straps may be taped or tacked down with thread to keep them out of the way between visits for adjustments.
9. Give the parents written instructions and be sure they have the name and phone number of the person to call if they have questions or problems

---

Nursing Management. Management of the child with developmental dysplasia is aimed at early detection and treatment. Information for the parents about the Pavlik harness can be found in Boxes 18–1 and 18–2. Parents need education on the purpose of the harness, and the need for the child to wear the harness as instructed should be reinforced during office visits. The nurse should check the harness straps periodically for any adjustments that may be needed.

The child who has undergone hip surgery will be in a hip spica cast. For the first day or two after surgery, the infant requires intravenous opioids for pain. This can be followed by the administration of oral opioids. Moleskin should be placed around the borders of the cast. A small diaper should be tucked inside the opening in the cast with a larger diaper over it to cover the outside of the cast.

The head of the crib should be slightly elevated to help the urine drain downward instead of up inside the cast.

Parents of the child who has undergone surgery and is in a hip spica cast must be instructed regarding care of the cast. In addition, it is helpful to inform parents in advance that car seats, strollers, and highchairs need to be evaluated because of the position of the child in the cast. Nursing diagnoses and interventions for the child in a spica cast or one undergoing surgery can be found in Chapters 11 and 12.

Summary. DDH ideally is diagnosed and treated in the newborn period. The later the diagnosis is made, the more complex the treatment required. Regardless of the treatment, educating the family, monitoring the child's progress, and supporting the parents are essential aspects of the treatment.

Congenital Dislocation of the Patella

Definition and Classification. Congenital dislocation of the patella is a condition in which the patella is dislocated at birth and cannot be reduced by closed manipulation. The patella is dislocated to the lateral side of the knee, and knee instability increases with growth. Diagnosis is often delayed because the condition is not apparent until the child starts walking. In addition, many of these children are late walkers because the condition is often associated with other congenital problems, such as Down syndrome.

Etiology. The most widely accepted cause of this disorder is failure of the myotome containing the quadriceps and patella to internally rotate during the first trimester of intrauterine life. The reason this occurs is unknown.

Pathophysiology. Failure of internal rotation of the myotome containing the quadriceps muscle results in the muscle remaining on the anterolateral aspect of the thigh and the patella dislocating laterally. If left untreated, genu valgus and external rotation of the tibia result from the continual pull of the quadriceps on the lateral aspect of the knee. The medial collateral ligament and the capsule on the medial and anteromedial aspect of the knee become hypertrophic from the valgus pull and external rotation. Intraoperative findings include contraction of the quadriceps with the insertion of the patellar tendon on the anterolateral aspect of the tibia, attachment of the iliotibial band on the lateral aspect of the tibia, a fixed, hypoplastic patella, a flattened appearance of the anterolateral femoral condyle, anterior and medial thickening of the capsule, and genu valgus and external tibial torsion. In addition, lateral subluxation of the tibia and flattening of the articular surface of the patella are often found (Langenskiold & Ritsila, 1992).

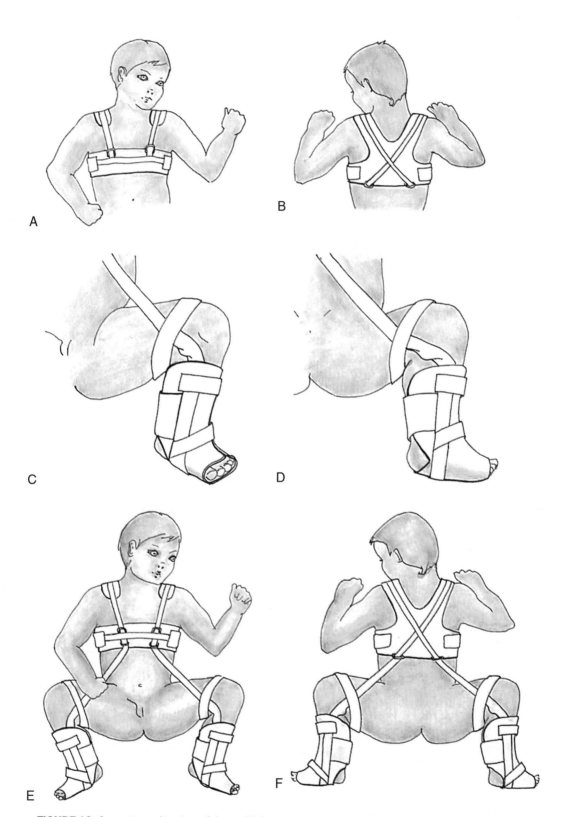

FIGURE 18–6. *A–F,* Application of the Pavlik harness. See Box 18–2 for explanation. (From Tachdjian, M. O. [1990]. *Pediatric orthopedics.* Philadelphia: WB Saunders.)

Assessment

Subjective Assessment: Nursing History. Difficulty with ambulation and late ambulation are common complaints from parents when a child has a congenital dislocation of the patella.

Objective Assessment: Physical Examination. Early diagnosis of this disorder is difficult. Dislocation may not be apparent until after the child is more mobile because of the smallness and late ossification of the patella.

The child may have an abnormal gait, or the gait may appear normal. Absence of active or passive knee extension from the flexed position is often diagnostic, particularly before the patella is ossified. Palpation of the patella (if ossified) shows it to be hypoplastic and laterally moveable. Subluxation of the tibia and valgus deformity of the knee, as well as flexion contracture, are common. With increasing age, the valgus deformity progresses to more than 40 degrees.

Diagnostic Evaluation.
Radiographs are not useful in diagnosis until ossification of the patella occurs, generally between ages 3 and 5 years. Ossification is often delayed in these children. X-ray films may show valgus deformity at the knee joint and changes in femoral and tibial condyles.

Treatment Modalities and Related Nursing Management.
Congenital dislocated patella cannot be reduced by closed manipulation, so most authorities advocate early operative intervention. Open reduction is achieved with release of the iliotibial band, medial rotation of the quadriceps mechanism, division and lateral release of the patellar tendon, and reattachment medially. Variations in the procedure are determined by individual findings. Detailed reports of the surgical procedures are provided by Stanisavljevic, Zemenick, and Miller (1976), Langenskiold and Ritsila (1992), and Warner, Canale, and Beaty (1994). A long leg cast with the knee in slight flexion is needed for 5 to 6 weeks after surgery. Nursing management focuses on preoperative and postoperative needs, cast care, and psychosocial concerns. Attention should be paid to other congenital problems that can affect the child's treatment or reaction to surgery.

Nursing Management. Nursing diagnoses applicable to the child with congenital dislocation of the patella include impaired mobility, self-esteem disturbance, and altered growth and development. Postoperative nursing diagnoses include pain and impaired mobility. See the section on common nursing concerns at the end of this chapter for more information.

Summary. Congenital dislocation of the patella requires early surgical intervention to prevent progressive deformity. Diagnosis is often difficult because of the smallness and late ossification of the patella. Other congenital dysplasias are commonly found with this disorder.

Congenital Dislocation and Subluxation of the Knee

Definition and Classification.
Congenital dislocation and subluxation of the knee are hyperextension deformities. Quadriceps shortening and fibrosis are routinely present, and flexing the knee past neutral is generally difficult. Hyperextension deformities generally are classified as severe genu recurvatum (group I), subluxation (group II), and complete dislocation (group III). Classification alone cannot be considered reliable in determining outcomes or needed treatment. Congenital dislocation of the knee is often associated with other congenital anomalies or syndromes, such as dislocated hips, arthrogryposis, and joint laxity syndromes.

Incidence and Etiology.
Congenital knee dislocation is a relatively rare deformity, its incidence being approximately 0.017 to 0.7 per 1000 live births. Congenital or developmental dislocation of the hip occurs about 40 to 80 times more often than congenital dislocation of the knee. There is a two to three time higher incidence in girls than in boys. At least 80% of children with this disorder have other congenital musculoskeletal abnormalities, usually of the hip or foot (Warner, Canale, & Beaty, 1994).

The etiology of congenital dislocation of the knee is unknown. A familial occurrence has been noted, but there is no clear genetic pattern. About 40% of these children are born in a breech presentation. Abnormal intrauterine positioning may play a role in the development of congenital dislocation of the knee, but it is generally not accepted as a definitive cause of this disorder.

Pathophysiology.
Fibrosis of the quadriceps is the major finding in congenital knee dislocation. It is unclear, however, whether this is a cause or an effect of the dislocation. Knee flexor weakness with strong extensors in utero causes differential muscle growth, with the stronger quadriceps becoming shortened. In children with laxity syndromes, a secondary muscle imbalance can occur because of hyperextension of the knee in utero. The hamstrings can subluxate anteriorly to the axis of flexion of the joint and serve as knee extensors, thereby resulting in a shortening of the quadriceps. Primary muscle imbalance can be seen in children with arthrogryposis and neuromuscular disorders, such as myelomeningocele.

Assessment

Subjective Assessment: Nursing History. Birth history, including type of presentation (e.g., breech), should be obtained. Familial history of congenital dislocation of the knee should be determined, as well as the presence of other congenital anomalies or syndromes.

Objective Assessment: Physical Examination. Hyperextension of the knee, often more than 45 degrees, is the key sign of this disorder. The knee generally cannot be flexed much past 0 degrees of extension. In the supine position, the hip laterally rotates because of the knee hyperextension and weight of the leg. An anterior skin fold is usually found, and prominent femoral condyles can be palpated in the popliteal fossa. The patella is generally not palpable. Signs of other congenital anomalies or syndromes are usually present.

Typical findings during surgery include quadriceps fibrosis, suprapatellar pouch ablation, hamstring tendon dislocation, dysplasia of the femoral and tibial articular surfaces, and elongation and attenuation of the anterior cruciate ligament.

Diagnostic Evaluation. Radiographs are taken to confirm clinical findings. Lateral flexion and extension views are taken to determine whether the dislocation is irreducible. Typical findings are anterior dislocation of the tibia to the femoral condyles and proximal displacement.

Arthrography can demonstrate flattening of the inferior femoral condyle and lack of suprapatellar pouch. Ablation of the suprapatellar pouch is associated with a poor outcome if treated by conservative measures.

Treatment Modalities and Related Nursing Management

Conservative Treatment. Early serial manipulation with splinting is the primary method of treatment for congenital dislocation of the knee. Gentle knee flexion is achieved through manipulation by applying an anterior force to the distal femur and a posterior force to the proximal tibia. Flexion is maintained by cast or splint application. Weekly manipulation and splinting are performed until knee flexion of 90 degrees is obtained. Splints are left on 4 to 6 weeks after completion of manipulation to maintain flexion. Generally, a 3-month course of treatment is expected. Vigorous manipulations are avoided because of the possibility of damage to the epiphyses and fracture of the distal femur or tibia. Radiographic evidence of knee reduction and flexion to 90 degrees is a key indicator of successful conservative management.

The family needs teaching and support about the proposed treatment plan. Care of the child's skin and the splinting device must be discussed with the family. (See Chapter 12 for information on casts and splints.) Additional support may be needed if no progress is made with conservative management.

Surgical Management. Operative treatment may be necessary for children for whom conservative management has failed. The age at which the surgery should be performed is not clearly delineated. Some advocate early intervention, that is, between 3 and 6 months of age

(Bensahel, Dal Monte, Hjelmstedt, Bjerkreim, Wientroub, Matasovic, Porat, & Bialik, 1989). Elongation of the quadriceps mechanism, usually by a V-Y quadricepsplasty, division of the iliotibial band, and relocation of the hamstring tendons, allows reduction of the tibia on the femur. Clients are generally casted in knee flexion for 4 to 6 weeks after surgery. Physical therapy to mobilize the knee is performed after cast removal. Potential complications from the procedure can include anterior skin necrosis and wound dehiscence (resulting from stretch) and loss of full active extension, as well as knee instability.

Nursing Management. Nursing interventions during the perioperative period include assisting the family to accept the failure of conservative treatment, helping the family to devise a means of ensuring mobility for the casted child, and providing support for the family and child during the hospitalization and the extended treatment period.

As with any congenital condition, there is a period of adjustment for the family. The nurse explaining the diagnosis to the family should remind them of the need for frequent visits to the physician and the possible need for surgery, as well as help them to cope with an infant in a splint or cast. The nurse should also remind the family that the problem is correctable.

Summary. Congenital dislocation of the knee is a hyperextension deformity that often can be treated successfully by serial knee manipulation and casting or splinting. Some cases may be resistant to conservative measures and require quadriceps lengthening.

Metatarsus Adductus

Definition. Metatarsus adductus is a positional deformity of the forefoot commonly seen in infants. The entire forefoot is adducted giving the foot a kidney-shaped appearance (Fig. 18-7). The foot often has an arch. The hindfoot is normal, and the heelcord is not tight.

Incidence and Etiology. Metatarsus adductus is a common pediatric foot deformity, with an incidence of approximately 1 to 2 per 1000 live births. It is often bilateral. Most cases are related to in utero positioning.

Pathophysiology. The effects of intrauterine positioning are thought to be the cause of metatarsus adductus. The feet are often in a tucked position in utero.

Assessment

Subjective Assessment: Nursing History. The chief complaint from the child's parents is that the feet turn in. If the child is walking, a history of an intoeing gait may be present.

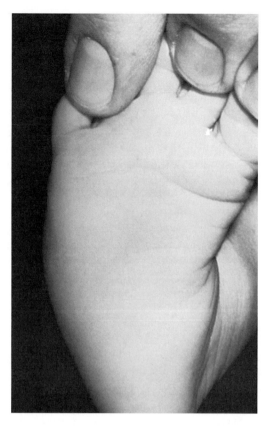

FIGURE 18–7. Metatarsus adductus. Deformity is confined to the forefoot with the hindfoot being normal.

Objective Assessment: Physical Examination. Metatarsus adductus is assessed by examining the plantar aspect of the foot. The nurse should note the overall shape of the foot and the presence of an arch, especially in infants and toddlers. The presence of a skin crease is indicative of a more rigid, congenital deformity. The kidney shape of the metatarsus adductus foot should be noted. The most important aspect of the examination is for the nurse to ascertain whether the forefoot can be actively or passively moved into neutral position. A supple or flexible deformity normally corrects on its own independent of intervention. If the infant can pull the foot into a neutral position upon stimulating the foot, no intervention is needed. A more rigid deformity may require further intervention. The motion of the foot should otherwise be good with full plantar flexion and no tightness of the anterior tibial tendon. The child should also be assessed for additional orthopaedic problems, such as DDH, which can be associated with foot deformities. The tibia should also be examined because these children often have an internal tibial torsion.

Diagnostic Evaluation. The diagnosis is made on physical examination; however, in the older child who has not spontaneously corrected, x-ray films may be used to visualize the bony deformity and decide whether surgical intervention is necessary.

Treatment Modalities and Related Nursing Management. Most cases of metatarsus adductus resolve without treatment. The key is flexibility of the forefoot. The child should have follow-up visits for observation of the deformity and to determine whether correction is taking place. Treatment may include stretching of the medial soft tissues. Parents are taught to hold the heel and stretch the forefoot gently toward the midline. These exercises can be done at each diaper change. A more significant deformity, such as one in which the infant cannot pull the foot into a straight position when stimulated, may require special reverse-last shoes. An extremely rigid deformity may need serial casting. Surgical correction is rarely necessary and performed only in cases of persistent deformity when the child is older.

Nursing Management. Metatarsus adductus often resolves without treatment. The parents may experience anxiety about the appearance of their child's foot and the prognosis. Reassurance and support should be given. Parents should be told that resolution usually occurs spontaneously. Information about the possible cause (i.e., in utero positioning) should be given. The parents should be taught how to properly exercise the child's foot. If manipulation and casting or bracing is necessary, see Chapter 12 for information on cast and brace nursing diagnoses and interventions.

Summary. Metatarsus adductus is a common foot disorder in the infant. It is thought to be the result of in utero positioning. The foot is usually flexible, and the deformity resolves in many cases without treatment.

Clubfoot (Talipes Equinovarus)

Definition and Classification. Clubfoot, or *talipes equinovarus,* is a combination of three deformities in the foot. The forefoot and heel are in varus (turned inward). The ankle is in equinus (points downward), and the entire foot is in supination (the foot rotates upwards) (Fig. 18–8). A postural clubfoot is easily corrected with manipulation or resolves spontaneously and is not associated with bony deformity. Soft tissue tightening may be present. A true clubfoot is often found in conjunction with other congenital anomalies, such as myelodysplasia, cerebral palsy (CP), or arthrogryposis. There is increased incidence of hip dysplasia in those afflicted with a clubfoot.

Incidence and Etiology. The incidence of clubfoot is 1 to 2 per 1000 live births. Boys are affected twice as often as girls. Bilateral clubfeet occur in 50% of the cases. The incidence is increased with a positive family history. Although the etiology is considered multifactorial, an autosomal-recessive pattern of inheritance has been noted. The incidence of clubfoot is lowest in the Chinese population and highest in individuals of Polynesian descent.

The postural clubfoot is believed to be the result of intrauterine positioning; the exact etiology of the true, rigid clubfoot is unknown. Alexander, Ackman, and Kuo (1999) have summarized the major theories regarding the cause of a clubfoot and have also described the pathology of the deformity.

The deformities resulting in a clubfoot are due to changes in the talocalcaneonavicular joint. In the clubfoot, the head and the neck of the talus angulate plantarly and medially. The talus is smaller in size. The hindfoot is

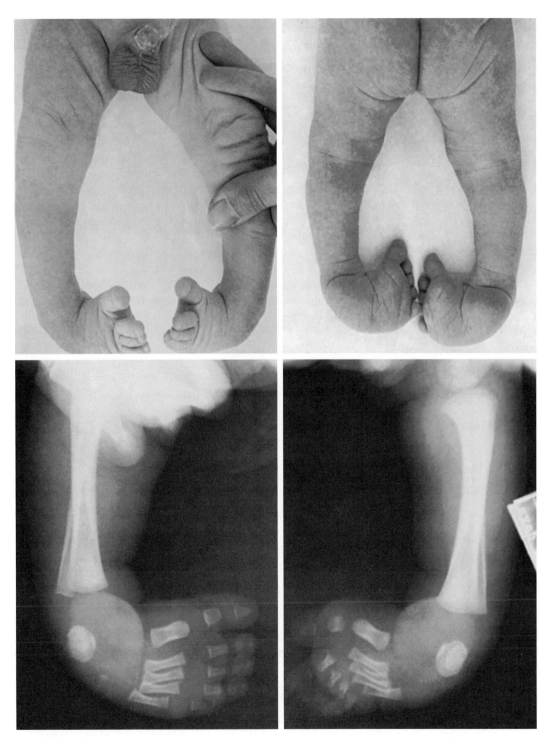

FIGURE 18–8. Bilateral talipes equinovarus in newborn. (From Tachdjian, M. O. [1990]. *Pediatric orthopedics.* Philadelphia: WB Saunders.)

in equinus and varus. The calcaneus is directed forward and outward and rests in an equinus position. Its posterior aspect rotates laterally and upward and is tethered to the lateral malleolus. The navicular, which normally articulates with the head of the talus, is shifted to the medial aspect of the foot. The navicular is smaller than normal in size. Changes in the soft tissue are also present. Shortening of the soft tissue occurs at the medial and posterior portions of the foot and ankle. The capsules of the posterior, ankle, subtalar, and talonavicular and peroneal tendons are contracted. The cavus deformity results from a tight plantar fascia, abductor hallucis, and flexor digitorum brevis.

Assessment

Subjective Assessment: Nursing History. The examiner should begin with a comprehensive history. Because clubfoot is often associated with chromosome defects, the clinician should determine whether the foot deformity is an isolated occurrence or whether other anomalies exist as well. A thorough health history can be obtained, and developmental milestones should also be assessed. A family history of clubfoot or other congenital anomalies should be included in the assessment.

Objective Assessment: Physical Examination. A complete musculoskeletal examination should follow the history. Because foot deformities are commonly associated with spinal dysraphism, the spine and reflexes should be examined. Because there is also an increased incidence of hip dysplasia in these children, a thorough hip examination should be incorporated into every follow-up visit the first year, and it is recommended that the child have a diagnostic study of both hips by the age of 3 months. The entire lower extremity should be examined. Knee ROM should be full. Leg lengths should be measured because clubfoot clients often have a limb length discrepancy.

The foot should then be examined for the severity of its deformities. How rigid are the deformities: ankle equinus, varus of the forefoot and hindfoot, and supination? Does a cavus deformity exist (high arch)? How small is the heel? In general, the smaller the heel, the more severe the deformity. Skin creases on the medial and plantar aspects of the clubfoot are deeply furrowed.

Muscle function should be tested by tickling the infant's foot. Ankle ROM is limited. The clinician should check for active function in the anterior and posterior tibialis, peroneal muscle, and toe extensors and flexors. The anterior and posterior tibial tendons are contracted but should provide active movement. However, the peroneals are usually weak, and motor function is absent in the preoperative stage. Generally, this function is gained after surgery, but in some cases, it may not and the child will require an additional procedure. The calf circumference on the affected side is decreased. This is the

trademark of the clubfoot and remains throughout life. Any leg length discrepancy should be documented so that it can be followed as the child grows.

Diagnostic Evaluation. Often, clubfoot is diagnosed before birth during an ultrasound examination. After birth, x-ray films are taken to fully evaluate the deformity.

Radiographs of the foot (anteroposterior and lateral stress views in the infant; standing in older children) can be used (1) to determine the severity of the deformity by assessing the subluxation of the talocalcaneonavicular joint, (2) to assess conservative treatment progress, (3) for preoperative planning, and (4) to determine correction and maintenance both intraoperatively and postoperatively.

Treatment Modalities and Related Nursing Management. The goal of treatment of the clubfoot is to achieve as normal a foot as possible. The child's foot should be pain free, supple, plantigrade, cosmetically acceptable in appearance, and capable of wearing normal shoes.

Treatment should begin as early as possible, preferably in the newborn nursery. During the first 2 to 3 weeks of life, the infant's ligamentous tissues are lax. This makes the newborn period an optimal time to begin treatment because the soft tissues are moldable. Initial treatment is always nonoperative, in the form of manipulation with the application of a cast. The manipulation is gentle to prevent damaging the bones of the foot, and correction is done over time. Casts (long leg) are applied to hold the foot in the corrected position. The casts are removed, and the foot is manipulated and recast every 1 to 2 weeks for approximately 3 months.

At age 3 to 6 months, the results of nonoperative treatment are evaluated and a decision is made about whether to continue with casting, wear a brace, or plan for surgical correction. Treatment decisions are based on clinical examination and radiographs.

If the foot is in a good position, the child is placed in an ankle-foot orthosis (AFO) and enters a holding pattern. At some point a decision is made regarding whether the foot requires surgery. The brace is worn 23 hours a day and is removed only for a daily bath. Occasionally, a Dennis–Brown Bar is prescribed for night use when the child has a severe internal tibial torsion.

Surgery is necessary to correct bony abnormalities. The timing of the surgery depends on the severity of the deformity. A study by Smith, Sirirungruangsarn, and Kuo (1997) suggests that 9 months of age is the optimal time of surgery, although milder deformities may be corrected closer to 1 year of age. In the infant and young child, surgical treatment usually consists of a one-stage release of all contracted tissues and a realignment of the foot. The surgery is progressive. The surgeon does as many releases as necessary to bring the foot into normal alignment without overcorrecting it. The realigned bones are held in position with percutaneous pins. Long leg casts are used for 6 weeks. Initially, the foot is brought as close to a plantigrade position as possible without overstretching the skin. Two weeks after surgery, the casts are removed to reposition the foot all the way to neutral. The casts are then reapplied. These casts then stay on for the remainder of the 6 weeks. There may be variations to this protocol depending on the nature of the deformity, the surgical procedure, and the surgeon's preference.

When the casts are removed, the child is fitted for an AFO. This maintains the foot in the corrected position and is an integral part of the treatment. The brace is removed only for bathing and for family members to check the skin for irritation. The brace is worn over a sock and can be worn under a shoe. The child will not have difficulty walking while wearing the brace.

Vascular compromise is the earliest complication that can result from clubfoot surgery. It has been reported by Sodre, Bruschini, Mestriner, Miranda, Levinsohn, Packard, Crider, Schwartz, and Hootnick (1990) that a deficiency of the anterior tibial and dorsalis pedis arteries occurs in 90% of clubfeet. Therefore, the foot is at greater risk for necrosis after surgery should any further disruptions compromise the vascularity. Infection and wound dehiscence resulting from the stretching of contracted tissues are also potential complications. Every precaution should be taken to prevent swelling. The child should have the lower extremity elevated on a pillow for 48 hours. A fever is normal 1 to 2 days postoperatively. After the third day after surgery, a fever of 101°F or higher may be indicative of a more serious problem.

Nursing Management. The child's feet should remain elevated for at least 48 hours after surgery, with as little disruption to that position as possible. It is helpful to tape the child's foot (or feet) to the pillow to maintain the elevation. Pain after a clubfoot procedure is of a limited duration. Short-term use of an intravenous opioid such as morphine may be used in the initial postoperative period. Usually, 24 hours after surgery an oral opioid can be used.

Before discharge, the family should be given instructions regarding cast care, signs and symptoms of infection, and neurovascular assessment. Parents may be advised not to let the infant's foot (or feet) hang in a vertical position for a short time after being released from the hospital.

As with any congenital deformity, the presence of clubfoot causes concern and anxiety on the part of the parents. Parents should be told that the affected foot may be smaller and the calf circumference will be smaller when compared with the unaffected leg but that this will not affect the child's overall function. From the time of diagnosis, parents require reassurance that with treatment the child will walk normally and be able to participate in all activities, including sports.

Summary. Congenital clubfoot is a congenital disorder in which the foot is in an equinus, varus, and supinated position. Parents must cope with the birth of a child with a congenital deformity, as well as comply with the treatment plan required to correct the deformity. The first line of management requires manipulation and casting as soon as possible after birth. Surgical treatment may be necessary. Parental support and education are important aspects of the treatment plan.

Talipes Calcaneovalgus

Definition. Talipes calcaneovalgus, or calcaneovalgus foot, is another common postural deformity of the neonate. The forefoot is in valgus and the ankle has an excessive amount of dorsiflexion.

Incidence and Etiology. The incidence of talipes calcaneovalgus is 1 per 1000 live births, with girls and first-born children being affected more often. It is caused by intrauterine positioning.

Pathophysiology. It is believed that the foot is compressed against the uterine wall late in pregnancy. Soft tissues on the dorsum and lateral aspect foot of the infant contract and limit plantar flexion.

Assessment

Subjective Assessment: Nursing History. Birth history and developmental and medical histories should be taken to uncover any additional deformities the child may have.

Objective Assessment: Physical Examination. The foot and heel are deviated laterally, and the foot dorsiflexes beyond 20 degrees. Occasionally, the foot dorsiflexes to touch the tibia. Passive plantar flexion may be limited to the neutral position. Active plantar flexion can be assessed by tickling the infant's foot.

Diagnostic Evaluation. No diagnostic tests are needed unless some other type of foot deformity is suspected. If the hip examination is abnormal, radiographs or ultrasound of the hips should be performed.

Treatment Modalities and Related Nursing Management. This problem resolves spontaneously with no treatment. Stretching exercises may be recommended. Education about the usual course of talipes calcaneovalgus should be given to the parents. If stretching exercises are recommended, demonstration and return demonstration should be done.

Summary. Talipes calcaneovalgus is a common foot deformity that is present at birth and usually resolves spontaneously.

Vertical Talus

Definition. Vertical talus is also known as *congenital pes valgus* and *congenital pes planus* (congenital flatfoot). It is a dorsal and lateral dislocation of the talocalcaneonavicular calcaneocuboid joints. The talus is locked into a plantar-flexed vertical orientation, the navicular bone is anteriorly dislocated relative to the talus, and the calcaneus is in equinus. The forefoot is in dorsiflexion and valgus. All this gives the bottom of the foot a rocker-bottom shape.

Incidence and Etiology. Congenital pes valgus is believed to occur during the first trimester of pregnancy. Boys are more often affected than girls are. Unilateral or bilateral deformity can occur and appear as a solitary deformity or in conjunction with central nervous and musculoskeletal system abnormalities, such as myelomeningocele. The cause of the congenital pes valgus as a single deformity is unknown.

Pathophysiology. The talus is locked into a vertical position as a result of the navicular articulating with the dorsal neck of the talus. Posterolateral displacement of the calcaneus from the talus occurs. Ligament, tendon, and muscle contractures are present.

Assessment

Subjective Assessment: Nursing History. The primary goal of the history should be to determine whether the deformity is an isolated finding or if it is occurring in conjunction with other congenital deformities.

Objective Assessment: Physical Examination. The deformity is usually diagnosed at birth. The foot is rigid with a rocker-bottom appearance. The heel is in equinus and the forefoot is in dorsiflexion and valgus.

Diagnostic Evaluation. On radiographs, the longitudinal axis of the talus (normally oblique) is vertical and almost parallel to the axis of the tibia. The calcaneus is in an equinus position. The key to diagnosis is the position of the navicular. In congenital pes valgus, the navicular is dislocated dorsally on the talus neck when the foot is plantar flexed.

Treatment Modalities and Related Nursing Management. The initial treatment, which consists of serial casting, begins in the newborn period. Manipulation and casting alone are not sufficient to correct the deformity but do stretch the soft tissues in preparation for surgery when the infant is older (at about 3 months of age) and the foot is larger. Various surgical options exist, and the method of correction depends on the degree of deformity and the age of the child. Options include closed reduction of the talocalcaneonavicular dislocation (often not successful), open reduction of the dislocation with tendon transfers, and arthrodesis.

Nursing Management. Nursing care is similar to that required for the child with clubfoot (see the section on clubfoot for nursing interventions). The importance of manipulation and casting, even though surgery may still be anticipated, should be reinforced with the family.

Summary. Congenital pes valgus is generally diagnosed at birth because of the rigid rocker-bottom appearance of the foot. Open reduction of the talocalcaneonavicular dislocation is usually necessary for treatment.

CHILDREN AND ADOLESCENTS

By the time the child has had his or her first birthday, the spine is straight. The postural deformities present at birth have begun to straighten and may continue to do so for several years. The bowlegged appearance of the infant gradually disappears, and at 18 months to 3 years of age, the child's lower extremities assume a valgus position. At 3 to 5 years, the legs straighten.

The child walks with a heel-toe gait and swings both arms when he or she walks. Occasionally, the toddler may be a toe-walker, but this should not persist, and the child should be able to stand and walk plantigrade. The hips and knees have full ROM. At the age of 2, the foot begins to form an arch. An infant, child, or adolescent should have 20 degrees of foot dorsiflexion, 40 degrees of plantar flexion, and 20 degrees of inversion and eversion in the ankle. The child and adolescent should be able to hold those positions against resistance and should have 5/5 strength in the ankle tendons.

Children and adolescents usually have few musculoskeletal problems or complaints. When a previously healthy child or teenager begins limping or complaining of pain, the discomfort should be assessed. The nurse should begin with a complete history and physical examination.

Hip Problems

Acute Transient Synovitis

Definition. Acute transient synovitis of the hip is the most common cause of a painful hip in children between the ages of 3 and 6. It is a nonspecific, self-limiting inflammatory condition. The problem is characterized by groin pain with weight bearing and decreased ROM of the hip. The onset is sudden; often, the child awakens in the morning refusing to bear weight. The child is either afebrile or runs a low-grade fever. Overall, the child appears well. The primary responsibility of the clinician is to distinguish the benign condition of synovitis from more serious problems such as septic arthritis, osteomyelitis, or juvenile rheumatoid arthritis. Trauma should also be ruled out.

Assessment

Subjective assessment: nursing history. The nurse should elicit information as to whether the child fell or experienced any injury that might be the cause of pain. Because synovitis is often associated with a recent upper respiratory infection or immunization, the parent should be asked if the child experienced either event within the last month. When the symptoms began and whether the child is getting better or worse are also important factors because synovitis generally runs a short course and other more serious problems have symptoms that do not improve and may worsen quickly. Whether the parent has noted any fevers, warmth, swelling, or redness is important because septic arthritis is characterized by all three of these symptoms. Often, the child with synovitis, unlike children with more serious conditions, has a normal appetite. Pain accompanies weight bearing but does not interfere with sleeping. Pain that awakens the child at night and pain and/or swelling in other joints should lead the clinician to think of other possible more serious problems.

Objective assessment: physical examination. ROM of the hips should be tested. The affected hip has a limited ROM, especially decreased abduction and internal rotation. Motion elicits pain. The nurse should closely examine the affected joint to observe any redness and swelling that might be indicative of infection. Because synovitis is an acute problem, there should not be any sign of atrophy that has affected the muscles in the lower extremity. The remaining joints should be examined for any limitation in movement, warmth, redness, or swelling that might indicate a rheumatologic condition.

Diagnostic Tests.

A complete blood count (CBC) and erythrocyte sedimentation rate (ESR) should be performed if the case is severe enough to warrant suspicion that the child may have a septic hip. The white blood cell (WBC) count and ESR are normal if the child has synovitis. An elevated WBC count and ESR often indicate the child has one of the more serious problems. An x-ray film of the hips can be performed to rule out the presence of a fracture or tumor. A bone scan can be used to rule out osteomyelitis and other problems.

Treatment Modalities and Related Nursing Management.

Treatment for synovitis usually consists of supportive care. The benign nature of the problem should be explained to the parents. The child should be allowed to rest until the condition resolves and until he or she can be given acetaminophen or children's ibuprofen for pain. The parent, however, should be instructed to notify the nurse or physician if the child does not show signs of improvement over the next 5 days, runs a fever of 101°F or higher, has increased redness or swelling around the affected joint, has other joints that become affected, or begins to manifest any other signs of a more serious illness.

Summary. Synovitis is a self-limited inflammatory disorder that resolves without intervention over the course of a few days. The problem can be similar to more serious conditions such as septic arthritis, which must be ruled out. Treatment consists of bed rest and nonsteroidal anti-inflammatory medication.

Legg-Calvé-Perthes Disease

Definition and Classification. Legg-Calvé-Perthes (LCP) disease (i.e., avascular necrosis of the femoral head in the child) is caused by the disruption of the blood supply to the femoral head and results in collapse of the femoral head. The disease runs its course over a number of years and is characterized by three factors: It affects children ages 3 to 9 years, it is of an unknown etiology, and it is a self-limiting process that eventually heals independent of medical intervention. It was first described in 1910 by three different physicians: Arthur T. Legg in the United States, Jacques Calvé in France, and Georg Clemens Perthes in Germany.

Incidence and Etiology. Boys are affected by LCP disease four times more often than girls. The incidence is higher among first-born children; those with low birth weights; and those of Japanese, Mongolian, Eskimo, or Central European heritage. Australians, Native Americans, Polynesians, and African Americans have the fewest reported cases. It occurs bilaterally in only 12% to 20% of cases and occurs more often in those with a lower socioeconomic status.

The cause of LCP disease is unknown, but theories about the cause of the avascular necrosis have related to hereditary, metabolic, chemical, and mechanical dysfunction. Metabolic bone disease, thrombi, vascular insults, trauma, infection, and transient synovitis have all been implicated. The actual cause is most likely multifactorial. One common factor that has been noted is that many of these children often have delayed skeletal age and short stature.

Pathophysiology. The primary feature of LCP disease is avascular necrosis of the proximal femoral epiphyseal region as a result of a temporary loss of blood supply. Collapse of the femoral head occurs, followed by resorption of the dead bone and replacement with newly formed immature bone cells—a process that takes place in stages.

The disease is grouped into four stages based on radiologic findings: (1) initial, or avascular; (2) fragmentation, or revascularization; (3) reossification, or reparative; and (4) healed, or residual deformity.

Avascular stage. In the initial, or avascular, stage, the earliest signs are a smaller ossific nucleus of the proximal femur and a widening of the medial joint space. Often, symptoms do not occur during this period, which can last from several months to a year. In some children, however, symptoms begin immediately.

Fragmentation stage. During the fragmentation, or revascularization, stage, the necrotic bone is resorbed and replaced with immature new bone cells. This new bone is laid down on the dead bone, making the original ossific nucleus more radiodense. This bone is easily molded at this stage into either a normal or an abnormal shape, depending on the forces exerted on it. At this point, the hip becomes painful, with effusion and decreased motion. This is a vulnerable phase, and progressive deformity can occur when suitable molding forces are not exerted. This stage lasts from 1 to 3 years.

Reossification stage. During the reossification, or reparative, stage, the necrotic bone is resorbed, new bone formation occurs, and remodeling continues until the femoral head is reconstituted. The bone is still biologically plastic during this stage, which lasts from 1 to 3 years.

Healing stage. The final stage is that of healing or residual deformity. The resorbing bone cells are replaced by normal bone cells. The femoral head and neck may be deformed as a consequence of the disease process, the repair process, or the premature closure of the growth plate. If there is residual deformity with its associated joint incongruity and decreased ROM, the hip is at risk for early degenerative joint disease. The amount of residual deformity is influenced by the promptness with which the initial diagnosis is made and treatment is instituted.

The three classification systems often used to describe the stages of LCP disease are outlined in Table 18–1.

Assessment

Subjective assessment: nursing history. LCP disease has an insidious onset, with a prolonged course of symptoms. The child describes pain in the groin, thigh, or knee. The pain is aggravated with activity and relieved with rest. In some children, parents note a limp before the child complains of pain. The child may have a history of synovitis in that hip. Because there are many childhood problems that can present with similar symptoms (e.g., synovitis, septic arthritis, osteomyelitis, juvenile rheumatoid arthritis), the practitioner should determine the duration of the symptoms, whether the child sustained an injury, and whether the symptoms are accompanied by a fever or rash. Children with LCP disease are in otherwise good health and afebrile. Any history of a rash, fevers, swelling or redness of the hip joint, or history of trauma should alert the examiner to other possibilities.

Objective assessment: physical examination. In LCP disease, ROM of the hip is painful and limited, particularly abduction and internal rotation. A flexion and/or adduction contracture of the hip can occur with atrophy of the thigh, calf, and gluteal muscles on the affected side. A leg length discrepancy may be present, with shortening of the femur on the affected side.

Diagnostic Evaluation. The easiest and least expensive method for diagnosing LCP disease are anteroposterior and frog lateral radiographs (Fig. 18–9*A* and *B*).

TABLE 18–1. *Catterall, Salter-Thompson, and Lateral Pillar Classifications of Legg-Calvé-Perthes Disease*

CLASSIFICATION	DESCRIPTION
Catterall	
I	Anterior portion of the epiphysis is involved. The epiphysis on the involved side is smaller. Prognosis is good.
II	Anterior superior and posterior portion of the epiphysis is involved. The medial and lateral margins are not involved. Prognosis remains good because the lateral margin is intact.
III	There is a loss of the lateral margin, which increases the risk of collapse and subsequent deformity. The prognosis is less favorable.
IV	The entire epiphysis is involved. The prognosis is poor because the growth plate is often severely damaged, further increasing the risk of residual deformity.
Salter-Thompson	
A	Less than half of the epiphysis is involved. Intact lateral margin of the capital femoral epiphysis. Individuals do well without treatment. Corresponds to Catterall I and II.
B	Greater than half of the epiphysis is involved. Lateral margin is not intact. Poor prognosis. Results are improved with containment treatment. Corresponds to Catterall III and IV.
Lateral Pillar	
Group A	Lateral pillar radiographically normal, with full height maintained. Corresponds to Catterall I and II.
Group B	Over 50% of lateral pillar height maintained. Corresponds to Catterall II and III.
Group C	Less than 50% of lateral pillar height maintained. Corresponds to Catterall III and IV. Results are significantly worse than for the other two groups. Longer fragmentation and reossification periods.

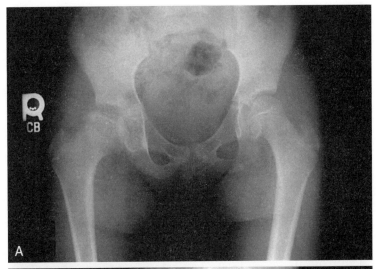

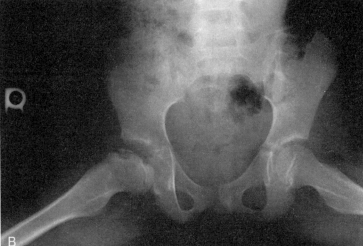

FIGURE 18–9. Legg-Calvé-Perthes disease in the right hip. Note the flattening and fragmentation of the femoral head. Anteroposterior *(A)* and frog-leg *(B)* radiographs. Magnetic resonance imaging scan *(C)*.

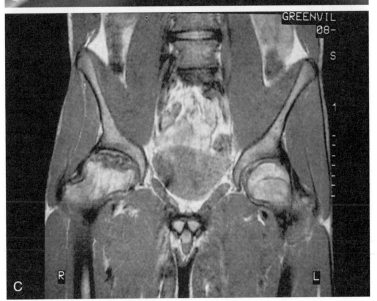

Magnetic resonance imaging (MRI; Fig. 18-9C) can be helpful in the evaluation and staging of LCP disease because it allows changes in the femoral head and epiphyseal plate to be seen. The ischemic area emits a weaker signal. MRI may provide an earlier and more detailed diagnosis than radiographs. Its disadvantages are its expense cand the need for sedation in children who cannot hold still for the necessary length of time.

Treatment Modalities and Related Nursing Management. The goals of treatment are to relieve symptoms, restore and preserve ROM, contain the femoral head, and maintain its sphericity (Herring, 1994). Treatment depends on the severity of the symptoms and x-ray findings. Some children have mild pain, with only a moderate decrease in ROM, and the femoral head remains well within the acetabulum. These children do not require any intervention and can be observed.

If the child initially presents with severe pain and limited ROM, the first step is to regain motion by relieving any synovitis, spasm, or tenderness around the hip joint. This is achieved through physical therapy and possibly nonsteroidal anti-inflammatory (NSAID) medication.

After motion has been restored, the physician decides whether the child is at risk for deformity or displacement of the femoral head. To prevent deformity of the diseased epiphysis or subluxation, the femoral head must be contained within the joint to allow acetabulum to mold the femoral head during the biologically plastic stages of the disease. Containment should first be tried by nonoperative means. The need for surgery depends on the extent of femoral head involvement and its ability to remodel. The younger the child, the better the potential for remodeling.

Containment is accomplished by bracing, casting, or surgery. A hip abduction brace maintains the hips in 30 degrees of abduction. Currently, the Scottish Rite orthosis is the most commonly used brace. It consists of two molded plastic thigh cuffs and a pelvic band and allows almost full hip flexion and extension while maintaining the abducted position. The knees are completely free to move. The position of abduction and flexion allows redirection of the compression forces across the hips to make them assist in the healing and remodeling process.

For bracing to be effective, there must be compliance on the part of the client during the time in which the orthosis must be worn. Most children tolerate the brace well and are able to participate in a wide range of sports and other activities while wearing the brace.

Surgical containment is accomplished by a pelvic osteotomy (most often the Salter innominate osteotomy), a proximal femoral osteotomy, or combined procedure. Surgery is the treatment of choice when the femoral head is flattened and deformed and no longer completely covered by the acetabulum.

Prognosis. There are two aspects to the prognosis in LCP. The short-term prognosis concerns the femoral head deformity at the completion of the healing phase. The long-term prognosis concerns the late development of secondary degenerative osteoarthritis of the hip in adult life.

The prognosis for femoral head deformity is determined in part by age at onset, extent of femoral head involvement, containment of the femoral head, and ROM. The younger the child, the better the prognosis. Extensive epiphyseal involvement, particularly of the lateral portion, is a poor prognostic sign. Loss of containment of the femoral head within the socket results in deformity and loss of motion.

Residual femoral head deformity and age at clinical onset are prognostic factors related to the development of late degenerative osteoarthritis. Clients with significant residual femoral head deformity not congruent with the acetabulum are at risk for developing degenerative osteoarthritis before the age of 50. If the age at onset is 5 years or less, the incidence of symptomatic degenerative osteoarthritis in adults with deformity is negligible (Herring, 1994).

Nursing management. The client and family initially require education about the disease process and treatment. Encouragement and support should be provided if the child must wear a brace. The nurse should check the brace once it is made to ensure it fits properly. The family should be instructed to check the skin for any signs of irritation from the brace. The child should be encouraged to participate in as many normal activities as possible. Nursing intervention with school and community caregivers may also be necessary for the child in a brace.

Summary. LCP disease is a self-limiting disorder, but it can cause significant deformity and osteoarthritis in adulthood if not treated appropriately. Treatment may be long term, and the child and family need ongoing support during this time.

Slipped Capital Femoral Epiphysis

Definition and Classification. Slipped capital femoral epiphysis is a displacement of the femoral head relative to the femoral neck occurring through the open growth plate.

The slipped capital femoral epiphysis is often classified as stable or unstable. The unstable type is a sudden slip of the femoral head resulting from trauma. In many cases, there is no prior history of pain. In other instances, progressive slippage may have occurred, and a traumatic incident causes the femoral head to be further displaced (often called an acute on chronic slip). In a stable slipped capital femoral epiphysis, the femoral head gradually slips off the femoral neck. Slipped capital femoral epiphysis can also be classified in terms of severity. Table 18–2 has a description of the classification.

Incidence and Etiology. The incidence of slipped capital femoral epiphysis has been reported to be 2 to 10 per 100,000, and it varies greatly with race, sex, and geographic location. Boys are affected two to five times more than girls, and there is an increased incidence in

TABLE 18–2. *Classification of Severity of Slipped Capital Femoral Epiphysis*

CLASSIFICATION	DESCRIPTION
Preslip (grade I)	Widening and rarefaction of the physis No displacement of the epiphysis
Minimal slip (grade II)	Extent of maximal displacement of the femoral head is up to one third of superior metaphyseal width of the femoral neck
Moderate slip (grade III)	Neck migration between one third and one half of upper metaphyseal diameter of the femoral neck
Severe slip (grade IV)	Displacement of the femoral head is more than 50% of the upper metaphyseal diameter of the femoral neck

African Americans. The highest incidence in the United States is in the northeastern states. A lower incidence is found in the southwestern states. The average age of onset is 13 to 15 years for boys and 11 to 13 years for girls. It rarely occurs after menarche. Obesity is reported in as many as 75% of clients. The incidence of bilateral involvement is 25%.

The exact cause of slipped capital femoral epiphysis is not known, although it is probably multifactorial. Biomechanically, during the adolescent growth spurt, the growth plate is weakened and less able to resist shear stresses as it approaches closure and takes on the configuration of the adult femoral head and neck. Because this disorder is primarily a disease of adolescence, the cause is believed to have an endocrine component. Furthermore, an imbalance is thought to exist between growth and sex hormones (either an excess in growth hormones or a deficit in sex hormones), which further increases the vulnerability of the growth plate. This hypothesis is supported by the fact that slipped capital femoral epiphysis occurs most often in obese, skeletally immature individuals. Trauma is also a factor in its development. In acute cases, trauma can cause a sudden slip of the weakened growth plate. In chronic cases, repetitive microtrauma can play a role. Slipped capital femoral epiphysis is also associated with a number of syndromes, such as trisomy 21 and hypothyroidism.

Pathophysiology. The changes found depend on the severity and stage of the disease. In the preslip stage, the physis is widened and the synovial membrane is engorged and edematous. The slip occurs in the layer of cartilage cells adjacent to the zone of provisional calcification. In the chronic case, the slip occurs gradually. With an acute slip, the perichondrium can be stripped from the femoral neck anteriorly and inferiorly. Hemarthrosis can be present with an acute slip. As the femoral head is displaced posteriorly, it slips inferiorly.

The synovium can remain edematous for several months. In 1 to 3 years, the physis ossifies, with a bony union occurring between the femoral neck and head. The residual findings depend on the integrity of the circulation to the femoral head, cartilage viability, amount of deformity, and joint mechanics.

Complications that can appear as a result of slipped capital femoral epiphysis include chondrolysis (acute necrosis of the hyaline articular cartilage) and avascular necrosis.

Assessment

Subjective assessment: nursing history. History of trauma, the duration and location of the pain, and how long the client has had a limp should be determined. As with most hip problems, the pain from a slipped capital femoral epiphysis can be in the groin, thigh, or knee. The exact symptoms and duration of complaints depend in part on whether the slip is thought to be preslip, acute, chronic, or acute on chronic. In addition to information about the pain and limp, the nurse also should elicit information regarding the client's overall health history, including renal and endocrine problems. This is especially pertinent in a girl younger than age 11 or a boy younger than age 13 because these types of medical problems are associated with slips in younger children.

The exact complaints help the practitioner determine whether the slip is stable or unstable. In the client with a preslip, the history consists primarily of complaints of leg weakness, limp with exertion, and pain. In the acute traumatic slip, the femoral head has been abruptly displaced by a traumatic incident. Clients with chronic slips usually have a history of dull or vague groin pain that is referred to the anterior thigh and knee that has been going on for weeks or months. The pain may be continuous or intermittent and is usually increased with activity. In the case of an acute on chronic slip, the client has a history of hip, thigh, or knee pain for the past several weeks or months but experiences a sudden onset of severe pain and decreased weight bearing after a traumatic incident.

Objective assessment: physical examination. Depending on whether the client has a stable or unstable slip, he or she will ambulate with a limp or may be unable to ambulate at all. If able to ambulate, the client has an antalgic gait, with the foot on the affected side externally rotated. ROM will be painful and severely limited. The client has no internal rotation of the hip on the side of the slip. This is marked by a positive figure four sign (flexion of the hip forces the leg into external rotation). Abduction and hip flexion are deceased. The client may have a leg length discrepancy and thigh atrophy depending on how long the symptoms have been present. This information is important because the longer the client has had the problem untreated, the greater the risk of complications.

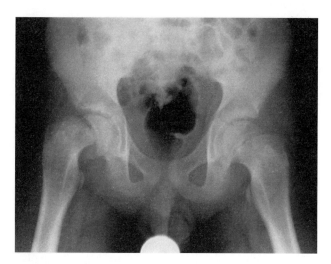

FIGURE 18-10. Slipped capital femoral epiphysis of the right hip.

Diagnostic Evaluation. Both anteroposterior views of the pelvis and frog lateral x-ray films of the hip should be obtained (Fig. 18-10). On the anteroposterior view of the hips, a line drawn along the outer margin of the neck should transect the head. In slipped capital femoral epiphysis, the line does not pass through the femoral head. The degree of slip is classified as in Table 18-2. In the chronic or acute on chronic slip, healing or remodeling is evident along the femoral neck. Other radiographic studies are not routinely used in the diagnosis. If the child is younger (younger than age 11 in girls and 13 in boys), a thyroid panel should be ordered to rule out a metabolic cause of the slip.

Treatment Modalities and Related Nursing Management. Treatment of slipped epiphysis is always surgical. From the time of diagnosis until surgery, the client is placed on crutches, non-weight bearing. The goal of surgery is to prevent further slippage. This is accomplished by in situ pinning to hold the femoral head in its present position until closure of the femoral physis. In the more severe slip that limits function and predisposes the client to early degenerative changes or in the hip that has suffered the complications of avascular necrosis or chondrolysis, a femoral or pelvic osteotomy may be needed to correct the deformity.

For the client who has undergone a simple in situ pinning, the postoperative period is generally uneventful. The incision is less than 1 inch long, and the client's pain is generally well managed with oral opioids for the first day or two and then acetaminophen if further discomfort persists. Persistent pain and limitation of hip motion in the postoperative period can indicate avascular necrosis or chondrolysis of the femoral head. The client with a stable slip can be bear full weight with crutches after the surgery. The client with an unstable slip cannot bear weight for 4 weeks.

Nursing management. Slipped capital femoral epiphysis is a problem that the client and parent may not have heard of before the child's incident. In addition, surgery is urgent. The client who has been walking around with a stable slip is often unaware of the serious nature of the problem, and the entire family is taken by surprise when the diagnosis and need for surgical intervention is discussed. In addition to a thorough explanation about the problem, treatment, and possible complications, reassurance that the child will walk and be able to participate in physical activities is necessary. (See the section on common nursing concerns for the child with an orthopaedic congenital or developmental disorder in this chapter, and perioperative care [Chapter 11], modalities for mobilization [crutches, Chapter 13], and modalities for immobilization [casts, Chapter 12] for nursing diagnoses and interventions.) In addition, when warranted, the nurse should discuss a weight loss program with the client and family and if possible initiate a dietary consult. There is a 25% chance that the problem will occur on the opposite side and a weight reduction program may decrease the chances of this occurring in an obese child.

Summary. Slipped capital femoral epiphysis is the most common hip disorder in adolescence. It can occur acutely as a result of trauma or can be a progressive slippage. Treatment must be instituted immediately on diagnosis to prevent further slippage and possible avascular necrosis of the femoral head. The nurse must assist the individual and family in dealing with the urgent need for treatment and the limitation in mobility after surgery.

Deformities of the Leg/Knee
Limb Length Discrepancy
Definition. A limb length discrepancy is a difference in length between the two upper extremities or the two lower extremities. In general, a limb length difference is more often problematic when the lower extremities are affected. A difference in the length of the lower extremities that is greater than 1 cm has the potential to cause low-back pain, limp, increased energy expenditure with gait, heelcord contracture, scoliosis, and degenerative joint disease. A limb length difference in the arms may not become disabling until the difference exceeds several inches.

Etiology. The etiology of a limb length discrepancy can be congenital; neurologic; vascular; or due to a tumor, infection, or fracture. In the child, any of these problems can cause a growth arrest or overgrowth depending on the specific nature of the problem and the portion of the bone involved. For example, an injury to the growth plate can result in decreased growth and a subsequent shortening of the affected limb. If, on the other hand, the insult involves the metaphysis or diaphysis, the client can experience up to 2 cm of overgrowth in the affected bone during the 2 years following the accident. The actual amount of shortening or overgrowth depends on the age of the child at the time of the trauma and the amount of growth left in the bone.

When determining the etiology of a limb length discrepancy, the practitioner should also keep in mind that other congenital problems such as clubfoot, Blount's disease, or hip dysplasia can also cause a limb length difference. Box 18-3 has a complete list of causes.

Assessment

Subjective assessment: nursing history. The first goal of the clinician should be to determine whether the cause of the leg length difference is acquired or congenital. The history should include information about the child's age when the discrepancy was first noted; history of trauma, pain, or infection; and whether there has been an increase of the leg length difference. The practitioner should also know about the child's activities, whether the problem interferes with participation in physical education or sports activities, and the presence of pain. Information about any previous treatment (including shoe lifts) should be obtained. Also, the nurse should elicit a thorough family history, placing an emphasis on musculoskeletal problems. From the beginning, assessing the maturity of the client, the family interactions, and available support systems is vital in planning future treatment.

Objective assessment: physical examination. A complete musculoskeletal examination is essential. The child's height should be measured and plotted on a growth chart. The spine should be examined in both the

---

BOX 18–3.
Causes of Lower Limb Length Inequality

I. Resulting from shortening by growth retardation
   A. Congenital anomalies of musculoskeletal system
      1. Proximal focal femoral deficiency
      2. Congenital short femur
      3. Congenital dislocation of the hip
      4. Congenital longitudinal deficiency of the long bones in the lower limb—fibular hemimelia, tibial hemimelia
      5. Congenital hemiatrophy
      6. Other severe congenital malformations of the foot, such as talipes equinovarus
   B. Developmental and tumorous affections of the skeleton
      1. Fibrous dysplasia—Albright's syndrome
      2. Enchondromatosis—Ollier's disease
      3. Multiple hereditary exostosis
      4. Punctate epiphyseal dysplasia
      5. Dysplasia epiphysealis hemimelica (Trevor's disease)
      6. Neurofibromatosis
   C. Infections of bones and joints (produce shortening by destroying the growth plate)
      1. Osteomyelitis—femur or tibia
      2. Tuberculosis of the hip, knee, or ankle
      3. Septic arthritis
   D. Trauma
      1. Injury to physis may cause its premature fusion and shortening
      2. Overlapping and malposition of fracture fragments of the shaft of the femur or tibia cause shortening
      3. Severe burns
   E. Neuromuscular diseases—asymmetrical paralysis causes shortening
      1. Poliomyelitis
      2. Cerebral palsy

   3. Myelomeningocele
   4. Lesions of brain and spinal cord, such as neoplasms or abscesses
   5. Peripheral nerve injuries, such as sciatic, femoral, or peroneal nerve palsy
   F. Others
      1. Slipped capital femoral epiphysis
      2. Legg-Calvé-Perthes disease
      3. Prolonged immobilization by weight-relieving orthoses
      4. Radiation therapy and arrest of physeal growth

II. Resulting from lengthening by growth stimulation
   A. Congenital anomalies of musculoskeletal system
      1. Congenital hemihypertrophy
      2. Localized gigantism with or without congenital vascular malformations
   B. Developmental and tumorous affections of skeleton and soft tissue malformations
      1. Neurofibromatosis
      2. Hemangiomatosis of soft tissues
      3. Arteriovenous fistulae
   C. Infections and inflammatory conditions of bones and joints (by increasing blood supply to the epiphyseal and metaphyseal regions)
      1. Metaphyseal or diaphyseal osteomyelitis
      2. Rheumatoid arthritis
      3. Hemarthrosis because of hemophilia
   D. Trauma
      1. Metaphyseal or diaphyseal fractures can increase blood supply to the physis and stimulate growth
      2. Traumatic arteriovenous aneurysm or fistula
      3. Operations on the diaphysis-metaphysis of the femur or tibia (iatrogenic trauma)
         a. Stripping of the periosteum
         b. Osteosynthesis
         c. Taking of bone graft

From Tachdjian, M. O. (1990). *Pediatric orthopaedics* (2nd ed.). Philadelphia: WB Saunders.

standing and sitting positions because leg length discrepancies may cause an apparent scoliosis. The hips should be examined for any decrease in ROM that might be indicative of hip dysplasia. The examiner should also assess both legs, looking for angular deformities or muscle atrophy. The presence of any deformity in the foot should also be noted. The muscle strength of each lower extremity, neurovascular status, and motion of the knee and ankle should be assessed. The examiner should also examine the upper extremities to determine whether one entire half of the body is longer than the contralateral side.

Leg lengths are measured from the anterior superior iliac spine to the bottom of the medial malleolus. If the examiner suspects that the foot is part of the limb length discrepancy, he or she should measure down to the bottom of the foot. This type of measurement can be difficult in an obese client and in that case, the clinician can ascertain the discrepancy by using measured blocks. A block of a known height is placed under the short leg to determine how much is needed to produce a level pelvis (Fig. 18–11). This part of the examination is useful because the client can tell the examiner at what point he or she is most comfortable and feels balanced. This method is also helpful in clients with complex deformi-

ties because the effect of lengthening on these other deformities can be assessed.

The examiner can evaluate whether the shortening lies in the femur or tibia (or both) by looking at both the Galeazzi and Allis signs. The Galeazzi sign tests for a difference in the length of the femur. The child lies supine, and both hips are flexed to 90 degrees. The examiner then notes the level of the knees. If the level of the knees is not symmetrical, the test is positive. The length of the tibia is assessed using the Allis test. The knees are flexed to 90 degrees, with the feet resting flat on the examination table. Again, the level of the knees should be examined. If one knee is lower, one of the tibiae is affected.

Diagnostic Evaluation. Radiographs can be used to measure leg lengths. Scanograms are x-ray films (Fig. 18–12) that consist of separate exposures of the hip, knee, and ankle on one film, allowing an individual to calculate the lengths of both lower extremities. Leg length measurements can also be obtained using computed tomography (CT). This provides a visualization of the entire pelvis and lower limbs. The technique is accurate, but the cost is significantly higher than the scanogram, without a substantial increase in precision.

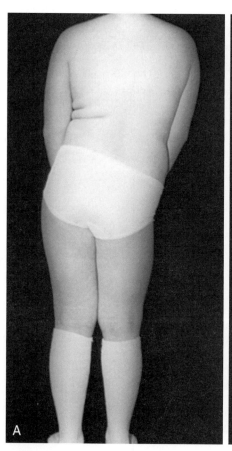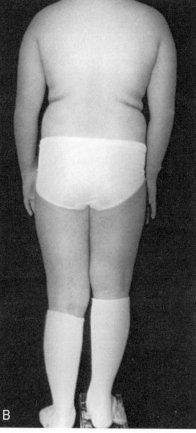

FIGURE 18–11. *A,* Leg length discrepancy after femoral fracture, which damaged the distal femoral growth plate. *B,* Blocks are used under the short side to level the pelvis and estimate the discrepancy.

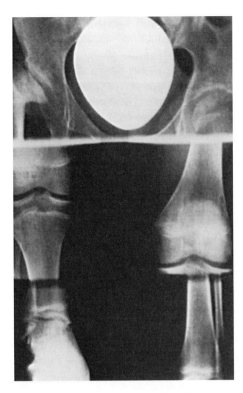

FIGURE 18–12. Example of a scanogram. The scanogram is an easy, inexpensive, and accurate method of determining limb length. (From Morrisy, R. T. [1990]. *Lovell & Winter's pediatric orthopaedics.* Philadelphia: Lippincott.)

Treatment Modalities and Related Nursing Management

Shoe lifts. The first line of treatment, for smaller discrepancies or before surgical intervention, is a shoe lift. A shoe lift can be used regardless of the child's age and is a painless and simple way of solving a leg length difference. However, children and adolescents usually do not react favorably to shoe lifts unless they are small enough to fit inside the shoe. For the client with a small discrepancy and low-back pain, a trial with a shoe lift can be helpful in determining whether equalizing the leg lengths would ease the discomfort

Surgical intervention. Several surgical options are available to reduce a leg length discrepancy. Most procedures take place close to skeletal maturity; however, large discrepancies may require earlier intervention. In the development of a treatment plan, the amount of discrepancy, age of the child, predicted height at maturity, predicted discrepancy at maturity, cause of the discrepancy, and skeletal maturity are all taken into account.

Leg-shortening procedures. There are several options available for the child who still has growth remaining in the physes of the lower extremities. One method is a procedure called an *epiphysiodesis*. This is the planned surgical arrest of growth in the longer leg. When the amount of growth remaining in one or more growth plates around the knee is calculated to equal the amount

of the leg length discrepancy, the surgery is performed. During this procedure, the growth plate at the proximal tibia or distal femur is disrupted. Growth no longer continues at that physis. (For larger discrepancies, the procedure may be needed at both the proximal tibial physis and the distal femur.) For example, if a child's left tibia is 2.5 cm shorter than the right, the procedure would take place when the child has 2.5 cm of growth remaining in the proximal tibial growth plate. During the surgery, the right proximal tibial physis is ablated. Over the next year, growth continues in the left proximal tibial physis, and at the time of skeletal maturity, the leg lengths should be equal. An obvious complication resulting from an epiphysiodesis is uneven leg lengths resulting from miscalculation of bone growth. The procedure can be performed on an outpatient basis, and a knee immobilizer or brace is used after surgery to provide immobilization.

The client and family need to understand that the results of an epiphysiodesis are not immediate. Changes take place over time. The goal is to have equal leg lengths at the end of growth. Regular follow-up examinations are needed until that time.

Another procedure, which can be done in skeletally mature clients to shorten the longer leg, is a shortening osteotomy. During this procedure, the surgeon removes as much of the bone on the long leg as is necessary to equalize the leg lengths. Up to 25% of the bone's original length can be removed. Nonunion is one possible complication, and many are hesitant to perform a procedure such as this on an unaffected leg.

The client must be made aware that there will be a loss in height after any leg shortening procedure. However, these procedures are generally less time-consuming and easier on the client than leg-lengthening procedures.

Leg-lengthening procedures. Leg-lengthening procedures are indicated for the client with a discrepancy of 2 cm or greater, for those who are skeletally mature and are no longer candidates for an epiphysiodesis, or for the shorter client who does not want to sacrifice any of his or her height from a leg-shortening procedure. In general, the bone can be safely lengthened up to 25% of its original length. In cases of severe discrepancies, leg-lengthening procedures are done in combination with the epiphysiodesis. Also, many clients who have severe discrepancies require staged procedures. The leg is lengthened in childhood and the procedure then repeated at skeletal maturity and/or both the tibia and the femur require lengthening.

Leg lengthening is accomplished through the use of an external fixator. These are devices that attach to the bone but lie on the outside of the limb. Depending on the problem and its location, several types of fixators can be used. Uniplane fixators lie on one aspect or side of the limb. These are useful for straight, uncomplicated lengthenings and are more comfortable for the client who is undergoing a femoral lengthening. The other method commonly employed is the use of a circular fixator. The Ilizarov external fixator consists of metal rings that circumscribe the limb and are connected by longitudinal threaded rods. The fixator attaches to the bone by thin 1.5- to 1.8-mm stainless steel wires that connect to the rings and cross at 90-degree angles (Fig. 18–13).

During the Ilizarov surgery, a corticotomy (cut through the cortex of the bone) is performed at the metaphysis. This area of the bone has a rich blood supply and is the primary site of osteogenic activity for bone growth and remodeling. The corticotomy site lies between two rings, which are separated during the procedure. The corticotomy site functions as a pseudogrowth plate and is the focus of the procedure as distraction occurs. The process of mechanically separating the two ends of the bone is known as distraction.

The distraction process in children begins 6 to 7 days after surgery. The delay in beginning the lengthening process is to allow some early callus formation and to let any intraoperative injury to the medullary circulation repair itself. The distraction process can take place either manually by turning clickers or automatically by a small computerized device that attaches to the frame. As the bone ends separate, undifferentiated bone cells migrate to the distraction site and proliferate to fill the ensuing gap. An osseous bridge forms between the two bone ends; this bridge is histologically identical to early bone formation at the node of Ranvier (the circular periosteal bridge surrounding the growth plate) (Aaronson, 1997). The lengthening proceeds at a rate of 1 mm/day. This slow rate of distraction gives the blood vessels and nerves time to adapt to the change in length and encourages new bone growth (Figs. 18–14*A* and *B*).

Once the client has distracted the bone to the desired length, he or she enters a latency period. During this time, differentiation occurs and collagen and matrix form. Eventually, the membranous network ossifies and a segment of bone is added to the limb. In addition, the stretching of the periosteum, vessels, nerves, muscles, and skin stimulates histogenesis of the soft tissues as well as angiogenesis (proliferation of new blood vessels) (Bianchi-Maiocchi & Aaronson, 1994). The fixator is removed when at least three of four cortices of the new bone show complete consolidation (Fig. 18–14*C*).

Nursing management

Preoperative preparation. A great deal of time is required to prepare the client and family for a leg-lengthening procedure. Instruction should include a description of the surgical procedure, care of the fixator, time commitment on the part of the client and family, and advantages and disadvantages of other options. It is often helpful to have an initial meeting with the family to introduce the procedure, allow the client and family to see the fixator, and briefly discuss the treatment plan. The family can be given written materials to take home and read. After they have had time to weigh their options and contemplate questions, they should return for an in-depth discussion of the entire process including risks and possible complications, pin care, the distraction process, frequency and importance of office visits, pain management, physical therapy, clothing modifications, and other details that the clinician deems important to the client's treatment. Emphasis should be placed on the goals of the procedure and the expected outcome. Also, if the client and family desire, they should be provided with the opportunity to talk with a similar client and family that has undergone the procedure.

One of the most important assessments the nurse can make before the procedure is the assessment of the compliance and reliability of the client and family. The technique requires a great deal of vigilance. If they are not conscientious, the child risks severe complications and problems. Because the child's cooperation is essential to the procedure, his or her psychological readiness, as well as family support, must be assessed.

Risks and complications of lengthening procedures include infection, knee subluxation, transient sensory or motor loss, nerve palsy (sciatic, peroneal), loss of motion, delayed consolidation, and fracture at the lengthening site. Careful pin care, neurovascular assessment, and aggressive physical therapy can help prevent or detect many of the potential complications in their early stages. Smoking has been shown to seriously impair bone growth. Adolescents should be warned of this and the procedure should be delayed until the client has been able to stop smoking.

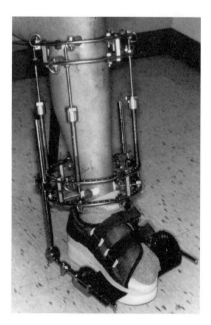

FIGURE 18–13. The Ilizarov external fixation device. A dynamic extension orthosis attaches to the fixator.

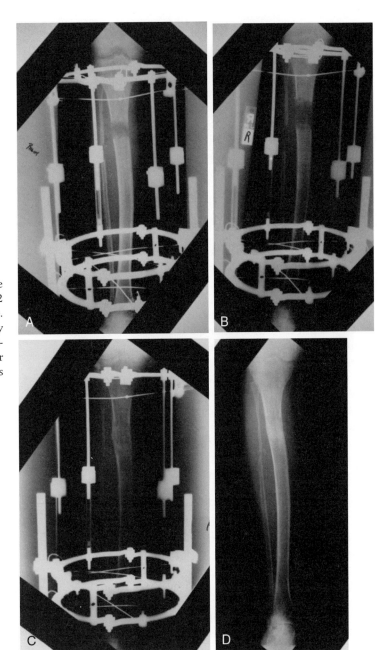

FIGURE 18–14. Limb-lengthening process. *A,* Three weeks postoperative. Client has lengthened the tibia 2 cm at the corticotomy site. *B,* Six weeks postoperative. Five centimeters of distraction has taken place. Early bone formation is visible. *C,* Twelve weeks postoperative. Consolidation of new bone. Client is ready for removal of fixator. *D,* Remodeling of the tibia 24 weeks after surgery.

Postoperative care. In the immediate postoperative period, the client's extremity should remain elevated to prevent undue swelling. Neurovascular checks should be performed every 4 hours. Although not a common occurrence, compartment syndrome can occur in the hours following surgery. Unless there are wires or rings that cross the ankle and foot, the client should have active dorsiflexion, inversion, and eversion. The client with an upper extremity fixator should have active dorsiflexion and radial and ulnar deviation of the wrist, as well as finger flexion, extension abduction, and adduction.

Whenever the client complains of sudden irretractable pain unrelieved by medication and interrupting his or her sleep, the possibility of infection or nerve impinge-ment should be considered. On occasion, a client may have an infection without the classic signs of inflammation, swelling, or purulence at the pin sites. The only adequate relief of pain for these clients is antibiotics. Nerve impingement is generally accompanied by numbness and/or decreased movement. Tapping on the affected wire with a metal object will send a feeling of electricity down the leg. The treatment for this is to remove the wire.

During the postoperative period, the family is taught pin care, neurovascular assessment, and the signs and symptoms of infection. Physical therapy is begun. Aggressive ROM exercises are an integral part of a leg-lengthening procedure. Equal leg lengths without functional motion is not an improvement over a short extremity. In the Ilizarov technique, weight bearing is begun immediately to stimulate development and consolidation of new bone.

The family and child need to be taught the distraction procedure. Written instructions and return demonstration are both important to ensure that the distraction proceeds as planned. With the Ilizarov device, distraction takes place manually by turning four clickers. One clicker is attached to each of the four longitudinal rods. Each set of four clicks (one click × four clickers) distracts the bone 0.25 cm. At the end of 1 day, the bone is lengthened 1 cm.

At follow-up visits, x-ray films are obtained to observe the gap created by distraction, to assess for the presence of new bone formation, and to ensure alignment and pin integrity. Pin sites are checked, as are motion and neurovascular status of the extremity.

Recently, the external fixators are being used to lengthen the limbs of children afflicted with one of the short stature disorders, such as achondroplasia. Many individuals are functionally impaired and unable to carry on normal activities of daily living (ADLs). Children with achondroplasia and other disorders that cause severe shortening of the upper extremities can have difficulty bathing and combing their hair. Short stature can also make using public transportation and restrooms difficult and can create other issues. Many believe that lengthening the extremities and correcting any angular deformities not only limit disability but also improve quality of life. These are issues that must be decided by the children and their families.

If a client is interested in increasing the length of both arms and/or legs, the procedure should be initiated when the child is between the ages of 11 and 16. After the age of 20, the psychological impact that results from changing one's body image can be overwhelming to the individual. The child must be an active participant in the decision-making process. Clients with short stature who are interested in undergoing a lower extremity lengthening must be aware that lengthening the legs may increase the need for an upper extremity lengthening because of the increase in body disproportion that may result from lengthening the legs.

Summary. Limb length discrepancies have multiple causes, but the goal of any treatment is to have equal or near equal leg lengths at skeletal maturity. A number of options are available to accomplish this goal. Care of children undergoing lengthening procedures is complex and challenging, and nursing assessment and support play an integral role in caring for these children.

Blount's Disease (Tibia Vara)

Definition and Classification. Tibia vara, or Blount's disease, was first described by Dr. Walter Blount in 1937. The tibiae are bowed secondary to a growth disturbance of the medial portion of the proximal epiphysis of the

TABLE 18–3. *Early-Onset versus Late-Onset Blount's Disease*

TYPE	DESCRIPTION
Early onset	Onset age 1–3 years
	Girls affected more than boys
	Blacks affected more than whites
	Obesity common
	Early walking history
	More severe varus deformity
	Bracing in early stages
	Tibial osteotomy in later stages or failed conservative treatment
Late onset	Juvenile onset 6–13 years
	Adolescent onset after 11 years
	75% affected are boys
	Obesity common
	More mild progressive deformity
	Pain or locking or popping of knee
	High tibial osteotomy or lateral tibial hemi-epiphysiodesis for progressive or significant deformity

tibia. The effects of this disease can be seen in three different age categories. The infantile type (early onset) occurs between the ages of 18 months and 3 years. The juvenile onset is between 4 and 10 years, and the adolescent type begins after 11 years. The disease characteristics and treatment of the juvenile and adolescent types (both considered late onset) are the same. Table 18–3 summarizes the key differences between the early-onset and late-onset types.

Incidence and Etiology

Infantile/early type. Infantile Blount's disease is more common than the late-onset type. Girls are affected more often than boys. The incidence is higher in black children than in white children. Repetitive stress of weight bearing on an already bowed leg is believed to be the cause of this disorder. The bowing may be exaggerated by obesity. Approximately 80% of children with infantile Blount's disease have bilateral involvement. Pain does not accompany this type of Blount's disease.

Late onset. The juvenile type of Blount's disease is generally found in children between the ages of 6 and 13 years. With late-onset Blount's disease, there is bilateral involvement in approximately one third of boys and in two thirds of girls. Of those affected, 75% are boys. Obesity is usually present (Loder, Schaffer, & Bardenstein, 1991).

Pathophysiology. Biologic and mechanical factors are thought to interact to produce Blount's disease. A varus angulation of the knee and weight bearing increases stress across the medial physis. This abnormal force damages the growth plate. Growth at the proximal medial aspect of the tibia is altered and results in further deformity.

In the late-onset type, fissuring and clefts in the physis and fibrovascular and cartilaginous repair at the physeal-metaphyseal junction are observed. An arrest or a partial disturbance of the endochondral growth mechanism is noted in the medial aspect of the physis. As described, a cycle of stress is believed to be responsible for the disorder. Obesity and persistent genu varus increase the medial physeal stress.

Assessment

Subjective assessment: nursing history

Early-onset type. Progressive bowing of the legs after the age of 18 months is the chief complaint that characterizes infantile Blount's disease. The clinician must rule out other metabolic causes such as rickets (a nutritional disorder) and vitamin D–resistant rickets (a hereditary disorder). Therefore, information must be elicited about the child's overall health and family history. This should be followed by a nutritional history, including information on how much milk the child drinks, how long the child was breast-fed, and the overall amount of calcium in the child's diet. If the bowing is unilateral, questions regarding infection or fracture in the affected leg should be included in the history because these problems can cause premature closure of an isolated portion of the growth plate and lead to a varus deformity.

Juvenile/adolescent Blount's disease. The examiner should begin by asking when the problem was first noted,

if one or both legs are affected, and whether the client is having pain. As in the infantile form, when the problem is unilateral, the clinician requires information regarding any history of trauma or infection in the bone. A health history and family history should be taken because bowed legs are also a symptom of certain skeletal dysplasias that are genetic disorders.

Objective assessment: physical examination

Early-onset type. The clinician should plot the child's height on a growth chart, and this can be followed if subsequent visits are needed. Any child who is below the fifth percentile should be examined carefully for a skeletal dysplasia. The clinician should also look at body proportions to make sure the limbs and trunk are proportionate. When the child's arms are at the side, his or her fingertips should touch the midthigh area. A child, who is below the fifth percentile for height, has bilateral bowing, and has a body disproportion between the trunk and limbs may have one of the skeletal dysplasias.

The clinician should thoroughly examine the child, with a specific emphasis placed on the rotation of the hips and tibiae. Often, a young child with excessive retroversion of the hips and a marked internal tibial torsion appears bowlegged even though both femurs and tibia are straight. These children can just be observed, and this should correct independent of intervention over time.

A prominent medial metaphyseal beak, often palpable, is characteristic of Blount's disease. A varus deformity of both tibiae is obvious (Fig. 18–15). A leg length discrepancy may be present if the problem is unilateral.

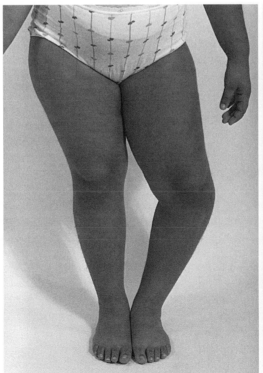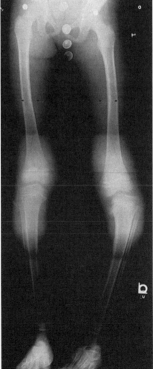

FIGURE 18–15. Child with Blount's disease.

Full ROM is present in the hips and knees. The clinician should also examine the child's wrists and ankles. Deformities resulting from rickets can be noted in joints other than the knees.

Juvenile/adolescent Blount's disease. Once again, the clinician should examine height and body proportions. The lower extremities should be examined, with the clinician noting the degree of varus present in one or both legs. The ROM of the hips and knees should be checked, although this is usually unaffected. Both legs should be measured because a limb length discrepancy may be present. An antalgic gait may be seen.

Diagnostic Evaluation. Anteroposterior standing radiographs of both lower extremities from the hip to the ankle are taken of the younger child. Medial angulation of the medial cortical wall of the proximal tibial metaphysis is noted on x-ray film (see Fig. 18–15). Fragmentation of the medial proximal tibial metaphysis may be observed with depression of the medial plateau. The medial proximal tibial physes are irregular.

If rickets is suspected, laboratory tests should be performed. Calcium and phosphorus levels should be drawn. Below-normal levels of calcium or phosphorus are indicative of rickets.

Juvenile/adolescent Blount's disease. Mechanical axis x-ray views are taken of the lower extremities in the older child or adolescent. Growth of the proximal medial tibial physis is slowed. A narrow area in the middle of the medial physeal line with sclerosis on both the epiphyseal and the metaphyseal sides of this area is characteristic.

Treatment Modalities and Related Nursing Management

Early-onset type. Bracing may be effective in correcting the deformity in the early stages. A knee-ankle-foot orthosis (KAFO) is recommended to reduce compressive forces on the medial physis. The brace is worn 23 hours per day until the deformity is corrected, which usually occurs in approximately 6 to 9 months.

The braces are locked in extension when the child bears weight. Parents should be taught to check the skin for irritation and about the importance of having the child wear the brace as prescribed.

A proximal tibial osteotomy is the procedure of choice for children who do not respond to conservative treatment or for those who have a more advanced stage of Blount's disease. This can be performed with internal or external fixation. If internal fixation is used, a long leg cast is usually applied for approximately 6 weeks.

Juvenile/adolescent Blount's disease. The deformity can be corrected in this age group only through surgical measures. A high tibial osteotomy is the recommended procedure. Internal fixation can be used to hold the corrected position as well as external fixation (uniplane or

circular). If a leg length discrepancy accompanies the deformity, both problems can be simultaneously corrected by using the Ilizarov external fixator.

Children with Blount's disease and their parents require teaching about the disease, its progression, and the usual treatment methods. In addition, cast care and bracing or external fixation care may need to be taught to the caregivers after surgery (see Chapter 11).

Postoperatively, neurovascular checks should be done every at least every 4 hours for the first 48 hours after surgery. Compartment syndrome is a postoperative complication from a tibial osteotomy. This is further addressed in Chapter 10. Pain management with intravenous opioids, followed by oral opioids, is necessary for several days to a week after surgery. Physical therapy consists of teaching the client to walk with crutches. If the child is in an external fixator, ROM exercises are important. The nurse should be sure that the client is medicated before therapy to maximize the child's progress.

For the obese child, a dietary consult should be initiated to provide information about weight reduction, sound dietary habits, and exercise.

Summary. Blount's disease is a varus deformity of the tibia that can occur in very young (younger than age 3) children (infantile form), in children ages 4 to 10 (juvenile late-onset type), or in children older than 11 (adolescent late-onset type). Although bracing is often successful in the toddler, surgical correction is necessary in children and adolescents.

Osgood-Schlatter Disease

Definition. Osgood-Schlatter disease, or tibial osteochondrosis, is a painful enlargement of the tibial tubercle in which the tibial tubercle apophysis separates from the proximal end of the tibia. The condition is self-limiting.

Incidence and Etiology. Osgood-Schlatter disease generally occurs in active children around the time of a growth spurt. Girls ages 9 to 13 and boys 10 to 15 years old are most commonly affected. The condition develops from repetitive microtrauma to the tibial tubercle, as secondary ossification centers are being formed.

Pathophysiology. The tibial tubercle is prone to strain during rapid growth from repetitive stress from the quadriceps. Quadriceps contraction transmits stress through the patellar tendon onto a small portion of the partially developed tibial tuberosity. The developing secondary ossification center is not able to withstand these tensile forces, resulting in partial avulsion fractures through the ossification center. Heterotopic bone formation occurs in the tendon near its insertion. In some cases, the avulsed segment of the tibial metaphysis fails to unite with the tuberosity.

Assessment

Subjective assessment: nursing history. When a child complains of knee pain, it is always helpful to begin by asking the child to point to where the pain is using one finger. With Osgood-Schlatter disease, the child does not point to the knee, but rather points below the knee at the tibial tubercle. The pain is aggravated by activity, and kneeling is difficult. The child often participates in sports or dance that requires repetitive quadriceps contraction, such as basketball, soccer, gymnastics, or ballet.

Objective assessment: physical examination. Swelling or an enlargement of the proximal tibial tuberosity can be noted. Palpation of the tibial tubercle elicits tenderness. Pain is usually present if the examiner extends the knee against resistance or if the individual squats with the knee in full flexion. The rest of the knee examination is normal.

Diagnostic Evaluation. In Osgood-Schlatter disease, radiographs can show thickening or calcification of the patellar tendon, soft tissue swelling, irregularities of the tibial tuberosity (although these occur in asymptomatic individuals also), or a superficial ossicle in the patellar tendon. Proximal displacement of the patella or a bony fragment may be apparent in a lateral radiograph.

Treatment Modalities and Related Nursing Management. Most cases of Osgood-Schlatter disease are self-limiting and the child can participate in physical activities according to his or her own tolerance. Activities that aggravate the condition should be avoided until the pain subsides. Exercises, such as quadriceps tightening, straight leg raising, and hamstring stretching exercises, may be needed before resuming sports. Kneepads can be of benefit in sports involving direct knee contact. Ice can be helpful in reducing pain in the acute phase.

In more resistant cases, immobilization in a knee immobilizer or walking cylinder cast may be necessary. Knee pain can be minimized by the use of analgesics, such as acetaminophen or an NSAID. Surgical management is rarely indicated; however, recurrent, disabling episodes of pain that are not amenable to conservative measures, formation of a discrete ossicle, and removal of a cosmetic deformity are indications for surgery. Excision of the ossicle is the most common procedure.

Anxiety about recurring pain or the need for further treatment can occur. Individuals and their families need to be reminded that pain may recur but that the process is generally self-limiting and stops when growth is complete.

Summary. Osgood-Schlatter disease is a painful enlargement of the tibial tubercle that typically occurs in active adolescents. Conservative treatment involves limitation of aggravating activities and is generally sufficient to alleviate symptoms. Symptoms resolve after growth is complete.

Chondromalacia Patellae

Definition. Chondromalacia is an irregularity of the articular surface of the patella. This occurs as a result of abnormal or repetitive mechanical forces (Fig. 18–16). Other names for this problem include anterior knee pain and patella femoral pain.

Incidence and Etiology. Chondromalacia patellae is a common problem in adolescents and young adults and is seen more often in females than in males (2:1 ratio). Activities that entail kneeling, bending, squatting, or overbending the knee exacerbate this condition, as do sports that involve continuous heavy impact on the knee (e.g., track, aerobics, dance).

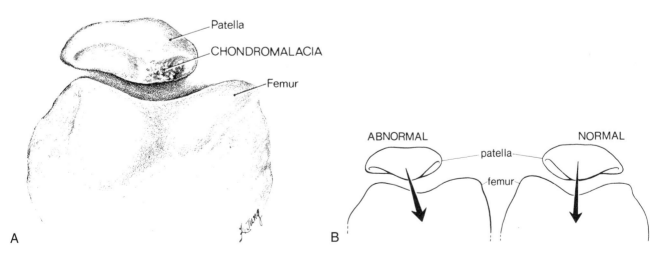

FIGURE 18–16. *A,* The undersurface of the articular cartilage of the patella is affected in chondromalacia. *B,* The patella in an abnormal position within the femoral groove and the normal position within the femoral groove. (From Komisarz, J. M. [1984]. Chondromalacia patellae. *Orthopaedic Nursing, 3*[3], 24, 25.)

Assessment

Subjective assessment: nursing history. The presenting symptom is pain around or under the kneecap. Pain is aggravated by activity, especially stair climbing, kneeling, squatting, and running. Occasionally, the client complains of pain after sitting for long periods. There may be a history of the knee "giving way" or of a dislocating kneecap.

Objective assessment: physical examination. The client's knee ROM is usually full, and this generally does not elicit pain. Crepitus can be felt in the knee joint with flexion and extension. Mild swelling may or may not be present.

The primary physical finding is that of a positive grind test. The client lies supine on the examination table and relaxes the quadriceps muscle. The examiner gently pushes down on the patella while asking the client to tighten the quadriceps. This maneuver should not elicit pain; however, the client with chondromalacia experiences pain upon tightening the quadriceps.

Quadriceps atrophy can be present on the affected leg. The client often has an increased valgus alignment of the knee, and the patella tracks laterally when the knee is flexed.

Diagnostic Evaluation. Radiographs are usually normal but are sometimes taken to rule out other problems that cause knee pain. Skyline views often show the individual has a patella tilt.

Treatment Modalities and Related Nursing Management. Treatment for chondromalacia patellae is usually nonoperative unless it is caused by a malalignment. Most clients respond to conservative measures. The client must avoid bending the knee past 90 degrees, kneeling, and squatting. Exercises, such as quadriceps setting, straight leg raising exercises, and hamstring stretches with the knee in full extension, strengthen the muscles without increasing patellofemoral compressive forces. Exercises must be done daily, and it may take as long as 3 months before the pain resolves.

Patella-stabilizing elastic knee braces may provide some support during activity. Ice can be applied before and after exercise to decrease discomfort. NSAIDs also diminish inflammation and pain.

Realignment procedures, including arthroscopic examination and lateral retinacular release, may be necessary in individuals with severe pain that cannot be managed with conservative measures or in those who have malalignment problems. Shaving of the patellar cartilage may be necessary in severe cases not responsive to conservative methods.

Nursing management. Information about the condition should be given. The nurse can often provide an exercise program for the client. The need for a consistent exercise regimen should be emphasized. Activities that aggravate the condition (e.g., kneeling, squatting, over-bending the knee) should be avoided, and this should be discussed with the client and parent.

Summary. Chondromalacia is common in the active adolescent. Individuals experience patellar pain. The majority obtain relief with conservative treatment, including quadriceps strengthening exercises and NSAIDs. Care must be taken not to unnecessarily restrict activity in the active individual.

Intoeing. Although the causes of intoeing are usually developmental and may be related to intrauterine posture, the condition often does not become apparent until the child begins to walk and run. The problem of intoeing can be caused by excessive internal rotation in the femur or tibia or a metatarsus adductus of the foot. The problem can be unilateral or bilateral. One foot may turn out while the other foot turns in (a windswept deformity). Excessive out-toeing can exist as well; however, treatment is sought less for out-toeing than intoeing.

Femoral Anteversion

Definition. Femoral anteversion is the forward, or anterior, angling of the femoral neck from the femoral shaft. The femoral head points too far forward in the acetabulum. To walk, the individual must rotate the hip medially. This causes the child to walk with an intoeing gait.

Incidence and Etiology. Femoral anteversion is most commonly seen in children 3 to 5 years of age. Girls are affected two times more often than boys. In most cases, femoral anteversion is a developmental condition associated with delayed lateral rotation of the lower extremities. Children afflicted with certain neuromuscular disorders such as CP or myelodysplasia often have an increased anteversion angle of the hips. It also can be indicative of developmental hip dysplasia.

Excessive out-toeing from the hip may occur as well. This problem is the exact opposite of femoral anteversion and is called *femoral retroversion.* The position of the femoral head lies too far posterior in the acetabulum. The clinician performs the same procedures during the physical examination; however, when the hip is rotated, there is an excessive amount of external rotation and limited internal rotation. This condition is expected to improve by age 8 years without intervention. In severe cases, surgery can be performed to internally rotate the femur to a better position.

Assessment

Subjective assessment: nursing history. The chief complaint is that the child walks with an intoeing gait. Another characteristic of the problem is the way these children sit on the floor with their legs in a W position. In addition to asking whether the problem is getting better, the nurse should assess whether the child trips and falls frequently, is able to participate in sports and physical education without difficulty, and is psychologically distraught by the way he or she walks. Any history of DDH should be noted.

Objective assessment: physical examination. The nurse should observe the child walking. The child with femoral anteversion turns the knees inward when he or she walks. The child should lie supine on the examination table. Then, the clinician rotates both legs at the hip joint and observes the patella. Normally, the child should have 45 degrees of internal and external rotation at the hip joint. The client who has an increased femoral anteversion angle has increased internal rotation of the hip, often as much as 90 degrees. Accompanying this is decreased external rotation of the hip (sometimes as little as 0 degrees). If the child has an external tibial torsion along with the femoral anteversion, the legs may appear bowed when the feet are pointed straight (Fig. 18–17). This increase in internal rotation can also be noted when the

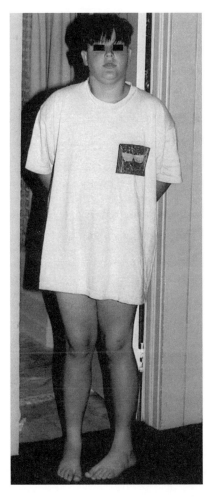

FIGURE 18–17. Femoral anteversion of the left side. Note how the left knee and foot point inward.

child lies prone and the knees are flexed to 90 degrees. The hips rotate inward excessively and have limited motion when rotated externally.

Diagnostic Evaluation. The clinical examination is of prime importance when diagnosing femoral anteversion. Plain radiographs can be helpful in ruling out hip dysplasia as a cause of intoeing. CT scans are used to determine the exact amount of anteversion when surgery is being considered in an older child.

Treatment Modalities and Related Nursing Management. Femoral anteversion often corrects spontaneously before 8 years of age. Braces and orthotic devices do not improve the condition. Sitting posture can be altered by encouraging the child to sit in a tailor's position (hips externally rotated, knees flexed, ankles crossed) rather than in a reverse tailor's, or W, position (hips internally rotated, knees flexed, ankles to the sides). Figure skating and ballet often improve the child's gait pattern because these activities help the child concentrate on turning the leg outward.

If the intoeing condition is so severe that it is disabling or causes the child to frequently fall or be ridiculed by other children, an external rotation femoral osteotomy can be performed. Because correction can occur spontaneously until age 8, surgery is indicated only in children older than 8 years of age.

Summary. Femoral anteversion is an anterior angling of the femoral neck from the femoral shaft. This condition usually resolves without treatment by age 8. The child and family need to feel free to discuss their concerns and be given adequate reinforcement about the self-limiting nature of the condition.

Tibial Torsion

Definition. Tibial torsion is a rotation of the shaft of the tibia around its long axis. A medial, or internal, torsion is a twisting of the tibia toward the body's midline, causing an intoeing gait (Fig. 18–18). Lateral or external tibial torsion is a twisting of the tibia away from midline, causing an out-toeing gait. A child may also have a combination of internal tibial torsion on one side and external tibial torsion on the contralateral side (windswept position).

Etiology. Tibial torsion is the result of fetal position. The degree of tibial torsion varies with age.

Assessment

Subjective assessment: nursing history. The child with internal tibial torsion usually has a history of an intoeing gait and/or of being bowlegged. The clinician should ask whether the child trips and falls frequently and whether the deformity is getting better or worse. An older child

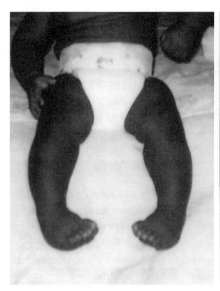

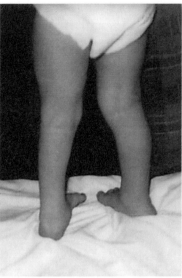

FIGURE 18–18. Bilateral internal tibial torsion.

should be asked how much the problem bothers him or her both physically and psychologically.

Objective assessment: physical examination. There are several methods for assessing for tibial torsion. The nurse should begin by observing the child's gait. The child with internal tibial torsion walks with an intoeing gait. The knees point straight, but the feet turn in. The problem may be worse on one side than it is the other.

The clinician should then observe the relationship of the knee to the foot. With the child in a sitting position, the knee and ankle are flexed to 90 degrees. The second ray of the foot should be in alignment with the center of the patella. In other words, the foot and the knee should point in the same direction. If the knee is pointing straight and the foot is internally rotated, the child has internal tibial torsion. If the foot is laterally rotated, the child has external tibial torsion.

Another test for internal tibial torsion is to examine the position of the malleoli. When the knee and ankle are flexed to 90 degrees, the examiner places the thumb and index finger over the medial and lateral malleoli and notes their position and relationship to one another. In the child with internal tibial torsion, the malleoli may be parallel or the medial malleolus may be slightly posterior to the lateral malleolus. As the child grows older, however, and the tibia begins to straighten, the medial malleolus should lie in front of the lateral malleolus.

One other method can be performed by having the child lie prone. The knee and ankle should be bent to 90 degrees. The clinician notes whether the foot points straight or is rotated inward. If there is no tibial torsion, a line drawn down the center of the thigh should be parallel to a line drawn down the center of the foot. If the foot points inward, the child has internal tibial torsion. If the foot points outward, the client has external tibial torsion.

When the parental complaints are of the child's feet turning outward, the clinician examines the child using the same methods; however, the foot points laterally, indicating an external tibial torsion.

Diagnostic Evaluation. Radiography is not generally used in infants and young children with tibial torsion because of its limited clinical value.

Treatment Modalities and Related Nursing Management. Most children with internal (medial) tibial torsion do not require treatment. This is another developmental condition that corrects spontaneously as the child grows. Children with severe cases should be followed to ensure that improvement is occurring. The Denis Browne bar (Fig. 18–19) is recommended when internal tibial torsion exceeds 35 degrees in a child between the age of 18 and 24 months and when the child is not experiencing spontaneous correction.

The Denis Browne bar is worn 12 hours at night. The bar is fixed between two straight-last open-toe shoes that attach to the bar. The bar is the width of the child's shoulder, and the shoes are externally rotated. The

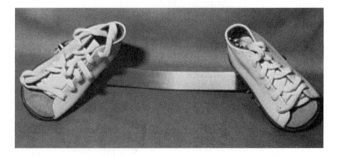

FIGURE 18–19. Denis Browne splint.

amount of external rotation depends on the severity of the internal rotation. Parents are taught to check the skin for redness and signs of irritation. Until the child is used to wearing the bar, the parent may need to gradually get the child accustomed to it. One method is to have the child wear only the shoes for a few nights and then attach the bar. The Denis Browne bar is worn for 6 months.

After age 5, spontaneous correction no longer occurs, and if the condition is still problematic, a tibial osteotomy may be required. The criterion for judging whether the surgical procedure is needed is similar to that for femoral anteversion: intoeing that causes the child to frequently fall or is psychologically distressing.

Summary. Medial tibial torsion generally resolves with growth. Treatment may be necessary if the tibia does not rotate laterally with time.

Foot Deformities

Physiologic Flatfeet

Definition. A flexible flatfoot (physiologic flatfeet) is a physiologic condition in which ligamentous laxity causes the longitudinal arch of the foot to flatten upon weight bearing.

Incidence and Etiology. A flexible flatfoot is a common disorder. Laxity of the joint capsules and ligaments of the plantar aspect of the foot is believed to be the cause.

Assessment

Subjective assessment: nursing history. The main objective when taking the history and examining the foot is to differentiate between the flexible flatfoot and one of the more rigid congenital disorders. The primary concern is whether the child is having pain. The child with a flexible flatfoot generally has no pain and no problem with wearing shoes. However, congenital deformities causing a flatfoot may be accompanied by severe discomfort during ambulation.

Objective assessment: physical examination. The child should be able to walk on his or her toes and heels. When the foot is evaluated with the child standing, the flexible flatfoot is pronated and the heel is in valgus. To distinguish a flexible flatfoot from other deformities, such as a peroneal spastic flatfoot or tarsal coalition, the child should be asked to stand on his or her toes. When non–weight bearing and standing tiptoe, the flexible flatfoot should form an arch. The child with a flexible flatfoot also has good muscle function in all directions and good subtalar motion.

When a congenital deformity is present, the foot is flat even when non–weight bearing, and generally, the child has difficulty walking on the toes. Subtalar motion

is limited, and stress on the peroneal tendon elicits severe pain.

Treatment Modalities and Related Nursing Management. No treatment is needed for flexible flatfoot. Corrective shoes, orthotics, and arch supports are not indicated. In most cases of flatfoot, recognition of the parents' concern and reassurance that the disorder generally needs no treatment and causes no discomfort are the primary nursing interventions. Many parents believe that expensive or corrective shoes are needed to prevent flatfoot. Parents can be assured that these shoes are not necessary. Shoes for toddlers are needed only for protection, and any well-fitting shoe will suffice.

Summary. Many parents have concerns about their child having a flatfooted appearance. In toddlers, a flatfoot is due to a fat pad that is present until the second or third year of life. If the child has a rigid flatfoot, further workup and treatment is necessary if the child is experiencing discomfort or is limited in his or her activities.

Tarsal Coalition

Definition. Tarsal coalition, also known as *rigid* or *peroneal spastic flatfoot,* is a failure of two tarsal bones to separate and a consequential lack of joint formation. Two bones of the foot are joined by a bony or fibrous bridge. The most common conditions are coalitions between the calcaneus and talus or the calcaneus and navicular.

Incidence and Etiology. Tarsal coalition is a rare condition, the exact incidence of which is not known but is probably less than 1%. The problem results from a failure of the primitive mesenchyme to differentiate and segment. Coalitions may be a solid bony bridge or may be divided by cartilage or fibrous tissue. They may be unilateral or bilateral.

Assessment

Subjective assessment: nursing history. The client typically is brought for an evaluation in late childhood or adolescence with complaints of pain in the foot. Younger children are usually asymptomatic. Greater body weight and sports participation may increase discomfort. Pain is relieved with rest and increased with activity.

Objective assessment: physical examination. The motion of the foot is limited, particularly at the subtalar and midtarsal joints. Gait disturbances may be present. A hindfoot valgus deformity, forefoot abduction, and peroneal tendon tightness are common findings. Muscle spasms may occur.

Diagnostic Evaluation. Conventional radiographs can be taken to rule out other problems, but generally, CT is necessary to demonstrate a tarsal coalition.

Treatment Modalities and Related Nursing Management. Treatment is based on age of the child, symptoms, location of the coalition, and presence of degenerative joint changes. If discomfort is not great, no treatment may be required. Immobilization for 3 to 4 weeks by casting can be tried initially. For severe deformity associated with pain and spasm, surgical intervention may be needed. Various procedures can be performed, and the decision often depends on the age of the child.

Regardless of the type of surgical procedure, the postoperative surgical care is the same. Foot surgery of this nature can be accompanied by a great deal of pain. The foot should be elevated on several pillows. The neurovascular status should be checked frequently. Intravenous opioids are recommended for the first 24 to 48 hours, followed by an oral opioid. The client should be given cast care instructions, and the parents taught neurovascular checks.

Summary. Tarsal coalitions are bridges formed between tarsal bones that are normally separated. Calcaneonavicular and talocalcaneal coalitions are the most common. Pain and limitation of motion can occur.

CHRONIC DISORDERS AFFECTING INFANTS, CHILDREN, AND ADOLESCENTS

Chronic disabilities can present both physical and psychosocial challenges that extend across an individual's life span.

When an infant is born with a musculoskeletal deformity, parents search for a cause for the occurrence. When the problem is severe and is indicative of a lifelong disabling condition, parents often experience feelings of loss, grief, and guilt. For this reason, repeated explanations may be needed before the family completely comprehends the full scope of the problem and the care that will be required. If this is the parents' first child, additional time may be needed because they are learning to cope with a newborn, as well as with a diagnosis that may be unfamiliar to them. Nurses not only share the responsibility of educating the family about the diagnosis and prognosis but may also be responsible for coordinating a multidisciplinary team that is often required to provide comprehensive care for the child and family. Advanced practice nurses may be involved in the initial assessment of the child, ordering diagnostic tests, providing genetic counseling, and of course, providing family education.

Siblings may encounter the same types of feelings as their parents. They may have difficulty explaining the problem to friends and may experience a loss of parental attention as the family focus shifts to the problems of the disabled child. The nurse should remind parents of the needs of siblings and the importance of spending time with the other children as the entire family adjusts to a new lifestyle.

Cerebral Palsy

Definition and Classification. CP is a nonspecific diagnosis used to describe any one of a group of disorders caused by a nonprogressive lesion within the brain. These disorders result from a known or unknown incident that occurs before, during, or after birth (Box 18-4) and that damages the brain or alters its development. Clients afflicted with CP experience disturbances in the motor areas of the brain. Voluntary muscle function, posture, movement, sight, speech, and hearing, as well as cognitive development, can all be altered depending on which portion of the brain is affected. The child may have difficulty acquiring fine and gross motor skills. CP is one of the most common causes of permanent physical disability in children.

CP is classified by the portion of the body that is affected and the specific type of involvement. The most common terms used for area of involvement are listed in Table 18-4. Terms used to describe the types of involvement are *spastic, athetoid, ataxic,* and *mixed.*

Approximately 70% to 80% of all clients with CP have the spastic form. Increased muscle tone, muscle contractures, and brisk deep tendon reflexes are all characteristic of this type of CP. In addition, some clients have clonus and a positive Babinski sign. Tendons, which function as flexors, adductors, and internal rotators, are stronger than extensors, abductors, and external rotators. The increased tone in these muscle groups can result in contractures, depending on the severity of the condition. At the same time, the antagonist muscle groups are

---

BOX 18-4.
Etiology of Cerebral Palsy

Prematurity (most common cause)
Breech delivery
Toxemia of pregnancy
Birth trauma
Anoxia
Rh factor incompatibility and kernicterus
Maternal rubella
Precipitate or cesarean delivery
Placenta previa and abruptio
Familial
Head injury
Cerebral maldevelopment
Encephalitis
Prenatal infections (toxoplasmosis, rubella, cytomegalovirus, herpes, syphilis)
Meningitis
Maternal drug use
Fetal alcohol syndrome

TABLE 18–4. *Common Terms and Areas of Involvement in Cerebral Palsy*

TERM	AREAS AND TYPE OF INVOLVEMENT
Monoplegia	One extremity involved, spasticity usually present; uncommon
Diplegia	Spasticity of both lower extremities, minor motor deficits in upper extremities
	Most common type
	Good prognosis for walking
	Intellect and speech usually normal or slightly impaired
Triplegia	Three extremities involved, spasticity usually present
	Usually variant of asymmetrical quadriplegia
Quadriplegia or tetraplegia	Total body involvement (may be spastic, athetoid, or mixed type)
	Legs usually more severely affected than arms
	Seizures are common manifestation
	Mental impairment common
Hemiplegia	Both extremities on same side of body involved, spasticity usually present
	Able to walk independently and perform activities of daily living
	Forty percent have seizure disorder
	Difficulty with written symbols and memory
Paraplegia	Lower limb involvement only, rare in spastic cerebral palsy

stretched and weakened. These individuals are the most likely to have orthopaedic deformities compared with individuals with other types of CP.

About 10% to 15% of clients with CP are athetoid, manifested by purposeless, involuntary, and uncontrollable movements of the face and all four extremities. These movements are exaggerated during attempts at voluntary movement or in stressful situations. Deep tendon reflexes are normal, and the involuntary movements are absent during sleep. Less than 5% of individuals with CP have the ataxic form, which is characterized by disturbed coordination and lack of equilibrium, resulting in an unsteady gait. The remaining individuals afflicted with CP have a mixed type such as spastic-athetoid.

Individuals with spastic CP are also classified according to the extent of neurologic involvement. If one side of the body (upper and lower extremity) is affected by paresis, the individual is described as having hemiplegia. If the lower extremities are both equally involved and affected more than the upper extremities, the individual has diplegia. Quadriplegia is used to describe involvement of all four limbs.

The oral motor muscles (including the jaw, tongue, lips, and throat) may be affected in any of the forms, resulting in drooling and difficulties with speech, swallowing, and feeding. Poor weight gain may result from a number of factors, including feeding difficulty, concomitant medical problems such as gastroesophageal reflux, disturbed parent-infant bonding, and feeding refusal. Choking, gagging, and extensor thrusting of the tongue are commonly seen in young children with CP. These symptoms are associated with brain injury and result in retention of primary sucking patterns. Children may have difficulty swallowing foods of specific thickness or texture. Food refusal may result because the child associates feeding with a negative experience such as choking. Parent-infant interactions may become increasingly difficult as mealtime becomes more and more stressful (Zickler & Dodge, 1994).

Other associated problems are seizures and sensory impairment. Approximately 25% to 35% of individuals with CP have some type of seizure disorder. Seizures occur most often in individuals with hemiplegia and spastic quadriplegia acquired postnatally. Approximately 25% of all CP clients exhibit speech disorders, 25% have auditory impairments, and 40% to 50% experience vision problems (Olney & Wright, 1994).

There is a great deal of variation in the amount of developmental delay or learning disorder that the child with CP can have. Although 50% to 75% of children with CP experience some type of developmental delay or exhibit a learning disorder, not all children are cognitively affected. The association between extent of motor involvement and developmental status is unpredictable. Some children with mild involvement of CP can exhibit significant developmental disabilities, whereas others who are severely affected have normal intelligence. Many individuals with CP attend regular schools, go to college, and lead normal productive lives. Of utmost importance are early intervention and periodic developmental and physical assessments to ensure that the child's maximum potential is achieved.

Incidence and Etiology. The incidence of CP is approximately 2.5 per 1000 live births. Premature birth is associated with 33% of all cases of CP (Olney & Wright, 1994). Despite the decreasing infant mortality rates, the number of cases of CP has remained constant. This is because of the increased survival of premature and low-birth-weight infants. Many infants, who would have died in the past, are now surviving with CP. The risk of developing CP rises as birth weight decreases. Infants under 2500 g are 20 times more likely to develop CP than infants of a normal birth weight.

There is a multitude of other risk factors for CP, including genetic abnormalities, intrauterine infection, birth asphyxia, intrauterine growth retardation, intraventricular hemorrhage, meconium aspiration, persistent fetal circulation, traumatic brain injury, and an early postnatal infection. In many cases, the exact cause is not possible to identify.

Pathophysiology. Spasticity is the result of an upper motor neuron disorder and results from lesions in the cerebellum and pyramidal pathways. When the lesion lies in the extrapyramidal system of the brain, the individual is affected by athetosis. Lesions of the cerebellum cause ataxia. In the mixed type spastic-athetoid, the individual has lesions in both the pyramidal and extrapyramidal systems.

CP associated with prematurity can be caused by hemorrhage into the lateral ventricles. The disruption in blood flow and subsequent hypoxia may cause a necrosis of the white matter and cystic changes that eventually lead to gliosis and ventriculomegaly. This permanent damage to the white matter is called *periventricular leukomalacia* and is the most common type of lesion seen in clients with CP attributable to prematurity. Neuronal connections of the white matter are involved in motor control and muscle tone, and damage to this area causes the motor deficits of spastic CP, along with varying degrees of intellectual impairment.

Some of the causes afflicting term infants with CP (e.g., meconium aspiration, persistent fetal circulation) may result in damage to the basal ganglia and cause the athetoid types of CP. In all cases, the underlying lesion is irreparable but not progressive.

Assessment. The diagnosis of CP is based primarily on the history and physical examination. An astute practitioner is alert to the subtle signs of CP as well as the major components. When examining any child, the practitioner should keep in mind that the diagnosis of CP is not always made during the first year of life. In some mildly affected children, the diagnosis of CP can be delayed for years. These children often present as toe-walkers or with parental complaints of the child being clumsy. The practitioner then must put many pieces of the puzzle together to determine whether a child's problems are caused by CP.

Subjective Assessment: Nursing History. Regardless of whether the child has been previously diagnosed, the nurse seeing the client for the first time should take a detailed history to effectively assess the client and family. Initial questions should focus on the child's birth history, development, overall health, and family history. Because CP can be caused by a complication before, during, or after birth, obtaining information about the pregnancy, labor and delivery, Apgar scores, and other postnatal events is extremely important. If any problem is identified, the practitioner should inquire whether the child experienced any anoxia, required time in a neonatal intensive care unit, had to be ventilated, or had any seizures after birth.

A family health history should be taken to help the clinician rule out a genetic disorder. Many genetic problems can present with symptoms that are similar to CP. If there is reason to suspect that the child has a genetic disease and not CP, a referral should be made to a geneticist for further evaluation.

Because there are other medical problems associated with CP, such as frequent pneumonia, gastroesophageal reflux, and seizures, the practitioner also must include a general health history in the assessment. This information not only is important for helping the families obtain any other referrals that may be necessary but is imperative for a child who may need to undergo surgery. Questions should also be asked about allergies, especially any past allergic responses to latex.

One of the first signs of CP may be a delay in achieving normal developmental milestones. For this reason, a developmental history must be a part of the assessment. Parents are extremely helpful in this regard because they are usually aware of delays in their child's progress. A simple scale to evaluate the approximate times of motor development is described in Table 18–5. Even after the diagnosis has been made, it is important to continue to monitor the client's development throughout childhood to plan appropriate interventions.

For the older child, information about school and age-appropriate activities can be elicited as part of the developmental assessment. The child should be asked questions about his or her ability to participate in physical activities. This information is helpful in identifying any psychosocial problems a child with CP may have, and the answers to these questions may provide a piece of the puzzle that will assist in diagnosing a child suspected of having a mild case of CP. The practitioner should determine whether a child is behind in school or has any problems learning. In addition, the child may be unable to keep up with peers in gym class or ordinary play activities. Simple questions, such as whether the child can ride a bike, play sports, and keep up with his or her friends when running, provide a great deal of information.

The overall well-being of the family of a child with CP should also be assessed. The family, including siblings, need support because many of the problems associated

TABLE 18–5. *Approximate Times of Motor Development*

DEVELOPMENT STAGE	APPROXIMATE AGE AT WHICH STAGE NORMALLY OCCURS
Head control	3 months
Pull to sitting without head lag	5 months
Sitting independently	6 months
Crawling	8 months
Pulling to stand	10 months

BOX 18–5.
Reflex Testing in the Infant

Asymmetrical Tonic Neck Reflex

Place the infant in the supine position, rotate the head to one side without neck flexion, and hold for 5 to 10 seconds. Then rotate the head to the other side. A positive response is flexion of upper and lower limbs on the "skull," or occiput, side and extension on the face side. This extension posturing is commonly known as the fencing position. This reflex may be present to some degree in normal children up to age 7 months but usually disappears by age 4 to 6 months.

Neck-Righting Reflex

With the infant supine, rotate the head and shoulder to one side and hold for a count of 10. If the trunk and pelvis rotate in the same direction as the head, the reflex is positive. This reflex is normally present between birth and 6 to 10 months of age.

Moro Reflex

This reflex should not be confused with the startle reflex elicited by a sudden loud noise in which the elbows are flexed and the hands closed. The Moro reflex is sudden abduction and extension of upper extremities with spreading of the fingers and extension of the spine, followed by flexion and adduction of the extremities as if in an embrace. This response can be elicited by any stimuli involving sudden extension of the neck. One way to elicit this response is to place the child supine, place the right hand under the thoracic spine, and the left hand under the head. Gently lift the child and then drop the left hand to allow for cervical spine extension. Presence of this reflex after 3 months is abnormal. The violence of this reflex in older children with cerebral palsy may throw the child out of a chair if adequate seat belt restraints are not used.

Symmetrical Tonic Neck Reflex

Place the child in a crawling position on the table or in a prone position over the examiner's knee. Flexion of the neck results in flexion of the arms and extension of the legs. Extension of the neck results in extension of the arms and flexion of the legs. This reflex is normal until age 6 months.

Parachute Reflex

This is also known as the *protective extension of the arms reflex*. Lift the child from the table in the prone position and suddenly lower or tip him or her toward the tabletop. By age 6 to 12 months, this maneuver should result in automatic extension of the arms toward the table. Spasticity prevents the child from putting his or her hands out as a normal protective mechanism. If this reflex does not appear, useful hand function will probably not be possible.

Foot Placement Reaction

Support the infant upright and bring the distal anterior tibia or dorsum of the foot against the edge of the table. The infant flexes the hip and knee spontaneously and steps on the tabletop. This response is normal in all infants and is voluntarily suppressed at age 2 to 4 months.

Extensor Thrust

Pressure applied to the ball of the foot with the limb in a flexed position results in extension of the leg. This is normal until age 2 months.

Labyrinthine Reflex

Another useful reflex for assessing the child is the labyrinthine reflex. When placed supine, the child assumes a posture with the shoulders abducted, elbows flexed, spine and lower limbs extended. When prone, the upper and lower limbs are flexed. Extensor tone is reduced when prone and increased when supine. This reflex is normally gone by 6 months. If it persists, whenever the child leans forward, he or she relaxes, the head falls forward, and he or she drools. When the child leans back, the hips extend and thrust him or her out of the chair.

---

with having a disabled child may place a stress on everyone.

Objective Assessment: Physical Examination. Observation is an important part of the physical examination. Rigid posturing of the infant, evidence of hand dominance before 18 months, asymmetry of movements between left and right sides of the body, tongue thrust, and the absence of any normal infant reflexes should all be noted. As the infant gets older, particular attention should be paid to the neurologic examination for the presence of primitive reflexes, such as the Babinski sign, that persist beyond the normal period or expected reflexes, such as the Landau reflex, that do not develop. Bleck (1987) suggests that the eight reflexes described in Box 18-5 be tested in the order listed. After the age of 12 months, these eight tests are used in determining the prognosis for walking. Table 18-6 describes the ages at which these reflexes are normally present. One characteristic of the child afflicted with CP is the development of a commando crawl in place of the normal reciprocal crawl. Deep tendon reflexes should also be tested. Children with spastic CP are hyperreflexive.

In both infants and older children, the physical examination should begin with the spine. The muscle imbalances caused by CP can cause scoliosis, and the child should be periodically monitored for this. For children who are able to walk, a great deal of information can be obtained from observing the child's gait pattern. When assessing gait, the clinician should focus on three

TABLE 18–6. *Neurologic Examination*

REFLEX	APPROXIMATE AGE AT WHICH REFLEX NORMALLY OCCURS
Asymmetrical tonic neck reflex	May be present from birth up to age 7 months; usually disappears between 4 and 6 months
Neck righting reflex	Present from birth to 6–10 months
Moro reflex	Present from birth to 3 months
Symmetrical tonic neck reflex	Present from birth to 6 months
Parachute reflex	Present by age 6–12 months
Foot placement reaction	Present in infants; can be voluntarily suppressed by age 2–4 months
Extensor thrust	Present from birth to 2 months
Labyrinthine reflex	Present from birth to 6 months

areas of the body: the position of the knees and feet and the arm swing. A crouched gait (walking with the knees bent) is caused by tight hamstring and hip flexors; scissoring (crossing the legs over one another) is the result of femoral anteversion (internal rotation of the hip) and tight adductors. A tight Achilles tendon causes toe-walking. Hemiplegics can manifest very subtle symptoms. One characteristic of hemiplegic clients is the lack of arm swing on the affected side. The upper extremity is often held with the elbow, wrist, and fingers flexed and the thumb adducted into the palm.

The nonambulatory child should be observed in the wheelchair for posture. Inability to maintain an upright comfortable position, such as from scoliosis or hip dysplasia, may be an indicator for bracing or surgery.

The clinician should examine the ROM of the extremities, muscle tone, and presence of abnormal movements and contractures. Differentiation of the types of CP based on physical examination are described in Box 18-6. Common orthopaedic problems seen in the individual with spastic CP are listed in Table 18-7. The examiner should note any contractures of the upper or lower extremity.

A common deformity of the spastic CP client is hip adductor contractures. These can lead to progressive subluxation and eventual dislocation of the hip. Problems resulting from the subluxed (partially displaced) or dislocated hip are decreased ROM (particularly abduction and extension), pelvic obliquity, and possibly pain. When severe, these problems can lead to difficulties in hygiene and in seating the client. In the ambulatory client, a subluxed hip can lead to early degenerative changes and disability. Excessive femoral anteversion that results in a severe intoeing gait in the ambulatory child can also be

---

BOX 18–6.
Signs and Symptoms of Cerebral Palsy

Spastic Type
Increased muscle tone
Increased deep tendon reflexes and clonus (sudden dorsiflexion of the ankle or rapid distal movement of the patella results in alternating spasm and relaxation of the muscles being stretched)
Flexor, adductor, and internal rotator muscles more involved than extensor, abductor, and external rotator muscles
Difficulty with fine and gross motor skills
Most common contracture is that of the heelcord
Hip adductor contractures lead to progressive subluxation and dislocation
Knee contractures
Scoliosis is common
Typical gait is crouched, intoeing, scissoring
Elbow, wrist, and fingers in flexed position with thumb adducted
Motor weakness of antagonist muscle groups

Athetoid Type
Purposeless, involuntary, uncontrollable movements of face and extremities
Movements are increased with stress and voluntary movements, absent during sleep

Rarely develop contractures
Deep tendon reflexes normal

Ataxic Type
Disturbed coordination
Lack of equilibrium
Unsteady gait
Few orthopaedic problems
Hyporeflexia
Loss of ability to gauge distance, speed, power of movement
Muscles hypotonic
Speech slurred, jerky, explosive
Nystagmus often present

Other Manifestations
Visual deficits (most common in spastic type)
Hearing impairment (most common in athetoid type)
Oral motor involvement resulting in drooling and feeding problems
Developmental delay (40% to 60%; most common in atonic and rigid types and spastic quadriparesis)
Sensory impairment
Seizures (approximately 40% of those with spastic hemiplegia affected)

TABLE 18-7. *Orthopaedic Problems in Cerebral Palsy*

AREA	ORTHOPAEDIC PROBLEM
Hip	Hip flexion deformities
	Hip subluxation
	Hip dislocation
Knee	Knee flexion deformities
	Contracture of knee capsule
	Recurvatum (hyperextension)
	Patella alta (high-riding patella)
Ankle and foot	Equinus deformity of ankle
	Valgus deformity
	Varus deformity
	Toe flexion deformity
Upper extremity	Contractures (elbow, wrist, fingers flexed, thumb adducted)
Spine	Scoliosis
	Kyphosis
	Pelvic obliquity

present. Frequent assessment of the hip allows the clinician to make judgments about the progression of the deformity.

Spasticity of the hamstrings can cause a flexion contracture of the knee. Testing of the hamstrings requires that the client lie supine with the hip and knee in extension. The leg should then be raised off the table by flexing the hip toward 90 degrees and keeping the knee in extension. Children with tight hamstrings cannot achieve a normal straight leg raise of 90 degrees. The tighter the hamstring, the greater the limitation in raising the leg.

The foot and ankle are often affected in spastic CP clients. Most common is an Achilles tendon contracture, producing an equinus foot and toe walking. The Achilles tendon can be tested for tightness by having the child lie supine with the leg in extension. The examiner should dorsiflex the foot. Although the amount of dorsiflexion a child's foot may have can vary, the normal amount is approximately 20 degrees. Many children with CP have tight Achilles tendons and have very limited dorsiflexion. For this reason, CP must be ruled out in any child older than 2 years of age who is a toe-walker. CP should also be suspected in any child who has tight hamstrings and a tight Achilles tendon affecting only one side of the body.

Diagnostic Evaluation. MRI of the brain may be performed to establish a definitive diagnosis of CP or to rule out other problems. All clients should undergo general screening x-ray films of the hips and of the spine (if any curvature is noted).

Gait analysis is becoming a popular method for evaluation of an ambulatory child with CP. The evaluation can be done by videotaping the child ambulating or by a more sophisticated means of motion analysis done through computerized gait studies. This type of formal

analysis may be helpful in determining the surgical plan to correct lower extremity abnormalities (Gage, 1993).

Treatment Modalities and Related Nursing Management. Care of the client with CP requires a holistic multidisciplinary approach (Table 18-8). Early recognition of CP is important to begin early intervention. Often, more than one physician (orthopaedic surgeon, neurologist, and pediatrician) is asked to evaluate the child before a firm diagnosis is reached. In addition to making the diagnosis, prognosis is important. An important issue for parents is whether the child will be able to ambulate. See Box 18-7 for ambulatory classification descriptions. By the age of 2 years, most children with CP are talking and pulling themselves around in some fashion if they are going to become ambulatory.

It is important to differentiate between ambulation and mobility. The process of walking may require such tremendous energy expenditure that the use of a wheelchair is more practical. A wheelchair rather than crutches frees the hands for other tasks. The concept of mobility is an important one for parents to grasp. However, the skill of ambulation is important and should be attained and maintained if possible. The community ambulator (see Box 18-7) can use nonadapted restroom facilities and public transportation and has more options for employment. The household ambulator can live in a less adapted environment with less assistance. When asked to rank their goals in order of importance, adults with CP rank communication, ability to perform ADLs, and mobility as being more important than walking, and it is important to maintain this perspective.

Wheelchair Adaptation. The goal for the nonambulatory child is to have a good sitting balance. To achieve this goal, a straight spine, stable hips, level pelvis, and hip motion with a flexion/extension arc of 90 degrees are needed. This can be accomplished through customized seating or orthotics or may need to be addressed surgically. Just as bracing changes with growth, wheelchair requirements also change and need to be reassessed regularly. Evaluation of the wheelchair itself and positioning devices as well as evaluation of the child's skill in propelling the chair should be carried out by a physical or occupational therapist. Chairs can be adapted so that the wheels can be gripped more easily or so they can be driven with one hand. Even the severely affected child can have enough function to handle a power chair if cognitive abilities are present. Independent mobility is an extremely valuable skill and should be obtained if possible.

Physical and Occupational Therapy. The orthopaedic needs of the child with CP are many, and the child should be involved in an early intervention program as soon as possible after diagnosis. Treatment plans must be individualized because of the many ways CP can be

TABLE 18–8. *Multidisciplinary Care and Teaching: Cerebral Palsy (CP)*

FOCUS	TEACHING POINTS
Normal growth and development	Physical
	Emotional/social (Erikson)
	Intellectual (Piaget)
Effects of CP on growth and development	Physical: gross and fine motor skills
	Emotional/social
	Intellectual
Nutritional needs	Feeding problems
	Increased caloric requirements
Entry into school	Laws: PL 94-142 (minimal restricted environment)
	PL 99-457 (early intervention)
	Special preschool programs available (i.e., Headstart)
	Testing: Denver Developmental
	Mainstreaming: pros/cons
	Special education classes
	Self-contained classrooms
	Interactions with school before child enters
	Interactions with school after child enters
	Physical environment of school (e.g., bathrooms, playground)
	Emotional impact of entry into school
Discipline	Consistency
	Limit setting
	Realistic expectations
Impact of CP on the family	Effect on siblings
	Effect on parents
	Parents: taking care of yourself
Mobility	Preparation for movement
	Facilitation of movement (e.g., orthotics, wheelchairs)
	Exercise: active and passive
	Adaptive devices: computers, eating utensils
	Spasms
	Uncontrolled movements
Community resources	Physical therapy/occupational therapy
	Orthotics
	Speech
	Vocational rehabilitation
	Early intervention
Latex	Sensitivity: symptoms
	Exposure
	Allergy versus alert

manifested. Short- and long-term realistic goals must be planned, taking into consideration growth and developmental changes. Short-term goals include prevention of deformities that limit mobility and inhibit function. The long-term goals are to assist the individual to reach maximum potential and achieve as much independence as possible.

The physical, occupational, and speech therapist are integral members of the child's multidisciplinary team. The goals of therapy vary according to the client and can include promotion of standing for transfers and ADLs, gait training, and prevention of contractual deformities of joints. Stretching is used to prevent contracture, and some activities promote balance, posture, and coordination. Activities should be geared to the promotion of independent mobility and daily living skills and should begin early. Home exercise programs that do not take an excessive amount of time are an important part of the therapy.

Bracing can be used in conjunction with therapy. The most common type of bracing used in the child with CP is an AFO. AFOs are used to maintain a plantigrade position in the foot with a tight Achilles tendon. They also serve to prevent further contracture of the ankle and provide lower extremity support for ambulation. However, even with appropriate bracing, surgical intervention (Achilles tendon lengthening) is often necessary.

Children with scoliosis and a curve of 25 degrees or greater may require a thoracolumbar orthosis (TLSO). Bracing for scoliosis in individuals with CP is not effective in preventing surgery; however, bracing can be useful in slowing the progression of some curves and/or allowing for growth before spinal fusion in these individuals. Parents and clients must be taught proper care and wearing of any type of orthosis.

Pharmacologic Measures and Other Modalities to Reduce Spasticity. Oral medications can be effective in decreasing spasticity. Commonly used drugs include baclofen (Lioresal) and diazepam (Valium). These can cause side effects such as sedation but have the advantage of exerting a systemic effect and decreasing spasticity throughout the body.

Intrathecal administration of baclofen is being used to control severe spasticity. Implanted subcutaneously into the abdominal wall with a catheter that attaches at the spine, programmable pumps infuse baclofen directly into the spinal canal. The dosage of medication can be

titrated to produce the desired affect. Complications can include infection, displacement of the catheter, and cerebrospinal fluid leaks (Dormans & Pellegrino, 1998).

Selective dorsal rhizotomy is a surgical procedure that involves selectively dividing the sensory nerve rootlets that cause spasticity. Muscle tone is deceased, preventing contractures and increasing normal movements. The outcome with rhizotomy varies. The desired result for the ambulatory client is that gait will be improved. For the nonambulatory client, the goal is improvement in positioning and ease in the performance of ADLs (Abbott, Johann-Murphy, Shiminski-Maher, Quartermain, Forem, Gold, & Epstein, 1993). Extensive physical therapy is necessary after surgery. Client selection is critical. Clients are generally 3 to 6 years of age. Ideally, the child will be able to walk and to follow directions. Rhizotomy is not indicated for individuals who have a fixed deformity, dystonia, or previous lower extremity orthopaedic surgery (Marty, Dias, & Gaebler-Spira, 1995).

Botox injections (botulinum toxin) are another type of treatment to reduce spasticity. The injections are given into the neuromuscular junction. The substance binds to the cholinergic terminal and inhibits the release of acetylcholine, which is essential for muscle contraction. Decreased muscle spasticity with improvement in gait have been reported (Cosgrove, Corry, & Graham, 1994). The disadvantages are cost and limited duration of effect, which lasts less than 6 months.

Surgery. Surgery is indicated when conservative methods, such as bracing, have failed to correct or prevent progression of a deformity. Surgery is performed to improve function; to ease the care of severely affected children; and to prevent life-threatening deformities, such as scoliosis. Children with spastic CP usually warrant surgery more often than do children with other types of CP. Surgery is usually not indicated in a child with athetoid CP because of the lack of muscle contractures. Table 18–9 is a summary of procedures performed to correct the various problems associated with spastic CP.

The goals of surgery for clients with spastic CP are as follows:

1. To diminish muscle contracture and overpull of selected muscles by release or lengthening
2. To make the motion of opposing muscles more effective by tendon transfers
3. To correct joint contractures and deformities
4. To improve positioning of hips, rotation of lower extremities, or correct spine deformity

Before surgery, it is important to have the family verbalize their expectations of the surgery. Goals should be discussed so that disappointment is avoided. For certain clients, a nutritional and pulmonary evaluation may be necessary. If major spine or hip surgery is planned, the child may require a gastrostomy tube placement so

---

BOX 18–7.
Classification of Ambulators and Nonambulators

Ambulators

The ambulatory child can be classified in one of three ways:

Community Ambulator

Able to walk, perhaps with braces or crutches, throughout the community, handling steps and public transportation. A wheelchair is needed only for long distances.

Household Ambulator

Can get around the home only. Can get in and out of the bed or chair with little or no assistance.
A wheelchair is needed for other activities.

Exercise Ambulator

Walks only in therapy sessions.

Nonambulators

A nonambulator requires a wheelchair at all times.
    Nonambulators can also be classified in three ways:

Independent Sitter

Can sit upright without support and can independently transfer in and out of the wheelchair.

Self-propped Sitter

Can maintain independent sitting balance momentarily. One person is needed to assist with transfers, but the child does not need to be lifted.

Propped Sitter

Requires special support to maintain an upright posture and must be lifted in and out of the wheelchair.

TABLE 18–9. *Common Procedures for Correction of Orthopaedic Disorders in Cerebral Palsy*

DISORDER	COMMON PROCEDURES
Hip flexion deformities	Release of rectus femoris tendon
	Iliopsoas tenotomy
	Soft tissue release
Hip subluxation	Varus osteotomy
	Pelvic osteotomy and varus osteotomy (if the acetabulum is deficient)
Hip dislocation (usually age 5–7 years)	Soft tissue release
	Open reduction
	Varus derotation osteotomy with femoral shortening
	Chiari pelvic osteotomy
Knee flexion deformity	Hamstring lengthening
Contracture of knee capsule	Posterior capsulotomy of knee joint with hamstring lengthening
Knee hyper-extension	Rectus femoris tenotomy with iliopsoas recession
Patella alta	Prevention or correction of knee flexion deformity
Equinus deformity of ankle	Achilles tendon lengthening
Valgus deformity of foot	Subtalar arthrodesis and bone graft with soft tissue procedures
	Triple arthrodesis with heelcord lengthening (if rigid deformity)
Varus deformity of foot	Split tendon transfer or tendon lengthening
Hallux valgus	Bunionectomy and metatarso-phalangeal joint fusion
Toe flexion deformities	Lengthening of toe flexors
Upper extremity contractures	Muscle and tendon releases
	Tendon transfers
	Joint arthrodesis
Scoliosis	Anterior or posterior fusions (or both)
Leg spasticity	Selective posterior rhizotomy

that the child is in optimal condition to undergo surgery. If frequent respiratory infections or episodes of aspiration pneumonia have occurred or if pulmonary function is compromised in some way, an anesthesiology consult before surgery is suggested. The child with seizures should have a recent neurologic examination, and seizure medication levels should be drawn to determine whether the current drug regimen is appropriate. The neurologist can also help in managing the medications in the postoperative period.

Spine. Surgical intervention for scoliosis can be successfully performed in individuals with CP. Surgical candidates must be chosen carefully, with potential gains evaluated against the risks of surgery. Surgery is generally indicated when other modalities have failed, when sitting balance or ambulation is being lost, or when pulmonary capacity is compromised from scoliosis. Spinal stabiliza-

tion may require an anterior and a posterior approach to the spine with segmental instrumentation to the pelvis (see Chapter 17).

Hips. Adduction contractures causing a subluxation of the hip may require releases. The hips are then placed in a cast and held in abduction for 4 to 6 weeks. The goal is to prevent or delay further hip subluxation. Hip dislocation may require procedures that relocate the femoral head and/or reconstruct the pelvis. The procedure used depends on the deformity present. Casting for 6 weeks is necessary following these procedures. To maintain the position of the hip after pelvic surgery, a hip abduction orthosis is used.

Knee. Surgical lengthening of the hamstrings may be performed on children with tight hamstrings. This procedure requires knee immobilization with casts followed by KAFOs to maintain the correction. Depending on the individual case, these may be worn only at bedtime or for a limited amount of time during the day.

Foot. Bracing or casting is first attempted for the tight Achilles tendon and if not effective, surgical lengthening of the heelcord is performed. The correction is maintained with short leg casts for 6 weeks, followed by an AFO and physical therapy.

Nursing Management. In addition to normal postoperative care, the nurse must be aware of the unique needs of the CP clients, especially for those who are unable to verbalize. In addition to postoperative incisional pain, the CP client often experiences intense muscle spasms. Diazepam or another muscle relaxant can be given in small doses in conjunction with an opioid to control spasms. Richtsmeier, Barkin, and Alexander (1992) have documented case reports of the efficacy of these drugs in reducing muscle spasms. As with any medication, the client should be monitored for side effects, especially sedation.

Another comfort measure is positioning. Placing the child who has undergone hamstring lengthening or hip surgery on pillows in the prone position helps relax him or her and decreases muscle spasms. (The prone position is not recommended for children younger than the age of 12 months because of the increased risk of sudden infant death syndrome, unless the child is advised to lie prone for some other reason such as gastroesophageal reflux.) Casts should be well padded, and the nurse should check the cast for any sharp edges or areas irritating or digging into the skin. Applying moleskin to the borders of the cast helps prevent this problem. For children who are incontinent and placed in a hip spica cast, a small diaper should be tucked inside the opening in the cast. A larger diaper can be placed over it to cover the outside of the cast. Slightly elevating the head of the bed helps the urine drain downward instead of up inside the cast.

Parents should be encouraged to have the child participate in as many normal activities as possible. A reclining wheelchair with leg extenders for the child in a hip spica cast facilitates this. Children should be included in family activities and should attend school. Laws require schools to make accommodations for children in casts, in wheelchairs, and on crutches.

Children with CP often undergo some type of physical therapy in the postoperative period. The child with spastic quadriplegia may continue to attend physical therapy while in a hip spica cast and receive trunk strengthening exercises. The child that has undergone hamstring lengthening should be encouraged to sit in an upright position to further stretch the hamstrings.

Children with spasticity may be very uncomfortable when the casts are removed. Analgesics and muscle relaxants should be administered. Soaking in a warm bath or whirlpool is soothing and parents can begin a gentle ROM. Physical therapy also helps loosen tight and sore muscles.

Summary. CP manifests itself in numerous ways, and care must be individualized. Identification of the child at risk and diagnosis are important so that early intervention can begin. A multidisciplinary approach is required to meet the many needs of the individual with CP. Treatment is aimed at prevention of deformities and encouragement of activities to maximize the potential of the individual.

Spina Bifida

Definition and Classification. Spina bifida, the most common congenital abnormality of the spine, involves a developmental defect of the spinal column characterized by failure of fusion between one or more vertebral arches. It can occur with or without a protrusion of the intraspinal contents and is associated with varying degrees of neurologic deficits. *Spina bifida* is a broad term used for all types of such defects and is often synonymous with *myelomeningocele* and *myelodysplasia*.

The defect in the spinal column can occur in any level but is most common in the lumbar and lumbosacral spine because these are the last areas of the neural tube to close. The most significant aspect is not the bony defect, but rather the neurologic deficits that may be associated with it. These can vary from mild muscle imbalance and sensory loss in the lower extremities to complete paraplegia. Terms commonly used in spina bifida are described in Box 18–8.

Spina Bifida Occulta. Spina bifida occulta, a localized defect of the vertebral arch without spinal cord or meningeal involvement, is the mildest form of spina bifida and is detectable only by x-ray film. It occurs so frequently that it can be considered a normal variation for which there often is no external manifestation. A dimple, hairy patch, hemangioma, subcutaneous lipoma, or increase in pigmentation may appear over the area, indicat-

ing an increased likelihood of a diastematomyelia (midline spur that splits the spinal cord) or a congenital neoplasm, such as a lipoma, hemangioma, or dermoid cyst. In the presence of these signs, neurologic damage may be evident at birth or may appear during spinal growth as the spinal cord and cauda equina are stretched. In most cases, spina bifida occulta is of little or no clinical significance. Surgery may be necessary for neurologic deficits or for aesthetic reasons (e.g., to remove hairy patches or skin nevi).

Spina Bifida with Meningocele. The meninges extruding through a bony defect in the spine and producing a sac is known as *spina bifida with meningocele*. The sac contains cerebrospinal fluid and occasionally some nerve roots, but the cord is not involved. There is usually little or no neurologic deficit evident at birth, but such a deficit may develop with spinal growth. This form of spina bifida is relatively uncommon and often requires surgical excision and closure.

Spina Bifida with Myelomeningocele. Myelomeningocele is the more severe form of spina bifida (Fig. 18–20). The sac contains not only cerebrospinal fluid but also nerve roots and the spinal cord itself. The exact neurologic deficits present depend on the level of the lesion. The deficits are exhibited as sensory, motor, reflex, and

---

BOX 18–8.
Terms Used for Spina Bifida

Spina Bifida Occulta
Bony defect seen on x-ray film
No spinal cord or meningeal involvement
Usually no neurologic deficits

Spina Bifida with Meningocele
Bony defect with sac containing meninges extruding
    through defect
Spinal cord is not involved
Usually little or no neurologic deficit

Spina Bifida with Myelomeningocele
Bony defect with sac containing nerve roots and spinal
    cord extruding
Neurologic deficits associated with level of defect
Often accompanied by hydrocephalus

Lipomeningocele
Sac contains lipoma, may involve sacral nerves
Neurologic function normal at birth, but progressive
    problems may occur with growth if not treated early

Rachischisis
Complete absence of skin and sac, neural tissues exposed

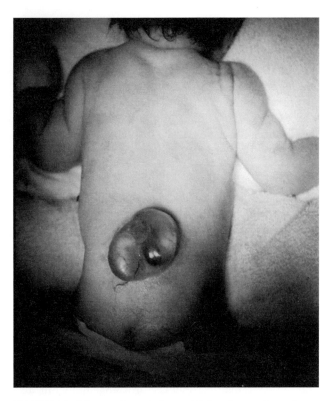

FIGURE 18–20. Newborn infant with lumbosacral myelomeningocele.

sphincter control problems. The sac is usually covered with thin, translucent skin or membrane, with no overlying muscles or subcutaneous tissue.

It was previously assumed that neurologic deterioration was the natural progression of the disease. Now, however, it is thought that deterioration should not occur and is usually the result of (1) Chiari II malformations, (2) tethering caused by scarring of the spinal cord to the closure site or hydromyelia (enlarged dilated cord), or (3) syringomyelia (cavities or outpouching in spinal cord).

Approximately 75% to 80% of individuals with a myelomeningocele have or develop hydrocephalus. The hydrocephalus results from an Arnold-Chiari II malformation or other developmental defects within the brain. An Arnold-Chiari malformation is a herniation of the lower brainstem and cerebellum, including the fourth ventricle through the foramen magnum into the spinal canal. The fourth ventricle becomes obstructed, passage of cerebrospinal fluid becomes impeded, and hydrocephalus results.

Lipomeningocele. Lipomeningocele is the sac containing lipomas involved with sacral nerves. There are usually no central nervous system abnormalities or hydrocephaly. Neurologic function is usually normal at birth, but progressive problems appear with growth.

Disability usually includes foot deformities and bowel and bladder incontinence. If lipomeningoceles are excised at birth and do not involve the spinal cord, no progressive neurologic deterioration occurs.

Rachischisis. Rachischisis is the complete absence of skin and sac over the defect. Neural tissues are exposed, and the spinal cord is dysplastic.

Because the orthopaedic nurse is primarily involved in the care of individuals with myelomeningocele, the focus of this section is on this type of spina bifida.

Incidence and Etiology. The incidence of myelomeningocele is approximately 0.6 per 1000 births in the United States (Yen, Khoury, Erickson, James, Waters, & Berry, 1992). The rate of occurrence varies considerably throughout the world, with the highest incidence being in northern Europe. It is slightly more common in girls than in boys.

The exact cause of myelomeningocele is unknown and can best be described as multifactorial. Family genetic studies are limited because, until recently, individuals with myelomeningocele generally have not lived to childbearing age. Preliminary case reports have not shown an increase in incidence of neural tube defects in children born to parents affected by myelomeningocele (Rauen & Aubert, 1992). It has been established that parents with a child with myelomeningocele have a greater risk of subsequent children being similarly affected than do parents in the general population. Environmental pollutants and the use of valproic acid (an anticonvulsant) have also been associated with an increased incidence of myelomeningocele. The use of folic acid before conception and during pregnancy decreases the risk of spina bifida.

Pathophysiology. Myelomeningocele is a malformation arising from an embryonic defect of the neural tube, but the exact embryologic defect is unknown. Two hypotheses currently exist to explain how it occurs. Normally, the neural tube is closed by the end of the fourth week of gestation. One hypothesis suggests that the neural tube fails to close. The second is that the neural tube closes, but then ruptures at a later time in development.

Assessment

Subjective Assessment: Nursing History. The clinician should begin by finding out as much about the child's condition as possible. A family and obstetric history, as well as problems occurring during the neonatal period, should be obtained. Attention should be paid to the review of systems, especially the central nervous system, genitourinary, and musculoskeletal systems because these systems are primarily affected by myelome ningocele. Changes in these systems are common with growth. Table 18–10 lists areas of concern and assessment parameters. Any reported changes in functioning or sensation are particularly important because they could indicate problems such as diastematomyelia or tethered cord. Developmental, educational, and social histories are also important to the assessment.

At the time of birth, the family unit should be assessed to determine their coping mechanisms and the resources available to them. Psychological evaluation of the family unit should be carried out periodically. (See Chapter 2 for more information on psychosocial assessment.)

The home environment and cultural background also should be assessed. It is important to determine the ability of the family to meet the special needs of the child with myelomeningocele on a regular basis because the home needs of the child change with growth and development. A home visit by the nurse, therapist, or social worker may be helpful in planning needed adaptations.

A high incidence of latex allergy has been reported in the myelomeningocele population. Approximately 10% to 40% of individuals with myelomeningocele develop this allergy, which can produce an anaphylactic response to products containing latex, such as gloves and catheters. The client and family should be asked if the individual has experienced any prior reactions to latex products.

Objective Assessment: Physical Examination. In the immediate postnatal period, observation of the newborn with myelomeningocele is an important part of the physical examination (see Table 18–10 for assessment guidelines). The external appearance of the lesion or the postoperative incision should be noted. Then, voluntary movement of individual muscle groups is evaluated. This is important information for determining the level of the lesion. A thorough neurologic examination should be performed, in addition to daily head circumference measurements. Any symptoms of hydrocephalus should be addressed immediately. Treatment for hydrocephalus is most effective if begun early.

The child should be examined for any associated defects. Clubfeet are a common deformity in myelomeningocele, and hip dislocation can also be present along with scoliosis and kyphosis. Although some deformities are present at birth, the majority are acquired through growth, muscle imbalance, positioning, and effects of gravity. A thorough neurologic examination and muscle testing should be performed regularly to detect any changes.

A consult for formal developmental testing may be initiated to determine the educational needs of the child with myelomeningocele. Learning disabilities and perceptual deficits may be present.

TABLE 18–10. *Assessment in Myelomeningocele*

AREA OF CONCERN	ASSESSMENT
Hydrocephalus	In infant: increased head circumference, dilation of scalp veins, downward deviation of eyes, tense fontanelles
	Irritability, vomiting, seizures, decrease in level of consciousness
	Upper extremity weakness
Arnold-Chiari malfunction	Apnea, stridor, vocal cord paralysis, gagging
	Upper extremity weakness or spasticity
Bowel and bladder	Infant: rectal prolapse, lack of rectal tone, lack of urinary control (intermittent dribbling increases with suprapubic pressure, maceration of perineal skin)
	Urinary tract infections
	Kidney failure
	Hard dry stool; abdominal palpation of stool mass
Neurologic	Degree and distribution of paralysis
	Skin problems related to decreased sensation
Tethered spinal cord	Progressive neurologic dysfunction; decreased urologic function
	Progressive orthopaedic deformity, particularly scoliosis
	Change in motor status, back or leg pain, alteration in gait
Musculo-skeletal	Clubfoot
	Muscle atrophy and osteopenia of affected extremities
	Joint contractures
	Hip subluxation and dislocation (may be present at birth)
	Scoliosis and kyphosis
	Knee flexion contractures
	Acquired foot deformities, such as talipes calcaneus, talipes cavus
Latex allergy	Status: latex alert versus allergy
	Knowledge regarding latex allergy
	Latex exposure
Nutrition	Gagging
	Obesity
Psychological	Family functioning
	Depression
	Chemical addiction
	Independence and self-care
Educational	Learning disabilities
	Client education and teaching of self-care, need to recognize limitations of child
	Appropriate school placement
	Individualized educational plan if appropriate

Diagnostic Evaluation

Prenatal Diagnosis. From 6 to 14 weeks of gestation, alpha-fetoprotein normally present in fetal tissues is present in the amniotic fluid and maternal blood. Closure of the abdominal wall and neural tube at 16 weeks prevents further alpha-fetoprotein release, and after this point, the maternal levels of alpha-fetoprotein should be undetectable. Increased levels of alpha-fetoprotein in maternal blood or amniotic fluid after 16 weeks of gestation can be indicative of myelomeningocele.

Diagnosis of neural tube defects can also be made prenatally by amniocentesis or chorionic villus sampling. Analysis of the amniotic fluid is more accurate than analysis of the maternal serum for alpha-fetoprotein. Most of the lesions that are not detected are low lumbar or sacral lesions, which are associated with less paralysis. Amniocentesis or serum analysis does not detect lesions covered with normal epithelial tissue.

A test for acetylcholinesterase can also be performed. This enzyme should be absent in maternal serum and at low levels in normal amniotic fluid. Therefore, a higher level of alpha-fetoprotein and acetylcholinesterase increases the level of confidence in diagnosing myelomeningocele prenatally.

Ultrasonography can be used to diagnose myelomeningocele and hydrocephalus. Nadel, Green, Holmes, Frigoletto, and Benacerraf (1990) recommend that level 2 sonography (targeted evaluation of fetal anatomy by a person experienced in the diagnosis of congenital anomalies with sophisticated equipment) instead of routine amniocentesis be used for clients with elevated serum alpha-fetoprotein levels.

Postnatal Evaluation. Radiographs of the vertebral column to define defects should be performed after birth. A urologic evaluation should be done to determine whether any renal pathologic condition exists. MRI or high-resolution spinal sonography can help detect occult dystrophic lesions, tethered cord, hemangioma, lipoma, tumor, hydromyelia, and diastematomyelia. CT scans or ultrasonography are performed to evaluate the status of hydrocephalus.

The neurologic examination yields information in planning the future functional goals for the child. The most common levels of the disorder and their effect on muscle function and mobility are summarized in Table 18–11. Many lesions result in mixed levels, so a pure level is unusual and each child must be evaluated individually.

Treatment Modalities and Related Nursing Management.

The majority (85%) of children born with myelomeningocele in the United States live to adulthood (McLone, 1989). Current management of myelomeningocele in most medical centers in this country is aggressive treatment from all involved specialties, beginning with

TABLE 18–11. *Common Levels of Myelomeningocele and Effects on Mobility*

LEVEL	EFFECTS ON MOBILITY
T12	Complete loss of motor and sensory function of both lower extremities
	Parapodium and reciprocating braces in early years, wheelchair dependent later
L1	Iliopsoas and sartorius muscles present
	Ambulatory with knee-ankle-foot orthosis early but wheelchair dependent in most cases as adolescent
L2	Strong hip flexion, moderate hip adduction
	Prone to develop hip flexion and adduction contracture and hip dislocation
	Knee-ankle-foot orthosis early, wheelchair dependent in most cases as adolescent
L3	Strong quadriceps
	Ability to extend knee
	Ambulatory with knee-ankle-foot orthosis or ankle-foot orthosis
	By adolescence, household or community ambulator
L4	Ankle dorsiflexion and inversion
	Prone to develop calcaneal deformities of foot
	Functional ambulator with ankle-foot orthosis or knee-ankle-foot orthosis and/or crutches
	May develop hip dislocation because of muscle imbalance around hip
L5	Lacks plantar flexion
	Also prone to development of calcaneal or valgus foot deformity and late hip dislocation
	Ambulatory with ankle-foot orthosis

early closure of the sac. In the case of a large thoracolumbar myelomeningocele, a latissimus dorsi myocutaneous flap closure has been recommended to preserve viability and prevent the development of pressure sores (Jaworski, Dudkiewicz, Lodzinski, & Lenkiewicz, 1992). A multidisciplinary team approach is imperative in the management of the client with myelomeningocele.

The goal of treatment of the child with myelomeningocele is to establish a pattern of development as near normal as possible. The primary aim of orthopaedic treatment is to provide for stable posture and ambulation or mobility. A stable posture for standing or sitting that allows one or both arms to be free for other activities is very important. More than half of the children with myelomeningocele have neurologic abnormalities of the upper extremities and need both hands to perform activities that unaffected children perform with only one hand. The ability to sit or stand without involving the hands is necessary in assisting the child to reach developmental goals and maximum potential. The goals are discussed with the family and child, who are included in the decision-making process.

Development and Interaction. Various means are used to assist the child in meeting developmental goals at the appropriate time. Development may be impeded as the result of decreased mobility. Some emotional delay may occur as a result of hospitalizations and illnesses. Special attention must be paid to handling, positioning, and interacting with the child to promote development. This awareness of special needs should begin at birth. From birth to 3 months, the child should be provided with a variety of forms of sensory stimulation. Care must be taken to avoid pressure on the infant's back; to alternate positions frequently; and to provide visual, tactile, and auditory stimulation. Children 3 months to 3 years old need to be encouraged to support their heads themselves, change positions frequently, and find means to become mobile (e.g., use of scooter boards). Toys and other means of stimulation should be provided to encourage movement, development, and independence.

Early intervention, therapy, and adaptive equipment can increase mobility and decrease developmental delays in children with myelomeningocele. Intellectual and motor development is assisted by ambulation even if it is limited to early childhood years.

Gaining Mobility. Upright posture decreases contracture formation, enhances bone density and growth, increases environmental input for cognitive development, enhances self-esteem, and prevents complications in other body systems. Neurologic level and functioning, intelligence, sense of balance, weight, and motivation all influence the achievement of ambulation. Excess weight can be the single greatest deterrent to ambulation, and intervention in this area should begin early to prevent future problems. Even if a child is primarily wheelchair dependent, minimal ambulatory ability aid in the number of school, employment, and recreational activities available by allowing the person access to facilities that may not be barrier free.

Bracing and Orthotics. There are various types of braces, standing frames, and parapodiums that can be used to assist children to stand. When the child can shift weight and swivel while holding the hands of an adult or using a walker, he or she is ready to proceed with bracing for ambulation. The type of bracing needed depends on individual assessment. Knutson and Clark (1991) provide an overview of various orthoses for individuals with myelomeningocele. AFO, KAFO, and hip-knee-ankle-foot orthoses and reciprocal bracing with walkers (Fig. 18–21), crutches, or canes allow almost any child who has achieved head and upper body control to ambulate for at least short distances. Children should be taught early the application and removal of their braces and the importance of skin care, including inspection and early attention to areas of breakdown.

Wheelchairs. Many children may still need a wheelchair. Frequent assessment by a therapist to ensure that the chair is appropriate for the growing child and his or her changing needs is important. The concept of ambulation versus mobility discussed in the CP section should be applied to these children as well. Many adolescents who

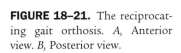

FIGURE 18–21. The reciprocating gait orthosis. *A,* Anterior view. *B,* Posterior view.

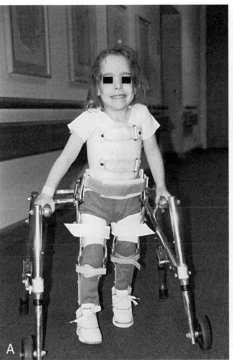
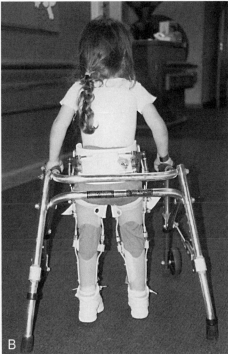

were ambulatory as children may not be able to tolerate the increased energy needed for ambulation as they grow and their weight increases. Skin care and wheelchair push-ups should be encouraged. Participation in sports, such as swimming, weight lifting, or wheelchair basketball, can aid in increasing mobility and self-esteem.

Spinal Deformities. Spinal deformities in myelomeningocele are common. Congenital scoliosis can occur, as can scoliosis or kyphosis resulting from vertebral instability consequent to the lack of posterior elements and paralyzed muscles. Congenital scoliosis is treated in the same manner as that in children without myelomeningocele by prompt fusion when progression is evident.

Paralytic curves at high levels can be expected to progress. Bracing is used to slow progression and to allow the trunk to grow. Surgical fusion is usually inevitable. Attainment of maximum trunk height is especially important to clients who are likely to be wheelchair dependent. Special attention must be paid to the insensate skin under the brace, and special linings for the orthosis can be helpful. Wheelchairs and braces may need to be modified to accommodate the spinal orthosis.

Spinal fusion is indicated to stop progression of a spinal deformity, improve ambulatory status, correct pelvic obliquity, relieve skin pressure, and establish independent sitting balance. The establishment of sitting balance is particularly important because if the hands are needed for balance, the child is a functional quadriplegic.

Kyphosis is an especially difficult problem. When present at birth, closure of the myelomeningocele is difficult and skin coverage obtained may be poor. Kyphosis is most common with thoracic lesions, and approximately one third of these children have severe kyphotic deformities by early adolescence. With progression, the child is forced to sit with the rib cage resting on the thighs. The skin becomes progressively more atrophic, and sitting balance is more difficult to attain without using the hands. The progressive kyphosis also is unsightly, and the adolescent can become self-conscious of it.

Bracing can be applied for a flexible kyphosis to allow for spinal growth. In the more rigid kyphosis, which is more common, bracing is poorly tolerated by the skin. Surgery is indicated to alleviate chronic skin breakdown, to improve sitting ability, and to alleviate back pain. Excision of the affected spinal segment (kyphectomy) is necessary to attain satisfactory spinal realignment in most cases. Because kyphosis is more severe in thoracic lesions with no neurologic function in the lower extremities, this is not a concern. If lower extremity function is present to some extent, attempts are made to spare the involved nerve roots; however, this cannot be guaranteed.

The exact procedures to correct spinal deformities depend on the degree and flexibility of the spinal curve, age of the child, neurologic level, and experience of the surgeon. Both anterior and posterior procedures and segmental instrumentation to the pelvis often are needed. New procedures are being developed using instrumentation without fusion to allow for continued growth when intervention cannot wait until spinal growth is complete.

Nursing Management. Care for the individual with myelomeningocele focuses on assisting the child and family in dealing with the disorder and helping the child reach maximal potential. Teaching about skin care, brace use, wheelchair use, and preoperative and postoperative instructions is needed. Thorough preoperative evaluation must be carried out. Shunts should be evaluated because problems can be encountered after spinal surgery.

After surgery, these children have the needs of any other children undergoing spine surgery plus the special needs of insensate skin; paralysis; and impaired bowel, bladder, and pulmonary function. Wound infections are more common. Therefore, wounds must be observed carefully.

In later years, the child is at risk for becoming overweight. Healthful dietary habits should be encouraged. The individual should also be as active as possible within physical limitations. Even wheelchair-dependent individuals can do aerobic exercise, such as swimming and racing.

Summary. Myelomeningocele is the most common congenital abnormality of the spine. A team approach is imperative in the care of these individuals. Orthopaedic goals are directed toward the establishment of a stable posture and the development of ambulation or mobility. A great deal of support is needed by the family and child as they face the multiple problems associated with this disorder. The orthopaedic nurse can act as coordinator, teacher, and support person to these clients and their families.

Osteogenesis Imperfecta

Definition and Classification. Osteogenesis imperfecta (OI), often referred to as "brittle bone disease," is a genetic connective tissue disorder marked by excessive fragility of the bones. In certain forms of this disease, the bones are so brittle that ordinary tasks such as throwing a ball or turning in bed can cause a fracture. Because this disease is caused by alterations in the production of collagen, many other organ systems and tissues are affected as well. Another manifestation of the disease exhibited by individuals afflicted with certain types of OI is a blue sclera. Many clients are of short stature.

For many years, clients with OI were considered to have one of two types: OI congenita was the severe form and present from birth. OI tarda was the milder form and became apparent sometime in the first few years of life. However, studies of a large series of cases and advancements in diagnostic and genetic methods have allowed for the development of the Sillence classification system that divides the disease into four types. The categories are based on mode of inheritance and clinical findings (Table 18–12).

Incidence and Etiology. OI affects all racial and ethnic groups, and there is no difference in the occurrence in males versus females.

As described in Table 18–12, some forms of OI are autosomal dominant and some are autosomal recessive, although new mutations occur in each type. Mutations in the collagen production genes *COLIA1* and *COLIA2* are responsible for the phenotype of OI. These two genes are responsible for the production of type I collagen. Disruptions in the formation of collagen can be catastrophic. In addition to bone, type I collagen is found in skin, ligaments, tendons, and the sclera among many other parts of the body.

The milder types of OI are thought to result from decreased synthesis of structurally normal type I procollagen molecules. More severe types of OI are thought to result from structural aberrations of type I procollagen molecules. Byers and Steiner (1992) provide a detailed description of the molecular basis of OI. As described in Table 18–12 several patterns of pathologic consequences of altered collagen synthesis occur.

Assessment

Subjective Assessment: Nursing History. The number of fractures a child has experienced and the type and magnitude of traumatic incidents associated with the fracture occurrence may lead the clinician to do a further workup. The nurse should also ask about the birth history and any fractures that occurred during delivery or the neonatal period. A history of several fractures at birth or sustaining fractures after minor traumatic incidents

TABLE 18–12. *Classification of Osteogenesis Imperfecta*

OI TYPE	INHERITANCE	CLINICAL FEATURES
I	Autosomal dominant	Mild type
		Normal or mild to moderate short stature
		Little or no deformity; bowing and angulation at knees and feet may be due to ligament laxity
		Fractures occur with moderate trauma, decrease at puberty
		Blue sclerae
		Hearing loss common in adolescents and young adults
		Dentinogenesis rare, present in type IB
II	Autosomal dominant or recessive	Most severe form
		Lethal in perinatal period because of respiratory or cardiovascular compromise; many are stillborn
		Numerous fractures present at birth
		Beaded ribs
		Compressed femurs
		Compressed skull
		Small extremities
		Marked long-bone deformity
		Kyphosis may occur (can be diagnosed prenatally)
III	Autosomal dominant or recessive	Moderately severe form
		Severe osteoporosis
		Progressive deformity of bones
		Frequent fractures associated with minimal trauma
		Scoliosis and kyphosis common
		Variable scleral hue
		Dentinogenesis common
		Very short stature
		Often nonambulatory by adolescence
		Large skull, triangular face shape
IV	Autosomal dominant	Mild type
		Normal sclera or bluish sclera that lightens with age
		Fractures may occur at birth or later in life
		Mild to moderate bone deformity, particularly bowing of the legs
		Stature variable
		Dentinogenesis in type IVB
		Often spontaneously improves at puberty
		No hearing loss

may be indicative of OI. Family history should also be elicited. In all cases, child abuse should be ruled out. See Table 18–12 for symptoms of specific types of OI. Information about development, vision, and hearing should be obtained. Hearing loss accompanies certain types of OI.

Objective Assessment: Physical Examination. Observation of the newborn and infant is an important part of the physical examination because the presentation of OI varies greatly, both between and within types (Fig. 18–22). See Table 18–12 for typical signs of OI by type. Differentiation between OI and battered child syndrome is partially dependent on the presence of other signs of physical abuse, such as bruises, welts, burns, lacerations, and abdominal and head injuries. X-ray films may help explore the type and number of current and old fractures.

The nurse should examine the child completely, beginning with the face and eyes, to determine the diagnosis and any intervention that might be needed. The presence or absence of the blue sclera should be noted, as should the shape of the child's face. Type IV individuals have a triangular-shaped face. The spine should be examined for scoliosis and/or kyphosis. The chest should also be examined. Type III clients manifest a conical-

shaped chest. The ROM of the hips and knees should be examined. The child's height should be plotted on a growth chart, and this can serve as a baseline, especially if treatment with growth hormone is initiated.

Diagnostic Evaluation. Prenatal diagnosis can be made with ultrasonography, in some cases as early as 15 weeks of gestation (Phillips, Shulman, Altieri, Wilroy, Emerson, Dacus, & Elias, 1991). Because the problem is genetic, amniocentesis can be used to diagnose the condition. Chorionic villus sampling can be used to analyze the collagen synthesized by the chorionic villus cells.

Radiographic findings vary and may not be evident at birth. Some degree of generalized osteoporosis is almost always evident. Bone densitometry can be helpful in diagnosing OI when the clinical examination is not clear-cut. Dent and Paterson (1991) caution that there are no distinct radiographic differences between the fractures seen in OI and those in nonaccidental injury (battered child syndrome). Therefore, a differential diagnosis cannot be made based solely on radiographs.

Quantitative analysis of cultured skin fibroblast collagen by electrophoresis can be performed. A decreased quantity of collagen in the affected individual cells is

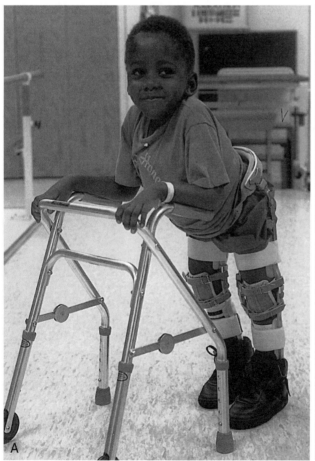 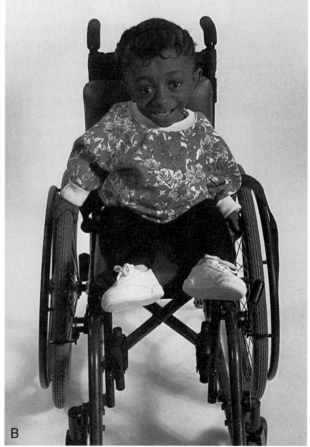

FIGURE 18–22. Osteogenesis imperfecta. Child with type I *(A)* and type III *(B)*.

indicative of OI. The parents are then tested to determine the mode of inheritance. Phillips et al. (1991) describe the inheritance pattern and findings.

Treatment Modalities and Related Nursing Management. The short-term goals of OI treatment are to reduce the number of fractures and resultant deformity and to promote the highest level of mobility, independence, and social interaction possible. After fracture occurrence, providing splinting for pain relief and prevention of deformity becomes the primary treatment goal.

Binder, Conway, Hason, Gerber, Marini, Berry, and Weintrob (1993) advocate early intervention, muscle strengthening, aerobic conditioning, and protected ambulation. Early intervention includes careful handling and positioning with head supports and devices, such as sandbags or custom-molded seats for lower extremity positioning. A swimming program has been successful for increasing muscle strength of the hips and spine. Orthoses (or casts or splints depending on age) can aid in ambulation. For nonambulatory children, orthoses can aid in decreasing fractures.

Fractures are unavoidable, and when they occur, they should be splinted or immobilized in such a way as to prevent deformity. Immobilization should be kept as minimal as possible to prevent further osteoporosis and decrease the risk of future fracture, resulting in a fracture-immobilization-refracture cycle. As much motion as possible should be maintained during immobilization.

Surgical intervention may be the treatment of choice for severe deformities or long-bone fractures. The technique of osteotomy, realignment, and intramedullary fixation has been of great value. This procedure not only corrects bony deformity but also provides internal support to prevent future fractures.

The spine is often involved in OI. The occurrence of scoliosis, kyphosis, or compression fractures with resulting pain and deformity has been reported in a high percentage of cases. Bracing can be used as support but rarely prevents progression and does not correct any deformity already present. Surgical correction is difficult because the poor quality of bone makes fixation with instrumentation difficult. Anterior and posterior procedures may be necessary. Despite the difficulties involved, surgical stabilization of severe curves is recommended to aid ambulation and improve pulmonary function.

Nursing interventions associated with perioperative care for the child undergoing intramedullary rodding can be found in Chapter 11 for general concerns and in Bender (1991).

Fractures are common in this population. Parents may be anxious about caring for their child and causing injury. Although it is important to prevent injury, it is also necessary for the child to be held and cared for to promote development.

Careful handling from the time of diagnosis or suspected diagnosis is imperative. Extremities should be supported fully at all times without twisting or hyperextension and the child's body should be moved as a unit. Pillows and other supports can be helpful in carrying out activities with the child. Demonstration of techniques to hold and care for the child, along with the opportunity for the parents to practice these techniques and voice their concerns, is beneficial. The parents need to receive a great deal of encouragement to handle and hold their newborn so that normal bonding can develop.

Recognition of a fracture can be difficult, particularly in the younger child. Irritability, lack of appetite, fever, and changes in respiration (for rib fractures) can be indicative of fractures. The parents should be reminded that fractures can occur even with cautious handling.

Teaching about the devices described previously is essential to increasing parental effectiveness and reducing anxiety. Providing information about the expected course of the disorder and referring the parents for genetic counseling are important interventions.

Socialization Enhancement. Parental education begins as soon as the diagnosis is made. The parents need to develop realistic goals, know how to set limits, and plan appropriate and safe activities for the child.

The importance of education should be stressed. The child with OI is of normal intelligence, and the school should make whatever accommodations are necessary to assist the child in attending school. The nurse can play a vital role in working with the school to educate others about the child with OI. Although there may be several limitations for the child, interaction and participation in school and extracurricular activities are important. Those who are fearful that the child will experience fractures may limit these opportunities for interaction.

Summary. OI is a relatively uncommon hereditary disorder of collagen formation that causes fragility of the bones. Treatment at this time is supportive and is aimed at preventing fractures and deformities, managing fractures as they occur, and assisting with normal development, with the goal of independence and gainful employment. Research continues to better define the exact mechanism of the collagen disorder so that prevention and perhaps medical treatment may be possible.

FUTURE DEVELOPMENTS

On the horizon are the technological developments that will allow in utero diagnosis of musculoskeletal disorders. Three-dimensional ultrasound imaging will allow a panoramic view of the fetus, providing for detailed study of the spine and limbs. Spine defects and more minor problems such as syndactyly or polydactyly will be diagnosed before birth. This will pave the way for in utero treatment, including surgery. Although in utero surgery has limited use currently, it is believed to play an important role in treatment in the future.

As the basic defects of a multitude of disorders are mapped within the human genome, DNA linkage analysis or specific mutation assays will be available for identifying a multitude of disorders that carry musculoskeletal problems.

Molecular genetic techniques are increasingly being used to diagnose DNA alterations. These techniques are being used to diagnose a variety of mendelian and mitochondrial disorders. Continued research will continually increase the number and type of disorders that can be diagnosed in the prenatal period. Specimens come from chorionic villi tissue or amniotic fluid cells. Newer techniques include harvesting fetal cells from maternal blood and analyzing DNA of the embryo or gamete before implantation or fertilization.

MRI is gradually coming into use for evaluating complex disorders such as spina bifida in utero. MRI may help in evaluating whether the lesion is open or closed, what the level of the lesion is, and whether cerebral or posterior fossa abnormalities exist. Currently, the technology is used as an adjunct with ultrasound for evaluating complex problems.

Although still in clinical trials, pamidronate, a bisphosphonate, is being used to treat clients with OI and offers hope in improving bone quality in these clients. More advanced therapies that may one day offer a cure for OI and other genetic disorders are stem cell and/or bone marrow transplants and gene therapy.

COMMON NURSING CONCERNS FOR THE CHILD WITH AN ORTHOPAEDIC CONGENITAL OR DEVELOPMENTAL DISORDER

Children with orthopaedic disorders have many of the same concerns as children with other disorders, including coping with hospitalizations and the effects of an acute or chronic condition.

Although specific nursing concerns are related to individual disorders and the exact treatment required, a number of concerns are applicable to any child with an orthopaedic congenital or developmental disorder. Each child's plan of care must be individualized to fit the needs of the child and those of the family. The following are potential problems.

Nursing Diagnoses

Pain

Pain management in children is an issue that has come to the forefront in recent years. Contrary to what was formerly believed, children do experience and remember pain. Because of limitations in experience and verbalization, children often express pain differently than adults. Orthopaedic procedures and surgery may be especially painful for children if accentuated by an underlying disease, such as CP. Therefore, the nurse must be astute in assessing and intervening to manage pain in children.

Pain Management. A key factor to consider when assessing pain in children is that indications of pain are often exhibited in different ways than in adults. Children often express pain by being irritable, uncooperative, withdrawn, or quiet. When questioned, they may deny pain if they feel it is "childish" to admit to being in pain, if they feel they would be judged as being a "bad client," or if they fear an injection to relieve the pain or dislike taking medicine.

Both pharmacologic and nonpharmacologic pain management modalities are beneficial for children. Intramuscular injections are rarely needed in the pediatric setting. Analgesics and anti-inflammatory nonsteroidal medication are helpful when dealing with mild or nonacute pain. Opioids are necessary to control severe pain and may be administered intravenously. Patient-controlled analgesia (PCA) devices have become popular mechanisms for pain control but often provide poor control pain because of a number of reasons: (1) Clients are often given instructions in the recovery room when they are still sleepy; (2) clients are told to press the button "when they have pain," and this results in too little medication, too late (the pain is sometimes already out of control); and (3) falling asleep for several hours may mean the child awakens in pain, unless he or she is on a continuous drip or a basal rate.

Nonpharmacologic modalities of pain management work quite effectively with children undergoing procedural pain or in conjunction with pharmacologic interventions. Successful interventions include diversional activities, such as TV or games; relaxation techniques, especially relaxation tapes heard through earphones; visualization; and comfort measures, such as rocking and cuddling. Play therapy techniques should also be used. These techniques can be very simple yet very effective in promoting understanding and comfort. Coping mechanisms also vary with children. Crying, rocking, and being held are often helpful for small children.

Impaired Mobility

Orthopaedic interventions with children often cause altered mobility because of casts or traction. Some congenital disorders result in immobility from birth or progressively limited mobility. Children are at a disadvantage in being able to understand the rationale for limited mobility and often are creative in finding acceptable and unacceptable methods to circumvent their immobility.

Activity Therapy. Mobility for children is more than a physical issue. Children need to attain and maintain a level of mobility to grow socially and developmentally. When physical issues must take precedence, the nurse should assist families to discover ways to meet the child's mobility needs. A variety of mobility aids are available to facilitate movement. These include staircars, scooter boards, strollers, and wheelchairs. For younger children who have limited ability to move, it is crucial that they are able to be placed in a semireclining or upright position. Infants can be placed in an infant seat and progress to a stander or parapodium as they become toddlers.

Limitations in mobility because of casting or traction, although short term, may be a great cause of frustration to children and result in feelings of isolation, loneliness, and even depression. It is important that the child not feel totally isolated from friends and family. When mobility aids are not available or practical, every effort should be made to bring family and friends to the child. This can be done by visits to the home or hospital, by moving the child and bed into a more central location, and by allowing specific playtime with parents and others. Pets are often a real comfort and provide a special level of companionship for children who are immobilized.

Mobility becomes a greater challenge as children get older and heavier, especially for children who have chronic conditions that affect their ability to ambulate. It is important to view walking as only one method of ambulation. Some teenagers are faced with the challenge of weighing the advantages of walking against their limited physical resources. Wheelchair ambulation may be a better alternative for some children with limited strength and endurance if this is viewed as an acceptable alternative.

Impaired Skin Integrity

Skin integrity can be a challenge specifically for the child with an acute episode that requires a cast and for the child with a chronic disorder that includes insensate skin. Special attention must be given to both of these situations.

Skin Surveillance and Pressure Management. Perhaps the greater challenge related to skin integrity comes with those children who have insensate skin, usually those with spina bifida. As the child grows and becomes heavier, skin integrity becomes an issue, particularly for those who are in a wheelchair. Teens seem especially vulnerable to problems with skin integrity.

Positioning: Wheelchair. The child who is confined to a wheelchair is also at high risk for skin breakdown. The child in a wheelchair who has adequate upper extremity function should be taught to perform wheelchair pushups to relieve pressure on the buttocks. Proper cushions for wheelchairs are imperative. A number of brands and types are available, and which is used depends on the individual needs and condition of the skin.

Alteration in Nutrition: More Than or Less Than Body Requirements

Weight management is a concern and a challenge for all children with congenital and developmental orthopaedic disorders. This is especially true for those with chronic conditions, such as osteogenesis and myelodysplasia. Being overweight or obese is readily identified as a common problem. Being underweight should also be considered, especially with those disorders such as CP, when a feeding disorder may be coexistent. Malnutrition may exist in either situation.

Obesity in children with chronic orthopaedic conditions often occurs as the child reaches the late school years and approaching adolescence. Children are heavier and larger at this point simply because of normal maturation. Hormonal changes may contribute to weight gain. The risk for children with orthopaedic conditions is that weight gain can result in significant limitations to mobility. Social isolation, lack of diversional activities, and ability or opportunity to be involved only in sedentary activities may result.

Obesity can occur relatively quickly and insidiously in children who are physically inactive. An increase in weight for these children has a spiral effect: The more weight that is gained, the less mobile they are and the more weight they gain. Although weight gain is not completely avoidable and limitations in mobility may be inevitable as the child grows, consideration should be given to maintaining a healthful weight.

Self-care Deficit

Self-care Assistance. Self-care deficit is present in varying degrees, depending on the diagnosis. As the child grows and develops, ways have to be found to allow as much independence as possible. Numerous adaptive aids are available to assist in feeding, dressing, and transfers. A number of companies offer special clothing lines designed for individuals with limited ability or those confined to a wheelchair. Often, the parents require encouragement to allow the child to be independent. It is often easier and quicker for the parent to perform tasks rather than wait for the child to do them.

Individual/Family Management of Therapeutic Regimen. Many devices and treatments for orthopaedic disorders are difficult for the child and family to tolerate. Parents can experience guilt about the disorder and are concerned that the child is uncomfortable in the device.

Anticipatory Guidance. If it is possible, allow the child to become adjusted to part of the appliance or device before adding other restrictive devices. For example, with the Denis Browne splint, it is helpful to first allow the child to become accustomed to sleeping in the shoes and then to add the bar. The parents should be told that if the child cries initially, it is important (after checking fit and application for appropriateness) that the parent not remove the device because this reinforces the crying behavior. If the parent persists, the child generally adjusts. If the child is able to remove or untie the device, straps or shoelaces can be taped over so that the child does not have access to them. The child's developmental stage can play a role in compliance. For example, the child may disregard treatment as a way to demonstrate independence and autonomy. Long-term care can also affect compliance. The parents must continually weigh the physical, medical, and psychosocial needs of the family and child.

The child and family should have the opportunity to openly discuss limitations they find in complying with the treatment program. Suggestions for increasing the comfort and ease of compliance with treatment, as well as consequences of noncompliance, should be addressed.

Knowledge Deficit

Teaching: Disease Process. The child and family may have a knowledge deficit about the disorder. The extent and accuracy of knowledge should be explored and assessed. Information must be given at a time when the family is ready to learn and in a manner appropriate to the family's level of understanding and the child's developmental level. As the child's condition or needs change, the nurse must assess the family's perceptions of the child's status, and parental knowledge must be updated. It is important that the following information be related to the child and family: understanding the disorder, its usual course, assessments or symptoms that the child or family need to note, treatment options and implications, follow-up care, and when to call the nurse or physician.

Impaired Psychosocial Adjustment

Family Integrity Promotion and Sibling Support. The entire family often feels the impact of the child's illness. Marital stability may be threatened. The nurse should encourage open communication between the parents and a regular schedule for the couple to have time away from their children. Referral for counseling may be indicated. Task sharing and discussion of problem issues are important for the entire family. Other siblings need to have their own activities and not feel pressured to care for the affected child. Social isolation may affect the child and family. Planning, additional assistance, and realistic expectations for outings make the event more successful.

Many children who previously would have been hospitalized for immobilization are now being taken care of in the home. Responsibilities associated with the care of a child in a body cast have a significant impact on the caregivers, especially the primary caregiver. Mobility, socialization, and often financial implications result from the need to care for a child in the home. Adjustments must be made in nearly every aspect of the caregiver's life, and support is needed for these parents. Innovative ways to address these concerns must be considered by the health care team.

If surgery is required, questions about expectations after surgery, changes that the child's needs impose on the family, and the ability of the family to care for the child at home need to be addressed.

Diversional Activity Deficit and Altered Growth and Development

Developmental Enhancement. Activities must be appropriate for the child's age and developmental status. Using toys and games to stimulate needed movements or to avoid unwanted movements is an effective strategy. For example, for the child with torticollis, alternating placement of toys to the left and right of an infant encourages movement of the head in both directions.

For the child who is ambulatory with crutches, braces, or wheelchair, accessible activities must be found. Getting the child in and out of the car and transporting the child are details that should be resolved by the family before the surgery. Special Olympics and wheelchair sports have promoted development and self-confidence for many children with congenital or developmental disorders. The nurse should provide information or the family should be referred to social services for information regarding available activities in the community.

TRANSITION TO ADULTHOOD

From 10% to 15% of all children born in the United States are born with a chronic or disabling condition. Of these, nearly one third have disabilities that limit independence. Over the past 20 years, improvements in neonatal life support technologies and medical-surgical interventions have led to a decrease in early childhood mortality. More than 85% of children born with chronic conditions and disabilities will survive to adulthood.

These children now face special challenges as they move through the life cycle, especially as they make the transition into adulthood and independence (Box 18–9).

BOX 18–9.

Transition Issues for Adolescents with Congenital and Developmental Disorders

---

Movement from pediatric to adult health care providers
Lack of knowledge about financial management and budgeting
Vocational and employment choices and limitations
Educational opportunities and challenges
Working within the public health care system
Transportation for work, school, socialization
Independent living or living independently
Socialization and intimacy; avoiding isolation and loneliness
Sexuality, reproduction, and healthful sexual behavior

Transition issues begin early in life and typically are a challenge for all children. However, physically challenged children and youth face additional and more complex transition issues.

Nursing interventions with these youth should begin in the toddler years with recommendations that encourage independence and self-esteem. Even very young children can gain self-esteem and a sense of mastery by assuming physically appropriate and age-appropriate responsibilities. As the child approaches adolescence, specific interventions should include socialization skills and identification of health care providers who are knowledgeable about caring for adults with the individual's condition.

SUMMARY

Caring for the child with an orthopaedic congenital or developmental disorder is both challenging and rewarding for the nurse. As more and more physically challenged children live into adulthood, the challenge to anticipate their needs as adults is great. The nurse plays a unique role in providing knowledge at all stages of care and treatment and emotional support to the child and family, as well as assessing growth and development and intervening when necessary. Assisting the child and family in planning for the future is an important role for the nurse.

INTERNET RESOURCES

Cerebral Palsy.com (a listing of numerous other websites and educational information for addressing almost every aspect of cerebral palsy): www.cerebralpalsy.com/

The Dupont Institute (educational modules for those wishing to lean more or test their knowledge in pediatric orthopaedics): http://gait.aidi.udel.edu/res695/homepage/pd_ortho/educate.htm

Health Resources and Services Administration, Maternal Child Health Bureau Division of Services for Children with Special Needs (contains documents relating to cultural communication needs, cultural and ethnic issues and the national agenda for children with special needs; also has a link to the Genetics Services Branch with information on newborn screening and the Genetic Research Center): www.mchb.hrsa.gov/html/dscshn.html

National Institutes of Health, Osteoporosis and Related Bone Diseases—National Resource Center (information on osteogenesis imperfecta): www.osteo.org/

Pediatric Orthopedic Society of North America (information for parents regarding common orthopaedic problems in children): www.posna.org/InfoParents/InfoParentsIndex.htm

United States Cerebral Palsy Athletic Association: www.uscpaa.org/about_purpose.htm

REFERENCES

Aaronson, J. (1997). Limb lengthening, skeletal reconstruction, and bone transport with the Ilizarov method. *The Journal of Bone and Joint Surgery, 79A*, 1243–1258.

Abbott, R., Johann-Murphy, M., Shiminski-Maher, T., Quartermain, D., Forem, S. L., Gold, J. T., & Epstein, F. J. (1993). Selective dorsal rhizotomy: Outcome and complications in treating spastic cerebral palsy. *Neurosurgery, 33*, 851–857.

Alexander, M., Ackman, J. D., & Kuo, K. N. (1999). Congenital idiopathic clubfoot. *Orthopedic Nursing, 18*, 47–58.

Alexander, M., & Kuo, K. N. (1997). Musculoskeletal assessment of the newborn. *Orthopaedic Nursing, 16*, 21–31.

Bender, L. H. (1991). Osteogenesis imperfecta. *Orthopaedic Nursing, 10*(4), 23–31.

Bensahel, H., Dal Monte, A., Hjelmstedt, A., Bjerkreim, I., Wientroub, S., Matasovic, T., Porat, S., & Bialik, V. (1989). Congenital dislocation of the knee. *Journal of Pediatric Orthopaedics, 9*, 174–177.

Bianchi-Maiocchi, A., & Aaronson, J. (1994). Indications. In A. Bianchi-Maiocchi (Ed.), *Advances in Ilizarov apparatus assembly* (pp. 3–4). Milan: Medical Publishing.

Binder, H., Conway, A., Hason, S., Gerber, L. H., Marini, J., Berry, R., & Weintrob, J. (1993). Comprehensive rehabilitation of the child with osteogenesis imperfecta. *American Journal of Medical Genetics, 45*, 265–269.

Bleck, E. (1987). *Orthopedic management in cerebral palsy.* London: Mac-Keith Press.

Byers, P. H., & Steiner, R. D. (1992). Osteogenesis imperfecta. *Annual Review of Medicine, 43*, 269–282.

Cosgrove, A. P., Corry, I. S., & Graham, H. K. (1994). Botulinum toxin in the management of the lower limb in cerebral palsy. *Developmental Medicine and Child Neurology, 36*, 386–396.

Dent, J. A., & Paterson, C. R. (1991). Fractures in early childhood: Osteogenesis imperfecta or child abuse? *Journal of Pediatric Orthopaedics, 11*, 184–186.

Dormans, J. P., & Pellegrino, L. (1998). *Caring for children with cerebral palsy.* Baltimore: Brooks.

Gage, J. R. (1993). Gait analysis: An essential tool in the treatment of cerebral palsy. *Clinical Orthopaedics and Related Research, 288*, 126–134.

Herring, J. A. (1994). Current concepts review: The treatment of Legg-Calvé-Perthes disease. *Journal of Bone and Joint Surgery, 76A*, 448–458.

Jaworski, S., Dudkiewicz, Z., Lodzinski, K., & Lenkiewicz, T. (1992). Back closure with a latissimus dorsi myocutaneous flap. *Journal of Pediatric Surgery, 27*, 74–75.

Knutson, L. M., & Clark, D. E. (1991). Orthotic devices for ambulation in children with cerebral palsy and myelomeningocele. *Physical Therapy, 71*, 947–960.

Komisarz, J. M. (1984). Chondromalacia patellae. *Orthopaedic Nursing, 3*(3), 24, 25.

Langenskiold, A., & Ritsila, V. (1992). Congenital dislocation of the patella and its operative treatment. *Journal of Pediatric Orthopaedics, 12*, 315–323.

Loder, R. T., Schaffer, J. J., & Bardenstein, M. B. (1991). Late-onset tibia vara. *Journal of Pediatric Orthopaedics, 11*, 162–167.

Marty, G. R., Dias, L. S., & Gaebler-Spira, D. (1995). Selective posterior rhizotomy and soft-tissue procedures for the treatment of cerebral diplegia. *Journal of Bone and Joint Surgery, 77A*, 713–718.

McLone, D. G. (1989). Spina bifida today: Problems adults face. *Seminars in Neurology, 9*, 169–175.

Morrisy, R. T. [1990]. *Lovell & Winter's pediatric orthopaedics.* Philadelphia: Lippincott.

Nadel, A. S., Green, J. K., Holmes, L. B., Frigoletto, F. D., Jr., & Benacerraf, B. R. (1990). Absence of need for amniocentesis in patients with elevated levels of maternal serum alpha-fetoprotein and normal ultrasonographic examinations. *New England Journal of Medicine, 323*(9), 557–561.

Olney, S. J., & Wright, M. J. (1994). Cerebral palsy. In S. K. Campbell (Ed.). *Physical therapy for children.* Philadelphia: WB Saunders.

Ozonoff, M. B. (1992). *Pediatric orthopedic radiology* (2nd ed.). Philadelphia: WB Saunders.

Phillips, O. P., Shulman, L. P., Altieri, L. A., Wilroy, R. S., Emerson, D. S., Dacus, J. V., & Elias, S. (1991). Prenatal counseling and diagnosis in progressively deforming osteogenesis imperfecta: A case of autosomal dominant transmission. *Prenatal Diagnosis, 11,* 705-710.

Rauen, K. K., & Aubert, E. J. (1992). A brighter future for adults who have myelomeningocele: One form of spina bifida. *Orthopaedic Nursing, 11*(3), 16-27.

Richtsmeier, A. J., Barkin, R., & Alexander, M. (1992). Benzodiazepines for acute pain in children. *Journal of Pain and Symptom Management, 7,* 492-495.

Smith, P. A., Sirirungruangsarn, Y., & Kuo, K. N. (1997). Result of clubfoot surgery: An analysis of failure. *Journal of Pediatric Orthopedics, 6B,* 294.

Sodre, H., Bruschini, S., Mestriner, L., Miranda, F., Jr., Levinsohn, E. M., Packard, D. S., Jr., Crider, R. J., Jr., Schwartz, R., & Hootnick, D. R. (1990). Arterial abnormalities in talipes equinovarus as assessed by angiography and the Doppler technique. *Journal of Pediatric Orthopaedics, 10,* 104-105.

Stanisavljevic, S., Zemenick, G., Miller, D. (1976). Congenital, irreducible, permanent lateral dislocation of the patella. *Clinical Orthopaedics and Related Research, May* (116), 190-199.

Tachdjian, M. O. (1997). *Clinical pediatric orthopedics: The art of diagnosis and principles of management.* Stamford, CT: Appleton & Lange.

Tachdjian, M. O. (1990). *Pediatric orthopedics* (2nd ed.). Philadelphia: WB Saunders.

Warner, W. C., Canale, S. T., & Beaty, J. H. (1994). Congenital deformities of the knee. In W. N. Scott (Ed.), *The knee.* St. Louis: Mosby.

Yen, I. H., Khoury, M. J., Erickson, D., James, L. M., Waters, G. D., & Berry, R. J. (1992). The changing epidemiology of neural tube defects. *American Journal of Diseases of Children, 146,* 857-861.

Zickler, C. F., & Dodge, N. N. (1994). Office management of the young child with cerebral palsy and difficulty in growing. *Journal of Pediatric Health Care, 8*(3), 111-120.

19

Fractures

CATHLEEN E. KUNKLER

Musculoskeletal conditions are the second most common cause of activity limitation in the United States, affecting 33% of adults annually. Injuries from accidents involve more than 58 million people a year and are the fourth most common cause of death for all ages. Trauma is the leading cause of death for Americans between the ages of 1 and 37; every 6 minutes someone in the United States dies from trauma (Brown, Henderson, & Moore, 1996). Motor vehicle accidents, farm accidents, falls, and gunshot wounds account for 30% of all trauma injuries, with open tibial fracture being responsible for 40% of annual trauma treatment costs.

Fractures constitute a high proportion of these injuries. Fractures occur in all age groups, at any point of the skeletal system, and they may result in a significant change in an individual's quality of life. They can cause activity restriction, disability, impairment, handicap, and economic loss. The incidence of fractures peaks in both males and females between the ages of 6 and 16 and then again in the older adult.

INJURY PREVENTION

Injury is a definable, correctable event, with specific risks for occurrence, and thus it is preventable. In *Health, United States, 1998*, 1 in 4 Americans (59 million) are injured annually. Of those injured, 36 million will require an emergency department visit and 2.6 million will be hospitalized. Of those, approximately 500,000 will die as a result of their injury. The estimate of the lifetime financial cost of injury exceeds $250 billion, 30% of which is spent for direct health care and the remainder in the indirect costs of lost productivity.

Therefore injury as such is preventable, diagnosable, treatable, survivable, and ultimately controllable. Patterns have been identified related to gender, race, substance abuse, and geographic and socioeconomic factors. Males, aged 15 to 40, have the highest incidence of preventable injury. Young children have the largest portion of deaths resulting from burns from fires, drowning, and homicides resulting from child abuse. Nearly half of all preventable injury deaths caused by motor vehicle incidents occur in young adults. The growing incidence of firearm injury in adolescents is a grave concern in our society. Injury-related fatalities in older adults from falls demonstrate the need for more fall-prevention interventions. Finally, the abuse of alcohol and other substances contributes to more than 50% of all injury-related preventable deaths. All of these somber facts combine to reinforce the fact that injury can largely be prevented. The American Academy of Pediatricians, the National Safety Council, and the American College of Surgeons Committee on Trauma are among the major medical organizations promoting injury prevention. Ongoing public health surveillance, education, and law enforcement will continue to be our best defense in the quest to eradicate preventable injury. See Chapter 1 for a more extensive discussion of injury prevention.

DEFINITIONS

Musculoskeletal trauma can result in fractures; joint dislocation; soft tissue edema; hemorrhage into muscle and joints; nerve, tendon, and vascular damage; and injuries to body organs. A *fracture* is any disruption, complete or incomplete, in the continuity of a bone. *Dislocation* occurs when there is complete displacement of the bone from its normal position at the surface of the joint and the articular surfaces are no longer in contact. *Subluxation* refers to the partial dislocation of the joint from its normal position, and *fracture-dislocation* is the

609

combination of fracture with dislocation of the involved joint.

PATHOPHYSIOLOGY

Predisposing Factors

Stress is the amount of force (load) applied to a bone. *Strain* is the reaction within the bone to the stress. The amount and frequency of stress applied and the number of repetitions play a part in determining when a fracture will occur.

The amount of force required to fracture a bone varies with the biologic, extrinsic, and intrinsic factors present. Biologic factors are conditions that alter the composition and strength of the bone. Age is one biologic factor affecting the amount of force required to produce a fracture. As age increases and bone becomes more brittle, the amount of force required to produce a fracture decreases. For more information on age-related musculo-skeletal changes, see Chapter 6. The amount of force required also varies with the size of the bone involved. Extrinsic factors include the magnitude, duration, and direction of the force, as well as the rate of loading. Intrinsic factors are properties of bone, such as its energy-absorbing capacity, elasticity, fatigue strength, size, and density. Behavioral factors that may predispose the individual to fracture include high-risk activities (e.g., parachuting, skateboarding) in which the individual engages for either recreation or employment.

Mechanism of Injury. A fracture occurs when bone is subjected to more stress than it can absorb. Fractures may be caused by direct or indirect force or by stress or fatigue of the bone. They may also be pathologic in origin.

Direct force causes tapping, crush, or penetrating fractures. A *tapping* fracture is caused by a small force applied to a small area, such as a kick or a blow with a blunt instrument. Most of the energy is absorbed by the bone, and there may be only a small bruise or laceration to the soft tissue overlying the fracture site. Tapping fractures usually result in a transverse fracture line and often occur in the forearm or leg.

Crush fractures are caused by a large amount of force being applied to a small area and are generally accompanied by extensive soft tissue damage. They result in comminuted or transverse fracture lines and often occur in the forearm or foreleg, with both bones being fractured at the same level.

Penetrating fractures are caused by a large amount of force acting on a small area, as in projectile injuries. The most common type of penetrating fracture is caused by a gunshot wound. Low-velocity gunshot fractures generally cause limited soft tissue damage, whereas high-velocity gunshot fractures are associated with a high degree of soft tissue damage.

Indirect trauma is force applied distant from the fracture site. Causes include traction or tension forces, angulation forces, rotational forces, vertical compression forces, or any combination of these. Traction or tension fractures (e.g., ankle sprain with avulsed fragment) result when a muscle contracts and force is exerted simulta-neously in the opposite direction. Traction fractures rarely occur in the shaft of a long bone but may occur in the patella or the olecranon. The fracture line in traction fractures is usually transverse.

Angulation fractures (e.g., nightstick fractures, Fig. 19-1) occur when the lever (bone) is forced into angula-tion. The fracture line begins on the side of the bone forced into convexity and progresses to the adjacent bone fibers. This produces a transverse fracture line and often causes a triangular (butterfly, see Fig. 19-1) fragment to break off on the convex side.

Rotational fractures produce a spiral fracture line either with or without splintering and commonly occur in the distal third of the tibia.

Compression fractures (see Fig. 19-1) (e.g., subcapital femoral fracture) of long bones produce T- or Y-shaped fractures and occasionally may cause a longitudinal non-displaced fracture. Compression fractures occur when there is compressive loading force along the long axis of the bone. Compression fractures commonly occur in the spine and are often associated with osteoporosis.

Stress fractures (see Fig. 19-1) occur after normal everyday activities when there is no evidence of trauma to explain the occurrence of the fracture. Stress fractures can be described as either fatigue fractures or insufficiency fractures. Fatigue fractures occur in normal healthy bones after repetitive use or loading. Insufficiency frac-tures occur in abnormal bones subjected to normal stress. Both meet the criteria for stress fractures because there is no preceding trauma.

One factor in the development of fatigue fractures is the ability of the muscles to absorb stress. With repeated loading or overuse, muscle fatigue occurs and the stress-shielding ability of the muscle decreases. More stress is passed to the bone, and fractures can occur more quickly. Additional predisposing factors for the development of fatigue fractures include variations in training or overtraining for a sport, new or increased activity, quality or change in footwear, and anatomic variations.

The normal ongoing process of bone metabolism provides a balance between new bone formation and old bone resorption. Normal bone is in a constant process of remodeling as it adjusts to the stresses applied to it. When bone resorption occurs more rapidly than bone replace-ment, the bone is weakened structurally. Under repetitive stress, weakened bone may develop cracks or microfrac-tures that can progress to complete fracture. Low-energy stress fractures are usually linear, with little displacement. As the amount of energy increases, the amount of

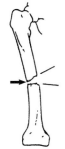

Angulated: Fracture with fragments at angles to each other *Cause:* Direct or lateral force, causing break and loss of anatomic positions

Angulated

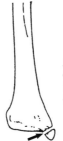

Avulsed: Fracture that pulls bone and other tissues from usual attachments *Cause:* Direct energy of force, with resisted extension of bone and joint

Avulsed

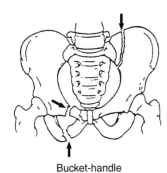

Bucket-handle: Double vertical fractures of pelvis on same side, resulting in pelvic dislocation *Cause:* Direct blow or anterior compression force, with or without sacral torsion

Bucket-handle

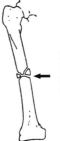

Butterfly: Butterfly-shaped piece of fractured bone, usually accompanying comminuted fracture *Cause:* Direct, indirect, or rotational force to bone

Butterfly

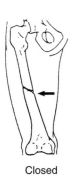

Closed: Skin intact over fracture *Cause:* Minor force or energy

Closed

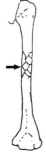

Comminuted: Fracture with more than two pieces; may have significant associated soft tissue trauma *Cause:* Direct crushing injury or force to tissues and bone

Comminuted

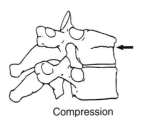

Compression: Fracture is squeezed or wedged together at one side *Cause:* Compressive, axial energy or force applied directly from above fracture site

Compression

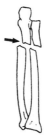

Displaced: Fracture with one, both, or all fragments out of normal alignment *Cause:* direct energy or force to site

Displaced

FIGURE 19–1. Types and causes of fractures. (From Thompson, J. M., McFarland, G. K., Hirsch, J. E., & Tucker, S. M. [Eds.]. [1997]. *Mosby's clinical nursing* [4th ed., pp. 392–394]. St. Louis: Mosby.)

Illustration continued on following page

TYPES AND CAUSES OF FRACTURES—cont'd

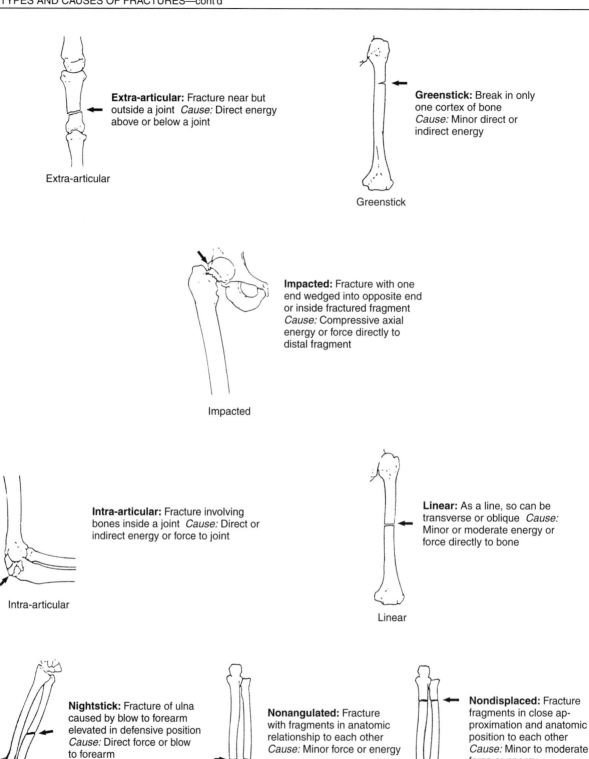

Extra-articular: Fracture near but outside a joint *Cause:* Direct energy above or below a joint

Extra-articular

Greenstick: Break in only one cortex of bone *Cause:* Minor direct or indirect energy

Greenstick

Impacted: Fracture with one end wedged into opposite end or inside fractured fragment *Cause:* Compressive axial energy or force directly to distal fragment

Impacted

Intra-articular: Fracture involving bones inside a joint *Cause:* Direct or indirect energy or force to joint

Intra-articular

Linear: As a line, so can be transverse or oblique *Cause:* Minor or moderate energy or force directly to bone

Linear

Nightstick: Fracture of ulna caused by blow to forearm elevated in defensive position *Cause:* Direct force or blow to forearm

Nightstick

Nonangulated: Fracture with fragments in anatomic relationship to each other *Cause:* Minor force or energy

Nonangulated

Nondisplaced: Fracture fragments in close approximation and anatomic position to each other *Cause:* Minor to moderate force or energy

Nondisplaced

FIGURE 19–1 *Continued.* Types and causes of fractures. (From Thompson, J. M., McFarland, G. K., Hirsch, J. E., & Tucker, S. M. [Eds.]. [1997]. *Mosby's clinical nursing* [4th ed., pp. 392–394]. St. Louis: Mosby.)

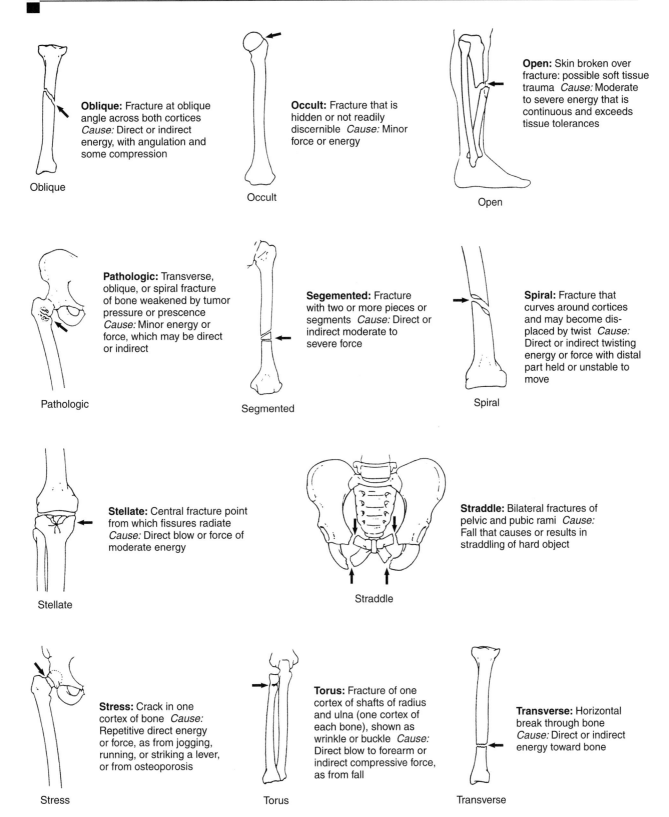

Oblique: Fracture at oblique angle across both cortices *Cause:* Direct or indirect energy, with angulation and some compression

Oblique

Occult: Fracture that is hidden or not readily discernible *Cause:* Minor force or energy

Occult

Open: Skin broken over fracture: possible soft tissue trauma *Cause:* Moderate to severe energy that is continuous and exceeds tissue tolerances

Open

Pathologic: Transverse, oblique, or spiral fracture of bone weakened by tumor pressure or prescence *Cause:* Minor energy or force, which may be direct or indirect

Pathologic

Segemented: Fracture with two or more pieces or segments *Cause:* Direct or indirect moderate to severe force

Segmented

Spiral: Fracture that curves around cortices and may become displaced by twist *Cause:* Direct or indirect twisting energy or force with distal part held or unstable to move

Spiral

Stellate: Central fracture point from which fissures radiate *Cause:* Direct blow or force of moderate energy

Stellate

Straddle: Bilateral fractures of pelvic and pubic rami *Cause:* Fall that causes or results in straddling of hard object

Straddle

Stress: Crack in one cortex of bone *Cause:* Repetitive direct energy or force, as from jogging, running, or striking a lever, or from osteoporosis

Stress

Torus: Fracture of one cortex of shafts of radius and ulna (one cortex of each bone), shown as wrinkle or buckle *Cause:* Direct blow to forearm or indirect compressive force, as from fall

Torus

Transverse: Horizontal break through bone *Cause:* Direct or indirect energy toward bone

Transverse

FIGURE 19–1 *Continued.* See legend on opposite page.

displacement, comminution, and soft tissue damage also increases.

Stress fractures occur most commonly in the lower extremity and are often related to military training programs or sports. Stress fractures in runners constitute approximately 10% of running injuries seen in sports medicine clinics.

Pathologic fractures occur when a bone weakened by preexisting disease fractures in response to an amount of stress that would leave a normal bone intact. Pathologic fractures may result from general systemic or local disorders (Box 19–1) and can occur with injury or during normal activity.

CLASSIFICATION OF FRACTURES

A concise and accurate description of fractures is essential for care and treatment. The type of fracture affects not only treatment but also the extent and complexity of the evaluation. Fractures are classified as open or closed; by the type of fracture line; by the anatomic location of the

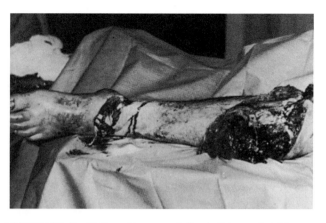

FIGURE 19–2. Oblique fracture of distal tibia, grade IIIB open ankle fracture, and grade IIIB open fracture of proximal tibia with extensive tissue loss. (From Browner, B. D., Jupiter, J. B., Levine, A. M., & Trafton, P. G. [1992]. *Skeletal trauma* [p. 317]. Philadelphia: WB Saunders.)

fracture on the involved bone; by the appearance, position, and alignment of the fragments; and by classic names (eponyms, e.g., Colles' fracture). When discussing a fracture or caring for a client with a fracture, one must understand the description and the mechanism of the injury.

An open fracture is one in which there is loss of continuity of the bone internally and an external wound communicating directly to the fracture site, that is, a fracture fragment protruding through the skin (Fig. 19–2). Open fractures are sometimes referred to as *compound* or *complex* fractures and can be further subdivided by the degree or severity of soft tissue damage, the size of the open wound, the amount of wound contamination, and the amount of soft tissue loss (Table 19–1). For open pelvic fractures, there is a direct tract between the fracture, vagina, rectum, perineal or other skin laceration, or a communication with the exterior as a result of drain or pack placement.

Closed fractures are those in which there is loss of bone continuity internally but no break in the skin. In the past, closed fractures were sometimes referred to as *simple* fractures. This term can be misleading because closed fractures are often as complicated as open fractures, and the term *simple* fracture is not used as often as it was in the past.

Types of Fracture

Classification by type of fracture line involves descriptive terms. A transverse fracture line (see Fig. 19–1) crosses the shaft of the bone involved at approximately a 90-degree angle and is usually caused by an angulation force. Transverse fracture lines are also common in pathologic fractures caused by Paget's disease, osteomalacia, and osteogenesis imperfecta. Transverse fractures are generally stable after reduction.

BOX 19–1.
Causes of Pathologic Fractures

General Systemic Disorders
Developmental
  Osteogenesis imperfecta
Nutritional and metabolic
  Rickets
  Osteomalacia
  Osteoporosis
  Hyperparathyroidism
  Cushing's syndrome
  Paget's disease
Neoplasm
  Metastasis from primary bone tumor
  Multiple myeloma
  Lymphatic leukemia
  Gaucher's disease

Local Disorders
Cystic bone disease
  Simple bone cyst
  Aneurysmal bone cyst
Primary benign bone tumor
  Giant cell tumor
  Hemangioma
  Chondroma
Primary malignant bone tumor
  Chondrosarcoma
  Osteogenic sarcoma
  Fibrosarcoma
  Ewing's sarcoma
Infection
Irradiation fracture

Oblique fracture lines (see Fig. 19–1) occur diagonally across the bone and are usually produced by a twisting force. Oblique fractures may slip following reduction unless traction is maintained or the fracture surfaces allow the fragments to interlock.

Spiral fracture lines (see Fig. 19–1) are caused by a twisting force with an upward thrust and are a continuation of an oblique fracture line coiling around the bone. These fractures are usually the result of indirect forces and may be associated with soft tissue damage. Reduction of spiral fractures is difficult to maintain without traction or internal fixation. Spiral fractures are a major cause of malrotation in fractures.

Greenstick fractures (see Fig. 19–1) are incomplete fractures that occur when the cortex of the bone bends on

TABLE 19–1. *The Gustilo-Anderson Classification of Soft Tissue Injury in Open Fractures*

TYPE	CHARACTERISTICS
Type I	Wound less than 1 cm long
	Minimal soft tissue damage, no signs of crush
	Usually simple transverse or short oblique fracture with little comminution
Type II	Wound more than 1 cm long
	Slight to moderate crushing injury, no extensive soft tissue damage, flap, or avulsion
	Moderate fracture comminution and contamination
Type III	Extensive wound and soft tissue damage, including muscles, skin, and (often) neurovascular structures
	Greater degree of fracture comminution and instability
	High degree of contamination
IIIA	Adequate soft tissue coverage of the fracture, despite extensive laceration, flaps, or high-energy trauma
	This subtype includes highly comminuted or segmental fractures from high energy, regardless of the size of the wound; type IIIA fractures do not require free flaps
IIIB	Open fracture associated with extensive injury to or loss of soft tissue, with periosteal stripping and exposure of bone
	Massive contamination and severe comminution
	After debridement and irrigation, bone is exposed and requires a local flap or free flap
IIIC	Any open fracture associated with an arterial injury that must be repaired, regardless of the extent of soft tissue injury
	Open fractures with arterial injuries have projected amputation rates ranging from 25% to 90%

From Russell, T., & Palmieri, A. (1995). Fractures of the pelvis, acetabulum and lower extremity. In S. Brotzman (Ed.), *Clinical orthopaedic rehabilitation* (p. 145). St. Louis: Mosby.

one side and buckles on the other. The cortex is intact on the side subjected to tension forces and fractures on the side forced into convexity. Greenstick fractures may be caused by a compression force on the long axis of the bone or by an angulatory force. They may require reduction or completion of the fracture line through the other cortex, followed by reduction to prevent an angulation deformity at the fracture site or a rotational deformity of the bone as growth occurs.

Compression fractures (see Fig. 19–1) are produced by a force applied parallel to the long axis of cancellous bone and usually result in a tubular bone changing rapidly in size and shape. Anatomic reduction of compression fractures is not usually possible.

Comminuted fractures (see Fig. 19–1) are produced by high-energy forces, such as crush or penetrating injuries, producing more than two fracture fragments. Comminuted fractures are commonly associated with severe soft tissue damage. It is generally difficult to achieve and maintain reduction in these fractures.

Impacted fractures (see Fig. 19–1) occur when a direct force causes a fracture and telescopes the fragment with the smaller diameter into the fragment with the larger diameter at the fracture line. Fragments of the fracture move in unison, and rapid union occurs.

Avulsed fractures (see Fig. 19–1) are those in which bone fragments and tissue are pulled away from bone at the insertion site. These fractures often occur in skeletally immature children, particularly in muscles originating on the pelvis and proximal femur.

Classification by Point of Reference

Terms to classify fractures by point of reference on the bone include *midshaft, proximal third, middle third,* and *distal third.* Point of reference may also refer to highly specific anatomic locations of the bone, for example, intra-articular, epiphyseal, metaphyseal, diaphyseal, or apophyseal. Table 19–2 lists fractures classified by anatomic location. Classification by appearance is a method of describing the appearance of the fracture and associated fragments. In Figure 19–1, examples of fractures described by appearance include butterfly, angulated and nonangulated, displaced and nondisplaced, segmental stellate, and torus. Classification by position is illustrated in Figure 19–1 by displaced and angular fractures and refers to the degree of displacement of fragments in reference to other fragments, including varus or valgus displacement. Displacement of a fracture may occur in any plane. *Alignment* refers to the rotatory or angular position of distal fragments in relation to the proximal fragment.

Classic and descriptive names for fractures may be derived from anatomic locations, the name of a person (eponyms), the method by which they occurred, or appearance of the fracture. Table 19–3 contains a selected list of the classic and descriptive names of fractures.

TABLE 19–2. *Classification by Anatomic Location*

NAME	DESCRIPTION
Apophyseal	Avulsion fracture of an apophysis (portion of the bone that contributes to growth but is not part of the joint) where there is strong tendinous attachment
Articular	Any fracture involving surface of a joint
Condylar	Fracture involving the condyle—the round bony projection of a long bone—at a hinge joint
Cortical	Fracture of the cortex of a bone (the thick outer portion of the bone)
Diacondylar	Fracture line across the condyle (transcondylar)
Diaphyseal	Fracture of the shaft of a long bone
Epiphyseal	Fracture involving the growth plate of a bone
Extracapsular	Any fracture near but outside the joint capsule
Intra-articular	Fracture involving the joint surfaces
Intracapsular	Fracture within the joint capsule
Metaphyseal	Fracture of a long bone between the diaphysis and the epiphysis
Periarticular	Fracture near a joint but not involving the joint surfaces
Subperiosteal	Fracture leaving the periosteum of the bone intact
Supracondylar	Fracture just above the condyle of a bone

DISLOCATIONS

Just as fractures can occur in any bone, dislocations can occur at any joint and at any age. Complete or frank dislocation (Fig. 19–3A) completely separates the articular surfaces of the joint. Subluxation (Fig. 19–3B) is an incomplete or partial dislocation of one bone from the joint surface. Recurrent or habitual dislocations are those that occur repetitively either with or without trauma. Congenital dislocations are those that exist at birth.

Dislocations are described as anterior or posterior and medial or lateral depending on the position of the distal bone relative to the proximal bone. Dislocations can be caused by either direct or indirect forces.

Knowledge of the mechanism of injury and proper handling are also important in the care of a client with a dislocation. The orthopaedic nurse must be aware of what actions and forces produced the dislocation so that the mechanism of injury is not reproduced during the care and treatment of the client.

Subluxations may be caused by loose surrounding support structures resulting from congenital problems, by trauma to tendons and ligaments, by joint effusions resulting from infection, or by disuse atrophy resulting from prolonged joint immobilization. The most commonly dislocated joints are small joints of the fingers, the patella, and the shoulder.

The symptoms of dislocation include pain, loss or change of normal contour of the joint, change in the length of the extremity, and loss of normal mobility. Diagnosis of dislocation is confirmed with radiographs, and there may often be an associated fracture. Treatment for dislocation includes immobilization of the joint and extremity until it has been reduced. Following reduction, if the joint is stable, gentle active range of motion (ROM) is begun as soon as possible to preserve joint motion. The joint is usually supported between the exercise sessions by immobilization devices (e.g., knee immobilizer, sling).

Nursing interventions include pain relief, assessment of neurovascular status, and instruction to the client or significant other on caring for any immobilization devices and prevention of reinjury.

GROWING BONES
Physiologic and Biomechanical Differences
The skeletal growth period lasts from conception until full skeletal maturity is reached at approximately age 25. During this period, bones in different regions of the body change in size and shape. Long bones increase in length and diameter, and other bones grow larger to meet the needs of the developing body. The process of bone growth is most obvious during the first months of life and again at puberty during the adolescent growth spurt. The slower growth of the head makes it smaller in proportion to the rest of the body, and the upper and lower extremities become relatively longer as skeletal maturity progresses. During the adolescent growth spurt, more growth occurs in the spine than in the limbs.

The immature skeleton is in a dynamic state of change as opposed to the mature skeleton, which is principally responding to the stresses applied to it. These structural and functional differences cause the immature skeletal system to be susceptible to a variety of injuries.

Congenital or acquired diseases can cause progressive deformities of the immature skeleton. Infection and skeletal dysplasia are examples of disease processes that can affect the immature skeleton. Abnormal patterns of cartilage and bone growth caused by these diseases may predispose to the development of injuries in the immature skeletal system. These injuries can result from the treatment of the disease or from the disease itself. An example of injury caused by the disease process is recurrent dislocation resulting from muscle spasm in children with cerebral palsy.

Injuries involving joints occur less commonly than fractures in the immature skeletal system because of the relative weakness of the growth plate (the ligaments are more elastic). An immature bone has a thicker periosteum than a mature bone. This results in less frequent disruption of the periosteum around the entire circumference of the bone. The bones deform more before breaking, so they may bend, buckle, or sustain incomplete (greenstick,

Text continued on page 624

TABLE 19–3. *Classic Names and Descriptions by Anatomic Location*

NAME	DESCRIPTION	COMMON TREATMENT	ILLUSTRATION*
Humerus			
Anatomic neck	Two-part fracture of the true neck of the humeral metaphysis at the area of tendon attachment with angulatory or rotational deformity usually less than 45 degrees	Sling and exercise program or collar/cuff and exercise program	
Surgical neck	Fracture occurring below the anatomic neck, usually angulated greater than 45 degrees or malrotated—may have associated nondisplaced linear fracture extending into humeral head	Closed reduction with sling and swathe to maintain reduction	
Diaphyseal	Fracture of the humeral shaft; middle third is most common site	Closed—hanging cast or coaptation splint (U-shaped plaster splint with collar/cuff) or sling and swathe Operative—compression plate and screws, intramedullary rods	
Elbow			
Condylar	Fracture of medial or lateral articular process of the distal humerus	Lateral: displaced (disrupts joint surface)—open reduction and internal fixation; undisplaced or minimally displaced—immobilization Medial: displaced—open reduction and internal fixation or pin fixation; undisplaced—aspiration of hemarthrosis and posterior splint application	
Epicondylar	Fracture through the medial or lateral epicondyle	Lateral—immobilization until pain subsides, displaced over 2–3 cm requires open reduction and internal fixation Medial—open reduction and internal fixation and immobilization	

Table continued on following page

TABLE 19–3. *Classic Names and Descriptions by Anatomic Location* Continued

NAME	DESCRIPTION	COMMON TREATMENT	ILLUSTRATION*
Elbow *Continued*			
Supracondylar	Fracture of distal humeral shaft	Closed reduction under general anesthesia and posterior splint, or percutaneous pinning Open reduction and internal fixation if reduction is unstable or fails Difficult to treat if displaced— watch for development of compartment syndrome	
Olecranon	Fracture of the olecranon process of the ulna (prominent portion of ulna at the elbow)	Displaced—anatomic reduction and internal fixation or primary excision Undisplaced—long-arm cast with 45–90 degrees elbow flexion	
Forearm and Wrist			
Colles'	Fracture through distal radial epiphysis within 0.5–0.75 inch of the articular surface with radial displacement and dorsal angulation of the distal fragment	Closed reduction and splint or cast Severely comminuted (uncommon)—external fixator	
Radial head	Fracture of the most proximal part of the radius	Undisplaced—long-arm splint or cast Displaced/single fracture line—open reduction and internal fixation Comminuted—excision with silastic implant	

TABLE 19–3. *Classic Names and Descriptions by Anatomic Location* Continued

NAME	DESCRIPTION	COMMON TREATMENT	ILLUSTRATION*
Hand			
Bennett's	Avulsion fracture of carpometa-carpal joint with displacement caused by pull of abduction	Closed—reduction and immobilization Operative—open reduction and internal fixation under direct visualization or percutaneous pinning under image intensification	
Boxer's	Fracture distal metacarpal (usually fourth or fifth) angulated or impacted	Closed reduction and short-arm cast with finger splint; seldom requires closed reduction with percutaneous pin fixation	
Mallet	Avulsion fracture of dorsal articular surface of distal phalanx of any digit involving extensor apparatus insertion, creating dropped flexion of distal segment	Closed reduction and dorsal splint, may require open reduction and internal fixation	
Spine			
Hangman's (C2)	Bilateral posterior pedicle fracture of axis (C2) with subluxation of C2 on C3	Avoid hyperextension, keep neck straight to achieve postural reduction, immobilize with halo	
Odontoid process	Fracture at base of odontoid process, which allows the skull, C1 vertebra, and the odontoid process of C2 to move relatively independently of the body of C2 vertebra	Reduction of displacement with skull traction and immobilization without distraction in halo or cervical brace Undisplaced—halo	

Table continued on following page

TABLE 19–3. *Classic Names and Descriptions by Anatomic Location* Continued

NAME	DESCRIPTION	COMMON TREATMENT	ILLUSTRATION*
Pelvis			
Central	Acetabular fracture with central displacement of femoral head	Traction, with or without closed reduction of femoral head Open reduction and internal fixation Primary arthroplasty or arthrodesis	
Malgaigne's (double vertical fracture dislocation)	Multiple fractures through the wing of the sacrum and ipsilateral pubic rami with associated upward displacement of the hemipelvis	Open reduction and internal fixation External fixation Skeletal traction	
Ring	Fracture through the pelvic circumference, must be at least two fractures for displacement to occur	Slightly displaced—pelvic sling and Buck's traction External fixation	
Proximal Femur			
Femoral neck	Fracture through midportion of femoral neck	Anatomic reduction and stable internal fixation or prosthesis	
Greater trochanter	Avulsion fracture of greater trochanter	Slight displacement—protected weight bearing (as an isolated injury) Displaced—open reduction and internal fixation	
Intertrochanteric	Fracture along a line joining the greater and lesser trochanter	Reduction and internal fixation of proximal femur—fixed or sliding nail/plate device, intramedullary device	

TABLE 19–3. *Classic Names and Descriptions by Anatomic Location* Continued

NAME	DESCRIPTION	COMMON TREATMENT	ILLUSTRATION*
Proximal Femur *Continued* Lesser trochanter	Avulsion fracture of lesser trochanter	Bed rest 2–3 days with hip flexed, then protected ambulation (as an isolated injury)	
Shaft	Fracture between subtrochanteric and supracondylar area	Skeletal traction Cast brace External fixation Intramedullary fixation Closed medullary nailing Interlocking nail, plate, and screws	
Subtrochanteric	Transverse fracture between lesser trochanter and a point 5 cm distally (may occur independently or as part of intertrochanteric fracture)	Open reduction and internal fixation Fixed-angle nail and plate AO blade plates Sliding compression hip screw Intramedullary devices	
Distal Femur, Knee, Tibia, Fibula Bumper (tibial plateau)	Fracture of tibial or fibular condyle resulting from direct blow in the area of the tibial tuberosity	Displaced—open reduction and internal fixation	

Table continued on following page

TABLE 19–3. *Classic Names and Descriptions by Anatomic Location* Continued

NAME	DESCRIPTION	COMMON TREATMENT	ILLUSTRATION*
Distal Femur, Knee, Tibia, Fibula *Continued*			
Patellar	Fractured kneecap	Undisplaced—cylinder cast Displaced or comminuted—operative fixation or excision	
Shaft, fibula	Diaphyseal fracture of fibula	As single fracture—cast	
Shaft, tibia	Diaphyseal fracture of tibia	Closed reduction, long-leg cast, or pin/plaster or external fixation Open reduction—compression plating or plate and screws	
Supracondylar	Fracture of distal femoral condyle	Open reduction and internal fixation Medullary fixation Blade/plates Skeletal traction	

TABLE 19–3. *Classic Names and Descriptions by Anatomic Location* Continued

NAME	DESCRIPTION	COMMON TREATMENT	ILLUSTRATION*
Distal Femur, Knee, Tibia, Fibula *Continued*			
Tibial plateau	Fracture of proximal tibial articular surface	Soft dressing Cast Traction Closed or open reduction	
Tibial tubercle	Avulsion and proximal dislocation of tibial tubercle	Minimal or nondisplaced—long-leg cast with full knee extension Displaced >5-7 mm—open reduction and internal fixation	
Ankle, Foot			
Boot top	Transverse fracture of distal third of tibia	Stable—closed reduction if possible Unstable—intramedullary fixation	
Paratrooper	Fracture distal tibial and malleolus	Open reduction and internal fixation	

Table continued on following page

TABLE 19–3. *Classic Names and Descriptions by Anatomic Location* Continued

NAME	DESCRIPTION	COMMON TREATMENT	ILLUSTRATION*
Ankle, Foot *Continued*			
Plafond	Fracture of tibial plafond extending in a spiral or longitudinal fashion into tibial shaft	Open reduction and internal fixation	
Pott's	Fracture of distal fibula, usually spiral/oblique, with distal tibial chipping or rupture of surrounding ligaments	Closed reduction or open reduction and internal fixation, followed by cast immobilization	

*From Connolly, J. (1981). *DePalma's the management of fractures and dislocations* (3rd ed.). Philadelphia: WB Saunders.

see Fig. 19-1) fractures. The thicker periosteum of immature bones also results in a decrease in the degree of displacement of fractures and tends to increase fracture stability.

Although many growth plate injuries can be evaluated by routine radiologic examination or ultrasound, magnetic resonance imaging (MRI) can clearly visualize unossified cartilage of the pediatric appendicular skeleton, especially of the elbow (Eustace, 1997). MRI is useful in the follow-up for growth plate injuries, particularly Salter 4 and 5 fractures.

Every age group from infancy through adolescence has its own typical fracture pattern (Della-Giustina & Della-Giustina, 1999). A plastic deformity in which bone is deformed beyond its ability to recoil, but not to the point at which any actual fracture will occur, is the precursor to greenstick fractures in which the bone fractures on the side opposite to the force of impact.

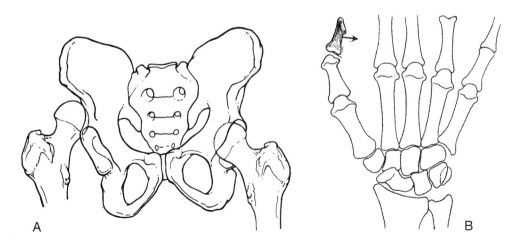

FIGURE 19–3. *A,* Dislocation. *B,* Subluxation. (From Connolly, J. [1981]. *DePalma's the management of fractures and dislocations* [3rd ed., pp. 1266, 1187]. Philadelphia: WB Saunders.)

Torus (buckle, see Fig. 19–1) fractures occur at the junction of the metaphysis and diaphysis as a result of compressive forces, whereas other fractures will directly involve the physis.

In pediatric fracture remodeling, new bone is laid down according to local forces, especially in the plane of motion in the joint. If a child has at least 2 years of growth remaining, a fracture adjacent to a hinged joint will remodel acceptably, if the angulation is less than 30 degrees in the plane of motion. Children rarely require physical therapy because they tolerate lengthy immobilization without resultant stiffness.

In children, approximately 10% to 15% of all injuries involve the skeletal system. If these injuries involve the growth plates in immature bones, acute or chronic growth disturbances may follow. There are two types of growth plates in the skeletal system. Those involved in the compression of weight bearing (epiphyseal growth plates) are responsible for longitudinal growth, and those subjected to distraction forces of muscles (apophyseal growth plates) assist in determining the general shape and proportion of the bone. Epiphyseal growth plates are located in long bones between the epiphysis and the diaphysis and control overall growth and limb length equality.

Growth plates are composed of cartilaginous tissue until growth is completed and bony fusion occurs. The growth plates of the lower extremities are probably the most significant in the immature skeletal system because they are primarily responsible for determining the height of the individual. They are also under the continual stress of weight bearing. Growth plates are also found in the long bones of the upper extremities and the vertebrae. There are bipolar growth plates (two growth plates next to each other) at the tibial tubercle and the innominate bone and spherical growth plates surrounding the nucleus of the ossification centers in smaller bones of the wrist and foot.

Treatment of fractures in children is determined by several factors: the probable mechanism of injury, short- and long-term treatment effects on the injured part, and treatment guidelines for the specific injury that are appropriate for the age of the client.

CLASSIFICATION OF EPIPHYSEAL INJURIES

Epiphyseal injuries have historically been grouped according to the Salter-Harris classification system. Ogden has expanded the original classifications and Figure 19–4 illustrates both classifications. Type I injuries have complete separation of the epiphysis without fracture. The injury is usually caused by shearing or avulsion forces and occurs during birth injuries or in early childhood. Type I (Fig 19–5*A, B*) injuries can also occur in children who have scurvy, rickets, osteomyelitis, or endocrine imbalance. Reduction of type I epiphyseal injuries is not

difficult, and the prognosis is good unless the epiphysis is entirely covered by cartilage. Damaged blood supply can cause premature closure of the epiphyseal plate and growth disturbances in these injuries.

Type II (Fig 19–5*C*) injuries are the most common epiphyseal injuries. Separation of the epiphyseal plate occurs, with a fragment of the metaphysis attached to the plate. The injury is produced by shearing or avulsion forces. Reduction is usually easily accomplished, and the prognosis is good if the blood supply is intact. The triangular metaphyseal fragment is commonly referred to as the *Thurston-Holland sign.* Treatment consists of a cast or splint immobilization (Della-Giustina & Della-Giustina, 1999).

Type III (Fig 19–5*D*) injuries involve an intra-articular fracture extending from the joint surface vertically to the epiphysis and then along the epiphysis to the edge of the bone. Type III injuries are relatively uncommon, but when they do occur, they are usually in the upper or lower tibial epiphysis. Accurate anatomic reduction is essential in these injuries, and open reduction may be necessary. The prognosis for type III injuries is good when reduction is accurate and the blood supply is intact.

Type IV (Fig 19–5*E*) injuries are also intra-articular fractures. The fracture line extends vertically from the joint surface through the epiphysis into the metaphysis yielding a significant incidence of growth disturbance. Anatomic reduction is necessary, and open reduction is usually required unless the fracture is undisplaced. If metallic fixation is used, the fixation device should be placed through the metaphysis if possible.

Type V injuries occur only rarely and are caused by a severe crushing force through the epiphysis to one area of the epiphyseal plate. This injury occurs only in joints that move in a single plane and has a poor prognosis for recovery. Premature growth cessation is common with type V injuries.

Type VI (Ogden) injuries involve the peripheral borders of the physis, which are sheared along with small portions of the adjacent metaphysis and epiphysis. An osseous bridge forms, causing deformity as growth is halted on one side of the physis and not on the other (Della-Giustina & Della-Giustina, 1999).

Type VII (Ogden) is an intra-articular fracture in which the ligament avulses a distal portion of the epiphysis only without any physeal involvement. Precise reduction is required to prevent future joint problems.

Type VIII (Ogden) fractures pass through the metaphysis only, without any physeal involvement. Temporary disruption of the bony circulation distal to the injury is significant with this injury.

Type IX (Ogden) involves significant loss or damage to the periosteum in association with the fracture and thus affects pediatric fracture healing. Parents should be counseled about the potential for growth abnormalities following physeal injuries, which may include asymmetri-

Type	Salter-Harris	Ogden

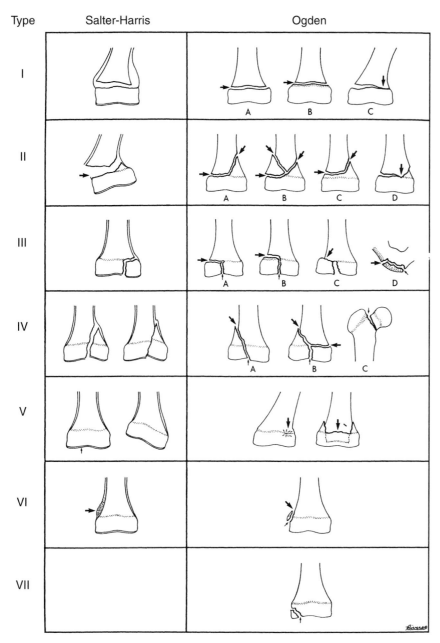

FIGURE 19–4. Classification of physical injuries by Salter-Harris and Ogden. Note that the Ogden classification adds more subclasses to the Salter-Harris system. (From Canale, S. T. [Ed.]. [1998]. *Campbell's operative orthopaedics* [9th ed., p. 2365]. St. Louis: Mosby.)

cal healing and growth, premature closure of the physis, and post-traumatic arthritis of any involved joints.

Epiphyseal injuries can cause transient acceleration or premature cessation of growth, resulting in progressive angular deformity or progressive shortening of a limb. Stimulation of the growth plate, causing bone overgrowth, is seen most often following distal femoral epiphyseal fractures, which are not anatomically reduced. Growth disturbance in an area with paired bones causes varus or valgus deformity in the joint nearest the involved plate, and disturbances in an area with a single bone cause leg length discrepancies. Significant disturbance of the growth plate function occurs in approximately 10% of injuries to epiphyseal plates, but the frequency of minor disturbances is higher.

CONSIDERATIONS IN THE IMMATURE SKELETON

Fracture healing occurs more rapidly in immature bones. The younger the age, the faster the rate of healing. Each day that passes makes reduction more difficult. After 10 days, it may be impossible to reduce a fracture in a child without using excessive force, which can damage epiphyseal plates. When one is considering the effect of trauma and its treatment on the immature skeleton, the determining factor is skeletal age, not chronologic age. Nonunion rarely occurs in children, and open reduction with internal fixation is usually unnecessary. The site, frequency, and nature of fractures in the immature skeletal system are age related.

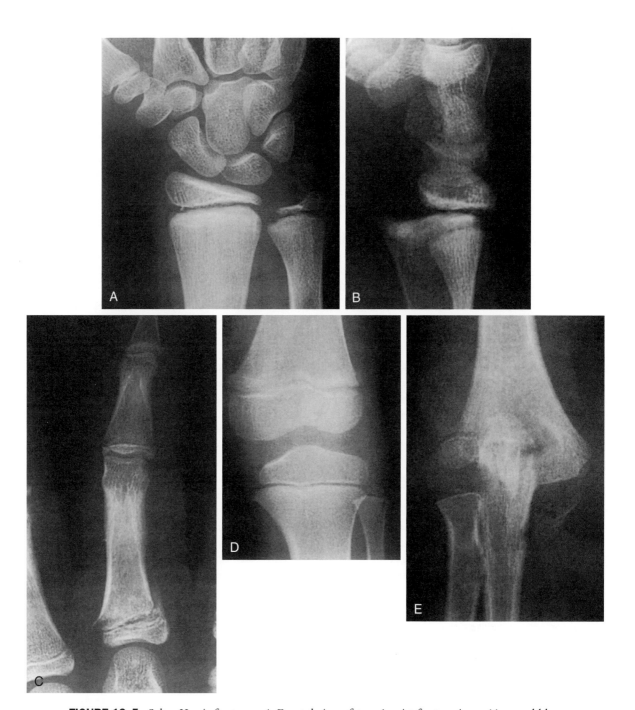

FIGURE 19–5. Salter-Harris fractures. *A,* Frontal view of type 1 wrist fracture in an 11-year-old boy shows metaphyseal sclerosis. *B,* Lateral view in same boy shows dorsal displacement of the distal radial epiphysis. *C,* Type 2 fracture of the proximal phalanx of the index finger in a 14-year-old boy. The fracture line passes through the epiphysis and separates a triangular metaphyseal fragment (corner sign). *D,* Type 3 fracture of the distal femur in a 4-year-old girl. The fracture runs obliquely through the epiphysis and then horizontally through the physis. *E,* Type 4 fracture of the lateral humeral condyle in a 4-year-old girl. The fracture extends from the nonossified portion of the epiphysis, through the physis, to the distal lateral humeral metaphysis. (From Kao, S., & Smith, W. [1997]. Skeletal injuries in the pediatric patient. *Radiologic Clinics of North America, 35,* 732–733.)

When multiple severe fractures occur in children, especially those younger than 1 year of age, they are usually the result of metabolic disorders, skeletal dysplasia, or more often, child abuse. The battered child may be brought to the emergency department some time after the injury occurs and for a complaint other than the injury. History about the injury or complaint may be vague or inconsistent with clinical findings. Parents of the battered or abused child may react inappropriately to the severity of injury and are often reluctant to provide specific, detailed information. Suspicion should be raised if the mechanism of injury is inconsistent with history or child's developmental stage. In addition, a changing history of mechanism of injury, evasiveness, or inappropriate anger with the child should be investigated.

Orthopaedic injuries, including soft tissue trauma, are the most common presentation of child abuse, otherwise known as *nonaccidental trauma*. Fractures from child abuse tend to occur in very young children. In fact, half of such skeletal injuries occur in babies 12 months old or younger. In addition, up to 30% of the head and limb injuries in children younger than 6 years who present to the emergency department are a result of child abuse (Della-Giustina & Della-Giustina, 1999). A complete physical examination must include a bone scan or ultrasonography, which can most accurately define the immature skeletal injuries. Findings of various stages of healing fractures of the posterior ribs, skull, scapula, sternum, spinous process, and vertebral bodies are highly specific for nonaccidental trauma.

The parents of a child with a fracture must be prepared to assume responsibility for the acute care required and for potential chronic problems. Possible complications, such as limping, decreased ROM, loss of reduction, and nerve deficits, should be fully explained. Emphasis must be placed on the need for long-term follow-up, especially when there has been an injury to the growth mechanism.

EMERGENCY MANAGEMENT

Emergency management of fractures is governed by basic principles of trauma care. Assessment and treatment are carried out simultaneously. Initial primary assessment at the scene of the injury includes the general condition of the client, including respiratory status (maintenance of airway with cervical spine stabilization), bleeding or shock (venous access and fluid replacement), and stabilization of any potential life-threatening injuries. Assessment of suspected fractures follows, beginning with neurovascular status and followed by splinting. When a closed fracture is suspected, a splint should be applied, if possible, before the extremity or the client is moved. Splinting minimizes bleeding, swelling, and pain and also helps prevent further damage to nerves, vessels, muscles, and tendons. Unnecessary handling should be avoided before splinting.

Improper handling of a fracture can complicate the care of the client and the fracture and may increase the degree of injury. Soft tissue injury, especially to nerves and vessels, may be increased, closed fractures may be converted to open fractures, pain may be significantly increased, and the incidence of fat embolism and shock increases. In addition, it is more difficult to transport the client and to perform x-ray examination if fracture sites are left unsplinted. Before splints are applied, open fractures should be covered with sterile compression dressings to help control bleeding and to prevent further contamination.

Methods available for controlling pelvic bleeding include pneumatic antishock garment, anterior external fixation, angiography with operative control of hemorrhage, and retroperitoneal packing.

ASSESSMENT OF FRACTURES

Trauma costs Americans more than $200 billion annually, with 150,000 deaths related to traumatic fractures in the 4 million or more treated (Mourad, 1997). Emergency department management of the trauma client with fractures follows basic trauma principles. Most fractures are not life- or limb-threatening injuries (Table 19-4), and their management is a secondary priority in the initial management of the multiple trauma client. Although many injuries result in single fractures, clients often sustain multiple fractures, especially when motor vehicle accidents are the cause of the injury. The mechanism of injury and accident history assist in determining the nature and extent of known injuries and may help in the identification of injuries that might otherwise be overlooked. Individuals at the accident scene assess level of consciousness, response to stimuli, orientation, position of the body and head, and movement of the limbs. Previous illnesses or injuries, allergies, the date of the last tetanus inoculation, and current medications should be determined and recorded.

Blunt trauma is the most common mechanism of injury in the client with multiple trauma. Blunt injuries

TABLE 19-4. *Life- or Limb-Threatening Emergencies*

CONDITION	POSSIBLE ADVERSE OUTCOME
Open fracture	Osteomyelitis
Fracture or dislocation with major vessel disruption (esp. popliteal)	Amputation
Major pelvic fracture	Exsanguination
Hip dislocation	Avascular necrosis of femoral head
Compartment syndrome	Ischemic contracture; myoglobinuria, renal failure

From Geiderman, J. (1998). Orthopedic injuries: Management principles. In P. Rose & R. Barkin (Eds.), *Emergency medicine concepts and clinical practice* (4th ed., p. 611). St. Louis: Mosby.

are caused by auto accidents, falls, and crush injuries. The degree of trauma sustained depends on the duration and degree of the force applied. Major points of impact include the head, chest, abdomen, and long bones. Following the primary survey to evaluate and treat life-threatening problems, a systematic secondary survey should be performed to assess the need for additional care. The secondary survey must include visual inspection of the entire body. All clothing must be removed to facilitate the visual examination. The secondary survey should not focus solely on obvious injuries or on client complaints but should be a thorough head-to-toe assessment to detect occult injuries that may have been missed during primary assessment.

The physical examination is the most important aspect of assessing the trauma client. Soft tissue damage, even a small bruise, may indicate a fracture site. Multiple fractures and joint injuries commonly occur in the same limb. Abnormal findings of the physical examination related to fractures include the presence of deformity, shortening of a limb, local swelling and discoloration, and soft tissue damage. Clinical findings include pain, loss of function, degree of deformity, restriction of posture and movement, abnormal mobility, crepitus, and neurovascular changes. Radiologic examination of a suspected limb fracture should include the joint above and the joint below the suspected fracture site. Neurologic examination of the trauma client should be related to the type of injury known or suspected. The multiple trauma client should always have x-ray films or computed tomography (CT) scans taken of the chest and pelvis. Spine films should be included if spinal injury is suspected or a possibility. Physical assessment of blood loss associated with fractures depends on the site of the fracture and the severity of the injury. A femoral fracture may cause a loss of 1 to 2.5 L of blood volume, and a tibial fracture may result in a loss of 0.5 to 1.5 L of blood. Displaced pelvic fractures usually result in a high volume of blood loss and may cause exsanguination.

Soft tissue damage and associated open fracture wounds should be covered with a sterile normal saline dressing. Irrigation of open wounds should never be performed in the emergency department but should be reserved for the operating room to avoid increasing contamination of the fracture site. All open wounds should be cultured, tetanus toxoid administered if needed, and all splints maintained. Antibiotic therapy is usually initiated in the emergency department.

Neurovascular assessment of the involved extremities should be performed and documented at frequent intervals. A comprehensive assessment includes the peripheral vascular assessment of color, temperature, capillary refill, peripheral pulses, and edema. The peripheral neurologic assessment includes sensation and motor function. Pain is the final element of a comprehensive assessment and is essential in the recognition of potential complications.

TABLE 19–5. *Nerve Injuries Accompanying Orthopaedic Injuries*

ORTHOPAEDIC INJURY	NERVE INJURY
Elbow injury	Median or ulnar
Shoulder dislocation	Axillary
Sacral fracture	Cauda equina
Acetabulum fracture	Sciatic
Hip dislocation	Femoral nerve
Femoral shaft fracture	Peroneal
Knee dislocation	Tibial or peroneal
Lateral tibial plateau fracture	Peroneal

From Geiderman, J. (1998). Orthopedic injuries: Management principles. In P. Rosen & R. Barkin (Eds.), *Emergency medicine concepts and clinical practice* (4th ed., p. 610). St. Louis: Mosby.

Table 19-5 describes the correlation of nerve injury to specific orthopaedic injuries.

A coherent, conscious individual should be asked about past injuries that may affect the neurovascular status of the extremity and assessed for prior injury. Peripheral tissue perfusion is an integral component of nursing care (Johnson, Mass, & Moorehead, 2000).

In the neurologically intact individual, a fracture always causes pain, although the intensity and severity of the pain differ from person to person. It is usually continuous, and the severity increases until the fracture is immobilized. Loss of function, if it does occur, may be due to the loss of the lever arm function or may be due to pain caused by the fracture. Deformity at a fracture site may be caused by swelling from local hemorrhage, angulation, or rotational deformity caused by the fracture or shortening resulting from muscle spasm. Muscle spasms, commonly seen with fractures, are a method of natural splinting to decrease further motion of fracture fragments. Restriction of movement and the assumption of certain postures are diagnostic in specific types of fractures. Abnormal mobility and crepitus are caused by motion in the middle of a bone or bone fragments rubbing together. Neurovascular injury occurs when there is damage to the vascular structures or to peripheral nerves.

ASSESSMENT OF DISLOCATIONS

A thorough account of the accident or incident causing the injury should be obtained, determining the mechanism of injury and the amount and direction of forces involved. The client should be questioned about previous injuries to the same joint and about whether the injury involved dislocation. Physical assessment reveals pain, which may be severe until the dislocation is reduced; deformity; and loss of motion. The incidence of neurologic damage in injuries involving dislocation is higher than in fractures.

DIAGNOSTIC EVALUATION

Diagnosis of fractures is based on the client's symptoms, history of trauma, physical examination, and radiologic findings. Physical examination may reveal deformity, mobility of bone fragments, crepitus, muscle spasm, edema, or ecchymosis. The major diagnostic mechanism used to evaluate fractures is radiology. X-ray films for suspected fractures must include the correct views to evaluate the fracture site adequately. An x-ray film is a two-dimensional representation of the bone and soft tissue. Single anteroposterior or lateral films are not adequate to evaluate a suspected injury. Two views at right angles are the minimum number required to evaluate a suspected fracture. Additional views, such as oblique films, may be necessary in some injuries to check for such things as rotation or overriding of fragments. The radiograph should include the joints above and below the suspected fracture to evaluate potential associated injuries, and good technical quality of the films with clear sharp images is essential. Some fractures may not be apparent immediately on x-ray film. Lack of evidence of a fracture on x-ray film does not take precedence over clinical evidence of a fracture.

The specific views ordered to evaluate fractures are determined by the type, severity, and location of the injury. In children, it may be necessary to obtain films of the normal extremity as well as the injured one for comparison. Stress films may be ordered, with the joint stressed during the film exposure to show some types of abnormalities. Stress films are commonly done under anesthesia.

Review of radiographs should be done in an orderly manner, beginning with analysis of soft tissue for edema or displacement. All bones should be scanned in a systematic manner so that an obvious fracture does not divert attention from less obvious problems. Radiologic findings in fractures include alterations in the normal contour of the bone and the appearance of fracture lines. Air may be seen in the soft tissue in compound fractures as well as in any compound dislocation or penetrating wound of the joint. Normal bone is smooth in appearance with even borders. Fracture lines appear as lines of increased radiolucency. Nondisplaced fractures have a normal anatomic appearance except for the fracture line. A deformity or change in the normal anatomic lines of a bone is seen in a displaced fracture. When joints are dislocated or subluxed, there is a change in the normal relationship of the two bones forming the joint. Box 19-2 lists abnormal radiologic findings.

Other findings that can be determined on the basis of radiologic examination include the density of the bone, the presence of lesions, the width of the joint space, and any previous injuries. On film, lighter areas indicate decreased density. Pathologic fractures may develop in localized areas in which the cortex is thin in comparison

---

BOX 19–2.
Abnormal X-ray Findings

Soft Tissue
Edema or displacement air in soft tissue

Bone
Alteration in normal contour of bone (normal—smooth with even borders)
Increased radiolucency of fracture line
Disruption of normal joint relationship
Punched-out holes—lytic lesions
Solid mass—tumor
Lighter areas—decreased bone density
Alteration in joint space width
Calcification
Bone cement—faintly white
Orthopaedic implants—solid white

---

with the medullary canal. Lytic lesions may appear as punched-out holes, and a tumor mass appears solid. Areas of calcification and changes that occur during the process of bone healing also show on x-ray films. Normal x-ray films do not necessarily ensure that there is no abnormality of the bone.

Additional radiologic, nuclear medicine, and ultrasound examinations may be ordered in special cases and include tomograms, CT scans, bone scans, fluoroscopy, MRI, and myelograms. See Chapter 9 for additional information on diagnostic procedures.

TREATMENT OF FRACTURES
Method of Treatment

The treatment method for fractures is governed by scientifically determined treatment options and by the wishes of the client. Treatment options for fractures are based on principles related to biomechanical and musculoskeletal factors. The specific choices available to a particular client depend on the type of fracture sustained, its location, and any associated injuries. Fractures may require closed or open reduction, traction, splinting, casts, internal fixation, external fixation, bracing, amputation, or combinations of these. After treatment alternatives have been reviewed with the client, he or she should be allowed to make the final determination of the method of treatment.

The preferred method of treatment for a specific fracture is closely related to the degree of associated injury. Early mobilization of the client is preferred to prolonged treatment by casting or traction, especially in the older client or the client with multiple injuries. Restoration of the upright position and early mobilization decrease cardiopulmonary and other immobility-related complications and are often accomplished by reduction with internal fixation.

The basis of the treatment of fractures is reduction and immobilization. For bony union to occur, the fragments should be in approximation and alignment and must be held relatively immobile during the period of healing. There are two objectives in the treatment of fractures. The first is to promote bone healing and restore function and appearance. The second is to return the client to his or her activities of daily living (ADLs), job, and lifestyle in the shortest time possible and at the least expense. These two objectives are not always compatible, and the desires and wishes of the client determine which is given more importance.

Closed Treatment. Closed treatment of fractures consists of reduction of the fracture, if needed, followed by immobilization. Closed reduction is the alignment of fracture fragments through manual manipulation or traction. The need for reduction is determined by x-ray film, and if necessary, it should be done as soon as possible after the injury occurs. Localized swelling at a fracture site increases for 6 to 12 hours after the injury. Edema and hemorrhage cause soft tissue to be inelastic and make reduction more difficult to accomplish if it is delayed. However, the reduction of a fracture is not an emergency procedure, and the client's life should never be jeopardized by attempts at early reduction.

Indications. There are three indications for reduction of a fracture. The first is to ensure recovery of limb function that has been threatened by fracture displacement. The second indication is to prevent or delay degenerative changes in joints, especially in weight-bearing joints that will undergo degenerative changes as a result of an unreduced fracture. The third indication for reducing a fracture is to minimize the deforming effects of the injury. Closed reduction is contraindicated when the degree of displacement is not significant for the type of fracture, when reduction is not possible or cannot be maintained, or when the fracture was caused by traction force.

Method. The method of closed fracture reduction is to apply traction force to the long axis of the limb and reverse the mechanism that produced the fracture. The fragment that can be controlled is aligned with the fragment that cannot be controlled. Closed reduction may be performed under general or local anesthesia, and traction force may be combined with manipulation of the fracture, either manually or as continuous traction.

Immobilization. Closed reduction of fractures is followed by immobilization. The purposes of immobilization are to relieve pain, prevent rotation and shearing at the fracture site, maintain the position of the fracture by preventing displacement or angulation until bony union occurs, permit active muscle contraction, and commonly, allow free movement of uninvolved joints. Immobilization may be accomplished by application of casts, traction, splints, braces, or external fixators. Casts may be of different materials, including plaster or fiberglass, and traction may be skin, skeletal, plaster, or combinations of pin and plaster. External fixators are indicated for immobilization following reduction when there has been extensive soft tissue damage or open wounds. External fixation may also be used whenever plaster immobilization is inappropriate for any reason (Box 19-3), in segmental comminuted fractures, when there are segments of bone missing, and in infected or nonunion fractures. In some cases, closed reduction may be followed by internal fixation to maintain proper alignment. The forms of external immobilization are covered in more detail in Chapter 12.

Open Treatment. Open reduction is indicated when the reduction cannot be attained or maintained by closed methods, for displaced intra-articular fractures, in certain types of epiphyseal fractures, and when there are major avulsion fragments with disruption of important muscles or ligaments. Open reduction may also be indicated in delayed union, multiple fractures, pathologic fractures, and fractures in which closed treatment is known to be ineffective (e.g., femoral neck fractures). It may also be the preferred treatment to allow early functional use of joints or extremities (Table 19-6).

Open reduction is usually contraindicated when the fracture fragment is too small for attachment by rigid fixation, the bone is too weak or soft to secure fixation devices (e.g., osteopenia), there are severe soft tissue abnormalities of surrounding tissue (e.g., burns), medical conditions preclude general anesthesia and spinal anesthetic is inappropriate, and fractures are undisplaced or impacted (except in special cases, e.g., femoral neck fractures). Active infection or osteomyelitis is generally

---

BOX 19–3.

Advantages of External Fixation

Rigid fixation when other forms of immobilization are
  inappropriate
Allowance for compression, neutralization, or fixed
  distraction of fragments
Direct visualization of soft tissue
Concurrent treatment of fractures and soft tissue
  damage
Immediate motion of joints above and below the fracture
Elevation without pressure on posterior soft tissue
Early client mobility
Insertion under general or local anesthetic
Suitable for use in infected, acute, or nonunion fractures

TABLE 19–6. *Summary of Indications and Contraindications for Open Reduction*

I. Absolute
    A. Fracture irreducible by manipulation or closed reduction
    B. Displaced intra-articular fractures
    C. Certain types of displaced epiphyseal fractures
    D. Major avulsion fractures with disruption of an important muscle mechanism or ligament
    E. Nonunions following either open or closed methods of treatment
    F. Replantations of extremities, either whole or part
II. Relative indications
    A. Delayed union
    B. Multiple fractures
    C. Loss of reduction following either open or closed methods
    D. Pathologic fractures
    E. To improve nursing care
    F. To reduce mortality or morbidity from prolonged cast or bed immobilization
    G. Fractures for which closed methods are known to be ineffective
III. Questionable indications
    A. Fractures accompanying blood vessel or nerve repair
    B. Open fractures
    C. Cosmetic considerations
    D. Economic considerations
IV. Contraindications to open reduction
    A. Active infection or osteomyelitis
    B. Fracture fragments of insufficient size
    C. Severe osteopenia
    D. Lack of surrounding soft tissue
    E. General health makes a poor surgical candidate

Adapted from Canale, S. (1998). *Campbell's operative orthopaedics* (pp. 2001–2002). St. Louis, Mosby.

considered a contraindication to open reduction, although in some cases, infected nonunion may be treated with open reduction and rigid immobilization.

Internal Fixation. Open reduction of a fracture is usually followed by internal fixation to stabilize the fracture and allow fracture healing to occur. The device used to provide internal fixation is dependent on the type of fracture, the reduction obtained, and the area involved in the fracture. Examples of different types of internal fixation devices are shown in Figure 19-6.

Wires and pins may be implanted to provide internal fixation either percutaneously or through open methods. They are usually used in small bone fractures that do not need compression. They provide the simplest form of internal fixation and are commonly made of stainless steel. Pins may be smooth, threaded, or a combination of smooth and threaded and may be used for temporary fixation of fractures, in skeletal traction, and in external fixation. Wire comes in several lengths and diameters and

is used in avulsion fractures, in tension band wiring, or as a supplement to other forms of fixation, such as cerclage. One advantage of wires and pins is that they can be left protruding through the skin and may then be removed easily with local anesthesia.

Bone screws may be used alone but most often are used with plates to provide internal fixation. Screws come in several different forms. They may be self-tapping with a fluted end, which cuts as the screw is inserted, or they may be threaded for their entire length or only partially threaded. Machine screws are threaded the entire length of the screw and are usually, but not always, self-tapping. They may be used alone to hold a reduced fracture fragment in position but are more commonly used to hold a plate on the shaft of the bone.

Cortical screws are threaded with a relatively small thread to allow solid fixation in dense cortical bone.

Cancellous screws have larger threads and are usually not fully threaded. They are used in the bone near joints, especially the hip, and in bones that are primarily cancellous.

Malleolar screws (another type of cancellous screw) are self-tapping and have a small thread extending halfway on the screw.

Plates are available in many different sizes and shapes and may have round or elliptical holes. They must fit the contour of the bone and be sufficiently long and rigid to provide adequate fixation of the fracture site. Plates may be used as tension band plates to provide compression at the fracture site, as neutralization plates to provide rigid fixation without compression, or as a buttress in cancellous bone to support the thin cortical wall and prevent deformity.

Nail and sliding screw-plate devices are commonly used for hip fractures and provide a combination of a large nail or screw, which permanently fixes to or interlocks with an angled side plate. The screw or nail fixes the femoral head and neck fracture, and the side plate and screws are attached to the femoral shaft. Impaction of the fracture occurs with weight bearing. There are three versions of the nail/plate devices: (1) the fixed nail/plate device, (2) the sliding nail-plate, and (3) the sliding screw plate, also known as the *compression hip screw*. Compression hip screws are used in femoral neck, intertrochanteric, and subtrochanteric hip fractures. Femoral neck fractures are primarily treated with prosthetic replacements because of interruption of the blood supply to the femoral head. Multiple pins may also be used in hip fractures to provide fixation and can be inserted percutaneously or through surgical incisions.

Intramedullary nailing uses one or more rods inserted into the medullary canal of a long bone (usually the femur) to provide internal fixation. Intramedullary nails must be strong enough to maintain alignment of the fracture and prevent angulation or rotation of the fragments. They should also allow compression of the fracture during weight bearing. Intramedullary nails may be supplemented with cortical screws or circumferential wiring to control rotation and movement of fracture fragments. Intramedullary nails may be straight, curved, rigid, or flexible. Rigid nails may be solid or hollow and can be inserted by closed or open methods. Flexible nails are curved, narrow, and cylindrical and do not provide rigid fixation. Intramedullary nails are used in midshaft femoral and long-bone fractures; pathologic fractures; and delayed union, malunion, or nonunion fractures. Their use is contraindicated if there is any indication of infection because they may spread the infection through the medullary canal.

Indications for Open Reduction and Internal Fixation

Fixation. Open reduction should be performed when closed methods have failed or would be ineffective, when articular surfaces are fractured and displaced, when the fracture is secondary to tumor metastasis, when there are associated arterial injuries or multiple injuries, when continued confinement in bed is undesirable, and when the cost of treatment might be significantly decreased. Open reduction is contraindicated in the presence of active infection, severe comminution of fracture fragments, and severe osteoporosis. Advantages of open reduction include early mobilization, restoration of the anatomic shape of the bone, decreased costs, and shorter hospital stays.

The objective of rehabilitation following treatment of fractures is to maintain and restore joint ROM. Stiffness of a joint following fracture is proportional to the extent of the injury and the length of immobilization. It is caused by shortening of the surrounding musculature and changes in the joint capsule. Methods of mobilizing joints during the rehabilitation period include the use of continuous passive motion, muscle exercise (isometric, isotonic, and isokinetic), gait training, and occupational

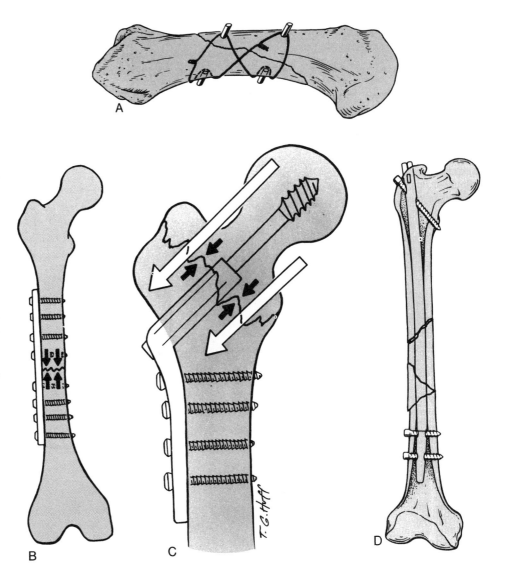

FIGURE 19–6. Examples of different types of internal fixation devices. *A,* Tension band wiring technique using Kirschner wires for fracture of a phalanx. *B,* Compression plate to the lateral aspect of the femur. *C,* Sliding hip screws. *D,* Static locked intramedullary nail fixed to both proximal and distal fragments of the femur. (From Browner, B. D., Jupiter, J. B., Levine, A. M., & Trafton, P. G. [1992]. *Skeletal trauma* [pp. 253, 254, 942, 1551]. Philadelphia: WB Saunders.)

therapy to provide purposeful exercise. (See Chapter 13 for detailed discussions of these methods.)

Treatment of Open Fractures

Open fractures present special problems in their care and treatment. They may occur as a result of the piercing of skin by a sharp bone fragment or through disruption of the tissue by the force that caused the fracture. Treatment is affected by the mechanism of occurrence, and soft tissue damage generally has priority over fracture treatment. Table 19–1 outlines the Gustilo-Anderson classification of soft tissue injury in open fractures. Contamination by bacteria from the external environment is a major concern in open fractures.

Open fractures should be covered with sterile dressings in the emergency department following preliminary examination and should remain covered until the client is in the operating room to prevent any additional contamination. If more than 8 hours have passed since the injury occurred or if there is excessive wound contamination, the fracture is always considered infected. The extent of soft tissue damage also correlates with the incidence of wound infection. Stripping of soft tissue makes bone and tissue susceptible to the establishment of active infection, and destruction or loss of soft tissue may affect the method used for immobilization as well as alter fracture healing. Loss of blood supply to the fracture may result in areas of bone necrosis. The effectiveness of the management of soft tissue damage may determine the ultimate outcome of the fracture. Box 19–4 lists risk factors for infections in open wounds.

To be most effective, antibiotic therapy should begin as soon as possible after the injury. The choice of which antibiotic to use is based on the organisms most likely to be present in the wound. Duration of therapy varies according to physician preference, but long-term administration may result in development of resistant strains of bacteria or superinfection by other organisms. In general, antibiotic therapy should continue for 2 to 3 days. An additional 3 days of antibiotics is repeated for any major surgical procedures.

Gas gangrene is a rare but extremely serious complication that may occur following open fractures. Gas gangrene can develop from the *Clostridium* spore in 72 hours, but onset may occur within hours if vegetative forms of the organism are present in the contaminating source. Symptoms of gas gangrene include severe pain, swelling at the fracture site, tachycardia, hypertension, fever, disorientation, and agitation. Muscle necrosis and crepitus are usually present.

Treatment for gas gangrene involves hyperbaric oxygenation or immediate surgical exploration, excision of all areas of necrosis, and intravenous administration of penicillin. Limb salvage may be possible, but amputation is often required. For a more complete discussion of gas gangrene, see Chapter 23.

BOX 19–4.
Infection Risk Factors

Host Susceptibility
Preexisting conditions
Age (<2 years—immune system immature)
Medications (steroids)
Disease processes (diabetes—impaired wound healing, compromised cardiovascular status)
Nutritional status (malnutrition)

Environment
Airborne or contact bacteria

Wound Contamination
Site and extent of injury
Type of injury and virulence of organism (soft tissue damage, bone loss)
Timing of treatment (delay increases risk)
Mechanism of injury (type of contaminating medium— organic compounds have higher bacteria counts)

Fracture
Amount of bone loss
Comminution
Displacement
Periosteal stripping
Soft tissue damage
Vascular injuries
Foreign bodies

An early objective in any open fracture is to convert it to a clean, closed wound. The initial decision made in severe open fractures with massive soft tissue damage is whether to attempt limb salvage or to perform amputation. If salvage is chosen, debridement of the wound should be performed in the operating room under sterile conditions and the fracture should be stabilized. Debridement of the wound includes detection and removal of all nonvital tissues and foreign material. This reduces bacterial contamination to create a wound capable of dealing with any residual bacterial contamination. Debridement is repeated in 24 to 72 hours.

Wounds may be closed by primary closure, or they may be left open for 5 to 7 days. Primary closure by suture, skin graft, or myocutaneous flap or graft is performed when all necrotic tissue and foreign material have been removed, vascular supply is essentially normal, the nerve supply is intact, and the client's general condition is satisfactory. The wound must be able to be closed without producing tension at the margins, and closure should not create a dead space with open space under a closed surface.

For wounds that are left open, soft tissue reconstruction is recommended 5 to 7 days after injury if the wound is clean and stable. Early stabilization in open fractures is generally considered advantageous for clients and may be accomplished by either internal or external fixation devices. External fixators are often used to immobilize type III open fractures.

Fracture Healing

Bone healing is a unique process in the human body. Healing occurs through regeneration of tissue rather than by scar tissue formation. The process of bone formation during fracture healing follows the same mechanism as bone formation during normal growth and maintenance. The sequence of bone formation involves organized mineralization of the bone matrix synthesized by osteoblasts, followed by remodeling to form mature bone. Bone formation may occur either as enchondral, intramembranous, or appositional formation. Enchondral formation occurs within cartilage, intramembranous formation occurs within an organic matrix membrane, and appositional formation occurs when new bone is deposited on existing bone.

The most important factors in bone healing are adequate circulation to the fracture site and adequate immobilization. The rate and effectiveness of the process of bone healing can be altered by the presence of systemic or bone diseases and are also affected by the age and general health of the individual, the character of the fracture, and the method of treatment. Fractures in an infant may heal in as little as 4 to 6 weeks, whereas the same fracture in an adolescent takes 6 to 10 weeks to heal. Age does not alter healing significantly after the age of 20 unless the individual has a metabolic disorder, such as

TABLE 19–7. *Stages of Fracture Healing*

STAGE	DESCRIPTION	LENGTH
I	Hematoma formation—fracture occurs and hematoma forms at site	1–3 days
II	Fibrocartilage formation—granulation tissue invades the hematoma	3 days–2 weeks
III	Callus formation—granulation tissue matures	2–6 weeks
IV	Ossification—callus bridges the gap between fracture fragments; callus gradually replaced by bone	3 weeks–6 months
V	Consolidation and remodeling—bone is reshaped to meet its mechanical requirements	6 weeks–1 year

osteoporosis. Box 19-5 lists factors that affect bone healing.

Two types of bone healing occur after fractures. The formation of periosteal or external callus is prevalent in fractures treated by closed methods. This type of healing is dependent primarily on the integrity of the blood supply to surrounding soft tissue and the degree of controlled motion at the fracture site. Medullary callus formation occurs with rigid immobilization of the fracture site. Healing relies on the process of bone turnover in which new bone growth from live bone enters the dead cortical bone adjacent to the fracture.

There are five stages (Table 19-7) in the process of bone healing. The stages do not occur independently in distinct and separate stages, but rather overlap as the healing process progresses.

Stage I occurs during the first 3 days after the injury and begins with the immediate formation of a hematoma at the fracture site. The size of the hematoma depends on the amount of damage to the bone, soft tissue, and blood vessels surrounding the fracture. The clot forms between the ends, surrounds the fracture fragments, and provides a small amount of stabilization to the fracture. Necrosis and death of the bone adjacent to the fracture occur in proportion to the loss of blood supply to the fracture and extend to the point where collateral blood supply begins.

Aseptic inflammation begins with the presence of dead cells and debris in the area of the fracture. Vascular dilation and exudation of fibrin-rich plasma initiate the migration of acute inflammatory cells to the region. Phagocytic cells begin the removal of tissue debris. Stage I of fracture healing is most affected by loss of the vascular supply to the fracture site.

Stage II is the formation of granular (or fibrocartilage) tissue containing blood vessels, fibroblasts, and osteoblasts and occurs from 3 days to 2 weeks after the

---

BOX 19–5.
Factors Affecting Bone Healing

Favorable
Location
  Good blood supply at end of bones
  Flat bones
Minimal soft tissue damage
Anatomic reduction
Immobilization
Weight bearing on long bones

Unfavorable
Wide separation of ends of fragments
Distraction of fragments by traction
Severe comminution
Severe soft tissue damage
Bone loss resulting from injury or surgical excision
Motion and rotation at fracture site resulting from inadequate fixation
Infection
Impaired blood supply to one or more bone fragments
Location (midshaft—decreased blood supply)

fracture. Fibroblasts, osteoblasts, and chondroblasts migrate to the area of the fracture as part of the inflammatory process. Organization of the hematoma provides the foundation for the reparative tissue and bone healing. The cells involved in repair of fractures come primarily from vessels surrounding granulation tissue but may also originate from the periosteum or the endothelium. The osteoblastic activity is stimulated by trauma, hematoma formation, periosteal stripping, and elevation. This early stage of organization of the hematoma and fibrous tissue formation is sometimes called *primary callus* and results in a gradual increase in the stability of the fracture fragments. Stage II is influenced by vascular and mechanical factors, such as motion and distraction of fragments.

Stage III, callus formation, occurs from 2 to 6 weeks after the fracture as the granulation tissue matures. The individual repair cells react to the environment, and this controls the development process of the cell. Variations in the surrounding environment and the stresses applied determine the eventual differentiation into collagen, cartilage, or bone. Tension or the absence of compression encourages the development of fibrous tissue. Cartilage is formed when the cells are distant from the blood supply and oxygen tensions are relatively low. Fibrous bone is formed when calcium is deposited in the collagen network of the granulation tissue. The size and shape of callus are proportional to the displacement of the fracture fragments and the amount of bone damage. Stage III is probably the most important in determining the final outcome of the fracture. If this stage is slowed or interrupted, the last two stages cannot occur and delayed union or nonunion results.

Stage IV, ossification, occurs from 3 weeks to 6 months after the fracture as the gap in the bone is bridged and union occurs. The callus, known as *bridging callus,* surrounds the ends of the fracture fragment and advances toward the other fragment. Medullary callus formation bridges the gap between fracture fragments internally and establishes continuity between the marrow cavities and the cortices of the fracture fragments. The callus is gradually replaced by trabecular bone along the lines of stress, and unnecessary or unneeded callus is resorbed. Bony union is eventually said to have occurred.

Stage V of the healing process is consolidation and remodeling, with reestablishment of the medullary canal. Wolff's law states that changes in the form or function of a bone are followed by changes in its external shape (remodeling). Following a fracture, bone continues to be resorbed and deposited along the lines of stress as the bone is reshaped to meet its mechanical requirements. Unnecessary or poorly placed trabeculae are resorbed, and new bone is laid down. This activity is thought to be controlled by a piezoelectric-type charge (the development of a small electric current induced by strain in crystalline substances). When bones are subjected to stress, a naturally occurring positive electric charge occurs on the convex side and a negative charge occurs on the concave side. The electropositive charge is thought to be associated with osteoclastic activity (bone formation), and the electronegative charge is thought to be associated with osteoblastic activity (bone resorption). This process causes change in the shape and design of the bone so that it can withstand the loads applied. The result of remodeling is that the bone is either returned to its original form or changed to accomplish its function in the most efficient way. The remodeling stage may begin as early as 6 weeks after the fracture and continue for as long as 1 year.

The goal of fracture healing is to achieve union of the fracture fragments and to restore the normal anatomy and function of the bone. *Clinical healing* refers to the point in the healing process when the fracture has achieved enough stability and strength to resume its function, the fracture site is pain free, there is no gross movement across the fracture site, and x-ray films show bone crossing the fracture site. *Biologic healing* is said to have occurred when the maximum strength of the bone is reached. Fractures are usually considered healed when the point of clinical healing is reached. Bony union is said to be clinically complete when there is no motion at the fracture site with gentle stressing, no tenderness is present when direct pressure is applied over the fracture site, and weight bearing is pain free in lower extremity fractures. Clinical evidence of fracture healing should always be supported by x-ray evidence, and stress films should be obtained if needed.

Factors Affecting Healing

Ehara (1997) states that 70% to 80% of all failures in fracture healing are technical failures and include infection, inadequate reduction, distraction, continued motion at the fracture, and compromised blood supply caused by the injury or treatment. The remaining 20% are biologic failures, which include failure of callus formation, failure of mineralization of callus (osteomalacia), abnormal differentiation (proliferation of fibroblasts and lipoblasts, instead of osteoblasts and chondroblasts), abnormal remodeling stage (delay in replacing callus with lamellar bone), abnormal modeling stage (osteogenesis imperfecta), and systemic disease such as diabetes mellitus and peripheral neuropathy.

Ruda (1998) categorizes factors affecting fracture healing into local or systemic factors. Local factors include severity of trauma, immobilization, intra-articular fracture, local stress, and metal implants. Infection, local malignancy or pathologic condition, avascular necrosis, age, and hormones are systemic factors.

Local Factors

Severity of Trauma. The amount of trauma to the soft tissues and area surrounding the fracture influences the rate of healing because the cells that differentiate into repair cells for the bone also provide cells to repair soft tissue damage. The hematoma surrounding the fracture can also spread into the surrounding tissue when there is severe soft tissue trauma resulting in a dispersion of the efforts of the repair cells. Fractures that have an intact soft tissue covering on at least one side and fractures that are not displaced heal faster than more complex fractures. This is partially a result of the increased number of repair cells available to heal the bone in simpler or undisplaced fractures. Displaced fractures have a greater amount of cartilage formation and less primary bone formation than do nondisplaced fractures. Loss of bone or excessive distraction of fracture fragments may slow the healing process or stop it completely if the repair cells are unable to bridge the gap between fracture fragments.

Type of Bone. The type of bone involved in the fracture can also affect the speed of healing. Cancellous bone is known to unite rapidly when there are points of direct contact between fragments. There is little callus formation during the healing process in fractures involving cancellous bone. Fracture healing is accomplished by direct new bone formation beginning at the contact points. Where there is no contact, the gap is filled by the spread of new bone from areas where there is contact.

Cortical bone unites by the repair process of external callus formation if there is wide displacement of the fragments or if immobilization is not rigid. If there is reasonably good alignment of fragments and rigid immobilization is maintained, a cortical bone fracture heals by a different process. If the ends of the fracture are in contact, the dead ends of the fracture are not resorbed. Instead, new Haversian canals are formed through the dead bone. Small gaps are healed by an ingrowth of bone. If the fracture has large amounts of necrotic cortical bone, the internal repair process takes place very slowly and necrotic areas can persist for long periods.

Immobilization. Adequate immobilization of fracture fragments is critical to the healing process. Repeated manipulation or motion of fracture fragments can result in the formation of pseudoarthrosis. This is thought to be related to the disruption of the fibrin platform by the motion of the fragments, resulting in failure of or improper formation of the bridge of external callus. Fracture fixation facilitates healing but does not accelerate bone repair. Immobilization that permits weight bearing stimulates the healing process.

Intra-articular Fractures. Fibrinolysin in synovial fluid can disrupt the initial clot and slow the rate of the first stage of fracture healing. Intra-articular fractures heal but are more difficult to treat than extra-articular fractures.

Local Stress. Stress across a fracture site through exercise or use of the extremity stimulates fracture healing. The mechanism thought to be involved is the generation of piezoelectric currents at the fracture site.

Local application of electric currents at fracture sites can also be used to stimulate fracture healing.

Metallic Implants. Open treatment of fractures causes additional soft tissue damage to the area surrounding the fracture. When metallic implants are used for fractures, there is an acute inflammatory response that is primarily the result of surgical trauma. Fibrous tissue is generated by the repair process to secure the implant in place. Although the metals used for implants are relatively inert, they do not remain totally inactive. Metallic particles are released from the metal, and a chronic inflammatory reaction can occur, with phagocytosis of the metallic particles. How much reaction occurs is directly proportional to the amount of metallic particles released. Table 19–8 outlines the general timetable for removal of metal implants following fracture fixation.

Systemic Factors

Infection. The presence of infection in a fracture slows or stops the fracture healing process because the cells that would normally be involved in the repair process are involved in the attempt to eliminate or contain the infection. This is true if the fracture results from an infection or if the infection occurs after the fracture.

Local Malignancy or Pathologic Condition. Fractures through primary or secondary malignancies do not usually heal unless the malignancy is treated. New bone

TABLE 19–8. *Timing of Metal Removal*

BONE FRACTURE	TIME AFTER IMPLANTATION (MONTHS)
Malleolar fractures	8–12
Tibial pilon	12–18
Tibial shaft	
Plate	12–18
Intramedullary nail	18–24
Tibial head	12–18
Patella, tension band	8–12
Femoral condyles	12–24
Shaft of the femur	
Single plate	24–36
Double plates	From month 18, in 2 steps (interval of 6 months)
Intramedullary nail	24–36
Pertrochanteric and femoral neck fractures	12–18
Pelvis (only in case of complaints)	From month 10
Upper extremity (optional)	12–18

These data essentially relate to recent fractures with uncomplicated healing processes and do not apply to osteosyntheses in pseudoarthroses, major fragments, or after infections, which must be considered on an individual basis.

From Canale, S. (Ed.). (1998). *Campbell's operative orthopaedics* (9th ed., p. 2015). St. Louis: Mosby.

formation may be seen microscopically, but adequate immobilization is not usually possible for completion of the healing process to occur. Fractures through bones involved in nonmalignant conditions may heal, but in many instances (e.g., Paget's disease), they may heal slowly or not at all.

Avascular Necrosis. Normal fracture healing progresses from both sides of the fracture. If there is avascular necrosis of one fracture fragment, all healing occurs from the other side of the fracture. Although the fracture heals, it heals slowly. If there is avascular necrosis of both fracture fragments, the chance for healing is very poor.

Age. Fractures heal more slowly in adults than in children. The younger the age of the individual, the faster the rate of healing. The remodeling process is also more active in children and allows the body to correct a greater degree of deformity than is possible in adults. Nonunion is rare in children. Some areas of the immature skeleton probably do not heal by the classic method of callus formation. These areas include the physis and the epiphyseal hyaline cartilage. When callus repair occurs in these areas, the result may be significant growth deformities because of the formation of a bony bridge between the secondary ossification center and the metaphysis. As the age of the child decreases, the extent and physiologic activity of the remodeling phase increase. Effects of epiphyseal growth dynamics can further complicate the remodeling phase in the immature skeleton.

Hormones. Corticosteroids slow the rate of fracture healing. Other hormones have been shown in experiments to affect the rate of healing, although they do not usually have an effect on clinical healing of fractures. Growth hormones, thyroid hormones, vitamins A and D, and anabolic steroids stimulate the rate of healing. Diabetes and hypervitaminosis A and D have been shown experimentally to slow the rate of healing.

Interventions to Stimulate Fracture Healing

Although most fractures heal adequately without any problems, assisting or improving the healing process may be useful in some situations. Biologic interventions include systemic and local approaches to stimulate fracture healing. Local approaches can be classified as osteogenic, osteoconductive, or osteoinductive.

Osteogenic methods to induce bone formation include the use of autogenous or allogeneic bone grafts. An additional osteogenic method currently under investigation is the injection or implantation of autogenous bone marrow or marrow-derived mesenchymal cells.

Osteoconductive methods involve the use of a three-dimensional structure, implant, or graft to provide a surface supporting the attachment, spreading, division, and differentiation of cells for bone growth. Material currently used includes ceramics, synthetic polymers, and bioactive glasses. Synthetic calcium-collagen graft materials are also currently being used to provide templates for bone formation and to treat fractures with loss of bone.

Osteoinduction involves the use of substances such as platelet-derived growth factor or peptide signaling molecules to stimulate or enhance bone healing.

Electric Stimulation. The first report of use of electric stimulation to enhance fracture healing occurred in 1841. There were no advances in the use of electric stimulation until the 1950s, when it was discovered that bone subjected to a bending load generated electric charges. The portion of the bone in compression becomes electronegative, and the bone under tension becomes electropositive. In 1966, it was discovered that non-stressed bone in areas of active growth or repair is electronegative. Following these discoveries, the effects of electric charges on bone and cartilage began to be studied. Three types of electric stimulation devices have been developed. Constant direct current stimulation devices are invasive, with implanted electrodes delivering the current. Electromagnetic devices use externally applied coils to provide a time-varying electric stimulation to the bone. In capacitive coupling, the electric field is produced by two charged metal plates attached to a voltage source that are placed on either side of the extremity. Although no one of these three methods is superior to the other, this noninvasive approach combined with a non–weight-bearing immobilization treatment is preferred by clients.

Low-intensity sonography has also been demonstrated to stimulate and promote bone healing (Cook, Ryaby, & McCabe, 1997).

Complications

Although many postfracture complications can be avoided by proper treatment and careful observation, there may be serious and unavoidable complications that exist by the time the fracture is seen or treated. Delays in treatment of skeletal trauma while other injuries are treated or while clients are transferred to alternative facilities increase the occurrence of wound infections. Fractures caused by high-energy forces may not allow anatomic restoration or functioning. The systemic status of the individual, including gender, advanced age, malnutrition, anemia, diabetes mellitus, hormone deficiency, and preinjury limb status (including oxygen tension, muscle quality, and adipose tissue thickness) are additional factors to be considered (Hayda, Brighton, & Esterhai, 1998).

Complications of fractures and immobility (Box 19-6) can be divided into immediate and delayed complications. Immediate complications include shock, fat embolism, compartment syndrome, deep venous thrombosis, pulmonary embolism, and infection. These complications are covered in Chapters 10 and 23.

BOX 19–6.
Complications of Fractures and Immobility

Fractures	Fat emboli syndrome
Hemorrhage	Immobility
Vascular injuries	Pneumonia
Nerve injuries	Deep venous thrombosis
Compartment	Pulmonary embolism
syndrome	Urinary tract infections
Volkmann's ischemic	Wound infection
contracture	Decubitus ulcers
Avascular necrosis	Muscle atrophy
Reflex dystrophy	Stress ulcers

From Geiderman, J. (1998). Orthopedic injuries: Management principles. In P. Rosen & R. Barkin (Eds.), *Emergency medicine concepts and clinical practice* (4th ed., p. 611). St. Louis, Mosby.

Delayed complications that occur after fractures may include joint stiffness, post-traumatic arthritis, complex regional pain syndrome (CRPS; reflex sympathetic dystrophy), myositis ossificans, malunion, delayed union, nonunion, loss of reduction of fracture fragments, refracture, and osteomyelitis. These complications are often preventable, or their effects can be minimized by proper care.

Joint stiffness may result from edema, from joint contractures caused by bursa or capsular adhesions, or from prolonged immobilization necessitated by treatment of the fracture. It can occur at the joint involved in the injury or at joints that are remote from the fracture but associated with the injury or its treatment. Joint stiffness following fractures is most common in the upper extremities in the shoulder, the elbow, and the finger. In the lower extremity, the knee is most often affected. The most common causes of joint stiffness are inadequate activity of the muscles and limb, prolonged dependent edema, infection, and prolonged immobilization of intra-articular fractures.

The degree of post-traumatic arthritis that develops is primarily determined by the severity of the initial trauma and by the effectiveness of reduction in weight-bearing joints. Articular surfaces in weight-bearing joints require anatomic reduction of the articular surfaces and long-bone fractures to prevent or delay the development of post-traumatic arthritis. The more severe the fracture, the sooner arthritic changes are likely to appear. To prevent further progression of post-traumatic arthritis, it is important to eliminate the stresses and strains on the joint or fracture site, to maintain the maximum level of efficiency of the muscles controlling the involved bone or joint, and to avoid exceeding the functional capacity of the joint or bone. Surgical replacement of joints may be required in severe cases of post-traumatic arthritis.

CRPS (reflex sympathetic dystrophy) is a painful dysfunction and disuse syndrome characterized by abnormal pain and swelling of the extremity and is usually precipitated by minor trauma. CRPS affects 5% to 30% of all fractures and has a classic clinical presentation of pain out of proportion to the injury, allodynia (pain with non-noxious stimuli), hyperalgesia (severe pain with mildly noxious stimuli), pain with movement, swelling, and edema, hyperhidrosis, and vasomotor instability (either flushed and warm or cool and pale) (Hoover & Siefert, 2000). The origin of the dystrophy syndrome is generally believed to be related to the sympathetic nervous system. Treatments for this syndrome include drug therapy, nerve blocks, physical therapy, and transcutaneous electric nerve stimulation.

CRPS II (formerly known as *causalgia*) is all of the previously discussed findings with the additional presence of an intractable pain after injury to a major nerve. Ehara (1997) identified three clinical stages. In clinical stage 1 (early phase), severe burning pain with no radiologic changes is present; this stage lasts 3 to 6 months. Clinical stage 2 (dystrophic phase) presents with edema, cold skin, restricted joint motion, and osteopenia. Clinical stage 3 (atrophic phase) exhibits progressive skin and muscle atrophy, fibrosis around joints, persistent pain, and marked osteopenia.

Myositis ossificans is the formation of heterotopic (abnormal or out of place) bone near bone and muscles, usually in response to trauma. The cause of heterotopic ossification is unknown, but it is generally agreed that the cause is local and involves systemic factors that are mostly unidentified. Although it can occur anywhere in the body, the most common sites are the arms, thighs, and hips. Heterotopic ossification is often seen in children, adolescents, young adults, athletes, and individuals with closed intracranial or spinal cord injuries causing paralysis. It has also been reported as a complication following blunt trauma, total joint replacement, and fractures. Prevention is the most effective treatment for myositis ossificans through avoidance of repetitive soft tissue injuries. Excision of heterotopic bone should be performed only when the bone is mature, never sooner than 6 to 12 months after the injury that precipitated it. Maturity of the bone can be determined by serum alkaline phosphatase levels. A return to normal levels indicates cessation of bone formation activity.

Malunion (healing in an abnormal position or alignment) occurs when unequal stress forces of muscle pull and gravity cause improper alignment of fracture fragments. It is often associated with fractures treated with skeletal traction followed by plaster immobilization. It can also occur when an ambulatory device is applied before the fracture is firm or if the client bears weight on the extremity against medical advice. The primary symptom of malunion is external deformity of the involved extremity, and it is diagnosed by x-ray film. Prevention of malunion is accomplished by adequate reduction and immobilization of the fracture and by being sure the client understands the importance of activity and position restrictions.

Delayed union is suspected from 3 months to 1 year after the injury when there is continuation of or increase in bone pain and tenderness beyond a reasonable healing period consistent with the degree of skeletal and soft tissue trauma. Clinically, motion at the fracture site is evident, and a radiologically persistent fracture line with deficient or scarce callus is noted (Ehara, 1997). Fractures of internal fixation devices may indicate delayed union. Delayed union may be caused by distraction of fracture fragments or systemic causes, such as infection. If the causative factors are identified early and corrected, the fracture, given additional time, usually heals.

Nonunion occurs when fracture healing has not taken place 4 to 6 months after the fracture occurs, and spontaneous healing is unlikely. Nonunion is said to occur in the client with multiple fractures when all other fractures have united, leaving all the stress on one unhealed fracture site. Nonunion is caused by insufficient blood supply and uncontrolled repetitive stress on the fracture site. This can be caused by interposition of muscle, tendon, and soft tissue between fracture fragments. It may also be caused by prolonged or excessive traction; insufficient, inappropriate, or inadequate immobilization (allowing motion at the fracture site); inadequate internal fixation; or wound infection following internal fixation. One of the most common occurrences of nonunion is after a segmental fracture in which there is impaired blood supply to one of the ends of the fracture fragments. In other instances, the outcome of bone healing may be related to local factors involving the injury site (e.g., shoulder fractures require early mobilization to prevent joint stiffness owing to the thickness of the shoulder capsule). Excessive use of steroids also compromises fracture healing. Nonunions are characterized by relatively narrow gaps between fracture fragments, with a nonrigid soft tissue bridge made of fibrocartilage and fibrous tissue. Delayed union or nonunion is most common in the tibia and fibula and the scaphoid and least common in the humerus, radius and ulna, and clavicle (Ehara, 1997).

Nonunion, once diagnosed, should be treated. Treatment may include bone grafting, internal fixation, external fixation, electric bone stimulation, or combinations of the methods. Bone grafts are used to bridge gaps in bone or nonunion sites to induce bone formation. In normal bone healing, when bone is compressed, it becomes electronegative and bone formation is stimulated. The application of negative current through the use of a bone stimulator is believed to induce the formation of bone in a manner similar to that of compression.

Fibrous union is characterized by a wide gap between fracture fragments, with fibrous tissue interposed. Loss of bone through injury or surgery predisposes to fibrous union. Pseudoarthrosis is the formation of a false joint at the fracture site, with synovial fluid filling the gap between the ends of the bones. In pseudoarthrosis, there is no tissue bridge between the ends of the bone.

Refracture is said to occur when the fracture is assumed healed or after the removal of rigid skeletal fixation when the fracture occurs again at the same site. Refracture can be prevented by the gradual increase of stress to the fracture site until full functional stresses are achieved. This should be done while the fracture is protected with internal or external support. Early application of stress may cause callus to fracture if the alignment of the fragments is random rather than according to functional stresses.

Post-traumatic osteoporosis can occur from 7 to 24 months after injury.

Osteomyelitis may occur in the femur or tibia following open fracture and internal fixation. *Staphylococcus aureus* remain the most common bacterial organism and can become a cause of chronic and recurring infection. In addition, osteonecrosis of the femoral head or scaphoid and secondary osteoarthritis can occur.

NURSING MANAGEMENT

After emergency management and treatment of the client with fractures, the continuing nursing management and treatment modalities are based on identified client problems that may accompany the disorder. The National Association of Orthopaedic Nurses (NAON, 1991) has identified the nursing care and interventions to prevent complications and restore independent function to the individual (Box 19-7). Prevention of complications occurs primarily in the acute and recovery phases following injury. Restoration of function is a process that must begin at the time of injury and that continues through the end of the rehabilitation phase.

Assessment factors that should be included in the determination of the actual or potential problems include both the history and the physical examination. The client interview and history should be obtained before physical assessment, if possible. This allows the practitioner to identify any previously unidentified potential problem areas rather than focusing on known injuries or problems. Occult injuries that were overlooked during the emergency management phase of care may be identified in trauma clients at this time.

The symptoms experienced by the client and the clinical signs present depend on the type of fracture, its location, and the amount of force involved in the trauma. The client should be questioned about the mechanism of injury and the sequence of the symptoms that were experienced (e.g., severe pain experienced before a fall is often associated with pathologic fractures). The medical history should be reviewed to determine any problems that need to be addressed and that could affect the care and treatment. Total physical assessment should then be

---

BOX 19–7.

NAON's Nursing Intervention Classification: Specialty Area Core Interventions

Analgesic administration	Medication administration
Autotransfusion	Medication administration: oral
Bathing	Medication administration: parenteral
Bed rest care	Pain management
Blood products administration	Patient-controlled analgesia (PCA) assistance
Cast care: maintenance	Physical restraint
Cast care: wet	Positioning
Constipation and impaction management	Preparatory sensory information
Controlled substance checking	Pressure management
Cough enhancement	Self-care assistance
Critical path development	Shift report
Delegation	Skin care: topical treatments
Delirium management	Skin surveillance
Discharge planning	Splinting
Documentation	Staff supervision
Embolus care: peripheral	Teaching: individual
Exercise promotion	Teaching: preoperative
Exercise therapy: ambulation	Teaching: prescribed activity and exercise
Exercise therapy: joint mobility	Teaching: prescribed medications
Fall prevention	Teaching: procedure and treatment
Heat and cold application	Traction and immobilization care
Incision site care	Tube care: urinary
Infection control	Urinary retention care
Intravenous (IV) insertion	Wound care
Intravenous (IV) therapy	Wound care: closed drainage

From McCloskey, J., & Bulechek, G. (2000). *Nursing intervention classification* (3rd ed., p. 819). St. Louis: Mosby.

---

performed, focusing on specific areas identified during the interview and history.

Common Nursing Concerns for the Client with Fractures

When caring for clients with fractures, it is essential that the nurse be familiar with the normal pathophysiology of the musculoskeletal system as well as other body systems. This knowledge enables the nurse to prevent or identify promptly potential complications resulting from fractures and promote early and complete rehabilitation. Common nursing diagnoses are listed in Box 19–8.

Risk for Peripheral Neurovascular Dysfunction

Neurovascular deficit following fractures may result from the injury itself or from the treatment of the injury. Factors that may contribute to neurovascular deficit at the time of injury include soft tissue disruption from the force or energy of the trauma, fracture fragments, hemorrhage, joint dislocation, body position assumed after the injury, and hypothermia. Neurovascular deficit occurring as a result of treatment may be caused by moving or splinting the fracture; manipulation at the time of reduction; application of casts, splints, traction, braces,

Ace bandages, dressings, or equipment (e.g., abduction pillow straps, continuous passive motion machine); hemorrhage; or edema.

Assessment, Decision Making, Prevention. Frequent monitoring, assessment, and documentation of the neurovascular status of clients with fractures must be

---

BOX 19–8.

Common Nursing Diagnoses in Fracture Management

Activity intolerance	Impaired mobility
Anxiety	Knowledge deficit
Altered tissue perfusion	Pain
Body image disturbance	Peripheral neurovascular
Disuse syndrome, risk for	dysfunction, risk for
Diversional activity deficit	Post-trauma response
Fatigue	Self-care deficit
Fluid volume deficit	Skin integrity, impaired
Hopelessness	and risk for impaired
Infection, risk for	Tissue integrity impair-
Impaired gas exchange	ment

linked to appropriate clinical decision-making skills. Neurovascular compromise, if unrecognized and untreated, may progress to limb-threatening status, with deformity, loss of function, disability, or amputation. Other common nursing interventions for individuals at risk for neurovascular compromise include elevation of the extremity above the level of the heart unless concern exists about compartment syndrome, the application of cold to minimize edema, and encouragement of finger or toe movement. For a detailed discussion of compartment syndrome, see Chapter 10.

Pain (Acute)

All fractures cause pain. The degree of discomfort experienced by individuals is related to the type of fracture and associated soft tissue injury as well as individual reaction to pain. Following fracture treatment, pain may be related to muscle spasm, the surgical procedure, immobilization devices, or the use of various orthopaedic equipment.

Pain Management. Pain management involves the use of traditional methods of analgesia, new technology, and delivery methods, as well as nontraditional methods of pain control. Each client must be assessed individually, and the team approach is vital in determining which interventions help prevent or relieve the pain caused by fractures. Inadequate pain management may put clients at risk for disuse syndrome. For a complete discussion of pain management, see Chapter 5.

Knowledge Deficit

Education: Disease Process/Procedure/Treatment. Knowledge deficit following a fracture may be the result of inexperience with trauma or hospitalization, care of immobilization devices (e.g., casts, splints, braces, external fixator, traction), immobility, or potential complications. Teaching must include preparation of the client and family for medical and nursing interventions that will be used in the treatment plan, normal bone healing, application and removal and care of equipment (e.g., braces, casts, splints), use of assistive devices, signs and symptoms of potential complications to report (e.g., neurovascular deficit, infection), and techniques to assist with ADLs. Chapter 13 outlines mobilization techniques, and immobilization techniques and devices are discussed in Chapter 12.

It is important to maintain an awareness of the client's and family's readiness to learn. The impact of trauma and the resulting changes in lifestyle and roles may alter coping mechanisms and learning ability. Learning can take place only when the client or family is ready to learn. Other factors that may affect learning include previous knowledge or experience, language and learning

skills, cultural beliefs, and psychomotor limitations. If learning is not completed during the period of hospitalization or the period of interaction with the client, outpatient referrals should be made.

Self-care Deficit

Self-care Assistance. Self-care deficits are commonly related to immobilization devices; activity intolerance; pain; anxiety; knowledge deficit; or restrictions on position, activity, and weight bearing. Clients with fractures may require assistance, assistive devices, teaching, and encouragement to strive for independence in ADLs as well as referrals to other health care professionals or community health services.

Impaired Physical Mobility

The degree of immobility caused by a fracture depends on the type of fracture, the amount of pain associated with the injury, and the method of treatment. Immobility may be related to activity or weight-bearing restrictions, immobilization devices, the age of the client, preexisting conditions, or inexperience with assistive devices.

Exercise Therapy, Positioning, Self-esteem Enhancement. The results of immobility include changes in self-esteem and a sense of powerlessness and increase the risk of secondary complications in all body systems. Examples of secondary complications that may occur with immobility are deep venous thrombosis, pulmonary embolism, renal calculi, skin breakdown, gastrointestinal problems, and pulmonary problems. Interventions are aimed at restoring early mobility and independence and at preventing the occurrence of secondary complications.

Infection

Infection Prevention. Following fractures, clients may be at risk for infection owing to factors related to the injury (e.g., open fractures) or to the surgical procedure (e.g., extensive time in surgery). Infection may be superficial or deep in a wound. It may cause delayed healing of fractures or soft tissue and result in postponement of rehabilitation.

Impaired Skin Integrity

Skin integrity may be compromised by open fractures, soft tissue injuries, pressure areas (e.g., from immobility or devices), or improper use of equipment. Additional factors that may contribute to impaired skin integrity are the age and general condition of the client and preexisting conditions, such as diabetes. For detailed information on skin integrity, see Chapter 4.

Fluid Volume Deficit

Fluid Management. All fractures result in blood loss. The amount of loss and its effect on the client depend on the type and location of the fracture as well as the age and general condition of the client before the injury. It may be difficult to estimate the amount of blood loss from fractures, but adequate volume replacement is necessary to prevent hypovolemic shock. A femoral fracture may cause a blood loss of 500 to 3000 mL, a pelvic fracture 750 to 6000 mL, an ankle fracture 250 to 1000 mL, a humerus fracture 500 to 1500 mL, and a tibia or fibula fracture 250 to 2000 mL. Fluid volume deficit may also result from third spacing (fluid shift to interstitial space of the injured extremity) without the client's having sustained a significant blood loss. This type of hypovolemia is treated with crystalloid fluids (normal saline or lactated Ringer's solution) rather than with blood administration. For more information on this topic, see Chapter 10.

Impaired Gas Exchange

Clients with fractures, especially those with multiple trauma, are at risk for impaired gas exchange from several causes. The client with a long-bone fracture, multiple rib fractures, pelvic fracture, or multiple fractures is at risk for the development of fat embolism. Additional trauma occurrences that may cause impaired gas exchange include chest trauma, immobility, and pain. Deep venous thrombosis and pulmonary embolism are two common complications that may cause impaired gas exchange. These are discussed in detail in Chapter 10.

Airway Management and Exercise Promotion. Interventions are aimed at minimizing or alleviating the risk factors that may preclude the development of impaired gas exchange. Early mobilization and the use of pulmonary toilet techniques are probably the two most effective interventions.

Ineffective Coping

Trauma resulting in fractures not only may cause physical complications but also may cause psychological complications. These complications may be related to the sudden unexpected nature of the trauma and injury. The client who enters the hospital as a result of trauma is not prepared for the experience and usually is in a state of crisis. Trauma clients generally have a high level of anxiety, with fear of pain, death, disfigurement, and loss of personal and financial independence. In addition, prolonged hospitalization, illness, disability, and rehabilitation cause changes in normal activities and activate a stress response. Clients may exhibit symptoms of anxiety; fear; depression; anger; hostility; regressive emotional

responses; or hypochondriacal, neurotic, or psychotic reactions to the injury. They may become uncooperative, noncompliant, and manipulative.

In helping trauma victims cope with these reactions, the nurse must assess the physical and emotional responses of the individual to the injury, the stage of grief over actual or perceived losses, and the usual coping mechanisms and responses to stressors. Post-traumatic stress disorder (PTSD) may also be a complication following traumatic injury. PTSD is a process of destabilization and adjustment to trauma with biologic and psychological components. Estimates of the incidence of PTSD vary from 10% to 75% depending on the nature and severity of the traumatic incident. Factors that have been identified as increasing an individual's vulnerability to PTSD include personality, history of trauma, history of psychological or behavioral problems, social support mechanisms, and life events at the time of the trauma.

PTSD may be acute or chronic. The main symptom is repeatedly experiencing the traumatic event, which may cause psychological numbing or decreased involvement in the external world. Nightmares, withdrawal from activities, decreased emotional responses, and fears of recurrence of the event are also common reactions. Symptoms such as insomnia, loss of concentration and memory, exaggerated startle response, anxiety attacks, chronic increase in the level of tension, decreased activity levels, and the development of phobias may accompany PTSD. For further information on this topic, refer to Chapter 2.

Coping Enhancement. Interventions should be directed toward helping individuals develop coping mechanisms that will allow them to resolve the crisis. The client may require assistance from occupational therapists and physical therapists to help channel energies in positive directions and to regain independence and control. Counseling may be beneficial in some cases, and social service personnel may be needed to help with financial needs and discharge planning.

Discharge Planning

Discharge planning for the hospitalized client with fractures involves many areas. Most of the information included under the nursing diagnosis knowledge deficit is related to client instruction required for discharge planning. In addition, many clients require the assistance of the social service department to help with arrangements for care, equipment, and financial needs after discharge. When assessing the client for discharge needs, the following areas need to be considered: ability to perform ADLs, mobility, orientation, memory and mood, and skilled nursing needs. Appropriate referrals should be made to enable the client to access the level of care required to complete rehabilitation. With an average length of stay of 3.85 days or less, transfer to a subacute or inpatient rehabilitation unit may be advantageous for some. Others may benefit from outpatient rehabilitation sessions or home-based rehabilitation services.

Individuals treated for fractures on an outpatient basis must comprehend the treatment prescribed by their physician. A thorough understanding of the restrictions of treatment and the potential complications are imperative. Client and significant other education must focus on the specifics of immobilization whether a splint, brace, or cast. The client and significant other must demonstrate a neurovascular assessment and state an understanding of the course of action should changes occur. Training with assistive devices must be completed before the client leaves the office or emergency department. Written discharge instructions and a follow-up phone call 24 to 48 hours later can help ensure that the client has an uncomplicated course of treatment. Routine outpatient follow-up should be undertaken to ensure that fracture healing is progressing at an acceptable rate.

EVIDENCE-BASED PRACTICE: WHAT ARE THE OPTIMAL TREATMENT OPTIONS FOR TIBIAL FRACTURES?

The tibia is the major load-bearing structure of the lower leg and lies just subcutaneous for most of its length.

The presence of a hinge joint at the knee and ankle allows no adjustment for rotary deformation after tibial shaft fracture (Whittle, 1998). Tibial fractures, the most common long-bone fracture, account for 77,000 hospitalizations annually and an estimated $20 billion in health care costs (Pacelli & Duwelius, 1998). Motor vehicle accidents and sports-related injuries are the primary mechanisms of injury. Treatment options range from casting and bracing to intramedullary nailing via open reduction and external fixation.

Motor vehicle collisions account for 1.2 to 1.6 million nonfatal open tibial fractures annually in the United States. The total cost of musculoskeletal treatment and rehabilitation and loss of productivity exceeds $20 billion annually (Brown, Henderson, & Moore, 1996). The major mechanism of injury identified is acceleration-deceleration when a seat belt is not used and the leg hits the dashboard or when the right lower leg is depressing the brake pedal upon impact.

Farm accidents disable more than 200,000 annually (Brown, Henderson, & Moore, 1996). Augers, balers, mowers, tractors, shredders, harvesters, grinders, and blowers are among the most common equipment involved. Human error, falls from heights, projectiles thrown from unshielded mechanical parts, and crush injures are the leading mechanisms of injury.

Gunshot wounds in civilian situations are classified as low-velocity (pistol) missile injury, high-velocity (rifle) missile injury, close-range shotgun injury, or long-range shotgun injury. Low-velocity injuries have bullet speeds of 600 to 1100 feet per second and produce a small entrance and exit wound. High-velocity injuries have small entrance but large exit wounds, with massive tissue necrosis. Close-range injuries have extensive soft tissue damage because the wadding material from the shotgun shell becomes lodged in the wound. Long-range injuries entail multiple low-velocity pellet injuries and require extensive wound management (Brown, Henderson, & Moore, 1996).

The tibia is the one bone in the body that is covered by only a thin layer of skin along most of its length, thereby causing many injuries to present as open fractures. The anteromedial surface and anterior crest of the tibia can be palpated from the tibial tuberosity to the medial malleolus. The fibula is palpable proximally in the area of the fibular head but then is covered by the peroneal muscle of the lateral compartment until the distal third, where it forms the lateral malleolus. The risk of compartment syndrome is great with tibia injury due to the four compartments that surround the tibia: anterior, lateral, superficial posterior, and deep posterior.

The anterior compartment (bounded by the tibia medially, fibula laterally, interosseous membrane posteriorly, and crural fascia anteriorly) contains the muscles (tibialis anterior, extensor digitorum longus, extensor hallucis longus, and peroneus tertius) primarily responsible for dorsiflexion of the foot, ankle, and digits of the foot. The anterior tibial and deep peroneal nerve are contained in the anterior compartment. The lateral compartment (lateral to the fibula and bounded by tissues of anterior compartment) contains the muscles (peroneus brevis and peroneus longus) responsible for plantar flexion and eversion of foot and the superficial peroneal nerve. The superficial posterior compartment contains the muscles to control plantar flexion of ankle and foot. The deep posterior compartment contains the muscle groups responsible for plantar flexion of foot and digits and inversion of foot, as well as the posterior tibial and peroneal arteries and posterior tibial nerve (Roberts & Stallard, 2000). The soleus, gastrocnemius, tibialis posterior, flexor hallucis longus, and the flexor digitorum longus muscles are located within the superficial and deep posterior compartments.

Initial clinical evaluation reveals a client with pain, inability to bear weight, and obvious deformity. A thorough history and physical examination will determine the mechanism of injury, assess neurologic and vascular integrity, assess open wounds, complete an ipsilateral assessment, and require anteroposterior and lateral roentgenograms. Direct nerve damage is rare in closed tibial fractures, but proximal tibial or fibular neck fractures can contuse or stretch the peroneal nerve, resulting in footdrop (Pacelli & Duwelius, 1998).

Four major types of tibial fractures (Roberts & Stallard, 2000) occur: stress fractures resulting from low energy repeated over time; crush injuries; torsional injuries; and three or four point bending forces resulting in oblique, transverse, or comminuted injuries. As previously discussed, the fractures should be described as open or closed; by their anatomic location (proximal, medial, distal); and if intra-articular or extra-articular, by pattern (e.g., oblique, spiral, transverse, comminuted) and by angulation (based on x-ray film; anterior/posterior or varus/valgus) (Pacelli & Duwelius, 1998).

Tibial Fracture Management Outcome

From 10% to 17% of open tibial fractures have life-threatening injuries and require advanced trauma life support protocols. In less severe injuries, initial treatment of tibial fractures requires immobilization above the knee to below the ankle, anaerobic and aerobic wound cultures, aggressive wound debridement, sterile dressing if indicated, determination of tetanus prophylaxis, and administration of antibiotics (first-generation cephalosporin, i.e., cefazolin) to treat wound contamination. Tetanus immune globulin should be administered at 250 units for most wounds or 500 units for severe or old wounds, with repeat administration advised if the wound is manipulated within 1 to 2 months. A second dose is advisable at 4 weeks and the third dose at 6 to 12 months following injury (Christian, 1998).

Wounds with heavy soil contamination require penicillin and an aminoglycoside (i.e., gentamicin) (Turen & Distasio, 1994). Infection rates for grade I is 0% to 2%, grade II 2% to 7%, grade III 10% to 25%, grade IIIA 7%, grade IIIB 10% to 50%, and grade IIIC 25% to 50%, with 50% or greater chance of amputation (Turen & Distasio, 1994). Wound management and infection control must concentrate on *S. aureus, Pseudomonas,* and *Clostridium.* A 2-g intravenous cefazolin loading dose followed by 1-g intravenously every 8 hours for 48 to 72 hours after the last surgical debridement is standard for grade II and III open fractures. In addition, an aminoglycoside and penicillin can be added to cover gram-negative and *Clostridium* contaminant. Vancomycin or ciprofloxacin is administered to clients with penicillin allergies. Trafton (2000) reminds us that clostridial myonecrosis and necrotizing fasciitis are life-threatening infections. The mechanism of injury may be significant to suspect high wound contamination following firearm wounds, tornadoes, or hurricanes (Christian, 1998). The use of antibiotic-impregnated polymethylmethacrylate (PMMA) bead chains is a new "infection-elimination-first" strategy in the treatment of septic nonunions (Ueng, Wei, & Shih, 1997). Tobramycin is often the antibiotic of choice for PMMA.

Tibial fracture complications, experienced in 5% to 40% of clients, include compartment syndrome and primary wound infection, especially osteomyelitis. For all tibial fractures, nonunion occurs in 2% to 3% and delayed union in 4% to 5% of clients. For open fractures, delayed union or nonunion occurs in 13% to 31% of clients, and a direct correlation exists between the energy absorbed by the fracture and by the surrounding tissue. The lack of overlying musculature results in a tenuous blood supply; thus, there is an increased risk of osteomyelitis and delayed union, malunion, and nonunion (Antosia & Lyn, 1998). Transection of the tibial nerve results in a nonfunctioning limb and is a criterion for primary limb amputation.

Pacelli and Duwelius (1998) defined the criteria for tibial union as the radiologic evidence of union between 20 and 26 weeks from injury, with malunion defined as more than 5 degrees of varus/valgus and/or 10 degrees of anterior/posterior malalignment and more than 1 cm of shortening. Two types of nonunion can occur. A hypertrophic nonunion has excessive callus formation resulting from excess motion at the fracture site. Atrophic nonunion has minimal callus formation and bone resorption at the fracture site resulting from little or no motion at fracture site (Pacelli & Duwelius, 1998). Treatment of either nonunion nonoperatively is with electrical stimulation or ultrasound, and surgical interventions include debridement or autologous bone grafting.

Resuscitation lines should never be placed in an injured extremity. When feasible, the femoral vein of an unaffected lower extremity should be spared from line placement because arterial reconstruction may necessitate harvesting the ipsilateral saphenous vein for an autogenous graft (Modrall, Weaver, & Yellin, 1998).

The integrity of the vascular structures of the lower extremity is assessed for frank hemorrhage, expanding hematomas, diminished or absent pulses, unexplained hypotension, bruits, peripheral nerve injury, and pulsatile external bleeding. Noninvasive diagnostic studies used are ultrasonic flow-detection Dopplers or duplex scanning B-mode (brightness modulation) (Shackford & Rich, 2000). Invasive studies consist of arteriography, intra-arterial digital subtraction angiography (IADSA), and venography. Geiderman (1998) estimates that 10% to 15% of significant arterial injuries have distal palpable pulses.

Closed Reduction

Pacelli and Duwelius (1998) state that the goal of closed tibial fracture management is to provide safe, inexpensive, accurate fixation that allows early ambulation and joint mobilization and that generates an acceptable long-term outcome of less than 1 cm of shortening and an angular alignment that is within 5 to 10 degrees of rotation or angulation in any plane. Treatment options include casting or bracing, plate and screw fixation, intramedullary fixation, external fixation, and amputation (Whittle, 1998). Russell and Palmieri (1995) state that a nondisplaced (low-energy) fracture with stable ligamentous structures is treated with rest, immobilization, and a castor brace with touchdown weight bearing.

TABLE 19–9. *The Tscherne Classification of Soft Tissue Injuries in Closed Fractures*

GRADE	DESCRIPTION
1	Soft tissue damage absent Indirect forces Torsion fractures
2	Superficial abrasion or contusion caused by fragment pressure from within Mild to moderate fracture severity
3	Deep, contaminated abrasion associated with local skin or muscle contusion from direct trauma Bumper injuries (pedestrian-motor vehicle) Increased fracture severity with comminution or segmental injury
4	Skin extensively contused with crushed muscle Muscle damage may be severe Compartment syndromes common

From Russell, T., & Palmieri, A. (1995). Fractures of the pelvis, acetabulum, and lower extremity. In S. Brotzman (Ed.), *Clinical orthopaedic rehabilitation* (p. 145). St. Louis: Mosby.

Soft tissue injury in closed tibial fractures has been classified (Russell & Palmieri, 1995) (Table 19–9). Closed reduction is the treatment of choice for closed tibial fracture with minimal comminution, less than 1 cm of initial shortening, little soft tissue damage, and minimal pain and swelling (Pacelli & Duwelius, 1998). Sarmiento (2000) researched the use of a cast or functional brace on 1000 clients and concluded that less than 12 mm of shortening and less than 6 degrees of angulation in any plane was obtainable. In addition, closed reduction can be provided at an acceptable cost level. Whittle (1998) prefers closed reduction and casting for stable low-energy tibial fractures, except for bilateral fractures, floating knee injuries, intra-articular extension of the fractures, and fractures in which the initial reduction is not achieved or is lost.

Open Reduction

Pacelli and Duwelius (1998) state that the goal of open fracture management is internal fixation to stabilize fracture fragments, afford repeated debridement, allow early soft tissue coverage, provide antibiotic therapy, and optimize reconstruction. Russell and Palmieri (1995) state that a displaced (high-energy) unstable fracture treatment plan is an open reduction and internal fixation (ORIF) with plate, screw, or combination with external fixation. ORIF provides immediate acceptable alignment and solid fixation and promotes early mobilization. Internal fixation is reserved for unstable closed fractures, open fractures, and any fracture involving significant soft tissue injury or in the multiple trauma victim. The Gustillo-Anderson classification is the most common classification used to grade open fractures (see Table 19–1).

Surgical intervention provides a temporary orthopaedic fixation for a grossly unstable fracture line, affords vascular repair followed by orthopaedic stabilization, can create a temporary vascular shunt or restore venous outflow, provides for graft harvesting, manages compartment syndrome via fasciotomy that is routine for grade IIIC, and most importantly provides for initial and ongoing debridement. The prevention of infection through irrigation and debridement procedures and the appropriate antibiotic therapy are essential. The ultimate client outcome is preservation and restoration of musculoskeletal function for weight bearing.

ORIF procedures routinely used for tibia shaft fractures include plates and screws (used for very proximal or distal fractures); external fixation (severe intra-articular proximal and distal tibial fractures, especially associated with compartment syndrome, head injuries, burns, or multiple injuries in which access to skin is important or for children with an open growth plate); or an intramedullary device, which is the most widely used and accepted fixation for most unstable fractures. Intramedullary devices have a 99% rate of union and 6% rate of complications (Pacelli & Duwelius, 1998). Intramedullary nailing of a "nonreamed" nail avoids disruption of endosteal blood supply and does not have the high complication rate of external fixation. Nailing with reaming destroys 70% of the cortical blood supply and results in a sixfold increase in periosteal flow, which may alter arterial circulation in adjacent tissues. In addition, the reaming procedure has been reported to increase the pressure in the deep posterior compartment and thus possibly alter the flow in the posterior tibial artery (Lindstrom, Gullichsen, Lertola, & Niinikoski, 1997).

Criteria for determining whether a fracture is unstable and requires ORIF include an initial postinjury x-ray film showing 100% displacement, shortening of at least 1 cm, and malalignment of more than 5 degrees in any plane; failure on one attempt at closed reduction in the operating room; and an intra-articular extension with joint line displacement of 2 mm or more (Pacelli & Duwelius, 1998). The only drawback of intramedullary nailing in closed tibial fractures is knee pain, with the overwhelming advantage being the speed of rehabilitation (McConnell, 2000).

Whittle (1998) states that most authors now recommend plating for tibial shaft fracture associated with displaced intra-articular fracture of the knee and ankle. Intramedullary fixation devices include ender pins, intramedullary nails, and interlocking intramedullary nails. Unreamed nailing for most open tibial fractures and locked intramedullary nailing currently is the preferred treatment for most tibial shaft fracture requiring operative fixation (Whittle, 1998).

Wounds created by high energy require extensive debridement, followed by subsequent soft tissue coverage day 5 to 7 via delayed closure, skin graft, or flap coverage (Whittle, 1998). The prognosis of tibial shaft fractures is more related to the severity of the soft tissue damage and primary dislocation than to the bone injury itself (Lindstrom et al., 1997).

Finkemeier, Schmidt, Kyle, Templeman, & Varecka (2000) report that the orthopaedic community is now debating the efficacy of small-diameter nails inserted without reaming. Reamed tibial nail insertion is the appropriate treatment for all closed fractures and for grade I to IIIA open fractures (Finkemeier et al., 2000).

External Fixation

External fixation provides realignment, wound access, and bone stabilization of complex fractures. After immediate debridement and irrigation, the decision to use intramedullary or external fixation is based on the proximal or distal extent of the fracture, the diameter of the isthmus, the nature of the wound after debridement, and anticipated difficulties with soft tissue coverage. Although intramedullary nails are limited to more diaphyseal fractures, external fixation can be applied to virtually all open fractures, including those with intra-articular extension (Whittle, 1998).

Small wire circular external fixators have several advantages. The wires are placed in a percutaneous fashion with minimal additional devitalization of bone and minimal disruption of the periosteal or endosteal blood supplies. The small tensioned wires allow capture of very small bone segments, which is good for comminuted periarticular fractures (Watson, 1994). Circular external fixators easily adjust to accommodate all plastic surgery procedures and do not hinder the ability of microvascular surgeons. External fixators offer advantages in the treatment of soft tissue injury associated with distal tibia fractures, but malunion continues to be a problem with this method of fixation (Pugh, Wolinsy, McAndrew, & Johnson, 1999). Complications associated with external fixation use include deep infection and serious wound slough requiring flap coverage or below-knee amputation as major complications and pin track infection or superficial wound problems as minor complications (Pugh et al., 1999). Bone grafting is often required to promote fracture union.

Limb Salvage versus Amputation

Historically, and as recently as the first half of the twentieth century, the open tibial fracture has been associated with infection, limb loss, marked morbidity, and high mortality rates resulting from sepsis (Turen & DiStasio, 1994). Whereas amputation and death were certain during the Civil War, subsequent military conflicts demonstrated that adequate immobilization, irriga- tion, debridement, and antibiotic therapy could salvage a complex tibial fracture. The debate today centers on the efficacy of external fixation versus intramedullary nailing and limb salvage versus early amputation.

Two absolute indications for primary amputation are the complete anatomic disruption of the tibial nerve in adults and crush injury with warm ischemia time of greater than 6 hours (Whittle, 1998). Secondary considerations include serious associated polytrauma, severe ipsilateral foot trauma, and a projected long course to full recovery. The client should also be evaluated relative to his or her age, occupation, medical conditions, the mechanism of injury, degree of fracture comminution and bone loss, extent and location of neurovascular injury, and severity and duration of shock. Postoperative nursing care following amputation is discussed in Chapter 20.

Crush injury, a delay in revascularization (warm ischemia time of 6 hours or longer), and a segmental tibial fracture equal a 70% chance of future amputation. Issues of futility associated with delayed amputation include prolonged treatment, multiple hospitalizations, and multiple surgical procedures. Grade IIIC limb salvage attempts may fail and result in delayed amputation. Amputation should be considered not as failure but as the preferred alternative to lengthy and expensive reconstructive procedures. Research has shown that limb salvage had more complications, more operative procedures, and longer length of stay than early below-knee amputation. Clients with successful limb salvage required more time to achieve a full-weight-bearing status, had more difficulty reentering the workforce, had higher hospital costs, and considered themselves more severely disabled than their below-knee amputee counterparts (Turen & Distasio, 1994). Georgiadis' research concluded that recovery time and long-term disability were reduced with early below-knee amputation (Whittle, 1998).

Primary amputation because of arterial injury is rarely necessary. In almost all cases of mangled extremities, arterial repair is technically feasible. Associated injuries, the magnitude of musculoskeletal injury, and the condition of the client are the primary determinants when one is considering a primary amputation. A hemodynamically unstable client who requires a lengthy arterial reconstruction may require a primary amputation to survive. A stable client with massive soft tissue or neurologic injuries that render the extremity functionally useless should also be considered for a primary amputation. Open tibial fractures with severe soft tissue and neurovascular insult result in high limb amputation rates. The decision to amputate should involve the client and his or her family when possible. In most instances, the client and physician are best served by delayed amputation, reserving primary amputation for extreme situations (Modrall, Weaver, & Yellin, 1998).

Blunt Injury. Limb salvage rates have improved dramatically with the widespread application of modern techniques of vascular repair. Permanent disability has decreased. Limb loss and disability have been minimized by expedient revascularization and primary arterial repair, routine heparinization, repair of popliteal venous injuries, aggressive wound debridement, and early soft tissue coverage (Modrall, Weaver, & Yellin, 1998). The goal is to provide the client with a functional limb or ultimately with a fitted prosthesis for the amputated limb (Brown, Henderson, & Moore, 1996).

Replantation, although rarely performed in the United States, can be accomplished with an anticipated functional achievement greater than that of prosthetic replacement through microsurgical techniques (Tooms, 1998). Judicious use of vascularized composite grafts and modern bone-lengthening techniques may allow preservation of severely traumatized limbs. Compromises the client may make for limb retention are multiple surgical procedures, extensive scarring of the noninvolved as well as the injured limb, prolonged hospitalization, and enormous financial costs. The ultimate functional capabilities of a salvaged limb compared with functional capabilities of modern prosthetics must be weighed. When all factors are considered, amputation may still be the preferred alternative. Limb amputation should not be viewed as trauma care failure because delayed limb amputation may cause a significant increase in sepsis, death, disabilities, the number of surgical procedures required, and hospital costs.

Faergemann, Frandsen, and Rock (1999) state the goal of open tibial fracture management as the restoration of function that will allow everyday activity. One approach to a final determination is the Sickness Impact Profile (SIP). The SIP includes body care and movement, mobility, ambulation, sleep and rest, home management, work, recreation and pastimes, eating, pain, and socioeconomic factors. The Eastern Association for the Surgery of Trauma (EAST) Practice Parameter Workgroup for Penetrating Lower Extremity Trauma (1999) has researched the literature to determine best practices. The following are their skeletal and arterial injury references for practice management guidelines for the management of penetrating trauma to the lower extremity.

INTERNET RESOURCES

The American Association for the Surgery of Trauma (AAST): www.aast.org
American College of Surgeons: www.facs.org
American Trauma Society: www.amtrauma.org
The Eastern Association for the Surgery of Trauma (EAST): www.east.org
Emergency Nurses Association: www.ena.org
Orthopaedic Trauma Association: www.ota.org

Society of Trauma Nurses: www.traumanursesoc.org
Trauma.org: www.trauma.org
Trauma Care: www.traumacare.com

REFERENCES

Antosia, R., & Lyn, E. (1998). Knee and lower leg. In P. Rosen & R. Barkin (Eds.), *Emergency medicine concepts and clinical practice* (4th ed., pp. 786-821). St. Louis: Mosby.

Brown, C., Henderson, S., & Moore, S. (1996). Surgical treatment of patients with open tibial fractures. *AORN Journal, 63*, 873-890.

Canale, S. (Ed.). (1998). *Campbell's operative orthopaedics* (9th ed.). St. Louis: Mosby.

Christian, C. (1998). General principles of fracture treatment. In S. Canale (Ed.) *Campbell's operative orthopaedics* (9th ed., pp. 1993-2041). St. Louis: Mosby.

Connolly, J. (1981). *DePalma's the management of fractures and dislocations* (3rd ed.). Philadelphia: WB Saunders.

Cook, S., Ryaby, J., & McCabe, J. (1997). Acceleration of tibial and distal radius fracture healing in patients who smoke. *Clinical Orthopaedics, 337*, 198-207.

Della-Giustina, K., & Della-Giustina, D. (1999). Emergency department evaluation and treatment of pediatric orthopedic injuries. *Emergency Medicine Clinics of North America, 17*, 895-922.

Eastern Association for the Surgery of Trauma. (1999). Practice management guidelines for management of penetrating trauma to the lower extremity. Available at www.east.org

Ehara, S. (1997). Complications of skeletal trauma. *Radiologic Clinics of North America, 35*, 767-781.

Eustace, S. (1997). MR imaging of fracture orthopedic trauma to the extremities. *Radiologic Clinics of North America, 35*, 615-629.

Faergemann, C., Frandsen, P., & Rock, N. (1999). Expected long-term outcome after a tibial shaft fracture. *The Journal of Trauma: Injury, Infection and Critical Care, 46*, 683-686.

Finkemeier, C., Schmidt, A., Kyle, R., Templeman, D., & Varecka, T. (2000). A prospective, randomized study of intramedullary nails inserted with and without reaming for the treatment of open and closed fractures of the tibial shaft. *Journal of Orthopaedic Trauma, 14*, 187-193.

Geiderman, J. (1998). Orthopedic injuries: Management principles. In P. Rosen & R. Barkin (Eds.), *Emergency medicine concepts and clinical practice* (4th ed., pp. 602-624). St. Louis: Mosby.

Hayda, R., Brighton, C., & Esterhai, J., Jr. (1998). Pathophysiology of delayed healing. *Clinical Orthopaedics and Related Research, 355*(Suppl), S31-S40.

Health, United States 1998.

Hoover, T., & Siefert, J. (2000). Soft tissue complications of orthopedic emergencies. *Emergency Medicine Clinics of North America, 18*, 115-139.

Johnson, M., Mass, M., & Moorehead, S. (2000). *Nursing outcomes classification (NOC)* (2nd ed.). St. Louis: Mosby.

Lindstrom, T., Gullichsen, E., Lertola, K., & Niinikoski, J. (1997). Leg tissue perfusion in simple tibial shaft fractures treated with unreamed and reamed nailing. *The Journal of Trauma, Injury, Infection and Critical Care, 34*, 636-639.

McConnell, T. (2000). Isolated tibial shaft fracture. *Journal of Orthopaedic Trauma, 14*, 306-308.

Modrall, J., Weaver, F., & Yellin, A. (1998). Diagnosis and management of penetrating vascular trauma and the injured extremity. *Emergency Medicine Clinics of North America, 16*, 129-144.

Mourad, L. (1997). Musculoskeletal system. In J. Thompson, G. McFarland, J. Hirsch, & S. Tucker (Eds.), *Mosby's clinical nursing* (4th ed., pp. 345-457). St. Louis: Mosby.

National Association of Orthopaedic Nurses (NAON). (1991). *Core curriculum for orthopaedic nursing*. Pitman, NJ: Author.

Pacelli, L., & Duwelius, P. (1998). Tibial fractures: Selecting the best treatment approach. *The Journal of Musculoskeletal Medicine, 15,* 4650, 55-58.

Pugh, K, Wolinsy, P., McAndrew, M., & Johnson, K. (1999). Tibial pilon fractures: A comparison of treatment methods. *The Journal of Trauma, Injury, Infection and Critical Care, 47,* 937-941.

Roberts, D., & Stallard, T. (2000). Emergency department evaluation and treatment of knee and leg injuries. *Emergency Medicine Clinics of North America, 18,* 67-84.

Ruda, S. (1998). Fracture biomechanics and healing. In V. Williamson (Ed.), *Management of lower extremity fractures* (pp. 23-29). Pitman, NJ: National Association of Orthopaedic Nurses.

Russell, T., & Palmieri, A. (1995). Fractures of the pelvis, acetabulum and lower extremity. In S. Brotzman (Ed.), *Clinical orthopaedic rehabilitation* (pp. 143-182). St. Louis: Mosby.

Sarmiento, A. (2000). On the behavior of closed tibial fractures: clinical/radiological correlations. *Journal of Orthopaedic Trauma, 14,* 199-205.

Shackford, S., & Rich, N. (2000). Peripheral vascular injury. In K. Mattox, D. Feliciano, & E. Moore (Eds.), *Trauma* (4th ed., pp. 1011-1046). New York: McGraw-Hill.

Tooms, R. (1998). General principles of amputation. In S. Canale (Ed.), *Campbell's operative orthopaedics* (9th ed., pp. 521-560). St. Louis: Mosby.

Trafton, P. (2000). Lower extremity fractures and dislocations. In K. Mattox, D. Feliciano, & E. Moore (Eds.), *Trauma* (4th ed., pp. 981-1010). New York: McGraw-Hill.

Turen, C., & DiStasio, A. (1994). Treatment of grade IIIB and grade IIIC open tibial fractures. *Orthopedic Clinics of North America, 25,* 561-571.

Ueng, S., Wei, F., & Shih, C. (1997). Management of large infected tibial defects with antibiotic beads local therapy and staged fibular osteoseptocutaneous free transfer. *The Journal of Trauma, Injury, Infection and Critical Care, 41,* 268-274.

Watson, J. (1994). High-energy fractures of the tibial plateau. *Orthopedic Clinics of North America, 25,* 723-752.

Whittle, A. (1998). Fractures of lower extremity. In S. Canale (Ed.), *Campbell's operative orthopaedics* (9th ed., pp. 2042-2180). St. Louis: Mosby.

20

Amputation

VERDELL WILLIAMSON

Approximately 135,000 to 150,000 amputations are performed each year in the United States, and it is estimated that in the United States there are about 350,000 to 2.5 million amputees (MossRehab ResourceNet, 2000; Winchell, 1995). Common causes for lower extremity amputation differ from upper extremity amputation. In lower extremity amputation, disease is the most common cause and accounts for 70% of cases. Trauma (22%), congenital or birth defects (4%), and tumors (4%) account for other causes. In contrast, disease accounts for only 6% of all upper extremity amputations, half of which are due to malignancies. Upper extremity amputation is largely due to trauma (70%) and birth defects (MossRehab ResourceNet, 2000).

Lower extremity amputations account for 90% of amputations performed in the United States, with 50% of these being transtibial (below the knee), 40% transfemoral (above the knee), and 10% hip disarticulations (Winchell, 1995). Recent statistics place the number of upper extremity amputees in the United States at approximately 100,000. Fifty-seven percent of all arm amputations are through the radius and ulna (transradial) (Esquenazi & Meier, 1996).

Advances in microvascular surgery, antibiotic therapy, treatment for musculoskeletal neoplasms, and orthopaedic reconstructive procedures and implants often make limb salvage a viable alternative to amputation. However, rather than being viewed as a failure, amputation should be seen as a reconstructive procedure aimed at restoring function and improving quality of life. The benefits of limb salvage in relation to amputation must take into consideration the potential for increased morbidity and possible mortality associated with prolonged limb salvage attempts.

The decision to amputate or the adjustment to sudden traumatic amputation or congenital limb deficiency is difficult and emotional for the client, significant others, and the surgeon. The nurse plays a vital role in assisting those involved to cope. A team approach is necessary to assist the client in returning to maximal activity and function. Other members of the team besides those already mentioned are prosthetists, physical and occupational therapists, the psychiatric advanced practice nurse, and the physical medicine and rehabilitation specialist.

INDICATIONS FOR AMPUTATION
Peripheral Vascular Disease

The primary indication for elective lower extremity amputation is ischemia secondary to peripheral vascular disease (PVD), and arteriosclerosis secondary to diabetes mellitus (DM) is the main cause of PVD. Clients with PVD make up approximately 80% of the lower extremity amputees in the Western world, and more than half of these clients also have DM (Smith & Fergason, 1999). The most common manifestation of chronic limb ischemia is a pain syndrome called *intermittent claudication*. Diagnosis of intermittent claudication is based on the presence of extremity pain in a definable muscle group (usually the calf muscles), which is precipitated by exercise and promptly relieved by rest. This pain is distinguished from pain resulting from diabetic neuropathy, which is distributed along dermatomes rather than confined to a specific muscle group and is constant and unrelated to exercise. Intermittent claudication is never a primary indication for amputation. As disease progresses, ischemic rest pain occurs in the toes and forefoot. There is no muscle involvement. Initially, the client experiences pain on elevation of the leg (usually when supine in bed), which is relieved by placing the leg in a dependent position, and the client may begin sleeping in a sitting position. As it becomes more severe, rest pain can occur even when the feet are in the dependent position.

Amputation is indicated only when previous reconstructive procedures (e.g., femoropopliteal bypass) have failed, pain can no longer be controlled by other means, and additional bypass surgery is not possible.

Trauma

As the ability to salvage severely injured extremities has developed, the burden on the surgeon to make appropriate decisions about which limbs to salvage has increased. Injury to a limb from a crushing or significant vascular injury can necessitate amputation if functional recovery is unlikely or if the client has suffered life-threatening trauma and cannot tolerate the operative time required for repair of the injured part.

In an effort to determine which mangled extremities are salvageable, the mangled extremity severity score was developed (Table 20–1). Using this scale, clients scoring 7 or more have limbs that are not salvageable and should undergo primary amputation (Kennedy, 1992). The decision to amputate also depends on whether an upper or lower extremity is in question. In the upper extremity, cervical nerve root injuries and extensive brachial plexus injuries result in a flail arm. This is a poor prognosis for recovery. However, even a severely compromised arm can

TABLE 20–1. *Mangled Extremity Severity Score (MESS)*

INJURY	SCORE
A Skeletal and Soft Tissue Injury	
Low energy (stabs, simple fracture, low-energy gunshot wound [GSW])	1
Medium energy (open or multiple fractures, dislocation)	2
High energy (close-range shotgun, high-energy GSW, crush injuries)	3
Very high energy (gross contamination, tissue avulsion)	4
B Limb ischemia	
Pulse reduced or absent, perfusion normal	1*
Pulseless, paresthesias, diminished capillary refill	2*
Cool paralyzed, insensate, numb	3*
C Shock	
Systolic blood pressure always above 90 mm Hg	0
Transient hypotension	1
Persistent hypotension	2
D Age (years)	
0–30	0
30–50	1
50+	2

*Double score for ischemia >6 hr.
Score less than 7 = salvageable extremity.
Score 7 or greater = nonsalvageable extremity.
Adapted from Kennedy, J. P. (1992). Traumatic amputation. In J. P. Kennedy & F. W. Blaisdell (Eds.), *Extremity trauma.* New York: Thieme.

function in an assistive capacity or be easier to use than any upper extremity prosthesis available to date. On the other hand, a severely compromised salvaged leg may not function as well as some of the lower extremity prostheses that are now available (Smith & Burgess, 1995). Amputation may be the most appropriate treatment when limb salvage conflicts with the primary goal of treatment—preservation of function. Occasionally, amputation may be delayed for several months as limb salvage is attempted, until the client can accept amputation as a viable option for treatment or the client is no longer willing to endure the interventions necessary for potential limb salvage.

Amputation can also be necessitated by thermal injuries (frostbite, burns, or electrocution). Frostbite is a thermal injury that can lead to gangrene in the digits and extremities. Exposure to cold temperatures can cause vascular impairment from vasoconstriction and endothelial vessel injury. Frostbite can occur in temperatures above freezing if wet extremities are exposed to cold. Treatment involves restoring core body temperature, then rewarming the injured body part in a water bath at 40° to 44°C for 20 to 30 minutes. Immediate amputation is avoided to allow for an area of demarcation to develop. The area of dry gangrene may be left in place for 2 to 6 months to allow for primary wound healing to take place. The affected tissue should be kept clean and dry (Smith & Burgess, 1995).

Metabolic Disease/Malignancy/Infection

Amputation can be necessitated by metabolic disorders (e.g., Paget's disease) and by massive muscle necrosis resulting from an acute embolic or thrombotic event. The 10- to 20-year-old group has the highest incidence of malignancy-related upper extremity amputations. Amputation for tumors of the bone or soft tissue is less common than in the past because of the development of sophisticated limb salvage procedures (see Chapter 22).

Gangrene. Gangrene can be acute or chronic. The type of onset (acute or chronic) is important because it helps establish the extent of the gangrene and the level of the amputation. Acute ischemia is generally the result of arterial embolism or thrombosis or major vascular injury. Because collateral circulation has not had time to develop, severe ischemia occurs rapidly, resulting in massive muscle necrosis. The significant muscle damage precludes salvage procedures, and most clients require amputation.

Chronic gangrene is usually caused by arteriosclerosis. As long as the gangrene is dry and not infected, it can be managed conservatively. *Wet gangrene* refers to gangrene with a superimposed infection. Tissue death is associated with severe pain, resulting in significant disability. Limb loss is likely from either progressive necrosis or superimposed infection that spreads through the ischemic tissue. Ischemic ulceration may be an indication for amputation, but amputation of a leg is rarely indicated for purely venous ulcers. When uncomplicated by arterial insufficiency, venous ulcers can be managed with conservative measures no matter how severe or infected.

Gas gangrene is an invasive, anaerobic infection of muscle characterized by extensive local edema, tissue necrosis, gas production, and toxemia. The cause is gram-positive bacilli (usually *Clostridium perfringens*). The incubation period is short (less than 3 days). Onset is sudden, with a rapidly progressive increase in severe pain. Localized edema and thin hemorrhagic exudate appear. Crepitus accompanies gas production but may not be prominent because of the infection and the deepness of the wound. If untreated, gas gangrene progresses rapidly and is usually fatal. Emergency treatment to surgically debride all involved muscle as well as to decompress involved muscle compartments by fasciotomy is essential. Amputation may be required to accomplish adequate debridement. For a detailed discussion of gas gangrene, see Chapter 23.

TREATMENT MODALITIES AND RELATED NURSING MANAGEMENT

Assessment

Nursing History. The client's history should include the mechanism of injury and the client's current and past health problems to ascertain the etiology of the present or impending amputation. Specific questions may include the following: Was the onset of symptoms sudden or chronic? Has the client undergone vascular or reconstructive surgery? Are draining, nonhealing ulcers or fistulas present? Is the client at risk for sepsis? Is the client able to ambulate? Are any assistive devices used? Is there any pain? Is the pain associated with walking? Is there a

pattern to the pain? Is the pain relieved by rest? Has the client noticed a loss of sensation or tingling in the feet? Is there a difference in sensation between the affected limb and the opposite limb? If the client is diabetic or has PVD, what is the current foot and lower extremity skin care? How does the client perceive the possibility or sudden necessity for amputation? Are there any religious or cultural constraints against amputation? Are there cultural or religious guidelines for handling the amputated parts? (Some cultural and religious groups require that amputated body parts be stored for burial with the body at the time of death.)

Physical Assessment. The physical examination should include determination of the neurovascular status of the affected extremity as well as evaluation of the functional status and condition of the opposite extremity. The nurse should observe the color and warmth of the extremity, palpate the pulses, and note capillary refill time. Further observation for discoloration of ankles, presence or absence and distribution of edema, skin integrity, ulceration, presence or absence and distribution of hair on the legs, and presence or absence of necrosis (gangrene) (Fig. 20-1) is also necessary. Capillary refill time may be difficult to evaluate in the older client because of thick, opaque nails. In this case, skin near the nail bed is assessed.

The elevation-dependency test is helpful in assessing collateral arterial blood supply. If there is rapid blanching with elevation and significant rubor when the leg is returned to a dependent position, poor collateral circulation is indicated (Haimovici, 1996).

If ulceration is present, the location, depth, and edges should be noted (Table 20-2). Arterial ulcers are usually deep, with well-defined margins, a pale interior, and some

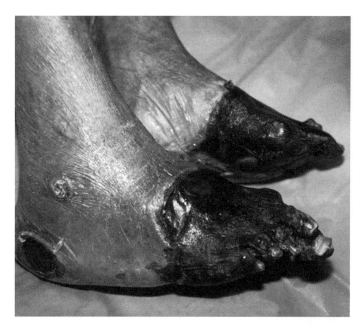

FIGURE 20-1. Bilateral lower extremity gangrene. Also note the dry, shiny, scaling skin; the absence of hair; and the pressure ulcers on the heel and malleolus. (Courtesy of V. Fahey, M.S., R.N., C.V.N., Advanced Practice Nurse, Vascular Service, Northwestern Memorial Hospital, Chicago, IL.)

TABLE 20–2. *Ulceration in Lower Extremities*

TYPE OF ULCER	CLIENT HISTORY	OBSERVATION	LOCATION OF ULCER	APPEARANCE OF ULCER	PHYSICAL ASSESSMENT	TREATMENT
Diabetic ulcer	Diabetes Peripheral neuropathy No complaints Claudication or rest pain Nonhealing, painless ulcer	Diminished capillary filling Thickened toenails Cellulitis (usually) Loss of hair on ankle, foot, and toes	Plantar area of foot Metatarsal heads Heel of foot (pressure points)	Same as arterial	Cool or warm foot Pulses may be present PVR shows normal arterial flow except distal (ankle transmetatarsal levels)	Rule out major arterial disease Control diabetes Provide client education Prevent infection Provide emotional support
Arterial	Less than two block claudication Rest pain Risk factors (2–3) Nonhealing, painful ulcer	Decreased or poor capillary filling Thickened toenail Ashen or blue foot Loss of hair on ankle, foot, and toes Dry, scaly skin Frank gangrene	End of toes Between toes	Deep, cavernous Pale Organized, even edges Minimal granulation tissue	Foot cold and blue Decreased or absent pulses at the DP and PT (palpable) with a Doppler PVR with decreased waveforms and pressures	Treat underlying cause (surgical revascularization angioplasty) Prevent infection Provide client education Provide emotional support
Venous stasis ulcers	No complaint of claudication or rest pain Complains of swelling No severe ulcer pain Previous history of ulcer	Normal capillary filling Edema at ankles Discoloration of ankle/ lower leg Hair present Dry, thin skin	Ankle area	Superficial, uneven edges Granulation tissue present	Warm foot Palpable pulses at DP/PT Normal PVR	Wound care (antibiotic ointment, Unna boot) Elevate extremity Provide client education Prevent infection Provide emotional support

DP, dorsalis pedis; PT, posterior tibial; PVR, pulse volume recordings.
From Waganer, M. M. (1986). Pathophysiology related to vascular disease. *Nursing Clinics of North America, 21*(2), 202.

necrotic tissue. Common sites are the toes, heels, and lateral malleolus. The client usually describes the pain as severe. With arterial involvement, expect to see dry, shiny skin without hair.

Venous stasis ulcers, located more commonly on the medial malleolus, tend to be shallow, with ragged edges, and often contain granulation tissue. Edema is typically present, and superficial veins are enlarged and tortuous. Pain is usually described as moderate rather than severe. Sensation in the affected limb should be assessed, comparing it with the opposite limb. Neurovascular assessment is discussed in detail in Chapter 8.

Diagnostic Evaluation. Diagnostic evaluation of the affected limb may include both invasive and noninvasive methods. Noninvasive modalities commonly used include measurement of the ankle-arm (ankle-brachial) index, Doppler ultrasonography, laser Doppler flowmetry, and transcutaneous oxygen pressure determination. The most common invasive method used is the angiogram. The ankle-arm index is the most widely used noninvasive test for evaluating PVD (Haimovici, 1996). Doppler ultrasonography evaluates blood flow to the extremities and can reliably distinguish exercise-related effects from severe ischemia. Angiography, Doppler studies, and transcutaneous O_2 pressure are among the most common diagnostic tests used. Angiography has not been helpful in predicting healing of amputations and is more useful if the client is a candidate for arterial reconstruction or angioplasty. Transcutaneous O_2 pressure and transcutaneous CO_2 have both been shown to be statistically significant in predicting amputation healing and are viewed by some clinicians as the gold standard for assessing blood supply and predicting healing potential of the residual limb (Smith & Burgess, 1995).

TECHNIQUES OF AMPUTATION

Amputation as a surgical procedure involves both plastic and reconstructive operations. Amputation may be open or closed. Open (guillotine) amputations are performed when the client has a fulminating infection that requires immediate treatment. The wound is left open, and skin flaps can be closed at a later time. Clients who are candidates for this procedure may have other debilitating illnesses that prevent the longer anesthesia time needed for a closed procedure. Traction can be applied to the skin flaps after open amputation to prevent retraction. If there are no tissue flaps, bone revision or skin grafting is necessary to obtain wound closure.

Closed amputation (also referred to as *flap,* or *myoplastic, amputation*) is the most common technique used when amputation is performed for vascular disease rather than trauma or infection. Skin flaps are prepared and closed over the site as part of the primary procedure. Complex reconstructive procedures, such as turn-up plasty to provide stump length and facilitate prosthesis wear, may be performed (Tronzo & Janek, 1995). Amputation may also be nonsurgical. Autoamputation involves allowing the gangrenous area to become well demarcated and eventually separate. This is usually reserved for small areas, such as individual digits or parts of digits. Physiologic freezing amputation is used for extremely unstable clients who are unable to undergo surgery. Once the client's condition stabilizes, a definitive amputation may be performed.

Selection of Amputation Level

Selection of the amputation level depends on both local factors (e.g., ischemia, gangrene) and systemic factors (e.g., cardiovascular status, renal function, severity of DM). The client's activity level, cognitive status, and ambulatory potential must also be considered. Although local signs provide the primary determination for level of amputation, poor or unstable general physical condition is an important consideration in the choice of surgical procedure. The objective is to amputate at the most distal level that will heal without infection and be functionally useful. More proximal amputations with the removal of more joints decreases the ability of the client to walk and live independently (Pinzur, 1997). In a child, amputation should be done with the goal of preserving all possible

epiphyses. If this is not done, progressive shortening of the stump follows. Figure 20–2 illustrates common amputation levels.

NURSING INTERVENTIONS IN THE PREOPERATIVE PERIOD

Esquenazi and Meier (1996) describe nine phases of amputee rehabilitation, beginning with the preoperative phase through acute postsurgical, preprosthetic, community integration, and follow-up phases. Interventions in the preoperative period fall under behavioral and physiologic (basic and complex) domains (McCloskey & Buelechek, 1995). This includes coping assistance, physical and psychological comfort promotion, activity and exercise enhancement, skin and wound management, and nutrition support.

Body Image Disturbance/Ineffective Individual Coping/Anticipatory Grieving Supportive Relationship

Coping Assistance

Whether the amputation is a result of trauma, an acute or chronic disease process, or malignant tumor, the client will need to adapt to the loss and change in body function and image. Anticipating surgery can be anxiety producing for any client. Therefore, each client should be given a basic explanation of what to expect and have their questions answered. Although there are common psychological adjustments all clients with amputation must make, there are specific issues and concerns that must be dealt with based on the reason for amputation (Fitzpatrick, 1999). The client's age, level of maturity, past experiences, resilience, personality traits, coping strategies, and quality of social support must be assessed. Preoperative preparation should include the introduction of a psychiatric advanced practice nurse or other mental health professional and information regarding type of procedure to be performed, how pain will be managed, the possibility of phantom sensations and phantom pain, rehabilitation strategies and goals, and sexuality (Fitzpatrick, 1999).

Clients with cancer and chronic disease have time before surgery to process the concept of amputation, which allows for the previously mentioned assessments to be done. Tumors requiring amputation usually occur in clients younger than 20 years of age when identity, sexuality, body image, and independence are most vulnerable. Peer support groups and honest straightforward communication about the situation and what to expect are strategies to use.

Clients undergoing amputation for disease (PVD) are usually older and may have significant comorbidities that will affect the psychological adjustment to amputation. It is best if the possibility of amputation is raised early to avoid suddenly raising the topic when the need for

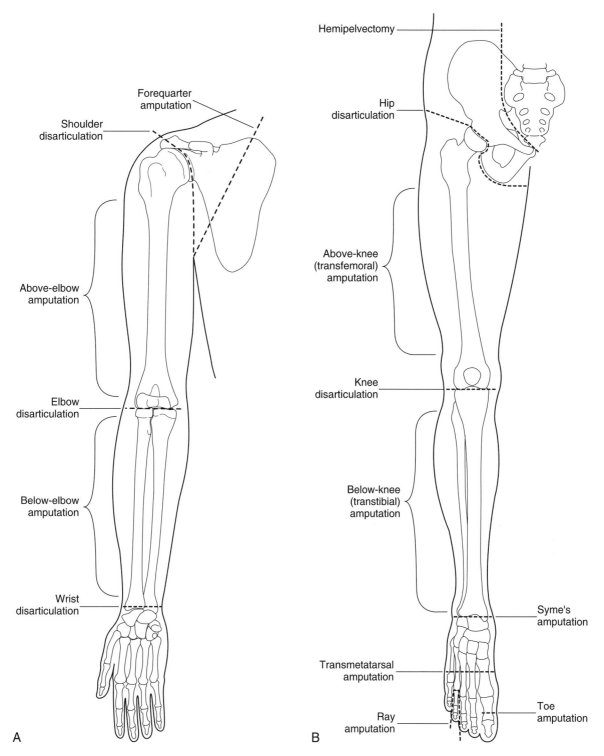

FIGURE 20–2. Levels of amputation. *A,* Upper extremity. *B,* Lower extremity.

amputation is impending so that the client is given time to work through the issues involved and come to a confident decision (Fitzpatrick, 1999). Grieving should be anticipated with all clients undergoing amputation. Clients can be expected to vacillate between the issues (stages) involved in grief and acceptance. Facilitating the grieving process promotes optimal recovery and rehabilitation of the client.

Pain

Physical and Psychological Comfort Promotion

Preemptive analgesia (i.e., administration of analgesics before incision) can prevent noxious stimuli from sensitizing the central cortex in the brain involved in the perception of pain (Katz, 1997). Studies have demonstrated that epidural analgesia before amputation, intra-operative epidural anesthesia, and postoperative analgesia for several days after surgery reduce the incidence and severity of stump and phantom pain (Jahanjiri, Jayatunga, Bradley, & Dark, 1994; Katz, 1997; Krane & Heller, 1995). However, Nikolajsen, Ilkjaer, Christensen, Kroner, and Jensen (1997) found that there was no difference in pain report for clients who received epidural analgesia 18 hours preoperatively and those who did not. Findings from studies about preemptive analgesia are summarized in the evidence-based practice table in this chapter. More research is needed in this area. Anxiety can contribute to pain intensity in all clients as they contemplate the potential effects of the amputation on their lives. For a discussion of pain management techniques, refer to Chapter 5.

Activity Intolerance/Disuse Syndrome

Exercise Promotion and Exercise Therapy: Joint Mobility

The client should be encouraged to perform regular active range-of-motion exercises in unaffected extremities and joints above the affected area so that muscle mass and mobility will be at optimal levels when rehabilitation begins. In this respect, clients can participate in a strengthening program for the upper extremities so that they are well conditioned for walker or crutch use after surgery. A physical therapist can also design a program for the client to correct or prevent contractures and to increase trunk mobility to assist with sitting balance, rolling, and moving in the sitting position.

High Risk for Impaired Skin Integrity

Skin Surveillance/Pressure Ulcer Prevention and Care

For clients with PVD, measures should be taken to minimize skin breakdown. Placing a cradle on the bed keeps the bed linen off the toes and allows less pressure on the heels. The client should be instructed to refrain from using the heels to push up in bed. The ulcerated areas should be covered with sterile dressings, and the heels should be kept off the bed by supporting the thighs and lower legs on blankets or pillows, leaving the heels free. Heel protectors that do not have elastic bands for securing them in place can also be applied. Pulses or arterial blood flows in clients with arterial disease should be checked every 6 months.

The feet and toes need to be inspected daily for any cracks or breaks in the skin. Preexisting ulcers or wounds should be monitored for changes in odor, color, and consistency of drainage. To control infection, systemic antibiotics are administered. Whirlpool treatments or dressing changes or both may be prescribed for debridement and wound cleansing. The client must be advised to always put on slippers when getting out of bed to prevent injury to the feet. The client care area should be kept as free of obstacles as possible.

Altered Nutrition: Less Than Body Requirements

Nutritional Management

Infection in the affected extremity, accompanied by systemic disease or multisystem injuries, can increase metabolic demands on the client, requiring more than the usual amount of calories. Proper nutrition is essential for maintenance of skin and tissue integrity as well as for wound healing. To promote adequate nutrition, monitoring protein intake, consulting with a registered dietitian, or providing nutritional supplements may be necessary. Serum albumin level less than 3.5 g/dL and total lymphocyte count less than 1500 cells/mm^3 are significant indicators for wound failure (Smith & Burgess, 1995). Vitamin C and iron are necessary for improving the oxygen-carrying capacity of the blood.

NURSING INTERVENTIONS IN THE POSTOPERATIVE PERIOD

Rehabilitation of the client begins within the first 24 hours of surgery. The goals are to (1) reduce edema and promote healing, (2) prevent contractures and the complications of bed rest, (3) increase strength and facilitate adjustment to the loss, and (4) maximize functional independence (Pandian & Kowalske, 1999). Interventions as described in the preoperative section may continue through the postoperative period.

Body Image Disturbance

Body Image Enhancement

Body image develops and changes as the physical body changes. Limb amputation requires body image reintegration. Adjusting to a traumatic amputation is often more difficult than adjusting to a planned one, and younger clients can find the task more difficult than do older clients. Body image concerns are related to fears about physical changes, pain, and mutilation. See Chapter 2 for a discussion of body image.

Alteration in Skin Integrity/Altered Peripheral Tissue Perfusion

---

Circulatory Care/Peripheral Sensation Management

Care of the Intact Lower Extremity. Because such a large percentage of lower extremity amputations are due to PVD with or without diabetes, protective measures must be taken to decrease the risk of amputation of the intact lower extremity. Many clients who have undergone amputations secondary to PVD require amputation of the opposite leg within several years. Therefore, protective measures, as described previously, must be taken.

Care of the opposite extremity is essential to maintain skin integrity and function of the remaining foot. Careful cutting of toenails, treatment of fungus infection, application of skin softeners to dry skin to prevent cracking, and placement of cotton wedges between toes to keep them separated and dry protect the foot. Shoes should be appropriately modified by an orthotist to include molded inserts and extra depth to evenly distribute body weight during ambulation.

Stump Care (Table 20–3). Stump hygiene, consisting of good skin care as well as maintenance of stump socks, elastic wraps, and sockets, is essential in avoiding breakdown. A daily routine of skin cleansing with soap and water, preferably at night, must be instituted. The stump must be dried thoroughly before any shrinkage device is applied. The client and family should be instructed to inspect the stump daily for redness, abrasion, and irritation.

Each client must learn how to massage the stump area to help desensitize the residual limb. Stump massage should begin 3 weeks after surgery. Clients with adherent scar tissue must learn techniques of friction massage to help break up the adhesions. It is essential that the skin be mobilized so that it does not adhere to the underlying tissue because it can tear when stressed by prosthetic wear.

Any open areas along the residual limb should be aired, for example, for 1-hour periods four times per day. If the area is infected, a whirlpool can be used for cleansing and debridement.

The stump socks and elastic wraps worn by the client must be changed daily and washed with mild soap and water. They must be allowed to dry completely before being worn again. Once prosthetic training begins, the socket must be washed regularly with soap and water and dried thoroughly before wearing. This should be done at night to allow thorough drying and should be done daily in hot weather.

A number of dermatologic lesions can occur with prosthesis wear. Epidermoid cysts are common. They occur at the prosthetic socket brim, are difficult to treat, and are usually the result of pressure. Socket modification is necessary to resolve this problem (Smith & Burgess, 1995). Verrucous hyperplasia can be a painful condition characterized by a wartlike overgrowth of skin that can progress to fissuring, oozing, and infection. It is caused by a lack of distal contact between the stump and the prosthetic socket (Smith & Burgess, 1995).

Abrasions, blisters, and hair follicle infections also occur as a result of pressure and an ill-fitting prosthesis (Stokosa, 1996). The nurse should observe for these skin lesions, especially in clients who wear prostheses but may not be seeking amputation-related treatment at the time of admission or contact. Clients should be instructed to watch for these complications and report them to the prosthetist.

TABLE 20–3. *Client Education: Amputation*

FOCUS	TEACHING POINTS
Care of the intact lower extremity	Do not use heel of intact lower extremity to push up in bed; use trapeze
	Protect heel of intact lower extremity with padding
	Careful foot care is essential. Cut toenails carefully, prevent or treat fungal infection, apply skin softeners to prevent cracking, place cotton wedges between toes to separate and keep dry
Stump care	Cleanse daily with soap and warm water; dry thoroughly before replacing shrinkage device
	Inspect daily for redness, abrasions, or irritation
	Massage stump end to help desensitize the residual limb and prevent scar tissue formation
	Any open areas on the residual limb should be aired for 1 hr qid
	Stump socks and elastic wraps must be changed daily and washed with mild soap and water
Phantom limb sensation and phantom limb pain	Almost all clients experience phantom limb sensation. It occurs in early postoperative period and is usually self-limiting
	Phantom limb sensation is usually felt in the phantom foot in lower extremity amputations and in the phantom hand in upper extremity amputations
	Phantom limb pain can occur immediately after surgery or 2–3 months after amputation. It is more severe in above-the-knee amputations and usually occurs when the amputation was delayed and the client was in severe pain preoperatively
	Almost 80% of amputation clients experience phantom limb pain, but it is severe in only about 1%
	Type of pain and precipitating factors vary
	Treatment includes drugs, measures to desensitize the stump, transcutaneous electrical nerve stimulation, biofeedback, hypnosis, imagery
	Surgery is considered only if conservative measures do not provide relief

Comfort Promotion/Medication Management

Postoperative Pain. The pain and anxiety experienced in the immediate postoperative period must be managed adequately. Opioid analgesics administered in a variety of routes are most effective at this time. See Chapter 5 for a discussion on the management of postoperative pain.

Chronic Stump Pain. Neuropathic pain due to neuroma formation can produce severe burning and lancinating pain. Clients may also experience allodynia (touch-evoked pain). This can be treated with opioids, antidepressants, anticonvulsants, phenothiazines, nerve blocks, transcutaneous electrical nerve stimulation (TENS), and even revision of the stump. Zuniga, Schlicht, Christian, and Abram (2000) report that intrathecal baclofen provides significant relief from neuropathic stump pain and allodynia with minimal use of adjuvant medications and no further need for opioids. Measures to desensitize the stump include superficial and deep kneading massage, progressively more vigorous tapping, and spraying the stump with ethyl chloride spray. Early prosthetic use can reduce the incidence of phantom limb pain (PLP). Therefore, early intensive rehabilitation is important. Sympathetic blocking agents, acupuncture, ultrasonography, and injection with local anesthetics are also helpful. Capsaicin cream has been used as a topical agent for the relief of residual limb pain (Cannon & Wu, 1998).

Phantom Limb Pain. PLP must be distinguished from phantom limb sensation. From 70% to 100% of amputees experience phantom limb sensation (i.e., the perception of the limb without pain). Sensations may include tingling, numbness, pins and needles, burning, cramping, squeezing, or itching (Montoya, Larbig, Grulke, Flor, Taub, & Birbaumer, 1997). Phantom limb sensation occurs early in the postoperative course and is self-limiting, although it can last for decades in some clients. In the case of lower extremity amputation, the client usually feels sensation in the phantom foot. In the upper extremity, sensation is felt in a phantom hand. Over time, the sensation diminishes, and the client feels as if the hand or foot is floating in midair. About 30% of clients experience the telescoping phenomenon, a shrinking or retraction of the amputated part into the stump (Montoya et al., 1997). The last sensation to disappear is that of the thumb or index finger or the great toe. If the phantom limb sensation is painful or unpleasant, it is referred to as *PLP.*

Most sources state that clients with congenital limb deficiencies or those who have had surgical or traumatic amputation before age 6 do not usually experience phantom limb sensation, but Melzack (1992) disputes this. He reports phantom sensations in children who have lost limbs at age 2 or younger, as well as in children with congenital limb deficiencies.

PLP occurs in 60% to 85% of clients (Montoya et al., 1997). The pain may diminish over time, but in 5% to 10% of clients, the pain may persist and even worsen over time (Nikolajasen et al., 1997). Nursing interventions for PLP include physical and psychological comfort promotion and medication management. PLP is a complication that can appear soon after surgery or as late as 2 to 3 months after surgery. It is more severe in above-the-knee amputation and usually occurs when the amputation is delayed and the client experiences severe pain associated with gangrene.

The pain experienced varies among clients and includes cramping, electric shocks, feeling of stabbing from knives or hot needles, and burning of phantom limb and foot. The pain can be triggered in a variety of ways. It may be precipitated or intensified by any contact, not necessarily painful, with the stump or a trigger point on the trunk, contralateral limb, or head. Other activities that can precipitate pain include urination, defecation, sexual intercourse, angina pectoris, and cigarette smoking.

Clients with an amputation resulting from trauma can experience severe, local, burning pain associated with trophic changes in the remaining part of the limb. These symptoms are considered part of the syndrome known as *complex regional pain syndrome* and should be treated as such. For a discussion of complex regional pain syndrome, see Chapter 5.

Theories of Phantom Limb Pain. No single unifying theory of pain satisfactorily explains PLP or predicts who develops it, but several theories have attempted to do so. These theories include the peripheral nervous system theory, the central nervous system theory, and the psychological theory.

The peripheral nerve theory states that PLP is the result of excitation of nerve endings in the stump and can be triggered by neuroma formation, scar tissue, or stump infection. However, neuroma excision or other local surgery is rarely successful in relieving pain.

The central nervous system theory that is most widely recognized is the one proposed by Melzack (1992). He states that phantom limbs originate primarily in the brain, but more than the somatosensory system is involved. He postulates a network of neurons that "in addition to responding to sensory stimulation, continuously generates a characteristic pattern of impulses indicating that the body is intact and unequivocally one's own." If somatosensory input was absent, this pattern of impulses, or neurosignature, would create the sense of an intact limb even after the limb had been removed. Such a matrix would be extensive, and Melzack proposes at least three major neural circuits in the brain: (1) sensory pathways passing through the thalamus to the somato-sensory cortex, (2) pathways leading through the reticular formation of the brainstem to the limbic system, and (3) cortical regions important to recognition of self and to the evaluation of sensory signals. The connections of the matrix are determined primarily genetically and are shaped by experience. This theory explains, for example, why clients who experience severe pain before amputation can suffer similar pain in the phantom—the matrix would have stored the pain memory.

The psychological theory is the most controversial as a major influencing factor. Early studies suggested that emotional factors contributed to the prolonged pain in a phantom limb, which could be prevented if clients were encouraged to express grief over their loss. Pucher, Kickinger, and Frischenschlager (1999) found that clients who coped better with the loss of the limb suffered less from PLP. Conversely, they also found that clients who saw their bodies as a complete undamaged entity suffered more PLP. Angrilli and Koster (2000) reported that PLP was associated with long-term emotional memory of painful experience of the amputation. Other researchers found no relation between the experience of pain and emotional distress (Fisher & Hanspal, 1998). It must be remembered, however, that there is an emotional component that is an integral part of the pain experience.

Pain Management (Phantom Limb Pain). As discussed previously, preoperative management of pain particularly via epidural analgesia will result in the client being less likely to experience severe PLP. Pharmacologic treatment for PLP includes beta-blockers, anticonvulsants, tricyclic antidepressants, and neuroleptics. They can be used alone or in combinations if a client experiences several kinds of pain (e.g., cramping pain and stabbing pain). Table 20–4 outlines dosage recommendations, monitoring parameters, and adverse reactions to these drugs.

Traditionally, opioids have not been recommended for chronic pain management and may provide little relief for PLP because they do not alter the response of afferent nerve endings to noxious stimulation. Their primary use should be for the management of early postoperative stump pain. However, they may be considered in the management of chronic pain. Beta-blockers, such as propranolol, are thought to increase serotonin levels, which in turn prevent pain transmission to the brain. They are given for pain that is a constant, dull, burning ache.

Anticonvulsants, such as phenytoin, carbamazepine, and gabapentin, are used for stabbing pain, and baclofen is used for control of spasms and cramps in the phantom limb. Tricyclic antidepressants, such as amitriptyline, doxepin, imipramine, desipramine, nortriptyline, and trazodone, improve mood and alleviate insomnia. They also increase serotonin levels in brain tissue. Controversy surrounds the use of neuroleptics, such as chlorproma-zine, the effect of which is sedative rather than analgesic. Neuroleptics alter pain centrally while acting peripherally to stabilize membranes, as local anesthetics do.

TENS can provide effective short-term relief. TENS is thought to activate afferent fibers within the nerve, which stimulates inhibitory activity from the brainstem. Some studies show TENS to be effective in 25% of clients. Poor efficacy of TENS may be due to depletion of the endorphin antinociceptive mechanisms (Gnezdilov, Syrovegin, Plaksin, Ovechkin, & Sul'timov, 1995). For more information on TENS, see Chapter 5.

A variety of surgical procedures, including cordotomy, deep brain stimulation, spinal cord stimulation, and sympathectomy, may be tried, but none provide permanent relief. Surgery should never be considered until all conservative measures are exhausted. Alternative interventions, such as biofeedback, hypnosis, imagery, and distraction therapy, may be helpful. Referral to a pain clinic for a comprehensive management program may be indicated.

Impaired Physical Mobility/Self-care Deficits

Promotion of Mobility. Key indicators of rehabilitation potential seem to be mental status and level of functioning before amputation. Most older clients should be considered appropriate for prosthetic training even though their ultimate level of functioning may not be as high as that of younger clients.

When considering clients with lower extremity amputations, those who can use walkers or crutches satisfactorily should be able to make good progress with prostheses. The increased energy requirements necessary for a lower extremity prosthesis must be considered in the overall decision-making process. The older client with a transfemoral amputation must put forth an effort equaling 68% to 100% above normal to walk at a reduced speed (Esquenazi & Meier, 1996). Older clients with bilateral transtibial and transfemoral amputations require overwhelming energy levels for ambulation, thereby making wheelchair locomotion a strong alternative. The energy expenditure associated with wheelchair locomotion is low and requires only minimal effort by the client. Because clients with PVD have a high incidence of coronary artery disease, exercise testing is indicated in all vascular disease amputee clients before beginning an exercise training and a prosthetic rehabilitation program (Roth, Park, & Sullivan, 1998).

For clients with upper extremity amputations, motivation is a strong determining factor in potential success. Because the upper extremity prosthesis is more difficult to use than the lower extremity prosthesis, can be cosmetically less appealing than the lower extremity prosthesis, and is less likely to be used functionally if the unaffected extremity is functional, motivation is key. For these reasons, many clients with upper extremity amputa-

TABLE 20–4. *Pharmacologic Treatment of Phantom Limb Pain*

DRUG	DOSAGE	MONITORING PARAMETERS AND ADVERSE REACTIONS
Beta-Blockers		
Propranolol metoprolol	40–240 mg/day 100–300 mg/day	Hypotension, atrioventricular nodal block or brady-cardia, nightmares, fatigue, bronchospasm in asthma clients, exacerbation of congestive heart failure, mask of hypoglycemic symptoms in diabetics, and decreased glomerular filtration rate in renal dysfunction
Anticonvulsants		
Gabapentin	100 mg bid or tid, titrate up as needed for pain relief	Somnolence, dizziness, ataxia, weight gain, nystagmus, tremor, edema. Most disturbing to patients is "feeling totally out of it"
Carbamazepine	Initiate at 100–200 mg bid or tid. Average dose: 400–600 mg/day. Titrate up to 1800 mg/day. When pain is relieved, the dosage should be decreased to the lowest effective dose. Drug withdrawal should be attempted because some clients do not have recurrence	Drowsiness, ataxia, confusion, hematopoietic disorders (monitor weekly for 1 mo, then monthly), aplastic anemia, agranulocytes, thrombocytopenia, and pancytopenia
Phenytoin	300–600 mg/day; levels greater than 20 g/m^2 associated with increased toxicity	Ataxia, nystagmus, hematopoietic disorders, and gingival hyperplasia. Drug serum levels are useful in determining toxicity and may be helpful in determining how high doses may be titrated. Levels are decreased with hypoalbuminemia
Clonazepam	Initiate at 0.5 mg/day orally at bedtime. Increase by 0.5-mg increments weekly to 2.5–4 mg/day orally at bedtime	Nonlancinating pain persists. Drowsiness, lethargy, and occasionally, changes in bladder control
Antidepressants		
Desipramine or nortriptyline	Initiate at 25 mg/day and titrate to lack of pain	Do not give if history of seizures or cardiac disease
Amitriptyline	Initiate therapy at 25–50 mg/day, and titrate to lack of pain. Maximum of 300 mg/day. Give dose at bedtime	Sedation and anticholinergic side effects are high; serotonin effects are high. Monitor for cardiac effects in older clients or those with arrhythmia
Doxepin	Initiate dose at 50 mg/day, and titrate to lack of pain. Maximum of 300 mg/day. Give dose at bedtime	
Imipramine	Initiate at 50 mg/day, and titrate to lack of pain. Maximum of 300 mg/day	
Trazodone	Initiate at 200 mg/day, and titrate to lack of pain. Generally, maximum of 600 mg/day	Increased antianxiety activity. Lower anticholinergic, cardiotoxic, and sedative effects. Efficacy may be lower than other agents, and dosage may be very cautiously advanced to 1200 mg/day

Adapted from Iacono, R. R., & Linford, J. (1989). Pain management after lower extremity amputation. In W. S. Moore & J. M. Malone (Eds.), *Lower extremity amputation* (p. 223). Philadelphia: WB Saunders.

tions opt for nonfunctioning prosthesis with a cosmetic hand. The energy expenditure necessary for upper extremity prosthetic wear is generally not an important factor to consider because most upper extremity amputations are traumatic and occur in people who are otherwise young and healthy. See the section "Prostheses" in this chapter for a detailed discussion of this topic.

Exercise Therapy

Exercises to increase the muscular strength and flexibility of the residual limb and the remaining extremities must be initiated as soon as possible after surgery. The client must be evaluated by the physical therapist to determine the level of muscle strength and flexibility, and the goals of exercise must be established accordingly. Exercises done two times per day in the supine and prone positions increase the strength and flexibility of the hip flexors, extensors, abductors, and adductors and knee flexors and extensors (for transtibial amputations).

Clients can also participate in a group exercise or a pool program for the upper and lower extremities. These exercise groups help add variety to the rehabilitation process and allow interaction among clients with similar problems. A pool program is an excellent means of

EXAMINING THE EVIDENCE: Moving Toward Evidence-Based Practice
In Lower Extremity Amputation, Does Preoperative, Perioperative, and Postoperative Epidural or Regional Analgesia Help Prevent Phantom Limb Pain?

AUTHOR(S), YEAR	SAMPLE SIZE	DIAGNOSIS	DESIGN	OUTCOME VARIABLE	MAJOR FINDINGS
Nikolajsen et al., 1997	60 patients	Lower limb amputation	Random assignment: Group I—epidural bupivacaine and morphine 18 hr before and during the operation Group II—epidural saline and oral or IM morphine All patients had general anesthesia	Rate of stump and phantom pain, intensity of stump and phantom pain, consumption of opioids at 1 week and 3, 6, and 12 months	Intensity of stump and phantom pain and consumption of opioids were similar in both groups at all four postoperative interviews
Jahangiri et al., 1994	24 patients	Lower limb amputation	Prospective controlled study: Study group—epidural of bupivacaine, clonidine, and diamorphine 24–48 hours preoperatively and 3 days postoperatively Control group—on-demand opioid analgesia	Pain intensity on visual analogue scale at 7 days and 6 and 12 months	At 1 year—1 patient in the study group and 2 patients in the control group had phantom pain
Pinzur et al., 1996	21 patients	Lower limb amputation because of ischemic necrosis secondary to PVD	Prospective, randomized: Regional anesthetic at sciatic or posterior tibial nerve Group A—postoperative continuous infusion of bupivacaine for 72 hours Group B—postoperative continuous infusion of normal saline for 72 hours	Use of opioids postamputation	Group A used less morphine during the first and second days after surgery No difference between groups on third day Intervention did not prevent residual or phantom limb pain at 3- and 6-month intervals
Elizaga et al., 1994	59 patients	Lower extremity amputation	Retrospective, unblinded, controlled (postoperative pain), and unblinded questionnaire and interview (phantom pain) 19 bupivacaine treated 40 nonbupivacaine treated 9 treated and 12 untreated patients interviewed for phantom pain assessment	Relief of postoperative pain and incidence and characteristics of phantom limb pain 6 months after surgery	No difference between the treated and control groups for opioid requirements and phantom limb pain
Katsuly-Liapis et. al., 1996	45 patients	Lower limb amputation	Random design, three groups: A—preemptive epidural analgesia 3 days before surgery with bupivacaine 0.25% and morphine Continued 72 hours postoperatively B—opioids and NSAIDs administered by nonepidural routes and postoperative epidural analgesia C—opioids and NSAIDs preoperatively and postoperatively	Incidence of phantom limb pain	1 week—3 patients in group A, 7 patients in group B, and 10 patients in group C reported phantom limb pain 6 months—1 patient in group A, 7 patients in group B, and 6 patients in group C reported phantom limb pain ($p < .01$) 1 year—2 patients in groups B and C reported phantom limb pain; none in group A

Box continued on following page

EXAMINING THE EVIDENCE: Moving Toward Evidence-Based Practice
In Lower Extremity Amputation, Does Preoperative, Perioperative, and Postoperative Epidural or Regional Analgesia Help Prevent Phantom Limb Pain? **Continued**

AUTHOR(S), YEAR	SAMPLE SIZE	DIAGNOSIS	DESIGN	OUTCOME VARIABLE	MAJOR FINDINGS
Bach et. al., 1988	25 patients	Lower limb (transtibial) amputation because of ischemia secondary to PVD	Prospective study Only patients with preoperative pain responsive to epidural analgesia were included Group 1—epidural analgesia with 0.25% bupivacaine and morphine begun 3 days preoperatively Group 2—opioids, NSAIDs, and other analgesics preoperatively All patients had epidural/spinal anesthesia	Presence of phantom limb pain, PLS, or stump pain	1 week–3 patients in group 1 and 9 patients in group 2 reported phantom limb pain (p < .10) 6 months–0 patients in group 1 and 5 patients in group 2 reported phantom limb pain (p < .05) 1 year–0 patients in group 1 and 3 patients in group 2 reported phantom limb pain (p < .20)

PVD, peripheral vascular disease; PLS, phantom limb sensation.

Discussion: The study by Bach et al. (1988) is a classic one that sparked ongoing research and discussion on preventing phantom limb pain (PLP) through preemptive analgesia. The study is based on Melzack's neuromatrix theory, which describes an integrated pathway that consists of both central and peripheral nervous system input contributing to "somatosensory memory" of pain. Katsuly-Liapis et al.'s (1996) study closely resembles Bach et al.'s study. A 72-hour postoperative epidural analgesia arm was added to the protocol. Results for both studies found preemptive epidural analgesia to significantly reduce or prevent PLP. Jahangiri et al.'s (1994) study resulted in similar findings, but the subjects were not randomized to groups. There are differences to note in the studies that do not support these findings. In Nikolajsen et al.'s (1997) study, the length of time for preemptive epidural analgesia was reduced to 18 hours. Pinzur et al. (1996) and Elizaga et al. (1994) investigated the effect of postoperative regional analgesia only. From this brief review, the conclusion is that preemptive analgesia for at least 24 to 48 hours before amputation is effective in reducing or preventing PLP and that postoperative efforts alone have no effect. Further randomized studies using larger sample sizes are needed to determine whether preemptive analgesia to prevent PLP is effective. This is particularly important because health care dollars are being reduced. The cost of hospitalization and an invasive and expensive procedure before amputation surgery must be evaluated against the cost of a lifetime of managing PLP. Further questions include the following:

How significantly does the presence of pain before amputation influence the development of PLP?

Does preemptive analgesia in the absence of preoperative pain prevent the development of PLP?

Is preemptive analgesia effective only for patients with ischemic lower extremities because of chronic PVD?

---

exercise for the client with an amputation. The water's buoyancy makes it an assistive device, but it can also be a means of resistive exercise. A pool can be used effectively to promote muscle endurance, strength, balance, coordination, and mobility.

Amputation Care

In the first 24 hours postoperatively, the lower extremity residual limb may be elevated to reduce swelling. Subsequently, the limb should remain fully extended to prevent hip and knee contractures. Contractures at the hip and knee can be the result of poor positioning and insufficient range of motion of the residual limb. Therefore, appropriate positioning techniques, including the avoidance of excessive hip abduction, flexion, and external rotation for clients with above-the-knee amputations and prolonged knee flexion in clients with transtibial amputations, must be instituted. Clients should lie prone at least 10 minutes twice a day and a knee immobilizer may be used to maintain knee extension in clients with transtibial amputations (Pandian & Kowalske, 1999). Clients should not be allowed to remain in semi-Fowler's or Fowler's positions for extended periods. In addition, stretching the musculature that crosses the remaining joints is essential. Flexion contractures of the elbow in transradial amputation should be prevented by initiating

physical or occupational therapy as soon as possible after surgery (Smith & Burgess, 1995).

Stump Shrinkage

Several types of shrinkage devices are available to decrease edema and shape the limb for prosthetic wear. Common shrinkage devices include elastic bandages, shrinker socks, and removable rigid dressings.

Elastic bandages are still the most commonly used support to control edema and shape the limb. They allow easy removal if frequent inspection of the wound is required. Unfortunately, they are probably the least effective of the shrinkage devices. They require frequent reapplication and often cause edema from proximal constriction because of improper application. Any client who has difficulty with the appropriate wrapping technique of the residual limb or who has visual or sensory limitations should choose another type of shrinkage device. If this technique of stump shrinkage is found to be feasible for the client, the appropriate size wrap must be used. For the below-the-knee stump, double-length 4-inch wraps are used, and for the above-the-knee stump, double-length 6-inch wraps are used to ensure complete coverage of the stump. Elastic wraps should be applied so that they provide the greatest compression at the distal end of the stump and decrease pressure proximally along

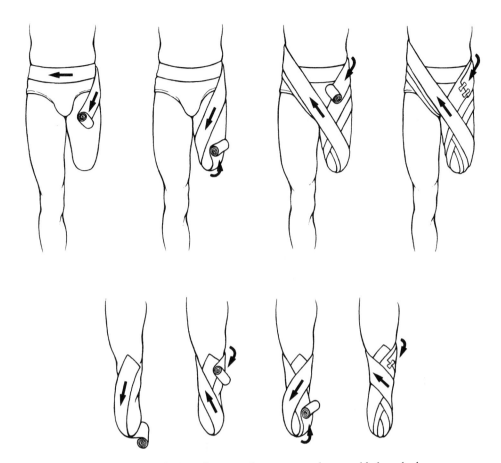

FIGURE 20–3. Technique for wrapping a stump above and below the knee.

the stump. The wrap should be applied in a figure-of-eight pattern, not in cylindrical rings, around the stump (Fig. 20-3). The advantages of this shrinkage method include low cost to the client and ease of availability for the rehabilitation staff.

Shrinker socks are another type of device used by clients with amputations. Stump shrinkers are useful with transfemoral amputation and on transtibial dressings after the rigid dressing has been removed (Pandian & Kowalske, 1999). The socks come in a variety of sizes, lengths, and materials for both transfemoral and transtibial residual limbs. These socks have the advantages of being relatively easy to apply and providing uniform compression of the stump (Fig. 20-4). Commercial shrinker socks have the disadvantages of being limited in available sizes and lengths and are not suitable for obese clients with short residual limbs or for children. They are difficult to size and must be changed as the residual limb shrinks. They are more expensive than elastic wraps.

Elastic stockinette, available in rolls in various sizes and traditionally used under casts, can be used effectively for controlling edema and shaping residual limbs. The advantages are that it is less expensive and is easily applied. Desired pressure gradients can be achieved by applying layers as needed (Wu, 1996).

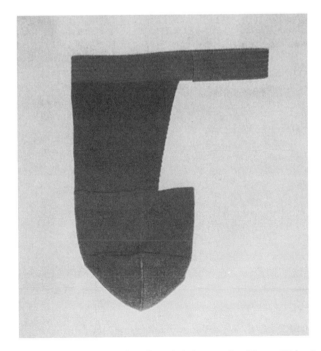

FIGURE 20–4. Example of a shrinker sock. (From Helt, J. [1988]. Amputation in the vascular patient. In V. A. Fahey [Ed.], *Vascular nursing* [p. 461]. Philadelphia: WB Saunders.)

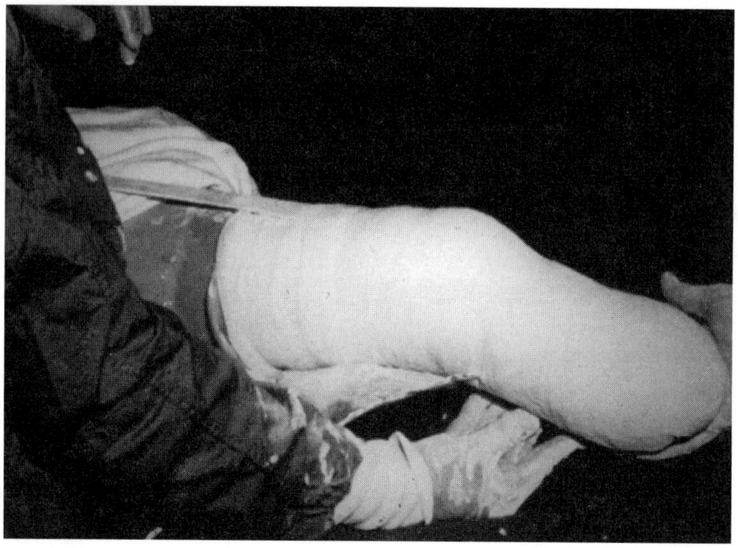

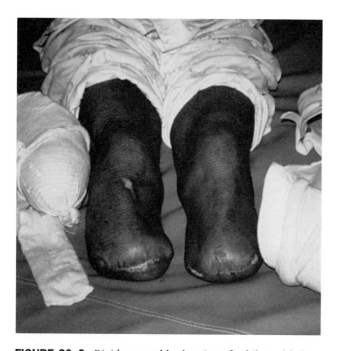

FIGURE 20–5. Rigid stump dressing applied in the operating room.

Another type of shrinkage device is the rigid dressing, which is made of a plaster cast and may be suspended by a stockinette, strap, or harness (Fig. 20-5). The advantages of this method include the elimination of the need for rewrapping (such as is necessary with elastic wraps), the reduction of distal edema, the prevention of trauma to the residual limb, and the ability to bear weight on the stump early. The stump also matures more rapidly, and hematomas are less likely to develop. Rigid removable dressings for transtibial amputation protect the limb and begin to shape it but also allow easy access for wound inspection (Wu, 1996) (Fig. 20-6).

For the shrinkage device to be of benefit to the client, it must be worn continuously and removed only for washing. Once prosthetic training has begun, the shrinkage device must be applied whenever the prosthesis is not being worn. Clients who have difficulty with skin irritation because of frequent applications of the shrinkage device should wear a nylon sock next to the skin.

The client should be observed when applying the shrinkage device to assess the technique and to provide further teaching if the technique is incorrect. Clients who will eventually have a prosthetic limb must continue wearing a shrinkage device until they are regularly wearing the definitive prosthesis. Clients who are not prosthesis candidates should continue to wear a shrinkage device until stump edema and pain are well controlled.

AMPUTATIONS IN CHILDREN

The prosthetic management of the juvenile client with an amputation is essentially the same as that of the adult. Prosthetic components are often scaled-down adult models. The amputation site in a child heals rapidly. By having an immediate postsurgical prosthetic fitting, the child feels little pain and is soon walking. Maturation of the stump is rapid, and definitive prosthetic fitting is done earlier than in the older client. Unique concerns with the growing child include skill development, psychosocial issues, family roles, and growth.

Children learn to ambulate quickly with lower extremity prostheses but require careful instruction with upper extremity prostheses so that they can derive maxi-

FIGURE 20–6. Rigid removable dressings for bilateral below-the-knee amputation. Note the prosthetic stump sock, below-the-knee plaster cast covered by suspension stockinette, and supracondylar suspension cuff. (Courtesy of Northwestern University School of Orthotics and Prosthetics and the Rehabilitation Institute of Chicago.)

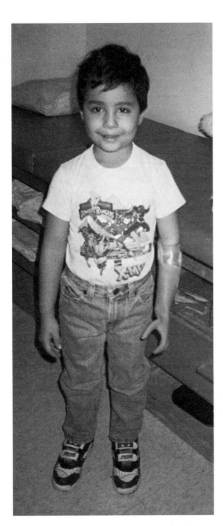

FIGURE 20–7. Child with myoelectric upper extremity prosthesis. (Courtesy of the amputee clinic, Rehabilitation Institute of Chicago.)

mal control and function. Parents should be included in therapy and instructional sessions so that they can reinforce proper use of the prosthesis. Few children are born with congenital absence of a hand. In this case, early fitting with a myoelectric hand prosthesis (Fig. 20–7) between the ages of 9 and 16 months is recommended to achieve the best results developmentally (Billock, 1995).

The major complication of juvenile amputation is bony overgrowth, which occurs most often in the humerus, fibula, and tibia. This disproportionate growth between the bone and skin is not related to longitudinal epiphyseal growth but rather to appositional bone growth. The earlier the amputation in life, the more likely this complication will occur. Treatment is by stump revision and removal of overgrowth. Other complications seen frequently in the older client, such as phantom pain, neuroma, and skin breakdown, are relatively rare in the pediatric client. For a more complete discussion of amputations in children, see Jain (1996).

PROSTHESES

Rehabilitation of the client with an amputation is a team effort by the client, nurse, physician, prosthetist, physical therapist, occupational therapist, social worker, psychologist, and vocational counselor. These specialized disciplines provide a comprehensive approach to the physical, emotional, financial, and social components of limb amputation. A detailed prosthetic prescription includes physical, surgical, and prosthetic factors; preprosthetic training; prosthetic fabrication; prosthetic training; and follow-up assessments of the fit, alignment, and appearance of the prosthesis.

Early walking aids (EWAs) are pneumatic devices that fit over the stump in the immediate postoperative period to allow for early walking, reduction of postoperative swelling, and improved client morale. An EWA device that allows for flexion and extension of the knee during walking allows the client to develop a more natural gait (Scott, Condie, Treweek, & Sockalingham, 2000). Immediate postoperative prosthetic fitting (IPOP) decreases the time to limb maturation and definitive prosthetic fitting (Fig. 20–8). In lower extremity amputations, clients may start weight bearing about 2 weeks after surgery if the wound demonstrates adequate healing. In the upper extremity, IPOP may be applied immediately. IPOP is believed to increase acceptance and use of the prosthesis (Smith & Burgess, 1995; Stokosa, 1996).

Determinants for prosthetic use include status of the residual limb, preoperative activity level, cardiopulmonary status, cognitive status, and motivation to use the prosthesis. Medicare has published a five-level classification system on which physicians and prosthetists must base the amputee's rehabilitation potential. This affects coverage for the type of prosthesis that is prescribed (Table 20-5). Special consideration must be made for bilateral amputees.

The type of prosthesis selected for the client with an amputation depends on the level of amputation and the client's lifestyle and occupation. The type of suspension system, artificial joints, and terminal device (for the upper extremity) or foot (for the lower extremity) depend on the age, agility, weight, endurance, and general medical condition of the client.

Each prosthesis is custom made for the client according to specific stump characteristics. In the past, prostheses have been fabricated out of wood, metal, and leather. Today, however, prostheses are generally fabricated of various plastic and foam materials.

Upper Extremity Prostheses

Upper extremity amputations are classified according to the length of the residual limb. The most important feature of the upper extremity prosthesis is the inner wall of the socket. If there is a poor fit, the prosthesis may not function appropriately and may not be comfortable to with the upper limb), shoulder disarticulations, and some humeral neck amputations. There are two types of shoulder units: a ball joint and two friction hinges or plates that make a universal joint. The shoulder units of the upper extremity prosthesis are moved only through prepositioning by the opposite extremity or by pressing against a solid object.

A harness is worn to hold the stump in the prosthesis and to provide an attachment for the control cable. This cable operates the elbow unit for those persons with above-the-elbow amputations as well as the terminal device of the prosthesis (Fig. 20–9). There are a variety of harnesses to choose from. Some clients with this high-level upper extremity amputation may desire only the padded cosmetic contour of the shoulder. The pad can be made of foam and held on with a chest strap.

Prostheses for Transhumeral Amputations. Clients with transhumeral amputations, except those with elbow disarticulations, use elbow units that lock at various ranges of motion between 5 and 135 degrees of flexion. There is also a friction plate turntable that is above the elbow and permits forearm rotation, which is likened to the natural internal and external rotation of the upper extremity. Elbow disarticulation stumps must use rigid hinges on the outside of the socket because if the elbow unit is installed distal to the socket, as is customarily done, the axis of elbow motion is approximately 5 cm distal to that of the opposite extremity. A variety of

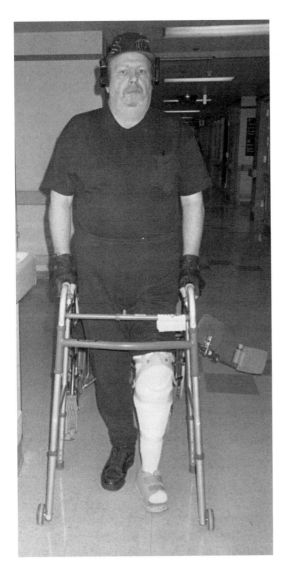

FIGURE 20–8. Patient ambulating with STAT-Limb immediate postoperative prosthesis (IPOP). (Courtesy of Veterans Administration Hospital, Hines, IL.)

wear. Most upper extremity sockets consist of two walls: an inner wall that fits the amputation stump and an outer wall that outlines the approximate contour of the upper extremity. Prostheses made for infants generally have a third middle wall. As the infant grows, the inner wall can be removed to accommodate the need for more space in the socket. This added feature extends the life of the socket and helps contain costs.

Early fitting of the client with an upper extremity amputation with a temporary prosthesis is beneficial because the client does not have sufficient time to become accustomed to one-handed activity, which ultimately decreases acceptance of the prosthesis.

Prostheses for Forequarter Amputations, Shoulder Disarticulations, and Humeral Neck Amputations.
Shoulder units are necessary for forequarter amputations (removal of part or all of the clavicle and scapula along

TABLE 20–5. *Prosthetic Function Levels (Medicare)*

LEVEL	CRITERIA
0	Does not have the ability or potential to ambulate or transfer safely with or without assistance, and a prosthesis does not enhance the person's quality of life or mobility
1	Has the ability or potential to use a prosthesis for transfers or ambulation on level surfaces at a fixed cadence; typical of the limited and unlimited household ambulator
2	Has the ability or potential for ambulation with the proficiency to traverse low-level environmental barriers, such as curbs, stairs, or uneven surfaces; typical of the limited community ambulator
3	Has the ability or potential for ambulation with variable cadence; typical of the community ambulator who is able to traverse most environmental barriers and may have vocational, therapeutic, or exercise activity that demands prosthetic use beyond simple locomotion
4	Has the ability or potential for prosthetic ambulation that exceeds basic ambulation skills, exhibiting high impact, stress, or energy levels; typical of prosthetic demands of a child, active adult, or athlete

Adapted from Oakbrook Orthopaedic Services, Ltd.

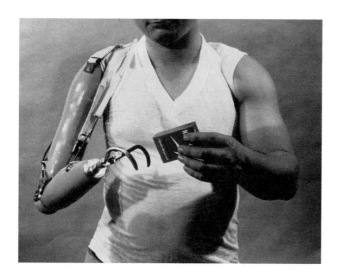

FIGURE 20–9. Upper extremity prosthesis. (Courtesy of Northwestern University School of Orthotics and Prosthetics and the Rehabilitation Institute of Chicago.)

electronic elbows are available, but myoelectric control systems are the choice of most of these clients.

Prostheses for Transradial Amputations.

Most clients with transradial amputations require a harness for suspension of the prosthesis and for control of the terminal device. Hinges attach the below-the-elbow socket to the harness. The hinges are made of either flexible or rigid material. Rigid hinges are made of metal and provide stability of the stump in the socket throughout elbow motion. Rigid hinges are available with a single pivot, polycentric pivot, multiple-action device, or locking device. Flexible hinges are made of some type of synthetic fabric, rather than leather, to avoid perspiration absorption and hinge stretching.

Wrist Components.

Wrist components of the upper extremity prosthesis provide a mechanism for the attachment of terminal devices. There are two basic types of wrist units. Most are threaded sockets that limit rotation of the hook or hand through the use of a friction ring. They do not lock into any particular position. The other type of wrist unit has a locking mechanism and a design that allows quick changes between terminal devices. Quick-change wrist units are preferred by those people whose occupation and daily activities require that they be able to lock the terminal device to prevent rotation when lifting or manipulating heavy objects. A special type of wrist unit that provides wrist flexion can be incorporated into the other standard units. The added wrist flexion allows the terminal device to be brought closer to the body, thereby aiding in dressing and grooming activities. Clients with bilateral transhumeral amputations find this additional feature very helpful. Most clients with unilateral amputations do not need it.

Terminal Devices.

The terminal devices of the upper extremity prosthesis are operated by either a voluntary opening or voluntary closing mechanism. Voluntary opening devices require tension on the control cable to open the hook or hand and close by rubber bands or springs. The voluntary opening device operates quickly with a minimum of control motions and is generally the terminal device preferred by clients with upper extremity amputations. Voluntary closing terminal devices generally consist of a four-cycle action that allows various degrees of tension at the hook or hand. By using slightly differing degrees of tension or pull on the control cable, the operator can partially or fully close the hook or hand, lock it into position or leave it unlocked, or spring it completely open (Fig. 20–10).

The most frequently prescribed hooks are the Dorrance utility-shaped type. They are made of either stainless steel or lightweight aluminum and come in a variety of sizes. Cosmetic hands are nonfunctional terminal devices made of a semirigid or rigid material covered by a cosmetic glove. The cosmetic hand is secured to the wrist unit of the prosthesis either with a screw mechanism or with a zipper attached to the palmar surface of the glove. The hands are made in a variety of colors to match the shade of the skin of the opposite hand.

Myoelectric Control of Upper Extremity Prostheses.

Myoelectric control is used to operate electric motor-driven elbow units, hooks, and hands. Electric hands provide a stronger grasp, and electric elbows make the control of raising and lowering the arm easier. Myoelectric arms eliminate the need for uncomfortable control cables. Surface electrodes are attached to the inner wall of the socket and press against the skin that

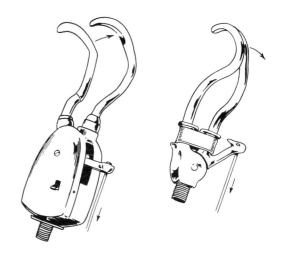

FIGURE 20–10. Voluntary closing (VC) *(left)* and voluntary opening (VO) *(right)* terminal devices. Tension applied to the control cable closes VC devices and opens VC devices. (From Bender, L. F. [1990]. Upper extremity prosthetics. In F. J. Kottke & J. F. Lehmann [Eds.], *Krusen's handbook of physical medicine and rehabilitation* [4th ed., p. 1013]. Philadelphia: WB Saunders.)

overlies the appropriate musculature. When the muscle contracts, the electromyographic signals detected by the electrodes can be amplified and used to control the flow of electric current from a battery to the electric motor.

Proportional myoelectric control allows the speed of motion to be regulated by the speed of the wearer's contractions. The disadvantages of myoelectric arms or hands include cost and amount of care required. Myoelectric control is most frequently used in transradial prostheses to control the electric hand or hook. Myoelectric devices can be very useful for clients with more proximal upper extremity amputations. Hybrid devices that use a combination of body power and myoelectric components are available and allow the amputee to operate the elbow and arm at the same time (Sears, 1999; Smith & Burgess, 1995).

Learning to Use the Prosthesis. Training a client with an upper extremity amputation to use a prosthesis is usually done by the occupational therapist on an outpatient basis. The client is often discharged before the upper extremity prosthesis has been received. The client must be taught to properly care for the prosthesis. The hook must be kept clean, and the socket should be washed with soap and water weekly. If a cosmetic hand is worn, the glove must be washed daily, and the glove and hand must be stored in a plastic bag in a dark place to avoid darkening of the glove with exposure to light. Care must be taken to avoid spilling food or liquids, such as gasoline, ink, or turpentine, on the glove because many liquids can permanently stain it. The client with an upper extremity amputation must first learn how to put on and take off the prosthesis.

Next, the method of operating the controls is taught. The client must learn to operate terminal devices with the hook first, then the hand. The client with a transhumeral amputation must also learn the dual-control technique for operating the elbow unit in conjunction with the terminal device. The client must also be trained in activity of daily living skills with the prosthesis. When the client is performing functional activities, the terminal device is always used for the static part of the activities. The uninvolved extremity performs the dynamic activities. For example, to iron a shirt, the hook or prosthetic hand holds the shirt in place while the intact extremity irons the shirt. When appropriate, the client should be trained in simulated job tasks related to the client's type of work to assess safety and efficiency in handling power tools and various other equipment or materials.

Lower Extremity Prostheses

The general goal for the client with a unilateral lower extremity amputation should be the ability to ambulate safely and independently on level surfaces, stairs, ramps, and curbs with or without assistive devices. Goals for clients with bilateral amputations vary depending on the level of amputations, but Torres and Esquenazi (1991) found that individuals with bilateral lower limb amputations can usually attain household ambulation and deserve a program that helps them attain and maintain this level of functioning. These researchers evaluated 47 amputation clients in a retrospective review at a regional rehabilitation center. The majority of clients achieved at least limited household ambulation at discharge and retained or exceeded this level at 3-month follow-up. Conversely, few of the clients discharged at wheelchair level progressed beyond this level.

The most important requirement of the lower extremity stump is that it be able to withstand weight in the standing position or with ambulation. The area of weight bearing on the stump depends on the level of amputation. Weight bearing can be end bearing (for an amputation performed through a joint level, i.e., ankle or knee disarticulation), at the tibial metaphyseal flare (side bearing), at the patellar tendon (patellar tendon bearing), or at the ischial tuberosity and gluteal fold. It is advantageous to have a stump with as large an area as possible for weight bearing, covered with skin that is free from scar tissue, and able to withstand the pressure of weight bearing. It is important for the client to maintain a steady weight. Weight gain or loss of 5 pounds compromises fit, as do volume changes caused by diuretics, hemodialysis, and moderate amounts of alcohol. Clients should expect to experience periodic changes in stump size over time.

Lower extremity prosthetic components include socket and ankle-foot components. For transtibial and higher, a shank is included. For knee disarticulation and higher, a knee component is needed; for transfemoral and higher, a thigh component is needed; and for hip disarticulation, a hip joint is needed (Schuch, 1998). Prosthetic components and systems are constantly evolving, and the discussion here is limited to the more common ones.

Gait Training. Beginning ambulation with a temporary prosthesis allows the client to learn proper weight-shifting techniques. This promotes a more energy-efficient gait that in turn increases the likelihood of prosthesis use. Walking is begun between parallel bars and is gradually progressed to crutches and then to a cane. Weight bearing is limited to 25 to 40 pounds to avoid pressure on the incision. The temporary prosthesis is generally worn for 3 to 4 months until stump shrinkage has stabilized (Pandian & Kowalske, 1999).

Gait training is initiated in the parallel bars, where the client can practice weight shifting, side stepping, balance techniques, and general transfer techniques to and from the wheelchair. The client must be taught to take steps of equal length, have equal stance phases on each extremity, and have equal arm swing. The client should progress to crutches or a cane as tolerated, paying continued attention to these components of gait.

As the client becomes adept at walking on level surfaces, training on uneven surfaces, stairs, and curbs must be initiated. The client should also learn to use public transportation as well as how to fall and get up from a fall. All of these movements are taught with the intent of making the client as functionally independent as possible (Pandian & Kowalske, 1999).

Prostheses for Hip Disarticulation. Hip disarticulation includes any amputation through the hip joint or up to 2 inches below the pelvic floor. It is usually done for cancer or traumatic injury, and both socket stability and weight bearing are at the pelvic level. This individual requires a cosmetically acceptable prosthesis that is suspended from the pelvis and that possesses both hip and knee joints that are relatively stable with standing and walking (Fig. 20–11) but that also allow sitting,

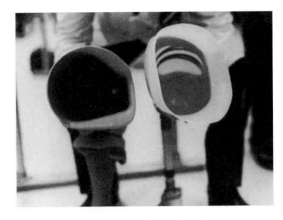

FIGURE 20–12. A down-into-the-socket view comparing the quadrilateral *(left)* with the CAT-CAM *(right)* socket design. (From Staats, T. B. [1989]. Lower extremity prosthetics. In W. S. Moore & J. M. Malone [Eds.], *Lower extremity amputation* [p. 289]. Philadelphia: WB Saunders.)

standing, or walking with minimum discomfort and expenditure of energy. The client must be motivated to learn to walk.

Prostheses for Transfemoral Amputations

Socket. There are two types of sockets available, the quadrilateral and the ischial containment socket. The quadrilateral socket resembles a rectangle from above (Fig. 20-12). Advantages of this system include a wide area for weight distribution, counterpressure to assist venous return and prevent distal edema, and sensory feedback that allows better control of the prosthesis (Edelstein, 1988). It is recommended for geriatric and debilitated clients (Schuch & Pritham, 1999). The ischial containment socket is said to be more comfortable and functional than the quadrilateral socket. The ischial containment socket uses a markedly reduced mediolateral diameter and an expanded anteroposterior diameter. The socket shape is oval in the anteroposterior direction (Fig. 20-12). These socket shape differences enhance mediolateral muscle forces during the stance phase of gait and allow more natural function of the flexor and extensor muscles. Most bilateral transfemoral amputees prefer this (Schuch & Pritham, 1999).

Suspension Devices. Suction suspension is a self-suspending system that calls for a precise socket fit. Socket skin contact and negative pressure act to hold the prosthesis on the stump (Fig. 20-13). It is most commonly used and is more cosmetic. It is not recommended for new amputees because the size of the stump is still fluctuating (Kapp, 1999). An alternative to suction is a roll-on silicone liner. It is easier to put on than suction suspension. A hyperbaric sock is also an alternative to hard socket suction. A silicone ring around the proximal sock makes it simple to put on and is recommended for geriatric and less active clients (Kapp, 1999).

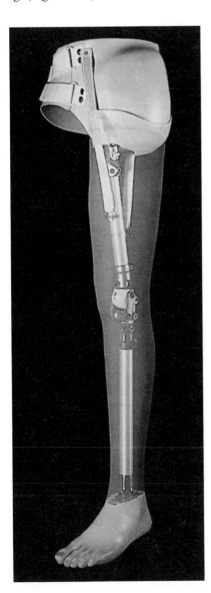

FIGURE 20–11. A modular hip disarticulation prosthesis. (Courtesy of Otto Bock Industries, Minneapolis, MN.)

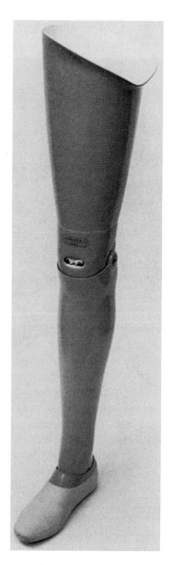

FIGURE 20–13. An above-the-knew prosthesis with a suction valve. (From Vitali, M., Robinson, K. P., Andrews, B. G., & Harris, E. E. [1986]. *Amputations and prostheses* [2nd ed., p. 170]. London: Bailliere Tindall.)

The total elastic suspension belt is easy to apply and spreads the pressure over a greater surface area. However, the wide band causes body heat retention. The Silesian belt is used to prevent socket rotation in limbs with significant redundant tissue when the total elastic suspension belt is inadequate. It can also be added to suction sockets to keep the prosthesis from slipping off when the person sits. It is not recommended for clients with significant hip instability, weak musculature, or a very short limb. For clients with short limbs and weak hip abductors, a hip joint and pelvic belt is used. This suspension system is weightier and less cosmetically appealing than the others (Kapp, 1999).

Belt suspension systems are contraindicated in clients who are pregnant or have had bypass surgery or shunt placement in the remaining lower extremity. Obese individuals may find the pelvic band uncomfortable because it pinches abdominal fat during sitting and requires more energy for ambulation. Shoulder suspension is necessary in these individuals.

Knee Component. Prosthetic knee joints must flex easily and provide stability under the load of weight bearing. Several different knee joint designs are available, some of which increase stability during the stance phase of gait, and others of which assist in the swing phase of the gait cycle. For more information on gait, see Chapter 8.

The conventional single-axis knee requires only simple maintenance and is low in initial cost. It can also be locked for extra stability. Polycentric-axis knees are also available but are expensive and less commonly used.

Once the amount of friction is set for a mechanical-friction knee unit, it remains constant. This type of component is useful for clients who do not require gait variation or who need a relatively lightweight and inexpensive knee unit. Older clients commonly choose this knee because it is helpful when stump musculature or balance is poor or if the client is generally weak. The primary advantage of this type of knee is its stability.

The fluid, or variable-friction, knee is cadence responsive and more flexible, allowing the client to ambulate with a more normal gait. It is heavier and more expensive than mechanical-friction units but provides the young client with a more cosmetically acceptable swing phase.

Prostheses for Transtibial Amputations

Socket. The patellar tendon-bearing (PTB) socket, introduced in 1959, is the most commonly prescribed socket for transtibial prostheses. It provides uniform proprioceptive feedback to all stump tissues and ensures moderate weight-bearing distribution over the weight tolerant areas of the limb but mostly the patella tendon. The total surface-bearing socket allows the pressure to be distributed more equally across the entire surface of the residual limb. The hydrostatic socket has no identified weight-bearing areas, and pressure is applied equally to all weight-bearing tissue on the residual limb. These are newer designs that are increasing in use (Fergason & Smith, 1999).

Suspension. The suspension system selected depends on the length and shape of the residual limb. Prosthetic sleeves are simple to apply and widely used. They allow for greater range of knee flexion and cosmesis. Gel liners with locking mechanisms are now being prescribed more than traditional suspension systems like the supracondylar cuff. Made of silicone, urethane, or thermoplastic elastomer, it results in unrestricted knee flexion and minimal pistoning of the stump. The supracondylar cuff is adjustable, durable, and one of the easiest to put on. However, it is not recommended for clients with vascular compromise or knee instability. Supracondylar suspension is useful for clients with short limbs. The supracondylar-suprapatellar suspension may also be used for short limbs but is used to control against recurvatum and increases medial lateral joint stability. It is not recommended for obese or very muscular limbs. A waist belt is used with a temporary or intermediate prosthesis because of limb volume and shape fluctuations. It can also be used as an auxiliary for higher levels of activity or for added comfort and security. It is useful for the client with vascular compromise. The thigh corset with joints is used for knee instability. It is the most cumbersome suspension system and should be used only if there is no other alternative (Kapp, 1999).

Prostheses for Syme's Amputation. Syme's amputation, first performed by James Syme in 1843, is an ankle disarticulation that retains the full length of the tibia, the heel pad, and the proprioceptive sense of the heel (Pinzur, 1999). The prosthesis comes to below the knee, incorporating the bulbous end of the stump within the foot portion. The medial wall of the prosthesis, at ankle level, is removable (Fig. 20–14). When in place, the prosthesis acts as a condylar suspension system over the malleolus. Energy consumption for ambulation is less than the requirements for a transtibial amputation. Hospitalization is not generally required for prosthetic gait training, and the best results are obtained when the prosthesis is combined with a dynamic response foot (Pinzur, 1999).

Ankle-Foot Components. Various prosthetic feet are available (Fig. 20–15). The same feet are available for transfemoral and transtibial amputations. The type of foot prescribed is determined by the client's ambulatory

level (Table 20–5). Clients must purchase all shoes with the same heel heights for a specific foot. If high heels are to be worn on occasion, the prosthetist must know this at the time of fabrication so that the prosthesis can be designed for interchangeable feet.

Feet can be classified as nondynamic and dynamic response. Nondynamic response feet include the solid ankle cushion heel (SACH) foot that was developed in the 1950s and is still the most widely prescribed. It has a rigid keel (the structural or load-bearing portion of the prosthetic foot). It is used for the household ambulator. The stationary ankle flexible endoskeleton (SAFE) foot can simulate inversion and eversion which makes it ideal for community ambulators who may walk on uneven terrain (Romo, 1999).

Dynamic response feet are either articulated or nonarticulated. Nonarticulated designs are further divided into long and short keel. Nonarticulated long keel feet deform under load but return to the original shape when the load is removed. This becomes like a spring that allows adequate dorsiflexion and push-off. It is used for moderate to highly active persons. Some examples are the Modular III (Flex-Foot) and the Springlite II. The nonarticulated short keel feet are not as responsive and provide less dorsiflexion. They may provide moderate inversion and eversion. They are also recommended for moderate to highly active persons but are used when financing is limited because they are less expensive than long keel designs. Some examples are Sure-Flex Carbon Copy II and Lightfoot II (Romo, 1999).

Articulated designs can be divided into true and other categories. They are available in several keel designs. True articulated designs allow smooth plantar-flexion and dorsiflexion and inversion and eversion because the prosthesis has axial joints rather that relying on keel deformation only. Therefore, the prosthesis is able to accommodate uneven surfaces and is excellent for outdoor activities. An example of this is the College Park True-Step. Golfers particularly benefit from this type of foot. The other articulation designs such as the Springlite Advantage, do not have a true axial joint but are composed of carbon coils or elastomeric joints. Because there are no moving parts, no maintenance is required for proper joint function (Romo, 1999).

TECHNOLOGIC ADVANCES IN PROSTHETIC DESIGN

Computer-aided design (CAD) and computer-aided manufacturing (CAM) are on the rise (Fergason & Smith, 1999). The CAD system uses stump measurements taken manually to modify a standard socket shape stored in a computer. The modified socket shape can then be graphically depicted on the computer screen, and the prosthetist can further refine the socket shape as necessary. All data are stored for further reference. The CAM technique

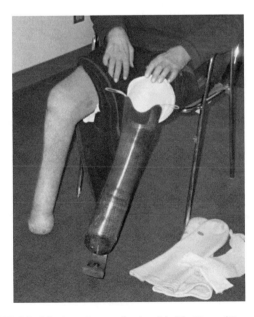

FIGURE 20–14. Syme's prosthesis with FlexFoot. (Courtesy of the amputee clinic, Rehabilitation Institute of Chicago.)

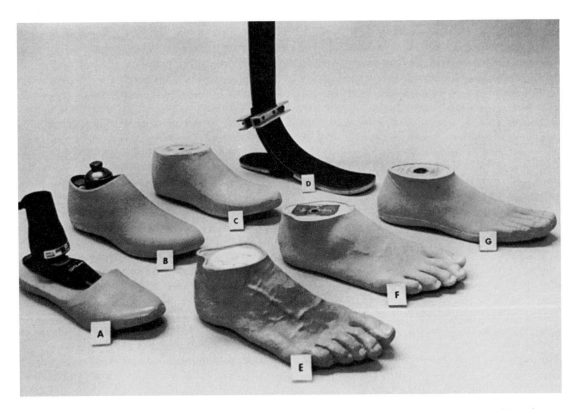

FIGURE 20–15. Designs of interchangeable prosthetic foot pieces: *A,* Multiflex. *B,* Multiaxial. *C,* Stationary and flexible endoskeleton (SAFE). *D,* FlexFoot. *E,* Seattle foot. *F,* Carbon Copy II. *G,* Stored Energy (STEN). (From Stokosa, J. J. [1989]. New developments in prosthetics. In W. S. Moore & J. M. Malone [Eds.], *Lower extremity amputation* [p. 316]. Philadelphia: WB Saunders.)

uses computer-controlled carving techniques for fabrication of the socket to individual stump specifications.

Advances are also being made in upper extremity prosthetics. New technology such as microcomputers and small sturdy circuit boards allows greater function than in previous years. These allow for electric wrist rotation and prosthetic hands that bend at the wrist. The majority of arm prostheses now use electric hands. Progress is being made in body-powered prostheses as well. New materials used in manufacturing result in lighter-weight and more natural-looking prostheses. Silicone hand covers are more sturdy and now make it possible to cover an electric hand so that high grip strength can be combined with an almost natural appearance (Sears, 1999).

In the lower extremity, microprocessor controlled prosthetic knees adjust the swing control of the knee allowing the amputee to easily vary gait speed and decrease the energy expended during ambulation. The development of polycentric knees allow greater stance stability and greater walking speed. There are hybrid hydraulic and pneumatic systems that also allow varying walking speeds (Michael, 1999). With all of these advances, amputation does not mandate an inactive or limited lifestyle. Many resources exist for advice and financing regarding prosthetics.

INTERNET RESOURCES

The Amputee Coalition of America: www.amputee-coalition.org; serves consumers and health care providers

Amputee Resource Foundation of America, Inc.: www.amputeeresource.org; provides information, performs charitable services, offers online consultation

Orthotics and Prosthetics: www.oandp.com; online resource for prosthetic information and facilities

RESOURCE FOR AMPUTEES AND HEALTHCARE PROFESSIONALS

Amputee Coalition of America, PO Box 2528, Knoxville, TN 37901-2528; telephone: 423-524-8772, e-mail: ACAOne@aol.com

REFERENCES

Angrilli, A., & Koster, U. (2000). Psychophysiological stress responses in amputees with and without phantom limb pain. *Physiology and Behavior, 68,* 699–706.

Bach, S., Noreng, M. F., & Tjellden, N. U. (1988). Phantom limb pain in amputees during the first 12 months following limb amputation, after preoperative lumbar epidural blockade. *Pain, 33,* 297–301.

Billock, J. N. (1995). Myoelectric hands for children—Are they appropriate? *In Motion, 5*(4), 26.

Cannon, D. T., & Wu, Y. (1998). Topical capsaicin as an adjuvant analgesic for the treatment of traumatic amputee neurogenic residual limb pain. *Archives of Physical Medicine and Rehabilitation, 79,* 591–593.

Edelstein, J. E. (1988). Prosthetic assessment and management. In S. B. Sullivan & T. J. Schmitz (Eds.), *Physical rehabilitation: Assessment and treatment* (2nd ed., pp. 404–433). Philadelphia: FA Davis.

Elizaga, A. M., Smith, D. G., Sharar, S. R., Edwards, W. T., & Hansen, S. T., Jr. (1994). Continuous regional analgesia by intraneural block: Effects on postoperative opioid requirements and phantom limb pain following amputation. *Journal of Rehabilitation Research and Development, 31,* 179–187.

Esquenazi, A., & Meier, R. H. (1996). Rehabilitation in limb deficiency. 4. Limb amputation. *Archives of Physical Medicine and Rehabilitation, 77* (3 Suppl), S18–S28.

Fergason, J., & Smith, D. (1999). Socket considerations for the patient with a transtibial amputation. *Clinical Orthopaedics and Related Research, 361,* 76–84.

Fisher, K., & Hanspal, R. S. (1998). Phantom pain, anxiety, depression, and their relation in consecutive patients with amputated limbs: Case reports. *British Medical Journal, 316,* 903–904.

Fitzpatrick, M. C. (1999). The psychologic assessment and psychosocial recovery of the patient with an amputation. *Clinical Orthopaedics and Related Research, 361,* 98–107.

Gnezdilov, A. V., Syrovegin, A. V., Plaksin, P. E., Ovechkin, A. M., & Sul'timov, S. A. (1995, March/April). Evaluation of the effectiveness of transcutaneous electroneuroanalgesia in phantom pain syndrome. *Anesteziologiia I Reanimatologiia,* 97–102.

Haimovici, H. (1996). Amputation of the lower extremity: general considerations. In H. Haimovici (Ed.), *Haimovici's vascular surgery: Principles and techniques* (4th ed., pp. 1317–1347). Cambridge, MA: Blackwell Science.

Jahanjiri, M., Jayatunga, A. P., Bradley, J. W., & Dark, C. H. (1994). Prevention of phantom pain after major lower limb amputation by epidural infusion of diamorphine, clonidine and bupivacaine. *Annals of the Royal College of Surgeons of England, 76,* 324–326.

Jain, S. (1996). Rehabilitation in limb deficiency. 2. The pediatric amputee. *Archives of Physical Medicine and Rehabilitation, 77*(3 Suppl), S9–S13.

Kapp, S. (1999). Suspension systems for prostheses. *Clinical Orthopaedics and Related Research, 361,* 55–62.

Katsuly-Liapus, I., Georgakis, P., & Tierry, C. (1996). Pre-emptive extradural analgesia reduces the incidence of phantom pain in lower limb amputees. *British Journal of Anesthesiology, 76*(Suppl 2), 125.

Katz, J. (1997). Prevention of phantom pain by regional anaesthesia. *Lancet, 349,* 519–520.

Kennedy, J. P. (1992). Traumatic amputation. In J. P. Kennedy & F. W. Blaisdell (Eds.), *Extremity trauma.* New York, Thieme.

Krane, E. J., & Heller, L. G. (1995). The prevalence of phantom sensation and pain in pediatric amputees. *Journal of Pain and Symptom Management, 10,* 21–29.

McCloskey, J., & Buelechek, G. (1995). Validation and coding of the NIC taxonomy structure. *Image: Journal of Nursing Scholarship, 27*(1), 43–49.

Melzack, R. (1992). Phantom limbs. *Scientific American, 266,* 120–126.

Michael, J. W. (1999). Modern prosthetic knee mechanisms. *Clinical Orthopaedics and Related Research, 361,* 39–47.

Montoya, P., Larbig, W., Grulke, N., Flor, H., Taub, E., & Birbaumer, N. (1997). The relationship of phantom pain to other phantom phenomena in upper extremity amputees. *Pain, 72,* 78–93.

MossRehab Resource Net. (2000). *Amputation fact sheet.* Available at www.mossresourcenet.org/amputa.htm

Nikolajsen, L., Ilkjaer, S., Christensen, J. H., Kroner, K., & Jensen, T. S. (1997). Randomised trial of epidural bupivacaine and morphine in prevention of stump and phantom pain in lower limb amputation. *Lancet, 350,* 1353–1357.

Pandian, G., & Kowalske, K. (1999). Daily functioning of patients with an amputated lower extremity. *Clinical Orthopaedics and Related Research, 361,* 91–97.

Pinzur, M. S. (1997). The metabolic cost of lower extremity amputation. *Clinics in Podiatric Medicine and Surgery, 14,* 599–602.

Pinzur, M. S. (1999). Restoration of walking ability with Syme's ankle disarticulation. *Clinical Orthopaedics and Related Research, 361,* 71–75.

Pinzur, M. S., Garla, P. G. N., Pluth, T., & Vrbos, L. (1996). Continuous postoperative infusion of a regional anesthetic after an amputation of the lower extremity. A randomized controlled trial. *Journal of Bone and Joint Surgery, 78A,* 1501–1505.

Pucher, I., Kickinger, W., Frischenschlager, O. (1999). Coping with amputation and phantom limb pain. *Journal of Psychosomatic Research, 46*(4), 379–383.

Romo, H. D. (1999). Specialized prostheses for activities. *Clinical Orthopaedics and Related Research, 361,* 63–70.

Roth, E. J., Park, K. L., & Sullivan, W. J. (1998). Cardiovascular disease in patients with dysvascular amputation. *Archives of Physical Medicine and Rehabilitation, 79,* 205–215.

Schuch, C. M. (1998). Prosthetics primer: A guide to lower limb prosthetics. *In Motion, 8*(2), 29–35.

Schuch, C. M., & Pritham, C. H. (1999). Current transfemoral sockets. *Clinical Orthopaedics and Related Research, 361,* 48–54.

Scott, H., Condie, M. E., Treweek, S. P., & Sockalingam, S. (2000). An evaluation of the amputee mobility aid (AMA) early walking aid. *Prosthetics and Orthotics International, 24*(1), 39–46.

Sears, H. H. (1999). Advances in arm prosthetics. *In Motion, 9*(3), 13–16.

Smith, D. G., & Burgess, E. M. (1995). Amputations. In H. B. Skinner (Ed.), *Current diagnosis and treatment in orthopaedics* (pp. 555–579). Norwalk, CT: Appleton & Lange.

Smith, D. G., & Fergason, J. R. (1999). Transtibial amputations. *Clinical Orthopaedics and Related Research, 361,* 108–115.

Stokosa, J. J. (1996). Prosthetics for lower limb amputees. In H. Haimovici (Ed.), *Haimovici's vascular surgery: Principles and techniques* (4th ed., pp. 1355–1371). Cambridge, MA: Blackwell Science.

Torres, M. M., & Esquenazi, A. (1991). Bilateral lower limb amputee rehabilitation. A retrospective review. *The Western Journal of Medicine, 154,* 583–586.

Tronzo, R. G., & Janek, A. M. (1995). The "turn-up" plasty: One solution to a complex problem. *Orthopaedic Nursing, 14*(3), 41–47.

Winchell, E. (1995). *Coping with limb loss* (pp. 7–12). New York: Avery.

Wu, Y. (1996). Postoperative and preprosthetic management for lower extremity amputations. In H. Haimovici (Ed.), *Haimovici's vascular surgery: Principles and techniques* (4th ed., pp. 1348–1354). Cambridge, MA: Blackwell Science.

Zuniga, R. E., Schlicht, C. R., Christian, R., & Abram, S. E. (2000). Intrathecal baclofen is analgesic in patients with chronic pain. *Anesthesiology, 92,* 876–881.

21

Athletic Performance and Injury

Sports medicine can be defined as the physiologic, biomechanical, psychosocial, and pathomechanical phenomenon associated with exercise and athletics. It is also the clinical application of the knowledge gained from this study to the improvement and maintenance of functional capacities for physical labor, exercise, and athletics and the prevention and treatment of disease and injuries related to exercise and sports. Because participation in sports itself is multidisciplinary, involving exercise physiology, biomechanics, and psychology, among others, the practice of sports medicine requires a team approach to provide optimal care to the athlete.

In some of the earliest Egyptian tombs of Beni-Hassam (c. 1991–1778 BC), sports, including archery, rowing, running, swimming, and wresting, were depicted. Comparatively, the first recorded association between medicine and sports was documented in the Hindu sacred text *Artharva Veda* at 1000 BC. The tenants in this sacred text advocated exercise to treat various ailments. The gladiators were thought to be the first professional sports competitors with Claudius Galen (AD 138–210) as the first team physician (Clendening, 1960; Garrison, 1967). In the 21st century, the Olympic motto, *citius altius fortius* (higher faster stronger), still brings forth the challenge and glory of competition. In the 21st century, "the thrill of victory, and the agony of defeat" are benefiting sports medicine by the study of the pathomechanics related to sports injury and the biotechnologic advances in treating sports-induced inflammatory conditions.

A joint statement released by the International Federation of Sports Medicine (FIMS) and the World Health Organization (WHO) advocates that physical activity increases longevity and protects persons against major noncommunicable and chronic diseases. FIMS and WHO urge governments to promote and enhance programs of physical activity and fitness as part of public health and social policy.

EQUIPMENT AND FACILITIES

Guidelines related to the quality, application, fit, and maintenance of athletic equipment has a direct relationship to injury prevention. Protective equipment is essential, particularly in direct contact and collision sports. Collision sports (e.g., football, hockey) create special need for protective equipment, especially helmets. Body surface areas exposed to high-impact forces in both direct contact and collision sports require padding. Extra padding about the chest/ribs, elbows, knees, shins, shoulders, and thigh helps prevent direct blunt traumatic injury to these regions. For example, cantilevered shoulder pads protect the shoulder girdle as well as the acromioclavicular (AC) joint. For more information on injury prevention in sports, see Chapter 1.

Other protective equipment includes socks. A variety of types of socks are marketed for their differing comfort abilities. Double-knit tubular socks without heels work best for baseball, whereas short ankle socks are worn for tennis. Improperly fitting socks can lead to wrinkles about joints and bony prominences causing blisters. Restrictive socks can inhibit proper biomechanics of the foot.

Improperly fitting shoes cause damage to the foot and ankle by interfering with foot biomechanics; calluses and blisters result from friction. Incorrect shoeing causes mechanical disturbances that affect postural balance and musculotendinous units and precipitate joint pathology and pain to the foot, ankle, and lower extremity. Pain may radiate to the lumbar spine from related lower extremity pathology.

The length and width of the sports shoe is important. Adequate toe box room allows freedom for the distal toes and metatarsals to function properly. Cleats on shoes for turf sports vary in length and should be evenly distributed on the two weight-bearing parts of the shoe (beneath the first and fifth metatarsals). Proper lacing of shoes can also prevent injury to the foot and ankle.

Facilities for athletes should incorporate injury protective equipment. Breakaway bases, deformable walls, padded backstops and goalposts, and stable soccer goalposts are suggested. The physical plant as well as outside playing surfaces should be routinely checked for erosion, rust, holes, rocks, and debris. The facilities should also have emergency resuscitative equipment and direct access via phone or walkie-talkie to emergency medical services.

PREPARTICIPATION PHYSICAL EXAMINATION

Preparticipation physical examination (PPE) is conducted before athletic performance and organized sports activities for the young and older athlete. For the young athlete, PPE has legal implications for school authorities. Although studies are equivocal, the benefits of gathering baseline physical data before competitive sports far outweigh the risks. The PPE should be performed well enough in advance that performance issues, biomechanical variances, and physical deficiencies may be identified and managed. Nouveau athletes should be cognizant of the risk factors associated with increased activity and exercise. When the health care provider performs the PPE, risk factors should be identified (Box 21-1). If potential risk factors are present and not already known by the athlete, the athlete should be referred to his or her primary care provider for further evaluation. Several factors should be considered when trying to decide on a sport, including physical ability, personal gain, and the ability to include the activity as part of a daily or life routine. Injury prevention is directly affected by participation in a safe environment with the proper equipment; adherence to guidelines for safe participation; and proper training for strength, endurance, flexibility, and technique. Choosing the right sport means having the correct

---

BOX 21–1.
Factors That May Predispose an Athlete to Injury

Age older than 40 years
Inactive lifestyle
Twenty or more pounds overweight
Personal and family history of cardiopulmonary disease
Undiagnosed pain/pressure in the chest, arm, throat
Prescribed medications that alter cardiopulmonary
   and/or peripheral vascular response
High cholesterol
Hypertension
Smoking and/or use of nonprescribed drugs that affect
   the cardiovascular system
Uncontrolled diabetes mellitus or other chronic disorders
History of joint disease, recent trauma, or injury
Hyperthyroidism

---

preparation and equipment. Attitudes about female participation in male-dominated contact sports as football, hockey, and lacrosse have undergone scrutiny. Although there is generally no reason why a sport must be segregated, there are gender characteristics that may place females at a greater risk for injury. Weight and size mismatch are factors to take into consideration before engaging in co-ed sports activities.

ATHLETES WITH DIFFERING ABILITIES

Sports competition within disabled populations has increased exponentially since the Paralympic movement began in 1960. Paralympic competition is geared to athletes with physical and sensory disabilities. These may include athletes with an amputation; athletes who are blind or visually impaired; or athletes with arthritis, cerebral dysfunction, short stature, or spinal cord injuries. Fourteen sports, including soccer, swimming, track and field, and volleyball, have Olympic equivalents that have the same regulations with modifications in the rules. Five sports are specific to those with a disability: bocce, goalball, lawn bowls, rugby, and sit volleyball.

Before beginning a program or permitting a challenged athlete to participate, several key factors need to be addressed. These factors include determining the athlete's physical condition, diagnosing the athlete's disability, identifying special needs in children, and setting realistic goals with the athlete. Certain contraindications apply to some sports, particularly those in which body contact with players is concerned. These contraindications include cardiac and respiratory conditions, bleeding diathesis, severe osteoporosis, recent trauma or surgery, seizure activity not fully controlled by drug therapy, unstable musculoskeletal conditions (e.g., C1–C2 instability), congenital spinal stenosis, dislocated hips, instability of major weight-bearing joints, and severe scoliosis. Injuries in the challenged athlete are generally musculoskeletal in nature. Preventing injury is paramount for all athletes with differing abilities.

Injury prevention stems from understanding the physical alterations and problems and precautions that must be taken before competition. Whether adaptive equipment, safety precautions, or field preparation are needed, key factors in injury prevention are proper conditioning and preparation. Certain populations have specific physical problems that predispose them to certain injuries (e.g., amputations, arthritis, cerebral palsy, Down syndrome, seizures, spinal cord injury, visual impairment, blindness). Athletes with special needs are classified according to functional and physical abilities before competition and play to ensure that play is equitable for each athlete.

The Special Olympics, a subset of the Paralympics, provides evaluation and guidance for athletes who have emotional difficulties and/or mental retardation. Cycling, swimming, table tennis, and track and field are popular sports for the Special Olympians. The Special Olympics team evaluates the physical function of the athlete and assists with placement of the athlete in sports that are best suited for his or her adaptive needs.

SPORT PSYCHOLOGY

An important component in "getting game" is physical conditioning. Yet aren't we forgetting something if we don't include mental conditioning? In 1921, Ty Cobb essentially said that the biggest part of a great ballplayer's body is above the shoulders, and one of Yogi Berra's famous statements was "90 percent of the game is ½ mental." The concept of sport psychology has been around for many years. However, the formal position of a sport psychologist is relatively new on the sports scene. Psychological conditioning is essential for any athlete. Even the ancient Greeks postulated "Mens sans in corpore sano"—a sound mind in a sound body.

Sport psychology is the study of the psychological and mental factors that influence performance and participation in exercise, sport, and physical activity. The sport psychologist assists athletes in improving performance, overcoming fears associated with competition, and enhancing the sports experience by assisting the athlete in developing a healthy self-esteem. In addition, the sport psychologist assists the athlete with postinjury rehabilitation to adjust to inability to play or compete and assists with pain control and adherence to physical therapy demands. The sports psychologist also provides information to individuals, groups, and organizations about behavioral, emotional, and psychosocial control skills for sports, exercise, and physical activity. The sport psychology professional helps prepare the athlete for his or her sport through emotional, behavioral, and psychological activities that encompass goal setting; visualization (seeing in the mind's eye completion of a kick, a throw, or coming across the finish line); and centering-balancing (literally, physically, and figuratively focusing energy through concentration to complete the pitch or throw, goal, kick, and so forth). Another key component to the mental routine advocated by the sport psychologist is deep breathing. Sport psychologists work with athletes at the amateur, elite, and professional levels to evaluate and suggest strategies for improving game preparation, communication skill, and team cohesion, and for dealing with other issues that affect team and personal performance (Singer, Hausenblas, & Janelle, 2001).

SPORTS MEDICINE ACROSS THE AGE CONTINUUM

Physiologic changes associated with the older athlete include alterations in the cardiovascular, metabolic, and musculoskeletal systems. Many of the changes that were previously considered specific to physiologic aging are now recognized as a function of disease, not age. Age-related decline in function is associated with a gradual loss of muscle mass both in number and size of muscle fibers. Loss of muscle mass is associated with loss of general strength and subsequently physical functioning. Age-related functional denervation leads to atrophy and selective loss of type II (fast-twitch) muscle fibers. Loss of muscle strength can lead to falls and fractures. Strength training can preserve independent functioning associated with activities of daily living (ADLs). Endurance training for older adults improves performance. Conditioning exercises help preserve energy, stamina, and vigor and also help reduce fatigue. Older adults should consult with their health care provider for exercise prescription and pre-exercise history and physical before beginning a strength and endurance program. Underlying medical morbidity and medications can affect exercise performance and therefore exercise prescription. The American Academy of Sports Medicine recommends that men older than 40 and women older than 50 have a graded exercise test before beginning a vigorous exercise program. Table 21–1 lists athletic injuries that are commonly seen in the older age group. Most of these injuries are associated with tendonitis secondary to overuse. Factors leading to overuse are biomechanical maladjustment, poor or inadequate footwear, improper equipment, training on nonyielding surfaces, decreased strength and flexibility, and sudden increase in duration of physical activity or sport.

Pediatric and adolescent athletes are training harder and for longer duration since the advent of sports training camps. The young athlete training for elite status at the national and Olympic levels is beginning at ages 4 and 5. Anatomic location of injury in the young athlete is related to skill demand of the sport not specifically age, yet age has a direct relationship on the maturity of the athlete's musculoskeletal system. For this reason, avulsion fracture is more common in children, whereas ligamentous damage is more common in adults. Table 21–2 lists injuries in children and adolescents. Organizations

TABLE 21–1. *Possible Sport Injury in the Older Adult Population*

BODY PART	TYPES OF CONDITIONS
Shoulder	Subacromial impingement syndrome
	Rotator cuff tear
	Attritional rotator cuff changes
	Secondary overuse/repetitive strain; deposition of calcium about tendons precipitating inflammation, fibrosis
	Adhesive capsulitis
Knee	Patellofemoral syndrome
	Degenerative osteoarthritic changes
	Meniscal injury
Ankle/foot	Achilles tendonitis
	Plantar fasciitis

TABLE 21–2. *Possible Sport Injury in Children and Adolescents*

BODY REGION	INJURY/CONDITIONS
Upper body	Ligamentous laxity of the shoulder
	Proximal humeral physeal injuries
	Little Leaguer's elbow (pitcher's elbow) medial/lateral epicondylitis
	Avulsion of medial/lateral epicondyles
	Osteochondritis dissecans
	Radial head overgrowth
	Chronic overuse of wrist
Lower extremity	Ankle sprains and tarsal coalition
	Avulsion of cruciate ligaments
	Distal femoral physeal fractures
	Musculotendinous overuse syndromes
	Osgood-Schlatter disease
	Osteochondritis dissecans
	Periostitis (shin splints)
	Physeal injuries of foot/ankle
	Slipped capital femoral epiphysis
	Tibial eminence fracture
Central body	Low-back pain
	Scoliosis
	Muscle strains
	Spondylolisthesis

such as American Academy of Pediatrics, American College of Sports Medicine, and many others advocate a PPE and cardiovascular evaluation for pediatric and adolescent athletes. Recommendations and guidelines have been published for the health care practitioner (Kenney, Humphrey, Bryant, & Mahler, 1995; Lyznicki, Nielsen, & Schneider, 2000).

THE FEMALE ATHLETE

With increased participation of women in organized sports, certain sports-related injuries and ailments have been identified that specifically relate to women athletes (Teitz, 1997). One ailment is the "female athlete triad," first identified by the American College of Sports Medicine in 1992. The triad consists of disordered eating, menstrual irregularities, and osteoporosis. The components of the triad are interrelated because disordered eating leads to amenorrhea, and eventually osteoporosis. These components are hormonally and metabolically related. The triad is associated with both endurance sports and sports with weight categories and subjective evaluation (e.g., gymnastics, cheerleading, horse racing).

Disordered eating entails extreme dieting, sporadic eating, poor nutrition, and sometimes, binging and purging. Restriction of calories while competing in a sport can lead to depleted energy and poor performance. A decreased metabolic rate disturbs musculoskeletal and cardiovascular performance. With continued inadequate carbohydrate, protein, and fat stores, endocrine function is altered, leading to amenorrhea. Fasting, binging, self-induced vomiting, and abusive use of laxatives and diuretics lead to potentially life-threatening metabolic imbalances.

Amenorrhea is associated with intense training. There are two types. *Primary* amenorrhea is complete absence of menstruation by age 16 in a girl with secondary sex characteristics. *Secondary* amenorrhea is the absence of 3 to 12 consecutive menses after menarche. Exercise-associated amenorrhea (EAA) is the most common cause of secondary amenorrhea. EAA results from decreased pulse frequency of gonadotropin-releasing hormone and decreased luteinizing hormone, which leads to a hypoestrogen state. In time, decreased estrogen results in decreased bone mineral density, which leads to osteoporosis. If left untreated, osteoporosis will increase fracture risk in competitive years and may have long-range consequences in later years. Diagnosis is based on the three components of the triad that are obtained during the history—diet and nutrition, menstrual irregularities, and recent fractures and/or excessive dental problems.

Treatment is individualized. Goal setting, good nutrition, and sometimes, drug therapy are needed to reverse amenorrhea. Public awareness and education regarding female athlete triad is crucial for young athletes and coaches.

Another concern for the female athlete is the increased incidence of knee injury particularly the anterior cruciate ligament (ACL). There is speculation as to the causes of ACL injury in the female athlete. Both intrinsic and extrinsic factors have been identified. Intrinsic factors are individual, affect both physical and sport biomechanics, and may have sex-specific implications. Specifically, intrinsics include hormonal influences, joint laxity (perhaps related to estrogen levels), ligament size, limb alignment (Q angle), and femoral notch dimension. Extrinsic factors concern environmental variables, conditioning of the athlete, type of sport, and sport equipment. Extrinsics tend to be modifiable and/or changeable. See the evidence-based practice question that examines the relationship between level of estrogen and ACL laxity in the female athlete. A paucity of empirical data exists, and the few studies examined demonstrated equivocal results. Recommendations for future research include the following: Would adjusting estrogen levels by using oral or injectable hormone replacements augment neuromuscular and proprioceptive athletic performance in the female athlete? Would preathletic jump-training programs benefit the female athlete, and what are the implications of screening female athletes for ACL laxity before they play collegiate and/or professional sports?

NUTRITION, MICRONUTRIENTS, ANTIOXIDANTS, ERGOGENIC SUPPLEMENTS, AND HYDRATION IN SPORTS MEDICINE

Athletes are instructed to eat a well-balanced diet consisting of adequate quantities of carbohydrates, protein, and

EXAMINING THE EVIDENCE: Moving Toward Evidence-Based Practice
Is There a Causal Relationship between Estrogen Level and Anterior Cruciate Ligament (ACL) Laxity in the Female Athlete?

AUTHOR(S), YEAR	SAMPLE	DIAGNOSIS	DESIGN	OUTCOME VARIABLES	MAJOR FINDINGS
Boden, Dean, Geagin, & Garrett, 2001	$N = 89$	Contact and noncontact ACL injury	Interview and video analysis in control and experimental groups	Noncontact injury cause more ACL injuries than contact; hamstring flexibility/laxity is greater in injured athletes compared with control group	Greater injury occurs to the knee when it is in extension Quadriceps may play an important role in ACL disruption Passive protection provided by hamstrings
Karogeanes, Blackburn, & Vangelos, 2001	$N = 26$	ACL laxity	Prospective, single-blinded; 5 groups used—basketball, gymnastics, soccer, tennis, and track	Measuring ACL laxity in 3 phases: follicular, ovulatory, and luteal by using the KT-1000 arthrometer	No statistical difference among menstrual phases No statistically significant variability in laxity among groups No single phase of menstrual cycle affected ACL laxity
Liu, Al-Shaikh, Panossian, Finerman, & Lane, 1997	Animal study $N = 144$	Fluctuation in estrogen during menstrual cycle induces changes in metabolism	In vitro study of estrogen receptors on rabbit ACL fibroblasts	Influence of estrogen on cellular metabolism of ACL	Significant dose-dependent effect on fibroblasts of ACL Fibroblast proliferation and rate of collagen synthesis are reduced by increasing estradiol concentrations Alterations of estrogen levels associated with menstrual cycle or oral contraceptives may induce changes in metabolism of ACL, resulting in compositional and structural changes, which predisposes female athletes to ligament injury
Wojtys, Huston, Linderfield, Hewett, & Greenfield, 1998	$N = 28$	Noncontact ACL injury	Test-retest	Association of noncontact ACL injury rate and phase of menstrual cycle (follicular, ovulatory, luteal)	Significant statistical association between menstrual cycle and likelihood of ACL injury More injuries occurred in ovulatory and luteal phases than in follicular phase
Yu, Liu, Hatch, Panossian, & Finerman, 1999	$N = 72$	Estradiol concentrations affect ACL physiology	Experimental in vitro primary cell culture	There is an inverse dose-dependent relationship between fibroblast proliferation and procartilage synthesis and estrogen concentrations	Relative decrease in procollagen synthesis with increased estradiol concentrations translating to ACL weakening Cumulative or acute fluctuations in estradiol (menses or oral contraceptives) may induce changes in metabolism of ACL Structural and compositional changes on molecular level could result in decreased strength of the ACL and predispose female athlete to ligamentous injury

---

EXAMINING THE EVIDENCE: Moving Toward Evidence-Based Practice
Is There a Causal Relationship between Estrogen Level and Anterior Cruciate Ligament (ACL) Laxity in the Female Athlete? Continued

AUTHOR(S), YEAR	SAMPLE	DIAGNOSIS	DESIGN	OUTCOME VARIABLES	MAJOR FINDINGS
Hewett, Lindenfeld, Riccobene, & Noyes, 1999	N = 1263	Knee injury	Prospective—3 groups (trained, untrained, and control)	Neuromuscular training in female athlete may decrease injury to ACL	Nontrained female athletes are predisposed to knee ligament injury Trained female athletes had a decreased overall incidence of serious knee injury Female athletes involved in pivoting, cutting, jumping (e.g., soccer, basketball, volleyball) may benefit by preparticipation knee training program (jump and progressive resistance) Decreased abduction/adduction moments and improvement of quadriceps/hamstring strength ratios will benefit knee performance in sports

---

fat; essential vitamins and minerals are also important. Nutrient requirements are determined by athletes' age-body habitus, environmental training conditions, gender, genetics, duration, frequency, and intensity of training. Energy requirement is determined by physical activity, resting metabolic rate, and thermogenesis (body heat production). Energy requirements can be calculated by specialized equipment in a laboratory (calorie versus carbon dioxide production) and by recording an accurate 3-day dietary intake.

Metabolic demands placed on the body by exercise and competitive sports are increased considerably compared with everyday metabolic needs. Good nutritional intake is needed for repair of injured tissues, recuperation of fatigued muscles, and replenishment of nutrients. Most of the essential elements needed for sports nutritional needs are contained in the foods that may be eaten every day.

High-intensity resistance exercise that causes increased oxygen consumption also increases free radical production. Free radicals are molecules that contain one or more unpaired electrons. These powerful oxidants damage proteins, lipids, nucleic acids, sugars, and cell membranes. In relation to musculoskeletal tissue injury and conditions, free radicals precipitate damage to skeletal muscle, bone, cartilage, synovium, meniscus, tendons, ligaments, and intervertebral discs. Antioxidants are metabolic substances that protect body tissues against oxidative stress. Vitamins B, C, and E are antioxidants and should be included as part of a balanced nutritional intake. Vitamins and minerals like macronutrients are essential for metabolic function (e.g., bone strength and stability) and muscle contraction. Deficiencies in trace minerals (e.g., magnesium, zinc, selenium, manganese)

may affect athletic performance. Minerals such as calcium, magnesium, phosphorous, selenium, and zinc are basic to physiologic functioning of the cardiovascular, musculoskeletal, and immune systems. When energy demands increase, certain vitamins, for example, B, C, and E, are very important for increased nutritional needs. Low-body-weight athletes such as cheerleaders, gymnasts, and jockeys may not consume enough foodstuffs containing essential macronutrients and micronutrients. Specialized ingestants such as liquid (often made with powder) nutritional supplements are popular with bodybuilders, weight lifters, college and professional teams, and those who wish to boost their nutritional intake. Some sports nutritionists believe that liquid supplements decrease pregame symptoms such as abdominal cramps, dry mouth, leg cramps, nervous defecation, and nausea. Pregame emotional upset can delay gastric emptying of undigested (solid) food. Nutrients are therefore not absorbed and are not available to the athlete during competition.

Ergogenic supplements are substances that increase work-exercise performance. Creatine phosphate, a popular ergogenic supplement, is advocated to boost energy and exercise capacity. The physiologic benefits of creatine are increasing both short- and long-term energy and resynthesis during rest intervals and modest increases in lean body mass. Another ergogenic aid is beta-hydroxy-beta methylbutyrate (HMB), a metabolite of leucine. It is believed that HMB inhibits catabolism of muscle. Glycerol is another supplement that is incorporated as a hyperhydrating agent to prevent alteration in performance secondary to hypohydration. Pyruvate is purported to increase endurance and decrease body fat percentages. Glucosamine and chondroitin are generally taken in combination to decrease pain and degenerative influences within joints. They are used preventively and prophylactically. As with all ergogenic supplements, further empirical data are warranted before these supplements are prescribed on a standard basis.

Fluids and hydration is a great concern for athletes. Up to 1 to 3 L of fluid may be lost with intense physical workouts and during competition. Fluid should be replaced before, during, and after competition. Water is the optimal replacement; however, sports drinks may be ingested. A secondary benefit of using sports drinks for replacement is the additional carbohydrates and electrolytes that are replaced. Fluids containing caffeine, carbonation, and alcohol are not recommended as fluid volume replacements.

Another concern for the athlete may be the pre-event meal. This still may be referred to as *carbohydrate* (CHO) *loading*. Adequate amounts of carbohydrate help maintain and replenish glycogen stores. CHOs with a low glycemic index (those that do not drastically affect blood glucose levels) are suggested; these may include pasta, oatmeal, rye bread, barley, lentils, apples, and oranges. Athletes should consume 1 to 4 CHO/kg 1 to 4 hours before a game and avoid foods such as beans, cabbage, cauliflower, nuts, seeds, onions, and bran.

ENHANCING ATHLETIC PERFORMANCE

The use of performance-enhancing substances, including drugs, has ethical as well as legal implications for those involved in athletic competition. The International Olympic Committee (IOC), the National Collegiate Athletic Association (NCAA), and the National Football League (NFL) are among the groups who have banned certain drugs and substances for their athletes. These groups may include collegiate athletes, professional major league and minor league sports teams, and Olympians. Examples of drugs and banned substances are listed in Box 21–2.

ATHLETIC INJURY AND CONDITIONS

Unless otherwise noted, inflammation, pain control, and physical rehabilitation treatment of sports injury is suggested by the acronym *PRICEMM*:

Protection by the use of padding about joints and bony prominences, braces, splints; altering techniques to avoid further aggravation of injury

Rest, literally sitting out of a game or refraining from competition for a period of time, avoiding activities or biomechanical limb or body postures that exacerbate pain and inflammation

Ice or application of cryotherapeutic techniques to decrease local effects of inflammation; increase central and peripheral endorphins; and decrease the effects of substance P, serotonin, leukotrienes, and kinins on perceptual pain response

Compression with elastic bandages (Ace wrap), Air Cast, splint, cast, direct-pressure ascending massage technique to assist and mobilize edema from tissues

Elevation of injured body part above level of heart to facilitate venous return and to decrease swelling

Medications—oral nonsteroidal anti-inflammatory drugs (NSAIDs), acetaminophen, narcotic analgesics, other analgesics; injectable corticosteroid preparations

Modalities—physical rehab, electric stimulation, ultrasound (phonophoresis and iontophoresis), whirlpool, pool therapy, strength, endurance training, heat

A phenomenon sometimes seen with persons beginning a physical training program or changing or increasing activities is delayed-onset muscle soreness (DOMS). DOMS occurs as a result of microscopic tearing of muscle fibers. The associated soreness is secondary to muscle inflammation and swelling from muscle fiber injury. Physical activities that require muscles to forcefully contract while elongating (eccentric muscle contraction) precipitate greater soreness. These activities may include running downhill, descending stairs, lowering weights, and performing downward motions (i.e., push-ups or squats). A few suggestions in preventing DOMS or decreasing symptoms are as follows:

- Warm up thoroughly before physical activity and cool down after exercise.
- Begin with mild to moderate exercises and build up the intensity slowly.

BOX 21–2.
Examples of Banned Drugs and Substances

Androgenic Steroids
Hormones and analogues

Nonsteroidal Enhancing Agents and Drugs
Alcohol (in school events)
Cardiovascular/antihypertensive agents (e.g., atenolol, propanolol, beta-blockers/agonists)
Dehydroepiandrosterone (DHEA) and androstenedione (AD)
Diuretics
Erythropoietin (used for blood doping—enhances the oxygen carrying capacity of hemoglobin)
Human growth hormone, chorionic gonadotrophin
Insulin
Stimulants (e.g., amphetamines, cocaine, caffeine—greater than 15 µg/mL excreted in urine, ephedrine, phenylpropanolamine)
Street drugs (e.g., heroin, marijuana, tetrahydrocannabinol—THC, PCP)

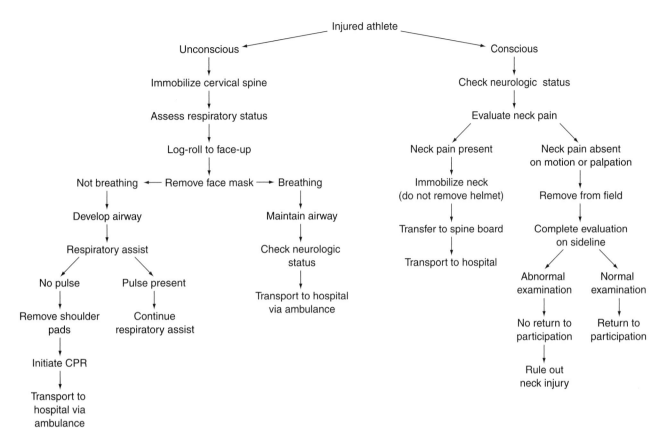

FIGURE 21–1. An algorithm for field decision making. CPR, cardiopulmonary resuscitation. (From Reider, A. B. [1996]. *Sports medicine: The school-age athlete* [p. 154]. Philadelphia: WB Saunders.)

• Avoid making sudden major changes in type of exercise or major changes in amount of time spent on exercise.

The PRICEMM principles can be used in the treatment of DOMS symptoms.

EVALUATION OF SPORTS INJURY

Obtaining a thorough history, including mechanism of injury, is mandatory in sports injury evaluation. If a sound understanding of the mechanism of injury is known, the health care provider can anticipate the type and level of injury as well as which diagnostic imaging study to order. Potential sequelae can also be anticipated. Acute injury assessment of the athlete commences with the basic ABCs (airway, breathing, circulation). The assessing health care provider should be certified in cardiopulmonary resuscitation (CPR) and basic and advanced first aid. After the ABCs have been evaluated, the assessment should next include a thorough neurovascular examination. If the mechanism of injury includes spine-related trauma, a spine evaluation is essential. If spine fracture is suspected or injury is associated with sudden loss of bowel or bladder function, loss of reflexes to the lower extremities, or loss of consciousness, the

athlete is stabilized in the field. The athlete is then transported to an emergency department (ED) or trauma center immediately. An injured extremity should be compared with the contralateral extremity, particularly in children. After an injured extremity is assessed, splinting or immobilization is performed, followed by transport to a medical facility for x-ray examination. In the case of a fracture, early immobilization leads to decreased sequelae and decreased functional disability. Sport injuries are rarely life- or limb-threatening; therefore, evaluation of an injured athlete can be performed in a unhurried manner (Fig. 21-1).

HEAD AND FACIAL TRAUMA

Protective sports equipment assists in decreasing the amount of head and facial trauma associated with collision and contact sports. However, some athletes do not wear protective gear, and injury to the integument and/or eyes may occur. Athletes with blunt and penetrating eye trauma are sent immediately to an ED. An athlete who is struck over a bony prominence (i.e., ocular ridge [eyebrow]) may sustain a laceration. Because of implications related to open wounds, blood, and body fluids, an athlete with a laceration or abrasion should receive treatment for suturing and wound management. Tetanus immunization status should be known for all athletes, and appropriate tetanus prophylaxis should be given if necessary.

Blunt head trauma may result in an open or closed head wound. Blunt-force closed head trauma can cause traumatic brain injury from acceleration-deceleration, rotational, and rotational-acceleration-deceleration mechanisms. Diffuse brain injury results from shaking the brain and can cause disruption of breathing, loss of consciousness, memory loss, and impaired cognition. Coup-countercoup injury from acceleration-deceleration creates maximum brain injury beneath the points of impact. The spinal fluid acts as a cushion for the brain, accepting some impact load; the skull also protects the brain tissue and decreases coup and countercoup injury. However, fractured skull fragments may penetrate the brain, compounding injury. Any athlete with open or closed head injury is stabilized and emergently transported to an ED.

CERVICAL SPINE INJURY

The cervical spine (C-spine) has extraordinary mobility compared with the thoracic and lumbar spines. Severe C-spine injury is rare in sports participation. When it occurs, it generally is from a freak injury in football or diving. However, the face mask on a football helmet may actually act like a lever to increase injuring forces to the C-spine. The mechanisms of injury that causes severe cervical injury are cervical flexion, forced hyperextension, hyperextension and hyperflexion, and forced rotational movements. Prevention of injury is accomplished by following good playing technique, using appropriate equipment, and being in a state of readiness before the snap. "Bulling the neck" is a protective muscular stance; it is performed by contracting the paracervical muscles and isometrically elevating the shoulders. Potentially disabling injury may be averted by this maneuver.

The most severe cervical injuries are fracture, dislocation, and spinal cord injury (SCI). These injuries are orthopaedic emergencies and require immediate C-spine immobilization and transport to an ED. Some injuries may cause partial or permanent paralysis.

Symptoms of fracture and dislocation of the C-spine may include pain, muscle spasm, swelling, and tenderness on palpation; initial neurologic deficits occur below the level of fracture or dislocation. Some neurologic deficits partially resolve after inflammation has decreased, leaving minimal dysfunction. Physical rehabilitation is mandatory to maintain muscle tone and preserve joint mobility. In some cases, permanent cord damage may precipitate life-long sequelae.

SCI, partial or complete transection, is devastating and causes complete areflexia below the level of injury. With high C-spine injury, interruption of brainstem function leads to cardiopulmonary arrest and death if

lifesaving activities are not implemented immediately. C-spine immobilization and basic and advanced life support are mandatory. In certain states, emergency medical services (EMS) personnel may institute "cord resuscitative measures" in the field while the athlete is stabilized and being transported to the ED. Athletic trainers and those qualified in emergency treatment need to establish an airway and protect the spine by immobilization in an unconscious athlete. Expect the worse until proven otherwise! Sandbags are placed laterally about the C-spine, adhesive tape across the forehead is used to immobilize the C-spine, and a hard cervical collar is applied. This immobilization prevents flexion, extension, rotation, and lateral bending of the C-spine. States with SCI specialty referral centers may use one of several drug therapy protocols. Ongoing research into the benefits of using drugs to prevent secondary damage from catecholamines, arachidonic acid metabolites, endorphins, free oxygen radicals, and deficient glucose utilization after injury are being studied. Some of the drugs under study are beta-blockers, high-dose methylprednisolone, naloxone, thyrotropin-releasing hormone, and synthetic corticosteroids or monosialotetrahexosylganglioside (GMI).

Cervical Sprains

Cervical sprains and strains are common injuries in sports. The mechanism of injury is similar to that which causes other types of sprains. Cervical sprain hyperextension, or whiplash, occurs when the neck is forcibly hyperextended. When cervical muscle-tendon-ligament structural forces reach their capacity, tearing occurs. Tearing and rupture of tissues precipitates bleeding, creating an inflammatory response and causing muscle spasm and pain. This inflammatory process ensues rapidly after the injury. One symptom of cervical sprain or strain is pain, usually on the side of the neck where the tear occurred. The pain usually starts out as a dull sensation and progresses to sharp pain. Range of motion (ROM) in the neck is decreased. The neck may be held in a rigid position because of spasm and pain. Sometimes, when palpating the muscles about the cervical spine, a localized region of tenderness can be isolated. Knots or painful points called *trigger points* are commonly palpated after cervical injury.

After the initial evaluation, including a neurologic examination, treatment consists of the application of ice or cryotherapy. Immobilization of the C-spine by a cervical collar is not recommended for longer than 24 hours. Treatment includes early physical therapy and the principles of PRICEMM. NSAIDs, analgesics, and muscle relaxants may be warranted.

Cervical Burner or Stinger Syndrome

Stretching of the cervical or brachial plexus that results in nerve root pathology causes cervical burner or stinger. Permanent nerve damage can result. The injury occurs when the athlete's head is forced away from the shoulder, stretching the nerves that descend from the brachial plexus and the spinal cord (Fig. 21–2). Nerve traction causes sensory and motor symptoms. A causalgia or burning sensation radiates down the arm. This injury causes a neurapraxia, which is a temporary cessation of peripheral nerve function without degenerative changes. This type of injury is most common in tackle football but may occur during hockey and wrestling. If this injury occurs frequently, fibrosis and scarring about the nerve roots can result in persistent or permanent weakness of the biceps, deltoids, and shoulder girdle muscles, as well as chronic neuritis and muscle atrophy.

Treatment for this injury begins with immediate application of ice or cryotherapy and temporary immobilization of C-spine and shoulder. If the pain is severe and associated with paralysis and loss of sensibility, the athlete may require x-ray examination to rule out dislocation, subluxation, or fracture of the C-spine. Strengthening of the paracervical muscles should be started early. As an adjunct, the athlete's technique should be examined to rule out improper methods of sport technique.

A cervical burner is a preventable injury. The rule prohibiting head spearing, a practice used by some football players in which the head is used as a battering ram, has decreased the incidence of cervical injuries and burners. In addition, cervical collars specially designed for play are placed between the neck and shoulder pads and are used to prevent lateral hyperflexion movements. Repeated burners may require surgical intervention to remove scar tissue and release entrapped nerves. Return to playing status depends on repeat or daily neurologic examinations. Return to unrestricted play may occur when ROM is full and no neurologic deficit is present.

UPPER EXTREMITY INJURIES
Shoulder

Injuries to the shoulder complex (bones, ligaments, tendons) usually result from a direct blow to the shoulder or a fall on an outstretched arm. Falling on an outstretched arm transmits axial loading forces directly against the scapula, resulting in various pathologies. Shoulder instability encompasses both subluxation and dislocation. Repetitive stretching of an injured shoulder with overhead activities and extremes of external rotation, such as swimming and throwing, stretches the anterior capsule and results in instability. Multidirectional instability creates serious performance problems for an athlete whose sport requires throwing, pitching, or swimming.

Assessment includes the apprehension test (Fig. 21–3). The affected shoulder is positioned to 90 degrees of abduction and external rotation with the elbow in 90 degrees of flexion. The shoulder is gently pushed into external rotation. Athletes with instability become apprehensive and feel a sensation of impending dislocation. X-ray film may reveal a Hill-Sachs lesion, a defect on the humeral head caused when the humeral head strikes the glenoid rim during dislocation. A Bankart lesion may also be detected. This defect is on the glenoid rim.

Glenohumeral dislocation or anterior shoulder dislocation happens 90% of the time in shoulder dislocation. The mechanism of injury is a fall on an outstretched hand and arm that is abducted, extended, and externally rotated. The humeral head is driven anterior and inferior to the coracoid. This is an acutely painful condition. The athlete is generally immobilized by pain and unable to move the shoulder. The affected shoulder is lower and the elbow is flexed and supported by the contralateral

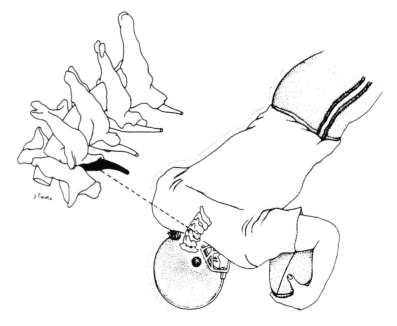

FIGURE 21–2. Acute lateral flexion of cervical spine causes brachial neurapraxia, known in football as a *burner*. (From Nicholas, J., & Hershman, E. [1995]. *The lower extremity and spine in sports medicine* [p. 1117]. St. Louis: Mosby.)

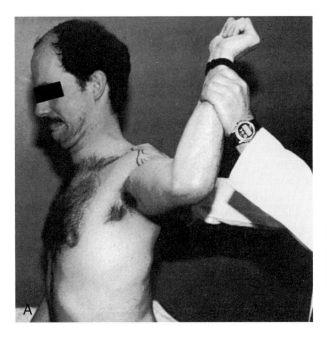

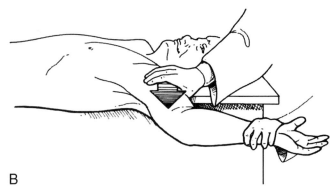

FIGURE 21–3. *A,* Apprehension test. The athlete fears pain and becomes apprehensive about the shoulder dislocating in this position. *B,* Relocation test. Anterior pressure on the proximal arm relocates the humerus and relieves apprehension. (From Miller, M. D., Cooper, D. E., & Warner, J. J. P. [1995]. *Review of sports medicine and arthroscopy* [p. 128]. Philadelphia: WB Saunders.)

extremity. Neurovascular assessment is important because axillary nerves as well as the radial artery can become impinged. Prompt reduction is necessary before excessive inflammatory swelling sets in. Posterior dislocation is less common but does occur. The mechanism of injury is axial loading onto an adducted, internally rotated, forward-flexed arm. Athletes are transported to an ED where x-ray equipment and analgesics are available. Rehabilitation consists of strengthening the shoulder girdle and reconditioning muscle-tendon units and the joint capsule.

Clavicle fracture is one of the most common fractures seen in sports. More than 80% occur over the middle third of the clavicle. Clavicle fractures in children are generally of the greenstick type. Treatment of fracture consists of PRICEMM, application of a sling and swath, or figure-of-eight sling. Rehabilitation is also instituted to maintain functional mobility of the upper extremity.

A sprain to the sternoclavicular joint happens after indirect traumatic force to the humerus, by a direct blunt injury to the clavicle, and by torsion of a posteriorly extended arm. Reducing the displaced clavicle is of primary concern. Treatment consists of immobilization and PRICEMM.

The AC joint is commonly injured in sports. The mechanism of injury is by a direct blow to the point of the shoulder driving the acromion process downward or by an upward force exerted against the long axis of the humerus. AC separations are classified into degrees of separation (Table 21–3). Protective taping of the AC joint allows movement of the shoulder while decreasing AC joint movement. Treatment consists of PRICEMM; surgery is rarely necessary.

Scapula fractures, which are rare, result from high-impact injuries. If a fracture occurs, it happens when the humerus pushes the scapula as the serratus anterior

TABLE 21–3. *Classification of Acromioclavicular (AC) Separation*

CLASSIFICATION	CLINICAL DESCRIPTION	CLINICAL EXAMINATION	X-RAY FINDINGS
First degree	Partial tear of AC joint but no actual separation of the bones	Pain about AC joint; difficulty elevating arm over head	Usually normal
Second degree	AC ligament completely torn; coracoclavicular (CC) ligament is intact	Pain, swelling at the site; actual separation can be palpated	Separation of AC joint demonstrated. Stress radiograph using weights, aggravates separation
Third degree	Complete tear of AC, CC, and joint capsule	Obvious deformity by inspection; severe swelling, tenderness, ecchymosis	Significant AC separation viewed without weights

Posterior

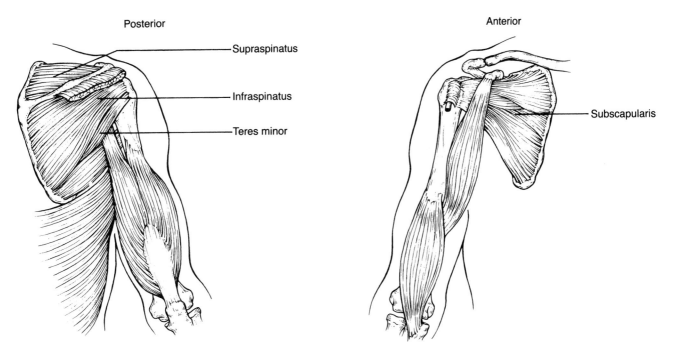

Supraspinatus

Infraspinatus

Teres minor

Anterior

Subscapularis

FIGURE 21–4. Rotator cuff muscles.

muscle violently forces the scapula forward. The athlete should be referred to an ED or orthopaedist for treatment.

Athletes with humeral fracture and suspected fracture about the shoulder are referred to an orthopaedist. Fractures are painful and may require cast or splint immobilization or possibly open reduction.

Rotator Cuff Disease

The supraspinatus, subscapularis, infraspinatus, and teres minor are called the *rotator cuff muscles* (Fig. 21–4). Repeated overhead activities, poor posturing, improper throwing technique, and direct injury causes swelling; repeated tears in the rotator cuff may result in scarring, swelling, and eventual rupture of the rotator cuff. Tears usually occur in the area between the supraspinatus and the coracohumeral ligament. This area is poorly vascularized, and degeneration often begins here. Repeated injury precipitates deposition of calcium into the tissues, which decreases the subacromial space and results in an impingement syndrome.

Impingement syndrome is an overuse injury caused by entrapment of the soft tissue structures between the acromion and the humeral head. Repetitive injury causes rotator cuff bursitis and tendonitis and chronically may lead to rupture of the rotator cuff. Athletes participating in sports that require overhead motion, such as racquet sports, throwing, and swimming, are more prone to this type of injury. When the arm is elevated over the head, the supraspinatus rubs against the acromion, causing irritation (Fig. 21–5). Note that the supraspinatus can be

isolated by placing the arm in the "empty can" position and examining for pain on resisted abduction (Fig. 21–6). During the assessment of the rotator cuff, the athlete may be able to abduct the arm to 45 to 60 degrees but will have difficulty abducting the arm from 60 to 121 degrees. This is the painful arc. It is painful because inflamed structures are being impinged or pinched by the acromion process. The athlete may have a positive drop arm test secondary to the painful arc phenomenon.

Diagnosis is based on clinical findings. Routine x-ray films are not usually warranted unless fracture or blunt trauma has occurred. Magnetic resonance image (MRI) is capable of revealing the severity of rotator cuff abnormalities.

Incomplete tears are treated with rehabilitation and PRICEMM, including NSAIDs. Injection of the subacromial space with lidocaine and a corticosteroid preparation may offer temporary relief of pain. Complete tears usually need surgical intervention, whereas partial tears and cuff inflammation are treated conservatively. The athlete begins a rehabilitation program to strengthen the rotator cuff complex. If a complete tear has occurred and all conservative methods have proved ineffective, surgical intervention is considered. Arthroscopy or an arthroscopy-assisted procedure can be performed for the purpose of direct examination and debridement of a rotator cuff tear. Arthroscopic debridement of the subacromial bursa and resection of the coracoacromial ligament and the inferior side of the acromion may be performed to increase the subacromial space and to prevent recurrence. Larger tears may require an open

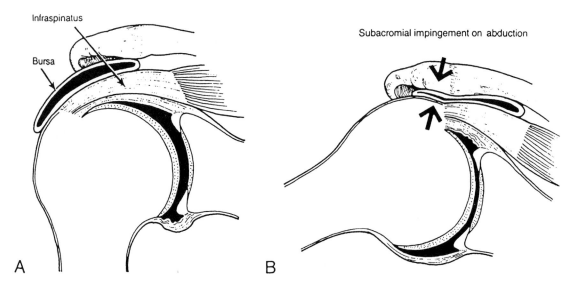

FIGURE 21–5. Subacromial impingement on glenohumeral abduction. *A,* The impingement interval and associated structures with the arm in neutral position. *B,* Subacromial impingement on abduction. (From Rowe, C. R., & Leffert, R. D. [1988]. Subacromial syndromes. In C. R. Rowe [Ed.], *The shoulder* [p. 106]. New York: Churchill Livingstone.)

surgical procedure followed by intensive rehabilitation that may last for several months. The rehabilitation program depends on the surgical repair performed. Most athletes perform shoulder shrugs; hand, wrist, and elbow strengthening exercises; and pendulum exercises progressing to flexion and external rotation. Most athletes are advised not to perform exercises that stress the supraspinatus. Undue stress on the supraspinatus may damage the surgical site and precipitate fibrosis. The goal is to enable the athlete to obtain full ROM of the shoulder.

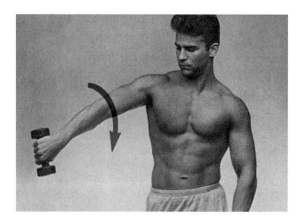

FIGURE 21–6. "Empty can" position as described by Jobe. (From Yahara, M. L. [1994]. Shoulder. In J. K. Richardson & Z. A. Iglarsh [Eds.], *Clinical orthopaedic physical therapy* [p. 195]. Philadelphia: WB Saunders.)

Lateral Epicondylitis

Lateral epicondylitis (tennis elbow) is caused by excessive irritation of the extensor carpi radialis brevis as it comes over the lateral epicondyle and radial head. Although most often associated with racquet sports, it does occur in other athletes who consistently pronate and supinate the forearm while using the wrists, such as pitchers and bowlers. The cause is often improper technique; however, the type of equipment must be considered. Symptoms include pain just below the lateral epicondyle (Fig. 21-7) and tenderness to palpation about this area. When the athlete is asked to hyperextend the wrist while the elbow is extended, increased pain is experienced because of the added stress on the tendinous structures. The athlete complains that lifting objects with the affected extremity is painful.

Treatment is usually cryotherapy, NSAIDs, and modification of technique. If NSAIDs appear to be ineffective, a local injection of a corticosteroid preparation may be indicated. Physical therapy with the application of ultrasound or iontophoresis may also be ordered. Several styles of tennis elbow splints are available. The device is fitted snugly just distal to the epicondyle, removing the stress from the epicondyle as the forearm is pronated and supinated (Fig. 21-8). Surgical intervention is rarely indicated for this problem.

In children, this injury is known as "Little Leaguer's elbow." The symptoms can occur as the result of attenuation of the medial structures, which increases the stress laterally. This commonly occurs in a child or an adoles-

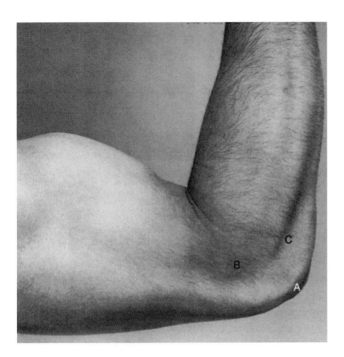

FIGURE 21–7. Lateral aspect of the elbow. *A,* Olecranon. *B,* Lateral epicondyle. *C,* Radial head. (From Reider, B. [1999]. *The orthopaedic physical examination* [p. 74]. Philadelphia: WB Saunders.)

cent because the epiphysis is extremely sensitive to compression stress before epiphyseal closure. Symptoms include pain in the lateral aspect of the elbow often accompanied by clicking and catching. The elbow may appear swollen, with tenderness palpated about the joint and a decrease in extension. In children, all throwing and pitching activities should be stopped. X-ray examination is usually performed to rule out displacement of the epiphysis. If displacement of the epiphysis has occurred and is still evident after conservative treatment, surgical intervention may be recommended to restore the growth center to anatomic position and to decrease the risk of permanent weakness or abnormal function. In more severe cases in which the ulnar nerve is impinged, surgical treatment to reroute the nerve away from the inflamed area may be indicated. In addition, removal of any loose bodies or calcifications may be performed. Surgery has a high failure rate and is avoided when possible.

Rehabilitation consists of stretching and strengthening the involved muscle-tendon group after a suitable period of rest. Adequate warm-up before a game is strongly recommended. It is also helpful to seek instruction to determine whether improper use of the equipment or improper technique is playing a part in increasing the stress. The principles of PRICEMM are also used.

Medial Epicondylitis

Medial epicondylitis usually occurs in pitchers and is caused by repeated stress on the muscle-tendon units used while throwing. It can also occur in golfers. The symptoms usually are pain and stiffness about the medial aspect of the elbow. The area is sensitive to touch and is sometimes swollen. Function of the elbow remains within expected limits. This injury in adults is treated with PRICEMM and NSAIDs. In some cases, a local injection of a corticosteroid preparation may be necessary to decrease the symptoms. Rehabilitation includes stretching and strengthening of the medial complex about the elbow.

Hand and Wrist Injuries and Conditions

Generally, finger injuries require immobilization with splints. Playing sports with an injured finger joint can be very cumbersome and can directly affect athletic performance. Fingertip injuries may include subungual hematoma, avulsed nails, paronychia, and felons (nail pulp infection). *Subungual hematoma* is a collection of blood beneath the nail bed, usually from a crushing mechanism. It is painful and requires trephination (puncture and letting) if bleeding is greater than 50% of the nail. If injury was caused by crushing, a radiograph is necessary. Distal tuft fractures are directly associated with subungual hematoma. Paronychia is an infection beneath the side of the nail. Warm soaks may help healing, however, and incision and drainage may also be necessary to clear the infection and create a healing environment. A felon is a

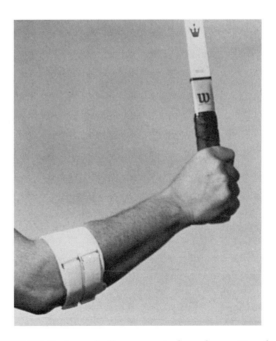

FIGURE 21–8. Lateral elbow counterforce brace. Nonelastic support is curved to fit conical forearm shape. Dual tension straps extend the width of the brace for full adjustments. Wide balanced support appears most effective for clinical pain control. (From Morrey, B. [Ed.]. [1993]. *The elbow and its disorders* [2nd ed., p. 543]. Philadelphia: WB Saunders.)

closed-space infection usually associated with puncture of the fingertip pulp. It requires referral for incision, drainage, and antibiotic therapy.

Distal Interphalangeal Joint. Mallet (baseball) finger is caused by direct forced flexion of the distal interphalangeal (DIP) joint. It may occur while attempting to catch a ball. The extensor mechanism is ruptured from the distal phalanx. The athlete is unable to extend the DIP joint. Treatment consists of ice or cryotherapy and splinting. Continual splinting is recommended for 6 to 8 weeks. ROM exercises are initiated after 6 weeks. If permitted by the health care provider, the finger can be taped and padded for playing.

Jersey finger is caused by a mechanism of injury opposite from mallet finger. Injury occurs after forced extension of a flexed DIP. It happens while an athlete attempts to grab an opponent's jersey causing avulsion of the long flexor tendon of the DIP. The athlete cannot flex the DIP. Splinting of the DIP is mandatory. Ineffective or delayed treatment may require surgery for tendon graft. The athlete is referred to a hand or orthopaedic specialist.

Proximal Interphalangeal Joint. Injuries to the proximal interphalangeal (PIP) joint occur from forced hyperextension and rupture of the volar plate; collateral ligament injury about the joint is not uncommon. Fracture of the joint may also occur. The athlete should be splinted and referred to a hand or orthopaedic specialist. Mild sprains are splinted and treated by PRICEMM.

Thumb. Forceful abduction injury to the thumb, or gamekeeper's thumb, is caused by sprain to the ulnar collateral ligament. It is seen in football and wrestling. The athlete complains of pain about the base of the thumb. During evaluation of the thumb, excessive laxity may be present compared with the contralateral thumb. The thumb should be splinted, an ice compress applied, and the athlete referred to a hand or orthopaedic specialist.

Dislocated finger joints should be promptly reduced. The athlete should be referred for an x-ray examination to rule out avulsion fracture. Treatment regimen includes PRICEMM and early rehabilitation.

Metacarpal Fractures. Fractured metacarpals require x-ray examination and accurate reduction, particularly in pediatric or adolescent athletes. A common finger fracture is the boxer's fracture (Fig. 21-9). It is fracture of the fifth metacarpal and happens after striking an object with a clenched fist, or when landing incorrectly after a fall. Oblique fractures affecting the articulating surface may require open reduction and internal fixation (ORIF). Athletes with metacarpal fractures should be referred to a

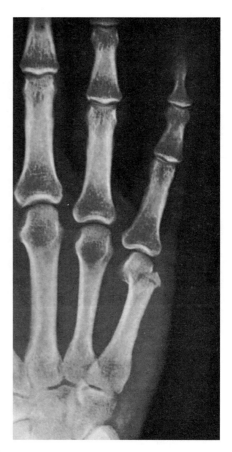

FIGURE 21–9. Boxers fracture. Displaced fracture, neck of fifth metacarpal (boxer's fracture). (From Gartland, J. J. [1987]. *Fundamentals of orthopaedics* [4th ed., p. 267]. Philadelphia: WB Saunders.)

hand or orthopaedic specialist. Open fractures are considered an orthopaedic emergency because of the potential for developing infection. Such athletes should be referred to a hand or orthopaedic specialist.

Wrist Injury. Wrist sprains are common in sports. They occur in football, basketball, soccer, and collision and contact sports. In children, swelling may not be as apparent as in an older athlete. Several wrist injuries may not be diagnosed promptly, which could lead to increased morbidity of an injured wrist. They include carpal scaphoid fracture (seen in basketball and football). The athlete complains of pain in the anatomic snuffbox (between the tendons of extensor pollicis longus and extensor pollicis brevis). The scaphoid has a tenuous blood supply, often resulting in avascular necrosis after injury. Hamate hook fracture results from strong twisting forces and may be seen in baseball, golf, and racquet sports. Anatomic position of the scaphoid and hamate are shown in Figure 21-10. Repeated strikes over the hypothenar eminence may cause a stress fracture. The athlete complains of pain about the hypothenar eminence. If conservative treatment is not successful, ORIF may be needed.

Fractures of the base of the second and third metacarpophalangeal (MCP) joint are considered wrist fractures because of the relationship to biomechanics, the volar retinaculum, and tendon-ligament structures. Falling on a flexed wrist is a common mechanism of injury. It is sometimes difficult to see these fractures on plain radiographs. Traumatic injury of the extensor carpi ulnaris tendon occurs after forceful flexion, supination, and ulnar deviation mechanisms. It may occur after a forced tennis forehand stroke. The athlete complains of a popping sound; this injury is usually treated conservatively with casting or molded splinting; however, surgery may be necessary.

Other Conditions. Dorsal ganglion about the scapholunate ligament is seen in the athlete, particularly the gymnast (Fig. 21–11). Repetitive stress from extremes of flexion or extension is thought to potentiate the formation of ganglia. Treatment includes splinting the wrist and using PRICEMM. If painful to the point of interfering with performance, surgical excision may be necessary.

Lacerations, abrasions, and puncture wounds are thoroughly cleansed with nonharsh solutions and covered to prevent contact with blood and serous fluid. Antibiotics and/or a tetanus booster may be warranted. These clients should be referred to their health care provider for necessary treatment. All fractures are referred for treatment.

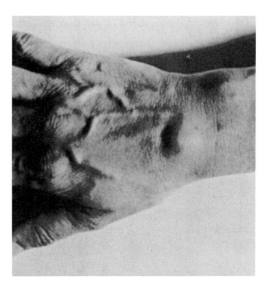

FIGURE 21–11. Ganglion. (From Jarvis, C. [1996]. *Physical examination and health assessment* [p. 700]. Philadelphia: WB Saunders.)

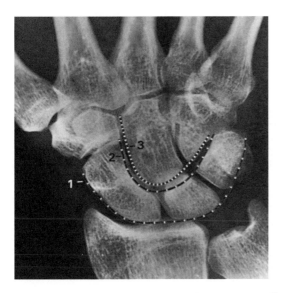

FIGURE 21–10. Wrist arcs. Three arcuate lines can normally be constructed along the carpal articular surfaces: (1) along the proximal margins of the scaphoid, lunate, and triquetrum; (2) along the distal aspects of the bones; and (3) along the proximal margins of the capitate and hamate. (From Weissman, B. N. W., & Sledge, C. B. [1986]. *Orthopaedic radiology* [p. 117]. Philadelphia: WB Saunders.)

LOWER EXTREMITY INJURIES

Injuries to the Hip and Groin

Iliac crest contusion, also known as a *hip pointer,* may be incapacitating. A hip pointer occurs from a direct blunt traumatic blow. Most often, this occurs in football, when a helmet comes in direct contact with the iliac crest, resulting in blunt soft tissue injury. Avulsion of muscles that insert along the iliac crest may cause significant soft tissue hemorrhage. The pain and tenderness are located about the iliac crest. Lateral bending, trunk rotation, and flexing the thigh may increase the pain. The young athlete may sustain an avulsion of the iliac crest apophysis. Fracture may also occur.

Initial treatment consists of application of ice or cryotherapy to control hemorrhage. A radiograph is taken of the pelvis to rule out a fracture of the iliac crest. Wearing hip pads can avert this injury. Hip pads are now mandatory for most collegiate games. The athlete usually must not participate in contact sports for 2 to 3 weeks and then can gradually return with the proper protective equipment. Heat may help speed the absorption of hematoma.

Avulsion Fracture of the Pelvis. Avulsion fractures occur when a tendon is forcefully pulled from the bone. In the pelvis, avulsion fractures may occur in the anterior superior iliac crest, sartorius, or anteroinferior iliac spine; it may also happen at the insertion of the superior head of the rectus femoris, at the ischial tuberosities, and at the insertion of the hamstrings. There is an increased incidence in young growing athletes because the tendons attached to these areas are weaker than mature bones. The sports in which avulsion fracture may be seen are football (especially the place kicker) and soccer. If the avulsion occurs at the insertion of the sartorius, the athlete feels pain over the anterior iliac crest. If the ischium is involved, pain, swelling, tenderness, and ecchymosis occur at the site (in the inferior aspect of the buttock). Sitting may be uncomfortable. X-ray films may show the avulsed bone.

The treatment of choice is usually conservative using crutches as necessary for 10 to 14 days. If avulsion is greater than 1 to 2 cm, open reduction may be necessary. As symptoms subside and healing progresses, a strengthening program for abdominal muscles, hamstrings, and lower spine muscles should be started. Return to full contact sports participation is possible when the muscles are rehabilitated to their previous level of strength and mobility.

Fractures of the sacrum, coccyx, and sacroiliac joint are not common, yet they do occur. Depending on the severity of the injury, treatment may be conservative or may require surgery.

Groin Strain. Sports that require extremes in cutting, quick starts and stops, running, and twisting, such as hockey, soccer, baseball, and football, can cause overexertion of groin structures causing strain. The groin musculature includes the iliopsoas, rectus femoris, and adductor muscles (gracilis, pectineus, adductor brevis, adductor longus, and adductor magnus). A severe strain can cause deep groin tenderness with radiation to the lower abdomen. The abdomen should be examined to rule out inguinal or femoral hernia and an acute abdomen. Symptoms of groin strain may range from mild to severe tearing of tissue structures, precipitating pain, hemorrhage, and weakness. Ecchymosis of muscle may be seen. ROM of the hip can increase pain.

Treatment of groin strain is sometimes difficult because the pain is diffuse. Treatment consists of the application of ice or cryotherapy and, after the initial inflammatory period of 3 to 5 days, heat and ROM. The athlete may need to modify activity until the pain has subsided. Preventive measures include warming up by flexibility and stretching exercises to the adductor group, iliopsoas, and rectus femoris muscles.

Dislocated Hip. Dislocation of the hip, although not common, does occur, particularly in contact sports. The hip is supported by ligamentous tissue, muscles, and a tough fibrous capsule made up of synovial tissue. Part of this capsule provides vascular supply to the femoral head. The mechanism of injury is traumatic force along the long axis of the femur. In a posterior dislocation, the athlete is found with the affected hip flexed, adducted, and internally rotated. In anterior dislocation, the hip is abducted and externally rotated. In both cases, the extremity appears shortened and the athlete complains of severe pain and spasm about the hip, thigh, and groin. Swelling and ecchymosis may be present.

Dislocation of the hip is an orthopaedic emergency. Sequela related to this injury is the development of avascular necrosis to the femoral head. If the head is not relocated within 12 hours, the chance of avascular necrosis increases. If the hip remains dislocated for more than 24 hours, the femoral head will suffer osseous death. Emergency treatment includes emergent transport of the athlete to an ED for x-ray examination and treatment. Relocation may require general anesthesia. Fracture of the labrum of the acetabulum is possible. Associated fracture of the femoral head requires surgical management. Splint the athlete's hip and do not manipulate the hip at the scene.

If no fracture is present, the femoral head is reduced and crutches are used for protected ambulation for 4 to 6 weeks. Rehabilitation is essential for strengthening and reconditioning of the hip.

Trochanteric Bursitis. Trochanteric bursitis is an inflammation of the bursa that lies posterior to the greater trochanter. The etiology may be related to broad pelvic structure seen in females (the pelvis in combination with wide Q angle of the knees) (Fig. 21–12), leg length discrepancy, poor running biomechanics, running on banked terrain and banked surfaces, tight tenor fas-

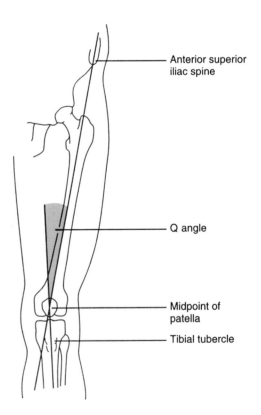

FIGURE 21–12. Q angle (quadriceps angle) of the knee. A normal Q angle is less than 21 degrees. An angle greater than 21 degrees predisposes the patella to problems such as subluxation/dislocation and patellofemoral syndrome. (From Magee, D. J. [1997]. *Orthopedic physical assessment* [3rd ed., p. 567]. Philadelphia: WB Saunders.)

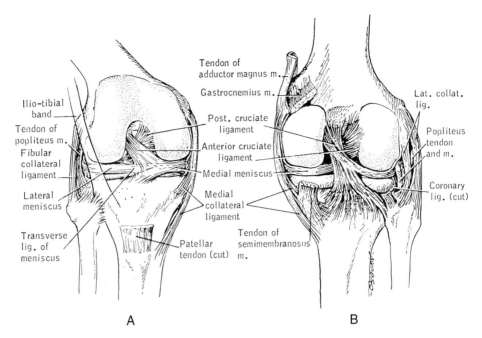

FIGURE 21–13. Anatomic drawings of knee. *A*, Anterior view, knee flexed. The patellar tendon is sectioned, and the patella is reflected upward. Note that the cruciate ligament rises in front of the anterior tibial spine, not from it. Note also that the medial meniscus is firmly attached to the medial collateral ligament. *B*, Posterior view, knee extended. Note that the posterior ligament has been removed. The two layers of the medial collateral ligament are shown diagrammatically, as is the tibial portion of the lateral collateral ligament. The posterior cruciate ligament rises behind the tibia, not on its upper surface. Observe the femoral attachment of the anterior cruciate ligament at the back of the notch. (From O'Donoghue, D. H. [1992]. *Treatment of injuries to athletes* [p. 669]. Philadelphia: WB Saunders.)

cialata, and tissue reaction secondary to a direct fall or blow to the trochanter.

When the bursa is inflamed, it may enlarge. Abduction of the hip, especially against resistance, is painful. ROM of the hip joint is usually within expected limits. X-ray films, although not generally indicated, may show calcification in the area of the bursa.

Rest from the sport with modification of activities; ice, cryotherapy, or heat; and NSAIDs are usually prescribed. An injection of a corticosteroid preparation into the bursa may be indicated if systemic drugs are ineffective.

For leg length discrepancies, orthotics, special shoes, or heel lifts can compensate for the discrepancy. The running surface should be evaluated. The athlete should be observed during performance. A flexibility and strengthening program is instituted. The athlete is allowed to return to full activity after the pain has decreased. For further information about bursitis and its treatment, see Chapter 14.

Myositis Ossificans. Myositis ossificans, or calcification within the muscle, sometimes occurs after a severe contusion and hematoma to a large muscle, commonly the quadriceps. In repeated injury, tissue undergoes a reactive process. With healing, the body deposits calcium

at the site of injury, creating heterotopic bone formation (particularly if the injury occurs about the periosteum).

Symptoms include swelling and inflammatory changes at the site of injury. The area may be tender to palpation and warm to the touch. Initial x-ray films may show a soft tissue mass. After the acute phase, the mass remains but is painless and eventually decreases in size. If the hematoma is contained within the muscle, it is usually resorbed. However, if the hematoma is closer to the insertion or origin of the muscle, there is a chance of functional impairment. Surgical excision may be necessary. On occasion, however, surgery has resulted in the formation of more heterotopic bone. An NSAID, such as indomethacin (Indocin) or long-term ibuprofen, may be helpful in decreasing the amount of heterotopic bone formation.

Myositis ossificans must be monitored closely because in the initial phase, the signs and symptoms may mimic those of malignant bone tumors. A thorough history and physical examination are essential.

Injuries to the Knee

The knee, the largest joint in the body, is complex and one of the most commonly injured joints during sports participation (Fig. 21–13). Because of its very nature, the knee is exposed to many injuries, some of which can be devastating to an athlete's career.

The ligaments in the knee provide four-plane stability to the knee joint. These planes consist of medial-lateral and anterior-posterior. The ligaments are the medial and lateral collateral ligaments and the anterior and posterior cruciate ligaments. The medial collateral ligament (MCL) provides stability to the knee by resisting valgus stress and external rotational forces of the tibia in relation to the femur. The lateral collateral ligament (LCL) is the primary static restraint against varus stress. The ACL provides knee stability against anterior translational forces. The posterior cruciate ligament (PCL) provides stability against stresses applied to the tibia. The ACL and PCL ligaments enable the knee to perform rolling and sliding movements.

Medial and Lateral Collateral Ligament Injuries.
The mechanism of injury related to an MCL/LCL injury occurs when an athlete's foot is firmly planted on the turf while sustaining valgus or varus stress to the knee joint. Torsional forces or a blow to the knee causes injury to the medial or lateral sides of the knee (Fig. 21–14). During the injuring mechanism, the athlete often feels a tearing sensation or hears a snap as the ligament is sprained. Immediate pain, swelling, and instability are experienced. Walking is difficult without assistance. Point and generalized tenderness at the site of injury is evident on examination of the knee. When valgus or varus stress is placed on the knee, as it is flexed approximately 30 degrees, the joint space widens either medially or laterally depending on which ligament is injured. This maneuver, as well as other provocative tests, also causes increased pain.

Immediate treatment consists of ice massage and PRICEMM. The athlete should be transported to a medical facility for x-ray examination to rule out associated avulsion fracture. A rehabilitation program begins early for strengthening the quadriceps and hamstrings. A reinforced brace may be recommended to protect grade II and III sprains and may be worn during sports play. Sports participation is permitted when stability and ROM is within expected limits, strength has returned, and pain has decreased.

Anterior and Posterior Cruciate Ligament Injuries.
The ACL and PCL are considered primary rotary stabilizers. The ACL and PCL cross each other within the knee; they are intracapsular but are extrasynovial.

The most common mechanism of injury for an ACL tear includes sudden deceleration, with some or no knee flexion, change in direction with the foot planted, and valgus force being applied to an externally rotated leg. It can occur during a "cutting" or "clipping" maneuver in football. The athlete often hears a pop and relates a feeling of something tearing and of the knee giving way. Immediate pain, moderate to severe hemarthrosis, instability, and difficulty walking are common symptoms of an acute ACL tear. An ACL tear may occur during basketball, gymnastics, football, skiing, soccer, and volleyball. Jumping, pivoting, and twisting maneuvers, often seen in noncontact sports, are associated factors. The ACL is injured more often than the PCL. Clinical diagnosis of an ACL tear can be accompanied by other injuries, especially torn menisci and collateral ligaments. A phenomenon known as "The Terrible Triad of O'Donoghue" (Brown & Neumann, 1995; Rosen & Barkin, 1998) consists of an ACL tear, MCL tear, and a torn medial

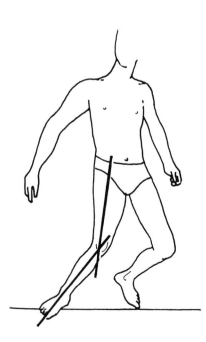
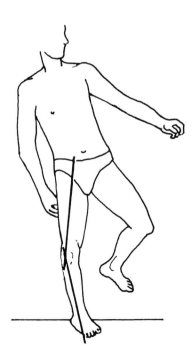

FIGURE 21–14. Mechanism of injury in capsule-ligament tears of the knee. (From Kuprin, W. [1995]. *Physical therapy for sports* [2nd ed., p. 275]. Philadelphia: WB Saunders.)

meniscus and is commonly seen during twisting and shearing mechanisms.

Immediate treatment of a torn cruciate ligament includes stabilization of the knee by a supportive dressing or splint and the application of ice or cryotherapy. The athlete is taken to a medical facility for x-ray examination to rule out associated fracture. Secondary to shearing mechanisms, there is a considerable amount of intracapsular and extracapsular hemorrhage that accompanies this injury.

Diagnosis of a torn ACL can be made on the basis of provocative tests during the clinical examination. Anterior drawer, Lachman's, and pivot shift test findings are positive (see Chapter 8). Clinical assessment that quantifies ligament laxity can be obtained by using an arthrometer instrument called a Kinemax or KT 1000. Both the athlete's knees are evaluated for comparative difference. A 3-mm difference demonstrates ligamentous dysfunction. These pieces of equipment provide the examiner with precise measurements (in millimeters) of the amount of anterior translation of the tibia onto the femur. One knee is tested against the other, assuming that both knees are comparable.

Similar to the Ottawa guidelines proposed for evaluation of acute ankle injury, the Ottawa Knee Rule (OKR) (Stiell, Wells, Hoag, Sivilotti, Cacciotti, Verbeek, Greenway, McDowell, Cwinn, Greenberg, Nichol, & Michael, 1997; Tandeter & Shvartzman, 1999) was developed to allow the treating health care provider to be more selective and efficient in when or if to order diagnostic imaging studies for acute knee injury. Incorporating the OKR is up to the discretion of the treating health care provider. The OKR postulates ordering plain radiographs for the following findings:

- Age 55 years or older
- Isolation of tenderness of the patella (no bone tenderness to other parts of knee)
- Tenderness at head of fibula
- Inability to flex knee to 90 degrees
- Inability to bear weight both immediately and in the ED (or if unable to transfer weight twice onto each lower limb regardless of limping)

Treatment for ACL injuries continues to be controversial among treating orthopaedists. Some physicians favor primary, immediate reconstruction, whereas others prefer delayed reconstruction after a period of 3 to 6 weeks of rehabilitation and after the hemarthrosis has subsided. Some surgeons prefer to treat athletes nonsurgically with physical therapy and bracing. Surgery in young children (prior to Tanner stage 3—a physical developmental guide) may be delayed because of surgical alterations of growth plates that are necessary. Surgical repair may include patellar tendon autografting or allografting techniques and reconstruction using a portion of hamstring. In some cases, using synthetic material,

such as Gore-Tex, augments repair of the ACL. Most ACL repair procedures are performed on an outpatient basis. Most current rehabilitation protocols (after patellar tendon graft) allow weight bearing as tolerated and encourage unrestricted ROM and an early strengthening and flexibility exercise program. After treatment of a ligamentous injury to the knee, whether surgical or conservative, rehabilitation is extremely important. This requires a commitment from the athlete to participate in a stringent therapy program. Some physicians require the athlete to wear a brace during vigorous sports activity, but this remains controversial.

Meniscal Injuries. The menisci are semilunar fibrocartilaginous structures that function by transmitting load forces across the knee. The meniscus increases and displaces surface area of bony contact between the femoral condyles and the medial tibial plateau. It is also prone to damage from varying mechanism of injury during running, cutting, and contact sports. The peripheral third of the meniscus has minimal blood supply, which gives that portion of the meniscus limited potential for healing when torn.

Signs and symptoms of a cartilage tear can include a popping or tearing sensation at the time of injury. Medial meniscus tears are symptomatic with medial joint line pain and mild to moderate effusion. If the tear is large a piece of cartilage may glide around inside the knee causing locking of the knee; that is, the athlete is not able to fully extend the knee. Other symptoms that may occur are catching, popping, and clicking while walking and with ROM of the knee. Stiffness (especially after sitting for long periods), periodic swelling, and giving way (buckling) may also occur.

Surgery may be indicated for a torn meniscus. Torn cartilage is a source of irritation in the knee and precipitates the buildup of an effusion. Chronic irritation can cause synovitis.

Physical examination includes palpating the joint line for tenderness. The menisci lie along the outer rim of the tibia and may be felt by palpating the space between the tibia and the femur. Tenderness is an indication of possible meniscal pathology. The amount of effusion is noted. Stability of the ligaments is tested to rule out tearing or stretching of those structures. Extreme flexion of the knee, as in squatting, often causes pain if the cartilage is torn. Pivot shift and McMurray's test, which is often positive for a torn meniscus, involves flexing the knee to allow the torn piece of cartilage to recede into the joint space. The examiner then attempts to fully extend the knee while rotating the tibia. The examiner places the fingers along the joint line (see Chapter 8). With this maneuver, the torn piece of cartilage can be felt popping back into place. This test may also cause locking and pain.

Routine x-ray films are of little value in diagnosing a torn cartilage but are of value in ruling out the presence of other types of pathology, such as bone cysts or osteochondritis dissecans, which may produce similar symptoms. If more definitive testing is indicated, an arthrogram or MRI scan may be ordered.

Conservative treatment for a torn meniscus includes PRICEMM. Once the initial swelling and pain decrease, quadriceps strengthening exercises are started. If the pain and swelling are persistent and the athlete continues to complain of transient locking, surgery is considered. This surgery is performed arthroscopically on an outpatient basis. Rehabilitation is started early postoperatively.

Rehabilitation consists of quadriceps strengthening and ROM exercises. Return to previous level of activity is allowed as soon as strength has returned to normal. If the meniscus has been repaired by osteochondral transplant technique, the client is kept non–weight bearing, and ROM of the knee is limited to protect the integrity of the repair. Isometric, active, and resistive exercises are performed to maintain the strength of the quadriceps and hamstrings. Progression to full weight bearing and full ROM is determined by the extent and location of the meniscal tear.

Osteochondritis Dissecans.

Osteochondritis dissecans is a focal area of necrotic subchondral bone. The cause varies; however, injury to end arterioles in subchondral bone from repetitive microtrauma causes local bone ischemia and eventual avascular necrosis. This condition is most commonly found on the medial femoral condyle and may also occur in the capitellum of the elbow and the talar dome of the ankle.

Symptoms of osteochondritis dissecans are clicking, popping, pain, swelling, and transient locking of the joint. The athlete often complains of something getting caught inside the knee, pain, and the inability to extend the joint. Plain radiographs may show a subchondral defect. MRI is sensitive and specific for diagnosis.

Conservative treatment includes quadriceps strengthening and avoidance of pain-producing sports in the young athlete. The occurrence of osteochondritis dissecans in the teenager or adult usually requires arthroscopic examination and coring of the stable fragment. This treatment attempts to stimulate healing. If the fragment is loose or very large, surgical intervention is considered. The goal of the surgery is to fix the fragment in place, using wires or screws or excision of the fragment. This procedure usually can be completed using arthroscopic techniques. On occasion, however, arthrotomy is necessary. Rehabilitation consists of quadriceps strengthening and ROM exercises. The athlete can usually return to full activity when strength and endurance have returned to preinjury status.

Osgood-Schlatter Disease.

Osgood-Schlatter disease (OSD) is a common traction apophysitis and exertional injury in knees of young adolescents. It is usually associated with jumping sports. It is thought to occur from repetitive microtrauma to the tibial apophysis. A prominence to the tibial tubercle may be palpated. The athlete complains of achy-type pain and swelling after acceleration/deceleration forces. Treatment consists of avoidance of aggravating sports, PRICEMM, hamstring strengthening, and a knee support. Casting in severe cases after surgical excision may be necessary.

Injuries to the Lower Leg and Foot

Shin splints (posterior tibial stress syndrome) or periostitis may occur in athletes who pursue activities that require a great deal of high impact on hard surfaces. It results from cyclic loading at the posterior tibial and talus muscle attachments onto the tibia causing periosteal inflammation. Shin splints are characterized by pain in the anterior portion of the lower leg, which can be caused by overuse, improper footwear, or high impact on hard surfaces.

This area can swell and be tender to palpation. The athlete is usually able to initiate running but has to stop because of increasing pain. This condition is not usually serious and often can be treated with conservative methods such as rest, cryotherapy, and NSAIDs. Athletic shoes should be examined for excessive or abnormal wear and replaced as needed. The athlete should be cognizant of excessive pronation of the foot because this increases the stress on the tendons and contributes to the problem. In addition, the training regimen, type of shoe, and running surface should be examined. A rapid increase in mileage, change in running surface, or lack of adequate shoe support can also contribute to the development of shin splints. If the symptoms persist, it may be wise to obtain an x-ray film of the tibia to rule out stress fracture. Stress fractures are usually seen on a plain x-ray film after 4 to 6 weeks, when evidence of healing is apparent. To confirm a stress fracture, a bone scintigraphy is the gold standard; however, MRI may be ordered instead of bone scan.

Achilles Tendon Injuries.

The Achilles tendon attaches the gastrocnemius and soleus muscles to the os calcis. The blood supply to the tendon is located in the anterior aspect of the tendon, with the poorest blood supply located in the area 2 to 6 cm above the os calcis, the most common area of injury for the tendon.

Achilles tendonitis is characterized by generalized pain in the tendon. Inflammation may occur after an athlete changes the height of the heel by wearing different shoes. An example of this is when a woman who wears high-heeled shoes almost exclusively begins an exercise program with athletic shoes. The abrupt and persistent change in tension on the tendon causes inflammation and pain. This condition can also occur in the athlete who runs uphill in stiff shoes or in the cyclist who exaggerates ankle motion when pedaling. Recent literature has postulated a correlation between taking fluoroquinolone antibiotics and rupture of the Achilles tendon. Apparently, these antibiotics affect the histopathology of the Achilles tendon, predisposing certain individuals to rupture of the Achilles tendon (Williams, Attia, Wickiewicz, & Hannafin, 2000).

Treatment of the problem includes elevating the heel with a heel insert or heel cup in the shoe and using the PRICEMM principles. NSAIDs are usually helpful. Early treatment is important in preventing the development of chronic tendonitis, whereby degeneration of the tendon predisposes it to rupture.

Partial rupture of the Achilles tendon may occur after tendonitis or during the push-off phase of activity. This injury causes pain, limping, and inability to continue in the athletic activity. Treatment includes examination of the tendon to evaluate for complete rupture of the tendon. Cryotherapy, taping or strapping the ankle in plantar flexion, and insertion of a heel lift in the shoe may be used to relax the tendon so that it can heal.

Achilles tendon ruptures usually occur in athletes older than 30 years of age. Athletes who experience this injury report a sudden sharp pain, like getting "shot," and a loud snap at the time of injury. The athlete experiences pain and has difficulty walking because of limited motion in the ankle. Examination of the ankle may demonstrate a gap between the ends of the tendon, which can be palpated about 1 to 1.5 inches (2.5 to 4 cm) proximal to the heel. X-ray films are usually not diagnostic but are necessary to rule out avulsion fracture. The Thompson test is used to assist with the diagnosis of Achilles tendon rupture. The athlete should kneel on a chair or lie prone on a table. The examiner squeezes the calf of the affected leg. When this is done, the ankle and foot should plantar flex, indicating that the tendon is intact. If the ankle and foot do not move, the tendon is most likely ruptured.

Initial treatment of this injury includes cryotherapy and compression. Conservative treatment may include casting, with the foot in plantar flexion for 6 weeks. The athlete is then required to wear a heel lift to help decrease the amount of stress on the tendon. If the conservative approach is used, the athlete has an increased chance of rerupturing the tendon on return to full activity. If the ends of the tendon have receded, surgical intervention may be necessary. Complete ruptures are surgically repaired.

Rehabilitation consists of gentle plantar flexion exercises. Dorsiflexion is cautioned. Athletes should not return to full activity until strength is approximately that of the unaffected extremity. Rehabilitation may take 5 to 6 months. One of the best ways to prevent injury is to warm up and condition before participation in strenuous or vigorous activity.

Ankle Sprains. The ankle is the most frequently injured joint in the body during sports participation. An ankle sprain most often occurs when the foot is inverted,

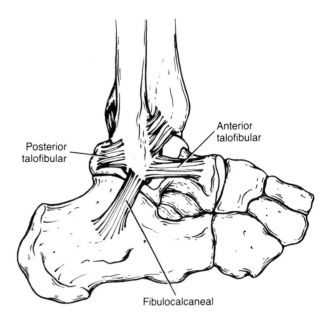

FIGURE 21–15. The three components of the lateral collateral ligament are the anterior and posterior talofibular and, between them, the calcaneofibular, which crosses the talus. The orientation of anterior talofibular and fibulocalcaneal ligaments is demonstrated. (From Browner, B. D., Jupiter, J. B., Levine, A. M., & Trafton, P. A. [1992]. *Skeletal trauma: Fractures, dislocations, ligamentous injuries* [p. 1874]. Philadelphia: WB Saunders.)

causing an inversion sprain. The main stabilizing ligaments supporting the lateral collateral complex are the anterior talofibular ligament (ATFL), calcaneofibular ligament (CFL), and posterior talofibular ligament (PTFL) (Fig. 21–15). The medial complex is the deltoid ligament and is made up of the ATFL/PTFL, tibionavicular ligament, and talocalcaneal ligament. A posterior ring structure provides stability. The ankle is a hinge joint articulating with the dome of the talus and the distal tibia and fibula. A strong retinacular capsule associated with powerful ligaments support the joint. Flexibility, proprioception, and strength are important for sound ankle function.

Pathomechanics associated with ankle sprain include plantar flexion and inversion of the lateral complex, which results in an inversion sprain. Associated fracture may include distal fibula and base of the fifth metatarsal. Ligamentous attachments have greater tensile strength at these regions. Significant twisting, torque, and shearing mechanisms can cause disruption of the anterior inferior talofibular ligament (AITFL), PTFL, inferior transverse ligament, and interosseous ligament (called the *syndesmosis*), causing a high ankle sprain (Childs, 1999). The tibiofibular syndesmosis creates a supportive ringlike structure about the ankle. Syndesmosis or syndesmotic sprain is a serious injury and causes ankle instability.

After a history is obtained and the mechanism of injury determined, a thorough evaluation of the ankle may proceed. The athlete complains of varying levels of

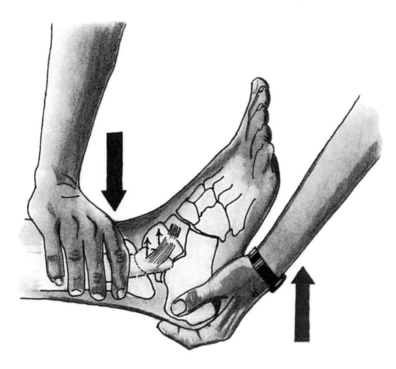

FIGURE 21–16. Anterior drawer testing of the right ankle, demonstrating anterior talar subluxation on the tibia. (From DiChristina, D., & Garth, W. P. [1996]. Ankle sprains. In V. R. Masear [Ed.], *Primary care orthopaedics* [p. 120]. Philadelphia: WB Saunders.)

pain, instability, and swelling. Provocative tests determine injury to certain anatomic structures. These tests include the anterior drawer test, talar tilt test, and squeeze test.

The anterior drawer (Fig. 21-16) test assesses the integrity of the ATFL. To perform this test, the examiner holds the foot in neutral, grasps the hindfoot while pulling the foot forward, and feels for an endpoint (tightness to ligamentous structures). The talar tilt test is done to detect ligamentous stability of the CFL. The ankle mortise is placed in inversion and eversion. To perform the talar tilt test, the examiner immobilizes the lower extremity, grasps the calcaneus, inverts and everts the foot, and feels for a tight endpoint. A significant difference between medial and lateral sides of greater than 25% or a soft endpoint with dimpling about the lateral complex compared with the contralateral ankle indicates a positive test. The squeeze test determines instability in the distal syndesmotic ligaments (AITFL, PTFL, inferior transverse ligament, and interosseous ligament). It is performed by squeezing the tibia and fibula at midshaft of the lower extremity. A positive test yields pain in the ankle.

Some health practitioners may incorporate the Ottawa Ankle Rule (Stiell, Greenberg, McNight, Nair, McDowell, & Worthington, 1992; Stiell, Greeenberg,

McKnight, Nair, McDowell, Reardon, Stewart, & Maloney, 1993) before ordering x-ray films (anteroposterior [AP], lateral, mortise views) after injury. In using these guidelines, x-ray examination should be the discretion of the health care provider treating an injured athlete. The Ottawa guidelines state that x-ray films are warranted in the following situations:

- Athlete is unable to bear weight on the affected ankle immediately and for four steps while being evaluated.
- There is bone tenderness at posterior edge or tip of lateral and medial malleolus.
- There is pain on palpation at base of fifth metatarsal (MTP).

If these findings are present, the athlete should be referred for definitive diagnostic imaging. Referral is made for treatment of fracture of the articulating surface, for moderate or severe ankle instability, or for locking of the joint. Sprains associated with open fracture are orthopaedic emergencies. These athletes should be referred.

Sprains are treated immediately using the PRICEMM principles and immediate rehabilitation. Rehabilitation is begun early for edema control and to maintain proprioception and ankle flexibility. Table 21-4 lists characteristics of sprains.

TABLE 21–4. *Ankle Sprain*

SIGN/SYMPTOM	GRADE I (FIRST DEGREE)	GRADE II (SECOND DEGREE)	GRADE III (THIRD DEGREE)
Pain	Mild/moderate	Moderate	Severe
Swelling	Mild/moderate	Moderate/severe	Severe
Range of motion	Normal	Abnormal	Positive anterior drawer test
Talar tilt sign	Normal	Normal/abnormal	Talar tilt > 21 degrees

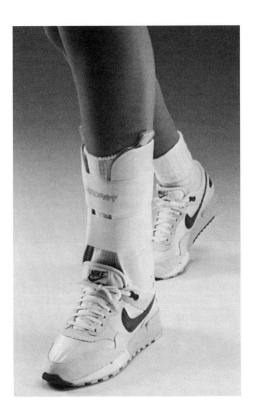

FIGURE 21–17. Air-Stirrup ankle brace. (Courtesy of Aircast, Inc.)

First-Degree Sprain. PRICEMM is used for 3 to 5 days and rehabilitation begun the day of injury with ROM and strengthening exercises. The athlete may be able to return to competition within 10 days to 2 weeks. Taping or bracing protection should be provided.

Second-Degree Sprain. PRICEMM is used; these sprains usually require immobilization with a splint or brace until the initial swelling has diminished, usually in 1 to 2 weeks. Pain and swelling usually mandate partial weight bearing with crutches and full weight bearing after the swelling has decreased. Active ROM and functional rehabilitation of the ankle should be performed daily during the initial stages of therapy. A brace (e.g., an Air-Stirrup splint) (Fig. 21–17) to prevent inversion and eversion of the ankle while permitting plantar flexion and dorsiflexion is used with full weight bearing as tolerated. Sporting activities may be prohibited for 2 to 3 weeks, and the ankle should be taped or braced before playing.

Third-Degree Sprain. PRICEMM is used; cast or brace immobilization is required for 3 to 6 weeks. Once the cast is removed, the athlete's ankle can be placed in an Air-Stirrup–type splint for support (see Fig. 21–17).

Gentle ROM, functional rehabilitation, and strengthening exercises can be started at this point. When strength and mobility return, the athlete can return to competition, provided that adequate taping and protection are worn.

Syndesmotic Sprain. Syndesmotic sprain creates an unstable ankle and is treated like a grade III sprain. PRICEMM is used; the athlete may require 4 to 8 weeks of rehabilitation before return to full activity. Nighttime splinting may also be necessary. Achilles tendonitis is a sequela of syndesmotic sprain.

Repeated inversion injury causes a condition known as *lateral instability of the ankle.* The athlete has repeated episodes of the ankle giving out secondary to ligamentous laxity. Chronic instability can be confirmed with stress radiographs. Ligamentous reconstruction of the lateral complex about the ankle may be recommended.

As with any injury, prevention is a key part of education for the athlete. Pregame conditioning and using proper technique and equipment are also essential.

Runner's Toe

Runners, joggers, and athletes participating in sporting activities requiring quick stops on nonslip court surfaces, such as tennis, may jam the great toe against the inside of the athletic shoe. This blunt-force trauma may cause the formation of a hematoma or a subungual hematoma. It is especially common in rock climbers and runners who run on hilly or uneven terrain.

This injury is painful because the hematoma creates pressure beneath the nail. The pressure can be relieved by trephination (puncturing a hole in the nail with a heated instrument). Secondary disruption or elevation of the nail plate from the matrix usually causes the nail to loosen and to need removal. In some cases, the nail plate is so loose it may fall off. Protecting the exposed nail matrix with a dry dressing is suggested. If the matrix has been disrupted, the nail may grow back with a deformed ridge. By wearing properly fitting athletic shoes, this injury can be prevented. The sport does not have to be discontinued during the healing phase unless there is excessive pain. Cryotherapy, good socks, and the right athletic shoe are important for treatment.

Turf Toe. Turf toe is an injury that is seen in tackling sports, particularly football. It is caused by hyperextension of the first MTP (with disruption of the joint capsule) while the ankle is mildly dorsiflexed. This may occur while being tackled (the forefoot is planted with the heel in the air). The athlete complains of difficulty walking (in the push-off stance), pain, and swelling about the first MTP. There is an increased incidence seen in athletes who play on Astroturf. Treatment consists of ice or cryotherapy and NSAIDs; injection with lidocaine and corticosteroid preparation may help. Placing a stiffening piece inside the athletic shoe to prevent hyperextension and supportive taping may also help.

Plantar Fasciitis. Plantar fasciitis is a common cause of heel pain in runners. It is an inflammation of the fascia that may extend from the heel to the toes. The plantar fascia (aponeurosis) supports the forefoot and midfoot arches. When the arch is flattened upon stepping or walking, the fascia is stretched. This constant tension can cause microscopic tears in the fascia at the point where the plantar aponeurosis attaches to the calcaneus. Recurrent tears at the insertion site may precipitate the formation of a heel spur. Although the heel spur is impressive on x-ray film, the pain experienced is from the fasciitis not the spur.

A symptom of plantar fasciitis is pain in the medial calcaneal region, especially at the insertion of the fascia onto the heel. The pain is common with the first steps of the day as the inflamed fascia is stretched. The pain generally diminishes with walking and stretching. Pain can also be demonstrated by palpating the area. The area may feel full, indicating an inflammatory process.

Treatment is for symptomatic relief. It includes stretching of the Achilles tendon five to seven times per day, NSAIDs, orthotics, and night splints for severe cases. Using extracorporal shock wave therapy as a conservative alternative to treatment in addition to stretching of the plantar fascia maybe beneficial in treating plantar fasciitis (Hammer, Rupp, Ensslin, Kohn, & Seil, 2000). To ensure that this condition does not recur, proper shoe support and cushioning are important. In certain instances, injection of the fascia with a corticosteroid preparation may be necessary. Surgical intervention to perform a plantar fascia release is offered as a last resort. Again, heel spurs found on x-ray film are incidental findings and should not be excised.

Interdigital Perineural Fibroma (Neuroma). Morton's neuroma is a common problem in athletes and is usually the result of excessive pressure placed on the interdigital nerve between the third and fourth toes. The pressure causes inflammation and swelling of the nerve yielding a neuroma.

Symptoms include pain to the dorsum and/or ball of the foot that can radiate distally into the toes. Paresthesia of the toes may accompany the pain. Tight-fitting shoes, high-heeled shoes, hyperextension of the MTP joints, and repetitive impact of the forefoot are conditions that may increase the pain.

Morton's foot (shortened first MTP and elongated second toe) causes forefoot weight-bearing misdistribution about the first MTP. Excessive first MTP loading and shifting of normal weight-bearing distribution precipitates repetitive stressing of the joint, leading to formation of osteophytes, ankylosis, and pain of the first MTP; increased pressure interdigitally and chronic friction causes local inflammation of the interdigital nerve, leading to causalgic pain.

Examination of the foot by inspection alone rarely reveals the problem. Palpation of the dorsum and third and fourth toes may increase pain. Squeezing the ball of the foot also causes increased pain. X-ray films may demonstrate a narrowing between the metatarsals that surround the nerve.

Treatment is to change to a shoe with a larger toe box, one that provides more room for the forefoot. NSAIDs and warm, moist compresses are prescribed; if oral NSAIDs are ineffective, a corticosteroid injection may be tried. If this does not result in long-term relief, surgical resection of the neuroma may be considered.

SPORTS AND THERMOREGULATION ISSUES
Heat-Related Injuries

Thermoregulation is maintained centrally by the anterior hypothalamus. Peripheral thermoreceptors in the skin and mucous membranes and vasoactive mediators (e.g., cytokines, histamine, prostaglandins) stimulate vasodilation or vasoconstriction, thus regulating heat loss or preservation through changes in skin and body temperature. Sport performance is affected by increased ambient (environmental) and body temperature from exercise. Maintaining heat acclimatization before competition is crucial.

With increased ambient temperature, the risk of heat-related problems increases. Other environmental factors, such as high humidity, low wind speed, and radiant heat from the playing surface, also contribute to a rise in core-body temperature. High humidity prevents heat evaporation from the surface of the skin. In addition, heat is produced by aerobic and anaerobic exercise. Core-body temperature may rise to 102° to 105°F (38.8° to 40.5°C). The body's main defense against hyperthermia (body temperature above 100.1°F [38.3°C]) is the evaporation of sweat from the skin. Prolonged hyperthermia can precipitate heat cramps, heat exhaustion, or heat stroke, all of which result from the loss of large amounts of fluid and electrolytes by profuse sweating during sports or exercise.

Heat Cramps. Excessive loss of sodium chloride (NaCl) and fluid in the sweat precipitates muscle cramps. Muscle cramping occurs in the legs or abdomen; it is temporarily disabling and generally subsides with rest and fluid or electrolyte replacement. Drinking large quantities of fluid without replacing NaCl causes hyponatremia. This condition is most commonly found in athletes who are not conditioned and acclimatized to a hot environment. To reduce cramps, treatment should consist of placing the athlete in a cool environment and replacing fluids that contain sodium. Prevention consists of progressive acclimatization and training in the competition environment before the event, wearing proper clothing that allows sweating and evaporation, and drinking fluids or sports drinks before and during the event.

Heat Exhaustion. Heat exhaustion is caused by a poor circulatory response to heat and reduction of blood volume secondary to increased sweating. The athlete sweats profusely, which causes the skin to become cool and feel moist; color is pale, and generalized weakness exists, as do dizziness and nausea. Core-body temperature may be elevated above normal range.

Treatment for heat exhaustion consists of having the athlete rest in a cool environment, ingest cool fluids (preferably containing electrolytes), and cool the body externally with cool water or ice applications. If feeling faint, the athlete may be placed supine with elevation of the lower extremities. With prior medical morbidity, one should monitor vital signs and refer or transport the athlete to an ED for further evaluation. The symptoms of heat exhaustion may mimic those associated with myocardial infarction. The athlete may or may not complain of chest discomfort.

Heatstroke. Heatstroke is life-threatening and increases the morbidity in a medically compromised athlete. Heatstroke requires *emergent* medical treatment; 911 or EMS should be called and the person transported immediately. The body's heating regulatory mechanisms have failed, and there is severe hyperpyrexia—core-body temperature is greater than 106°F (41.1°C). The athlete's skin is red, hot to touch, and dry, and sweating ceases; the athlete is tachycardic. The athlete may become disoriented, violent, and/or lose consciousness. The athlete should be brought to a cool place while awaiting transportation to the ED. If possible, intravenous fluid resuscitation is begun at the scene. Vital signs are monitored closely. A cooling blanket is used or cool compresses are applied to the axilla, back of neck, forehead, groin, and popliteal regions; sips of cool water can be given if the athlete is conscious and able to swallow.

The best treatment for all hyperthermic conditions is prevention. The athlete and coach should monitor ambient temperature and percentage of humidity before training and competing. Performance in a controlled environment (e.g., gym, school, athletic center) is suggested. Early morning or late evening workouts are also suggested. The athlete should drink plenty of fluids and should avoid high-glucose, sodium-laden, or alcoholic beverages. Other tips include the following:

- Slow the pace, decrease the duration of activity when ambient temperature is above 80°F or relative humidity is greater than 50% to 60%.
- Train indoors.
- Find a shady trail or road on which to run.
- Wear lose fitting white or light-colored clothing.
- Protect the head from intense sun exposure.
- Drink 6 to 8 ounces of fluid every 15 to 21 minutes during intense exercise or sport.
- Avoid excess protein intake before training or the event; protein metabolism produces extra heat.
- Acclimatize with changing environments.

Cold-Related Injuries

In cold weather, the athlete should wear protective clothing to prevent hypothermia (decreased core-body temperature). A few examples of cold-barrier clothing are polypropylene, Thinsulate, and Gore-Tex. In addition, athletes competing in water sports should be aware of water temperature and avoid prolonged exposure in cold bodies of water unless wearing a diving wet suit or insulated material.

Hypothermia. Humidity and wind chill increase the adverse affects of cold ambient temperatures. When the hypothalamus senses heat loss, vasoconstriction occurs. Shivering can increase metabolic demand fivefold; it increases myocardial workload, oxygen consumption, and carbon dioxide production. Glycogen stores are decreased.

Systemic body cooling causes several stages of hypothermia. Systemic hypothermia is a medical emergency that requires management at a facility capable of advanced cardiac life support; this type of management is necessary for athletes with moderate to severe hypothermia. Cardiac arrhythmias and reperfusion shock are two potential sequelae related to severe hypothermia. Cooling of the body's temperature to 95°F (35°C) causes shivering, which in turn causes the body to create heat. When the core temperature drops below 94°F (34.4°C), in mild hypothermia, the brain slows the respiratory rate, resulting in hypoxia.

Mild hypothermia occurs most often in the athlete. Treatment for mild hypothermia consists of active rewarming of the body. Wet clothing should be removed and replaced, and external heat should be provided in the form of a heating blanket, hot water bottle, campfire, or extra clothing. If the athlete is conscious, he or she should be given hot liquids; caffeinated beverages and alcohol should be avoided. Submersion in a constant or controlled warm water bath between 105° and 110°F (40.5° to 43.3°C) may assist with rewarming. Breathing warm, moist air from a humidifier aids in rapidly warming the core temperature. The athlete should be removed from wind. Direct wind and cool temperatures have an inverse relationship. The greater the wind speed (mph) the lower the temperature feels as a result of wind chill.

Frostbite. Frostbite is damage to the tissues as a result of exposure to cold ambient temperatures. It is categorized as superficial or deep. Several factors influence the level of severity of frostbite, including the degree of cold penetrating the tissues, duration of exposure to the elements (wind, humidity, ice), inadequate clothing, poor nutritional status, substance abuse, medical morbidity, and homelessness.

Initial treatment of frostbite should include rapid rewarming with warm water between 104° and 112°F (40° and 44.4°C). This treatment should be continued until the affected tissues are deep red. Blisters are not punctured, and loose dry sterile dressings are applied over frostbitten areas. The affected tissue should *not* be rubbed because this may increase tissue damage. If the frostbite is deep, treatment should be provided at an ED where essential equipment; supplies; and drugs, such as antibiotics, tetanus immunization, and analgesics, are available. Analgesics should be given to the athlete during active rewarming.

COMPLEMENTARY AND ALTERNATIVE MEDICINE IN SPORTS MEDICINE

Sports medicine has traditionally used conventional Western medical practices to treat injury and tissue damage. A popular trend now used by athletes and practiced by advanced practitioners, AT-C, and sports medicine specialists is using complementary and alternative medicine (CAM) to augment personal healing. CAM juxtaposes the mind/body relationship. CAM coalesces systems of treatment and thought that may seem alien to those that routinely use Western medicine to treat sports-related injury. Many athletes are using CAM when conventional allopathic medicine has not afforded relief of pain. Most users of CAM are between 25 and 49 years old, tend to have higher education, subscribe to a holistic lifestyle with spirituality and transformational thinking as part of their consciousness, desire culturally creative experiences, and may or may not have been distrustful or lost hope in conventional Western medicine (Alspach, 1998). CAM techniques include homeopathic medicine, acupuncture/meridian therapy, qigong, magnet therapy, hyperbaric oxygen therapy (HBOT), chiropractic care, Ayurvedic medicine, and many more.

Homeopathic medicine uses remedies and formulas in gel, liquid, ointment, pill, and spray forms to treat musculoskeletal problems. These remedies or formulas are natural herblike preparations that are prescribed for purposes of tissue repair and to speed healing, particularly in soft tissues (e.g., ligaments, tendons), in the periosteum, and in connective tissues.

CAM practices include acupuncture or more accurately meridian therapy; this technique uses very fine needles to stimulate meridians to better equalize and focus healing energy (chi or qi). Qigong is another chi healing modality that the athlete can use to concentrate healing chi for therapeutic tissue restoration. It is believed that a blockage in chi can cause disease or conditions within the body.

Magnet therapy involves wearing high-powered magnetic disks on various parts of the body and sleeping on a mattress with magnetic pads. Bioelectromagnetism involves very-low-voltage electrical currents and magnetic fields and is used for pain relief and soft tissue wound healing. There has been some evidence that using magnets for pain relief in fibromyalgia (Salerno, Thomas,

Olive, Blotman, Picot, & Georgesco, 2000) and using pulsed-electromagnetic fields (PEMFs) to stimulate osteogenesis postfracture has been therapeutic (Darendeliler, Darendeliler, & Sinclair, 1997; Matsunaga, Sakou, & Ijiri, 1996).

HBOT is postulated to speed healing in tissues by hyperoxygenating damaged tissues, stimulating angioneogenesis (new blood vessel growth), and increasing the healing time of sprained ligaments and muscle injury.

Chiropractic care is increasing in popularity. It provides hands-on treatment through spinal manipulation, exercise, and rehabilitation. Chiropractic care is one of the most well-established CAM practices. A large group of chiropractors are members of the American Chiropractic Association's Council on Sports Injury and Physical Fitness.

Ayurvedic medicine prescribes meditation, yoga, and herbal preparations combined with diet and sleep to correct imbalances. This type of medicine has been practiced for more than 5000 years.

Other types of CAM practices advocate mind/body techniques such as guided imagery, meditation, yoga, biofeedback, and hypnosis. Emotions and thoughts influence the neuromuscular and immune systems. This field of study is called *psychoneuroimmunology*.

Other CAM treatments use bee therapy, chelation therapy, shark cartilage, herbs, and diet or nutrition therapies to treat illness and medical conditions. As CAM practices are being accepted and used within the Western medical community, more empirical studies are necessary. The National Institutes of Health (NIH) has a Center for Complementary and Alternative Medicine, which has an annual budget of $50 million. This NIH center is funding studies in many states concerning CAM.

FUTURE TRENDS IN SPORTS MEDICINE

Scientific research has recently produced a plethora of data regarding advances in the human genome project and using this biotechnologic information for the treatment of musculoskeletal diseases and conditions (Jeffers & Evans, 1998). Basic science related to the musculoskeletal system has not changed; however, these new genometric data and their relationship to disease juxtapose new diagnostic tools, treatment conditions, and decisions and have spurred updated guidelines for preventive care of the athlete with musculoskeletal problems. The implications for human gene research affect many human biologic systems.

Eventually, genes responsible for the growth, regeneration, and repair of tissues such as bone, cartilage, ligament, muscle, marrow, and tendons can be manipulated to prevent unfavorable outcomes in tissue healing (e.g., tissue response after allograft surgery, postfracture care, trauma, prenatal genetic counseling) (Evans, Ghiviggani, & Robbins, 2001). Mesenchymal stem cells harvested from adult tissue sources (e.g., marrow, muscle connective tissue, periosteum) also hold great potential. Stem cell applications will be used for cellular regeneration of damaged or diseased musculoskeletal tissue such as bone graft for fracture nonunion, segmental bone defects, and spinal fusions. Other conditions that will benefit from stem cell applications are articular resurfacing secondary to degenerative and postinjury articular defects.

Genetic coding pattern alterations in individuals precipitate differences in the metabolism of drugs. Genetic mutations or polymorphisms, in certain persons, affect enzymes subsequently causing drug reactions or subtherapeutic responses while undergoing drug therapies for disease or conditions. Genotyping determines polymorphisms and drug-altering phenotypes. Genotyping could become a standard before prescribing drug treatments. For more information on the role of genetics in musculoskeletal health, see Chapter 7.

Acknowledgment

This chapter is dedicated to the honor of Officer Matthew C. Childs, the greatest athlete I have known, and to Dr. William H.B. Howard the finest sports medicine physician that I had the pleasure to work with at the Sports Medicine Center, Union Memorial Hospital, in Baltimore, Maryland.

INTERNET RESOURCES

American College of Sport Medicine: www.acsm.org
The American Orthopaedic Society for Sports Medicine: www.sportsmed.org
The Physician and Sportsmedicine Online: www. physsportsmed.com
International Federation of Sports Medicine: www. fims.org
American Sports Medicine Institute: www.asmi.org

REFERENCES

Alspach, G. (1998). Alternative and complementary therapies: Treading tentatively out of the mainstream. *Critical Care Nurse, 18*(5), 13–16.

Boden, B., Dean, G., Feagin, J., & Garrett, W. (2001). Mechanisms of anterior cruciate ligament injury. *Orthopaedics, 23,* 573–578.

Brown, D., & Neumann, R. (1995). *Orthopaedic secrets.* Philadelphia: Hanley & Belfus.

Childs, S. (1999). Acute ankle injury. *Lippincott's Primary Care Practice, 3,* 428–437.

Clendening, L. (1960). *Source book of medical history.* New York: Dover.

Darendeliler, M., Darendeliler, A., & Sinclair, P. (1997). Effects of static magnetic and pulsed electromagnetic fields on bone healing. *International Journal of Adult Orthodontia Surgery, 12,* 43–53.

Evans, C., Ghiviggani, S., & Robbins, R. (2001). Potential applications of gene therapy in sports medicine. *Physical Medicine Rehabilitation Clinics of North America, 11,* 405–416.

Garrison, F. H. (1967). *An introduction to the history of medicine* (4th ed.). Philadelphia: WB Saunders.

Hammer, D., Rupp, S., Ensslin, S., Kohn, D., & Seil, R. (2000). Extracorporal shock wave therapy in patients with tennis elbow and painful heel. *Archives of Orthopaedic and Trauma Surgery, 120,* 304–307.

Hewett, T., Lindenfeld, T., Riccobene, J., & Noyes, F. (1999). The effect of neuromuscular training on the incidence of knee injury in female athletes. *American Journal of Sports Medicine, 27*(6), 1–19.

Jeffers, D., & Evans, C. (1998). The human genome project: Implications for the treatment of musculoskeletal disease. *Journal of the American Academy of Orthopaedic Surgeons, 6,* 1–14.

Karogeanes, S., Blackburn, K., & Vangelos, Z. (2001). The association of menstrual cycle with the laxity of anterior cruciate ligament in adolescent female athletes. *Clinical Journal of Sports Medicine, 10*(3), 162–168.

Kenney, W. L., Humphrey, R. H., Bryant, C. X., & Mahler, D. A. (Eds.). (1995). *American College of Sports Medicine guidelines for exercise testing and prescription* (5th ed.). Baltimore: Williams & Wilkins.

Liu, S., Al-Shaikh, R., Panossian, V., Finerman, G., & Lane, J. (1997). Estrogen affects the cellular metabolism of the anterior cruciate ligament: A potential explanation for female athletic injury. *American Journal of Sports Medicine, 25,* 704–709.

Lyznicki, J., Nielsen, N., & Schneider, J. (2000). Cardiovascular screening of student athletes. *American Family Physician, 62,* 765–774.

Matsunaga, S., Sakou, T., & Ijiri, K. (1996). Osteogenesis by pulsed electromagnetic fields (PEMFs): Optimum stimulation setting. *In Vivo, 10,* 351–356.

Reider, B. (1999). *The orthopaedic physical examination.* Philadelphia: WB Saunders.

Rosen, P., & Barkin, R. (1998). *Emergency medicine: Concepts and clinical practice. Vol. 1.* St. Louis: Mosby.

Salerno, A., Thomas, E., Olive, P., Blotman, F., Picot, M., & Georgesco, M. (2000). Motor cortical dysfunction disclosed by single and double magnetic stimulation in patients with fibromyalgia. *Clinical Neurophysiology, 111,* 994–1001.

Singer, R. N., Hausenblas, H. A., & Janelle, C. M. (Eds.). (2001). *Handbook of sport psychology* (2nd ed.). New York: Wiley.

Stiell, I. G., Greenberg, G. H., McKnight, R. D., Nair, R. C., McDowell, I., Reardon, M., Stewart, J. P., & Maloney, J. (1993). Decision rules for the use of radiography in acute ankle injuries. Refinement and prospective validation. *Journal of the American Medical Association, 269*(9), 1127–1132.

Stiell, I. G., Greenberg, G. H., McKnight, R. D., Nair, R. C., McDowell, J., & Worthington, J. R. (1992). A study to develop clinical decision rules for the use of radiography in acute ankle injuries. *Annals of Emergency Medicine, 21,* 384–390.

Stiell, I. G., Wells, G. A., Hoag, R., Sivilotti, M., Cacciotti, R., Verbeek, R., Greenway, K., McDowell, I., Cwinn, A., Greenberg, G. H., Nichol, G., & Michael, J. (1997). Implementation of the Ottawa Knee Rule for the use of radiography in acute knee injuries. *Journal of the American Medical Association, 278,* 2075–2079.

Tandeter, H., & Shvartzman, P. (1999). Acute knee injuries: Use of decision rules for selective radiograph ordering. *American Family Physician, 60,* 2599–2608.

Teitz, C. (1997). *The female athlete.* Park Ridge, IL: American Academy of Orthopaedic Surgeons.

Williams, R., Attia, E., & Wickiewicz, T. (2000). The effect of ciprofloxacin on tendon, paratendon, and capsular fibroblast metabolism. *American Journal of Sports Medicine, 28,* 364–369.

Wojtys, E., Huston, L., Linderfield, T., Hewett, T., & Greenfield, M. (1998). Association between the menstrual cycle and anterior cruciate ligament injury in female athletes. *American Journal of Sports Medicine, 26,* 614–619.

Yu, W., Liu, S., Hatch, J., Panossian, V., & Finerman, G. (1999). Effect of estrogen on cellular metabolism of the human anterior cruciate ligament. *Clinical Orthopaedics and Related Research, 366,* 229–238.

Neoplasms of the Musculoskeletal System

KIM HAYNES

ORTHOPAEDIC ONCOLOGY

The diagnosis and treatment of musculoskeletal neoplasms have advanced markedly since the 1970s, largely because of the advent of computed tomography (CT), magnetic resonance imaging (MRI), radiation therapy, and chemotherapeutic agents. Because of biomedical technology and the advancement in diagnostic and therapeutic modalities, radical changes have taken place in the surgical and medical treatment of malignant and benign bone and soft tissue tumors. Surgical procedures using osteochondral allografts with the articular cartilage, tendons, and ligaments still attached; synthetic and cadaver bone graft material; and custom-designed implantable prostheses, including expandable prosthesis, have allowed the option of limb-sparing surgical procedures (Fig. 22–1). Chemotherapy protocols and treatment regimens for the different types of sarcomas are continually being tested and evaluated in hopes of finding the combination of medications to kill the circulating cancer cells. Before these new surgical and chemotherapeutic developments, the only treatment option for a malignant tumor of the extremity, such as osteosarcoma, was amputation. The survival rate was approximately 17% after amputation. Currently, the survival rate for this type of tumor is approximately 70% with the use of chemotherapy in combination with limb-sparing surgery.

A neoplasm of the musculoskeletal system is either benign or malignant. A malignant neoplasm is called a *sarcoma*. Sarcomas arise from tissues derived from mesoderm or primitive mesenchyme, such as muscle, bone, fat, fascia, and cartilage. Sarcomas differ from carcinomas by the cell origin. Common carcinomas are of the breast, lung, prostate, thyroid, and kidney; they are derived from ectodermal and endodermal tissues. By convention, nerve tumors, which arise from ectodermal

and endodermal structures, are categorized as sarcomas because of their behavior. The most common sarcomas are listed in Table 22–1.

Musculoskeletal neoplasms are divided into two categories: malignant bone and soft tissue sarcomas and benign bone and soft tissue tumors. However, an orthopaedic nurse may also care for clients with metastatic bone disease or multiple myeloma, which is a malignancy of the bone marrow that destroys the structure of the affected bones. Because of the rarity of musculoskeletal neoplasms, their diagnosis is often difficult and the care of clients with these types of tumors is complex. To facilitate delivery of quality nursing care to clients with a musculoskeletal neoplasm, especially high-grade malignant musculoskeletal tumors, the nurse must understand surgery, chemotherapy, and radiotherapy. The nurse's clinical knowledge should include basic principles of orthopaedics, surgery, the cancer disease process, the developmental process of the client and the family, the treatment plan, the management of treatment side effects, discharge planning, and long-term follow-up.

SARCOMAS

Primary sarcomas are tumors that originate in the bone or soft connective tissue. The incidence of primary sarcomas is low. According to the American Cancer Society, it was estimated that 10,600 new cases of bone and soft tissue sarcomas would be diagnosed in 2000. Approximately 6000 deaths will be attributed to primary sarcomas (Greenlee, Murray, Bolden, & Wingo, 2000). Sarcomas are known to affect males and females of any age equally. Table 22–1 lists common malignant musculoskeletal tumors and the body tissues from which they arise.

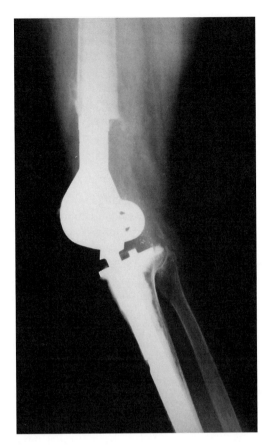

FIGURE 22–1. Distal femoral replacement prosthesis.

Primary Malignant Bone Tumors

A primary bone sarcoma originates from bone cells or forms within the bone. Approximately 2500 new cases of primary bone tumors are diagnosed each year. The most common malignant bone tumor is osteosarcoma, and it is usually found around the knee. Osteosarcoma is generally considered a pediatric cancer and is usually diagnosed in children between 12 and 16 years of age. However, it has been found in children as young as 2 years old and in young adults in their 20s. It also is seen as a primary bone tumor in persons between 40 and 60 years of age, but it occurs much less frequently in this population. Other primary bone tumors include chondrosarcoma, malignant fibrous histiocytoma (MFH) of bone, and Ewing's sarcoma. These tumors are locally aggressive, will recur locally if not completely excised, and will metastasize to the lungs, especially if they are high-grade tumors. The most common sites of sarcomas of bone are in the metaphysis of long bones (distal femur, proximal tibia, proximal humerus) and the pelvis.

Primary Malignant Soft Tissue Tumors

Malignant soft tissue tumors arise from extraskeletal soft connective tissues (muscle, fat, cartilage, fibrous tissue, tendosynovial tissue, vessels, and peripheral nerves). These tumors are locally aggressive, are capable of recurrence, and have the propensity to cause distant metastases. Soft tissue sarcomas occur more frequently in males,

TABLE 22–1. *Common Malignant Musculoskeletal Tumors and Their Body Tissue Origin*

TUMOR	ORIGIN
Osteosarcoma	Primary malignancy of bone that produces osteoid. Commonly arises in epiphyses of long bones. May occur as extraosseous lesion but rarely.
Ewing's sarcoma	Primary malignant bone tumor characterized by primitive round cells. Tumors commonly found in flat bones and diaphyses of long bones, with prominent soft tissue component.
Chondrosarcoma	Primary malignant tumor of bone that produces cartilage and no osteoid. May occur extraskeletally in soft tissue. May occur secondarily in prior benign lesion. Often arises in pelvis, femur, and shoulder.
Malignant fibrous histiocytoma	Most common soft tissue sarcoma characterized by cells of fibroblastic origin. Can be found in bone also but much less common.
Liposarcoma	A common soft tissue sarcoma that varies in characteristic and behavior. Commonly found in the thigh or retroperitoneum. Lipoblasts or small round cells are present.
Fibrosarcoma	Primary malignant tumor of bone that originates from intermuscular and intramuscular fibrous tissue, fascia, tendons, or aponeuroses.
Synovial sarcoma	Epithelial and spindle cells characterize this soft tissue sarcoma, which arises around the knee involving the joint capsule, bursae, and tendon sheath.
Neurofibrosarcoma	Soft tissue sarcoma that arises from tissues of ectodermal embryologic origin and commonly extends within major nerve sheaths in the proximal extremity or trunk.
Angiosarcoma	A malignancy of vascular endothelium that arises in the skin; soft tissues; or organs, including breast, liver, heart, and lungs. These rare tumors may arise in sites of previous radiotherapy.
Leiomyosarcoma	A primary sarcoma derived from malignant smooth muscle, most commonly found in the gastrointestinal tract, retroperitoneum, and skin.
Rhabdomyosarcoma	A primary sarcoma of striated muscle, rhabdomyosarcomas have three variants that can occur: the embryonal variant of the orbit is common at age 4 years, and the gastrointestinal tract variant occurs in childhood and adolescence; alveolar variant arises in the extremities of adolescents and young adults; and pleomorphic variant occurs most often in the older adult.

and the most common age range is 55 years or older. Approximately 40 different types of soft tissue sarcomas exist. The most common soft tissue sarcoma is MFH and is usually found in the large muscles of the extremities, the chest wall, the mediastinum, and the retroperitoneum (Enzinger & Weiss, 1995). Other more common soft tissue sarcomas include liposarcoma, synovial sarcoma, fibrosarcoma, leiomyosarcoma, angiosarcoma, neurofibrosarcoma, hemangioendothelioma, hemangiopericytoma, and rhabdomyosarcoma.

Prognosis

The most commonly used indicator of prognosis for sarcomas is the assigned grade. Bone and soft tissue sarcomas are graded I, II, or III. A grade I tumor is considered low grade, with a low propensity to spread to the lungs. Higher-grade lesion (grades II and III) tend to metastasize to the lungs early in their clinical course (Mirra, 1989; Sugarbaker & Malawer, 1992). The site and size of the primary lesion are other indicators that affect prognosis, either through local control issues, metastatic behavior, or response to adjuvant therapy. Generally, a client with a sarcoma of the extremity does better than a client with a sarcoma located in the trunk. Also, a client with a sarcoma measuring less than 5 cm has a tendency to do better than a client with a tumor greater than 5 cm.

Etiology

Primary Sarcomas. The exact cause of primary sarcomas remains largely unknown. Several factors have been thought to play a role in the development of sarcomas, and these factors are still being researched. Environmental factors, such as trauma or past injury, have been associated with the development of sarcomas. Environmental carcinogens, such as asbestos, dioxin, and radium, have also been implicated in the development of sarcomas. A past practice of painting watch dials with radium is known to have caused osteosarcoma. The painters ingested cumulative amounts of radium as they moistened their paintbrushes with their tongues.

Secondary Sarcomas. Secondary sarcomas may develop from an existing benign medical condition, such as enchondromatosis or neurofibromatosis (von Recklinghausen's disease) or from an existing metabolic condition, such as Paget's disease. Sarcomatous transformation in clients with Paget's disease most often occurs in clients with polyostotic disease and usually results in osteosarcoma. However, fibrosarcoma and osteoclastic sarcoma have also been diagnosed (Mirra, 1989). Squamous cell carcinoma has been known to occur at sites of prolonged (approximately 20 years) chronic osteomyelitis. Therefore, clients with these diseases must be monitored closely to detect malignant transformation.

Secondary sarcomas also can be induced by therapeutic procedures that may have carcinogenic side effects, such as chemotherapeutic agents or radiation. Considering the frequency of use of radiotherapy, radiation-induced soft tissue sarcomas are definitely uncommon. There is no doubt that the benefit of radiation in the treatment of malignant neoplasms outweighs the risk of developing sarcomas (Enzinger & Weiss, 1995). Radiation sarcomas can occur 4 to 20 years after high doses of ionizing radiation have been delivered. They are found most frequently in the pelvis and shoulder. The most common postradiation soft tissue sarcoma is MFH, which accounts for nearly 70% of cases, followed by osteosarcoma, fibrosarcoma, malignant peripheral nerve sheath tumor, chondrosarcoma, and angiosarcoma (Enzinger & Weiss, 1995). The prognosis with this type of tumor is usually poor because these tumors are generally high-grade sarcomas and are detected late in their course of development.

Less than 5% of all malignancies are known to have a hereditary cancer predilection. For example, neurofibromatosis is an autosomal-dominant disorder. In 1% to 5% of cases, malignant peripheral nerve sheath tumors develop as a result of malignant degeneration of neurofibromas (Enzinger & Weiss, 1995). Retinoblastoma is another disease that is associated with the development of sarcomas. The inherited or bilateral form has been associated with the development of osteosarcoma. Other soft tissue tumors have been reported to have familial tendencies, but these tumors are so rare that they account for an insignificant proportion of the cases.

Immunodeficiency and therapeutic immunosuppression have been reported to be associated with the development of soft tissue sarcomas. Sarcomas of various types may be associated with therapeutic immunosuppression (long-term administration of cyclosporine and other immunosuppressive drugs) used with organ transplantation, especially liver and renal transplant (Enzinger & Weiss, 1995).

Translocation, an exchange of material between two or more chromosomes, has characterized some cytogenetic developments in human solid tumors. Cytogenetic studies have demonstrated consistent chromosome translocation in Ewing's sarcoma and synovial sarcoma (Bridge, Sanger, Shaffer, & Neff, 1987; Griffin & Emanuel, 1987; Smith, Reeves, Wong, & Fisher, 1987). Other reports have shown chromosomal translocations in alveolar rhabdomyosarcoma, myxoid liposarcoma, and extraskeletal myxoid chondrosarcoma (Mertens, Johansson, Mandahl, Heim, Bennet, Rydholm, Willen, & Mitelman, 1987; Sandberg, 1987; Smith, Reeves, & Wong, 1987; Turc-Carel, Dal Cin, & Sandberg, 1987). A trisomy, or extra chromosome, has been found in clients with MFH (Bridge et al., 1987). Osteosarcomas carry a long chromosome arm originally seen in retinoblastomas. Children with familial retinoblastoma have about a 7% incidence of osteosarcoma developing both in radiation ports of the original tumor site and in long bones outside the ports, suggesting a hereditary susceptibility to osteosar-coma (Antman, Eilber, & Shiu, 1989). For a detailed discussion of the role of genetics in disease development, see Chapter 7.

BENIGN BONE AND SOFT TISSUE TUMORS

Benign Bone Tumors

The exact prevalence of benign bone tumors is unknown. Many of these tumors go undiagnosed because they cause no pain and therefore are unknown to the client. Many times, these tumors are found incidentally on x-ray film when the client is being evaluated for another problem, for example, a client with a fracture through a unicameral bone cyst. The cyst may have been present for a long time but did not cause pain, although it weakened the bone. The client may have fallen and fractured the humerus through the unicameral bone cyst, which was then found by x-ray examination.

The most common benign bone tumor is a fibrous cortical defect, which may be considered a developmental anomaly rather than a true tumor. These tumors rarely cause pain or problems, and the majority are found incidentally. Therefore, the exact number is unknown. An osteochondroma (exostosis) is more easily detected because of its direction of growth outward near joints (Fig. 22–2). The most common locations for this tumor are the

distal femur, proximal tibia, pelvis, and shoulder. This tumor enlarges with skeletal growth and may reach a large size. Osteochondromas can occur in multiple locations, and this disease process is known as *multiple hereditary exostosis* (Table 22–2).

Many benign bone tumors can be monitored by interval x-ray films. However, some of these tumors can be locally aggressive and can cause bone pain, weakness, fracture, and destruction. They can also grow to large sizes and become unsightly. Surgical intervention is then warranted.

Benign Soft Tissue Tumors

Benign soft tissue tumors outnumber malignant tumors by a margin of about 100:1 in a hospital population, and their annual incidence is approximately 300 per 100,000 population (Suit, Mankin, Wood, Gebhardt, Harmon, Rosenberg, Tepper, & Rosenthal, 1988). The most common benign soft tissue tumor is a lipoma. These benign tumors can grow to reach very large sizes and can be locally aggressive. Many of these tumors can be monitored without surgery if they are not causing any pain, changing in function, or changing in size. However, certain tumors have a small chance of turning into malignancies and therefore must be watched closely or removed.

METASTATIC BONE DISEASE

More prevalent than sarcomas are metastatic lesions that have spread to the bone from primary carcinomas. In a large autopsy series, the ratio of skeletal metastases to primary bone tumors was about 25:1 (Mirra, 1989). Metastatic carcinoma is the most common malignant tumor of the bone and occurs usually in the sixth and seventh decades of life. The most common primary carcinomas to metastasize to bone are breast, prostate, lung, and kidney. Other malignancies that metastasize to bone are thyroid, bladder, uterine, colorectal, and vaginal cancers. Bone is the third most common site for metastases, after the lung and liver. Common sites of bone metastases are the vertebral bodies, pelvis, proximal femur, proximal humerus, and ribs. Less common sites of metastases are the tibia, foot, radius, and hand. Metastasis may occur by direct spread within a body cavity or by hematogenous or lymphatic spread.

Surgical treatment for metastatic skeletal disease has progressed over the last 20 years and includes several different surgical techniques. Depending on the location and type of tumor, methods such as intralesional curettage, cryosurgery, prophylactic internal fixation, cementation, segmental resection and reconstruction with a prosthesis, or total joint replacement procedure can be performed. The primary goals of treatment for metastatic disease are pain relief, restoration of function, and facilitation of nursing care.

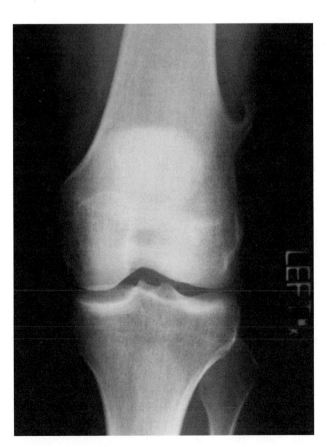

FIGURE 22–2. Osteochondroma, left distal femur.

TABLE 22–2. *Common Benign Musculoskeletal Tumors and Their Body Tissue Origin*

TUMOR	ORIGIN
Osteochondroma	Cartilage-capped bony protuberance of the metaphysis or diaphysis, continuity of the cortical and cancellous bone. Most common bone tumor. Most common locations are distal femur, proximal tibia, shoulder, pelvis. Can have multiple osteochondromas or exostosis, a condition known as *MHE* (multiple hereditary exostosis).
Giant cell tumor	Solitary lesion characterized by benign-appearing osteoclast-like giant cells and stromal cells that originated within the epiphysis of adults. Can be locally aggressive and can spread to the lungs even though it is benign.
Enchondroma	Solitary bone tumor, also called central chondroma, is a benign hyaline cartilage growth, found within the medullary cavity of a single bone. Multiple enchondromas are called Ollier's disease. Most common tumor arising in the hand. Also found in proximal humerus, distal femur, and proximal tibia.
Osteoid osteoma	Benign osteoblastic lesion characterized by well-circumscribed core (nidus) of usually <1–2 cm and by distinctive surrounding zone of reactive bone formation. Classic symptom is pain, which is worse at night and is relieved by aspirin. Most common locations are proximal femur and region of femoral neck.
Fibrous dysplasia	Developmental anomaly of the bone-forming mesenchyme. Bone maturation is arrested at the immature woven-type stage. Abnormal bone growth may result in deformity. Can be monostotic (one bone) or polyostotic (multiple bones). Most common locations include skull, jaws, ribs, and femoral neck.
Chondroblastoma	Benign tumor arising in epiphyses consisting of polygonal chondroblasts, small foci of chondroid production, osteoclast-like giant cells, and often small foci of calcification. Common locations are proximal humerus, distal femur, and proximal tibia.
Aneurysmal bone cyst (ABC)	Multilobulated spongy mass filled with blood, commonly found in metaphysis of long bones, pelvis, and spine.
Unicameral bone cyst (UBC)	An intramedullary cavity, usually unicameral (one compartment), filled with clear, yellow, or serosanguineous fluid, commonly located in the metaphysis or proximal femur or proximal humerus.
Fibrous cortical defect	Probably the most common benign tumor, usually solitary and found incidentally. The lesion is cortically based and is most commonly found in long bones around epiphyseal cartilage plate. Most common site is the cortex of the lower femoral metaphysis, often bilateral.
Nonossifying fibroma	A fibrous cortical defect that did not become sclerotic but proliferated. Seen mainly in older children and adolescents. May provoke pain, swelling, and fracture.
Lipoma	Benign tumor composed of mature fat and represents by far the most common mesenchymal neoplasm. Occurs most frequently in the upper back and neck, shoulder, and abdomen, then in upper arms, buttocks, and upper thigh.
Leiomyoma	Benign smooth muscle tumor relatively common in the genitourinary and gastrointestinal tracts, less common in the skin, and rare in deep soft tissue.
Neurofibroma	Benign nerve sheath tumor, can occur solitary or multiple, which is associated with neurofibromatosis.
Hemangioma	Benign but nonreactive process in which there is an increased number of normal- or abnormal-appearing vessels. May be capillary (located in skin and subcutaneous tissue) or cavernous (upper portion of body).
Arteriovenous malformation (hemangioma)	Partial persistence of fetal capillary bed, causing abnormal connections between arteries and veins. May be located in any portion of the body but most frequently affects the head, neck, and lower extremity.

MULTIPLE MYELOMA

Multiple myeloma, a malignancy of the bone marrow, will account for approximately 13,600 new cancer diagnoses in 2000. Of those diagnosed, it is estimated that 11,200 will succumb to the disease (Greenlee, Murray, Bolden, & Wingo, 2000). It is not considered a sarcoma, but the symptoms and radiographic findings are very similar. Malpas, Bergsagel, Kyle, and Anderson (1998) defined multiple myeloma as a "clonal proliferation of idiotypic B lymphoid cells, characterized by infiltration of the bone marrow, bone destruction, infiltration of lymphoid and other soft tissues with malignant plasma cells, and suppression of normal hematopoiesis" (p. 187). Symptoms of multiple myeloma are fairly diagnostic, but the disease can be difficult to diagnose, especially in the older adult population. Common symptoms and complaints include bone pain, weakness, fatigue, fever, and infection.

Also, a client may experience renal, neurologic, cardiac, pulmonary, and hematologic symptoms (Malpas et al., 1998). Myeloma is more common in men and among blacks and is found mainly in persons 60 to 75 years of age.

Plasma cell malignancies can present in different forms and develop at different paces. Multiple myeloma is considered a slow-growing neoplasm. A long time may elapse before a client becomes symptomatic. The most common symptom is bone pain, and the pain usually is described as incapacitating. Multiple myeloma can affect any bone but most often involves the thoracic and lumbar vertebrae. Individuals may experience hypercalcemia and a pathologic fracture through the area of bone destruction. Multiple myeloma also affects the kidneys, the immune system, and the circulatory system. Workup is extensive and includes blood and urine tests as well as bone scan or skeletal survey to diagnose the extent of the bone involvement. The diagnosis of the exact type of myeloma is crucial so that the correct treatment can be initiated.

Treatment for multiple myeloma varies depending on the extent of the disease. If the client is asymptomatic, no treatment is given. When signs of progression become evident, such as an increase in bone pain, elevated serum and urinary M-proteins, weight loss, anemia, or renal failure, treatment should be initiated. Treatments include chemotherapy, corticosteroids, and interferon-alfa-2a. Plasmapheresis and radiation are other treatment options for this disease, depending on the symptoms and type of myeloma. Radiation may be used both palliatively to relieve bone pain and as an adjuvant because myeloma is highly radioresponsive.

There is no cure for multiple myeloma. The most common complication related to multiple myeloma is renal failure secondary to protein deposits in the kidneys, which causes obstruction problems. Nursing interventions must include pain management, prevention of pathologic fractures, maintenance of adequate renal function, prevention of infection, prevention of cardiovascular problems, and maintenance of emotional support. The nurse's role in client and family teaching is vital for this multifaceted disease.

NURSING HISTORY AND SUBJECTIVE REVIEW
Bone and Soft Tissue Sarcomas, Metastatic Bone Tumors, Multiple Myeloma

Clients with bone and soft tissue sarcomas and clients with metastatic carcinomas to bone have similar histories and subjective reviews. Table 22–3 lists common sites, history, possible symptoms, and diagnostic findings of musculoskeletal tumors. Most clients with a malignant bone or soft tissue tumor come to a physician's office or ambulatory clinic with complaints of enlarging mass, deep progressive pain, fever, weight loss, and malaise. An

acute episode of severe pain and fracture brings the client into the emergency department. At this time, a comprehensive physical assessment should take place.

A person with a primary sarcoma commonly complains of a painless enlarging hard mass or progressive deep bone pain. A mass may also be brought to attention by some incidental trauma. Although the malignancy is not caused by trauma, there is commonly an occurrence, such as a fall or blow to the extremity, that brings the mass to the client's attention. Masses confined within a compartment or invading surrounding structures often become painful. Clients may report limited range of motion (ROM) or joint swelling if the mass is near a joint. Masses adherent to muscle or bone may also cause limitation of motion of the joint and weakness of the extremity.

The onset of symptoms is often described as gradual. Pain is more common with bone sarcomas than soft tissue sarcomas, in part because of inflammation and weakness of the bone. Initially, the pain is mild, but it worsens over time. Night and rest pain are common. As opposed to pain with arthritis, pain from tumor does not necessarily worsen with activity. Pain may radiate and become severe. Another source of pain is direct extension of the tumor into surrounding nerves, such as the brachial or lumbosacral plexuses. This pain is commonly described as a radiating, burning pain in the nerve's distribution.

Metastatic bone lesions from a previously known or newly diagnosed carcinoma or bone marrow condition, such as multiple myeloma, often cause multiple areas of progressive pain. Some may even cause an impending or actual pathologic fracture brought on by tumor invasion of the medullary canal. This pain may be both acute and chronic. Malignant chronic pain, more prevalent with metastatic bone disease, is often a trying challenge to the client and all health care providers. Unresolved pain causes the client to limp, limits joint motion, and eventually results in muscle weakness. In addition, chronic unresolved pain often leaves the client psychologically depressed and interrupts sociocultural subsystems.

Clients may have other symptoms depending on the severity, location, and type of tumor or mass. Masses invading nerves can cause paresthesia or anesthesia. Anorexia, weight loss, or malaise may occur. Fevers, although rare, may occur in clients with large necrotic tumors.

Alteration in the ability to perform activities of daily living (ADLs) can occur because of underlying pain, limp, limited joint ROM because of a mass, muscle weakness because of neurovascular compromise, or generalized weakness caused by weight loss or malaise. Pulmonary symptoms are rare, although shortness of breath may occur in clients with metastatic pulmonary disease.

The personal history is completed with questioning about signs or symptoms that may trigger signs of metastatic disease (e.g., pain, weight loss) or history of another malignancy. Some clients are susceptible to more than one malignancy. A history of previous exposure to ionizing radiation or precancerous conditions is deter-mined. The client is questioned about a family history of musculoskeletal neoplasms. Conditions such as neurofi-bromatosis are congenital neurologic disorders in which multiple tumors are found under the skin.

TABLE 22-3. *History and Assessment of Bone Sarcomas, Soft Tissue Sarcomas, and Metastatic Disease to Bone*

SITE	HISTORY	SYMPTOMS	DIAGNOSTIC FINDINGS
Bone Sarcomas			
Upper or lower extremity or pelvis Commonly, metaphysis of distal femur, proximal tibia, proximal humerus, and pelvis	Progressive deep bone pain Acute episode of pain or pathologic fracture may bring client to physician	Worsening deep bone pain because of inflammation or weakness of bone Night or rest pain common Pain may radiate and become severe Muscular weakness or atrophy because of pain Soft tissue mass extending from bone is possible Limited ROM from mass adhering to bone Joint effusion or overlying swelling Overlying erythema or warmth of skin Palpable local lymph nodes because of inflammation or tumor Alteration in ability to perform ADLs Antalgic gait Anxiety, depression, malaise, or weight loss because of severe pain Fever	Elevated alkaline phosphatase levels with osteosarcoma Plain x-ray film shows cortical destruction, bony expansion, calcifications, sunburst appearance, medullary irregularity, or pathologic fracture CT or MRI shows cortical and medullary irregularities and possible bone mass extending into soft tissue Bone scan shows increased uptake at tumor site Biopsy identifies malignancy
Soft Tissue Sarcomas			
Upper or lower extremity and pelvis Commonly, thigh, shoulder, and pelvis	Enlarging, usually painless mass Incidental trauma often brings mass to client's attention	Enlarging firm mass with irregular borders Erythema or warmth overlying skin Venous dilation of overlying skin Initially painless; pain with tumor invasion of surrounding soft tissue structures Invasion of nerve plexus causes radiating, burning pain and weakness in nerve distribution Joint effusion Muscular weakness or atrophy Limited ROM Paresthesias with neurologic involvement Distal swelling Palpable local lymph nodes because of inflammation or tumor Alteration in ability to perform ADLs Altered gait	Plain x-ray film may show soft tissue shadow CT or MRI shows soft tissue sarcoma invading surrounding structures (muscle, nerve, vessels, bone) Bone scan may show inflammation near bony structures Angiogram demonstrates increased vascularity of mass Biopsy identifies malignancy
Pelvis	Enlarging mass with or without pain	In addition to above mentioned, the client may have altered bowel or bladder habits or pain with intercourse Weakened muscles because of lumbosacral nerve involvement	CT or MRI shows large mass abutting rectum, bladder, or vagina Myelogram, CT, or MRI may show nerve impingement

ROM, range of motion.

TABLE 22–3. *History and Assessment of Bone Sarcomas, Soft Tissue Sarcomas, and Metastatic Disease to Bone* Continued

SITE	HISTORY	SYMPTOMS	DIAGNOSTIC FINDINGS
Metastatic Disease to Bone			
Commonly, vertebral bodies, pelvis, proximal femur, proximal humerus, ribs Less commonly, tibia, foot, radius, and hand	Commonly, a history of breast, prostate, lung, or kidney cancer Acute episode of severe pain signaling impending pathologic fracture	Pathologic fracture Multiple areas of acute or chronic pain Multiple areas of progressive pain Antalgic gait or limp Alteration in ability to perform ADLs Depression because of chronic pain Anorexia, weight loss, or malaise because of chronic pain Generalized muscle weakness and atrophy secondary to pain	Decreased hemoglobin and hematocrit values because of underlying anemia Elevated serum calcium level Elevated alkaline phosphatase level Elevated acid phosphatase level with prostate cancer Monoclonal spike on electrophoresis and Bence Jones protein concentration in urine with myeloma Elevated CEA level Plain x-ray films show multiple osteoblastic or osteolytic areas with possible pathologic fracture Focal increase on bone scan in skull, pelvis, scapula, or diaphysis of long bone MRI or myelogram shows vertebral body or spinal cord involvement

ROM, range of motion.

Benign Bone and Soft Tissue Tumors

Most benign bone and soft tissue tumors are found incidentally. The client may need to be evaluated because of an injury, and the bone tumor is found on x-ray film or the soft tissue mass is found by palpation. The client may already be aware of the tumor but states that it has been there for several years and has not changed or caused pain. The personal history still should be completed and should include questioning about the signs or symptoms the client may be experiencing. The questioning should include a family history of tumors, benign or malignant, because of the heredity aspect of some tumors, such as multiple exostosis (osteochondromas) or neurofibromatosis. Table 22-2 lists common benign musculoskeletal bone and soft tissue tumors and the body tissues from which they arise.

PHYSICAL ASSESSMENT AND OBJECTIVE REVIEW

Malignant Bone and Soft Tissue Tumors, Metastatic Disease, Multiple Myeloma

The initial physical examination consists of an inspection of the overlying skin, a gentle palpation of the mass or painful area in question, and an evaluation of the affected extremity or adjacent structures and other areas suggestive of metastatic disease. Inspection of the overlying skin is done to assess tumor involvement. Erythema or warmth indicates inflammation, and venous dilation over the mass indicates displaced veins caused by tumor growth, emboli, or impingement of the vessel. Highly vascular tumors may pulsate. Nodules or cutaneous lesions, such as café-au-lait spots, may indicate conditions such as neurofibromatosis (Fig. 22–3).

After the skin is carefully inspected, the mass, if present, is very gently palpated for its consistency, mobility, shape, and size. Most malignant masses are firm or hard and are usually located deep to fascia. They become adherent to underlying structures, such as bone, causing immobility of the mass (Fig. 22–4). Malignant masses normally have irregular borders because of infiltration into surrounding structures (Fig. 22–5). Sarcomas can invade surrounding nerves, vessels, bone, or any other connective tissue. If left untreated, they can even invade the skin and ultimately become necrotic. Sarcomatous masses may or may not be painful to palpation. Next, the tumor is palpated and measured in 1-cm increments so that future growth or shrinkage can be objectively assessed. Generally, a bone tumor or mass measuring 5 cm is suspicious for a malignancy. Review of plain x-ray films, CT scans, MRI, and bone scans confirms the size and exact location of the tumor. Finally, the affected extremity or adjacent structures are examined. Distal swelling can occur because of vascular disturbances. Muscle atrophy or weakness can result from disuse of the extremity.

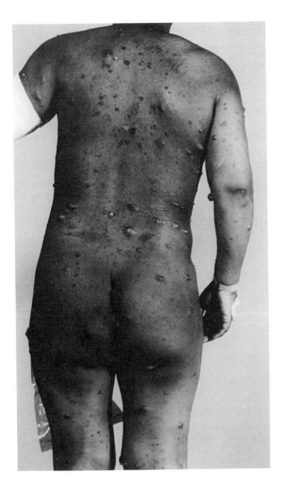

FIGURE 22–3. Neurofibromatosis.

ROM of joints proximal and distal to the tumor may be limited because of pain or tumor encroachment on the joint. Joint effusions may be present if the tumor invades the joint capsule. Neurovascular compromise, such as peripheral paresthesia or decreased peripheral pulses, may indicate neurologic invasion or arterial involvement. Palpable, enlarged, firm lymph nodes, especially peripheral to the tumorous area, may indicate metastatic lymph node disease. Clients with pathologic fractures may have any of these symptoms.

The extremity is measured to detect any alterations in limb length, and circumferences are measured to detect any decreases resulting from muscle wasting or any increases resulting from tumor, swelling, or edema. Muscle strength is tested using a scale of 1 to 5. Involved joints are tested for their ROM using goniometric measurements. Deep tendon reflexes are elicited, and peripheral pulses are palpated for patency. Light and deep sensation is grossly checked. Lymph nodes are palpated for signs of inflammation or metastatic disease. The client is assessed for alteration of gait pattern, and often, the client demonstrates an antalgic gait associated with the presence of pain. This is common with bony sarcomas, multiple myeloma, and metastatic carcinomas to

bone. Any other areas in question, especially unexplained masses or sites of pain, are examined for signs of malignancy.

Benign Bone and Soft Tissue Tumors

The initial physical examination is the same as that for a malignancy, that is, inspection and palpation of the area of involvement. However, differences in the examination results can be diagnostic. The overlying skin of benign conditions is most often normal. Benign masses are usually soft and mobile and located in the subcutaneous tissue. Benign tumors are normally encapsulated, have smooth borders, and generally are not painful to palpation. The tumor is measured and usually found to be smaller than 5 cm. The exact size and location of the tumor are determined by plain x-ray films, CT scans, MRI, and bone scan.

Distal swelling and muscle atrophy or weakness may occur but are much less likely with a benign tumor. Joint effusion and neurovascular compromise may occur because many benign bone tumors occur near joints, especially the knee and hip. For the same reason, ROM may be affected.

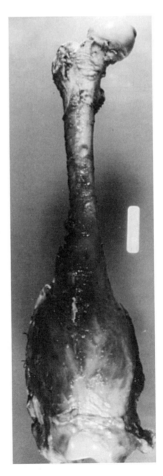

FIGURE 22–4. Osteogenic sarcoma of the right femur.

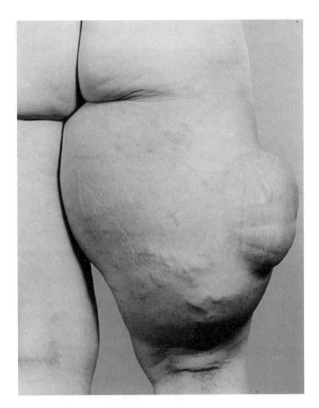

FIGURE 22–5. Malignant hemangiopericytoma of the right thigh.

The extremity is measured to detect any alterations in limb length, and circumferences are measured to detect any decreases resulting from muscle wasting or any increases resulting from tumor, swelling, or edema. Muscle strength is tested using a scale of 1 to 5. Involved joints are tested for their ROM using goniometric measurements. Deep tendon reflexes are elicited, and peripheral pulses are palpated for patency. Light and deep sensation is grossly checked. Lymph nodes are palpated for signs of inflammation or metastatic disease. Last, the client is assessed for alteration of gait pattern, and often, the client demonstrates an antalgic gait associated with the presence of pain.

PSYCHOLOGICAL AND SOCIOCULTURAL ASSESSMENT

The diagnosis of a malignancy and its effects on a client's sociocultural and psychological subsystems can be a major disruption of life. Emotional distress caused by anxiety, sleep disturbance, depression, or pain affects the client's social environment and response to treatment. Behavioral problems related to anticipatory nausea or pain can be barriers to treatment. Marital relationships can be strained because of issues of self-esteem and body image. The entire family is disrupted, especially when a child is diagnosed with cancer. See Chapter 2 for more in-depth information on assessment of these areas.

DIAGNOSTIC EVALUATION

Laboratory Tests

After a thorough history and physical examination are performed, laboratory and radiographic studies are conducted. To rule out infection, the Westergren sedimentation rate and glycoprotein, fibrinogen, and C-reactive protein levels are checked. If infection is present, these test values are usually elevated.

A complete blood count is done to detect any abnormalities. An elevation in the white blood cell count is observed in cases of inflammation, hematologic malignancy, and myeloproliferative disorder. A decrease in the white blood count is noted with replacement of bone marrow by tumor.

As a result of the malignant process or blood loss during surgery, the hemoglobin and hematocrit values may be decreased. The platelet count may be increased with advanced malignancies or may be decreased with tumors that have metastasized to bone marrow.

Calcium may be increased in the blood and urine as a result of malignancies with bone involvement, mainly those of the breast, lung, and kidney. Hypercalcemia (serum calcium levels greater than 11 mg/dL) can be an oncologic emergency because of possible cardiac arrhythmias.

Although laboratory values add to the clinical diagnosis, management, and follow-up evaluation processes, they are not diagnostic in and of themselves. Some laboratory tests, however, are used as tumor markers. An elevation in the serum alkaline phosphatase level may be present with osteoblastic (bone-forming) tumors, and lactate dehydrogenase (LDH) may act as a marker of tumor progression for Ewing's sarcoma. Common diagnoses in which alkaline phosphatase levels are elevated are osteogenic sarcoma, myeloma, Hodgkin's lymphoma, and metastatic cancer to bone and liver. An elevation in acid phosphatase levels may be seen in men with metastatic prostate cancer to the bone.

Serum electrophoresis determines the amounts of various serum proteins. With multiple myeloma, levels of serum total protein, albumin, and globulins are commonly elevated. Serum calcium levels may be increased, with a subsequent decrease in serum phosphorus levels. Calcium and Bence Jones protein are commonly present in the urine.

Carcinoembryonic antigen (CEA) is often used to monitor response to therapy or to indicate recurring disease. CEA is monitored in clients with metastatic carcinomas, such as those of the colon, breast, and lung. Urine analysis is done to assess for hematuria, which may be present in renal cell carcinoma, and a prostate screening antigen (PSA) test is used to check for and monitor prostate carcinoma.

Laboratory studies are done initially at the time of diagnosis and periodically throughout adjuvant therapy.

Some findings, such as increased serum alkaline phosphatase in osteosarcoma or an elevated PSA, may indicate a recurrence or progression of the disease process.

Radiographic Studies

Radiographic studies most commonly performed to diagnose a musculoskeletal lesion or mass include a plain x-ray film, CT scan of the involved area and of the lung, MRI, and bone scan. Angiograms, myelograms, and tomograms are performed as needed.

The plain radiograph is the most important study and usually provides the diagnosis. Anterior and posterior views of plain radiographs are done to show the extent of bone involvement and location of tumors. The x-ray film may show cortical destruction, bony expansion, calcification (Fig. 22-6A), or sunburst appearance (Fig. 22-6B), which are characteristics of malignant bone tumors. Pathologic fractures or impending pathologic fractures (those that destroy more than 50% of the diameter of the bone and are painful) are also detected on plain radiographs. Soft tissue outlines or shadows may be seen with soft tissue sarcomas or soft tissue extension from bone sarcomas that have eroded through the cortex. Posteroanterior and lateral chest x-ray films, in addition to lung CT scans, are done to assess metastatic lung disease. Bone lesions that are benign in radiographic

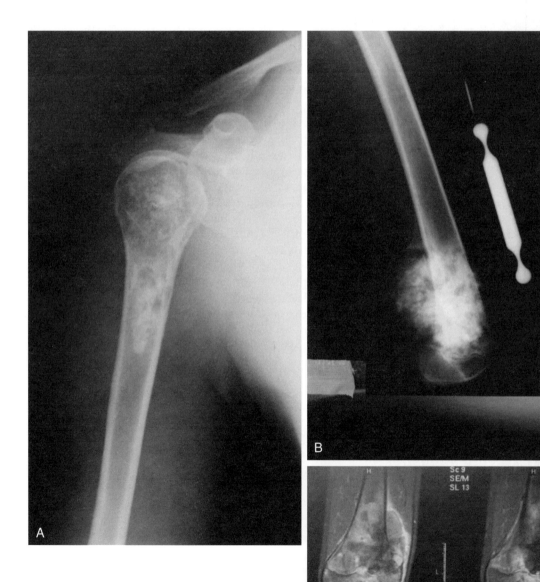

FIGURE 22–6. *A,* Chondrosarcoma, right proximal humerus. *B,* Osteosarcoma, left distal femur. *C,* MRI of Figure 22-6B osteosarcoma, left distal femur.

appearance may be either watched or treated with elective surgery. Suspicious or malignant-appearing lesions are further evaluated.

CT scans demonstrate multiple cross-sectional views of tumor involvement. They delineate tumor invasion into bone, soft tissues, and neurovascular structures. They are used as a diagnostic tool and to help plan further treatments. CT scans are particularly beneficial for diagnosing intraosseous tumors and tumors of the trunk (shoulder, spine, pelvis). Positive scans show the extent of the lesions and anatomic abnormalities of the matrix. They are most often done preoperatively but are also done periodically after surgery to detect local recurrences, especially in areas that are hard to examine, such as the pelvis. Scans of the lung are performed initially during the staging process and periodically to monitor for lung metastases. Pulmonary nodules may be detected in either lung on the CT scan, which is more sensitive than a plain chest radiograph. The drawback of the CT scan is its limited sensitivity. Tomographic scans are sensitive only to 3-mm lesions; lesions smaller than 3 mm are undetectable by this method.

In addition to CT scans, MRI can be used to demonstrate multiple sagittal and coronal views of tumor involvement. It delineates tumor invasion into bone, soft tissues, and neurovascular structures (Fig. 22–6C). MRI is particularly beneficial in delineating extraosseous lesions, such as those occurring in the thigh and those invading the sciatic nerve or brachial plexus. Although both CT and MRI can demonstrate soft tissue masses, many physicians find MRI superior in contrasting soft tissues and other areas, such as growth plates in children. Positive scans show the extent of the tumor and anatomic abnormalities. MRI scans are done preoperatively to plan surgery and are used postoperatively in long-term follow-up to detect any local recurrence.

A bone scan may be ordered to detect the skeletal extent of the disease process. Bone scans are very sensitive but are not specific. A radioactive isotope is injected intravenously and concentrates in areas that are metabolically active or in an area of increased blood flow. An area of activity is called a *hot spot* because it appears very dark on the scan because of an accumulation of the isotope (Fig. 22–7). Tumors, fractures, bone infections, arthritis, and hyperemia make the bone scan results positive, or hot. Bone scans are done during the staging process for a primary malignancy as well as to detect any bone metastases, which are often signaled by unexplained, persistent, deep pain. Clients should be informed of the two-stage procedure of injection and scanning.

To detect vascular involvement of a tumor, an angiogram can be performed. Angiograms demonstrate vascularity of tumors, such as aneurysmal bone cysts or angiosarcomas. Angiograms can also help determine patency of arteries for vascularized muscle flaps when coverage is necessary after surgery or for access for

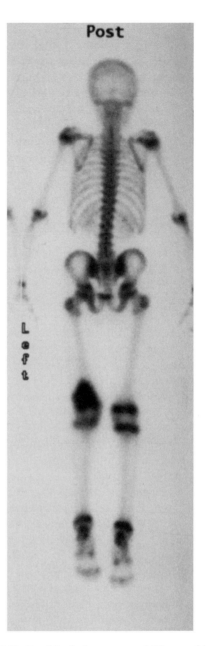

FIGURE 22–7. Total body bone scan of 13-year-old boy with osteosarcoma, left distal femur (same client as Figure 22–6B and C).

intra-arterial chemotherapy. Other uses for angiography are infarcting arteries that supply vascular tumors and demonstrating the effects of chemotherapy. A common sign of successful intra-arterial cisplatin therapy is sclerosis of the mass. Clients undergoing angiography should be warned that the test can take several hours and causes discomfort at the catheter site. Postprocedure care includes pushing fluids to facilitate excretion of dye and ensuring recumbency for at least 8 hours to prevent bleeding at the catheter insertion site.

When spinal cord involvement or nerve route impingement is suspected as a result of a malignancy, a myelogram can be performed. Myelograms demonstrate blockage of the spinal canal by a mass, as demonstrated by incomplete flow of dye. MRI is being performed more often to detect spinal involvement.

Less commonly performed tests include tomography and ultrasonography. Tomography can be helpful for some benign osseous lesions, and ultrasonography can differentiate fluid-filled cysts from solid masses. Because radiographic studies are nonspecific for histologic status, pathologic studies are done. For detailed information about diagnostic tests and related nursing responsibilities, see Chapter 9.

CYTOLOGIC AND PATHOLOGIC DIAGNOSIS

The staging process is completed by cytologic and pathologic studies. Tissue type and behavior are determined by pathologic study. Tissue specimens are retrieved in several ways. Bone marrow aspirations by needle biopsies are often performed to reveal abnormal or immature cells, such as those seen in multiple myeloma. Fluid aspirations for cytologic examination can be done to confirm a suspected metastatic tumor (malignant cells are seen on cytologic examination). However, needle biopsy is rarely used when the most likely diagnosis is a sarcoma. Needle biopsy tissue specimens often are too small to allow for accurate tissue diagnosis. Needle biopsies should be done only at institutions where the pathologists reading the tissue samples are well trained in diagnosing sarcomas.

Tissue samples are obtained in a sterile fashion, usually under general anesthesia. The initial step in obtaining a sample is to perform an open biopsy in the operating room. Several tissue samples are excised and sent immediately to the pathology department. The pathologist freezes the tissue, which allows the sample to be looked at immediately under the microscope. This procedure may take 10 to 15 minutes. If the preliminary diagnosis is a benign bone or soft tissue tumor, the surgeon will remove the tumor in the appropriate fashion. If the preliminary result is questionable or definitely a sarcoma, the surgeon will close the wound and wait for the definitive diagnosis; this is necessary because in many cases, chemotherapy may be needed before the surgical resection is performed. Care is taken intraoperatively to control bleeding because tumor cells can seed wherever

bleeding has occurred. The incision and biopsy track are later excised during the definitive surgical procedure.

Cytologic and pathologic studies to determine tissue type and behavior and to distinguish between benign and malignant conditions are the last steps in the staging process. It is often an anxious time for the client and family as they await the final results. Soft tissue masses can often be diagnosed the same day, but specimens from bone normally take 5 to 7 days for diagnosis because of the need to wash calcium from the bone before slides can be made, a process known as *decalcification*. After all radiologic and tissue studies are completed, an alphanumeric stage, which serves as a method of classification and communication, is assigned to the client's condition.

Tumor Staging

Staging is a method of classifying a condition according to pathologic diagnosis, size of tumor, anatomic structural involvement, and presence or absence of metastasis. Staging helps direct medical and surgical treatments and predict prognosis. It also contributes to cancer research by ensuring reliable comparisons. Staging is done at the conclusion of the diagnostic workup and is updated as the client's condition changes. The surgical staging system of musculoskeletal sarcomas describes the grade (G), the local tumor site (T), and the presence or absence of metastasis (M) (Table 22–4). This method of staging was described by Enneking, Spanier, and Malawer in 1980 and is a commonly used staging system for planning the surgical management of sarcomas, specifically those arising from mesenchymal connective tissue. Lesions derived from bone marrow, such as leukemias, plasmacytomas, Ewing's sarcomas, and metastatic carcinomas, are excluded from this staging system because their natural history, surgical management, and response to treatment are different. The stage provides guidelines for the type of surgical margin required to achieve local control.

From the viewpoint of surgical management and according to the surgical staging system, neoplasms of any histology are divided into two grades, low (G1) and high (G2). Low-grade lesions are well differentiated and have few mitoses and moderate cytologic atypia. Marked by a rather indolent course, low-grade lesions can be managed with relatively conservative procedures because

TABLE 22–4. *Surgical Staging System of Musculoskeletal Sarcomas*

STAGE	GRADE	SITE	METASTASES
IA	Low (G1)	Intracompartmental (T1)	None (M0)
IB	Low (G1)	Extracompartmental (T2)	None (M0)
IIA	High (G2)	Intracompartmental (T1)	None (M0)
IIB	High (G2)	Extracompartmental (T2)	None (M0)
IIIA	Low (G1)	Intracompartmental or extracompartmental (T1–T2)	Region or distant (M1)
IIIB	High (G1)	Intracompartmental or extracompartmental (T1–T2)	Regional or distant (M1)

From Enneking, W. F. (1983). *Musculoskeletal tumor surgery* (p. 81). New York: Churchill Livingstone.

they pose a low risk of regional or distant metastasis. Examples of common low-grade sarcomas include adamantinoma, chordoma, secondary chondrosarcoma, and clear cell sarcoma of tendon sheath.

High-grade lesions are poorly differentiated, have a high mitotic rate, frequently necrotize, and invade surrounding vasculature. Characterized by a highly active clinical course, high-grade lesions are managed with aggressive procedures to achieve control because they pose a significantly higher risk of metastasis. High-grade lesions have a more unfavorable prognosis than low-grade lesions. Examples of common high-grade sarcomas include intraosseous osteosarcoma, radiation sarcoma, Paget's sarcoma, primary chondrosarcoma, MFH, angiosarcoma, neurofibrosarcoma, Ewing's sarcoma, and rhabdomyosarcoma.

The extent of local tumor or setting in which the tumor lies describes the surgical site (T). If the lesion is confined within the natural barriers to extension of a well-delineated anatomic compartment, it is an *intracompartmental* lesion. Natural barriers where microextension of tumor is unlikely include cortical bone, articular cartilage, outer fibrous layer of joint capsule, major fascial septa, tendinous origins of muscle, and sites of muscle insertions. Intracompartmental sites include lesions within a bone or joint; lesions superficial to deep fascia; paraosseous lesions; and lesions of intrafascial compartments, such as the posterior calf, anterior thigh, buttock, anterior arm, and periscapular area.

In contrast, if the lesion extends along fascial spaces and planes between compartments or if the lesion extends into this loose tissue from an original intracompartmental site, it is *extracompartmental*. Within extracompartmental spaces lie all major neurovascular structures. Therefore, if a lesion involves any of these major neurovascular structures, it is by definition extracompartmental. Other extracompartmental sites include lesions originally from bone or joints extending into soft tissues; lesions into the deep fascia; intraosseous or extrafascial lesions; and lesions of extrafascial planes or spaces, such as the midfoot, popliteal space, groin or femoral triangle, intrapelvic tumors, axilla, and paraspinal tumors.

Factors such as the size of the lesion, the distance between vital neurovascular structures and the lesion, and whether the lesion is contained by natural barriers within a well-defined anatomic compartment are taken into consideration when planning a surgical resection. Large, high-grade tumors and those located anatomically deep are considered prognostically unfavorable. Small, low-grade tumors and those located superficially are prognostically more favorable.

The third component of the surgical staging system is the presence or absence of metastasis, either regionally to lymph nodes or distant to the lung via hematogenous spread. The presence of metastasis indicates failure of local control and implies a decreased chance of survival

(Enneking, 1983; Enneking et al., 1980; Enneking & Spanier, 1982).

Another staging system, the TNM method of the American Joint Committee on Cancer (AJCC), is a widely used and universally recommended staging system for many cancers, especially for soft tissue tumors. In the TNM system, the *T* refers to the tumor's size, skin involvement, ulceration, or other tumor changes. Tumors range in size and character from noninvasive to invading surrounding structures. The *N* refers to the characteristics and extent of regional lymph node involvement, and the *M* refers to extent of metastasis. Nodal involvement or metastasis is either absent or present. Combinations of T, N, and M are grouped to describe tumors of various stages from 0 to IV. The AJCC also considers histologic grade, either low or high, in correlating the prognosis of clients with primarily soft tissue sarcoma (Holleb, Fink, & Murphy, 1991). Orthopaedic surgeons who are treating musculoskeletal tumors and those who are members of the Musculoskeletal Tumor Society more commonly use and support the surgical staging system, especially for bone tumors.

TREATMENT MODALITIES AND RELATED NURSING MANAGEMENT

The treatment goal for clients with primary tumors is to eradicate the tumor completely to promote long-term survival. Treatment goals for clients with metastatic disease are palliation, extension of life, and remission. Palliation includes relief of such symptoms as pain and anorexia. Goals should be mutually established with the client and family, keeping in mind the client's biophysical, sociocultural, and psychological needs. The nurse's role is to support goals and plans according to the client's wishes.

Treatments for clients with malignancies are commonly chemotherapy, surgery, radiation therapy, and supportive therapy. Experimental protocols are under way with biologic response modifiers. However, these have not thus far proved effective in the eradication of sarcomas. Treatment for most benign lesions is either observation or surgery.

Nursing interventions supporting medical treatments are directed toward prevention of normal cellular breakdown, maintenance of homeostasis, and restoration of function. In the initial diagnosis stage, biophysical needs most commonly focused on are knowledge deficit, alteration in comfort, impaired physical mobility, ineffective individual and family coping, fear, and anxiety. During the treatment phase, interventions also focus on impaired home maintenance management, altered protective mechanisms, disturbance in self-concept, alteration in nutritional status, and prevention of complications from treatment and disease. During the maintenance phase, when all treatment modalities have been completed and the client is seeing the doctor for follow-up only, knowledge deficit regarding the treatment plan and anxiety related to scheduled radiologic examinations to rule out recurrence or metastatic disease must be dealt with. Clients with malignancies may become disabled, temporarily or permanently, because of lengthy treatment or progressive disease. With disability, sociocultural and psychological needs are predominant and are addressed by nurses in the home or hospice or rehabilitative facility.

Chemotherapy

A dramatic increase in survival of clients diagnosed with a sarcoma has occurred because of the advances made in chemotherapy since the early 1970s. However, the success of chemotherapy depends on several factors, such as the dose and route of administration, the relative antitumor activity of the agent, the biology of the tumor, the drug's interactions with other drugs and modalities of treatment, the drug's mechanism of action, and the drug's acute and chronic toxicity (Yasko & Lane, 1991). The goals of chemotherapy are curative treatment with total eradication of the malignant cells; control of the disease and its symptoms; or palliation to reduce tumor size, extend life, and improve quality of life (Groenwald, Frogge, Goodman, & Henke, 1992). Chemotherapeutic drugs work by displaying selective toxicities on cells that proliferate rapidly. Tumor cells divide rapidly, as do many normal cells, such as hematopoietic cells, gastric epithelial cells, hair follicles, and embryonal and germinal cells. Therefore, besides the tumor kill effect desired from the chemotherapy, the most common side effects, such as bone marrow suppression or myelosuppression, nausea and vomiting, alopecia, and infertility, are unavoidable in most clients.

Chemotherapy for soft tissue and bone sarcomas is administered according to a protocol that is a standard regimen. Chemotherapy regimens in the treatment of primary sarcomas cause controversy and may vary widely among such institutions and cancer study groups as the Intergroup Sarcoma Study Group, Eastern Cooperative Oncology Group, South West Oncology Group, Memorial Sloan-Kettering Cancer Center, St. Jude Children's Research Hospital, and the National Cancer Institute. Research into the effectiveness of chemotherapy protocols is an ongoing process worldwide. However, it takes several years of testing the drugs before they can be used on humans. The key is to follow a known protocol consisting of multidrug therapy. According to Yasko and Lane (1991), "The effectiveness of a regimen of chemotherapy can be enhanced by the combination of individually active agents possessing different mechanisms of action to achieve synergistic antitumor activity, abrogate resistance to drugs, and address heterogeneity of the tumor" (p. 1265).

Chemotherapy may be given preoperatively (neoadjuvantly) or postoperatively as adjuvant therapy. Chemotherapy is most often administered intravenously. If it is administered by continuous intravenous infusion instead of intravenous bolus, chemotherapy causes less toxicity. Chemotherapy (cisplatin or doxorubicin hydrochloride) can be administered intra-arterially before resection to provide a higher concentration of active drug directly to the tumor site. However, research has not shown this method to increase overall survival.

Neoadjuvant chemotherapy is the standard of care for cancer clients because it allows assessment of tumor kill. See the evidence-based practice question for a review of the results of neoadjuvant chemotherapy trials. During neoadjuvant chemotherapy, which may last up to 3 months or longer, the tumor activity is monitored by assessing parameters, such as size of the tumor and pain. The goals of neoadjuvant chemotherapy are to see a decrease in tumor size radiographically and a decrease in pain. A decrease in tumor size allows for a less radical surgical procedure. The amount of tumor necrosis on pathologic examination is key. The amount of tumor necrosis is generally used as a prognostic factor. If the amount of dead tumor exceeds 95% of the tumor, a good chemotherapy response is achieved and the chemotherapy regimen is continued postoperatively. Prognosis for 5-year survival is high. If less than 95% of the tumor specimen is necrotic, a poor response has occurred and the chemotherapy may be changed. The chance of metastatic disease or recurrence is considered higher, and a less favorable long-term survival is expected. Finally, neoadjuvant chemotherapy is also given to eradicate possible microscopic disease already present and to treat metastatic disease.

The systemic effects of the chemotherapy may promote complications such as delayed wound healing and infection after surgery. Therefore, postoperative or adjuvant chemotherapy is not resumed for at least 2 weeks after surgery. This delay allows for wound healing and surgical recuperation time for the client. The chemotherapy protocol that the client was following preoperatively is resumed. Commonly used chemotherapeutic agents in the treatment of sarcomas are listed in Table 22–5.

Currently, regimens that bring about the highest response rates in soft tissue sarcomas include doxorubicin hydrochloride (Adriamycin) as their common denominator in combination with other agents, including dacarbazine, cyclophosphamide, vincristine, dactinomycin, and methotrexate. Ifosfamide, a cyclophosphamide analogue, is being used for some clients with sarcomas who have not responded to a regimen containing doxorubicin hydrochloride. However, the use of chemotherapy for soft tissue sarcomas remains controversial because the long-term efficacy has not been shown, except in the

EXAMINING THE EVIDENCE: Moving Toward Evidence-Based Practice
Examine the Evidence: The Effect of Neoadjuvant Chemotherapy and Resulting Tumor Necrosis on Event-Free Survival

AUTHOR(S), YEAR	SAMPLE SIZE	DIAGNOSIS	DESIGN	OUTCOME VARIABLE	MAJOR FINDINGS
Ferrari et al., 1999	N = 95 clients with biopsy-proven, classic, high-grade osteosarcoma of extremity, <40 yr, no metastasis by bone scan, <1-month interval between biopsy and start of chemotherapy, normal renal and liver function, no prior chemotherapy or surgery for bone lesion	Osteosarcoma	Preoperative chemotherapy Methotrexate (MTX) Cisplatin (CDP) Doxorubicin (Adriamycin, ADR) 72 clients randomized to receive CDP IV or intra-arterial (IA) Week 8—surgery Postoperative chemotherapy For good histologic response (GR) = ADR, MTX, CDP/ADR; repeat 3 times For poor response, (PR) = ADR, ifosfamide (IFO), MTX, CDP/ADR; repeat 3 times	Efficacy of protocol with reduced cumulative dose of ADR Role of route of infusion (IV vs. IA) CDP on histologic response Use of IFO as salvage chemotherapy in PR	Decreased dose of ADR avoided cardiotoxicities without consequences IA had better histologic response but disadvantages of this treatment outweigh the benefits IFO represents an effective salvage therapy for PR
Fuchs et al., 1998	N = 171 clients with high-grade extremity osteosarcoma, ≤40 yr, registered within 3 weeks from biopsy, no metastasis, negative bone scan	Osteosarcoma	Study COSS-86 Low-risk group = tumor size ≤⅓ bone involved 20% chondroid ground substance in biopsy ≤20% reduction of activity in sequential bone scans ADR—4 courses MTX—2 courses CDP—4 courses High-risk group = any of 3 risk factors listed above ADR—5 courses MTX—14 courses CDP—5 courses IA or IV IFO—5 courses Surgery week 10 Stat analysis Kaplan-Meier	Adding IFO preoperatively to ADR, MTX and CDP to increase event-free survival (EFS) and overall survival (OS) in high-risk clients CDP given IA or IV to test benefits	10-year OS was 72% and disease-free survival (DFS) was 66% No benefit to IA CDP
Bacci et al., 2000	N = 44 clients with peripheral neuroectodermal tumor (PNET) N = 138 clients with typical Ewing's sarcoma (TES) 182 clients were in original sample Retrospective review found 44 to have actually had PNET not TES	Nonmetastatic PNET	6-drug chemotherapy to all clients = vincristine, ADR, dactinomycin, cyclophosphamide, IFO, and etoposide Local treatment of surgery in 20 clients Surgery followed by radiotherapy in 13 clients Radiotherapy only in 11 clients	Comparing OS and EFS of clients with PNET with clients with TES following same treatment protocols	In this study, clients with PNET diagnosis carry a worse prognosis than TES clients and this conclusion was attributed to the neural differentiation Authors noted other studies have found no difference in OS or EFS when comparing the same tumors
Bacci et al., in press	N = 23 clients >39 yr with Ewing's sarcoma of bone (ES)	ES	Retrospective comparison of 23 clients >39 yr, with 327 clients <39 yr with ES and treated with same protocol	Behavior of ES in adults >39 yr is the same as or different than ES in clients <39 yr	Treatment protocol for the two groups was the same, and the study concluded that the behavior in ES in adults is no different than that in children and that all adult clients should be included in the multidisciplinary treatment trials of this tumor

Box continued on following page

EXAMINING THE EVIDENCE: Moving Toward Evidence-Based Practice
Examine the Evidence: The Effect of Neoadjuvant Chemotherapy and Resulting Tumor Necrosis on Event-Free Survival Continued

AUTHOR(S), YEAR	SAMPLE SIZE	DIAGNOSIS	DESIGN	OUTCOME VARIABLE	MAJOR FINDINGS
Szendroi, Papai, & Illes, 2000	N = 96	High-grade osteosarcoma of the extremities treated between 1986 and 1997	3 groups Group I, N = 75, all with nonmetastatic osteosarcoma, received intensive chemotherapy (ADR, MTX, CDP, IFO) and underwent surgery Group II, N = 9, had metastases at time of referral Group III, N = 12, received chemotherapy in delayed or suboptimal form	Surgical results and survival, prognostic factors and survival	Favorable 5-year EFS rate of 65%-75% can be achieved with appropriately wide or radical surgical margins and intensive chemotherapy given per protocol Positive prognostic factors were tumor volume ≤60 cm^3, side or radical surgical margins, far distal location of tumor, 20% cartilage content of tumor, and 90% tumor necrosis
Rytting et al., 2000	N = 30 <11 yr for boys and <10 yr for girls	Osteosarcoma of the pelvis or extremity treated between 1978 and 1995	Retrospective analysis 4 treatment and investigation of osteosarcoma (TIOS) treatment groups TIOS I, 1978-1982; randomized to receive high-dose MTX with leucovorin rescue or cisplatin II for treatment of primary tumor If >60% tumor necrosis, continued preoperative agent plus ADR, CDP, MTX If preoperative treatment was ineffective, <60% tumor necrosis, preoperative agent was eliminated TIOS II, 1982-1986; 7-course IA CDP TIOS III, 1986-1989; 7-course IA CDP TIOS IV, 1989-1996; preoperative IFO, ADR, and IV CDP	Determine EFS and OS and prognostic indicators that could influence therapy in preadolescent children vs. adolescents and older children	No statistical difference in EFS and OS when comparing ages No significance in clients who relapsed and elevated alkaline phosphatase levels No significant difference in survival of clients who had increased height for age Slight improvement in DFS for females Small increase in OS if >95% tumor necrosis Review of preadolescent clients with osteosarcoma did not reveal any significant prognostic variable in gender, height, serum alkaline phosphatase, serum lactic dehydrogenase, tumor histologic features, tumor site, and tumor necrosis induced by preoperative chemotherapy

DFS, disease-free survival; EFS, event-free survival; OS, overall survival.

treatment of rhabdomyosarcoma in children. Surgery and radiation remain the primary treatment.

Chemotherapy prescribed for osteosarcomas consists primarily of doxorubicin hydrochloride, cisplatin, and high doses of methotrexate, with leucovorin calcium rescue and ifosfamide. Chemotherapy for Ewing's sarcoma consists of combination chemotherapy with doxorubicin hydrochloride, vincristine, cyclophosphamide, VP-16 (etoposide), or ifosfamide. Unless metasta-

sis has occurred, chemotherapy for high-grade cartilage tumors, such as a chondrosarcoma, is normally not given because it is usually not effective. Chemotherapy for metastatic carcinomas is specific to the type of cancer.

Nursing care of the client undergoing chemotherapy is multidisciplinary and covers the psychological as well as the physiologic needs of the client and family. Coordination of care among inpatient, outpatient, home health, and hospice nursing is essential. Nursing interventions cover the following areas:

1. Educating the client and family about the goal of chemotherapy, potential side effects, and symptom management
2. Monitoring hematologic studies
3. Monitoring renal, hepatic, neurologic, vascular, muscular, immune, and integumentary systems
4. Administering prescribed antiemetics before therapy
5. Providing information about nutrition during chemotherapy
6. Supporting the emotional responses of the client and family
7. Assisting with the use of coping mechanisms
8. Assisting with methods to increase the client's self-esteem
9. Ensuring compliance of treatment scheduling

Nursing management includes understanding the pharmacologic agent's mechanism of action, dose, method of administration, and potential side effects. Most side effects occur as a result of the action of chemotherapy on normal cells. Normal cells that are most affected by chemotherapy are those that rapidly multiply and are located in the bone marrow, gastrointestinal tract, hair follicles, and gonads. Some potential side effects that should be considered in nursing management of the client include bone marrow suppression, stomatitis or mucositis, esophagitis, nausea and vomiting, anorexia, taste changes, constipation, alopecia, cutaneous reactions, and sexual dysfunction. Toxicities resulting from chemotherapy mandate intermittent therapy whereby the body's tissues can recover.

Radiation Therapy

Radiation therapy, as defined by Perez and Brady (1998), is a "clinical modality dealing with the use of ionizing radiations in the treatment of clients with malignant neoplasias (and occasionally benign diseases)" (p. 1). The goal of radiation therapy is to deliver safe doses of radiation to malignant cells while sparing normal cells from damage. Radiation can be given for curative intent or for palliation. The desired effect is eradication of the tumor with a prolonged high quality of life. However, if cure is not possible, palliative therapy can help control the size of the tumor or prevent fracture, therefore easing the pain. Radiation affects normal tissue and tumor. Radiation works best on rapidly dividing cells, both normal and cancer cells. These rapidly dividing cells, which are most sensitive to radiation, are referred to as *radiosensitive*. Mucosa is an example of a radiosensitive tissue. Cells that divide slowly are considered radioresistant, or less radiosensitive, and include tissues like muscle and nerve cells.

Side effects of radiation therapy stem from damage to normal cells in the treated fields. Major advancements in this field have been brought about by refinements of radiation machines that spare skin sensitivity, by a better understanding of cancer and radiobiology, and by the use of computers in planning treatments—a process known as *simulation*.

In general, large spindle cell sarcomas, including osteosarcomas, chondrosarcomas, and rhabdomyosarcomas, are not sensitive to radiation. Radiotherapy can be used in some small, round cell tumors, such as Ewing's sarcoma, in combination with chemotherapy. It also is used in myxoid liposarcomas. When administered

TABLE 22–5. *Common Chemotherapy Drugs Used in Sarcoma Treatment*

AGENTS AND ROUTE	ACTION
Antitumor Antibiotics	
Bleomycin SC, IM, IV	Bind to DNA to inhibit synthesis of RNA and DNA. Formation of toxic oxygen-free radicals
Doxorubicin IV	results in single- and double-stranded DNA breaks with subsequent inhibition of DNA
Dactinomycin IV	synthesis and function.
Alkylating Agents	
Cisplatin IV	Forms cross-links with DNA resulting in inhibition of DNA synthesis and function. Acts in all
Cyclophosphamide PO, IV	phases of the cell cycle.
Dacarbazine IV	Ifosfamide is activated by the liver cytochrome P450 system.
Ifosfamide IV	
Antimetabolites	
Methotrexate	Folic acid analogue that interferes with DNA and RNA synthesis by inhibiting enzyme activity;
PO, IM, IV or IT (intrathecal)	acts on rapidly dividing cells that are synthesizing DNA.
Plant Alkaloids	
Vincristine IV	Binds to substance necessary for formation of mitotic spindles, preventing cell division. It works
VP-16 IV	on cells in the mitosis phase in which the parent cell divides into two new daughter cells.

From Chu, E., & DeVita, V. (2001). *Cancer chemotherapy drug manual 2001*. Boston: Jones and Bartlett.

preoperatively for a myxoid liposarcoma, radiation will shrink the fatty tissue tumor and make the surgical resection easier. Radiation therapy is sometimes indicated for those rare occurrences of metastatic disease from sarcomas to lymph nodes, such as with clear cell sarcomas. Quite effectively, radiation therapy is used in metastatic carcinomas to the bone as a method of pain control, to eradicate bone lesions, or to eradicate remaining tumor in a lesion previously resected, such as with an intralesional excision and intramedullary rodding of the femur for metastatic renal cell carcinoma.

Radiation for sarcomas can be given in several ways: (1) external beam radiation therapy (EBRT), preoperatively, postoperatively, or both; (2) brachytherapy; and (3) intraoperative radiation therapy (IORT). There are advantages and disadvantages of each and particular tumors where one method is superior.

EBRT is used preoperatively if the tumor is radiosensitive and is close to or touching vital structures such as blood vessels and nerves. As in the case of a myxoid liposarcoma, radiation shrinks the tumor away from these structures, allowing for wider tumor-free surgical margins. Part of the allowable dose may be given before surgery and then if the surgical margins remain close or questionable, completion of the dose may be given after wound healing (approximately 2 to 3 weeks).

Another approach to the management of clients with soft tissue sarcomas is surgical excision and intraoperative implantation of radioactive sources. Known as *brachytherapy,* a radioactive isotope can be chosen for surface, interstitial, or intracavitary application. Implantation of the isotope allows for a high dose of radiation to be delivered to the tumor with decreasing amounts to adjacent normal tissues. Brachytherapy is becoming more widely used because of its advantages when used with surgery. Benefits include a shorter treatment time for the

client (4 to 5 days) and possibly less extensive surgery because of the ability to place the catheters directly on the wound bed (Fig. 22–8). This aggressive treatment kills the malignant cells before they have a chance to become attached to underlying soft tissues or scar. Special attention to wound closure is needed to avoid tension at the incision site. Radiation slows healing. Therefore, extra planning for wound closure with a possible muscle and skin flap may be needed. The use of brachytherapy is increasing, and it is the treatment of choice in conjunction with surgery at some major institutions.

The last method of delivering radiation is IORT. The main benefit of this method is that the radiation can be concentrated to an area where the cancer is located while the remaining tissue is surgically mobilized out of the radiation field. Intraoperative radiation can be used only at institutions that have a dedicated operating room with a linear accelerator. These suites are usually located in the radiation departments of larger facilities.

As with all cancer treatments, there are benefits and side effects. The benefits of radiation therapy include its ability to assist with local tumor control, shrink tumors before surgery, and relieve bone pain caused by tumor invasion. Side effects of radiation include permanent tanning of the skin over the radiated area, possible skin breakdown, possible joint fibrosis, and possible growth disturbance in a child if the radiation field includes the growth plate.

The nurse's role in radiation therapy is to educate the client and family about radiation and its potential side effects, provide information on nutrition during treatment, monitor for impaired skin integrity and the overall response to radiation therapy, and facilitate compliance of treatment schedules. Depending on the dose, site, and preexisting state of the client receiving radiation therapy, systemic effects can occur from treatment. Clients with

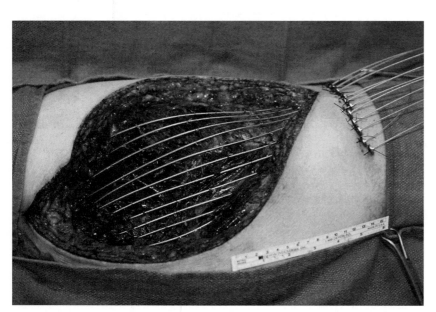

FIGURE 22–8. Brachytherapy catheters in the surgical wound bed.

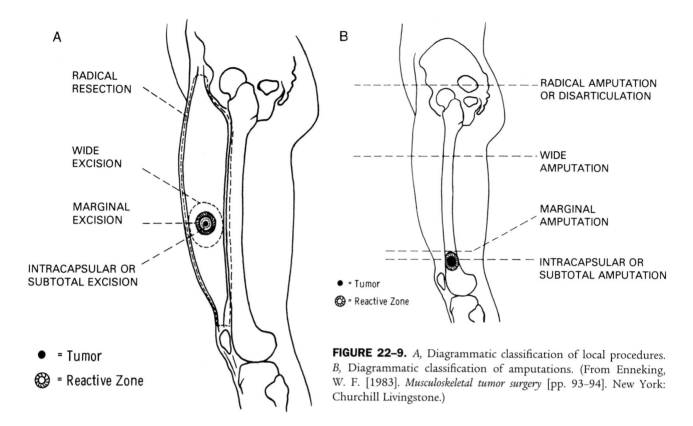

A

RADICAL
RESECTION

WIDE
EXCISION

MARGINAL
EXCISION

INTRACAPSULAR OR
SUBTOTAL EXCISION

● = Tumor

⊛ = Reactive Zone

B

RADICAL AMPUTATION
OR DISARTICULATION

WIDE
AMPUTATION

MARGINAL
AMPUTATION

INTRACAPSULAR OR
SUBTOTAL AMPUTATION

● = Tumor

⊛ = Reactive Zone

FIGURE 22–9. *A,* Diagrammatic classification of local procedures. *B,* Diagrammatic classification of amputations. (From Enneking, W. F. [1983]. *Musculoskeletal tumor surgery* [pp. 93–94]. New York: Churchill Livingstone.)

malignancies are prone to a declining nutritional status and anemia. Consequently, normal tissue maintenance is lessened, and wound healing can be retarded. Uncorrected anemias and negative nitrogen balance impair healing. Infections can occur in nonhealing wounds. Care is taken to commence radiation therapy after all surgical wounds are well healed. Hematologic studies performed during radiation treatments include measurement of uric acid, platelet, hemoglobin, and hematocrit levels, and white and red blood cell counts.

Surgery

Principles. The goal of surgery for the treatment of primary sarcomas is to eradicate the tumor completely. To do this, the mass or lesion along with a wide zone of normal tissue is surgically excised. Tumors are eradicated either by en bloc excision or by amputation. Current methods of treatment are aimed at sparing the limb (limb sparing or limb salvage) with optimal tumor eradication. Limb-sparing surgery became prominent after the advent of CT and MRI, which enabled surgeons to determine more precisely the tumor site and surrounding involved structures. Resections instead of amputations allowed removal of the malignancy while preserving limbs and function. If complete tumor eradication is deemed impossible, an amputation is often recommended and performed. Today, fewer amputations are being done. Four types of procedures are described according to the type of surgical margin achieved at the time of operation:

intracapsular or intralesional excision, marginal or simple excision, wide excision, and radical resection. These margins are more commonly recognized with limb-sparing procedures but are also used to describe the type of margin achieved through amputation (Fig. 22–9).

Intralesional excision, sometimes referred to as *curettage,* is the subtotal removal of a lesion. It is done for a presumably benign lesion or for a metastatic bone lesion in which total removal is not possible.

With marginal excision, the surgeon dissects through the reactive zone of the tumor, a zone where neoplastic cells are still present. Marginal excisions are reserved for benign lesions because dissection through the reactive zone of a malignant tumor leaves behind malignant cells.

Removal of the tumor with dissection through a wide zone of normal tissue is known as *wide excision.* Because the reactive zone of malignant cells is removed, the wide excision is the most common margin for the treatment of primary sarcomas when total tumor eradication is the goal. However, although preserving the limbs, the wide excision can result in local tumor recurrence.

Radical resection, the removal of the tumor and the entire bone or muscle in which it lies, from origin to insertion, is reserved for much more extensive cases in which the tumor consumes the majority of the muscle compartment or bone. Radical resection can also be done when function, resulting from a wide excision, will be no greater than if a radical excision is performed. An example of a radical resection is the removal of the entire quadriceps femoris muscle for a soft tissue sarcoma. Another example is the complete resection of the proximal femur and reconstruction with a megaprosthesis for high-grade osteosarcoma of the femoral head and neck.

A common procedure for the treatment of soft tissue sarcoma is wide excision. If the overlying skin is involved in the tumor, the skin is excised. The soft tissue defect is filled with skin grafts, local muscle flaps, myocutaneous free flaps, or vascularized flaps.

Bone sarcomas are most often treated by radical resection of the involved bone. Muscles commonly used to reconstruct soft tissue defects are the rectus abdominis, gastrocnemius, and latissimus dorsi. Bone defects around a joint can be replaced by using a total joint arthroplasty prosthesis or endoprosthesis. However, depending on the size of the defect, a megaprosthesis may be needed. Bone grafts with internal fixation can also be used for bone defects around a joint or for segmental defects. Allografts are cadaveric whole bones or segments of bone, whereas autografts are bone grafts taken from the client at another anatomic site. Allografts and prostheses can be used together to form an alloprosthesis during reconstruction of a bone defect. Allografts can be ordered from a bone bank with all the tendons and ligaments still attached to allow for better soft tissue reattachment during reconstruction.

The choice of reconstruction depends on the client's age, level of activity, location of tumor, and expected functional result after surgery. The advantage of the allograft is that large bone defects can be reconstructed using biologic tissue. However, the bone does not have a blood supply at the time of transplantation, making the allograft more prone to infection. Other disadvantages are the fear of transmission of hepatitis or acquired immunodeficiency syndrome (AIDS) and the risk of fracture. The advantage of autograft is the ability to use the client's own tissue. The disadvantages are that it is difficult to obtain enough bone from the client when large areas need to be reconstructed and it creates another surgical site that is very painful. With both allograft and autograft, healing is prolonged. Sufficient time is needed for bone union, from 6 weeks to 1 year. During this time, protected weight bearing is enforced with crutches and an orthosis. A cane may be needed for an extended time.

Although total joint arthroplasty provides quicker mobilization and return to activities than bone grafting, the disadvantages are the potential loosening of the prosthesis and the need for additional surgery in the future. Some segmental defect-replacement prostheses are being used to replace large bone defects resulting from diaphyseal tumors.

Benign soft tissue masses normally are treated with simple marginal excisions. Benign bone lesions commonly are treated with intralesional excisions and filling of the defects with autograft or allograft tissue. Depending on the location and size of the lesion, internal fixation

can provide stability. Protective weight bearing and immobilization are required until bone union is evident. The amount of allowable weight bearing and extent of immobilization depend on the particular surgery.

Metastatic lesions of bone cause pain and have the potential to fracture. Whether impending or actually fractured, metastatic lesions to the long bones commonly are managed with intralesional excision followed by intramedullary rodding and insertion of methylmethacrylate cement. Cement provides immediate fixation of the weakened area. Immediate fixation is necessary because metastatic lesions of the bone are difficult to heal. Weight bearing is protected until the excision is healed.

Once controversial, resection of lung metastases is now common. In general, surgical or laser resection of metastatic lung lesions produces a better prognosis if lesions are smaller than 3 cm and are located in only one lobe and the primary tumor site is controlled. Surgery for lung lesions ranges from wedge resection to lobectomy or pneumonectomy. Defects in the chest wall can be reconstructed with surgical mesh.

The last area of common procedures for clients with musculoskeletal tumors is that of palliation. When all other noninvasive means of pain relief are exhausted, neurosurgical procedures may be considered. Procedures such as chordotomies, in which the anterolateral tracts of the spinal cord are severed, provide relief of intractable pain to the area innervated by these nerves.

Intraoperative Care. The operating room nurse is challenged with the following:

1. Protecting the affected extremity or tumorous area from undue stress
2. Maintaining peripheral circulation and tissue perfusion
3. Promoting optimal gas exchange
4. Maintaining skin integrity
5. Preventing neurologic complications
6. Promoting infection control
7. Obtaining, safely handling, and maintaining quality control for all bone grafts, implants, and orthopaedic hardware

Specific nursing interventions can include the following:

1. Applying and monitoring alternating compression hose for lower extremity perfusion
2. Inserting a Foley catheter and monitoring output
3. Weighing sponges and measuring suction bottle contents to analyze blood loss
4. Positioning the client for optimal chest expansion while preventing injury from pressure and nerve compression over bony prominences
5. Applying alternating pressure mattress or similar pads to the operating room table

6. Maintaining strict aseptic technique and controlling traffic in the operating room throughout the procedure
7. Monitoring the laminar air flow system
8. Handling all tissue grafts, implants, and hardware with care and ensuring correct selection and size, adherence to sterilization expiration, and quality control measures for allografts related to hepatitis and human immunodeficiency virus (HIV) testing

Operating room nurses may collaborate with the surgeon in ordering, tracking, and receiving custom implants. For a more detailed discussion of perioperative issues, see Chapter 11.

COST OF TREATMENT

With health care costs continually on the rise and physician and hospital reimbursement down, the need for cost-effective health care is crucial. Limb-salvage surgery is expensive because of the length of surgical and operating room time, cost of the prosthesis, and cost of the grafting material. The price range for a titanium prosthesis can vary from $3500 to $15,000. An osteochondral allograft such as a distal femur may cost $8000 or more if soft tissue attachments are needed. The demineralized bone graft used to fill bone defects ranges in price from $650 to more than $1000 for a 30-mL vial. Plates and screws used to secure allografts or fix pathologic fractures vary from $200 to $2000. Therefore, the need for careful surgical planning is imperative.

Not only is there the surgical cost, but chemotherapy and radiation therapy are also costly. Chemotherapy may range from $80,000 to $100,000, which includes all laboratory costs, medication, and hospitalization. Infusion of chemotherapy has moved to the outpatient clinic setting and to the home, which has helped keep the hospital costs down for the client. Radiation therapy costs start at $40,000 for the 6-week EBRT and vary for brachytherapy and IORT depending on the amount and time the radiation is delivered.

COMMON NURSING DIAGNOSES AND INTERVENTIONS IN THE INITIAL DIAGNOSIS PHASE

The challenge of managing the care of orthopaedic oncology clients is the ability to customize the care of clients of all ages and to direct the nursing process in which complicated surgical and medical modalities are implemented. The care is multidisciplinary and may involve all of the following health care providers: family practice physician; general orthopaedists; surgical, medical, and radiation oncologists; orthopaedic oncology and mental health clinical nurse specialists; office nurses; inpatient and outpatient staff nurses; social workers; nutritionists; physical therapists; occupational therapists;

home health nurses; and hospice nurses. The initial care for these clients may start in the client's general or family practitioner's office and then move to a general orthopaedist's office. The orthopaedist, on recognizing a probable bone or soft tissue tumor, will contact the nearest orthopaedic oncologist for definitive care. There are only about 75 orthopaedic oncologists in the United States, and they are spread around the country. Clients may have to travel up to 8 to 10 hours to be seen by this specialist. Usually, these orthopaedic oncologists are located in major cities at comprehensive cancer centers.

When care is then transferred to the orthopaedic oncologist's office, further workup and definitive treatment planning take place. Consultation with the physician may last up to an hour, and then a biopsy is scheduled to get a tissue diagnosis. The clinic nurse has client and family teaching to do regarding the upcoming radiology scans that may be scheduled as well as the biopsy. The orthopaedic staff nurse has only a brief opportunity to work with the client at this time because the client's stay in the hospital for the biopsy or excision may only be 1 to 2 days. The client returns to the clinic in approximately 1 week for the postoperative visit and discussion of the results of the biopsy. Depending on the diagnosis, the clinic nurse may have to schedule an appointment for the client to see the medical oncologist for neoadjuvant chemotherapy or the radiation oncologist for preoperative radiation treatment. If surgery to completely remove the tumor is the next step, a surgical date is scheduled. Therefore, in the initial diagnosis phase, knowledge deficit, anxiety, fear, pain control, mobility, and coping take precedence and must be addressed by the office nurse and briefly by the staff nurse. If amputation is required as the surgical procedure, grief work will need to be discussed also.

Knowledge Deficits

Teaching: Disease Process/Procedure/Treatment. Knowledge deficits are related to the new diagnosis of a malignancy and multiple treatment modalities (Table 22–6). Issues relating to diagnosis, radiologic evaluation, biopsy, staging, surgery, chemotherapy, radiation therapy, potential complications, alternatives of care, risks, benefits, nursing management, discharge plans, home care, and long-term follow-up and treatment are addressed with the client and family.

After the physician discusses the diagnosis with the client, the nurse often must explain it in simpler terms. Radiologic tests are described according to their purpose, procedure, client preparation, and expected outcome (either positive or negative) in differentiating the diagnosis. The biopsy procedure is explained, along with what the results can indicate, such as a benign or a malignant tumor.

After all the information is obtained from the workup, a tumor stage is identified. A stage can be

TABLE 22–6. *Client Education: Knowledge Deficit: Bone or Soft Tissue Tumor*

FOCUS	TEACHING POINTS	FOCUS	TEACHING POINTS

Assessment	History
	  Symptoms
	  Antecedent trauma
	  Pain
	Physical
	  Palpation
	  Range of motion
	  Strength
	  Neurovascular assessment
	  Deep tendon reflex
	  Size (measurement)
		Surgical options for complete removal of tumor	Explain surgical options for soft tissue mass
			  Excisional biopsy (for benign mass)
			  Wide resection
			  Radical resection
			  Amputation
			Explain surgical options for bone tumor
			  Intralesional curettage, cryosurgery, with bone graft and internal fixation
			  Radical resection bone, reconstruction with use of osteochondral allograft with soft tissue attachments or megaprosthesis (custom) or both
			  Rotationplasty
			  Amputation
			Discuss
			  Length of procedure
			  Length of stay
			  Placement of incision
			  Risks and benefits
			  Expected functional outcome

Diagnosis	Explain
	  Benign vs. malignant
	  Etiology of probable diagnosis
	  Incidence		

Radiologic evaluation	Discuss
	  Films client has
	If no films or if not sufficient, order and explain (reason for and preparation required)
	  Plain x-ray film (extremity affected and chest)
	  MRI (extremity affected)
	  Bone scan (whole body)
	  CT scan chest (rule out metastatic disease if diagnosis suspicious for high-grade malignancy)
		Postoperative routines	Explain
			  Nursing care of
			    Wound
			    Drains
			    IV
			    Catheter
			    Thrombosis embolism deterrent stockings (TEDS)
			  Incentive spirometry
			  Possible ICU stay
			  Physical therapy consultation
			  Occupational therapy consultation

Biopsy	Explain
	  Types: open vs. needle
	  Length of procedure
	  Placement of incision and reason
	  Preliminary diagnosis report
	  Immediate if soft tissue tumor
	  Touch preparation only if bone tumor
	  Final pathology report
	  3–5 days if soft tissue
	  Up to 7 days if bone because of decalcification that must occur to be able to cut the specimen
		Rehabilitation	Explain
			  Reasons for physical therapy
			  Ambulation training with assistive device
			  Exercises
			  Inpatient and probable outpatient
			  Reasons for occupational therapy
			  Assistive devices for ADLs

Staging	Explain
	  Purpose of medical staging for sarcomas
	  Inclusion of pathology and radiology studies in staging process
	  Meaning of stage
	  How stage is used in planning of treatment		

explained as a label or level given to the client's condition concerning the grade of the tumor, its location, and evidence of metastasis in the body. It also is used as a prognostic indicator.

Once surgery has been decided on, teaching focuses on explaining the surgical procedure itself, the timing of the procedure, and the length of the operation. Postoperative expectations relating to dressings, drains, and placement of the incision, as well as postanesthesia care, are discussed. Expected functional results, especially if large muscle masses or motor nerves are excised, and length of recovery are other issues that must be addressed.

Should chemotherapy or radiation therapy be indicated, issues relating to their purpose, expected results, method of administration, timing of the treatments, potential side effects, and health maintenance during therapy are discussed.

Knowledge deficits relating to nursing management are best addressed by the primary caregivers. Management of needs is a team approach by ambulatory, surgical, postanesthesia, intensive care, and floor nurses. Clinical specialists, clinicians, or case managers may coordinate total care from an ambulatory or inpatient setting. Knowledge deficits regarding discharge plans and home care are reduced by centering on the type of facility (home versus rehabilitation center or extended care facility), home care providers (family, significant other, visiting nurses, hospice nurses), special needs for equipment or supplies, and ADLs in relationship to the home setup. A social worker is often consulted to assist with home care arrangements.

Knowledge of long-term follow-up care and treatment is paramount. Regular evaluations with the physician are necessary to check for any evidence of local recurrence or metastasis. Routine chest x-ray films, CT, bone scans, or MRI may be performed to determine evidence of recurrent tumor.

Further client teaching focuses on alternative forms of care, risks, benefits, and potential complications of treatment. The nurse should be knowledgeable about experimental protocols and help alleviate myths concerning cancer and various unproven regimens. Information about alternatives must be based on objective measures of care. Risks of treatment are more prevalent with many adjuvant therapies. Complications, such as cardiomyopathy, can occur and are irreversible. Benefits of treatment are usually many, but they are not always predictable. Clients often want to be assured of a cure, but a cure is not always certain. Much hope and encouragement must be given at the time of client teaching.

Potential complications of treatment are many. Clients undergoing extensive orthopaedic surgeries are prone to wound infections and deep venous thrombosis. Each surgical procedure has its own peculiar potential complications. A client undergoing a proximal-third total hip replacement for a hip joint sarcoma is prone to dislocation of the prosthesis. Clients receiving large allografts are subject to nonunions at the graft sites, fracture of the allografts, or bony resorptions of the allografts. Clients undergoing amputation are prone to flexion contractures and neuromas. Myocutaneous flaps are subject to impaired healing of skin grafts, requiring additional procedures.

Client education is a long-term process requiring repetition by many nurses involved in the care of the client. During this time, the client with a newly diagnosed malignancy is very anxious. Discussions should be short and frequent and involve family members. Anatomic models, x-ray films, booklets, and pictures are helpful in implementing the teaching plan.

Anxiety

Anxiety Reduction. In the acute stage of illness, anxiety related to diagnosis, potentially terminal illness, lengthy hospital stays, and extended treatments is a problem needing attention. Sufficient time must be allowed for interaction among the client, family, physician, nurse, and others. Outbursts of anger or hostility are often results of high anxiety. The nurse should help the client recognize the issue and provide reassurance. While helping the client and family set short- and long-term goals, concentration should be given to shorter-term activities so as not to overwhelm the client with instructions and thoughts. The nurse must gain the client's confidence and trust over time to be able to help alleviate anxiety. If the problem of anxiety is not addressed, biophysical changes may result. The psychiatry liaison is often consulted to assist with measures to relieve anxiety.

Fear

Coping Enhancement. Fear related to upcoming surgery, chemotherapy, or radiation must be addressed by the physician and nurses. Giving the client information is a necessity but should be done in increments. A client and his or her family may be able to understand only small amounts of information and instructions at a time. Repeating information in a calm and assuring manner and allowing the client time to ask questions is imperative. Giving clients informational handouts as well as allowing clients to talk with other cancer clients is helpful.

Pain

Pain Management. The goals for pain management—to relieve pain while awake, with activity, and while asleep—should include strategies for controlling both acute pain from surgery, fracture, or inflammation and chronic pain from progression of the disease. In the treatment of cancer pain, it is important to individualize the pain management regimen to the client. According to the *Management of Cancer Pain: Adults, Quick Reference Guide for Clinicians* (Agency for Health Care Policy and Research [AHCPR],1994), a three-step hierarchy developed by the World Health Organization (WHO) should be used for analgesic pain management. First-line management of pain from sarcoma or metastatic disease is most often with analgesics combined with nonpharmacologic methods of pain control. Therefore, when acute and chronic malignant pain is mild to moderate in nature, it is best managed with a prostaglandin inhibitor, such as NSAIDs, acetaminophen, or aspirin (unless contraindicated). If pain persists or increases, one should progress to step two, which includes an opioid, nonopioid, and the adjuvant or nonpharmacologic means of pain relief. If pain continues or becomes severe, one should progress to step three, which involves increasing the opioid potency or the dose.

When analgesics are prescribed, attention must be given to allowances for incremental increases, round-the-clock dosing, and long-term or sustained-released dosing. Occasionally, other drugs, such as antidepressants or antianxiety drugs, may be needed. The preferred method of administration of pain medications is orally. It is the most convenient and usually the most cost-effective way to manage pain. However, if the client is unable to take oral medications because of nausea, stomatitis, difficulty swallowing, or decreased level of consciousness, other routes of administration, such as rectal, transdermal, intravenous or subcutaneous infusion, patient-controlled analgesia, and intraspinal, are available.

In a few cases when the conventional methods of pain management are not effective, the more invasive palliative methods may need to be explored. Procedures such as local or whole-body radiation may be initiated. Treatment with radiation is effective in relieving some bone pain because of metastasis. Once pain is relieved (in approximately 10 days) after completion of therapy, medication dosages are adjusted. Assistive gait devices, such as canes, walkers, and crutches, can lessen the pain caused by weight bearing while ambulating. Surgery (curative or palliative), nerve blocks, or ablation of pain pathways are also available.

Effective pain management is best achieved by a team approach involving clients, their families, and health care providers (AHCPR, 1994). Immediate and long-term control is often best managed by specialists in pain management, followed by home care or hospice nurses.

Nursing strategies concurrently used to assist with pain management include changing the client's position; applying cutaneous stimulation by heat, cold, or massage to a nontumorous area; providing distraction through music therapy and imagery; and teaching and encouraging regular methods of relaxation. Nursing interventions must also be aimed at monitoring the client for potential side effects of opioid use, including nausea, vomiting, sedation, urinary retention, respiratory depression, and constipation. A bowel program should be instituted to prevent constipation, which is the most common and persistent side effect. Gradual increase of opioid dosages may be needed to control chronic malignant pain. Therefore, the client should be reassured that, with the exception of constipation, tolerance to side effects of

sedation and respiratory depression will develop. A side effect of NSAIDs is gastrointestinal bleeding. Nurses should be familiar with equivalency dosages of various opioids to ensure maximization of pain relief. See Chapter 5 for equivalency tables. Health care providers must be alert to new symptoms of pain that can indicate new tumor growth. Deep, persistent, and worsening pain should draw the immediate attention of health care providers.

Impaired Physical Mobility

Preoperatively, impaired physical mobility is related to a mass invading a joint, pain, or systemic disease that causes fatigue.

Exercise Therapy: Ambulation and Joint Mobility/ Pain Management/Energy Management. Postoperatively, impaired mobility is related to the response from surgery (namely, swelling and discomfort) or restrictions imposed by the procedure (namely, excision of muscle or motor nerves). The nurse assesses the ROM of the involved joints, muscle strength, and the ability to ambulate. In addition, the ability to perform ADLs is assessed in relation to impaired mobility. For example, will the client be able to ascend and descend stairs to use the bathroom? The need for assistive gait devices is determined and implemented after surgery.

In collaboration with the client, physician, and physical and occupational therapists, goals are set and a plan is developed to achieve the maximum potential function. Therapy should be instituted at a time of maximum comfort for the client to allow for increased mobility. Analgesics or other pain-relieving modalities should be provided at least 30 minutes before beginning exercise. Although the physical therapist initiates the exercise program, the nurse reinforces the program on the patient care unit and for home care. Significant to the client with metastatic bone disease is the need to conserve energy. Proper use of body mechanics is discussed and demonstrated in the plan for functional improvement. In conjunction with reinforcing the physical component of mobility, the nurse should assess the physiologic and psychological effects of immobility and teach the client and family how to recognize these effects should they occur.

Problems such as pressure sores, disuse atrophy, flexion contractures, constipation, decreased peripheral perfusion, and hypercalcemia resulting from immobility are preventable. Measures to prevent depression related to prolonged immobility are initiated with ongoing communication about the client's illness and the effects of the illness on biophysical, psychological, and sociocultural subsystems. Interactive counseling is instituted and carried through to the home setting as needed.

Ineffective Individual Coping

Coping Enhancement. Ineffective coping is common and may be related to fear of the unknown, expected or real loss of body parts resulting in self-care limitations, change in self-concept, alteration in physical appearance, inadequate support systems, potential for social isolation, fear of resocialization, anxiety, and pain. The nurse must assist the client in recognizing the problem and in assessing the ability to cope. Fears, which are very common with the new diagnosis of a malignancy, should be identified and discussed. The nurse is often in a position to dispel myths concerning cancer.

Decision-Making Support/Support Group. When one is faced with the diagnosis of a malignancy, ineffective coping mechanisms are common. The individual may never have been faced with this type of problem in the past. The nurse can assist by encouraging participation in the decision-making process and facilitating the problem-solving process. Allowing the client control over decisions is an effective strategy. The adequacy of support systems is assessed. Support groups, such as I Can Cope, are led by health care professionals for the benefit of the individual and the family or significant others. These groups discuss topics such as coping with the illness by giving time for dialogue among participants. Children and adolescents often find support from their peers. Members of the clergy provide spiritual support and comfort.

Socialization Enhancement. At the time of diagnosis, clients are often overwhelmed with well-wishers. However, as time passes during treatment, support may diminish. Clients then feel isolated from social functions.

Concomitant with feelings of isolation are potential fears of returning to previous socialization activities. The stigma carried with the diagnosis of cancer is a problem for those wishing to return to their previous lifestyles. Employers may be hesitant when considering workloads and future promotions, even though the client may be free of disease. Chemotherapy treatments can necessitate loss of workdays, which may prohibit formalization of the social process. The nurse can assist with scheduling treatments to accommodate the client's work schedule. Encouraging verbalization of feelings about socialization brings forth the problem so that solutions can be offered.

At this time, other spiritual strategies, such as prayer, may be helpful. In the chronic, disabling state, psychological and spiritual need is even more pronounced. Lifestyle changes, and the client may experience discrimination on the job or with insurance carriers. However, issues relating to resocialization and the cost of cancer care are encouraging. As more care is being given on an ambulatory basis, efforts to return to one's prior state of activity is facilitated. Ineffective coping is resolved by helping the individual integrate the new body image and status into the daily lifestyle.

Ineffective or Compromised Family Coping

Family Involvement/Mobilization/Support/Process Maintenance. Assessing the family's mental health can assist the nurse in determining their ability to cope. The nurse should assess the degree of autonomous and independent actions, the manner of conflict resolution and problem solving, the degree of flexibility and adaptability to change, the relationships among family members, and the presence of sibling despair or parental guilt. Families reacting to situational stress can show negative processes, such as cognitive disorganization and emotional lability. However, these negative processes are short or sporadic and are followed by attempts to overcome the unfavorable responses. Strategies to promote family functioning include alleviating anxiety, strengthening effective family dynamics, reframing negative behaviors as positive, and modeling and promoting communication. The adequacy of the family's support system is also assessed. Although family members comfort the client, the family may be left without their own support system. Families needing extra support can be referred to social services or practitioners trained in counseling families in distress. Families may also benefit from support groups.

COMMON NURSING DIAGNOSES AND INTERVENTIONS IN THE TREATMENT PHASE

During the treatment phase, the client is undergoing chemotherapy or radiation treatments. The clients follow a protocol, which is a time schedule stating what chemotherapy drugs are given and at what dose. For radiation, the client receives the recommended amount of radiation over the appropriate amount of days or weeks. At this time, the orthopaedic nurse has little contact with the clients. The clients are followed closely by the medical and/or radiation oncologist and their office nursing staff. If the client is admitted to the hospital during this phase, he or she will be admitted to the medical oncology unit and cared for by the oncology trained and certified nurses. Client care problems at this time include altered nutrition, home health maintenance management, protective mechanisms, impaired skin integrity, self-concept, and prevention of complications, in addition to those problems encountered in the initial stage. Clients at this time may be able to attend work, may be hospitalized intermittently, may reside in their own home with the assistance of family, have additional home care providers or visiting nurse agencies, or may live in an extended care facility or nursing home.

Altered Nutrition: Potential for Less Than Body Requirements

Nutrition Management/Weight Gain Assistance. Alteration in nutrition, the potential for less than body requirements, may be a problem in the acute phase. Obtaining less nutrition than body requirements can result from loss of appetite caused by the disease, pain, depression, or side effects of chemotherapy agents. The nurse must first identify the source of the problem. Baseline height and weight are obtained. The current body weight is compared with the ideal body weight to determine deficiencies. A daily caloric and nutrient intake is assessed. Electrolyte balance and hydration status are assessed because dehydration can occur secondary to diarrhea or vomiting. Laboratory values for total protein and albumin levels are evaluated to assess protein stores. The condition of the oral mucosa, teeth, and mouth is assessed to determine whether a problem with mastication exists.

Food preferences are discussed. In collaboration with a licensed nutritionist, the client, and significant others, a dietary plan that considers likes, dislikes, and nutritional requirements is prepared. With surgery, requirements for carbohydrates and protein usually increase. In the event of large intraoperative blood losses, the need for iron and vitamins B and C increases. The nurse should encourage the client to eat foods rich in these nutrients. Small, frequent meals may be more palatable than large ones. When moderate deficits exist, oral nutritional supplements that provide essential amino acids are often required.

In addition to providing a diet conducive to the individual's health, the nurse should assist in providing a pleasant environment during mealtime. If alteration in taste is a problem because of some chemotherapeutic agents, hard candy, seasonings, or sauces may be helpful. If anorexia is a problem, light exercise before meals may help stimulate the appetite. In addition, cool beverages, such as lemonade, beer, and wine, between meals may also help. If nausea is a problem, antiemetics are administered 30 minutes before mealtime. Alteration in nutritional status affects not only the biophysical system but also the psychological and sociocultural systems. Should the client's physical status become greatly impaired because of deficiencies, problems with depression or alterations in mood can occur. The family can become obsessed with trying to encourage an anorexic client to eat, which may result in their own discouragement.

Altered Nutrition: More Than Body Requirements

Nutrition Management/Weight Reduction Assistance. The client undergoing a lower limb amputation is prone to weight gain because of decreased mobility and the consequent postoperative change in nutritional requirements. Excessive weight gain in this client can lead to disturbance in body image and alteration in overall health status. A program customizing nutritional intake requirements with energy expenditure is planned. Nursing interventions are aimed at arranging a consultation with a nutritionist, physical therapist, or exercise physiologist; evaluating dietary intake; teaching the risk of weight gain; describing basic food groups; encouraging modification of eating behaviors; monitoring weight control; and observing for signs of potential disturbance in body image because of weight gain.

Impaired Skin Integrity

Skin Surveillance/Pressure Ulcer Prevention. In the acute stage, potential for the impairment of skin integrity is related to large surgical incisions, devascularization of the skin from underlying soft tissue resection, radiation, and immobility. Nursing intervention is aimed at observing the wound after surgery for signs of tissue necrosis and infection. Skin problems related to immobility are more prevalent with clients undergoing plastic surgery reconstruction because an initial period of bed rest (7 to 14 days) is required for grafts to adhere and heal. Diets sufficient in protein and calories are encouraged to promote healing. Over the long term, clients should be instructed not to expose the grafted areas to direct sunlight because sunburns may result. A minimum sunscreen number of SPF 22 should be applied during any potential sun exposure.

Impaired Home and Health Maintenance Management/Self-care Deficit

Support System Enhancement/Home Maintenance Assistance. Impaired home and health maintenance management and self-care deficit may be caused by impaired mobility, difficulty for family members in providing adequate client care, unavailable resources, financial crisis, or unsuitable environment. When home and health maintenance is an issue, social services and home care nurses are involved. Resources, including financial, extended family and friends, living arrangements, community or agency resources, and transportation, must be identified. Needs are recognized, and information is provided. Alternatives are established with home care provisions, transportation, and meals. Adaptive equipment is arranged via the occupational therapist, nurse, social worker, and medical supplier. Assistive gait devices, wheelchairs, oxygen, suction equipment, bedpans, urinals, and a hospital bed with a trapeze are some devices that may be needed.

Securing adequate assistance must be accomplished before the client's discharge from the acute care facility.

Nurses, physical therapists, or social workers often provide home care assistance. Agencies such as the American Cancer Society and Meals on Wheels should be contacted to assess their ability to help. Living arrangements are assessed for ease of mobility and safety. Orthopaedic clients may require such measures as removal of throw rugs, rearrangement of furniture to allow for wheelchair access, motorized stairway carriers, and handrails. Financial concerns are often a problem when a disease becomes chronic. Financial status is assessed to ensure that suitable health care is provided despite financial difficulties.

Altered Protection

Infection Protection/Pressure Ulcer Prevention/ Chemotherapy Management. Alterations in protective mechanisms are related to the immune system, hematopoietic system, integumentary system, and sensorimotor system. Protective mechanisms are compromised by disease and treatment, and the client must be regularly evaluated by a health care professional for signs and symptoms of alterations in protective mechanisms. Nursing interventions in the chronic stage are aimed at preventing impaired skin integrity, infection, neurologic deficit, and bleeding resulting from chemotherapy. Pressure sores caused by immobility, local or systemic infections resulting from neutropenia, neurologic alterations resulting from disease or treatment, and bleeding resulting from thrombocytopenia are some problems that the client may encounter when at home with a chronic illness. Home care providers should be included in client education regarding recognition of problems and measures of protection.

Clients with neutropenia from chemotherapy or those receiving prolonged antibiotic therapy are monitored for skin infections at injection or venipuncture sites, respiratory infections, and urinary tract infections. Caregivers must be cautious of transferring infections to the neutropenic client. Peripheral neuropathy may be caused by high doses of chemotherapy agents, such as vincristine, cisplatin, and methotrexate, or by tumors impinging on nerves. Nursing interventions are aimed at teaching and monitoring the client for changes in neurologic status, such as tingling, numbness, paresthesia, diminished motor strength, altered sensation, or pain. Thrombocytopenia can be caused by chemotherapy agents that suppress bone marrow function, by radiation therapy to long bones or a large body surface area, or by tumors invading the bone marrow. Nursing interventions focus on monitoring and teaching the client the following signs of spontaneous or excessive bleeding because of thrombocytopenia: petechiae; bruises; hematomas; bleeding from orifices or venipuncture sites; and blood in the urine, feces, or emesis.

Body Image Disturbances

Body Image Enhancement/Grief Work Facilitation/Self-esteem Enhancement. As the disease becomes chronic or disability ensues, disturbances in body image can occur. In the orthopaedic oncology client, this is often a result of loss of an extremity from amputation or alteration of a body part, such as a shoulder joint defect from a large tumor resection. Because of its permanency, this disturbance is longer lasting than a disturbance caused by a temporary loss of hair from chemotherapy.

Strategies should center on enhancing the client's physical appearance through dress and hygiene and promoting self-esteem. Counseling services and support groups can help address issues of self-esteem, such as physical appearance, social and intimate relations, and personal and professional achievements. Maintaining a positive self-concept affects the client's functioning within groups. Interventions are key factors of sociocultural adaptation.

Grief Work Facilitation/Body Image Enhancement. The inability to cope with the expected loss of a limb is common with individuals about to undergo amputation. Strategies to promote acceptance of amputation should focus on potential cure of the tumor rather than loss. However, a normal grieving period should be allowed for the loss of a limb. Changes in self-concept are inherent with any physical change caused by surgery and by side effects related to adjuvant therapy, especially the loss of hair caused by some chemotherapy agents. Biophysical changes are directly related to psychological effects. Inability to cope with one's self-concept can ultimately result in depression or noncompliance with therapy, especially in accepting chemotherapy when hair loss is the issue. Physical changes imposed by surgery can cause problems with self-concept. Ineffective individual coping is of special concern with the adolescent. The nurse can be very supportive in discussing ways to enhance appearance with accessories and dress.

Sexual Dysfunction or Infertility

Sexual Counseling/Family Planning: Contraception. Sexual dysfunction or infertility is possible as a result of the side effects of treatment. Drugs commonly causing oligospermia, azoospermia, or amenorrhea are the alkylating agents chlorambucil, cyclophosphamide, doxorubicin hydrochloride, procarbazine, vinblastine, and cytarabine. Long-term cyclophosphamide treatment can cause ovarian failure. The degree of dysfunction is related to dosage, the use of combination drugs, length of treatment, and age. The degree of genetic damage to the ovaries or testes is unpredictable. In addition to the side effects of chemotherapy, surgical ablation of sacral nerves entwined in a tumor can cause dysfunction, such as impotence. Clients should be assessed for their current fertility status, desires for future childbearing, and contraceptive use. Contraception with the postponement of childbearing for a minimum of 2 years after completion of cancer treatment is sometimes recommended. Before chemotherapy is initiated, sperm banking with subsequent artificial insemination may be an option. Nursing interventions are aimed at assessing the possibility of dysfunction and the effect on the client and partner, teaching aspects of contraception and reproductive planning, and addressing issues related to self-esteem. Reproductive counseling is strongly encouraged for clients of childbearing age.

Surgical Excision to Remove the Tumor

After the client has completed the neoadjuvant chemotherapy or radiation, the definitive surgical planning and procedure take place. Again, the clinical nurse specialist, nurse practitioner, or clinic nurse is responsible for coordinating the client's surgery and answering questions the client and family may have. The staff nurses on the orthopaedic unit or on the oncology unit will care for these clients postoperatively. The clients stay may last anywhere from 2 to 10 days in the hospital. Client care problems to be addressed during this phase include knowledge deficit, pain management, alteration in skin integrity, mobility, alteration in nutrition, anxiety, and compromised immune system from chemotherapy. Approximately 2 to 3 weeks postoperatively, the client will resume chemotherapy if neoadjuvant therapy had been given. If the preoperative radiation dose was only part of the total dose allowed to that area, radiation will be resumed also. Following and completing the standardized protocol will provide the best outcome.

MAINTENANCE PHASE

After any combination of surgery, chemotherapy, and radiation has been completed for the particular sarcoma, the client will continue follow-up with the orthopaedic oncologist for life. Follow-up visits with the medical oncologist and radiation oncologist occur for a few months after surgery, but then the care is turned back over to the orthopaedic oncologist for management. The clinic visits range from every 6 to 8 weeks for the first year, every 2 to 3 months the second year, every 3 to 4 months the third year, every 4 to 6 months the fourth year, and then yearly for the next 5 years. At the 10-year mark, the orthopaedic oncologist may see the client every 2 years. This schedule may vary from physician to physician and also may vary from client to client. Radiographic examinations occur frequently during this maintenance phase. CT scans and chest x-ray films are used to watch for metastatic disease; MRI scans of the surgical bed, if the

sarcoma was soft tissue, and plain x-ray films as well as a MRI, if the sarcomas was a primary bone tumor, are used to monitor for local recurrence. Bone scans may be ordered if the client complains of pain in another area. Even though sarcomas, if they metastasize, usually do so to the lungs, metastatic deposits to the bone and other soft tissues have been documented. Client care problems to be addressed during this time include knowledge deficit related to long-term follow-up treatment plan and anxiety and fear related to follow-up radiologic examinations to rule out recurrence or metastatic disease.

DISABLED STAGE

The orthopaedic oncology client may become chronically disabled as a result of above-the-knee amputation or hip disarticulation, chronic lymphedema, or widespread metastatic disease to bone and lung. Some clients with an amputation, especially older or obese clients, can experience impaired mobility or inability to ambulate altogether. Lymphedema of the leg may be pronounced in some clients after resection of lymphatic channels or as a complication of radiation therapy to the leg. Activity intolerance and self-care deficits related to hygiene, grooming, and feeding are prevalent in the client with metastasis, often resulting from chronic pain, muscle weakness, fatigue, and ineffective breathing patterns. Nursing interventions focus on defining the extent of self-care tasks the client is able to perform, soliciting assistance from others to maximize function, providing a safe physical environment, strengthening functional muscles as feasible, arranging for assistive devices to maximize independence, and promoting effective coping mechanisms. Coping and teaching a client to cope with role changes in the presence of impaired function, sexual dysfunction, pain, and weakness are challenging to the client and caregiver. Restoring or improving appearance helps boost spirits. Should the disability be a result of spinal cord compression, bowel and bladder function and maintenance of skin integrity are addressed.

Complications

Prevention or early detection of complications of disease or treatment is a major role of home care providers for the client with a musculoskeletal tumor. The home care providers may be family members, friends, visiting nurses, or hospice nurses. Conditions requiring urgent attention are infection, hypercalcemia, and spinal cord compression, which happens rarely in sarcomas but is a potential life-threatening problem.

A postoperative infection can be minor or catastrophic depending on the location and type of surgical wound. If a wound becomes infected after a soft tissue tumor removal, it will delay restarting adjuvant therapy such as chemotherapy or radiation. Because both treatments delay wound healing, resuming either treatment would cause further wound breakdown. When a client has been treated for a malignant bone tumor with a metal prosthesis or plates and screws, an allograft, or alloprosthesis, an infection is catastrophic because the hardware or allograft must be removed and cannot be replaced until all evidence of infection is gone. Chemotherapy and radiation must also be delayed in this situation. Unfortunately, if chemotherapy and/or radiation are delayed, the client may be at risk for metastatic spread of the tumor or local recurrence because no treatment is being given.

Hypercalcemia, detected by calcium levels greater than 11 mg/100 mL of blood, is more common with carcinomas of the breast, lung, kidney, and esophagus; multiple myeloma; and squamous cell carcinoma of the thyroid, head, and neck. More than 80% of clients with hypercalcemia have bone metastases. The degree of hypercalcemia, however, does not always correlate with the extent of bone involvement. The most common cause of hypercalcemia associated with cancer is increased bone resorption secondary to increased osteoclast activity (Itano & Taoka, 1998). Common signs and symptoms in varying degrees are muscular weakness, decreased deep tendon reflexes, lethargy, fatigue, anorexia, nausea, vomiting, constipation, polyuria, and polydipsia. Late signs are seizures, stupor, and coma. A hypercalcemic crisis can result in death from cardiac arrhythmias. Therefore, hospitalization is warranted. The client may be admitted to the orthopaedic or medical oncology unit.

Interventions include hydration with 3 to 5 L of normal saline per 24 hours; accurate recording of intake and output; diuretics, such as furosemide with potassium replacement, to increase urine flow; and mobilization. Medications, such as mithramycin, phosphates, calcitonin, and steroids, to lower serum calcium are used. Dietary intake of calcium is restricted. Cardiac monitoring; laboratory monitoring of serum calcium, albumin, potassium, blood urea nitrogen, and creatinine levels; and careful observation for confusion are necessary. Education of the client and home care providers is essential, including the prohibition of medications that can potentiate hypercalcemia: thiazide diuretics and vitamins A and D.

The occurrence of spinal cord compression is more common with metastatic carcinoma of the breast, lung, prostate, and kidney and lymphoma but can be caused by a primary bone or soft tissue tumor. Spinal cord compression is a result of direct tumor extension to the spinal cord or collapse of the vertebral body because of destruction from the tumor. Clients having metastatic disease to the spine should be educated about early signs of pain, sensory impairment, and weakness. Spinal cord compression requires immediate radiologic diagnosis (plain radiograph, CT scan, MRI or myelogram, lumbar puncture). Dexamethasone to decrease edema, spinal immobilization, treatment by surgery (laminectomy to decompress the spinal cord), radiation therapy (alone or

postoperatively), or chemotherapy (if tumor is chemosensitive) may be necessary depending on the extent of the disease.

COMPLEMENTARY THERAPY FOR THE TREATMENT OF SARCOMAS

Over the last few years, questions regarding the use of complementary medicine, in conjunction with or as an alternative to modern medicine, has become commonplace. Most patient information sheets in doctors' offices and in the hospital setting have a section of questions regarding the use of herbal medicines and other nontraditional treatment therapies. Many alternative or complementary treatments may interfere with traditional medicine and treatments; therefore, it is imperative to have an accurate history on the client's chart.

Shark cartilage and green tea are two alternative treatments that clients are taking with hopes of fighting off cancer. Other practices such as mega dosing with vitamins and using other herbal therapies are common. The most important issue for the health care professional is to encourage clients to discuss all treatments that they may be using and to teach and inform clients of situations that are nontherapeutic and may be life-threatening.

Health care professionals must be open to learning more about complementary and alternative health practices. Clients may want to try massage or acupuncture for pain control or may want to try biofeedback, imagery, meditation, and prayer for relaxation. Music, art, and play therapy and laughter are other forms of therapy being offered for clients with acute or chronic illnesses.

INNOVATIONS AND FUTURE TRENDS

Because the cure for cancer has yet to be found, the constant battle to improve quality of life for cancer clients continues. Research into better prostheses and limb reconstruction techniques and stronger and more effective chemotherapy protocols and radiation techniques is occurring all over the world. Also, the completion of the Human Genome Project will promote continued research into oncogenes and cancer vaccines.

INTERNET RESOURCES

Because the Internet is so widely accessible, clients have resources and information at their fingertips. Clients who use the Internet should be cautioned to use websites and addresses from nationally known research centers, hospitals, and agencies. Clients should also be encouraged to discuss the information found on the Internet with their health care professionals. For a list of Internet websites, see "Internet Resources" following the summary.

SUMMARY

Care of the orthopaedic oncology client is a collaborative approach by the nurse, surgical oncologist, medical oncologist, radiation oncologist, family physician, occupational and physical therapists, social worker, prosthetist, nutritionist, clergy, pain management specialist, hospice and home care nurse, and most of all, the client, family, and significant others.

Musculoskeletal neoplasms cross all ages and involve the whole individual in the biophysical, sociocultural, and psychological subsystems. Overall medical goals are to eradicate the tumor or achieve remission or palliation. Nursing goals are aimed at promoting comfort, maximizing function, increasing knowledge, preventing complications, and restoring the individual to a state of self-care.

Nursing interventions in the initial diagnosis phase are aimed at knowledge, coping mechanisms, communication, and measures to alleviate anxiety and fear. Nursing interventions in the treatment phase are aimed at facilitating home maintenance management, maintaining nutritional status, educating the family about protective mechanisms against disease and side effects, promoting the client's functioning and roles within groups and society, preventing complications of disease and treatment, and educating the client and family about complications of disease and treatment.

In the maintenance phase, the nursing interventions must focus on teaching the client the follow-up treatment protocol and reassuring the client when he or she is fearful and anxious about upcoming CT chest scans and MRI scans to rule out metastatic disease or local recurrence. Finally, in the disabled stage, the nurse's role focuses on maximizing support systems and maintaining equilibrium of the interrelated subsystems.

Although client care management before and at the time of diagnosis is the role of the family physician, it is often transferred to other physicians who specialize in the comprehensive care and treatment of orthopaedic malignancies in tertiary care settings that are equipped with facilities for special diagnostic techniques, surgery, chemotherapy, and radiation therapy. Community and other professional resources are ultimately solicited to provide comprehensive, quality care while clients progress through the various stages of wellness, acute and chronic illness, and disability.

INTERNET RESOURCES

American Cancer Society: www.cancer.org
Cancer Guide: http://cancerguide.org
OncoLink: www.oncolink.upenn.edu/
National Cancer Institute (CancerNet): http://cancernet.nci.nih.gov
Look Good . . . Feel Better: www.lookgoodfeelbetter.org/

REFERENCES

Agency for Health Care Policy and Research (AHCPR). (1994, March). *Management of cancer pain: Adults. Quick reference guide for clinicians. No. 9.* (AHCPR Publication No. 94-0593). Rockville, MD: Agency for Health Care Policy and Research, U.S. Department of Health and Human Services, Public Health Service.

Antman, K. H., Eilber, F. R., & Shiu, M. H. (1989). Soft tissue sarcomas: Current trends in diagnosis and management. *Current Problems in Cancer, 13*, 337–367.

Bacci, G., Ferrari, S., Bertoni, F., Donati, D., Bacchini, P., Longhi, A., Brach del Prever, A., Forni, C., & Rimondini, S. (2000). Neoadjuvant chemotherapy for peripheral malignant neuroectodermal tumor of bone: Recent experience at the Istituto Rizzoli. *Journal of Clinical Oncology, 18*, 885–892.

Bacci, G., Ferrari, S., Comandone, A., Zanone, A., Ruggieri, P., Longhi, A., Bertoni, F., Forni, C., Versari, M., & Rimondini, S. (in press). Neoadjuvant chemotherapy for Ewing's sarcoma of bone in clients older than thirty-nine years. *Acta Oncologica*.

Bridge, J. A., Sanger, W. G., Shaffer, B., & Neff, J. (1987). Cytogenetic findings in malignant fibrous histiocytoma. *Cancer Genetics Cytogenetics, 29*, 97.

Chu, E., & DeVita, V. (2001). *Cancer chemotherapy drug manual 2001.* Boston: Jones and Bartlett.

Enneking, W. (1983). *Musculoskeletal tumor surgery* (Vol. 1, pp. 3–99). New York: Churchill Livingstone.

Enneking, W., & Spanier, S. (1982). In L. Straub & P. Wilson (Eds.), *Clinical Trends in Orthopaedics* (pp. 125–129). New York: Thiemme-Stratton.

Enneking, W., Spanier, S., & Malawer, M. (1980). Current concepts review. The surgical staging of musculoskeletal sarcoma. *Journal of Bone and Joint Surgery, 62A*(6), 1027–1030.

Enzinger, F. M., & Weiss, S. W. (1995). *Soft tissue tumors.* St. Louis: Mosby.

Ferrari, S., Mercuri, M., Picci, P., Bertoni, F., Brach del Prever, A., Tienghi, A., Mancini, A., Longhi, A., Rimondini, S., Donati, D., Manfrini, M., Ruggieri, P., Biagini, R., & Bacci, G. (1999). Nonmetastatic osteosarcoma of the extremity: results of a neoadjuvant chemotherapy protocol (IOR/OS-3) with high-dose methotrexate, intraarterial or intravenous cisplatin, doxorubicin, and salvage chemotherapy based on histologic tumor response. *Tumori, 85*, 458–464.

Fuchs, N., Bielack, S., Epler, D., Bieling, P., Delling, G., Korholz, D., Graf, N., Heise, U., Jurgens, H., Kotz, R., Salzer-Kuntschik, M., Weinel, P., Werner, M., & Winkler, K. (1998). Long-term results of the co-operative German-Austrian-Swiss osteosarcoma study group's protocol COSS-86 of intensive multidrug chemotherapy and surgery for osteosarcoma of the limbs. *Annals of Oncology, 9*, 893–899.

Greenlee, R. T., Murray, T., Bolden, S., & Wingo, P. (2000). Cancer statistics, 2000. *CA-A Journal for Clinicians, 50*(1), 7–33.

Griffin, C. A., & Emanuel, B. S. (1987). Translocation (X;18) in a synovial sarcoma. *Cancer Genetics Cytogenetics, 26*, 181.

Groenwald, S. L., Frogge, M. H., Goodman, M. Y., & Henke, C. (1992). *Comprehensive cancer nursing review.* Boston: Jones & Bartlett.

Holleb, A., Fink, D., & Murphy, G. (1991). *American Cancer Society textbook of clinical oncology.* Atlanta: American Cancer Society.

Itano, J. K., & Taoka, K. N. (1998). *Core curriculum for oncology nursing* (3rd ed.). Philadelphia: WB Saunders.

Malpas, J., Bergsagel, D., Kyle, R., & Anderson, K. (1998). *Myeloma: Biology and management* (2nd ed.). Oxford, England: Oxford University Press.

Mertens, F., Johansson, B., Mandahl, N., Heim, S., Bennet, K., Rydholm, A., Willen, H., & Mitelman, F. (1987). Clonal chromosome abnormalities in two liposarcomas. *Cancer Genetics Cytogenetics, 28*, 137.

Mirra, J. M. (1989). *Bone tumors, clinical, radiologic and pathologic correlations* (Vols. 1 & 2). Philadelphia: Lea & Febiger.

Perez, C. A., & Brady, L. W. (1998). *Principles and practice of radiation oncology* (3rd ed.). Philadelphia: Lippincott-Raven.

Rytting, M., Pearson, P., Raymond, A., Ayala, A., Murray, J., Yasko, A.,

Johnson, M., & Jaffe, N. (2000). Osteosarcoma in preadolescent clients. *Clinical Orthopaedics and Related Research, 373,* 39–50.

Sandberg, A. A. (1987). The usefulness of chromosome analysis in clinical oncology. *Oncology, 1*(5), 22, 30.

Smith, S., Reeves, B. R., & Wong, L. (1987). Translocation t(12;16) in a case of myxoid liposarcoma. *Cancer Genetics Cytogenetics, 26,* 185.

Smith, S., Reeves, B. R., Wong, L., & Fisher, C. (1987). A consistent chromosome translocation in synovial sarcoma. *Cancer Genetics Cytogenetics, 26,* 179.

Sugarbaker, P. H., & Malawer, M. M. (1992). *Musculoskeletal surgery for cancer.* New York: Thieme.

Suit, H. D., Mankin, H. J., Wood, W. C., Gebhardt, M. C., Harmon, D. C.,

Rosenberg, A., Tepper, J. E., & Rosenthal, D. (1988). Treatment of the patient with stage Mo soft tissue sarcoma. *Journal of Clinical Oncology, 6,* 854.

Szendroi, M., Papai, Z. S., & Illes, T. (2000). Limb-saving surgery, survival, and prognostic factors for osteosarcoma: The Hungarian experience. *Journal of Surgical Oncology, 73,* 87–94.

Turc-Carel, C., Dal Cin, P., & Sandberg, A. A. (1987). Nonrandom translocation in extraskeletal myxoid chondrosarcoma. *Cancer Genetics Cytogenetics, 26,* 377.

Yasko, A. W., & Lane, J. M. (1991). Current concepts review chemotherapy for bone and soft-tissue sarcomas of the extremities. *Journal of Bone and Joint Surgery, 73,* 1263–1271.

23

Infections of the Musculoskeletal System

SUSAN WARNER SALMOND and CYNTHIA FINE

Musculoskeletal infections can be severe and difficult to treat because they are relatively inaccessible to the body's protective macrophages and systemic antibodies. As a result, small numbers of microorganisms may be sufficient to establish infection. Bone infections have a potential for serious sequelae, such as chronic infection, loss of function, alterations in quality of life, and even death.

Most orthopaedic infections are caused by infectious agents that elicit the body's inflammatory and immunologic responses. This chapter presents the body's general response to infection, followed by a specific discussion of osteomyelitis, septic arthritis, tuberculosis (TB) of bones and joints, and orthopaedic complications of postpolio sequelae and Lyme disease.

INFLAMMATORY RESPONSE

Inflammation is a nonspecific response to tissue damage that can be caused by mechanical injury, autoimmune reactions, and infections. Following injury or microbial invasion, histamine and kinins are released, which results in immediate vascular changes. A brief period of vasoconstriction is followed immediately by vasodilation. This increased blood flow to the area (hyperemia) elicits the characteristic redness and warmth of inflammation. Capillary permeability increases, resulting in cellular and fluid exudation. Fluid exudation (most active in the first 24 hours) produces swelling, leading to pain and impaired function. The inflammatory process can produce both local manifestations (redness, heat, pain, swelling, and loss of function) and systemic manifestations. Classic systemic manifestations include fever, leukocytosis, cardiovascular changes (increased pulse and respiration), malaise, and anemia. The extent and severity of the injury along with the reactive capacity of the person determine the intensity of the inflammatory response.

IMMUNOLOGIC RESPONSE

The body responds to infection by mobilizing leukocytic systems, which defend the body from foreign material by phagocytosis and antibody formation. The leukocyte and differential counts can provide clues to the type and severity of the infection. The normal white blood cell (WBC) count usually ranges from 4000 to 10,000/mm^3. Leukocytosis accompanies most acute infections caused by bacteria, fungi, or protozoa, and the total WBC count may increase to three to four times the normal value. Viral infections are generally accompanied by a normal or slightly decreased WBC count. Examining the percentiles of the various types of WBCs found in the blood can provide additional clues to the type of infection.

The concentration of blood neutrophils increases in response to most acute bacterial infections, except TB, brucellosis, and typhoid fever. These levels may not persist as the infection becomes chronic. Immature neutrophils, called *bands,* are often seen at the very early stages of an infection as the bone marrow struggles to release phagocytes to the infected site. This is described as a "shift to the left" in the differential. Tissue damage, inflammation, and hydrocortisone can also produce an increase in the neutrophil count.

Monocytes are released into the blood at a slower rate than neutrophils and are phagocytic. They tend to be seen in more chronic infections such as TB and Rocky Mountain spotted fever.

Eosinophils are commonly elevated in allergic reactions and parasitic infections. They may disappear from the blood in acute infections.

Basophils are rich in histamine and play a role in delayed allergic response. Basophil concentration may increase in chronic inflammatory disorders.

Lymphocyte elevations can be seen in chronic infections such as TB and viral infections such as mononucleosis. These cells are involved with antibody production rather than phagocytosis.

NURSING MANAGEMENT

Transmission and Risk of Infection

Infection Control: Intraoperative, Infection Protection, Nutrition Management. Because orthopaedic infections may be debilitating or life-threatening, it is imperative that the nurse assess for the general and specific risk factors that may predispose the client to infection. Orthopaedic injuries, procedures, and individual risk factors may lead to musculoskeletal infection. The nurse must identify clients with potential for infection and initiate measures to reduce risk. Table 23–1 identifies general variables that place the client at greater risk for infection as well as procedures commonly used to detect and alleviate these risks.

Careful handwashing and scrupulous management of invasive devices form the foundation of nosocomial infection prevention. Table 23–2 describes interventions and protocols designed to prevent infection. It must be stressed to health care personnel, the client, and the family that handwashing is the single most effective mechanism for preventing the spread of infection. Hands should be washed before and after client contact. Gloves should be worn if contact with blood or body fluids is anticipated. When caring for clients at high risk of infection (e.g., those who are immunocompromised), antimicrobial solutions should be used for handwashing. Standard precautions blend the major features of universal (blood and body fluid) precautions that were designed to protect the health care worker from transmission of pathogens from moist body substances, and apply them to all clients regardless of their diagnosis or presumed infection status. Standard precautions apply to (1) blood; (2) all body fluids, secretions and excretions except sweat, regardless of whether they contain visible blood; (3) nonintact skin; and (4) mucous membranes.

Three types of transmission-based precautions are used in addition to standard precautions. These are airborne precautions, droplet precautions, and contact precautions. A special mask is required when caring for clients who have suspect or known infectious pulmonary TB. Masks of this type are called *respirators*. The respirator that has been approved by the National Institute for Occupational Safety and Health (NIOSH) and Occupational Safety and Health Administration (OSHA) for protection from TB is called an *N-95 respirator*. This type of respirator effectively screens the wearer from at least 95% of particles the size of the TB droplet nuclei.

Maintaining an optimal aseptic environment during bedside insertion and maintenance of intravenous catheters, orthopaedic hardware, and urinary drainage devices is critical to minimize risks of infection. Careful aseptic technique and standard precautions are essential when dealing with all aspects of wound care to protect a client from contamination as well as to protect the caregiver. The nurse provides the client and family with guidelines for infection control so that necessary precautions are implemented when the client goes home.

Accurate and early assessment for systemic and localized signs and symptoms of infection allows prompt intervention to eliminate the invading organisms. Documentation of temperature patterns, skin conditions, wound healing, and client behaviors indicating progress or lack of improvement is fundamental in monitoring the infectious process.

Laboratory diagnostic evaluation of infections includes complete blood count (CBC) with differential, erythrocyte sedimentation rate (ESR), and culture and sensitivity. Table 23–3 lists common laboratory studies. The nurse must ensure that laboratory specimens are collected appropriately and results reported promptly.

Antibiotics are ordered according to the culture and sensitivity results. Empiric antibiotic therapy, based on infection site and likely organism, is usually initiated after the culture is obtained but before sensitivities are obtained. Antibiotic changes are then determined by culture and sensitivity results.

Nutritional Considerations with Infection. Nutritional deficits may delay wound healing and increase the individual's susceptibility to infection. Metabolic demands are increased (elevation of body temperature of just 1 degree increases the body's metabolic rate by 13%), and additional calories, protein, carbohydrates, and vitamins are required. This is especially important for major orthopaedic infections, such as gas gangrene or acute osteomyelitis associated with an open fracture, in which metabolic needs may be increased by as much as 75%. A 24-hour caloric intake monitoring may be required to ensure sufficient intake of carbohydrate and protein. If the oral diet is not sufficient, supplemental feedings, either orally or enterally, should be considered. Parenteral nutrition may be needed in the presence of protein-calorie malnutrition.

Wound Management and Infection. When a wound is present, the nurse must assess the wound and the surrounding area for redness, swelling, and warmth. Although a certain amount of inflammation is part of the healing process, an increase in inflammation, especially if accompanied by purulent drainage, is indicative of infection. Wounds should be evaluated carefully for necrotic tissue, which can provide favorable conditions for anaerobic growth. Wet-to-dry dressings may be ordered to remove necrotic tissue or the physician may debride the wound to remove suspicious-looking tissue.

TABLE 23–1. *Factors That Increase Susceptibility to Infection*

RISK FACTOR	RATIONALE
Age	
Older adults	Decreased immune response
	Increased nutritional deficits
	Increased chronic illness
Children (younger than 1 year)	Immature immune system
	Decreased body mass
Sex	Hormonal and hereditary sex-linked characteristics (e.g., female has greater resistance to infection)
Heredity	Certain hereditary conditions impair response to infection (e.g., agammaglobulinemia)
Socioeconomic/cultural status	Unsanitary living conditions
	Insufficient income or no health insurance
	Delay in seeking medical treatment
Medications	Drugs such as chemotherapy, steroids, and frequent use of antibiotics may impair immune response
Obesity	Inadequate blood supply to fatty tissues for delivery of nutrients and essential cellular elements (visceral protein depletion)
	In surgical client, obesity associated with poor subcutaneous wound closure and healing
Malnutrition	Adversely affects humoral and cell-mediated immunity, impairs neutrophil chemotaxis, diminishes bacterial clearance, and depresses neutrophil bactericidal function, the delivery of inflammatory cells to infectious foci, and serum complement components
	Results in delayed wound healing
Alcoholism	Impaired nutrition
	Delayed hypersensitivity
	Depressed neutrophil activity
	Suppresses bone marrow function
Smoking	Decreased tissue oxygenation
Diabetes	Impaired tissue perfusion
	Depressed phagocytosis and T-cell functions
AIDS and altered immuno-competence	Impaired immune response
	Susceptibility to a microorganism depends on the specific defect in immunity (neutrophil response, humoral immunity, cell-mediated immunity and reticuloendothelial cells)
Wound stress (unexpected tension to an incision)	Impairment of wound layer and inhibition of formation of endothelial cell and collagen network
Invasion of skin integrity (IV lines, Foley catheters, decubiti)	Direct access for introduction of abnormal pathogens
Invasion of skin integrity (trauma, surgery)	Previous surgery in same site
	Clients undergoing orthopaedic implant surgery are at greater risk for infection, with average reported deep wound infection of 2%
Arthroscopic surgery	Direct introduction of microorganisms into joint via contaminated equipment
Joint injections/aspirations	Microorganisms may be introduced directly into joint via contaminated syringes, needles, medications, or fluids
Casts	May create pressure sores and not permit direct access to open wounds
	Casting material applied over an open wound or operative site may create environment that supports microbial growth
	Contaminated plaster cast padding or contaminated water may produce nosocomial infection
Tape	Tape may be contaminated when left adhering to bed rails, countertops, or IV poles before application

TABLE 23–2. *Prevention and Management of Infection*

FOCUS	INFECTIONS/PATHOGENS INVOLVED	NURSING INTERVENTIONS
Identify high-risk client and high-risk factors	Laboratory monitoring for infection	Assess for high-risk factors (see Table 23–1) Institute infection control and infection protection routines Change open containers routinely (q24h) Isolation measures (standard precautions) in accordance with type of organism present and additional precautions as indicated
Surgical management	Skin bacteria Airborne bacteria	Proper skin preparation decreases contamination caused by bacteria present on the skin Shaving operative site the night before surgery is not recommended because of local trauma favoring bacterial reproduction Use of laminar airflow systems or personnel isolator systems reduces risks from airborne bacteria Ultraviolet light reduces the number of airborne bacteria

Peripheral/ central lines	Organisms
	  Staphylococcus epidermidis
	  Staphylococcus aureus
	  Candida albicans
	Infections
	  Bacteremias
		Strict handwashing and aseptic technique
		Change tubing no more frequently than at 72-hour intervals unless clinically indicated
		Replace tubing used to administer blood, blood products, or lipid emulsions within 24 hours of initiating infusion
		Rotate peripheral venous catheters q72h*
		Replace peripheral catheters inserted in emergency and insert new catheter at different site within 24 hr
		Monitor peripheral/central sites†
		Replace dressing when catheter is replaced or when dressing becomes damp, loosened, or soiled; replace more frequently in diaphoretic clients

Urinary drainage system	Organisms
	  Gram-negative rods
	  Group D enterococci
	Infections
	  Urinary tract infections
		Strict handwashing
		Aseptic technique for catheter insertion
		Maintain closed system
		Keep drainage bag lower than bladder to prevent urinary reflux
		Tape catheter to client
		Avoid irrigation of catheter
		Remove as soon as possible
		Use separate measuring container for each client

External fixator/pin care	Organism
	  Staphylococcus aureus
	Infections
	  Pin tract infection (can lead to sequestrectomy)
		Strict handwashing
		Clean pins/fixator according to established protocol
		Observe skin for redness, tenderness, swelling, exudate; report
		Do not impede flow of serous drainage fluid
		Avoid tenting of skin around pin
		Avoid occlusive dressings/thick ointments at pin care site
		Minimize stress on pin tracts/external fixator devices

Skin care and wound care	Infection protection	Keep skin surfaces dry, intact Avoid preoperative shaves; use clipping or depilatory for hair removal Standard precautions and aseptic technique for wound care and dressing change Consistent monitoring for signs of infection Debridement as needed to minimize anaerobic growth
Antimicrobial therapy	Specific to organism cultured	Observe for suprainfection development in clients receiving antimicrobial therapy
Nutritional management		Nutritional assessment to identify high-risk client Enteral or parenteral replacement as indicated

Table continued on following page

TABLE 23–2. *Prevention and Management of Infection* Continued

FOCUS	INFECTIONS/PATHOGENS INVOLVED	NURSING INTERVENTIONS
Client education	Infection control and infection protection	Teaching to include the following:
		Signs and symptoms of infection
		Method of infectious agent transmission
		Importance of good handwashing, especially after toileting, after contact with wound drainage and before touching IV site
		Rationale behind any infection control precautions (standard precautions, category-specific isolation procedures)
		Need to complete prescribed dosage of antibiotics
		Factors that may increase client risk of infection
		Avoidance of visitors who may have a cold
		Importance of adequate rest periods in the recovery period
		Application of infection control to home environment
		Use of 1:10 dilution of household bleach for disinfection
		Adaptation of clean or sterile techniques as needed
		Proper disposal of articles contaminated with drainage
		Importance of maintaining an adequate fluid intake

*Many facilities are increasing the dwell time of peripheral IV catheters to 96 hours. There are no recommendations for the frequency of catheter replacement or removal of catheters under emergency conditions in pediatric clients.

†Peripherally inserted central catheters should not be routinely replaced. No recommendation for the frequency of replacement of tunneled catheters, totally implantable devices, or the needles used to access them.

Hyperthermia

Fever Treatment, Environmental Management.
Fever, defined as a temperature greater than or equal to 38.5°C, is part of the body's complex physiologic response to disease. Fever is an inconsistent sign in bone infections, and it must be remembered that it is possible to have an infected joint without the presence of fever.

Fevers may be beneficial in limiting growth of organisms and enhancing cellular destruction of pathogens. Measures to reduce fever, such as removing excess clothing or covers, giving tepid baths, reducing ambient temperature, encouraging fluid intake, and administering antipyretics, may be used to increase client comfort. However, a recent study (Gozzoli, Schotter, Suter, & Ricou, 2001) concluded that systemic suppression of fever may not be useful unless the client has severe cranial trauma or significant hypoxemia. When evaluating a client's fever, one must observe for chills and rashes, determine the WBC count, and monitor the response to treatment. These characteristics may assist with diagnosis.

Pain

Pain Management. Because there is often pressure or stretching of tissues with the edema of inflammation, analgesics and anti-inflammatory agents often are required. Medications commonly given include aspirin, acetaminophen, nonsteroidal anti-inflammatory drugs (e.g., ibuprofen, naproxen, indomethacin), and narcotic analgesics. Skeletal muscle relaxants, such as diazepam

and chlorzoxazone, may be helpful in promoting client comfort during the acute phase of infection. Maintaining the joint in a position of function as well as comfort is an integral part of pain management in the orthopaedic client.

Activity Intolerance

Energy Management. Clients with an infection often report the accompanying symptoms of malaise and easy fatigability. Although the client may require bed rest during the acute phase of the infection, range of motion (ROM) is needed for the orthopaedic client. Specifics of activity intolerance are discussed later in the chapter within the specific infection section.

OSTEOMYELITIS

Osteomyelitis is a severe infection of the bone and surrounding tissues that requires immediate treatment. Sophisticated diagnostic methods and antibiotic therapies have lowered the complication rate to about 5%, and the mortality rate is negligible. However, delayed or inadequate treatment of osteomyelitis may result in progression to chronic disease, with significant morbidity, including symptoms of continuing pain, chronically draining sinuses, loss of function, amputation, and death.

The client presents initially with bone pain, fever, swelling, and restricted movement of the affected bone. Further assessment may reveal systemic signs of infection or a recent history of bacteremia. If osteomyelitis is suspected, treatment with empiric antibiotics may be initiated before a definitive diagnosis is made. The components of osteomyelitis treatment include client evaluation, identification and sensitivity of the microorganism or microorganisms, administration of antibiotics, debridement surgery, dead space management, and if necessary, stabilization (Mandell, Bennett, & Dolin, 2000).

Epidemiology

Although osteomyelitis can occur at any age, children younger than the age of 12 are commonly affected. Males have a higher incidence than females because of the increased incidence of blunt trauma. Osteomyelitis may be more difficult to contain in the presence of other disorders, such as malnutrition, alcoholism, acquired immunodeficiency syndrome (AIDS), and kidney or liver failure, all of which interfere with the body's ability to fight infection.

Although generally bacterial in origin, osteomyelitis may also be caused by viral or fungal organisms. *Staphylococcus aureus* is the most common infecting microorganism, causing 60% of hematogenous and introduced infections, and is a principal agent when osseous sepsis spreads by contiguity. *Staphylococcus epidermidis* has become a major pathogen in bone infections associated with indwelling prosthetic materials, such as joint implants and fracture fixation devices. *Salmonella* organisms have an increased incidence in clients with sickle cell disease or neonatal osteomyelitis. Prominent pathogens vary with the client's age group and are presented in Table 23–4.

TABLE 23–3. *General Laboratory Information for Infection*

TEST	RESULTS
White blood cell (WBC) count	Elevation >10,000 U/L indicates acute infection but is not consistently reliable and may be normal even when infection is present
	Decreased values may reflect viral infection
WBC differential count	Provides details of morphology and distribution of white cells; helps identify type of infection
Neutrophils	Value elevated rapidly with inflammation and tissue injury
	First line of defense with an acute infection
Monocytes	Value elevated with bacterial infections and foreign substances
	Second line of defense; phagocytize bacteria
Basophils	Value elevated with inflammatory process
	Function not fully understood; help body to resist systemic allergic reactions
Lymphocytes	Value elevated with chronic and viral infections
	Important to humoral and cell-mediated immunity
Eosinophils	Value increases in allergic conditions
	Provide differential diagnoses between allergic response and infection
Erythrocyte sedimentation rate (ESR)	Nonspecific test; early indication of inflammation and bacterial infection
	Also elevated after surgery and in chronic conditions, such as rheumatoid arthritis and gout
	ESR is unreliable in neonates, clients with sickle cell disease, clients taking steroids, and clients whose symptoms have been present for less than 48 hours
	Peak elevation of ESR occurs at 3–5 days after infection and returns to normal about 3 weeks after treatment is begun
C-reactive protein (CRP) (abnormal specific glycoprotein produced during acute inflammation)	Value elevated with bacterial infections and tissue destruction (necrosis)
	Detects generalized inflammation
	Increases more rapidly with an acute inflammation response than ESR
	CRP increases within 6 hours of infection, reaches a peak elevation 2 days after infection, and returns to normal within 1 week after treatment has begun
	Note: Test results may be positive in the absence of inflammation with pregnancy, oral contraceptives
Hemoglobin	Value decreased with bacterial toxins
Culture and sensitivity (blood, wound, stool, urine, sputum, throat)	Isolates specific microorganisms that are causing clinical infection
	Initially may do smear to classify organism
	Cultures provide definitive diagnosis of organism but may require several days to weeks for sufficient growth of pathogen
	Sensitivity testing determines the microbes' susceptibility to specific antibiotics; crucial to effective treatment
	Note: Follow prescribed protocols for collection of specimens; improper technique negates results

TABLE 23–4. *Assessment and Management of Osteomyelitis*

AGE/ COMMON SITES	TYPE/ HISTORY	MOST COMMON ORGANISMS	SYMPTOMS	DIAGNOSTIC FINDINGS	MANAGEMENT
Neonates Epiphyseal and joint involvement resulting from presence of transphyseal vessels	Prematurity Treatment in intensive care unit	Group B streptococci, *S. aureus*	Hard to detect: systemic symptoms may be mild or absent, making diagnosis difficult Edema Decreased motion in limb Crying when extremity passively moved Multiple bones are commonly infected May see osteomyelitis in association with septic arthritis because of the way the epiphyseal-metaphyseal junction is actually positioned inside the joint	↑ ESR (may be unreliable) ↑ C-reactive protein ↑ WBC count ↓ Hemoglobin Blood cultures positive in 50% of cases 7–14 days before x-ray films show changes Bone scan not helpful in the neonate CT or MRI with pelvis or vertebral involvement or before surgical intervention Aspiration or bone biopsy to determine organism	Administration of empiric antibiotics before culture and sensitivity: nafcillin/oxacillin for *S. aureus,* penicillin for streptococci Duration of antibiotics minimally 2 weeks, often 4–6 weeks Surgical intervention to drain purulent material, remove sequestra or infected foreign material, debride and drain puncture-associated infection In neonate early drainage of bone and joint is critical
Children Long bones Femoral metaphyses Tibial metaphyses Less frequent Humerus Radius Ulna	**Hematogenous spread:** Recent infection (upper respiratory infection, genitourinary infection, otitis, boils) Recent soft tissue injury or bruising (trivial trauma) Recent childhood viral disease (chickenpox or measles) **Contiguous spread:** Puncture wounds through sneakers	*S. aureus* Streptococcus *Haemophilus influenzae* in children younger than 3 years Children with sickle cell disease: *S. aureus* or *Salmonella* *Pseudomonas* from puncture wound	Generally an acute onset of symptoms Infection and inflammation signs: Fever Leukocytosis Local erythema Localized swelling Heat/warmth Pain: throbbing and severe; in early stages may not be well localized (in some children, acute infection signs are absent, and child presents with limb pain) Limitation in movement secondary to pain: limping, fear of walking; in severe cases, pseudoparalysis Malaise and sleep disturbances Anorexia, nausea, emesis	As with neonates Bone scan: increased tracer uptake reflects inflammatory process in bone lesion Needle aspiration or open bone biopsy: bacteriologic diagnosis and evaluation of presence of abscess	Outcome most favorable if treated within 3 days of symptoms Children more responsive to antibiotic administration Administration of empiric antibiotics before culture and sensitivity to include the following: *Older than 3 years of age:* nafcillin or oxacillin for gram-positive organisms *Younger than 3 years of age:* add a third-generation cephalosporin for possible *H. influenzae* *With sickle cell disease:* third-generation cephalosporin or ampicillin to cover *Salmonella* Continue antibiotic administration for 3–6 weeks If compliance can be ensured and after response to IV antibiotics, can switch to high-dose oral antibiotics; monitor blood levels to ensure bactericidal activity Surgical decompression if pus found on bone aspiration or x-ray film shows metaphyseal cavity

TABLE 23–4. *Assessment and Management of Osteomyelitis* Continued

AGE/ COMMON SITES	TYPE/ HISTORY	MOST COMMON ORGANISMS	SYMPTOMS	DIAGNOSTIC FINDINGS	MANAGEMENT
Adults Vertebrae Pelvis	**Hematogenous spread:** *Adults:* IV drug use, Pott's disease, fungal infection, immunocompromised host *Older adults:* urinary tract involvement, respiratory infection (including tuberculosis), soft tissue infection Contiguous spread: Invasion of organisms to bone from deep soft tissue infection, periodontal infection, or infected, irradiated tumor or infected pressure ulcer **Direct infection:** Penetrating wounds Compound fractures Complication of surgery (e.g., open reduction of fracture)	*S. aureus* (40%–60%) Streptococci Older adults: *Candida* may cause hematogenous osteomyelitis in this age group Enteric gram-negative bacilli: *E. coli, Klebsiella, Enterobacter* IV drug addicts: *Pseudomonas aeruginosa, Candida* Implantation of orthopaedic prostheses: *Staphylococcus epidermidis* Immunocompromised host: fungi, mycobacteria	Can have an acute inflammatory response but more commonly insidious onset with minimal systemic signs Vertebral: back pain or neck pain, spine tenderness, and possible low-grade fever Pain can be mild to excruciating, commonly described as throbbing or intermittent; may intensify with movement, coughing, sneezing, straining Pain generally not relieved by analgesics, bed rest, heat 20%–40%: signs of nerve root or spinal cord involvement (weakness, paralysis, abnormal reflexes) Paravertebral and hamstring spasms Abdominal pain with lumbar involvement Low-grade fever when associated with hematogenous spread for other infectious site Night sweats may be found with vertebral osteomyelitis, especially with tubercular pathogen Direct osteomyelitis: increased pain at operative site, poor incision healing and protracted wound drainage	Possible leukocytosis ↑ ESR Blood cultures positive in low percentage of cases (10%) Culture specimens from percutaneous or operative bone biopsy vs. sinus tract, because tracts may be colonized with organisms not found in bone Plain x-ray films: takes 2–4 weeks for changes to be visualized Vertebral: disc space narrowing followed by cortical destruction at the adjacent endplates Radionuclide scans: diagnostic in many cases and may reveal signs of disease within several days of onset of infection; however, may be unable to differentiate from other inflammatory and degenerative processes in adjacent tissues, recent orthopaedic surgery, bone fractures, and neoplasms MRI: greater than 90% specificity; helps determine the extent of vertebral osteomyelitis and delineation of sinus tracts and soft tissue abscesses CT scanning is better for detecting sequestra	Administration of empiric antibiotics before culture and sensitivity: generally start with nafcillin or cephalosporin, then change based on culture and sensitivity Gram-negative bacilli: use two drugs that give synergistic activity against offending organism (first-generation cephalosporin plus an aminoglycoside—cefazolin plus tobramycin) *Candida:* treat with amphotericin B followed by indefinite course of fluconazole Tuberculous osteomyelitis: treat with the same regimen as for pulmonary tuberculosis IV antibiotic therapy duration: 4–6 weeks parenteral therapy followed by PO therapy for at least 2 months Surgical: removal of dead bone, devitalized tissue and foreign material; drainage of abscess; obliteration of dead space
With pressure ulcers, greater trochanter, or sacrum	Immobility Malnutrition	Polymicrobial Staphylococci Streptococci Anaerobes: *Enterobacteriaceae* and *Pseudomonas*	Stage 2 or 3 pressure ulcer Drainage from ulcer Local inflammation Tenderness, pain	In clients with deep chronic skin ulcers from which infection has spread to bone, curettage cultures from the base of the ulcer correlate with osseous tissue 75% of the time Screening for malnutrition (albumin, serum transferrin, total protein)	Mixed flora more common with contiguous infection: combined antimicrobial therapy such as cefoxitin, ciprofloxacin, and metronidazole Nafcillin, gentamicin, and clindamycin regimen also common

Table continued on following page

TABLE 23–4. *Assessment and Management of Osteomyelitis* Continued

AGE/COMMON SITES	TYPE/HISTORY	MOST COMMON ORGANISMS	SYMPTOMS	DIAGNOSTIC FINDINGS	MANAGEMENT
Foot Small bones of the foot	Osteomyelitis with vascular insufficiency seen with diabetes mellitus or atherosclerosis Puncture wounds Prolonged skin ulcers Draining sinus	Generally polymicrobial, with *S. aureus* most frequently isolated from sinus tracts and ulcers Other pathogens: gram-negative bacilli and anaerobes	Long-standing insulin-dependent diabetes or other vascular disease is a risk factor Due to vascular insufficiency, few systemic signs Local evidence of inflammation or necrosis at site Painful extremity but variable with underlying neuropathy Limp Mild temperature; frequently afebrile Ulcers, sinus tracts	Leukocytosis and ↑ ESR may or may not be present Screening for malnutrition (albumin, serum transferrin, total protein) Culture of multiple organisms from ulcer: if possible take deep cultures including bone biopsy X-ray film: mottled lytic lesions	Mixed flora: select a second-generation cephalosporin that has good activity against both *S. aureus* and anaerobes—cefoxitin or cefotetan—or a third-generation cephalosporin, such as ceftriaxone, which has activity against gram-positive organisms and *P. aeruginosa* Metronidazole (Flagyl, Protostat) or clindamycin can be added to improve coverage of anaerobes Prolonged use of aminoglycosides should be avoided because of increased risk for ototoxicity and nephrotoxicity in older clients Quinolones: good activity against gram-negative bacilli and penetrate well to the bone Diabetic foot: local hyperbaric oxygen therapy; vascular surgery to improve blood flow
Chronic, all ages	Chronic osteomyelitis Brodie's abscess Reformation of sinus tracts History reveals continuous or intermittent symptoms and functional deficits	Variability in infecting organisms, necessitating isolation of microorganism for culture Commonly associated with gram-negative organisms	Systemic signs generally absent, afebrile Mild local tenderness, warmth, swelling, erythema Drainage from sinus tracts Pain on movement	Normal WBC count ↑ ESR Possible anemia X-ray film: radiolucent area indicating abscess with adjacent soft tissue inflammation	Surgical therapy is mainstay of treatment Multiple surgical procedures may be needed: sequestrectomy, saucerization, followed by bone grafting and myocutaneous flaps or skin grafting for wound coverage Amputation in more severe cases Hyperbaric oxygen therapy

The infecting organisms reach the bone by one of three routes: through the bloodstream (hematogenous spread), by extension from adjacent soft tissue infection (contiguous focus), or by direct introduction of microorganisms into the bone.

Hematogenous osteomyelitis is the most common. It occurs predominantly in children before the age of epiphyseal closure but also has a peak incidence during advanced middle age and older adulthood. In hematogenous osteomyelitis, there is usually a single organism (most commonly *S. aureus*) that enters the bone from remote sites of infection via the bloodstream. Common sources of infection include urinary tract infections, skin and soft tissue infections (furuncles, impetigo), upper respiratory tract infections, and acute otitis media. When these sources are not present, it is possible that the initiating source may be trivial trauma. Therefore, the history should include inquiry about ordinary cuts and bruises of the skin.

Hematogenous osteomyelitis generally involves bones with rich red marrow. The anatomic location of hematogenous osteomyelitis is age dependent. In children and infants, the long bones (especially the femur and the tibia) are involved, and the infection usually begins as an acute onset in the metaphyseal region of the bone. The blood-borne bacteria are carried to the marrow space by way of the nutrient artery. When infection follows blunt trauma, a hematoma develops and creates a pathway for organisms into the bone. In the adult population, the infection may begin insidiously and is usually secondary to a primary bacteremia caused by genitourinary tract, soft tissue, and respiratory infections or infections contracted by intravenous drug abusers. The blood-borne organisms seed vertebral bodies because the vertebrae become more vascular than other skeletal tissue with maturation.

Osteomyelitis secondary to a contiguous infection may be related to soft tissue infection from burns, sinus disease, trauma, malignant tumor necrosis, periodontal disease, or pressure ulcers. The onset is insidious, and infection spreads to adjacent bone through the soft tissue. Clients with diabetes mellitus or severe atherosclerosis are at greater risk for developing the condition because of vascular insufficiency. In contrast to hematogenous osteomyelitis, osteomyelitis secondary to contiguous infection is primarily a disease of adults.

Direct invasion of the bone by microorganisms can occur at any age. Microorganisms gain entrance to the bone through open fractures, penetrating wounds (bullets or foreign bodies), or contamination during a surgical procedure. Any implanted item, such as metal plates, prostheses, or screws can act as a focus for bacterial growth. Indwelling foreign bodies decrease the quantity of bacteria necessary to establish infection in bone and permit pathogens to persist on the surface of the avascular material, sequestered from circulating immune factors and systemic antibiotics.

Chronic osteomyelitis may occur following undiagnosed or inadequately treated osteomyelitis. In chronic osteomyelitis, the avascular dead tissue, pus, and bacteria may remain isolated within an area of bone fibrosis and sclerosis, giving rise to recurrent episodes of acute osteomyelitis.

Pathophysiology

Bacteria generally seed in the more vascular bones. The tortuous course of nutrient vessels in bone can trap bacteria in the metaphysis. The inflammatory and immunologic responses to bacteria cause pus formation, edema, and vascular congestion. Pressure increases as the pus collects and is confined within the rigid bone, contributing to vascular occlusion, ischemia, and eventually bone necrosis. The Volkmann and haversian canals, although allowing minimum exudation of the pus, permit the infection to travel to other segments of the bone. The increasing pressure results in further compromise of the vascular supply, supporting the process of necrosis. Blood and antibiotics cannot reach the bone tissue once the pressure within the vascular system reaches the arteriolar pressure, thus influencing the course and virulence of the osteomyelitis. Even with aggressive treatment, recurring trauma to the area or immunosuppression may cause the organism to proliferate years after apparently successful treatment.

If initial treatment is omitted or inadequate, suppurative and ischemic injury causes the necrotic bone to separate from the living bone into devitalized segments (sequestra) (Fig. 23-1A). Sequestra become a medium for microorganism growth, and chronic osteomyelitis results. The sequestra continue to enlarge, with possible extrusion through the bone into surrounding soft tissue (subacute osteomyelitis) if surgical removal does not occur. It is possible that the sequestra, once outside the bone, will revascularize and resolve owing to the effects of normal defense mechanisms.

The osteoblasts, in an attempt to heal the infected bone, isolate the dead fragments, forming the involucrum (a layer of new bone around the old dead bone). The involucrum interferes with normal phagocytosis and antibiotics and becomes a reservoir of chronic infection.

Soft tissue abscesses and cutaneous sinus tracts can develop once the infection reaches the periosteum. The cutaneous sinus tracts develop when pressure increases and erosion of the soft tissue occurs. The sinus tracts offer a route for chronic wound drainage and a port of entry for new microorganisms (Fig. 23-1B).

The infection may become walled off by fibrotic tissue reaction and remain localized. This formation is referred to as a *Brodie's abscess.* Pathologic fractures can occur at sites of severe cortical bone destruction.

Age can affect the progress of osteomyelitis. In children, the overlying periosteum is loosely attached, allowing for subperiosteal collection of exudate. Unarrested infection eventually disrupts the cortex, causing a joint infection—septic arthritis. In adults, the periosteum is firmly attached, and subperiosteal collections are rare.

Vertebral osteomyelitis, most common in adults, generally begins near the anterior longitudinal ligament and spreads to adjacent vertebrae by direct extension through disc space or by communicating venous channels. Extradural abscesses form when purulent material accumulates between the vertebrae periosteum and dura mater. Compression of the spinal cord by abscesses or rupture of abscesses into subarachnoid space can cause paralysis and meningitis.

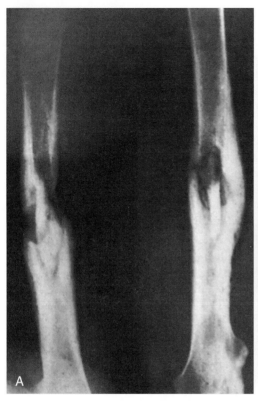
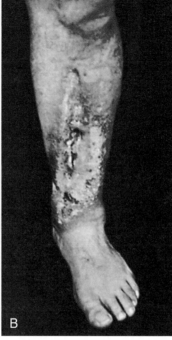

FIGURE 23–1. *A,* Chronic osteomyelitis of the femur with large retained sequestrum. *B,* Chronic osteomyelitis of the tibia. Note the marked scarring of the overlying skin and draining sinuses. (From Gartland, J. [1987]. *Fundamentals of orthopaedics* [pp. 153, 157]. Philadelphia: WB Saunders.)

Complications of osteomyelitis are common and can have long-term implications for growth and development in the child. In the neonate, the osteomyelitis starts in the metaphyseal area and therefore can damage the growth plate, resulting in stunted growth and angular deformities. Osteomyelitis adjacent to the joint can result in septic arthritis, with resulting loss of articular cartilage and development of osteoarthritis early in life. In adults, squamous cell carcinoma has been reported (rarely) to arise in the tracts of chronically draining sinuses.

Assessment: History and Physical

Early diagnosis of osteomyelitis is necessary to prevent progression of the disease to the disabling chronic stage. Comprehensive history and assessment are critical to this process.

Table 23–4 outlines key areas for history and assessment according to the site of involvement and age. Generally, the child presents with a sudden onset of the classic symptoms of pain and acute septic reaction. Vomiting and dehydration may be present. The parents should be questioned to gather information about recent infections or diseases as well as recent trauma. It should be determined whether the child has been limping or showing hesitation or fear when ambulating.

Presenting symptoms and typical history vary in the adult according to the site of involvement. Acute pain and signs of sepsis accompany infection of long bones. Generally, however, systemic symptoms are not as pronounced as in the child, and the disease manifests as a clinical picture of subacute or chronic illness. History may reveal recent trauma or newly acquired prosthetic devices. Malaise may be present, but adults are not acutely ill with other systemic signs. Localized pain and drainage may be the first indications of a problem. Osteomyelitis in the older adult is often subtle or atypical in presentation.

Involvement of the vertebral body or foot is not generally accompanied by systemic septic symptoms, but pain and accompanying mobility or movement deficits dominate. Clients with vertebral involvement often have a history of genitourinary involvement or drug abuse, and these infections follow the hematogenous route. Foot involvement is most commonly associated with vascular insufficiency.

After a thorough history has been obtained, a detailed physical assessment, with the emphasis on the manifestations of inflammation and infection, is performed. Pain assessment and evaluation of accompanying functional deficits are integral to this examination. Physical examination of the affected area reveals localized pain, extreme tenderness on palpation, redness, and warmth to touch. Muscle spasms may be observed over the affected area. The client may demonstrate an unwillingness to move the affected limb and guard against any movement because the pain is aggravated with motion. ROM above and below the diseased segment should be noted. Soft tissue swelling and tenderness at the site of the infection in a child generally indicate the elevation of the periosteum by pus.

Diagnostic Evaluation

Laboratory tests and x-ray films or scans are also important tools to assist in the early diagnosis of acute osteomyelitis (see Table 23-4). The diagnosis of acute osteomyelitis is often made based on the initial clinical signs (history, physical examination, complete cell count, and ESR) of the client and is not delayed by waiting for further laboratory or x-ray evidence. Diagnostic tests help differentiate this diagnosis from acute rheumatic fever, early juvenile rheumatic arthritis, acute cellulitis, and abscess formation.

Routine laboratory tests in the diagnostic phase include CBC, ESR, and both aerobic and anaerobic blood cultures. The ESR is elevated, indicating the presence of an inflammatory process. Marked leukocytosis may be present in a child yet may be absent in an adult. Low hemoglobin and WBC counts may be the result of bacterial toxins. Leukocyte counts and elevated sedimentation rates may fall in response to therapy.

A definitive diagnosis requires isolation of the responsible organism. Cultures should be done before the initiation of antibiotic therapy or after the client has been off antibiotic therapy for at least 24 hours. A Gram stain should be ordered and can provide initial information about the organism's identity and optimal empiric antibiotic therapy.

Superficial cultures of open wounds or skin ulcers and cultures of cutaneous sinus tracts are usually polymicrobial and are unreliable indicators of deep-seated bone infections. Needle aspiration, a percutaneous needle biopsy of infected bone, or open bone biopsy in surgery yields a specimen for culture and sensitivity testing. Surgical culture specimens are especially desirable with neonates and infants, children with a history of chronic osteomyelitis or altered host defenses, and children with osteomyelitis secondary to wound extension.

In clients with chronic osteomyelitis, post-traumatic osteomyelitis, or osteomyelitis from a contiguous site, culture specimens can be obtained during surgery. In addition, apparent sources of sepsis, such as boils, should be cultured. Cultures of material obtained from a draining sinus usually reflect bacteria present on the skin but often fail to identify organisms present in the infected bone. These cultures may act as guidelines for initial antimicrobial therapy, but definitive therapy is based on bone tissue biopsy.

Radiographic evidence of osteomyelitis lags behind the symptoms and pathologic changes by at least 7 to 10 days despite large medullary pus collections. Most cases do not manifest plain film evidence of infection until 3 to 4 weeks because 30% to 50% of the bone matrix must be lost to show a lytic lesion on x-ray films. At this point, the disease may have progressed to the chronic stage. X-ray films are done initially to rule out the possibility of a fracture.

Early changes of acute osteomyelitis seen on x-ray film usually reflect changes in the adjacent tissue and not the bone. Soft tissue changes on the x-ray film may be displacement of fat lines, evidence of subcutaneous edema, or swelling of the area adjacent to the metaphysis. Periosteal elevation or an irregularity in the cortex is seen 2 to 4 weeks after onset (Fig. 23-2).

Evidence of bone necrosis appears on radiographic evaluation between the 10th and 14th days. At this point, the bone shows spotty, irregular areas of decalcification, most prominent in the metaphyseal area of bone. Ultimately, this may extend throughout the entire shaft of the bone. Periosteal new bone formation can be seen. As sequestra form, they may appear as pieces of dead, separate bone.

Early x-ray changes associated with vertebral osteomyelitis are erosion of the subchondral bone plate and narrowing of the intervertebral disc space, with possible involvement of the adjacent vertebrae. Later, the vertebrae may show a loss of height, anterior osteogenesis, and soft tissue densities representing paravertebral abscesses.

Radionuclide bone scans (technetium diphosphonate bone scans, gallium citrate scans, and indium-

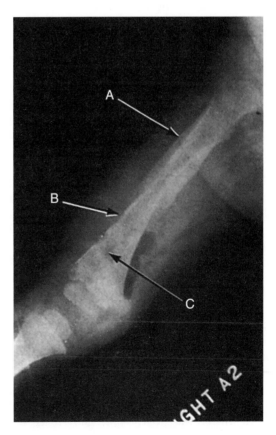

FIGURE 23-2. Acute osteomyelitis of the femur in a young child. *A*, Reactive periosteal bone. *B*, Multiple cortical defects. *C*, Areas of bone destruction. (Courtesy of Dr. Roshen Irani, Thomas Jefferson University Hospital, Philadelphia, PA.)

labeled scintigraphy) are more efficient in the diagnosis of early acute osteomyelitis and usually reveal increased radionuclide uptake when symptoms begin. Lesions in the spine or long bones can be detected within 24 to 72 hours after onset. Areas of increased uptake identify neovascularization. Areas of decreased uptake reflect an infarcted bone. Although more efficient, these techniques often have inadequate specificity and spatial resolution, so they are not conclusively diagnostic. Inflammatory and degenerative processes in adjacent tissues, recent orthopaedic surgery, and neoplasm produce abnormal scans in the absence of osteomyelitis.

Magnetic resonance imaging (MRI) has been recognized as a useful modality for diagnosing the presence and scope of musculoskeletal sepsis. MRI is able to distinguish between bone and soft tissue infection, thus making a diagnosis more definitive. MRI can detect osteomyelitis earlier than CT scans and x-ray films with equivalent or greater sensitivity, specificity, and spatial resolution when compared with scintigraphic methods.

Treatment Modalities and Related Nursing Management of Acute Osteomyelitis

With prompt treatment of the early manifestations of acute osteomyelitis, full recovery with minimal loss of function is possible. Chronic osteomyelitis develops with an ineffective or inadequate course of antibiotics or delayed treatment.

The major treatment goal for acute osteomyelitis is elimination of the microorganisms locally from the bone and systemically from the body. Prevention of further bone deformity and injury, maintenance of comfort, avoidance of the complications of impaired mobility and complications of the disease process, and psychological support are other goals that must be achieved.

The comprehensive treatment plan of a client, child or adult, includes medical, surgical, and nursing interventions. In the adult client, antibiotic therapy alone rarely results in resolution of infection, and surgery is considered a mainstay of therapy. Initial treatment involves surgical intervention to ensure adequate drainage, thorough debridement, obliteration of dead space, and adequate soft tissue coverage. This provides an environment in which antibiotics can work more effectively.

Surgical Intervention. A needle aspiration or a percutaneous needle biopsy of the infected bone may be done initially. However, these techniques are only 60% effective in detecting the specific causative agent.

Surgical intervention may be required to obtain a specimen for culture and sensitivity. By releasing the pressure within the bone, rapid pain relief may be obtained. Under a general anesthetic, the periosteum is excised, allowing access to the purulent material in the infected area. If pus is not apparent, several holes may be drilled into the bone to release the pus under pressure.

Culture specimens are obtained for immediate analysis. The wound and bone are irrigated with sterile saline before closure.

Surgical decompression is also considered when a client has demonstrated lack of improvement after 36 to 48 hours of antimicrobial therapy, prolonged bacteremia, or evidence of an abscess formation or suspected joint sepsis. Surgery to drain an abscess, release bone pressure, or debride the bone is indicated.

Debridement may leave a large bone defect, and this dead space is managed by local tissue flaps or free flaps to fill the space. Antibiotic-impregnated polymethyl methacrylate (PMMA) beads may be used to sterilize and temporarily maintain dead space. Used after debridement, PMMA beads have improved the outcome of osteomyelitis treatment in both experimental models and clinical trials. This approach provides high local concentrations of antibiotic while systemic levels of antibiotic remain low. Wallenkamp (1998) reported treating 100 clients with osteomyelitis using debridement and gentamicin-PMMA beads. Healing was achieved in 92 clients. Healing was more difficult to achieve when the infection was chronic. The major disadvantage of the PMMA beads is the need for their surgical removal at the completion of antibiotic release, which usually takes place 4 weeks after their implantation. A cancellous bone graft may be used after removal. External braces or casts may be used to protect the limb following surgical intervention.

Pharmacologic Intervention. Pharmacologic therapy must be instituted shortly after the onset of symptoms to prevent progression to the chronic stage. An effective therapeutic blood level of the antimicrobial agent must be reached promptly to ensure that the medication reaches the site of the infection. The blood supply to the affected area may be insufficient or completely absent as a result of pathologic changes. Thus, the antibiotic must reach the area largely by diffusion.

Parenteral antimicrobial therapy should be ordered based on results of the blood or wound culture specimens. Treatment should be initiated as soon as possible and antibiotics may be administered before cultures are taken, based on empiric understanding of infection site and likely organism. In this instance, the regimen is based on coverage for the most commonly occurring organisms for that age group and type of osteomyelitis. For example, cefazolin or a semisynthetic penicillin (e.g., oxacillin, nafcillin) may be given initially until the culture and sensitivity results are obtained because of the high incidence of osteomyelitis caused by *S. aureus;* however, if the child or adult has sickle cell disease, a third-generation cephalosporin (cefotaxime) may be added because of the possibility of *Salmonella* infection.

Large, frequent doses of antibiotics are administered parenterally for several weeks (4 to 8 weeks) to ensure a bactericidal level of the antibiotic in the bone tissue. Children are typically more responsive to the antibiotic regimen then are adults, and the duration of their parenteral therapy is generally 2 weeks.

To evaluate the client's response to pharmacologic therapy, serial bone scans and ESR measurements are done. A decrease in the ESR denotes a positive response. The radiographic changes of healing osteomyelitis lag considerably behind the clinical situation. Thus, they cannot be used to evaluate the client's response effectively. Once the client demonstrates the beginning of a resolution of the infectious process and is afebrile, oral antimicrobials may be initiated. Continuation and initiation of oral antibiotics depend on the ability of the specific medication to penetrate the tissue adequately.

Oral antibiotic therapy is continued for 4 to 8 weeks after intravenous therapy is completed. Accurate assays of the serum concentration of the antimicrobial agent are required to ensure a therapeutic level of oral antimicrobial. A peak serum bactericidal dilution of at least 1:8 should be maintained. To ensure the maintenance of a therapeutic blood level, the nurse or the client must administer the antibiotics according to schedule.

Parenteral therapy is generally administered via a long-term access device, such as a peripherally inserted central catheter (PICC). This decreases hospitalization time and allows for administration at home by the client, a family member, or a visiting nurse. The duration of parenteral antimicrobial therapy is one of the major variables influencing resolution of the osteomyelitis. An adequate duration of an antimicrobial at a therapeutic level may prevent the development of or progression to chronic osteomyelitis.

With prompt, adequate treatment of acute osteomyelitis, the infection may resolve, and the client has minimal or no loss of function. The client may return to normal activities of daily living (ADLs) and not have a recurrence.

Nursing Management

Nursing diagnoses associated with acute osteomyelitis target infection transmission, comfort, mobility deficits, and knowledge deficits.

Infection, Knowledge Deficit: Disease and Medications

Infection Control, Infection Protection, Teaching: Medication Administration, Catheter Management. In children and in some adults, initial symptoms manifest as an acute inflammatory and infectious process. Nursing care measures target infection control, infection protection, nutrition management, and fever management.

Administration of intravenous antibiotics is the mainstay of therapy in the acute phase. The purpose of

the medication, the rationale for the intravenous route, and the duration of the medication therapy should be discussed with the client. Because the client will be discharged from the hospital to home antibiotic therapy, intravenous catheter care should be discussed from the onset.

Infection control, infection prevention, and antibiotic administration are the focus of instruction in preparing clients for discharge. Table 23–2 reviews necessary client teaching about infection control and prevention. Special attention is given to the importance of handwashing and safe handling of wound drainage. Families should be reassured that routine laundering and drying of bedding and soiled clothes is sufficient to kill organisms. Ongoing monitoring and recognition of recurring or advancing problems are reviewed.

The client (or appropriate family member) is instructed, either in the hospital or at home, on administration of intravenous medication through an intermittent infusion catheter. Monitoring of adherence to parenteral or oral antimicrobial therapy is critical to effective treatment and optimal outcomes. Clients and families should be counseled about the need to continue therapy even after symptoms are alleviated. It is hard for clients and families to understand the need for (especially in light of the expense) continuing antibiotic administration weeks after symptoms disappear, and it is certainly easy to forget the medications when symptoms diminish. Clients and families should be helped to understand the ramifications of inadequately treated osteomyelitis. One must work to arrange incorporation of cultural health beliefs into the regimen. Referral to social services for financial support to purchase the medication might be needed. The nurse should interact with clients in a nonjudgmental fashion so that they will be forthcoming if problems exist.

Long-term administration of antibiotics requires monitoring for signs of superinfection. The nurse monitors or instructs the client to carefully assess for the signs of superinfection, as evidenced by changes in the oral cavity, genitourinary and gastrointestinal tract, and vaginal mucous membranes. Older, debilitated, or immunosuppressed clients are at the highest risk for superinfection.

Pain

Pain Management. The individual with osteomyelitis may experience mild to severe pain, as well as localized joint pain. The area may be tender to touch, and muscle spasms may occur.

Narcotic analgesics may be administered for acute pain. Pain medications (narcotic or non-narcotic) should be ordered around the clock rather than on an as-needed basis so that constant blood levels are achieved. Because bed rest may be required, the need for diversional activities and nonpharmacologic approaches to pain management become essential. Support should be given to the affected extremity to minimize pain. In some situations, the involved area may be immobilized with a splint or traction to alleviate the spasm and pain.

Impaired Physical Mobility and Activity Intolerance

Bed Rest Care, Energy Management, Exercise Therapy, Positioning, Distraction. In the acute phase, the client is often on complete bed rest. Diversional activities are important for both pain and mood management. The limb should be placed in good functional alignment or kept in alignment through bracing, splinting, or casting. Scheduled position changes are very important because movement may increase pain and it is unlikely that the client will adequately self-position to relieve pressure. ROM and other exercises should be implemented (and taught to client) to keep nonimmobilized joints problem free. Passive ROM may be done to the involved joint if approved by the physician to prevent contractures.

Active ROM to the involved joint and tolerance of increased joint stress (with ambulation) are achieved gradually and as ordered by the physician. Stress on the diseased bone may cause pathologic fractures or other musculoskeletal problems, so the involved area may be immobilized with the use of braces or casts. Assistive devices for mobilization may decrease the weight stress on the involved area.

Anxiety

Anxiety Reduction. The acute, painful process, as well as fear of long-term implications, can be frightening to the client. Providing consistent communication about what to expect, tests ordered, results of tests, and expected progress of symptoms is important in reducing anxiety. Fear regarding prognosis or the uncertainty of the outcome is present, as is anxiety over the long-term nature of the treatment. Role disruption, self-concept disturbance, and family disruption all contribute to the anxiety experienced.

Providing thorough client education and allowing the client as much control in decision making as possible may alleviate some of the anxiety. Stress reduction interventions (e.g., relaxation, guided imagery) may be indicated. Age-appropriate diversional activities can be stimulating and helpful. Family members should be encouraged to remain with the client if possible, especially when the client is a child.

Treatment Modalities and Related Nursing Management in the Chronic or Rehabilitative Phase

Chronic osteomyelitis is an acute osteomyelitis that has progressed to the point at which a Brodie's abscess or sequestrum has developed or there is a re-formation of sinus tracts (see Fig. 23–1). It is also defined as the recurrence of an acute febrile course related to one or more sites of infected bone tissue. Chronic cases may appear as continuous problems, or the client may have periods of exacerbation and quiescence. The incidence of chronic osteomyelitis is 2 in 10,000 people. Risk factors for chronic osteomyelitis include diabetes, hemodialysis, and intravenous drug abuse.

In chronic osteomyelitis, there is infected necrotic bone that has a poorly perfused surrounding soft tissue envelope. To arrest the infection, the focal point for the persistent contamination must be removed. Adequate drainage, thorough debridement, obliteration of dead space, hardware removal, wound protection, and antimicrobial therapy are the mainstays of treatment (Mandell, Bennett, & Dolin, 2000).

Assessment and Diagnostics. Manifestation of chronic osteomyelitis differs from that of acute osteomyelitis. The client is no longer acutely ill but demonstrates local manifestations of infections. Physical examination of the affected area reveals localized warmth, swelling, pain on movement, tenderness, and a possible draining sinus. The client is usually afebrile, with a normal WBC count and ESR. CBC may demonstrate anemia as a result of chronic infection. The history may reveal that the exacerbation was precipitated by trauma or a decrease in the client's resistance. X-ray films may show a radiolucent area, which is identified as an abscess with adjacent soft tissue inflammation.

The variability of the infecting organism in chronic osteomyelitis is much broader than in acute osteomyelitis. Because of this increase in variety, isolating the microorganism is especially important.

Surgical Management. Surgical debridement is the primary treatment, with antimicrobial therapy as an adjunct in the treatment of chronic osteomyelitis. Intravenous antibiotics are commonly used for 4 to 6 weeks, followed by oral antibiotics for an additional 1 to 2 months.

In preparation for surgical treatment, a sinogram or computed tomography (CT) scan of the bone may be ordered. The sinogram involves injecting a radiopaque dye into the external sinus, followed by x-ray films. The sinogram can reveal sinus tracts, abscess cavities, and sequestra.

The surgical objective is complete removal of all necrotic bone and poorly vascularized tissue and elimination of dead space. A sequestrectomy (surgical removal of the dead bone) is indicated when x-ray films show that the necrotic bone is well separated and that an involucrum has been formed.

A saucerization is indicated when the x-ray film or the CT scan shows that the chronic infection involves most of the bone. A Brodie's abscess may be treated with this procedure. This decompression type of surgery includes removal of all the scar tissue, infected tissue, sequestra, sclerotic bone, and overhanging bone edges, thus leaving a flat depression (saucer appearance) in the bone.

Systemic antibiotics are ineffective in the necrotic tissue because of poor circulation. PMMA such as gentamicin or tobramycin may be cemented into the area to deliver antimicrobial concentration directly to the bone (see the section on surgical intervention in "Treatment Modalities and Related Nursing Management of Acute Osteomyelitis").

In contrast to soft tissue, rigid bone does not collapse around a site evacuated by pus. This results in a cavity (dead space) that collects blood, debris, and microorganisms. After surgery, the dead space created by the surgery may be obliterated by open packing of the wound, allowing secondary healing to occur, or by bone grafting to fill the defect. Myocutaneous (musculocutaneous) flaps or skin grafting is used for wound coverage. If the dead space cannot be managed immediately, the cavity is kept clean with an irrigation suction system until grafting or packing can be done. Amputation is appropriate only when infection, bone destruction, or surgical resection is so extensive that the disability of the amputation with prosthesis promotes better client function than the alternatives.

Free microvascular bone transfers are indicated when bone resection creates a skeletal defect longer than 6 cm. The surgery involves the resection and transfer of a segment of bone with or without the attached muscle or skin. Because of the restoration of the blood supply, antibiotics have access to the wound, making the infection potentially controllable. The fibula and the iliac crest are the most common donor sites, although the rib, lateral scapula, metatarsal, and lateral aspect of the radius can also be chosen. Pulverized bone may also stimulate the growth of healthy bone.

Musculocutaneous (myocutaneous) flaps are another approach to the obliteration of the dead space while promoting increased blood supply and bone coverage. This approach allows for more radical debridement of the infected soft tissue and bone, permitting coverage of the large wound. Myocutaneous or musculocutaneous flap involves moving or rotating a muscle and the section of the skin fed by the arteries from that muscle into the cavity created by the surgery. With muscle rotation, the dominant blood supply to the muscle remains intact, increasing and maintaining a good blood supply. The muscle without the skin (muscle flap) is useful when contouring is a concern to prevent deformity. A skin graft is done at a later date. A local flap should be considered first, but if the blood supply is not adequate, a distant flap with a pedicle flap (with later division of the pedicle) or a free flap should be created. The advantage of a local flap (using rotation of the muscle) is long-range resistance to osteomyelitis through the blood supply to provide the

normal mechanisms of infection surveillance (antigen-antibody reactions). When the muscle cannot be used, the omentum is an option if the client can tolerate a laparotomy. Before surgery, the vasculature of the muscle, skin, and wound may be evaluated with an arteriogram.

Preoperative nursing care for the client undergoing a myocutaneous or musculocutaneous flap is routine surgical preparation physically and psychologically. Routine wound care should be completed, and the wound should be dressed. Clear antibiotic solutions or normal saline should be applied to avoid wound discoloration before surgery. Postoperative care for the client undergoing a myocutaneous and musculocutaneous flap focuses on promoting adequate blood supply to the flap by avoiding pressure from the dressing or from edema. During the neurovascular assessment, movement of the extremity should not be done until a physician's order has been obtained.

Adjunctive Management. Currently, hyperbaric oxygen (HBO) treatment is being used as adjunctive therapy with debridement and antibiotics in osteomyelitis that has remained refractory to standard treatment and in which borderline or low oxygen tensions are present. The recommended protocol for adjunctive HBO therapy for refractory osteomyelitis is 2.4 ATA for 95 minutes with appropriate air breaks. Sessions are usually once or twice daily for at least 15 days.

HBO treatment does not directly affect aerobic organisms. The effect is chiefly on the WBCs of the body, which require at least 30 mm Hg partial pressure to kill bacteria. In osteomyelitic bone, oxygen tensions fall to about 17 to 23 mm Hg, rendering the bone hypoxic. Increasing the oxygen tension in osteomyelitic bone to normal or supranormal increases the phagocytic killing ability of the WBCs. Some data suggest that HBO may stimulate neovascularization in the infected area and that it enhances antibiotic efficacy of aminoglycosides, which require oxygen to move across the bacterial wall.

HBO also has an effect on wound healing. There must be adequate oxygen tension for wound healing to proceed. In the ischemic or infected wound, HBO provides oxygen to promote collagen production, angiogenesism, and ultimately, wound healing.

There is a paucity of comparative clinical trials evaluating the efficacy of HBO treatment in clients in whom standard treatment has failed. Most reports are limited to single-site outcome data (Davis, 1986; Morrey, Dunn, Heimbach, & Davis, 1979), and in these studies, the results demonstrate efficacy of HBO. However, in comparative studies, HBO therapy has not been definitely shown to be effective (Esterhai, Pisarello, Brighton, Heppenstall, Gellman, & Goldstein, 1987). Currently, recommendations are to use adjunctive HBO to treat the most difficult stages of osteomyelitis (localized and diffuse) in the compromised host. It is not suggested for routine management of osteomyelitis, but rather for refractory cases.

Nursing Management. The client with chronic osteomyelitis faces frequent and prolonged hospitalization, extreme pain, ongoing expenses from treatment protocols, possible loss of financial support, and role changes within the family. The disease becomes more frightening to the client even with continual treatment because the prognosis is uncertain, with no guarantee of resolution of the disease process. Depending on the bone involved, functional deficits may occur. Amputation is a constant fear if the disease is not controlled.

Exercise promotion and exercise therapy are critical to supporting uninvolved muscles and joints and strengthening the involved area. Assistive devices for ambulation are critical because the client experiences ongoing pain and functional deficits. Immobilization of the limb or joint is used for pain management and support. Immobilization serves to prevent further stress on the weakened skeletal structure. If weight is placed on an infected bone before formation of a sufficiently mature involucrum, as may occur with chronic osteomyelitis, a pathologic fracture may develop.

With prolonged or frequent hospitalization, nursing emphasis expands beyond physiologic problems. Often, the nurse must deal with other nursing diagnoses relative to the client's personal, family, or economic problems. Increased psychological support is important for the client with chronic osteomyelitis because he or she may become hostile after repeated failure of treatments. Instillation of hope, emotional support, and coping support are all appropriate interventions. Promotion of the client's participation in the decision-making process concerning care is important.

SEPTIC ARTHRITIS

Septic arthritis, also known as *pyogenic arthritis, infectious arthritis, bacterial arthritis, septic joint disease,* and *suppurative arthritis,* is the most rapidly destructive form of joint and bone disease. The synovial membrane is invaded by pus-forming organisms that extend into the joint space, producing a closed-space infection. Monoarticular involvement is the typical presentation, with the hip being the most commonly involved joint in children and the knee in adults. The individual generally experiences an acute systemic reaction with chills and fever possible and on examination has a painful, tender, swollen joint.

Acute septic arthritis is a medical emergency requiring prompt diagnosis and treatment to prevent permanent joint damage or death. The mortality rate of nongonococcal bacterial arthritis is 5% to 15%, with a 25% to 60% rate of chronic joint damage and disability (Goldenberg, 1998). Susceptibility and mortality and morbidity rises with extremes of age.

Epidemiology

Bacterial infection of the joint space occurs most commonly via hematogenous spread. Organisms reach the joint from a remote site, such as an upper respiratory infection, otitis media, furuncle, or impetigo, and lodge in sites where conditions favor it, such as a previously traumatized or diseased hip joint. The causative organism suggests the site for hematogenous spread.

Extension from adjacent osteomyelitis is the second mechanism of infection. Osteomyelitis adjacent to a joint may lead to septic arthritis. Its mechanism of spread is influenced by the age of the client. In the infant (Fig. 23–3), a bone abscess near the growth plate may extend into the joint space via small capillaries that cross the epiphyseal plate. In the adult, anastomosis of metaphyseal-epiphyseal vessels permits spread of osteomyelitis to the subperiosteum and into the joint.

Direct inoculation is a less common mechanism of infection. Diagnostic and surgical procedures, such as arthrocentesis, arthrotomy, and arthroplasty, allow direct introduction of the pathogen into the joint cavity. The overall incidence of joint infection complicating a primary arthroplasty is 0.5% to 2%, but it is much greater for revision arthroplasty.

All age groups may develop septic arthritis. It occurs most commonly in adults; however, the most serious sequelae from infection occur in children, especially if the hip joint is involved. In these young age groups, infections are especially likely to occur near the growth plate and may extend into the joint cavity.

Traumatic injuries involving the joint foster development of septic arthritis. Risk factors for septic arthritis parallel those for other orthopaedic infections as presented in Table 23–1. In the adult client, the most significant risk factors include rheumatoid arthritis, prosthetic joint infections, old age, and immunocompromised host defenses. Males are more likely to acquire septic arthritis than females because of their increased incidence of trauma. Clients with systemic connective

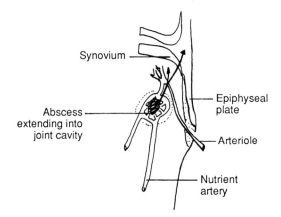

FIGURE 23–3. Route of transmission in infant with acute septic arthritis. Small capillaries across the epiphyseal plate allow entrance of the pathogen into the joint.

tissue disorders are more prone to bacterial arthritis, and there is a rising incidence among intravenous drug users. In these cases, bacterial arthritis often involves unusual joints, such as the sternoclavicular or sacroiliac joints.

There are two major classes of bacterial arthritis: arthritis resulting from *Neisseria gonorrhoeae* or other *Neisseria* species and nongonococcal bacterial arthritis. The nongonococcal pyogenic bacteria most often implicated are *S. aureus* and various *Streptococcus* species. *Haemophilus influenzae* type B is common in children younger than 2 years of age. Prosthetic joint infections most often are caused by skin flora such as *S. epidermidis* and other coagulase-negative *Staphylococcus* and gram-negative bacilli that are transient skin colonizers (Canale, 1998).

The incidence of septic arthritis is increasing with the development of resistant strains of organisms, the greater use of intra-articular injections, increased incidence of intravenous drug abuse, the increased incidence of AIDS, and the decreased mortality rate of premature infants, in whom the incidence of septic arthritis is relatively high owing to immature immune systems.

Less common causes of infectious arthritis include tubercular, fungal, and viral arthropathies. TB and mycotic infections rarely cause septic arthritis. Many common viral diseases—including hepatitis, infectious mononucleosis, and rubella—have associated arthralgias or arthritis. Viral arthritis generally terminates spontaneously and produces no permanent joint damage.

Any articulation may become infected, but the joints most often involved are, in order of frequency, the knee, hip, ankle, elbow, and small joints of the hand and wrist. In children, the hip and the knee are particularly susceptible. The knee is more commonly involved in adults. Monoarticular involvement is most common. Polyarticular involvement (nongonococcal) may occur in 10% to 20% of clients and is usually seen in clients with serious underlying chronic illness or rheumatoid arthritis. Other associated rheumatic conditions include gout or crystal-induced arthritis, Charcot's arthropathy, and systemic lupus erythematosus. The mortality of polyarticular septic arthritis is twice as great as with monoarticular involvement.

Delay in diagnosis is the single most critical factor affecting prognosis and long-term disability. Early recognition and initiation of appropriate therapy are critical to preventing long-term complications. Chronic septic arthritis may result from untreated or unsuccessful treatment of acute septic arthritis. Joint destruction is the outcome. The primary pathogenic organism, most commonly pyogenic cocci, gram-negative rods, and other drug-resistant bacteria, is likely to remain.

Pathophysiology

Most often, the portal of entry for the primary infection is distant from the involved joint cavity. When joint infec-

tion develops, it usually reflects the failure of multiple host defense mechanisms. Systemic diseases such as diabetes, uremia, sickle cell anemia, and rheumatoid arthritis predispose clients to joint infections. Intravenous drug use and gonorrhea may also result in septic joints. The bacteria or virus must travel from its point of entry and enter the joint cavity for full-blown septic arthritis to develop. Damaged joints from conditions such as arthritis seem to be more susceptible to bacterial seeding and infection.

In the early stages of acute septic arthritis, the synovial membrane is edematous and infiltrated by neutrophils. A purulent effusion containing neutrophils distends the joint and releases lysosomal proteolytic enzymes, which destroy articular cartilage, subchondral bone, and joint capsule. Enzymes released by polymorphonuclear leukocytes, as found in septic arthritis, can readily digest hyaline cartilage within 3 to 24 hours. Other abnormalities within the joint and synovial fluid include increased pressure, decreased pH, increased protein, and decreased glucose. Abscesses may appear within the synovium and subchondral bone, and necrotic debris may accumulate in the joint space. Eventually, the cartilage is destroyed, especially at articular surface contact areas. Granulation tissue replaces the synovial membrane. As healing progresses, the growth of fibroblasts may lead to fibrous or bone ankylosis, with ultimate joint destruction.

Other complications include avascular necrosis (which may be related to local septic embolization and vascular compression by effusion), early osteoarthritis (resulting from cartilaginous destruction), and spread of the infection to the subjacent bone (osteomyelitis).

Assessment and History

The focus of assessment is identification of factors that predispose the client to joint infection, including recent surgery, diagnostic procedures, injuries, intravenous drug abuse, and systemic disease. Special attention should be paid to identification of portals of entry for infection, including the skin, middle ear, urethra, and pelvis. Table 23–5 outlines key data to assess in the nursing history.

The health history should search for possible causative agents for septic arthritis. A female is often unaware of the presence of a cervical gonococcal infection and should be questioned about the presence of a skin rash or pustules, as well as recent sexual exposure. Asking the client "Have you noticed any pimples on your arms or legs?" assesses for the vesicular pustular rash. Often, by the time the client comes for treatment, there is no evidence of the rash or only a small lesion with a tiny scab remains. History taking is therefore essential.

The child with septic arthritis often has a recent history of ear infection, upper respiratory infection, or joint trauma. History of other viral infections, such as hepatitis and rubella (including rubella vaccination),

TABLE 23–5. *Assessment and Management of Septic Arthritis*

AGE	HISTORY, COMMON ORGANISMS	PRESENTING SYMPTOMS	DIAGNOSTIC FINDINGS	MANAGEMENT
Child	Recent trauma Recent infection, including impetigo, otitis media, upper respiratory infection Nongonococcal bacteria *S. aureus* *P. aeruginosa* *Escherichia coli* *Streptococcus* spp. Most common sites of involvement: knee, hip, ankle, elbow In child, most frequently monarticular; in neonate, multiple joints and contiguous osteomyelitis are common	Generally acute onset of fever, 104°–105°F Irritability, lethargy, anorexia Newborn infant may lack systemic response Impaired mobility: refusal to walk or limp Crying when diaper is changed or position of baby moved Localized swelling, warmth, erythema of joint Abduction and external rotation is typical with hip	Blood culture is positive in about 40% of cases Synovial fluid analysis: culture and Gram stain Synovial fluid WBC count >50,000/mm^3, 90% polymorphonuclear leukocytes; glucose low; blood may be present Plain x-ray film: soft tissue swelling, joint space widening (lag time for appearing) Bone joint Tc-99m scan	Empiric antibiotics *Neonate:* nafcillin *Child:* nafcillin or oxacillin *Adolescent with presumed gonococcal infection:* ceftriaxone Duration of antibiotics: ≥3 weeks Surgical management when repeat aspiration of the joint is done and remains swollen and erythematous All hips should be drained and many recommend same for shoulders Bed rest Optimal joint positioning to prevent joint deformation and contractures
Adult	Family/client history of arthritis History of trauma Intravenous drug abuse Recent acute illness: Infections, including gonorrhea, hepatitis, rubella Recent sexual exposure Recent antibiotic use Nongonococcal organisms: *S. aureus* Group B streptococci Gram-negative bacilli Gonococcal arthritis *N. gonorrhoeae* Nongonococcal monoarticular involvement: Involves large weight-bearing joints: knee, hip, shoulder Gonococcal arthritis: Polyarticular and may involve small joints of the wrist and hands and feet	Systemic: shaking, chills, fever (acute or low grade), malaise, tachycardia Local: migratory arthralgia; mono-articular or poly-articular painful, red, hot, swollen joint(s); muscle spasm Joint motion limited: decreased active and passive ROM; extremity held in protective flexion Antalgic gait; resistance to movement Gonococcal: rash (skin pustules), vaginal Purulent discharge, tenosynovitis	Increased leukocytosis with increased percentage of immature leukocytes (some adults may present with minimal or no elevation of peripheral blood leukocyte count ↑ ESR, CRP Positive blood culture for anaerobes and aerobes Decreased hemoglobin if condition secondary to underlying joint disease Synovial fluid aspiration shows elevated joint leukocytes >50,000/mm^3, elevated protein; decreased glucose to <40 mg/dL, Synovial fluid may be turbid, purulent, or serosanguineous Synovial cultures positive in up to 90% of those with nongonococcal bacteria; <50% of those with gonococcal arthritis Blood cultures positive in 10%–60% of cases Immunoelectrophoresis to detect bacterial antigens X-ray film changes—initial: Joint space narrowing, takes 2–3 weeks, soft tissue changes resulting from distention of joint space CT scan and MRI more useful: CT able to define contiguous bone lesions and guide needle aspiration; MRI better defines soft tissues, reflect bone and joint destruction Radioisotope scans detect early inflammation (not specific)	Empiric antibiotic treatment before culture as indicated with child Duration of antibiotic administration 2–6 weeks; less time with gonococcal septic arthritis Joint protection Pain management Drainage: needle aspiration, arthroscopy, surgical drainage

should be ascertained because they can cause transient septic arthritis.

A history of symptom progression reveals a common pattern. The adult client usually describes an acute onset. High temperatures and chills generally are present in those cases in which the blood cultures are positive. However, in at least half of clients, fever and chills are not present and the presenting pattern may be a low-grade fever and malaise. The client may experience an acute onset of migratory arthralgia, with eventual localization of pain in one (monoarticular) or a few (polyarticular) joints along with associated muscle spasm. The client generally describes the joint as being extremely painful, impossible to move, warm to the touch, and swollen. In the young child or infant, history taking is likely to reveal increasing irritability, high fever, and anorexia with the onset of sudden pain in the affected joint. Because of a lack of systemic response, the newborn may lack generalized manifestations. The caregiver in this case may note only alterations in appearance, movement, and positioning of the involved joint.

The client with gonococcal arthritis presents with differing symptoms. These clients are predominantly young, healthy, and sexually active. The client generally has migratory polyarthralgias, tenosynovitis, dermatitis, and fever. Tenosynovitis is most often present over the dorsum of the hand, the wrist, the ankle, or the knee (Goldenberg, 1998). Skin lesions are usually present on the extremities and trunk and may be macular, papular, vesicular, or pustular (Fig. 23–4). Approximately 25% of clients have local genitourinary symptoms.

The manifestations of septic arthritis vary depending on the pathogen present, client age, joint involvement, and time interval since onset. On examination, the nurse usually notes an acutely painful, hot, edematous joint. The large joints are most susceptible, but any joint may be involved, including the spine and small peripheral joints. ROM activities increase the severity of pain. Most often, the involved extremity is maintained in a flexed position, which allows for expansion of the joint cavity and enhances client comfort. Spontaneous movement of the involved limb may be decreased or absent. Weight bearing may be avoided or accompanied by an altered antalgic gait.

The hip joint is most often affected because of its large size, constant use, and vulnerable body position. With hip involvement, the pain is in the groin, lateral and upper thigh, or buttocks. The thigh is held in flexion, adduction, and internal rotation. On examination, the nurse notes an edematous thigh, swollen joint, and tenderness on palpation. ROM is markedly decreased, and weight-bearing activities are impaired. Without proper treatment, destruction of the hip joint may occur.

Involvement of the knee joint is more obvious because of its greater visibility and accessibility. The knee may be distended with fluid and is generally held in a

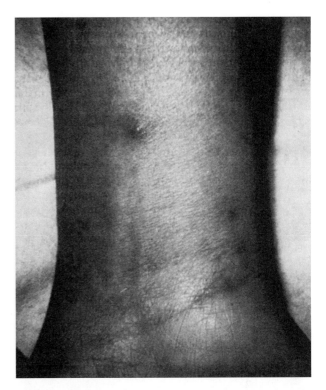

FIGURE 23–4. Skin lesions of disseminated gonococcal infection. The major lesion is vesicopustular, surmounting a hemorrhagic base. The other two, smaller lesions appear more necrotic and probably represent older lesions. (From Kelley, W. N., Harris, E. D., Ruddy, S., & Sledge, C. B. [Eds.]. [1993]. *Textbook of rheumatology* [4th ed., p. 1461]. Philadelphia: WB Saunders.)

flexed position. The joint is hot to touch, and inspection shows redness. The joint is quite tender to palpation, and splinting may be present.

Diagnostic Evaluation

Treatment of septic arthritis requires accurate identification of the causative agent. Initial laboratory studies are important in differentiating this condition from autoimmune diseases with joint involvement, especially rheumatoid arthritis. Table 23–5 summarizes diagnostic findings in septic arthritis.

Laboratory studies include CBC, ESR, C-reactive protein (CRP), serum calcium, phosphorus, alkaline phosphatase, and blood cultures for identification of aerobic and anaerobic organisms. Table 23–3 describes general laboratory information related to infections. The antinuclear antibody (ANA) test, rheumatoid factor (RF) titer determination, and complement-fixation test are performed to rule out the presence of autoimmune diseases. When infectious arthritis is present, CBC generally reveals leukocytosis, with an increased percentage of immature leukocytes. The ESR and CRP are elevated, indicating an inflammatory process. The serum calcium, phosphorus, and alkaline phosphatase levels are generally within normal limits. Approximately 50% of clients with

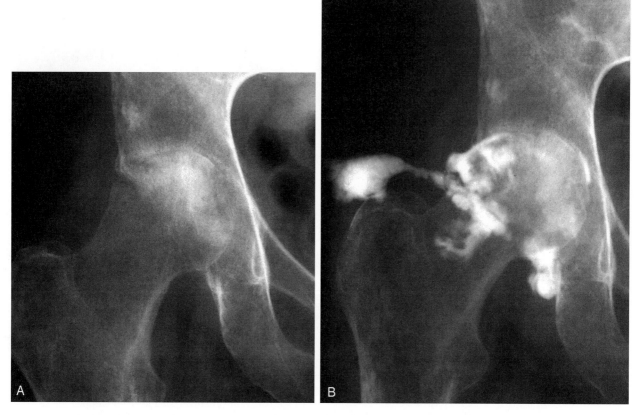

FIGURE 23–5. Septic arthritis. *A,* An anteroposterior view of the hip shows complete cartilage loss with loss of most of the subchondral bone of the femoral head and acetabulum. *B,* An arthrogram shows tracts of contrast material extending from the joint. The contrast agent is adjacent to the bone of the femoral head and acetabulum, confirming complete cartilage loss. (From Ruddy, S. [2001]. *Kelley's textbook of rheumatology* [6th ed., p. 643]. Philadelphia: WB Saunders.)

nongonococcal bacterial arthritis have positive blood cultures, and the blood culture may be positive even when the synovial fluid culture is negative. Gram stain and culture of possible sites of extra-articular infection (e.g., urine, skin lesions) should be examined and can assist with selection of appropriate antibiotic therapy.

Aspiration of joint fluid for analysis and synovial biopsy are the techniques for definitive diagnosis of bacterial arthritis. Joint fluid specimens and synovial tissue are obtained by arthrocentesis or arthroscopy using strict aseptic technique. The causative agent may be identified by Gram stain or culture. A positive result may not be obtained if an antibiotic was administered before fluid culture. Other studies of joint fluid include cell count and differential count. Although not definitive, synovial fluid leukocyte count and differential leukocyte count provide strong support for the clinical suspicion of bacterial arthritis.

Initially with septic arthritis, the joint fluid may be serosanguineous, but within a few days, it becomes cloudy and thick. It demonstrates an elevated cell count (often 1,000,000 WBCs/mm^3) and a high polymorphonuclear leukocyte differential count (98% to 100%). The synovial fluid glucose level is low in the presence of a normal serum glucose level. The protein count is generally elevated. The complement level in synovial fluid is decreased, but not as much as in rheumatoid arthritis. Antigen assays are helpful in cases in which antibiotic therapy has been instituted before joint aspiration. The synovial biopsy may yield positive results in cases in which synovial fluid results were negative.

Radiographic studies reflect destructive changes within the joint attributable to the infectious process. Initially, radiographic findings are negative except for distention of the joint capsule owing to increased synovial fluid. Within approximately 2 weeks of onset, there may be bone erosion, narrowing of the joint space, and evidence of osteomyelitis and synovitis. Progressive untreated septic arthritis may result in destruction of the articular surface and subchondral bone (Fig. 23–5). Comparison films of involved and noninvolved sites help detect subtle joint changes. Sequential films over several months are helpful in evaluating the effectiveness of treatment.

In joints that are difficult to evaluate clinically or those that have a complex anatomic structure (the hip, shoulder, sternoclavicular, and sacroiliac joints), CT scans, MRI, or radionuclide imaging may be of diagnostic value. CT may identify bone and joint destruction as well as soft tissue abscesses associated with the infectious process.

Radioisotope scanning techniques—technetium-99m (Tc-99m) diphosphonate and gallium-67 (Ga-67) citrate scintigraphy—are helpful in early detection of infection. However, results are not specific because other inflammatory and degenerative joint diseases can produce the same results. Scan results should be evaluated in conjunction with radiologic findings for accurate interpretation.

Treatment Modalities and Related Nursing Management (Acute Phase)

For the adult or child with septic arthritis, a comprehensive treatment plan incorporates medical and surgical intervention and nursing care. Prompt diagnosis and treatment, within the first week of onset, generally allow full recovery, with normal joint function or minimal loss of joint function. Goals of treatment include elimination of the pathogen from the joint cavity and body system, removal of joint debris associated with infection, and prevention of deformity. Treatment combines antimicrobial therapy, drainage of joint fluid, and early immobilization of the affected joints. The nurse plays a crucial role in the maintenance of comfort, alleviation of infection, avoidance of complications of impaired mobility, control of hyperthermia, and support of effective coping mechanisms.

Surgical Intervention. Prompt and adequate drainage of purulent synovial effusions is an essential aspect of treatment (Goldenberg, 1998). Needle aspiration, arthroscopy, and surgical intervention are all methods for drainage. Surgical intervention is used in joints, such as the hip and shoulder, where it is anatomically difficult to drain through needle aspiration or where it is difficult to assess the adequacy of the drainage. Hips in children should be immediately drained surgically, and many recommend similar action with shoulder involvement.

With early recognition and treatment of the disease, repeated joint arthrocentesis often provides adequate drainage. In some cases, daily needle aspirations may be necessary. Joint aspiration is required when the hip is involved because of potentially diminished blood supply to the femoral head. Accumulation of purulent fluids distends the joint cavity and deprives the femoral head of its blood supply. If treatment is delayed, the purulent material within the joint becomes excessively thick and fibrous. Continual fluid accumulation in a joint after repeated aspirations may necessitate open surgical drainage and irrigation with a physiologic saline solution.

Septic arthritis in the hip of newborns and infants poses special problems. The diagnosis is often difficult to make, and delay in recognition of the disease may demand surgical intervention rather than more conservative measures. The joint is entered posteriorly and is widely exposed to allow for irrigation and instillation of appropriate antibiotic solution.

Appropriate postoperative care and active rehabilitation programs are essential to restoration of joint function following surgical intervention. The infant requiring open drainage of a hip may be placed in traction with wide abduction. The traction provides separation of hip joint surfaces and thus decreases pressure on the articular cartilage. Several weeks of traction may be required. Throughout this time, the nurse prevents complications associated with immobility and the traction itself. (See Chapter 12 for care of the client in traction.) Drainage and wound healing are carefully monitored. Physical therapy is used to promote return of normal joint ROM.

Pharmacologic Intervention. Antibiotic therapy is crucial to successful treatment and must be readily initiated to prevent permanent joint destruction. Antibiotics are initiated when bacterial arthritis is suspected and when the synovial fluid is purulent. Specimens are obtained for cultures, and antibiotic therapy is initiated based on the Gram stain and clinical picture. After specific identification of the microorganism and its sensitivities, antibiotic therapy may be altered.

Initial administration of empiric agents such as cefazolin or nafcillin is often given intravenously because of the high incidence of infection with staphylococci, pneumococci, and gonococci (see Table 23–5). Studies indicate that with adequate parenteral dosage, the bactericidal agent penetrates the joint cavity and synovial fluid, thus eliminating the need for direct instillation of the antibiotic into the joint. The nurse must carefully monitor the client for toxicity associated with high antibiotic dosages.

The length of time required for intravenous antibiotics is variable depending on duration of symptoms, causative agent, and immune system status. Most clients with septic arthritis, without associated osteomyelitis, require systemic antibiotics for 2 to 3 weeks. Oral antimicrobials are initiated once there is clinical evidence of disease resolution and are continued for an additional 1 to 2 weeks. In older clients and in more complex cases, the duration of therapy may be 4 to 6 weeks. Clients with gonococcal arthritis require a somewhat shorter duration of therapy, with 7 to 10 days of intravenous antibiotic administration followed by 1 week of oral antibiotics. The presence of associated osteomyelitis prolongs treatment with parenteral antibiotics.

Nursing Management

Impaired Physical Mobility

Pain Management, Exercise Therapy: Joint Mobility. Management of septic arthritis requires meticulous attention to joint position, exercise, and rehabilitation. During the acute phase, the client often holds the joint in a position of slight to moderate flexion, which can lead to flexion deformities. Slings, immobilizers, or splints can be used temporarily to hold the joint in optimal position. When the inflammation begins to resolve, passive ROM is initiated to preserve joint function. Continuous passive motion may be used. When clinical symptoms permit and inflammation has almost completely disappeared, active motion and weight bearing can be initiated. Muscle tightening and muscle strengthening exercises are incorporated into a plan of care. Quadriceps sets are especially important in knee infections to help prevent muscle atrophy. Management of pain is essential to supporting the client both with comfort and with participation in the planned exercise regimens.

Chronic Septic Arthritis

Chronic septic arthritis rarely develops but may result from inadequate and delayed treatment. Joint contractures, bone ankylosis, and articular destruction lead to long-term complications that require surgical intervention and even joint replacement.

The manifestations of chronic septic arthritis disease may be continuous or can recur. Following open surgical drainage and antibiotic therapy, multiple new pathogens may appear in addition to the original pathogen. With continuous septic arthritis, the client experiences persistent localized pain and swelling, limited motion, increasing deformity, and sinus tract formation. Radiologic examination reflects destruction of cartilage, narrowing of joint space, and erosion of bone. The presence of a persistent joint infection may eliminate the potential for implants or other corrective surgeries.

Treatment for chronic septic arthritis incorporates therapies similar to those for chronic osteomyelitis (see the discussion of chronic osteomyelitis). Chronic septic arthritis must be differentiated from other forms of arthritis, including rheumatoid arthritis, and degenerative joint disease. As mentioned, antibiotic therapy is selected according to sensitivity study results. Various surgical procedures, including debridement, bone saucerization, or bone resection (when osteomyelitis is present), may be required to alleviate the persistent joint infection. Septic disease occurring in joints with implants generally requires removal of the implants and may eliminate the possibility of future replacements. (See Chapter 16 for a discussion of joint replacement procedures.)

The individual with chronic septic arthritis has multiple psychosocial disturbances. Depending on the severity of symptoms and personal coping mechanisms, the individual's role function and self-concept may change. The nurse must intervene to help the client and family to cope with long-term illness. (See Chapter 2 for nursing concerns relative to chronic illness.) Nursing diagnoses for the client with septic arthritis are similar to those for the client with osteomyelitis.

As with osteomyelitis, client education is vital to management of chronic septic arthritis and its complications. The nurse should instruct the client or caregiver about factors that precipitate joint infections, including infection elsewhere in the body and joint trauma. Other instructions include review of signs and symptoms indicating recurring joint infection, adequate nutrition, adherence to prescribed exercise program, completion of antibiotic therapy, and regular follow-up care.

TUBERCULOSIS OF BONES AND JOINTS

TB of bones and joints (skeletal TB) is a localized destructive disease caused by *Mycobacterium tuberculosis*. A chest x-ray film and complete history and physical should rule out pulmonary TB infection and the need for airborne isolation. As an extrapulmonary manifestation of TB, it cannot be transmitted to others unless the organisms are exposed and aerosolized by debridement or surgical manipulation. TB osteomyelitis or, more commonly, septic arthritis may develop secondary to an active or inactive primary lesion, generally in the respiratory tract. Skeletal TB occurs most frequently in the spinal column (Pott's disease) and in the bone and joint structures surrounding the hip and knee. TB of the spine is the most common and dangerous form. The onset of skeletal TB is insidious, and years may pass without diagnosis while the destructive process continues. Unrecognized and untreated, skeletal TB may produce long-term disability, including pain and paralysis.

Epidemiology

Among infectious diseases, TB is the leading killer of adults in the world today and poses a serious challenge to international public health work. Declared a "global emergency" in 1993 by the World Health Organization (WHO), fully one third of the world's population is now infected with the tubercle bacillus. It is estimated that between 2000 and 2020, nearly 1 billion people will be newly infected, 200 million people will get sick, and 35 million people will die from TB if control is not further strengthened (WHO, 2000).

The disease is especially devastating in developing countries, where it accounts for more than a quarter of all preventable adult deaths. In concert with the AIDS pandemic, TB has overwhelmed health services and devastated urban populations in parts of Africa and is of great concern in Eastern Europe. The biggest burden of TB is in southeast Asia.

In the United States, pulmonary TB has markedly declined in the last 40 years, primarily because of effective drug therapy. However, beginning in 1985, there was a resurgence of TB in the United States, associated with the AIDS epidemic, the influx of immigrants from underdeveloped parts of the world, emergence of multidrug-resistant TB, international travel, and perhaps some increased complacency in the medical community (Cesario, 1995).

Since 1993, there has been a decrease in the incidence of TB in certain geographic regions (New York, California, New Jersey) and certain populations (25- to 44-year age group and people born in the United States). These changes are attributable to improvements in community TB control and treatment programs serving populations at greatest risk for TB (older adults, persons with AIDS, and homeless individuals). Despite this decline, the number of foreign-born people with TB continues to increase, and targeting control of TB in this immigrant population is essential if the current downward trend is to be maintained (McCray, Weinbaum, Braden, & Onorato, 1997).

Skeletal TB occurs in approximately 10% of extrapulmonary TB or 2% to 3% of all cases. Evidence of pulmonary TB is present in fewer than half of skeletal TB cases. The incidence of extrapulmonary and osteoarticular disease has risen during the last decade at a rate exceeding that of lung involvement (Harrington, 2001).

Persons with debilitating disease or compromised immune systems have increased risk because there is depression of natural defense mechanisms that normally prevent dissemination of *M. tuberculosis* from primary lesions to other body parts. Additional risk factors that favor development include untreated primary TB, diabetes mellitus, and end-stage renal disease with hemodialysis treatment. TB remains a disease associated with conditions of inner-city social deprivation.

Manifestations of skeletal TB vary depending on the age of the affected individual and the location of bony involvement. In endemic countries, the incidence of infection is greater in children and young to middle-aged adults, and multifocal skeletal involvement of the ribs, pelvis, vertebrae, feet, and long bones is common. In contrast, in nonendemic countries, the incidence is higher in older and debilitated individuals. Vertebral involvement is most common in the older age group and multifocal involvement, including peripheral joint involvement, may be present in debilitated individuals.

Overall, vertebral TB (Pott's disease) is the most common form of skeletal TB in both adults and children. Lower thoracic and upper lumbar lesions appear most often. In the child, the TB lesion is usually upper thoracic.

Nursing responsibilities associated with skeletal TB include awareness of disease possibility, interventions to prevent disease transmission, health teaching to reduce the incidence of primary TB, and follow-up care for clients diagnosed with the disease. In children it is essential to do a contact investigation to locate and treat the infectious adult source client. Individuals with diagnosed skeletal TB require interventions specific to disease manifestations and treatment protocols. Nursing responsibilities include implementation of rest and exercise programs, dietary teaching, and instruction in medication administration.

Pathophysiology

TB of bones and joints develops secondary to primary TB. Dissemination of *M. tuberculosis* to bone occurs by hematogenous spread, lymphatic transmission from chronic extrapulmonary foci (renal, pleural, or lymph node), or reactivation of a tuberculous lesion. After the initial dissemination, the organism may lie dormant in the skeletal system for long periods before disease is detected. The metaphyseal side of growing ends of long bones is most often affected. Articular TB generally results from a hematogenous source or from an adjacent tuberculous osteomyelitis.

Characteristic alterations appear in bones and joints affected by TB. *M. tuberculosis* produces bone destruction. In contrast to other pyogenic organisms, bone tissue infected with TB makes little or no attempt to defend or protect itself, and very little new bone formation occurs. This process produces the characteristic x-ray appearance of skeletal TB: the presence of bone destruction associated with the relative absence of bone repair.

Bone destruction starts centrally, spreads outward, and may eventually erode into an adjacent joint. If invaded, the synovial membrane responds with excessive secretion, proliferation, and thickening. Tuberculous granulation tissue forms and covers hyaline articular cartilage and subchondral bone.

As the disease advances, caseous necrotic material and tuberculous exudate are produced, causing a buildup of pressure within the bone or joint, which may rupture through the joint capsule or bony cortex as a cold abscess. A cold abscess is filled with necrotic debris, as compared with a hot abscess, which is filled with pyogenic pus. Without effective therapy, the cold abscess may burst through the skin, leading to a draining tuberculous sinus. This process creates a risk for secondary infections in adjacent tissue and bone, leading to complete bone and joint destruction.

The spine is the most common site of TB of bone, with the lower thoracic and upper lumbar regions being most typically involved. This segment of the spine possesses the greatest mobility. Spinal lesions typically begin in the anterior subchondral bone of a single vertebrae adjacent to the intervertebral disc (Fig. 23–6). Progression to bone changes takes 2 to 5 months and begins first from cancellous to cortical bone and then across the disc space to adjacent vertebrae (Fig. 23–7). Bone destruction leads to anterior wedging of the vertebral bodies and, ultimately, to vertebral collapse. Vertebral bodies collapse anteriorly but maintain posterior articulations, producing the typical gibbus deformity (Fig. 23–8*A*) characterized by marked spinal angulation. Multiple vertebral

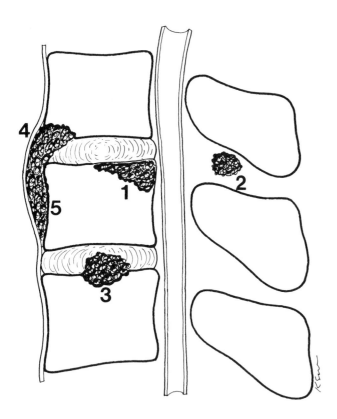

FIGURE 23–6. Tuberculous spondylitis: sites of involvement. Tuberculous lesions can localize in the vertebral body *(1)* or, more rarely, the posterior osseous or ligamentous structures *(2)*. Extension to the intervertebral disc *(3)* or prevertebral tissues *(4)* is not uncommon. Subligamentous spread *(5)* can lead to erosion of the anterior vertebral surface. (From Resnick, D. [1995]. *Diagnosis of bone and joint disorders* [3rd ed., p. 2464]. Philadelphia: WB Saunders.)

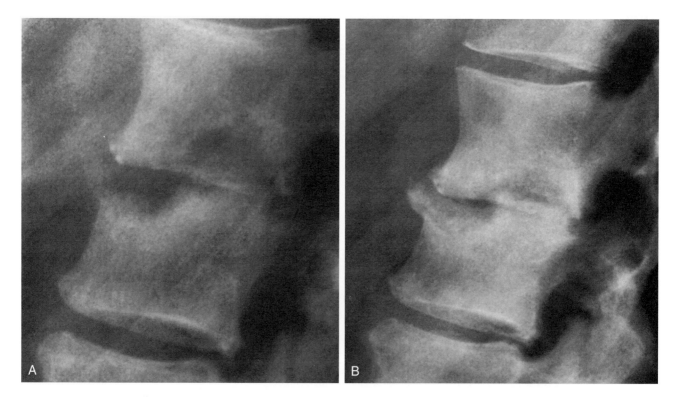

FIGURE 23–7. Tuberculous spondylitis: discovertebral lesion. *A,* The initial radiograph reveals subchondral destruction of two vertebral bodies with mild surrounding eburnation and loss of intervertebral disc height. The appearance is identical to that in pyogenic spondylitis. *B,* Several months later, osseous response is evident. Note the increased sclerosis. Osteophytosis and improved definition of the osseous margins can be seen. (From Resnick, D. [1995]. *Diagnosis of bone and joint disorders* [3rd ed., p. 2465]. Philadelphia: WB Saunders.)

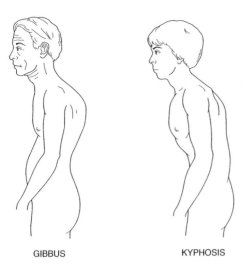

FIGURE 23–8. *A,* Gibbus deformity. *B,* Kyphosis. (From Magee, D. J. [1997]. *Orthopaedic physical assessment* [3rd ed., p. 703]. Philadelphia: WB Saunders.)

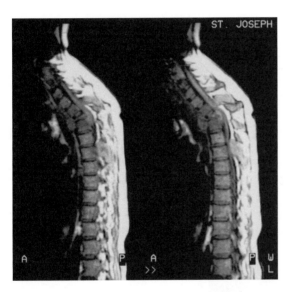

FIGURE 23–9. Kyphotic deformity at T2 pathologic fracture; posterior compression at T1–T2 (just above T2) and T4–T5, there is spinal cord compromise at T2 and T5. (From Huelskamp, L., Anderson, S., & Bernhardt, M. [2000, July/August]. TB of the spine: Pott's disease. *Orthopaedic Nursing, 19*[4], 33.) Reprinted with permission of the publisher, the National Association of Orthopaedic Nursing [NAON], East Holly Avenue, Box 56, Pitman, NJ 08071-0056.)

body collapse may cause a significant kyphotic deformity (Figs. 23–8*B* and 23–9).

With the collapse of the vertebral bodies, the necrotic material may be discharged into the soft tissues, forming a paravertebral abscess. Abscess formation and spinal collapse lead to pain, stiffness, and potential alterations in sensory and motor function.

Appendicular TB occurs primarily within weight-bearing joints, with involvement of the hip joint being most common, followed by knee or ankle involvement. As

with spinal TB, the majority of clients are young children. The disease may occur in a localized area, but eventually it progresses to the entire joint (Fig. 23–10*A*). TB granulation tissue spreads over the articular cartilage of the joint,

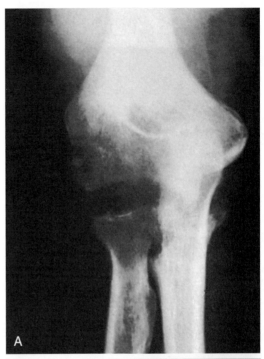

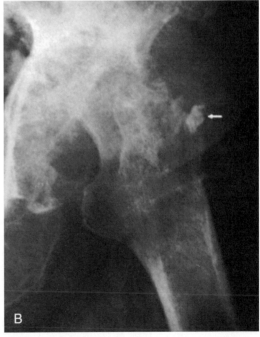

FIGURE 23–10. Tuberculosis arthritis. *A,* Osteopenic and ill-defined osseous destruction involves nearly the entire articular surface. *B,* Chronic tuberculosis infection has resulted in widespread destruction of the femoral head, enlargement and erosion of the acetabulum, prominent osteopenia, and soft tissue calcification *(arrow).* (From Mitchell, M., Howard, B., Haller, J., Sartoris, D. J., & Resnick, D. [1988]. Septic arthritis. *Radiologic Clinics of North America, 26*[6], 1305.)

similar to the pannus formation of rheumatoid arthritis. This process eventually destroys the cartilage and sub-chondral bone. With continued growth of synovial pannus and extravascular formation of fibrin, amorphous fragments—rice bodies—may separate from the margins of synovial granulation (Fig. 23-11). Ultimately, joint collapse may occur with weight bearing (Fig. 23-10*B*).

There are unique differences in manifestations of skeletal TB in the adult and child. Children are likely to develop growth deformities because of the proximity of lesions to growth plates. Lesions tend to heal, however, and bony fusion occurs spontaneously. The adult develops abscesses more frequently and earlier than the child does. Skeletal lesions in the adult rarely show evidence of healing with bony fusion.

Assessment

Data for a comprehensive nursing history are provided in Table 23-6. A history of pulmonary TB in the client or family members and other illnesses that compromise the immune system may be present. The nurse should assess for a history of long-term corticosteroid use or coexisting debilitating diseases, such as diabetes, alcoholism, or chronic renal failure, that compromise resistance.

The onset of skeletal TB is insidious. Signs and symptoms are vague, making an early diagnosis difficult. The disease may have been present for years before the individual seeks treatment. The most common early symptoms are pain, weakness, malaise, fever, chills, night sweats, anorexia, weight loss, and local swelling.

In advanced stages of skeletal TB, muscle atrophy and local tenderness develop. Abscess formation leads to development of sinus tracts, which extend from affected bone to the skin. There may be moderate swelling and redness, with periodic episodes of purulent discharge. Activation of the primary lesion produces classic signs of TB, including low-grade fever, night sweats, anorexia, cough, and weakness.

Spinal involvement (Pott's disease or tuberculous spondylitis) leads to rigidity of the spine, with alterations in posture. There is slight heat, tenderness of the involved area, and decreased joint motion. Disease progression leads to increased pain, with referred pain along nerve roots. The client may report weakness, back and leg pain, and altered sensation. Kyphosis with typical gibbus deformity (see Fig. 23-8) may develop. In very late stages, paraplegia may result from cord compression by abscess or vertebral collapse.

Cervical involvement may cause hoarseness because of recurrent laryngeal nerve paralysis, dysphagia, and respiratory stridor. Torticollis, neck pain, stiffness, and cervical lymphadenopathy may be present (Huelskamp, Anderson, & Bernhardt, 2000).

The sacroiliac joint is involved in up to 10% of cases and is generally unilateral. Buttock pain on the involved side is the presenting symptom and is often accompanied by proximal leg or radicular pain. Sacroiliac tenderness is present (Harrington, 2001).

Diagnostic Evaluation

Skeletal TB must be differentiated from other diseases affecting bones and joints. Diagnostic tools include synovial fluid analysis; biopsies of synovium, bony lesion, or associated lymph node; CBC; and radiologic studies. Table 23-6 summarizes laboratory and radiologic findings.

Initial laboratory studies reveal evidence of chronic illness, including hypochromic anemia, slight leukocyto-

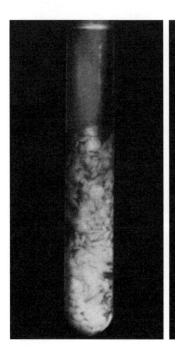
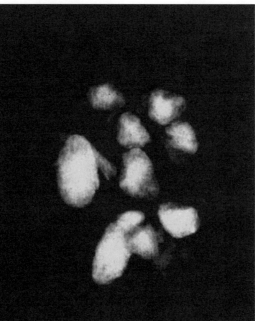

FIGURE 23–11. Rice bodies removed from the knee of a client with systemic lupus erythematosus and *Mycobacterium avium* infection. (From Kelley, W. N., Harris, E. D., Ruddy, S., & Sledge, C. B. [Eds.]. [1993]. *Textbook of rheumatology* [4th ed., p. 1469]. Philadelphia: WB Saunders.)

TABLE 23–6. *Assessment and Management of Skeletal Tuberculosis*

TYPE	HISTORY	PRESENTING SYMPTOMS	DIAGNOSTIC FINDINGS	MANAGEMENT
Skeletal tuberculosis	Pulmonary tuberculosis (often no history of skeletal tuberculosis) Drug abuse Crowded, poor living conditions Diseases that depress immune system Immigration from a country with endemic tuberculosis	Early stages: vague signs and symptoms of long duration Night pain, muscle spasms, swelling of involved joints Minimal local redness and warmth Most often evidence of monoarticular involvement Late stages: develop muscle atrophy May have low-grade fever, night sweats, anorexia, cough if pulmonary tuberculosis reactivated Children may show evidence of growth deformities because of proximity to growth plates	Slight leukocytosis ↑ ESR Anemia Synovial fluid analysis of involved joint: elevated leukocytes (primarily polymorphonuclear), elevated protein, decreased glucose, poor mucin clot PPD may not always be positive Biopsy positive for tubercle bacilli X-ray film changes nonspecific for months to years; late changes include bone decalcification, subchondral osteoporosis Chest x-ray film may reveal evidence of pulmonary tuberculosis	Multidrug approach generally selecting from isoniazid, rifampin, pyrazinamide, ethambutol, streptomycin, or cycloserine Conservative management: Bed rest, traction Surgical management: Synovectomy with curettage removes the focus of infection With severe bone destruction: Focal fusion may be needed to provide bone or joint stability and relieve pain An arthrodesis surgically fuses a joint and eliminates pain Joint replacement is generally not performed as an initial surgical intervention but may be required years later
Spinal tuberculosis (Pott's disease, tuberculous spondylitis)	Same as above	Early stages: similar to initial signs and symptoms for peripheral involvement, except discomfort and decreased ROM in spine Late stages: increased spinal and leg pain, weakness, and altered sensations Spinal deformity (kyphosis) Paraplegia from cord compression or abscess formation	X-ray film evidence: initial changes in anterior portion disc space; late destruction of disc space with anterior wedging Spinal deformity (gibbus or posterior prominence) Other pulmonary changes same as for skeletal tuberculosis	Antitubercular drug regimen as above Conservative management with rest Surgical intervention for the spine is reserved for cases complicated by neurologic abnormality, spinal instability, or large abscess formation Spinal fusion prevents vertebral collapse and neurologic sequelae in the majority of cases

PPD, purified protein derivative.

sis, and elevated ESR. In about 10% of cases, the person presents with a normal WBC count and normal ESR.

Synovial fluid analysis reveals an elevated leukocyte count, with predominance of polymorphonuclear cells, elevated protein, reduced or absent glucose, and poor mucin clot. The most significant finding is tubercle bacilli, which can be seen only with special staining called *acid-fast stain.* The most accurate diagnostic method is biopsy of the synovium, bony lesion, or lymph node to identify the tubercle bacillus. Several samples collected at regular intervals may be required to isolate tubercle bacilli from the affected site.

Tuberculin skin tests may be negative in up to 14% of clients with active disease, but history of a past positive test can provide an important piece of information (Boachie-Adjei & Squillante, 1996). Skin testing is contra-indicated in clients with prior tuberculous infection because of the risk of skin slough from an intense reaction and is therefore not of use in clients with suspected reactivation of the disease. Clients presenting with TB that has disseminated to the joint should also be tested for human immunodeficiency virus (HIV).

Radiologic examination findings are negative in the initial stages of skeletal TB, even though the client reports symptoms. Early findings are nonspecific and include bone atrophy, soft tissue swelling, and destruction of the joint capsule. MRI evaluation provides more exact ana-tomic localization of vertebral and paravertebral ab-scesses.

Radiologic studies may not show evidence of skeletal changes until the disease has been present for months to years. Bone decalcification may be extensive near the involved joints. There is little evidence of new bone formation until late stages of disease, when some healing occurs. Joint space narrowing and joint fusion develop late as a result of the slow destruction of hyaline cartilage by the tuberculous granulation tissue. Bone destruction is more often in peripheral aspects of bone because of the pattern of disease progression.

Spinal TB produces minimal early radiographic changes. There may be evidence of compression of the anterior part of the vertebral body with joint space narrowing and localized osteopenia. With progression of the disease, radiologic studies may demonstrate loss of the disc space and anterior collapse of the vertebral body and posterior spinal prominence (see Fig. 23–9). Ab-scesses may be visualized as soft tissue calcification or loss of the normal psoas shadow. Bone scans are negative in 35% of these clients, and gallium scans are negative in 70% (Huelskamp, Anderson, & Bernhardt, 2000).

MRI helps delineate the soft tissue mass and amount of bony destruction (Boachie-Adjei & Squillante, 1996). Vertebral destruction involving two consecutive levels with sparing of the intervertebral discs suggests the likelihood of TB. Use of a CT-guided biopsy is the best way to confirm the diagnosis (Huelskamp, Anderson, & Bernhardt, 2000).

Chest x-rays films are important when skeletal TB is suspected. The findings of the chest radiographic study may be negative in more than half of the cases, but if positive, it indicates the need for client isolation to protect other clients and health care workers. X-ray films may demonstrate active disease, with multinodular lymph node involvement. Calcified lung lesions indicate previous TB infection. Clients with abnormal chest x-ray films or pulmonary symptoms must be placed in negative-pressure airborne isolation to protect other clients and staff. In the outpatient setting, the client can be masked with a standard surgical mask. Precautions should be continued until infectious pulmonary TB has been ruled out by three negative sputum smears and cultures.

Treatment Modalities and Related Nursing Management in the Acute Stage

Medical and nursing interventions used in skeletal TB are directed toward elimination of underlying TB. General health must be improved, deformities must be mini-mized, and specific antituberculosis drug therapy must be used to eliminate the causative organism. Surgical inter-vention is controversial and is generally reserved for cases of advanced joint involvement with spinal cord compres-sion. The healing process is slow and requires adherence to the established treatment program.

Pharmacologic Management. Generally, regimens that are adequate for treating pulmonary TB in adults and children also are effective for treating bone and joint TB. Treatment should be continued for a minimum of 12 months. The long treatment period is required to prevent relapse of disease and is thought to reflect the fact that some of the bacteria are able to persist in a quiescent or dormant phase in which they are refractory to drug action.

The initial regimen for treating TB should include a multidrug approach generally selecting from isoniazid, rifampin, pyrazinamide, ethambutol, streptomycin, or cycloserine. Regimens for the treatment of TB must contain this multidrug approach to prevent the develop-ment of a bacterial population resistant to the drugs. Multiple drugs kill multiplying organisms by different mechanisms. Use of pyrazinamide potentiates the activity of isoniazid and rifampin. Streptomycin and ethambutol accelerate killing when they are added to isoniazid and rifampin. Isoniazid and rifampin eliminate the slowly multiplying "persisters" that most often cause late re-lapses.

The prevalence of isoniazid resistance is high in many developing countries and generally among Asians and Hispanics. In clients more likely to have drug-resistant strains, therapy should be initiated with at least two drugs that have not been previously used and preferably with three or four drugs for at least 24 months. Directly observed therapy (DOT) is widely advocated.

Surgical Management. Uncomplicated bone and joint TB usually is treated effectively with pharmacologic management. Surgical intervention for the spine is re-served for cases complicated by neurologic abnormality, spinal instability, or large abscess formation. Spinal fusion prevents vertebral collapse and neurologic se-quelae in the majority of cases. (See Chapter 17 for a complete discussion of nursing care for the client undergoing spinal surgery.) Because surgical intervention can aerosolize infectious TB droplet nuclei, all operating personnel must wear N-95 respirators.

Tuberculous synovitis may be treated with surgery in cases of exuberant synovial pannus, loose bodies, and progressive neurologic impairment. Bed rest and traction are used initially to manage the muscle spasm and pain that are present. Combined with antitubercular chemotherapy, this conservative management may induce healing and preserve joint mobility. If conservative therapy is not effective, however, surgical management may be required. A synovectomy with curettage removes the focus of infection. This is generally performed for TB of the knee joint before damage occurs. With severe bone destruction, focal fusion may be needed to provide bone or joint stability and relieve pain. An arthrodesis surgically fuses a joint and eliminates pain (see Chapter 16). Joint replacement is generally not performed as an initial surgical intervention but may be required years later.

Treatment Modalities and Nursing Management in the Chronic or Rehabilitative Phase

Recovery from skeletal TB takes from 1 to 2 years. Drug therapy must be continued during this time. In many cases, the disease has been present for years before its recognition and treatment. Severe bone and joint damage may be present. Loss of normal ROM and potential bony ankylosis is common. Severe kyphosis in spinal TB (Pott's disease) causes discomfort, potential respiratory difficulties, and altered body image. In addition, there is a social stigma associated with the disease of TB.

Nursing has important responsibilities in the recovery phase of skeletal TB. Generally, recovery takes place in the home over a long period. Hospitalization is generally needed only during the diagnosis and initial treatment phase and when surgical intervention is required. A prolonged medication regimen, lengthy hospitalization, or immobilization stresses the client or caregiver and challenges financial and personal resources. The client's living conditions are often not conducive to optimal well-being and must be evaluated for appropriate supports.

Potential for Nonadherence to Long-Term Pharmacologic Management

Teaching: Prescribed Medications, Disease Process, Health System Guidance. Skeletal TB may be considered a chronic disease because of its slow onset and prolonged treatment. Psychological concerns for the client with this disease are similar to those for the client with chronic osteomyelitis, with a special focus on the potential for nonadherence. Medications must be continued for as long as 2 years, even though the client does not feel acutely ill. The client may have few, if any, personal or financial resources. These factors also contribute to nonadherence.

On average, 25% of persons receiving treatment for TB do not complete a recommended regimen within 12 months. Consequently, the client is likely to experience relapse, can be a continued source of transmission, and contributes to the development of drug-resistant strains. Client teaching and guidance are critical to minimizing the risk of nonadherence. If possible, a nurse with the same cultural and linguistic background as the client should be assigned to help develop an individualized treatment adherence plan. One possible strategy is to have the client visit a clinic or be visited by a public health nurse to receive DOT. DOT can be administered intermittently, thereby reducing the total number of doses a client must take. Most DOT regimens are set up so that the client receives medication two or three times per week.

Nursing assessment identifies the client's personal resources and support system, community services, nutritional status, effects of disease and related health problems, educational level, environmental surroundings, and ability to comply with treatment plans. In long-term care, the nurse must emphasize the need for follow-up visits at regular intervals, usually every 6 weeks to 2 months, repeated radiographic evaluation of skeletal changes, and diagnostic workup for anemia or possible alteration in liver and kidney function secondary to medication.

Impaired Physical Mobility

Exercise Therapy: Joint Mobility. Emphasis in care of the client with skeletal TB is on control and eradication of infection, with maintenance of optimal joint function. Manifestations of impaired mobility vary widely, ranging from joint stiffness of the affected part to possible paralysis with spinal involvement. Immobilization of the involved joint may be required initially, often followed by physical therapy to promote optimal joint mobility. Resources are identified to help the client meet his or her particular needs.

Pain

Pain Management. Mild to moderate pain may be experienced by the client with skeletal TB. In addition to positioning the extremity in a position of comfort, immobilization measures may help reduce the pain. Narcotic analgesics are required after surgical intervention. Non-narcotic analgesics are used in the chronic phase to control the pain and increase the client's ability to perform needed exercises and activities.

POSTPOLIO SEQUELAE

Postpolio sequelae is a term used to encompass a group of poliomyelitis-related symptoms that develop anytime from 10 to 70 years after the original onset of polio. The more severe the acute polio, the earlier new symptoms are likely to occur. These symptoms include unaccustomed fatigue; return of weakness and pain to the muscles previously involved; development of weakness and pain in additional muscles; joint pain, respiratory, swallowing and speech difficulties; and heat or cold intolerance. In clients whose acute disease included bulbar involvement, difficulty in swallowing or change of voice may occur. Nomenclature for these symptoms includes postpolio syndrome (PPS), postpolio muscle atrophy (PPMA), late effects of polio, and progressive postpolio muscular atrophy.

Epidemiology

The epidemiology of PPS remains unclear. Data regarding the incidence and prevalence of PPS is quite variable (Jubelt & Drucker, 1999). Estimates of prevalence suggest that between 25% and 75% of those who experienced paralytic poliomyelitis now have PPS. Falconer and Bollenbach (2000) predict that all people who had paralytic poliomyelitis will develop some degree of PPS.

Risk factors that predispose clients to the development of PPS include a more advanced age at acute polio infection, a greater length of time since acute polio, a greater severity of initial polio and resulting paralysis, a greater recovery in muscular strength after poliomyelitis, and presence of permanent impairment after recovery from poliomyelitis (Jubelt & Drucker, 1999). In those who do recover totally or partially, overexertion or overuse appears to be a factor in the development of PPS.

It has recently been recognized that PPS can occur in individuals who had subclinical, abortive, or nonparalytic poliomyelitis (Bruno, 2000; Halstead & Silver, 2000). The threat of PPS therefore lies with all survivors of polio no matter its initial extent (Saxon, 2001).

Pathophysiology

The pathogenesis of PPS remains unknown. Several hypotheses have been formulated. Following the acute polio stage, it is postulated that neuronal sprouts are developed by surviving motor neurons to replace destroyed neurons (Fig. 23–12). It is thought that enlarged motor units that develop via sprouting may never fully stabilize and become unstable later in life because of (1) inability to sustain their function because of increased metabolic demands over several decades, (2) decreasing number of sprouts over time, and (3) breakage of axonal sprouts following chronic stress and exercise over a period of years without the ability to regenerate. Electromyographic (EMG) studies show a correlation between the decreasing number of sprouts and their ability to function within the number of years since the polio onset.

Some researchers have proposed that normal aging alone can explain the appearance of the syndrome in the older adult. After the age of 60 to 70, there is a decrease in

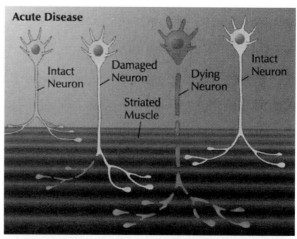

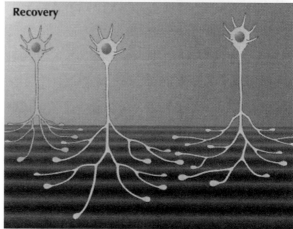

FIGURE 23–12. Changes in a muscle's motor innervation during and after acute paralytic poliomyelitis amount to a remodeling of motor units (the constellation of muscle fibers governed by a given motor neuron). In the acute disease, some motor neurons die entirely, and others lose axon collaterals but may otherwise survive. During recovery, distal sprouting from the axons of both damaged and intact motor neuronals may resupply denervated muscle fibers, thus enlarging the muscle's motor units and contributing to restoration of function. Continued reshaping of motor units may maintain functional stability for many years. (From Bartfeld, H., & Ma, D. [1996]. Recognizing post-polio syndrome. *Hospital Practice, 31*[5], 95. © 1996 the McGraw-Hill Companies, Inc. Reproduced with permission.)

the number of motor neurons in the spinal cord. The polio survivor enters this aging period already having lost a considerable number of motor neurons. It is proposed that additional age-related loss may further contribute to previously existing muscle weakness. However, the fact that many polio survivors develop PPS before their sixth decade refutes this theory.

Another proposed mechanism is motor neuronal loss resulting from reactivation of a persistent, latent virus. It is proposed that poliovirus may persist in the central nervous system (CNS) and cause delayed or chronic disease; however, this mechanism has not been supported with consistent empirical data. Immune-mediated responses, hormonal deficiencies, and environmental toxins are other mechanisms that are being investigated (Saxon, 2001).

Some PPS symptoms may occur because residual weakness leads to joint and muscle misuse and overuse, placing secondary strains on muscles, ligaments, and joints. This may lead to both arthritis and overuse syndromes.

Fatigue, the most prominent symptom of PPS, has been postulated to result from age and polio-related attrition of neurons in the substantia nigra and possible degeneration of reticular formation neurons (Bruno, Sapolsky, Zimmerman, & Frick, 1995) or from diffuse deterioration of the motor unit at the neuromuscular junction (Packer, Martins, Krefting, & Brouwer, 1991).

New onset of progressive muscle weakness appears to be related to a disintegration of the lower motor neuron unit and can occur in muscles previously affected and partially or fully recovered or in unaffected muscles (Jubelt & Drucker, 1999).

Assessment

In the diagnostic phase, an accurate, comprehensive nursing history targeting the common cluster of symptoms is vital (Box 23-1). Because there is no definitive test and because some of the symptoms are nonspecific, it may be difficult to diagnose PPS and differentiate it from other syndromes and diagnoses with similar symptoms.

On questioning, the client generally reports a gradual deterioration in functional capacity. The onset of this deterioration has been reported to be insidious, although

---

BOX 23-1.

Clinical Concerns in Postpolio Syndrome: An Approach to History Taking

Onset

Can be insidious or acute. Question about presence of increased stress, weight gain, or recent injury or illness.

Fatigue

Determine presence of muscle fatigue. When does it occur, and what muscles seem most affected? Central fatigue should be assessed by determining presence of overall sense of fatigue with inability to stay awake, attention deficits, inability to concentrate, and memory impairment.

Muscle Weakness

Determine location, extent, and precipitating factors. Is the weakness in new or previously affected muscle groups? Assess for presence of atrophy accompanying the weakness. Does the client report any falls or other motor limitations resulting from the weakness? Has endurance been affected and to what extent?

Pain

Describe location, scope, severity, and characteristics of pain. Note sensitivity to pain.

Pulmonary Dysfunction

Question about dyspnea on exertion and dyspnea at rest. Assess for prolonged or recurring respiratory infections that may indicate difficulty clearing respiratory secretions.

Sleep Disorders

Does client report awakening feeling refreshed or still tired? Does client awaken frequently at night for no apparent reason?

Dysphagia

Any problems with eating or swallowing? Does client complain of food sticking, making it difficult to swallow? episodes of coughing, choking? Has client modified diet or eating patterns?

Dysphonia

Any hoarseness, slurring of words, difficulty maintaining vocal tone and modulation?

Cold Intolerance

Does client experience limb coldness? Does client feel increased weakness in the presence of cold?

Functional Abilities

Determine the extent to which symptoms have affected the client's functional abilities. Have occupational modifications been needed? Are assistive devices being used that were not previously used? Have recreational or social activities been interrupted? Is there a need for assistance with cooking, cleaning, shopping, or other activities of daily living? Is there a need for assistance with hygiene care?

Emotional Status

Assess for levels of frustration, anxiety, grief reaction, presence of depression.

Coping Strategies

How did person cope with residual effects of polio—normalizing, minimizing, or identifying? What adaptations and accommodations has the person used to adapt to the new symptoms—adaptive aids, energy conservation, rests or naps, job modification, eating changes, support groups, activity pacing? What are the client's strategies for dealing with emotions?

acute episodes of injury, illness, or other stressors may precipitate the onset. The most common symptoms are fatigue, pain, and weakness. Fatigue is the most common manifestation and is generally described as a disabling generalized exhaustion or what is termed the "polio wall." It follows even minimal physical activity. The fatigue can be perceived as generalized (overall exhaustion, difficulty concentrating, tiredness, lack of energy) or muscular in origin (increasing loss of strength during exercise). It may be severe enough to interfere with normal role activities.

New, slowly progressive muscle weakness is the most important neurologic problem. The distribution of new weakness correlates with the severity of paralysis at the time of acute poliomyelitis and with the amount of recovery and thus with the number of surviving motor neurons (Jubelt & Drucker, 1999). Initial symptoms are most frequent in the lower limb that was most affected by the acute illness. In a small number of cases, upper motor neuron signs can occur such as hyperreflexia, Babinski's sign, and occasionally spasticity. Muscle pain or myalgia may occur presumably from overuse of weak muscles. The pain is a soreness or aching feeling and may appear with even minimal exercise or exposure to the cold. Atrophy may accompany the weakness.

Muscle weakness can involve specific muscle groups and is associated with symptoms of respiratory insufficiency, bulbar muscle weakness, and sleep apnea. Respiratory insufficiency, in part resulting from weakness of the diaphragm and intercostals muscles, is more likely to occur in those individuals who required respiratory support during the acute disease. Dyspnea on exertion and, less commonly, dyspnea at rest may be reported. The nurse should inquire about recurring or prolonged respiratory infections and the ability to cough and clear sputum because poor clearance of respiratory secretions may occur with muscular weakness. In severe cases, nighttime respiratory support may be required and, in the worst-case scenario, total ventilator support. Sleep disorders (sleep apnea) have been reported as a significant problem. Poor sleep quality and frequent awakenings have been described. This may result from pain and pharyngeal and respiratory muscle weakness, or there may be a central sleep apnea condition resulting from residual damage to the brainstem reticular formation.

Dysphagia, dysphonia, or choking may be present in clients with previous bulbar involvement but may also occur as a new symptom. The nurse should inquire about difficulty with eating or swallowing. It is important to determine whether the client has made modifications in the diet and eating processes. Clients with dysphagia also frequently report dysphonia with progressive speech difficulty marked by increased hoarseness, vocal weakness, or slurring.

Some clients with PPS report cold intolerance. The limbs may be cold, and cold is noted to produce weakness and fatigue. This is thought to be a result of intermedio-lateral column involvement causing vasoparesis, venous pooling, and excessive heat loss.

The nurse should determine the extent to which symptoms have challenged the individual's functional abilities. The main impact of disability for most clients is in mobility-related activities and instrumental ADLs, such as cooking, transportation, cleaning, and shopping. Falling and an increase in the use of assistive devices (e.g., cane, crutches, respirators) may also be identified.

Musculoskeletal concerns in the PPS client relate to pain from joint instability. The long-term overstress of joints because of residual weakness eventually results in joint deterioration (Jubelt & Drucker, 1999). Progressive scoliosis, poor posture, unusual mechanics because of deformed joints, uneven limb size, failing tendon transfers, and failing joint fusions can all contribute to joint pain. These problems may interfere with mobility and necessitate a return to using old assistive devices.

Psychological stress accompanies the reemergence of a supposedly resolved problem. The nurse should explore the coping strategies the client uses to adapt to the new set of symptoms. It is important to keep in mind that renewed disabilities rekindle old emotions and old fears and create a new sense of disillusionment. These clients have survived and learned to cope with their original disability and believed that they were cured and that it was "over with." Now, they must cope with the new deficits and find new ways of coping because many of the old mechanisms of fighting through the fatigue, persisting through pain, and not giving in are counterproductive in face of the new disabilities.

Physical Examination and Diagnostic Evaluation

No diagnostic test exists for PPS, and the diagnosis is predominantly one of exclusion. Box 23-1 shows the common symptoms that require assessment. Careful evaluation and exclusion of medical, musculoskeletal, neurologic, and psychiatric illnesses that may cause health problems similar to PPS is essential.

The physical assessment of the client is directed at the strength of the muscle groups. A complete neurosensory evaluation is done to assist in ruling out neurologic disease. The neurologic examination should identify atrophy or weakness and verify that reflexes are normal. Because of the insidious onset of PPS, the client may be unaware of significant weakness of the good limb. Careful emphasis should be given to evaluating vital capacity and swallowing.

Electrophysiologic testing can be helpful in the differential diagnosis to rule out neuropathy, radiculopathy, and myopathy or to confirm previous anterior horn cell disease. Nerve conduction studies generally show normal sensory nerve conduction, but motor nerve conduction shows slowing because of a loss of motor units from the original polio infection. Needle EMG assessment may show signs of denervation and muscle reinnervation in which axon sprouting increases the size of motor units. Muscle biopsies of newly weakened muscle may show histologic evidence of denervation.

Blood and spinal fluids are analyzed to evaluate immunologic status and to rule out other neurologic disease. Oligoclonal bands (IgG) and elevated antibodies to poliovirus in serum with no accompanying elevation in spinal fluid indicates no reactivation of the original poliovirus. X-ray films are used to rule out joint and spinal column disease. Pulmonary function testing is done if the client exhibits respiratory problems.

Treatment Modalities and Nursing Management in the Rehabilitative Phase

There is no specific treatment for PPS. The major focus is on rehabilitation to promote optimal function of the client while minimizing fatigue. The rehabilitative phase after diagnosis must emphasize education about the disease, counseling regarding the client's involvement, integration of the rest-activity regimen, and increasing muscular endurance.

The focus of physical therapy is to increase muscle capacity by achieving increased strength or endurance. Screening for inefficiency in movement resulting from deformity or weakness is the first step in evaluation. The muscles are carefully evaluated; muscles already functioning at their maximum should not be taken through isometric development because this may produce injury. An individualized exercise plan supervised by a physical therapist is developed so that specific muscles and exercises are selected for training and the regimen avoids exercise-induced fatigue by the incorporation of intervening rest as needed. Muscle capacity can also be increased by bracing, orthotics, or other aids that extend, amplify, or substitute for muscle strength. Anti-inflammatory medications, heat, and massage may be beneficial.

Pharmacologic management is primarily symptomatic. Respiratory insufficiency can be managed with noninvasive intermittent positive-pressure treatments using nasal masks and mouthpieces. Fatigue can be managed by rest and paced physical activities. Medications such as amantadine, amitriptyline, pyridostigmine, and pemoline have been found useful in some cases, but additional controlled studies are needed. Acupuncture (auriculotherapy) has been used with some clients.

Anxiety, Fear, Grief, Defensive Coping

Anxiety Reduction, Coping Enhancement, Environmental Management, Emotional Support, Cognitive Restructuring. Recurrence of symptoms has been likened to being hit with a sledge hammer because individuals must face new disabilities while continuing to manage memories of past polio-related experiences. They are continuing to cope with the original disability and now must go through the process of accepting a second

disability that is similar in symptoms but different in management from the initial one. Emotional reactions are understandably variable and may include denial, anger, fear, sadness, frustration, hopelessness, and powerlessness. Fear is a common emotion with PPS because the course and extent of symptom progression is unknown. The client may picture himself or herself moving from needing a brace, to needing crutches, to needing a wheelchair and being dependent.

Understanding how the person coped with the initial polio disability may be helpful in understanding the individual's current response to symptoms. Maynard's (1986) description of three patterns of coping with chronic disability—passers, minimizers, and identifiers—applies to the client with PPS. Described in detail in Chapter 2, one can anticipate coping problems based on the identified style. Passers have a mild disability that they actively work to keep hidden and may experience great distress at having to adjust to the late effects of polio. Minimizers are those with a moderate disability that can easily be recognized by others and who have coped using overachievement as a strategy. Such persons may have difficulty recognizing new changes because they are insensitive to their own pain, sadness, weakness, and anger. Identifiers had more severe deficits and fully identified with their disability to make lifestyle adaptations and cope successfully. Many of these individuals used wheelchair mobility before the onset of PPS and now must confront the loss of their independence as functional changes occur. These changes challenge their freedom to control their life activities and purpose for living.

Psychological support may be achieved by sharing emotions and providing information about essential community resources to help meet their needs. Attention to various psychosocial needs, such as health insurance, home care, accessible housing, transportation, vocational counseling, and treatment for grief, is an important component the client's care. Hope is instilled by helping individuals see that decline and deterioration are not inevitable and can be modified by energy management, physical therapy, and weight management techniques. Staying in the present rather than focusing on comparing present function to past function or projecting future deterioration is critical. Clients must be helped to focus on what can be done rather than what cannot be done. Clients should write down tasks they have accomplished during the day to illustrate all that gets accomplished. The nurse should give clients recognition for what they accomplish (including giving credit for rest), and the clients will begin to give themselves credit. Clients should be assisted in setting realistic expectations that allow them to feel success. Support groups can provide information sharing that is helpful in setting realistic expectations. Other informational resources include the Easter Seal Society, March of Dimes, and many Internet sources for polio and postpolio resources.

For many clients, one of the most difficult parts of the coping process is restructuring their understanding and approach to their symptoms. Clients must reverse everything they were told during the acute phase of the disease to cope with its late effects (Foster, Berkman, Wellen, & Schuster, 1993). The initial paradigm of treatment was "Use it or lose it" or "Push till it hurts—then push a little harder." These individuals adopted the values of pushing hard and having a hard work ethic. Now, clients are hearing a contradictory paradigm: "Slow down; don't push so hard; don't work so hard." This seems to go against the nature of many individuals because slowing down is equated with giving up. Understandably, this paradigm shift is stressful. Support with fatigue management and pacesetting is critical to this adjustment process.

Fatigue and Activity Intolerance

Energy Management, Sleep Enhancement, Weight Management. The new golden rule for postpolio is "If something you do causes fatigue, weakness, or pain, you should not be doing it." Protection of quality of life requires decreasing physical and emotional stress through moderation and pacing of activities, the use of appropriate assistive devices, and reducing hard-driving type A behavior (Bruno & Frick, 1991). Clients must be told that research shows that progression of PPS is at least halted and symptoms are reduced when clients start to take these measures.

Energy management involves regulation of energy expenditure to treat or prevent fatigue and to optimize function. Careful history taking can identify the individual's peak performance and factors that contribute to fatigue. Activity plans are made starting at about 50% of peak performance, modifying fatigue factors, and incorporating rest. A slow increase in performance is managed according to client tolerance.

Pacing of activity is the foundation of successful lifestyle modification. Box 23-2 describes work simplification techniques that will be helpful to clients. The nurse should suggest that clients keep a log of daily activities and the length of time they participate before experiencing fatigue. This provides the information needed to suggest breaking up activities into smaller units of activity followed by rest. Energy budgeting is another emphasis where clients are assisted to determine what their personal priority activities are. Recognizing that there is a relatively fixed amount of energy (that may increase with management), clients are encouraged to spend it in activities of high personal value.

Weight management may be needed to decrease muscle load. Use of orthotics to improve mechanical efficiency and use of wheelchairs or scooters to save energy expenditure may be recommended, but the nurse must be sensitive to the meaning of these interventions to the client.

BOX 23–2.
Postpolio Syndrome Energy Conservation and Work Simplification Measures

Observe proper body positioning at work and at rest. Use firm chairs with arms and full back support. Adjust work surface heights to encourage good posture. Wear low-heeled shoes that provide good arch support.
Periodically change position (stand, move around in the chair). Avoid staying in one position for long periods because this can fatigue muscles. If required to stand for long periods, stand on a soft surface. Be sure to take rest breaks when driving or standing for long periods.
Use proper body mechanics. When holding an object, hold it close to the body. When possible, place items in a cart or on counter rather than holding objects for any length of time.
Try to get enough rest; 8 to 10 hours of sleep per night and naps during the day may help. When possible, lie down because sitting requires two thirds more energy. Pace activities with rest times. Alternate light and heavy tasks. During stressful times, increase your rest periods and use stress reduction techniques (e.g., deep breathing, relaxation exercises).
Choose and prioritize your activities. Make a list of activities you wish to accomplish. Prioritize these tasks considering what must be done and what is enjoyable to do. Evaluate each activity to determine consequences if the activity is delayed temporarily or done by another individual. Are you the best person to do this task? Is the activity necessary? When choosing tasks, make a balance between enjoyable and required tasks. Plan activities to eliminate unnecessary motion.
Each activity done should be broken down into steps. Each step should be evaluated to see if energy expenditure could be decreased. Small appliances or assistive devices may help decrease energy expenditure. Use appliances (electric mixers) and utensils that do not require holding. Position tools before activity so they are easy to grasp and start work immediately.

Clients experiencing chronic pain and weakness are likely to have sleep deficits that contribute to the fatigue and changes in cognitive functioning. Nighttime sleep difficulties may be associated with daytime napping, needed for energy restoration. Pain management, muscle relaxation, and other comfort measures, along with environmental regulation may be helpful in promoting sleep.

Impaired Swallowing

Swallowing Therapy. In postpolio clients who experience swallowing difficulty, an interdisciplinary team, including occupational therapist, speech therapist, and nutritional therapist, is essential. A swallowing exercise program is initiated. Clients should be instructed on eating/swallowing techniques that prevent complications. Postural techniques include sitting in an erect position to eat with the head positioned in forward flexion. Eating or dietary modifications require all solid foods to be cut into small pieces (a soft diet may be required for some), reinforcement of the need to eat slowly and chew thoroughly, and emphasis that small sips of liquids should be taken and straws should be avoided.

Ineffective Airway Clearance and Breathing Patterns

Respiratory Monitoring, Ventilatory Support. Maximizing respiration is the goal in treating the client with PPS who experiences respiratory insufficiency. General pulmonary toilet including positioning for effective breathing, ensuring adequate fluid intake, and coughing and deep breathing should be practiced regularly by the client. Mouthpiece intermittent positive-pressure ventilation, nasal intermittent positive-pressure ventilation, manually and mechanically assisted coughing, and monitoring oxygen saturation at home can become the mainstays of care. Clients should be aware of medications that can depress respiratory function. Smoking cessation and prevention of respiratory infection with annual vaccines and by avoidance of people with infections are important practices for respiratory health.

Alteration in Comfort, Pain

Physical Comfort Promotion, Positioning, Pain Management. Clients must adapt a new mindset that recognizes pain as a potential problem, which should be managed or relieved. Polio survivors are twice as sensitive to pain as the normal population. This increased sensitivity occurs because endogenous opiate-secreting cells in the brain and spinal cord were damaged by the poliovirus. To achieve adequate pain relief, higher dosages of pain medication may be required (Bruno, 1997). Pain can be aggravated by cold, so appropriate climate control and layered clothing may be helpful.

Impaired Physical Mobility

Exercise Promotion, Joint Protection, Weight Loss, Assistive Support. Decreasing mechanical stress on joints and muscles with lifestyle changes such as losing weight, decreasing activities that cause overuse, and using assistive devices (including orthoses, wheelchairs, and adaptive equipment) can all contribute to maximizing mobility and function. Stretching exercises and nonfatiguing strengthening exercises (submaximal, short duration) can improve strength and should be planned with the physical therapist.

LYME DISEASE

Lyme disease is a complex, immune-mediated, multisystem disorder. It is caused by infection with a bacterial spirochete, *Borrelia burgdorferi*, which is transmitted to humans by a bite from an infected tick of the genus *Ixodes*. An early symptom is a distinctive skin rash referred to as *erythema migrans* (EM). In later stages, the disease may progress to include cardiac, neurologic, and arthritic complications. Lyme disease can usually be treated successfully with standard antibiotic regimens.

Epidemiology

In 1975, several cases of what appeared to be juvenile rheumatoid arthritis were noted to have occurred within a small area in and around Lyme, Connecticut. As a result of the investigation into this unusual clustering of cases, the disease was first described as Lyme arthritis. Since 1975, the incidence of Lyme disease has steadily risen and the geographic areas in which it is known to occur have widened considerably. In 1984, it surpassed Rocky Mountain spotted fever as the leading tick-borne illness in the United States.

Based on records kept by the Centers for Disease Control and Prevention (CDC), there was a 25-fold increase in reported cases of Lyme disease between 1982 and 1995. In examining prevalence data from 1992 to 1998, the CDC reports an increase in cases from 9896 in 1992 to 16,802 in 1998 (CDC, 2000c). This increased incidence likely results from both a true increase in incidence as well as from improved reporting systems. It is believed that the disease remains underreported, with 7 to 12 unreported cases for each reported case. This corresponds with the seasonal feeding activity of nymphal *Ixodes scapularis*.

Those affected with the disease range in age from 1 to 81 years, with the highest mean annual incidence occurring among children (5 to 9 years) and adults (45 to 54 years). Males are affected slightly more often than females. A majority of cases occur in the 4-month period from May through August, with the peak incidence in June and July.

A total of 92% of Lyme cases have been reported from three endemic geographic regions of the United States: the coastal areas of the Northeast (from Massachusetts to Maryland), the North-central states (Minnesota and Wisconsin), and the West Coast (especially northern California). The disease, however, continues to spread beyond these endemic areas and has been reported in 49 states and the District of Columbia.

The main vector for transmission of the disease is the *Ixodes* tick. In the Northeast and Midwest, the main vector is *I. scapularis*, commonly called the *deer tick*. In the West, it is *Ixodes pacificus*. The major endemic areas correlate well with the range of *Ixodes*. The natural 2-year life cycle of *I. scapularis*, with its implications for the transmission of infection to humans, is illustrated in Figure 23–13. Adult

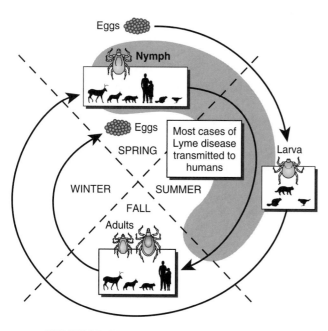

FIGURE 23–13. Life cycle of Lyme disease ticks.

ticks feed and mate on large animals, especially deer, in the fall and early spring. The female tick drops off the animal to deposit eggs on the ground. Larvae hatch the following early summer and feed on white mice, who serve as a reservoir for the spirochete *B. burgdorferi.* The larvae are inactive until the next spring, when they enter the nymphal stage. Tick larvae are not considered important in the transmission of Lyme disease to humans.

In the nymphal stage, the tick clings to the underside of vegetation, which may be tall grass or brush located in sand dunes, lawns, or at the edge of woods. It is during this stage that humans are most likely to encounter the tick. There must be direct contact with the nymph because nymphs cannot jump or fly. Its small size at this stage makes it difficult to see or feel. Consequently, the nymph may attach to a human without it being noticed, giving it ample time to feed and transmit the infection. The nymph is most active from May through July, when outdoor activities are at their peak.

The nymphs become adults in the fall, completing the 2-year life cycle. Adult ticks are easier to detect and remove because of their size. They are also most active in cooler weather, when there is less outdoor activity. For these reasons, the danger of adult ticks transmitting infection to humans is much less than in the nymph stage.

Pathophysiology

The spirochete *B. burgdorferi* is transmitted by the bite of an infected tick. Passage of *B. burgdorferi* to humans is delayed for many hours after the initial attachment of the tick. Attachment for less than 24 hours is rarely associated with *B. burgdorferi* transmission, whereas attachment for 72 hours or more uniformly transmits the disease

(CDC, 1992). The disease is not spread person to person or by direct contact with an infected animal.

EM, a characteristic red circular rash, usually appears at the site of the bite by an infected tick. The patch expands and may clear in the center, resembling a bull's-eye. Allergic reactions to tick saliva may be mistaken for EM but usually occur within hours to days after the tick bite, do not expand, and disappear in a few days. The organism may then spread to the lymph nodes, and from there disseminate, via the blood, to other organs of the body (CNS, liver, spleen, skin, synovial joints).

The complications of Lyme disease arise from the body's immune response to the invading organism. The later manifestations may actually mimic several immune-mediated disorders, such as juvenile rheumatoid arthritis, Reiter's syndrome, rheumatic fever, Guillain-Barré syndrome, and multiple sclerosis. There is evidence that by the time EM appears, almost all clients have abnormal circulating immune complexes. These complexes are the result of an intense reaction between antibody (of the IgM class) and the presence of antigen. The source and nature of this antigen have not been clearly identified. It may be part of *B. burgdorferi* itself, or it may be a substance endogenously produced by the body in response to the presence of *B. burgdorferi.*

It is postulated that the initial clinical manifestation (the appearance of EM) is the result of an immune-mediated inflammatory reaction that is initially associated with these circulating immune complexes. Either tissue deposition of these complexes or more widespread dissemination of the spirochete causing the formation of more immune complexes throughout the body is responsible for subsequent cardiac and neurologic dysfunction. Localization of the spirochete to joints, with a subsequent immune activation forming immune complexes in the joints, accounts for arthritic manifestations.

Often, three clinical stages are described in Lyme disease: stage 1 (localized), stage 2 (disseminated), and stage 3 (late or persistent). Table 23–7 describes the three stages and the signs and symptoms associated with each. Stage 1 occurs within 1 to 30 days of the initial bite. During this stage, *B. burgdorferi* spreads locally in the skin. EM, seen in up to 90% of cases, may appear within 4 to 21 days after a tick bite and generally fades within 3 to 4 weeks; however, it may recur. The rash is often mistaken for tinea corporis. Within several days of the onset of EM, almost half of the clients develop multiple secondary annular lesions. These lesions are less migratory. They may occur anywhere but the palms and soles. Sometimes, the characteristic and distinctive rash (EM) is absent. Flulike symptoms, such as headache, fever, and chills, and regional lymphadenopathy (with or without fever) may be present. Generalized aches and in some cases complaints of slight joint pain may be present.

Stage 2 occurs within weeks to months after the initial infection. During this stage, *B. burgdorferi* spreads via lymph and blood to many sites within the body. Secondary annular lesions may appear. These lesions resemble the primary lesion but are smaller. Generalized lymphadenopathy, sore throat, abdominal pain, cough, severe malaise and fatigue, conjunctivitis, mild or recurrent hepatitis, and microscopic hematuria or proteinuria may also be present. These symptoms are often intermittent and changing and are therefore easily confused with a number of viral illnesses. During the second stage, cardiac, neurologic, and musculoskeletal complications may arise.

Neurologic complications of stage 2 include a triad of meningitis, cranial neuritis, and radiculoneuritis. Meningitis is characterized by headache and stiff neck, but Kernig's and Brudzinski's signs are absent. The cranial neuritis usually involves cranial nerve VII, resulting in facial palsies (Bell's palsy). Often, Bell's palsy is the only neurologic manifestation. Neurologic symptoms may recur or become chronic. In some instances, more serious neurologic complications may occur. There is now some indication that neurologic demyelination syndromes may appear as later sequelae in some clients.

The cardiac complications of stage 2 occur in about 4% to 8% of clients with Lyme disease. The most common finding is acute onset of atrioventricular block. Myopericarditis and left ventricular dysfunction may occur. Cardiac manifestations may last for months but usually resolve completely, although they may recur.

TABLE 23–7. *Stages of Lyme Disease*

STAGE	ONSET	POSSIBLE SIGNS AND SYMPTOMS
Stage 1: localized (*Borrelia burgdorferi* spreads locally in the skin)	1–30 day after initial bite (mean, 7–10 days)	Erythema migrans (usually fades within 3–4 weeks but may recur) Regional generalized lymphadenopathy (may be accompanied by fever) Fatigue, malaise, lethargy Generalized aches, myalgias, arthralgias

Stage 2: disseminated (*B. burgdorferi* spreads via lymph and blood to many sites)	Occurs days to 10 months after the tick bite	Secondary annular lesions (occur in about 50% of cases, resemble primary lesion but are generally smaller)
		 Generalized lymphadenopathy
		 Severe malaise and fatigue
		 Conjunctivitis, iritis, choroiditis
		 Mild or recurrent hepatitis
		 Microscopic hematuria or proteinuria
		 Carditis (8%–10% of untreated clients)
		    Conduction defects: atrioventricular block
		    Mild cardiomyopathy
		 Neurologic (10%–12% of untreated individuals)
		    Meningitis
		    Cranial neuritis (especially Bell's palsy or shoulder-girdle neuritis)
		    Photophobia
		    Memory loss
		    Radiculoneuritis
		    Encephalitis
		 Musculoskeletal (about 50% of untreated individuals)
		    Migratory pain in joints (especially knees), tendons, bursae, muscle, bone
		    Brief arthritic attacks

Stage 3: late or persistent	Occurs months to years after the tick bite	Musculoskeletal
		    About 50% of untreated cases develop migratory polyarthritis
		    About 10% of untreated cases develop chronic monoarthritis, usually of the knee
		 Cutaneous
		    Localized scleroderma-like lesions
		    Keratitis
		 Neurologic
		    Chronic encephalomyelitis
		    Chronic peripheral neuropathy
		    Ataxia, dementia, sleep disorder

The musculoskeletal complications of stage 2 include migratory pain in joints, tendons, bursae, muscle, and bones and brief arthritic attacks. Arthritic involvement is characterized by recurrent, brief attacks (lasting weeks to months) of swelling in one or a few large joints. The brief attacks preceding a chronic, progressive arthritis are the critical parameter in differentiating Lyme arthritis from other forms of arthritis.

Stage 3, often referred to as *chronic Lyme disease,* occurs 1 year or more after the initial bite. This stage may be marked by the presence of fatigue, localized scleroderma, keratitis, chronic encephalomyelitis, prolonged arthritic attacks, and chronic arthritis. Arthritic attacks persist into stage 3 in a majority of the individuals initially infected. At this point, a characteristic pattern usually develops. In this pattern, each episode of arthritis lasts longer than the previous one. These attacks may range in length from weeks to months and can occur for several years. Eventually, however, the frequency of attacks begins to decline.

The stages of Lyme disease may overlap, and almost any clinical feature may occur alone or may recur at intervals. Symptoms are found to flare about every 4 weeks, which is thought to represent the organism's cell cycle, with the growth phase occurring once per month. Antibiotics are effective only during the growth period, which is why the minimum treatment duration should be at least 4 weeks. Some clients may never develop the symptoms of a particular stage. It is estimated that 15% of clients develop neurologic symptoms, about 8% develop cardiac dysfunction, and about 60% develop the arthritis characteristics of stage 3.

The number of clients who have recurrences decreases by 10% to 20% each year. It is not understood why in some clients with late Lyme disease symptoms eventually diminish or disappear, whereas in other clients the symptoms persist. It is thought that in some cases the spirochete may evade the immune system. It then survives in numbers too low to be detected by conventional tests yet high enough to produce illness. Persistent symptoms also may be the result of an overactive immune response that continues to injure the host's tissues long after the organism has been eradicated. Randomized, controlled studies of clients who remain unwell after standard courses of antibiotic therapy for Lyme disease are in progress, and interpretation of findings is complicated by lack of a standard criterion for diagnosis and the large number of diagnosed cases who do not meet the surveillance case definition. To date, no cause or effective treatment has been discovered for chronic Lyme disease.

Lyme Arthritis

The arthritis of Lyme disease is characterized by asymmetrical pain and swelling affecting primarily the large joints. Arthralgia and arthritis can start in the first few days of infection. Muscle pain may accompany the joint pain. Usually, only one or a few large joints are affected, with the knee joint being the most commonly affected. In children, the oligoarticular manifestations of Lyme disease can easily be mistaken for pauciarticular juvenile rheumatoid arthritis. Pediatric Lyme disease arthritis is typically less severe and more responsive to antibiotics than adult arthritis. Pediatric Lyme disease resembles that seen in adults, with 98% of children having arthralgias early in the course of Lyme disease.

Chronic arthritis may occur after arthralgia or migratory arthritis and typically occurs months to years after the start of infection. In about 10% of clients with Lyme arthritis, the disease may become chronic, causing erosion of cartilage and bone with pannus formation. In these extreme cases, permanent joint disability occasionally occurs. In these individuals, the pathologic changes are similar to those occurring in rheumatoid arthritis, except that no RF is present. Large effusions are common and reaccumulate rapidly after arthrocentesis, resembling Reiter's syndrome. The fluid is inflammatory, with 10,000 to 25,000 WBCs/mm^3, and contains mostly neutrophils (Ruddy, Harris, Sledge, & Kelley, 2001).

History and Physical Examination

For individuals who live in an endemic area and whose symptoms are nonspecific but suggestive of Lyme disease, a complete health history is essential. It is easy to overlook or misdiagnose Lyme disease because the disease is so complex. Yet, early diagnosis and treatment are essential if the morbidity of the disease is to be decreased.

It should be determined whether the client or the client's family has been in a tick-infested area within the last few months and whether they have participated in outdoor activities, such as hiking, fishing, camping, gardening, or hunting. The nurse should ask whether pets in the household have had ticks. If the client recalls having had a tick bite, the nurse should attempt to establish the date and how and when the tick was removed.

Careful history and physical examination for the presence of a rash are essential. EM is the unique clinical marker for Lyme disease and is sufficient criterion for diagnosis. It occurs in the majority of clients infected. Clients should be asked whether they remember having a bull's-eye rash or any other type of rash that may indicate secondary annular lesions (Fig. 23–14). The EM lesion usually begins as a red macule (a small red spot) that expands over days to weeks. It may appear as a red patch with varying intensities of redness or as a clear center surrounded by red annular rings (bull's-eye appearance). Occasionally, the central regions may give way to varying shades of blue, leaving only a narrow red peripheral band. These lesions have an average diameter of 15 cm (6 inches) but may spread up to 20 cm (8 inches) across. The thigh, groin, and axilla are common sites of involvement. EM appearing on clients with dark skin or a suntan may

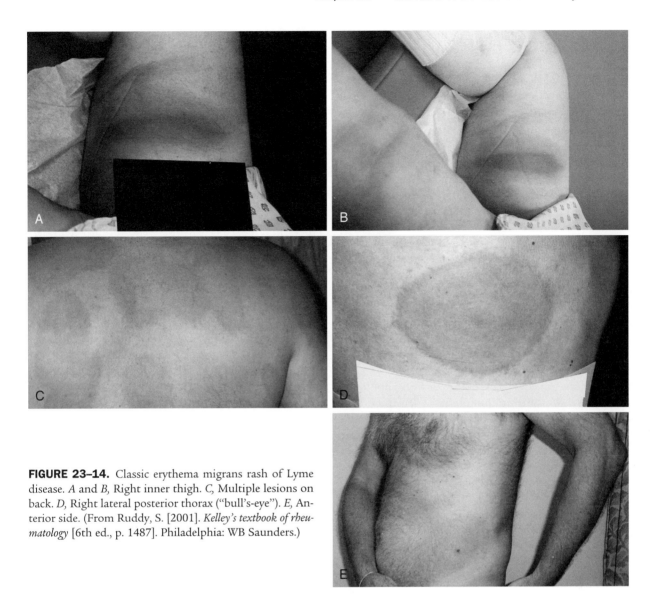

FIGURE 23–14. Classic erythema migrans rash of Lyme disease. *A* and *B,* Right inner thigh. *C,* Multiple lesions on back. *D,* Right lateral posterior thorax ("bull's-eye"). *E,* Anterior side. (From Ruddy, S. [2001]. *Kelley's textbook of rheumatology* [6th ed., p. 1487]. Philadelphia: WB Saunders.)

be more difficult to identify. Postinflammatory hyperpigmentation is more common on dark-skinned clients.

Question the client about any sensations that accompanied the rash. Although generally considered to be nonpruritic and nontender, about half of clients report a burning sensation and the lesion is warm to the touch. Occasionally, it is pruritic. The nurse should determine how long the rash was present. EM lesions usually fade within 3 to 4 weeks, even in untreated individuals, although they may recur. It is also important to determine whether the rash was accompanied by flulike symptoms. Specifically, the nurse should inquire about unexplained fevers, sweats, chills, flushing, swollen glands, sore throat, fever, headache, stiff neck, body aches, and fatigue. These symptoms tend to persist or may occur intermittently in the client with Lyme disease.

Table 23-7 categorizes symptoms that may occur in stage 2 or stage 3 of Lyme disease. Careful history and physical examination should focus on the presence of arthritic, neurologic, and cardiac symptoms. The client should be questioned and examined about other less commonly seen symptoms, including eye inflammation, hepatitis, and severe fatigue.

The arthritis of Lyme disease is characterized by asymmetrical pain and swelling affecting primarily the large joints. The client should be questioned about the presence of joint pain and stiffness. Is it monoarticular or migratory? Is muscle pain present?

Diagnostic Evaluation

B. burgdorferi is difficult to isolate or culture from body tissues or fluids. Consequently, serologic results are used in combination with clinical history, objective presentation, and an understanding of the antibody response in Lyme disease. It should be noted that laboratory confirmation is not required for diagnosis of an early case of Lyme disease in a client who presents with EM in an endemic area.

The CDC recommends early testing using either an enzyme-linked immunosorbent assay (ELISA) or through indirect immunofluorescence assay (IFA). The sensitivity of these tests varies with the stage of the disease. Early in infection, when only EM is present, as many as 50% of clients have negative test results with IFA. The ELISA test is somewhat more sensitive. Therefore, a negative test finding does not rule out Lyme disease. The probability that a client is seropositive increases the longer EM is present and the more marked the clinical manifestations. It is suggested that clients with a low pretest probability of Lyme disease, as judged by incidence in the community and absence of objective clinical signs, not be referred for laboratory testing.

False-positive test results may be encountered in clients with other spirochetal illnesses (e.g., syphilis, yaws, pinta) or other infectious processes (e.g., infectious mononucleosis, endocarditis) or in the presence of auto-immune disease. Other positive laboratory correlates, especially in stage 1, might be an elevated ESR, elevated serum glutamic-oxaloacetic transaminase (SGOT; aspartate transaminase, AST), or elevated serum IgM.

All positive or equivocal ELISA or IFA should be confirmed by Western immunoblot (WB) to aid in distinguishing true positive ELISA results. WB should not be used as a screening test. This test detects the presence or absence of antibody. Specific criteria for a positive IgM immunoblot and an IgG immunoblot have been established through the National Institute of Allergy and Infectious Diseases (NIAID) and the CDC. Antibody can be detected with WB years after successful treatment. Detectable IgG antibody may persist for years despite successful antibiotic treatment. To date, neither ELISA nor WB have been standardized and comparisons across laboratories remain problematic.

In certain situations, spirochete detection studies are used. Culture of *B. burgdorferi* from the EM lesion or cultures of blood, cerebrospinal fluid (CSF), and synovial fluid may be done. Although skin cultures provide the highest yield, efficacy in detecting the organism in the other culture materials is significantly lower.

Polymerase chain reaction (PCR) detects extremely small quantities of the genetic material of the spirochete in blood, CSF, synovial fluid, and skin biopsies. Because it is thought that *B. burgdorferi* is not found in blood in later phases of infection, PCR is best used on inflammatory fluids or biopsy specimens. PCR positivity in inflammatory fluid suggests that the neurologic or articular findings result from local *B. burgdorferi* infection. PCR becomes negative after treatment. Persisting positive findings in subsequent fluid specimens suggests persistence of infection and further antibiotic treatment should be considered. PCR is not recommended for routine clinical use because it is not yet standardized. Its extreme sensitivity can lead to false-positive serologic test results.

Treatment Modalities and Related Nursing Management

Prevention is considered paramount in the control of Lyme disease. Avoiding endemic areas, using protective clothing (e.g., wearing light-colored clothing, tucking pants into socks), using tick repellents, and performing tick checks after coming from outdoors are suggested. Host-targeted acaricides at deer feeding sites may be used. A Lyme disease vaccine (LYMErix) is now available and suggested only for high-risk populations.

Lyme disease can usually be treated successfully with standard antibiotic regimens. When disease is advanced, there may be a need to intervene to correct underlying problems. Synovectomies have been performed for clients with advanced Lyme arthritis. Insertion of transvenous cardiac pacing may be required for severe cardiac symptoms.

Active involvement in a personal rehabilitation program is essential for clients with Lyme arthritis or in those clients deconditioned as a result of ineffective treatment or post-Lyme syndrome.

Pharmacologic Intervention
Prophylactic Immunization. LYMErix (GlaxoSmithKline), the first vaccine against Lyme disease, was approved by the U.S. Food and Drug Administration (FDA) in 1998. LYMErix is made from recombinant OspA—the outer surface protein of *B. burgdorferi*—with alum. The vaccine is administered intramuscularly in three doses. The efficacy of the Lyme disease vaccine after three doses is 76% (95% confidence interval, 58% to 86%) and it offers no protection against other tick-borne diseases (CDC, 1999c). The CDC and the Advisory Committee on Immunization Practices recommendations for use of LYMErix are reported in Box 23–3. Because the vaccine does not protect all individuals and because it does not prevent other tick-related illness, individuals should be instructed to continue personal protection measures (Box 23–4) despite vaccination.

The decision to administer Lyme disease vaccine should be made on the basis of an assessment of individual risk, which is based on the likelihood of being bitten by tick vectors infected with *B. burgdorferi*. Thus, geographic location (narrowed to state and county) as well as the extent of outdoor activity (recreational, property maintenance, occupational, or leisure pursuits) in which the individual partakes in these geographic areas must be considered.

Initial clinical trials using LYMErix reported on the safety of vaccine use. The phase III clinical trial included 10,936 participants randomly divided into a vaccine group and placebo group. The most common adverse effect noted was soreness at the injection site. Myalgia, flulike illness, fever, and chills were more common among

---

BOX 23–3.
CDC Guidelines for Use of LYMErix

Persons Who Reside, Work, or Recreate in Areas of High or Moderate Risk

Lyme disease vaccination *should be* considered for persons aged 15–70 years who engage in activities (e.g., recreational, property maintenance, occupational, or leisure) that result in frequent or prolonged exposure to tick-infested habitats.

Lyme disease vaccination *may be* considered for persons aged 15–70 years who are exposed to tick-infested habitat but whose exposure is neither frequent nor prolonged. The benefit of vaccination beyond that provided by basic personal protection and early diagnosis and treatment of infection is uncertain.

Lyme disease vaccination is *not* recommended for persons who have minimal or no exposure to tick-infested habitats.

Persons Who Reside, Work, or Recreate in Areas of Low or No Risk

Lyme disease vaccination is *not* recommended for persons who reside, work, or recreate in areas of low or no risk.

Travelers to Areas of High or Moderate Risk

Because of the limited time of exposure, travelers to Lyme disease–endemic areas within the United States are generally expected to be at lower risk for Lyme disease than those who permanently reside in endemic areas. Vaccination should be considered for travelers to areas of high risk if frequent or prolonged exposure to tick habitat is anticipated.

Children Younger Than 15 Years

Until the safety and immunogenicity of rOspA vaccines in children have been established, this vaccine is not recommended for children younger than 15 years.

Persons Older Than 70 Years

The safety and efficacy of LYMErix have not been established for persons aged older than 70 years.

Persons with Immunodeficiency

Persons with immunodeficiency were excluded from the phase III safety and efficacy trial and no data are available regarding Lyme disease vaccine use in this group.

Persons with Musculoskeletal Disease

Persons with diseases associated with joint swelling (including rheumatoid arthritis) or diffuse musculoskeletal pain were excluded from the phase III safety and efficacy trial, and only limited data are available regarding Lyme disease vaccine use in this group.

Persons with a Previous History of Lyme Disease

Vaccination should be considered for persons with a history of previous uncomplicated Lyme disease who are at continued high risk.

Persons who have treatment-resistant Lyme arthritis should not be vaccinated because of the association between this condition and immune reactivity to OspA.

Boosters

Whether protective immunity will last longer than 1 year beyond the third dose is unclear. Data regarding antibody levels during a 20-month period after the first injection of LYMErix indicate that boosters beyond third dose might be necessary.

---

vaccine recipients than placebo recipients but reported only by 3.2% of recipients. Reports of arthritis were not significantly different between vaccine and placebo recipients, but vaccine recipients were significantly more likely to report arthralgia or myalgia within 30 days after each dose. Since that time, there has been growing anecdotal reports that LYMErix can trigger severe autoimmune arthritis. An FDA advisory committee (Beck, 2001), convened in February 2001 to hear concerns, recommended establishing a registry of all vaccines and suggested that client education efforts be increased. Studies are ongoing to determine whether LYMErix is associated with triggering autoimmune arthritis.

Prophylaxis/Treatment Post-Tick Attachment. Prophylactic administration of antibiotics to all persons who remove attached vector ticks is generally not recommended. A meta-analysis of three prospective, randomized, double-blind clinical trials involving persons bitten by *I. scapularis* ticks (more than 600 cases) and then treated with placebo, penicillin, tetracycline, or amoxicillin concluded that antimicrobial prophylaxis was not warranted (Warshafsky, Nowakowski, Nadelman, Kamer, Peterson, & Wormser, 1996).

Factors favoring the use of prophylaxis include the duration of tick attachment (more than 48 hours) and the engorgement status of the attached nymphal or adult tick when removed from an individual in an endemic area. *B. burgdorferi* is rarely transmitted by *I. scapularis* within the first 48 hours of attachment. Thus, ticks that have been attached for less than 48 hours theoretically cannot transmit *B. burgdorferi* infection. The option of

BOX 23–4.
Strategies to Limit Lyme Disease

Personal Precautions

1. Wear long pants with cuffs tucked into the socks so that any ticks that get on shoes or socks will crawl on the outside of the pants and be less likely to bite.
2. Wear light-colored clothing to facilitate visualization of any ticks (*I. scapularis* looks like a small brown freckle).
3. Smoother materials, such as windbreakers, are harder for ticks to grab onto and are preferable to knits.
4. Tick repellents that contain permethrin (Permanone) are meant to be sprayed onto clothing. Spray the clothes before putting them on and let them dry first. The chemical should not be applied directly to the skin.
5. Skin insect repellents that contain DEET are somewhat effective when applied to the arms, legs, and around the neck. Do not use over wide areas of the body because they can be absorbed and cause toxicity. Skin repellents should contain less than 50% DEET and 25% concentrations are preferred.
6. Monitor yourself and your children immediately after coming inside or every 2 to 3 hours while outside. Perform a tick check by inspecting clothes and undressing and looking for ticks. (It takes at least 18 hours for the spirochete to be transmitted from the tick.) Ticks can attach to any part of the human body but often attach to the more hidden and hairy areas such as the groin, armpits, and scalp.
7. Ticks are very intolerant to being dried out. After being outdoors in an infested area, place clothes in the dryer for a few minutes to kill any ticks that may still be present.
8. Check pets carefully.

Strategies for Reducing Tick Abundance

1. Remove leaf litter, brush, and woodpiles around houses and at the edges of yards.
2. Clear trees and brush to admit more sunlight, thus reducing deer, rodent, and tick habitat.
3. Apply pesticides to residential properties (insecticide Damminix in wooded areas and pesticides Dursban, Tempo, and Sevin at perimeter of lawn).
4. Investigate community-based interventions to reduce deer populations.
5. Investigate community-based interventions to kill ticks on deer such as pesticide application at deer feeding stations.

selectively treating these high-risk individuals assumes that the species, stage, degree of engorgement, and infection status of the tick, as well as the probability of transmission of infection, can be readily ascertained, which generally does not hold true. Many different tick species bite humans, and some "ticks" removed from humans are actually spiders, scabs, lice, or dirt and thus

pose no risk of Lyme disease (Warshafsky et al., 1996). To date, no study has demonstrated that antimicrobials are effective in reducing the risk of infection after a tick bite in this group.

Persons who present with EM or an elevated temperature within 30 days of tick removal should receive routine antibiotic administration. For early, localized Lyme disease or early disseminated Lyme disease with associated EM in the absence of neurologic symptoms or third-degree heart block, oral administration of antibiotics for 14 to 21 days is suggested. Doxycycline (100 mg twice a day) or amoxicillin (500 mg three times a day) is suggested. Doxycycline is relatively contraindicated for women who are either pregnant or breast-feeding, as well as for children younger than 8 years of age. In children, amoxicillin, erythromycin, or penicillin G may be used. Less than 10% of infected individuals fail to respond to antibiotic therapy.

In Lyme disease with acute neurologic disease such as meningitis or radiculopathy, third-generation cephalosporins (e.g., ceftriaxone, cefotaxime) or penicillin G are recommended to be administered intravenously for 2 to 4 weeks. Children with disseminated or late-stage disease are similarly treated with third-generation cephalosporins or penicillin G (Wormser, Nadelman, & Shapiro, 2000).

Following antibiotic therapy, many clients report continuing symptoms, such as headache, fatigue, and achiness. These symptoms have been referred to as nonspecific complaints, minor complaints, Lyme sequelae, post-Lyme syndrome, postinfectious fatigue syndrome, and as a continuation of Lyme active disease manifestations. Many sources contend that this malaise may take months to subside but that symptoms spontaneously subside without requiring additional antibiotic therapy.

Lyme arthritis usually can be treated successfully with antimicrobial agents administered orally or intravenously. Administration of doxycycline or amoxicillin for 28 days is the normal course. For individuals with persistent or recurring joint swelling after recommended courses of antibiotics, repeat treatment with another 4-week course of oral antibiotics or a 2- to 4-week course of intravenous ceftriaxone is recommended (Wormser, Nadelman, & Shapiro, 2000). The repeat course should be delayed several months to allow for the slow resolution of inflammation after treatment. Continuing arthritic symptoms may also be treated with anti-inflammatory drugs, such as aspirin or prednisone. Vitamin and nutritional supplements are generally recommended. Antidepressants, analgesics, or muscle relaxants may be helpful as adjunctive therapy.

Surgical Management. In the presence of persistent synovitis associated with pain and limitations in joint movement, synovectomy may reduce the joint inflammation.

Nursing Diagnoses

Activity Intolerance

Energy Management, Emotional Support, Exercise Therapy, Pain Management, Nutritional Counseling. Clients experiencing long-standing Lyme disease generally become deconditioned, with a resulting inability to tolerate activity. In late stages of the disease, muscle atrophy occurs, and because of extreme fatigue and body pain, the client finds it difficult to get the necessary exercise. For severe cases, physical therapy using massage, heat, transcutaneous electrical nerve stimulation, or ultrasonography may be recommended along with aggressive ROM exercises. In milder cases, the client can be instructed in a stretching and mild muscular toning exercise routine, which should lessen joint pain and increase mobility and stamina.

Management of fatigue and weakness should include a nutritional assessment. A balanced diet is extremely important, and a multivitamin is usually recommended. Essential fatty acids may be supplemented to help manage fatigue, and magnesium supplementation may be added for muscle cramps, soreness, and weakness. Many clients experience weight gain with Lyme disease, in part because of activity intolerance. Fad diets may contribute to the fatigue. Following a diabetic diet or general guidelines for weight reduction in arthritis clients may be helpful.

Infection, Risk for

Intravenous Administration: Medication Administration. Clients with diagnosed Lyme disease require treatment with antibiotics that may expose them to additional risks for infections. The client should be monitored for and instructed about the risk of suprainfection, especially of yeast infections. Incorporating live-culture yogurt into the daily meal plan may help prevent this, but antifungal agents are often required. Clients on long-term antibiotic administration may have a PICC line in place. The client and family must be educated on care of the line and signs of infection.

Environmental Management, Health Education. A large part of the nursing management of Lyme disease is focused on prevention. Surveillance of Lyme disease incidence and communication of the risks to community members in endemic areas is an important public health nurse responsibility. In nonendemic areas, public health programs can benefit by focusing on educational messages regarding the limited risk of acquiring Lyme disease; this effort may relieve public anxiety and reduce the occurrence of inappropriate testing and treatment of Lyme disease.

If residing in or going to areas where ticks are likely to be found, the personal precautions listed in Box 23–4

are recommended. Unfortunately, these measures are not consistently used, and their effectiveness in preventing Lyme disease has not been demonstrated conclusively (Orloski, Hayes, Campbell, & Dennis, 2000).

Strategies for reducing tick abundance are summarized in Box 23–4. Most Lyme disease cases occur during the summer months, and it is advisable to avoid tall grass, sand dunes, brush, and the edge of woods in the known endemic areas from April through October. It is important to point out that open areas, such as the parking lot and the beach itself, which are devoid of vegetation, are safe. Residential clearing of brush and trees may be helpful. Insecticides, such as Damminix, placed in the wooded areas of property and pesticides, applied at the perimeter of the lawn, may be helpful in reducing the risk of Lyme disease; however, if not used by neighbors, its overall efficacy is limited. Spring (late May) and fall (September) applications help eliminate both nymphs and adults.

Clients should be taught how to remove a tick correctly. The recommended procedure is to use tweezers to grasp the tick as close to the skin as possible and pull it straight up and out (part of the tick may remain embedded in the person's skin, but it will still be destroyed and unable to transmit the spirochete). After the tick is removed, the area should be disinfected by cleansing with alcohol or povidone-iodine (Betadine). The tick should be saved for future reference, if possible, by placing it in a jar. The bite area should be checked occasionally (for up to 2 weeks) to see if a rash forms. If either a rash or flulike symptoms develop, professional health care must be obtained.

Many people have the misconception that the best way to remove ticks is by suffocating them with Vaseline or butter or by applying either gasoline or a lighted match directly to the tick. It is important to reinforce the notion that these methods not only are ineffective as a means of tick removal but also may be counterproductive. Lyme disease is not transmitted from person to person. If one member of the family develops Lyme disease, other members of the family are not at risk unless they also were bitten by the tick.

Anxiety

Anxiety Reduction, Coping Enhancement, Emotional Support. Because of the variety of symptoms that may occur as a result of infection with Lyme disease and the difficulty of laboratory confirmation, diagnosis is often complicated or delayed. Symptoms may persist and grow worse before a diagnosis of Lyme disease is made. Once the diagnosis is made, some clients may experience a feeling of relief, but others may be angry and frustrated that the diagnosis took so long and that chances for early treatment were missed. For some clients, the disease, once diagnosed, is curable; for others, it might create chronic health problems. Because of the bewildering nature of the disease, clients may need psychological support.

The goals of care appropriate for the client with Lyme disease include early recognition and treatment, reduction in severity and duration of symptoms, and prevention of complications. The nursing interventions focus on educating the client, encouraging rest, providing comfort measures and symptomatic treatment, and administering and monitoring appropriate medications.

INTERNET RESOURCES

American Lyme Disease Foundation: www.aldf.com

Arthritis Foundation: www.arthritis.org

Centers for Disease Control and Prevention: www.cdc.gov

icanPrevent: www.icanprevent.com

Lyme Disease Network: www.lymenet.org

Morbidity and Mortality Weekly Report: www.cdc.gov/mmwr/

National Institute of Arthritis and Musculoskeletal and Skin Diseases: www.nih.gov/niams/

REFERENCES

Beck, E. (2001, February 2). FDA committee says safety of Lyme disease vaccine needs more study. *icanPrevent News and Commentary.* Available at www.icanprevent.com

Boachie-Adjei, O., & Squillante, R. G. (1996). Tuberculosis of the spine. *Orthopedic Clinics of North America, 27,* 95–103.

Bruno, R. L. (1997). *Preventing complications in polio survivors undergoing surgery.* PPS monograph series, Vol. 6, No. 2. Hackensack, NJ: Harvest.

Bruno, R. L. (2000). Paralytic vs. "nonparalytic" polio: Distinction without a difference? *American Journal of Physical Medicine and Rehabilitation, 79*(1), 4–12.

Bruno, R. L., & Frick, N. M. (1991). The psychology of polio and prelude to post-polio sequelae: Behavior modification and psychotherapy. *Orthopedics, 14,* 1185–1193.

Bruno, R. L., Sapolsky, R., Zimmerman, J. R., & Frick, N. M. (1995). Pathophysiology of a central cause of post-polio fatigue. *Annals of the New York Academy of Science, 753,* 257–275.

Canale, T. (1998). *Campbell's operative orthopaedics* (9th ed.). St Louis: Mosby.

Centers for Disease Control and Prevention. (1999c, June 4). Recommendations for the use of Lyme Disease, vaccine recommendations of the Advisory Committee on Immunization Practices (ACIP). *Morbidity and Mortality Weekly Report, 48*(RR07), 1–17.

Centers for Disease Control and Prevention. (2000c). *NNIS semiannual report.* [On-line]. Available at www.cdc.gov/ncidod/hip/SURVEILL/NNIS.htm

Cesario, T. C. (1995). Orthopedic implications of tuberculosis. *Western Journal of Medicine, 163*(6), 565.

Davis, J. C. (1986). The results of refractory osteomyelitis treated with surgery, parenteral antibiotics, and hyperbaric oxygen. *Clinical Orthopaedics and Related Research, April*(205), 310.

Esterhai, J. L., Jr., Pisarello, J., Brighton, C. T., Heppenstall, R. B., Gellman, H., & Goldstein, G. (1987). Adjunctive hyperbaric oxygen therapy in the treatment of chronic refractory osteomyelitis. *Journal of Trauma, 27*(7), 763–768.

Falconer, M., & Bollenbach, E. (2000). Late functional loss in nonparalytic polio. *American Journal of Physical Medicine and Rehabilitation, 79,* 19–23.

Foster, L. W., Berkman, B., Wellen, M., & Schuster, N. (1993). Postpolio survivors: Needs for and access to social and health care services. *Health and Social Work, 18*(2), 139–148.

Goldenberg, D. L. (1998). Septic arthritis. *Lancet, 351*(9097), 197–202.

Gozzoli, V., Schotter, P., Suter, P. M., & Ricou, B. (2001). Is it worth treating fever in intensive care unit clients? *Archives of Internal Medicine, 161,* 121–123.

Halstead, L. S., & Silver, J. K. (2000). Nonparalytic polio and postpolio syndrome. *American Journal of Physical Medicine and Rehabilitation, 79*(1), 13–18.

Harrington, J. T. (2001). Mycobacterial and fungal infections. In W. Kelly (Ed.), *Textbook of rheumatology* (6th ed., pp. 1493–1495). Philadelphia: WB Saunders.

Huelskamp, L., Anderson, S., & Bernhardt, M. (2000). TB of the spine: Pott's disease. *Orthopaedic Nursing, 19*(4), 31–35.

Jubelt, B., & Drucker, J. (1999). Poliomyelitis and the post-polio syndrome. In D. Younger (Ed.), *Motor disorders.* Philadelphia: Lippincott Williams & Wilkins.

Mandell, G. L., Bennett, J. E., & Dolin, R. (2000). *Mandell, Douglas, and Bennett's principles and practice of infectious diseases* (5th ed.). Philadelphia: Churchill Livingstone.

Maynard, F. (1986). Late effects of polio create large demand for re-habilitation. *Rehabilitation Report, 2,* 2–3.

McCray, E., Weinbaum, C., Braden, C., & Onorato, I. (1997). The epidemiology of tuberculosis in the United States. *Clinics in Chest Medicine, 18,* 99–113.

Morrey, B. F., Dunn, J. M., Heimbach, R. D., & Davis, J. (1979). Hyperbaric oxygen and chronic osteomyelitis. *Clinical Orthopaedics and Related Research, Oct*(144), 121–127.

Orloski, K. A., Hayes, E. B., Campbell, G. L., & Dennis, D. T. (2000, April 28). Surveillance for Lyme disease: United States, 1992–1998. *CDC MMWR Surveillance Summaries, 49*(SS03), 1–11.

Packer, T. L., Martins, I., Krefting, L., & Brouwer, B. (1991). Post-polio sequelae: Activity and post-polio fatigue. *Orthopedics, 14,* 1223–1226.

Ruddy, S., Harris, E. D., Sledge, C. B., & Kelley, W. N. (2001). *Kelley's textbook of rheumatology* (6th ed.). Philadelphia, WB Saunders.

Saxon, D. (2001). Another look at polio and post-polio syndrome. *Orthopaedic Nursing, 20*(3). Available at www.ajj.com/services/pblshng/onj/abstr1.htm

Walenkamp, G. H. (1998). Osteomyelitis treated with gentamicin-PMMA beads: 100 clients followed for 1–12 years. *Acta Orthopaedica Scandinavica, 69,* 518–522.

Warshafsky, S., Nowakowski, J., Nadelman, R. B., Kamer, R. S., Peterson, S. J., & Wormser, G. P. (1996). Efficacy of antibiotic prophylaxis for prevention of Lyme disease. *Journal of General Internal Medicine, 11,* 329–333.

World Health Organization. (2000). *Tuberculosis Fact Sheet.* Geneva: Author.

Wormser, G. P., Nadelman, R. B., & Shapiro, E. D. (2000). Practice guidelines for the treatment of Lyme disease. *Clinical Infectious Diseases, 31*(suppl 1), S1–S14.

Appendix: Computers As a Resource for Education

NANCY MOONEY

The 30th birthday of the Internet was celebrated in 1999, and in this short time, it has revolutionized the computer and communications world like nothing before (Leiner, Cerf, Clark, Kahn, Kleinrock, Lynch, Postel, Roberts, & Wolff, 2000). Few can argue with the fact that the Internet has changed how we think, work, and communicate. It has been instrumental in moving society from the industrial era to the information era. This information era is, in part, characterized by ease of rapid global communication and access to huge stores of information. The challenge to workers in the information era is to learn to manage large amounts of information. It is necessary for nurses to be computer savvy to keep in pace with knowledge areas, databases, and communication with others.

The Internet was originally designed to facilitate communication among government scientists. European physicists who needed to send information to each other created what we now know as the World Wide Web. They developed the hypertext markup language (HTML), which can be used to send and receive documents, sound, and pictures. As a result of the High-Performance Computing Act of 1991, Internet access was made public through telecommunication companies, information services, and other public access systems (Frandsen, 1999).

The size and scope of the Internet highlights its impact on society and health care today. Approximately 72 million adults, representing 35% of United States adults ages 16 and older, have been online "surfing" any of the estimated 43 million Internet host sites (Wright & Neill, 1999). Detwiler (2000) reports that by mid-1999, 36% of all Internet users had searched for health and medical information online. That these people are acting on some of this information is demonstrated by questions asked of health care providers. Detwiler informs us that as of mid-1999, 3.4 million Americans had requested a particular drug from their doctors based on information they found on the Internet.

Several authors (Cravener, 2000; Detwiler, 2000; Silberg, Lundberg, & Musacchio, 1997) remind us that although the Internet is affecting almost all aspects of health care delivery, we need to use caution in using the information that is brought to us so easily. The principles of basing health care on the best available evidence applies, and potential users need to critically appraise any information they wish to use. Nothing replaces the human interaction between client and practitioner;the Internet is meant merely to be an adjunct to knowledge.

THINKING CRITICALLY ABOUT WEB RESOURCES

Given the enormous amount of information in the World Wide Web, everyone, from the orthopaedic nurse doing research for a nursing class, to the orthopaedic client wanting more information about a chronic illness, can easily be confused by the sheer amount of information. What makes a website "good"? What makes it correct? Does a professional organization, a commercial venture, or the government sponsor it? Who put that information there? How do you know what is right? Often, more questions are evoked than are answered by finding that "perfect" site.

Professionals in library science offer some solutions on how to evaluate a website. Table 1 lists five criteria for evaluating web pages (Kapoun, 2000). Orthopaedic nurses should use these criteria in evaluating websites not only for professional sites but also for client/consumer sites. Tillman (2000) offers a quick list of items to consider when evaluating a website:

- Keep in mind how you best identify the quality of an Internet resource in this volatile, continually changing environment.

TABLE 1. *Evaluating Web Pages*

EVALUATION OF WEB DOCUMENTS	HOW TO INTERPRET THE BASICS
Accuracy of Web Documents Who wrote the page and can you contact him or her? What is the purpose of the document and why was it produced? Is this person qualified to write this document?	**Accuracy** Make sure author provides e-mail or a contact address/phone number. Know the distinction between author and webmaster.
Authority of Web Documents Who published the document and is he or she different from the webmaster? Check the domain of the document; what institution publishes this document? Does the publisher list his or her qualifications?	**Authority** What credentials are listed for the authors? Where is the document published? Check URL domain.
Objectivity of Web Documents What goals/objectives does this page meet? How detailed is the information? What opinions (if any) are expressed by the author?	**Objectivity** Determine whether page is a mask for advertising; if so, information might be biased. View any web page as you would an infomercial on television. Ask yourself why was this written and for whom.
Currency of Web Documents When was it produced? When was this updated? How up-to-date are the links (if any)?	**Currency** How many dead links are on the page? Are the links current or updated regularly? Is the information on the page outdated?
Coverage of the Web Documents Are the links (if any) evaluated and do they complement the document's theme? Is it all images or a balance of text and images? Is the information presented cited correctly?	**Coverage** If the page requires special software to view the information, how much are you missing if you do not have the software? Is it free, or is there a fee to obtain the information? Is there an option for text only, or frames, or a suggested browser for better viewing?

Source: Kapoun, J. (2000). Teaching undergraduates Web evaluation: A guide for library instruction. *College & Research Libraries News* [On-line]. Available at www.ala.org/acrl/undwebev.html

- Learn when to turn to an intermediary tool such as a guide or when to maneuver a search engine.
- Compare Internet resources with their competitors' content no matter what the format.
- Evaluate the resource yourself.
- Use the Internet's feedback capabilities to communicate. If you see shortcomings, speak up!

Beredjiklian, Bozentka, Steinberg, and Bernstein (2000) examined how orthopaedic clients looked up the words *carpal tunnel syndrome* in five commonly used search engines. The goal of their study was to assess the type, quality, and reliability of information about carpal tunnel syndrome that is available on the Internet. They combined the top 50 websites from each of the five searches, and created a master roster of 250 website addresses. The sites were then evaluated for authorship and content and were given an informational value score ranging from 0 to 100 points. They found the following:

- Thirty-three percent sold commercial products for the evaluation or treatment of carpal tunnel syndrome.

- Thirty percent were commercial websites that did not sell products.
- Twenty-three percent were authored by a physician or an academic organization.
- Less than 50% offered conventional information.
- Twenty-three percent offered unconventional or misleading information.
- The mean informational value of the websites was 28.4 of a possible 100 points.

These data suggest that the information about carpal tunnel syndrome on the Internet is of limited quality and poor informational value. We need to be aware of this, especially for our consumers and our students. More research on such topics is needed to make the information available both valid and reliable for clients and their families, as well as for practitioners.

Accrediting Websites

According to Winkler (2000), deputy editor of the *Journal of the American Medical Association,* effort is under way to develop standards for accrediting health websites. She said, "Health and medical information on the web has huge potential to benefit clients and the public, but inaccurate and biased information and potential breaches of client privacy may cause more harm than good." The 27-member committee will consider standards in a variety of areas ranging from privacy and professionalism to candor and accountability. For a complete review of the guidelines the American Medical Association has used to govern their website, see Winker (2000).

NURSING AND THE INTERNET

For nurses, the explosion of information has influenced how we study, work, use resources, and obtain continuing education credit. In a recent study done by Mediamark Research, Inc., the following was reported: 78% of nurses have Internet access, 55% reported being on-line in the past week, and 22% reported daily usage. This study reflects a significant increase in nurse Internet access from previous surveys, which reported a usage of 44% of nurses online in 1997, 54% in 1998, and 69% in 1999.

As the web grows, many sites are devoted to nurses specifically. Most of these sites have similar purposes and generally provide the following: information; full-text journal articles (some are free; others for a fee); current health news; an e-store where nurses can purchase items; a career center where nurses can search for jobs; and community access, bulletin boards, or chat rooms.

Some of the nurse-specific sites are listed at the end of this appendix. This list is not exhaustive and just represents some of the websites available to professional nurses.

Nursing Informatics As a Specialty

The American Nurses Association (1994, 1995) has identified the practice of those nurses who work in informatics through the publication of standards of practice and a scope-of-practice statement. Nursing informatics focuses on the methods and tools of information handling in nursing practice. Information handling includes identifying, naming, organizing, grouping, collecting, processing, analyzing, storing, retrieving, communicating, transforming, or managing data or information.

These standards are authoritative statements in which the nursing profession describes the responsibilities for which nurses are accountable. They provide the direction for professional nursing practice and a framework for the evaluation of practice. According to the American Nurses Association, the daily use of a word processor by the nurse giving care to clients is not, by itself, an instance of nursing informatics practice, nor is the use of a computerized client classification system.

If the integrated systems are to service clients and health professionals successfully by ensuring that the nursing perspective is available in such systems, the services of informatics nurses are required. It is the responsibility of the informatics nurse to protect the integrity of nursing information and nurses' access to information necessary for client care within an integrated, computer-based client record. The core phenomena of nursing informatics are all data, information, and knowledge involved in nursing. The core operations of nursing informatics takes all these data, information, and knowledge and makes them meaningful and useful to nurses. The technology that facilitates these operations is, of course, also of concern to nursing informatics. Navigating the Internet, and the integration of the information on the Internet into nursing practice, is just a part of the practice of the nursing informatics professional. The profession has identified nursing informatics as a specialty; nurses can become certified as a Nursing Informatics nurse through the American Nurses Credentialing Center (www.nursingworld.com).

THE WEB AS A RESOURCE TO CLIENTS

Health issues are a major reason people log onto the Internet (Brody, 1999). An increasing number of clients and consumers are using the Internet to research their illnesses or conditions. Ahmann (2000) reminds us that in some sense, the accessibility of health-related information on the Internet is revolutionizing client education and the client/provider interface. In the past, consumers received most of their health care information from nurses and doctors. Now those same individuals and families can easily research their own health concerns and can come to medical appointments with increasingly sophisticated questions and an awareness of treatment options. This certainly has been a long-term goal for health care professionals—to have informed consumers who know the treatment options that are available and who can make decisions based on that information.

Medical professionals apply the term *Internet syndrome* to people who independently research their illness, find the answer they are looking for, then try to convince their practitioner of the best way for them to be treated (Detwiler, 2000). This is a new way of interacting with clients. Biermann, Golladay, Greenfield, and Baker (1999) point out the advantages of clients being informed: "The patients who have done extensive searches are often well informed and you can spend less time on the basics, and more time on the finer points of treatment." The challenge is to assist individuals to critically evaluate Internet-based information and the relevance of different options in light of their own particular health care needs.

The utility of the Internet in learning about and managing illness is tremendous. Families with children with special needs or any illness can obtain information about the child's diagnosis, find service providers, share personal experiences, research treatment options, negotiate school regulations, get financial information, improve coping skills, and meet other families dealing with the same or similar issues. For parents who use chat rooms and listservs, many practical matters can be discussed and worldwide information can be shared easily.

Through its information sources and the opportunity to pose questions to other individuals who also are using the Internet, the Internet allows people access to information that is not readily available elsewhere. Brody (1999) reported the story of a gentleman who had several surgeries for recurrent respiratory papilloma. After his third surgery, through an inquiry on the Internet, he was able to learn about other remedies unknown to his physician, which led to a successful removal of his polyps.

With aging, seniors encounter multiple health problems and benefit from access to a wide range of reliable health care information quickly. In a National Institutes of Health pilot study conducted from September 1997 to July 1998, senior citizens were taught how to search for credible and useful health care information on the Internet. One hundred seniors were taught how to conduct health information searches and to share their information with family and friends. The average age of the senior trainees was 69 years. The study revealed a positive impact of the training, both in using a computer and using the Internet. In a 90-day post-training follow-up, two thirds of those who searched for health information on the Internet talked about it with their physicians, with more than half reporting that they were more satisfied with their treatment as a result of their search and subsequent discussion with their practitioners. This leads to challenges for nurses and nurse practitioners to examine how nursing can redesign client education and transform nursing practice (Leaffer & Gonda, 2000).

Limitations to Internet Health Research

Although the list of advantages to the access to information is long, there are some caveats regarding Internet health research. First, access is not available to every person. Although most homes have a personal computer, not all do. Access generally is available in public libraries; however, this is not equal access. Second, Internet information may not be in the language of origin for the individual or family. Medical terminology may confuse those who are not familiar with it. Moreover, individuals may find information that is upsetting to them, which may lead to jumps in assumptions, when the information may not be pertinent to their personal situation. A healthy skepticism and a willingness to be open minded about the information is needed for everyone looking on the Internet. The consumer needs to evaluate the contents on the Internet for sound medical content.

QUALITY ON THE INTERNET

With the multiple sources of information available online, it is possible to evaluate the quality of information by critiquing the site for quality certifications and by comparing the information with information acquired from known reputable sites. Several resources are available for individuals to check when determining whether information is accurate.

Health on the Net (www.hon.ch/HONCode)

The Health on the Net Foundation is a source of independent certification of health-related sites. The Foundation has established a voluntary code of conduct (HONCode) for medical and health websites. Close to 3000 sites adhere to this code, which is voluntary and is available in 17 languages. The principles guiding the HONCode are listed in Table 2. Sites that adhere to the code of conduct are permitted to display the HONCode seal. The presence of this seal provides consumers with some assurance that the site adheres to a basic code of ethical conduct. Searches can be done through the HONselect database (www.hon.ch/HONselect/Search.html).

TRUSTe (www.truste.org)

TRUSTe awards its trust mark only to websites that adhere to established privacy principles and agree to comply with ongoing TRUSTe oversight and dispute resolution procedures. This site is based on two principles:

1. Users have a right to informed consent.
2. No single privacy principle is adequate for all situations.

TRUSTe has been in business since 1997 and includes sites such as America Online, IBM, Microsoft, and Netscape. Of interest, the TRUSTe website provides the consumer with a mechanism to report violations of posted privacy policies, if not resolved with the sites that are members of TRUSTe. (They do not provide this service for nonmember sites.) An example of this would be, "I have requested to unsubscribe from a site's mailing list three times without success." TRUSTe has a "Watchdog Report" that can be used if there are any unresolved concerns with a member site.

QUICK (The Quality Information Checklist)

QUICK was a project of the National Health Service Health Education Authority (now the Health Development Agency) and the Centre for Health Information Quality in the United Kingdom. It is a resource for children and young people to evaluate information on the Internet. It is set up as a tutorial rather than as a site checker. It offers an easy to read format, with simple language that could benefit not only young people but also the elderly or those with low literacy. The format is eight simple questions, much like the ones the other

TABLE 2. *Principles of the Health on the Net Foundation Code of Conduct for Medical and Health Websites*

Authority	Any medical or health advice provided and hosted on this site will be given only to medically trained and qualified professionals unless a clear statement is made that a piece of advice offered is from a non–medically qualified individual or organization.
Complementarity	The information provided on this site is designed to support, not replace, the relationship that exists between a client/site visitor and his or her existing physician.
Confidentiality	Confidentiality of data relating to individual clients and visitors to a medical/health website, including their identity, is respected by this website. The website owners undertake to honor or exceed the legal requirements of medical/health information privacy that apply in the country and state where the website and mirror sites are located.
Attribution	Where appropriate, information contained on this site will be supported by clear references to source data and, where possible, will have specific HTML links to those data. The date when a clinical page was last modified will be displayed clearly.
Justifiability	Any claims relating to the benefits/performance of a specific treatment, commercial product, or service will be supported by appropriate, balanced evidence.
Transparency of Ownership	The designers of this website will seek to provide information in the clearest possible manner and provide contact addresses for visitors who seek further information or support. The webmaster will display his or her e-mail address clearly throughout the website.
Transparency of Sponsorship	Support for this website will be identified clearly, including the identities of commercial and noncommercial organizations that have contributed funding, services, or material for the site.
Honesty in Advertising and Editorial Policy	If advertising is a source of funding, it will be stated clearly. A brief description of the advertising policy adopted by the website owners will be displayed on the site. Advertising and other promotional material will be presented to viewers in a manner and context that facilitates differentiation between it and the original material created by the institution operating the site.

sites ask, but in simple language, using cartoon-like characters.

CINAHL (www.cinahl.com)

Detwiler (2000) interviewed many individuals knowledgeable about evaluating health and medicine websites. All agreed that CINAHL (Cumulative Index to Nursing and Allied Health Literature) is the most useful website for nursing. CINAHL started in hard copy as a nursing index in the late 1950s. It went electronic in 1983. From the start, it was multiformat. Although most people think of it as a journal article database, this is not its primary function. It also covers books, audiovisuals, software, government documents, and now websites.

The government documents (generally with the suffix ".gov") are in full text. This is all in the public domain and can be used by anyone. The CINAHL database has a field for website addresses, so if an article discusses websites in depth, the addresses are included. CINAHL also lists all the cited references for cooperating journals, so there is a whole field of bibliographies that can be searched.

An asset of CINAHL is that the language is in controlled vocabularies, meaning it is "tree" structured, so you can go broader with your search if you are not getting what you want with your search. For orthopaedic

nurses, the topic may be as broad as osteoporosis and as narrow as prevention of osteoporosis in teenagers.

Medscape (http://orthopedics.medscape.com/Home/Topics/orthopedics/orthopedics.html)

Medscape offers orthopaedic nurses an integrated, multispecialty information and education tool. You may choose a personal Medscape home page (both orthopaedics and nursing are available), and after a simple, free registration, you will get a tailored site for your selected specialty. It is built around practice-oriented content, including abstracts and full-text articles, next-day summaries of major medical meetings, and more. The goals of Medscape are as follows:

- To provide clinicians and other health care professionals with the most timely source of clinical information that is highly relevant to their clients and practice
- To make the clinician's task of information gathering simpler, more fruitful, and less time-consuming
- To make available to a broad medical audience clinical information with the depth, breadth, and validity needed to improve the practice of medicine

Medscape provides an integrated search tool that can run searches on databases of more than 30,000 articles, drug information, MEDLINE, and more. Information about specific evidence-based practice is listed in Medscape.

Medscape also has three separate resource centers listed under the orthopedics section. These are collections of the latest news, references, and other resources on major medical conditions. For orthopaedics, the following resources are listed:

- Joint replacements
- Osteoporosis
- Olympics/Sports medicine

There are, of course, many specific sites for both orthopaedic clinicians and consumers. Most of the subspecialties in orthopaedics have a site for client information and support, as well as an update on the newest therapies for these conditions. These sites also tend to contain information about the spectrum of illness, from the acute phase through rehabilitation, home care, and the illness trajectory for chronic illness. Table 3 summarizes many orthopaedic resources for clinicians and consumers.

THE FUTURE OF THE INTERNET IN ORTHOPAEDICS

Most authors agree that the Internet holds great promise as a tool for the collection and dissemination of medical information. McGrory (2000) suggests that the Internet will accelerate the effort to quantify orthopaedic outcomes. For example, just as periodicals such as *US News and World Report* rank hospitals for a variety of health settings (based primarily on physician polls), there are websites that rank specific interventions. Healthgrades.com is one site that rates total hip replacements, using partial MEDPAR (Medicare) files purchased from the Health Financing Administration for its raw data. These data are incomplete; they exclude non-Medicare clients (an important population), and complications are documented only for the hospital stay. This lack of a standardized approach to documenting complications (rare in

total hip replacement surgery and occurring months or years after the surgery) has implications for ratings in comparing institutions because the time and site (home or rehabilitation facility) of transfer are not consistent.

Orthopaedists (and orthopaedic nurses) find it cumbersome, time-consuming, and expensive to collect the data necessary for meaningful outcome reports and comparisons. With the advent of Internet outcome sites and the use of many standardized outcomes assessment instruments (such as the SF-36 Health Survey and the Musculoskeletal Function Assessment Instrument), it is possible to use standardized outcome assessment models in individual practices and institutions. This provides an opportunity to improve the quality of musculoskeletal care for clients and communities.

For nursing, two organizations provide a structure for nurses to register their research in progress with an abstract. The Sigma Theta Tau International's Registry of Nursing Research (www.stti.iupui.edu/library/registry.html) is a free service to members and is subscription based for others. The Canadian-International Nurse Research Database (http://nurseresearcher.com) is a free resource where nurses can register their research interests and contact information. Organizations should be looking toward promoting and developing this type of service (Lewis, 2000).

Leiner et al. (2000) remind us that the Internet, although a network in name and geography, is an entity of the computer, not the traditional network of the telephone or television industry. It must continue to change and evolve at the speed of the computer industry if it is to remain relevant.

SUMMARY

The Internet certainly has affected all of our lives, both personally and professionally. In our role as client advocates, orthopaedic nurses need to be familiar with the resources available to our clients and their families. This section reviews the history of the Internet, how to critique web resources, and what to look for when evaluating a

---

TABLE 3. *Orthopaedic Resources for Clinicians and Consumers*

American Academy of Orthopaedic Surgeons	www.aaos.org
Arthritis Foundation	www.arthritis.org
Journal of Orthopaedic Nursing	www.harcourt-international.com/journals/joon
National Association of Orthopaedic Nursing	http://naon.inurse.com
National Osteoporosis Foundation	www.nof.org
Wheeless' Textbook of Orthopaedics: full text on-line	www.medmedia.com/Welcome.html
Assorted Orthopaedic Sites	
About Orthopedics	http://orthoguide.com/ortho/
Orthogate: International Society of Orthopaedic Surgery and Trauma	www.orthogate.com
Orthopaedics.com	www.orthopaedics.com
OrthoSeek.com	www.orthoseek.com
Spine Universe	www.spineuniverse.com

website. Knowing who sponsors the site (commercial venture, professional organization, or government site) is important, as is knowing how often (and who) is updating the information on the site.

Quality is a common denominator for the practice of every orthopaedic nurse, wherever that practice might be. Nursing has been a major player in the development of standards of practice, and we now have the added challenge of ensuring that our clients get the right information. There is a vast quantity of useful information on the Internet, and the principles of basing health care on the best available evidence applies.

Potential users need to approach this information with a critical eye toward accuracy, timeliness, and conclusions based on valid research findings. The Internet sites listed in this section were correct at the time of publication, but sites and addresses may have been changed by the provider without notice. Readers are encouraged to check these sites personally before sharing any information with clients.

Internet sites for each chapter precede the bibliography and are listed in alphabetical order at the end of this appendix.

INTERNET RESOURCES: NURSING-SPECIFIC SOURCES

Allnurses.com: www.allnurses.com
Cumulative Index to Nursing and Allied Health
    Literature (CINAHL) Information Systems:
    www.cinahl.com
American Nurses Association: www.nursingworld.org
International Council of Nurses: www.icn.ch
Medscape (has nursing "channel"): www.medscape.com
National Association of Orthopaedic Nurses: http://
    naon.inurse.com
NursingCenter: www.nursingcenter.com
NursingHands: http://nursinghands.com
Sigma Theta Tau International Honor Society of
    Nursing: www.nursingsociety.org
The "Virtual" Nursing Center:
    www-sci.lib.uci.edu/HSG/Nursing.html

REFERENCES

Ahmann, E. (2000). Family matters: Supporting families' savvy use of the Internet for health research. *Pediatric Nursing, 26*(4), 419–423.

American Nurses Association. (1994). *The scope of practice for nursing informatics.* Washington, DC: American Nurses Publishing.

American Nurses Association. (1995). *Standards of practice for nursing informatics.* Washington, DC: American Nurses Publishing.

Beredjiklian P. K., Bozentka, D. J., Steinberg, D. R., & Bernstein, J. (2000). Evaluating the source and content of orthopaedic information on the Internet. The case of carpal tunnel syndrome. *Journal of Bone and Joint Surgery, 82A*(11), 1540–1543.

Biermann, J. S., Golladay, G. J., Greenfield, M. L., & Baker, L. H. (1999). Evaluating cancer information on the Internet. *Cancer, 86*(3), 381–390.

Brody, J. (August 31, 1999). Of fact, fiction, and medical web sites. *The New York Times* [On-line]. Available at www.nytimes.com/library/national/science/083199hth-brody.html.

Cravener, P. A. (2000). The world wide nursing web. *American Journal of Nursing, 100*(11), 75–77.

Detwiler, S. M. (2000). *Super searchers on health & medicine: The online secrets of top health and medical researchers.* Medford, NJ: CyberAge Books.

Frandsen, J. L. (1999). Pain resources on the Internet. In M. McCaffery & C. Pasero (Eds.), *Pain: Clinical manual* (2nd ed., pp. 745–748). St. Louis: Mosby.

Kapoun, J. (2000). Teaching undergraduates Web evaluation: A guide for library instruction. *College & Research Libraries News* [On-line]. Available at www.ala.org/acrl/undwebev.html.

Leaffer, T., & Gonda, B. (2000). The Internet: An underutilized tool in patient education. *Computers in Nursing, 18*(1), 47–52.

Leiner, B. M., Cerf, V. G., Clark, D. D., Kahn, R. E., Kleinrock, L., Lynch, D. C., Postel, J., Roberts, L. G., & Wolff, S. (2000). A brief history of the Internet. Internet Society (ISOC) All About the Internet: History of the Internet [On-line]. Available at www.isoc.org/internet-history/brief.html.

Lewis, D. (2000). Direct to consumer. *Reflections on Nursing Leadership, 26*(4), 24–26.

McGrory, B. J. (2000). Guest editorial: Orthopaedic outcomes on the Internet: Too good to be true? *Medscape Orthopaedics & Sports Medicine, 4*(4).

Silberg, W., Lundberg, G., & Musacchio, R. (1997). Assessing, controlling, and assuring the quality of medical information on the Internet: caveat lector et viewor—Let the reader and viewer beware. *Journal of the American Medical Association, 277*(15): 1244–1245.

Tillman, H. N. (2000). Evaluating quality on the Net. [On-line]. Available at www.hopetillman.com/findqual.html.

Winker, M. (October 2, 2000). Committee to develop accreditation program for health web sites. *Reuters Medical News* [On-line]. Available at www.medscape.com/reuters/prof/2000/10/10.02/20000929 ethc002.html.

Wright, S., & Neill, K. (1999). Using the world wide web for research data collection. *Clinical Excellence for Nurse Practitioners, 3*(6), 362–365.

Chapter 1

The Administration for Children and Families: www.acf.dhhs.gov/
Administration on Aging: www.aoa.dhhs.gov/
Agency for Healthcare Research and Quality: www.ahrq.gov
American Academy of Orthopaedic Surgeons: www.aaos.org
American Academy of Orthopaedic Surgeons: Prevent Injuries
    America: http://orthoinfo.aaos.org/prevention.cfm?category=
    Prevention
American Association of People with Disabilities: www.aapd.com/
American Disability Association: www.adanet.org/
American Public Health Association: www.apha.org
The Bone and Joint Decade: www.boneandjointdecade.org
Centers for Disease Control and Prevention (CDC): www.cdc.gov
CDC National Center for Chronic Disease Prevention and Health
    Promotion: www.cdc.gov/nccdphp
CDC National Center for Environmental Health: www.cdc.gov/nceh
CDC National Center for Health Statistics: www.cdc.gov/nchs
CDC National Center for Injury Prevention and Control:
    www.cdc.gov/ncipc
CDC National Center for Injury Prevention and Control: Acute Care,
    Rehabilitation Research, and Disability Prevention: www.cdc.gov/
    ncipc/dacrrdp/dacrrdp.htm
CDC National Institute for Occupational Safety and Health:
    www.cdc.gov/niosh/homepage.html
The Council on Quality and Leadership in Supports for People with
    Disabilities: www.accredcouncil.org/
Departments of Health and Human Services and Agriculture: Nutrition and Your Health: Dietary Guidelines for Americans: http://
    odphp2.osophs.dhhs.gov/dietaryguidelines/

Environmental Health Clearinghouse: www.infoventures.com/
e-hlth/

Health Resources and Services Administration: www.hrsa.dhhs.gov

Healthfinder: www.healthfinder.gov/

Healthtouch: www.healthtouch.com/

Healthy People 2010: http://odphp2.osophs.dhhs.gov/healthypeople/

HealthWeb: healthweb.org

Job Accommodation Network: http://janweb.icdi.wvu.edu

Magic Stream: Emotional Wellness Journal: http://fly.hiwaay.
net/~garson/

Mobility International USA: www.miusa.org/

Morbidity and Mortality Weekly Report: www.cdc.gov/mmwr/

National Health Information Center: http://nhic-nt.health.org

The National Information Center for Children and Youth with Disabilities: www.nichcy.org/

National Institutes of Health (NIH): www.nih.gov/

National Organization on Disabilities (NOD): www.nod.org/

National Osteoporosis Foundation: www.nof.org

The National Parent Network on Disabilities (NPND): www.npnd.org/

NIH National Institute on Aging: www.nih.gov/nia

NIH National Institute of Arthritis and Musculoskeletal Diseases and
Skin Diseases (NIAMS): www.nih.gov/niams/

NIH National Institute of Environmental Health Sciences: www.
niehs.nih.gov

NIH National Institute of Nursing Research (NINR): www.nih.
gov/ninr/

Occupational Safety and Health Administration (OSHA): www.
osha.gov/

Office of Disease Prevention and Health Promotion: www.odphp.
osophs.dhhs.gov

Office of Minority Health: www.omhrc.gov/

OSH-Link: An Online Resource Summarizing Current Literature on
Occupational Safety and Health: www.infoventures.com/osh/

United Nations: The UN and Persons with Disabilities: www.un.org/
esa/socdev/enable/

The Virtual Hospital: www.vh.org

The Virtual Office of the Surgeon General: www.surgeongeneral.gov/
sgoffice.htm

The World Health Organization: www.who.int

Chapter 2

Arthritis and Sexuality: http://arthritis.about.com/health/arthritis/
library/weekly/aa072299.htm

Center for Loss and Life Transition: www.centerforloss.com/

Coping with Major Illness: www.susankramer.com/coping/html

Crisis, Grief, and Healing: www.webhealing.com/

ElderWeb: www.elderweb.com

GriefNet: www.rivendell.org/

Integrative Medicine Reference Suite: www.library.ucsf.edu/sc/altmed/

International Society for Traumatic Stress Studies: www.istss.org/

Mental-Health-Matters.com: www.mental-health-matters.com/loss.
html

National Center for Complementary and Alternative Medicine: http://
nccam.nih.gov/

National Center for PTSD: www.ncptsd.org/

National Mental Health Association: www.nmha.org/

Online Resources for Coping with Chronic Illness: http://
victorian.fortunecity.com/cezanne/518/copinglinks.htm

Psych Web: www.psychwww.com/

PTSD Alliance: www.ptsdalliance.org/home2.html

PTSTD.com (Post traumatic stress disorder resources): www.ptsd.com/

Prescription for Power: Coping with Chronic Illness: http://
members.core.com/~echoes/

Selfhelp Magazine: www.shpm.com/

Sexual Health.com: www.sexualhealth.com/

Sexuality and People with Disabilities: www.iidc.indiana.edu/~cedir/
sexuality.html

Chapter 3

American Academy of Orthopaedic Surgeons: www.aaos.org

Cornell University Ergonomics Web: CUErgo: http://ergo.human.
cornell.edu/

Ergonomics Society: www.ergonomics.org.uk/

ErgoWeb: www.ergoweb.com/

Human Factors and Ergonomics: Usernomics: www.usernomics.com/
hf.html

Human-Computer Interaction Resources on the Net: www.ida.liu.se/
labs/aslab/groups/um/hci

Human-Computer Interaction Site Links: www.hcibib.org/hci-sites

Injury Control Resource Information Network: www.injurycontrol.
com/icrin/

National Institute of Occupational Safety and Health: www.cdc.gov/
niosh/

Occupational Safety Engineering: http://turva.me.tut.fi/english/
indexeng.html

Chapter 4

The National Decubitus Foundation: www.decubitus.org

World Wide Wounds: www.worldwidewounds.com/index.html

WoundCareNet.com: www.woundcarenet.com

Chapter 5

American Academy of Pain Medicine: www.painmed.org

American Pain Foundation: www.painfoundation.org

American Pain Society: www.ampainsoc.org

American Society of Pain Management Nurses: www.aspmn.org/

International Association for the Study of Pain: www.halcyon.com/iasp

Wisconsin Cancer Pain Initiative: www.wisc.edu/wcpi

Chapter 6

Index of Bone Disorder Images: http://medstat.med.utah.edu/
WebPath/BONEHTML/

Wheeless' Textbook of Orthopaedics: www.medmedia.com

Chapter 7

Centers for Disease Control, Office of Genetics & Disease Prevention:
www.cdc.gov/genetics

Genetic Alliance: www.geneticalliance.org

Human Genome Project Information: www.ornl.gov/hgmis

International Society of Nurses in Genetics, Inc. (ISONG):
www.nursing.creighton.edu/isong

March of Dimes: www.modimes.org

National Coalition for Health Professional Education in Genetics
(NCHPEG): www.nchpeg.org

OMIM: Online Mendelian Inheritance in Man: www.ncbi.nlm.nih.gov/
entrez/query.fcgi?db=OMIM

Chapter 8

American Academy of Family Physicians: www.aafp.org

American Academy of Orthopaedic Surgeons: www.aaos.org

American Academy of Pediatrics—Intensive Training and Sports
Specialization in Young Athletes: www.aap.org/policy/RE9906.
html

National Association of Orthopaedic Nurses: http://naon.inurse.com

Virtual Hospital: www.vh.org

Virtual PNP: home.earthlink.net/~emgoodman/cases/htm

Chapter 9

Radiological Society of North America: www.radiologyinfo.org/
content/mr_musculoskeletal.htm

Spine Universe: www.spineuniverse.com

Chapter 10

Blood Transfusions: Knowing Your Options; Pall Corporation: www.
bloodtransfusion.com

National Guideline Clearinghouse: http://text.nlm.nih.gov/ngrelease.html

Chapter 11

A.L.E.R.T., Inc. (a national nonprofit, tax-exempt organization website that provides educational materials, support groups, publications, and product information about natural rubber latex allergy): www.latexallergyresources.org

American Academy of Orthopaedic Surgeons: www.aaos.org/wordhtml/papers/advistmt/wrong.htm

American Society of PeriAnesthesia Nurses: www.aspan.org/PosStmts2.htm

Association of Operating Room Nurses, Inc.: www.aorn.org/patient/rnfafact.htm

Chapter 13

American Physical Therapy Association: www.apta.org

Life@Home: www.lifehome.com; home modification products and services for senior citizens and the disabled

McBurney Disability Resource Center: www.dcs.wisc.edu/mcb

National Institute on Disability and Rehabilitation Research: www.ed.gov/offices/OSERS/NIDRR

Chapter 14

Arthritis Foundation: www.arthritis.org/

Lupus Foundation of America: www.lupus.org/

National Databank for Rheumatic Diseases: www.fibromyalgia.org

Rheumatology Resources: www.rheumatology.org

Scleroderma Foundation: www.scleroderma.org/

Sjögren's Syndrome Foundation: www.sjogrens.org/

Chapter 15

American College of Rheumatology: www.rheumatology.org/patients/factsheet/gout.html

National Institutes of Health: www.nih.gov/niams/healthinfo/avnecqa.htm

National Osteoporosis Foundation: www.nof.org

Osteoporosis Prevention, Diagnosis, and Therapy: NIH Consensus Statement: http://odp.od.nih.gov/consensus/cons/111/111_statement.htm

Chapter 16

American College of Rheumatology: www.rheumatology.org

Arthritis Foundation: www.arthritis.org

FocusOnArthritis.com: www.aboutarthritis.com

Mayo Clinic: www.mayoclinic.com

Medical College of Wisconsin Physicians and Clinics: HealthLink: www.healthlink.mcw.edu

National Institutes of Health/National Institute of Arthritis and Musculoskeletal and Skin Diseases: www.nih.gov/niams/healthinfo

National Library of Medicine/MEDLINEplus Health Information: www.nlm.nih.gov/medlineplus

PodiatryNetwork.com: www.podiatrynetwork.com

Chapter 17

Scoliosis Research Society: www.srs.org

Spine Universe: www.spineuniverse.com

Spine-health.com: www.spine-health.com

Chapter 18

Cerebral Palsy.com: www.cerebralpalsy.com/

The Dupont Institute: http://gait.aidi.udel.edu/res695/homepage/pd_ortho/educate.htm

Health Resources and Services Administration, Maternal Child Health Bureau Division of Services for Children with Special Needs: www.mchb.hrsa.gov/html/dscshn.html

National Institutes of Health, Osteoporosis and Related Bone Diseases—National Resource Center: www.osteo.org/

Pediatric Orthopedic Society of North America www.posna.org/InfoParents/InfoParentsIndex.htm

United States Cerebral Palsy Athletic Association: www.uscpaa.org/about_purpose.htm

Chapter 19

The American Association for the Surgery of Trauma (AAST): www.aast.org

American College of Surgeons: www.facs.org

American Trauma Society: www.amtrauma.org

The Eastern Association for the Surgery of Trauma (EAST): www.east.org

Emergency Nurses Association: www.ena.org

Orthopaedic Trauma Association: www.ota.org

Society of Trauma Nurses: www.traumanursesoc.org

Trauma.org: www.trauma.org

Trauma Care: www.traumacare.com

Chapter 20

The Amputee Coalition of America: www.amputee-coalition.org

Amputee Resource Foundation of America, Inc.: www.amputeeresource.org

Orthotics and Prosthetics: www.oandp.com

Chapter 21

American College of Sport Medicine: www.acsm.org

The American Orthopaedic Society for Sports Medicine: www.sportsmed.org

The Physician and Sportsmedicine Online: www.physsportsmed.com

Sports Medicine: www.sportmed.org

International Federation of Sports Medicine: www.fims.org

American Sports Medicine Institute: www.asmi.org

Chapter 22

American Cancer Society: www.cancer.org

Cancer Guide: http://cancerguide.org

OncoLink: www.oncolink.upenn.edu/

National Cancer Institute (CancerNet): http://cancernet.nci.nih.gov

Look Good . . .Feel Better: www.lookgoodfeelbetter.org/

Chapter 23

American Lyme Disease Foundation: www.aldf.com

Arthritis Foundation: www.arthritis.org

Centers for Disease Control and Prevention: www.cdc.gov

icanPrevent: www.icanprevent.com

Lyme Disease Foundation: www.lyme.org/

Lyme Disease Network: www.lymenet.org

Morbidity and Mortality Weekly Report: www.cdc.gov/mmwr/

National Institute of Arthritis and Musculoskeletal and Skin Diseases: www.nih.gov/niams/

Appendix

Allnurses.com: www.allnurses.com

Cumulative Index to Nursing and Allied Health Literature (CINAHL) Information Systems: www.cinahl.com

American Nurses Association: www.nursingworld.org

International Council of Nurses: www.icn.ch

Medscape (has nursing "channel"): www.medscape.com

National Association of Orthopaedic Nurses: http://naon.inurse.com

NursingCenter: www.nursingcenter.com

NursingHands: http://nursinghands.com

Sigma Theta Tau International Honor Society of Nursing: www.nursingsociety.org

The "Virtual" Nursing Center: www-sci.lib.uci.edu/HSG/Nursing.html

Index

Note: Page numbers followed by the letter f refer to figures; those followed by t refer to tables; and those followed by b refer to boxed material.

ISBN 0-7216-9302-4